MW01105145

Textbook of Intravenous Anesthesia

Paul F. White, Ph.D., M.D., Editor
Professor and Holder of the Margaret McDermott Distinguished Chair in Anesthesiology
Department of Anesthesiology and Pain Management
University of Texas Southwestern Medical Center
Dallas, Texas

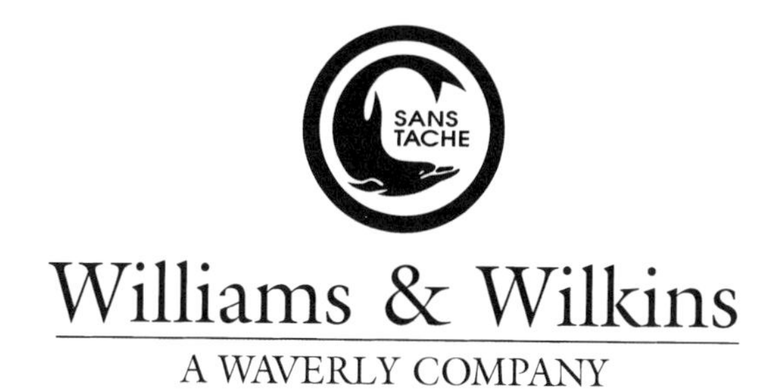

BALTIMORE • PHILADELPHIA • LONDON • PARIS • BANGKOK
BUENOS AIRES • HONG KONG • MUNICH • SYDNEY • TOKYO • WROCLAW

Editor: Sharron R. Zinner
Managing Editor: Tanya Lazar
Production Coordinator: Cindy Park
Book Project Editor: Robert D. Magee
Illustration Planner: Cindy Park
Cover Designer: Karen Klinedinst
Typesetter: University Graphics, Inc.
Printer: Edwards Brothers
Digitized Illustrations: University Graphics, Inc.
Binder: Edwards Brothers

351 West Camden Street
Baltimore, Maryland 21201-2436 USA

Rose Tree Corporate Center
1400 North Providence Road
Building II, Suite 5025
Media, Pennsylvania 19063-2043 USA

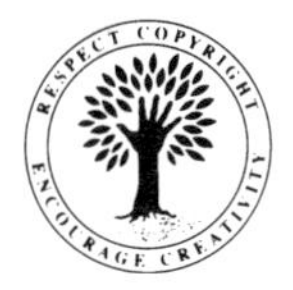

Printed in the United States of America

First Edition, 1997

Library of Congress Cataloging-in-Publication Data

Textbook of intravenous anesthesia / edited by Paul F. White. — 1st ed.
p. cm.
Includes bibliographical referenes and index.
ISBN 0-683-09000-3
1. Intravenous anesthesia. 2. Intravenous anesthetics.
I. White, Paul F., 1948– .
[DNLM: 1. Anesthesia, Intravenous. 2. Anesthetics, Intravenous—pharmacology. WO 285 T355 1997]
RD85.I6T49 1997
617.9'62—DC20
DNLM/DLC
for Library of Congress 96-15025
CIP

97 98 99
1 2 3 4 5 6 7 8 9 10

To the memory of Professor John Dundee

To my family and friends around the world

FOREWORD

In 1983, John Norman stated in an editorial that "one of the delights of anesthesia is that the administrator of the drugs observes the nature and duration of the effects produced" (1). In fact, every anesthesiologist is a practicing pharmacologist and physiologist. Drug administration and observation form a major part of our specialty. Every day in operating rooms and intensive care units, practitioners titrate intravenous drugs to achieve an effect, observe drug responses and interactions, and, if necessary, respond to adverse drug reactions. As a result, the majority of articles published in the anesthesia literature are related to drugs, delivery systems and monitoring devices. The most important reason for the use of intravenous anesthesia is that the essential components of anesthesia—namely, hypnosis, amnesia, analgesia, muscle relaxation and suppression of the "stress response"—can be managed independently. This is essential because their requirements during surgery depend on the needs of the individual patient. The clinician must also be able to reliably achieve the optimal "depth of anesthesia" for a specified period of time, a task that in the past was more easily managed with the volatile anesthetics. However, during the last decade many new intravenous agents with enhanced pharmacokinetic and pharmacodynamic properites have been developed. With these new drugs, therapeutic plasma and receptor ("effect") site concentrations are quickly achieved, providing for a more rapid onset of their actions on the central nervous system. These drugs may have small distribution volumes and/or high metabolic clearance rates, with elimination independent of the hepatic and/or renal system, characteristics which can lead to a rapid recovery after the drug is discontinued. It is now much easier for practitioners to rapidly adjust the depth of anesthesia in response to changes in the severity of the surgical stimulus. In addition, computer simulations and the development of target-controlled drug delivery systems has facilitated the use of intravenous anesthetic techniques in clinical practice. All these enhancements have allowed total intravenous anesthesia (TIVA) to become a routinely used technique. Thus, intravenous anesthesia has finally become a real option to inhalation anesthesia!

The Oxford English dictionary defines a "specialist" as an "authority who particularly or exclusively studies a single branch of his profession or subject." The editor of this textbook, Professor Dr. Paul F. White, is one of the founders of the Society of Intravenous Anesthesia and has devoted much of his professional career in academic medicine to becoming a master in the field of intravenous anesthesia. By choosing some of the leading authorities from around the world to contribute chapters to this text, Paul has created a book which will undoubtedly become the "gold standard" for the practice of intravenous anesthesia.

I am certain that this important textbook on intravenous anesthesia will become an indispensable source of up-to-date knowledge and practical advice for all practitioners of anesthesiology and critical care medicine.

Prof. Dr. Hugo Van Aken, MD, PhD, FRCA
Chairman, Department of Anesthesiology and Surgical Intensive Care
University Hospital
Westfälische Wilhelms–Universität
Munster, Germany

1. Norman J. Editorial: The intravenous administration of drugs. Br. J. Anaesth 1983;55:1049–52.

PREFACE

The history of intravenous anesthesia dates back to 1656, when Christopher Wren described the use of a feather to introduce a tincture of opium into the vein of a dog. Although the availability of the syringe and needle in 1853 greatly facilitated the administration of intravenous drugs, the use of intravenous anesthesia has only become popular in the last decade. Currently, intravenous anesthetic techniques are used in combination with local anesthetics as part of a so-called monitored anesthesia care technique, during regional anesthesia, as well as general anesthesia. The reasons for the slow progress in the field of intravenous anesthesia related to several factors, including the lack of drugs with appropriate pharmacokinetic and pharmacodynamic profiles, as well as inconvenient delivery systems and inadequate central nervous system (CNS) monitoring devices. With the availability of more rapid and shorter-acting intravenous anesthetics (propofol), analgesics (alfentanil, remifentanil), and muscle relaxants (mivacurium, rocuronium), it is now possible to achieve optimal intraoperative control of the patient's somatic and autonomic responses while attaining the desired level of CNS depression with total intravenous anesthetic (TIVA) techniques. Intravenous anesthetics produce dose-dependent depression of CNS function ranging from minimal sedation to deep coma. Improved cerebral function monitoring devices (e.g., EEG-bispectral index [BIS], auditory evoked potential monitors) should further improve the ability of practitioners to titrate intravenous anesthetics and analgesics to achieve the desired clinical endpoints. Finally, the availability of user-friendly, computerized drug delivery systems (e.g., Diprifusor™) has made intravenous anesthesia a viable option to inhalation-based anesthetic techniques in the 1990s.

For this textbook, the leading investigators in the field of intravenous anesthesia were invited to contribute chapters in their area of expertise. In the first section of the book, the background and scientific basis for intravenous anesthesia and analgesia are discussed. In the second, third, and fourth sections, the pharmacokinetics and pharmacodynamics of each of the major intravenous drug groups are extensively reviewed. In Section V, the clinical uses of these pharmacologic agents are described when they are administered alone, as well as in combination with other intravenous and inhaled anesthetic drugs. In Section VI, the applications of intravenous techniques in specific patient populations are discussed. Finally, in Sections VII and VIII, controversial issues related to drug delivery, CNS monitoring, and the effects of intravenous anesthesia on patient outcome are reviewed.

It is my hope that this comprehensive textbook on **Intravenous Anesthesia** will improve the clinical use of intravenous drugs for sedation and general anesthesia during the perioperative period. Pioneers in the field of intravenous anesthesia such as the late Professor John Dundee were clearly ahead of their time. With the recent pharmacologic and biotechnologic advances in our specialty, it should become safer, more convenient, and less costly to utilize intravenous anesthetic techniques in the future. However, more widespread acceptance of intravenous anesthesia will require further scientific evidence to support the notion that these techniques can facilitate recovery and improve patient outcome compared with traditional inhalation-based techniques. Organizations such as the **Society for Intravenous Anesthesia (SIVA)**, which support research and education related to the use of intravenous anesthetic drugs and techniques, will contribute to furthering our understanding of the basic concepts, as well as clinical applications of these techniques.

As editor of this textbook, I would like to express my sincere appreciation to the many outstanding contributors. In addition, the valuable editorial assistance of my wife, Linda, is graciously acknowledged. Without the generous support of Margaret Milam McDermott (whose Distinguished Chair of Anesthesiology I am honored to hold) and Dennis F. Landers, M.D., Ph.D. (my Departmental Chairman at the University of Texas Southwestern Medical School), it would not have been possible to find the time to undertake this major endeavor. Finally, the encouragement of my friends and colleagues was important in completing this project in a timely fashion. My early mentors in pharmacology, Professors Tony Trevor, Skip Way, and Ted Eger, provided a wonderful environment for research at the University of California in San Francisco and furnished the stimulus that led me to pursue a career in academic anesthesia. The insights gained from my clinical experiences at the University of California San Francisco, Stanford University, Washington University, and the University of Texas Southwestern Medical Center have also provided me with a unique perspective on the field of intravenous anesthesia.

Finally, I would like to acknowledge the editorial support and encouragement of the publisher, Williams & Wilkins (in particular, Sharron Zinner), as well as my secretary, Ms. Rebecca Sanchez. Without their dedication and tenacity, this book would never have been completed. As always, my family—Linda, Kristine, Lisa, and "Cuddles"—have been very supportive and understanding throughout this project.

Paul F. White, Ph.D., M.D., FANZCA
Dallas

CONTRIBUTORS

Peter Bailey, M.D.
Associate Professor
Department of Anesthesiology
University of Utah Health Sciences Center
Salt Lake City, UT

James G. Bovill, M.D., Ph.D., FFARCSI
Professor
Department of Anaesthesiology
University Hospital Leiden
The Netherlands

Scott S. Bowersox, Ph.D.
Director
Pharmacology
Neurex Corporation
Menlo Park, CA

Douglas V. Brown, M.D.
Assistant Professor
Department of Anesthesiology
Rush-Presbyterian-St. Luke's Hospital
Chicago, IL

Ann E. Buttermann, M.D., Ph.D.
Assistant Professor
Department of Anesthesiology
University of Minnesota Hospital and Clinics
Minneapolis, MN

Frederic Camu, M.D., Ph.D.
Professor
Chairman, Department of Anesthesiology
Flemish Free University of Brussels
Brussels, Belgium

Robert Litz Coleman, M.D.
Assistant Clinical Professor
Director of Quality Assurance
Department of Anesthesiology
Duke University Medical Center
Durham, NC

David P. Crankshaw, FANZCA, Ph.D.
Professor
Department of Anaesthesia
Royal Melbourne Hospital, Parkville
VIC 3050 Australia

Alfred Doenicke, M.D.
Professor
Institut fur Anaesthesiologie
Ludwig-Miximillians-University of Munich
D-8000 Munchen 2
Munich, Germany

Talmage D. Egan, M.D.
Assistant Professor
Department of Anesthesiology
University of Utah School of Medicine
Salt Lake City, UT

Jere Fellman, Ph.D.
Director Project Management
Neurex Corporation
Menlo Park, CA

Ron Flaishon, M.D.
Assistant Professor
Department of Anesthesiology
Emory University School of Medicine
Atlanta, GA

Atsuo Fukunaga, M.D.
Professor
University of California at Los Angeles
UCLA School of Medicine
Los Angeles, CA

Tong J. Gan, M.D., B.S. FRCA, FFARCS (I)
Assistant Professor
Department of Anesthesiology
Medical Director
Post Anesthesia Care Unit
Duke University Medical Center
Durham, NC

Brooks Gentry, M.D.
Assistant Professor
Department of Anesthesiology
University of Arkansas
Little Rock, Arkansas

Peter S.A. Glass, M.D.
Professor
Department of Anesthesiology
Duke University Medical Center
Durham, NC

Jeanette Harrington, M.D.
Associate Professor
Department of Anesthesia
University of Iowa Hospital and Clinics
Iowa City, IA

Thomas K. Henthorn, M.D.
Associate Professor
Department of Anesthesiology
Northwestern University Medical School
Chicago, IL

Michael B. Howie, M.D.
Professor and Vice Chairman
Department of Anesthesiology and Pharmacology
Ohio State University
Columbus, OH

Girish Joshi, MBBS, M.D., F.F.A.R.C.S.I.
Assistant Professor
Department of Anesthesiology and Pain Management
University of Texas Southwestern Medical Center
Dallas, TX

Gavin N.C. Kenny, B.Sc., M.D., FFARCS
Professor and Chairman
Department of Anesthesia
University of Glasgow
Glasgow, Scotland

Igor Kissin, M.D., Ph.D.
Professor
Department of Anesthesia
Brigham & Young Women's Hospital
Boston, MA

Alice Landrum, M.D.
Assistant Clinical Professor
Department of Anesthesiology
University of Missouri-Columbia
University of Missouri Medical Center
Columbia, MI

Eric Lang, M.D.
Assistant Professor
Department of Anesthesiology
Emory University School of Medicine
Atlanta, GA

Marilyn Lauwers, M.D.
Associate Professor
Flemish Free University of Brussels
Brussels, Belgium

Cynthia Lien, M.D.
Associate Professor
Department of Anesthesiology
Cornell University Medical Center
Cornell Medical College
New York, NY

Stephen P. Lordon, M.D.
Clinical Assistant Professor
Department of Anesthesiology
University of Utah School of Medicine
Salt Lake City, UT

Robert R. Luther, M.D., F.C.P.
Clinical Pharmacologist
Neurex Corporation
Menlo Park, CA

Dawn McGuire, M.D.
Assistant Clinical Professor
Department of Neurology
UCSF Medical Center
Neurex Corporation
Menlo Park, CA

Mervyn Maze, Ch.B., M.R.C.P.
Professor
Department of Anesthesiology
Veterans Affairs Palo Alto Health Care System
3801 Miranda Avenue
Palo Alto, CA

Robert J. McCarthy, Pharm.D.
Associate Professor
Department of Anesthesiology
Rush Medical College
Rush-Presbyterian-St. Luke's Medical Center
Chicago, IL

Dori Ann McCulloch, M.D.
Consultant Anesthetist
Stafford District General Hospital
Stoke-on-Trent, United Kingdom

John M. Murkin, M.D., F.R.C.P.C.
Professor
Director of Cardiac Anaesthesia
Department of Anaesthesia
University Hospital
London, Ontario, Canada

Peter Ostwald, M.D.
Associate Professor
Department of Experimental Anesthesia and Pain Research
University of Munich
Munich, Germany

Burdett R. Porter, M.D.
Associate Professor
Department of Anesthesia
University of Iowa College of Medicine
Iowa City, IA

John J. Savarese, M.D.
Professor and Chairman
Department of Anesthesiology
Cornell University Medical Center
Cornell Medical College
New York, NY

Jurgen Schüttler, M.D., Ph.D.
Professor and Chairman
Klinik Fur Anathesiologie
Friedrich-Alexander-Universitat Erlangen-Nurnberg
91054 Erlangen, Germany

John Sear, M.A., B.SC., M.B., B.S., Ph.D.
Professor and Associate Dean
Nuffield Department of Anaesthetics
University of Oxford
The John Radcliffe Hospital
Headington Oxford, OX3 9DU
United Kingdom

Peter S. Sebel, MB, BS, Ph.D.
Professor and Chief
Department of Anesthesiology
Grady Memorial Hospital
Emory University
Atlanta, GA

Steven L. Shafer, M.D.
Associate Professor
Stanford University
Veterans Affairs Palo Alto Health Care System
Stanford, CA

Ian Smith, B.Sc., M.B. B.S., F.R.C.A.
Senior Lecturer
University of Keele
North Staffordshire Hospitals
Market Drayton, Shropshire TF9 4BQ, United Kingdom

Martin D. Sokoll, M.D.
Professor
Department of Anesthesiology
University of Iowa School of Medicine
University of Iowa Hospital
Iowa City, IA

Andrew J. Souter, M.D.
Senior Lecturer
University of Oxford
Oxford, OX4 1TQ United Kingdom

Theodore H. Stanley, M.D.
Professor
Department of Anesthesiology
University of Utah School of Medicine
Salt Lake City, UT

James Temo, C.R.N.A., M.S.N.
Director of Nurse Anesthesia Services
Department of Anesthesiology
Duke University Medical Center
Durham, NC

Nancy Tich, Ph.D.
Senior Scientist
Neurex Corporation
Menlo Park, CA

Kenneth J. Tuman, M.D.
Max Sadove Professor and Vice Chairman
Department of Anesthesiology
Rush Medical College
Rush-Presbyterian-St Luke's
Chicago, IL

Jan Van Hemelrijck, M.D., Ph.D.
Professor
Department of Anaesthesiology
University Hospital K.U. Leuven
B-3000 Leuven, Belgium

Eric Vandermeulen, M.D., Ph.D.
Associate Professor
Department of Anaesthesiology
University Hospital K.U. Leuven
B-3000 Leuven, Belgium

Caroline Vanlersberghe, M.D.
Associate Professor
Flemish Free University of Brussels
Brussels, Belgium

H. Ronald Vinik, M.D.
Professor and Chief
Department of Anesthesiology
Eye Foundation Hospital
University of Alabama at Birmingham
Birmingham, AL

Meheno F. Watcha, M.D.
Associate Professor
Department of Anesthesiology
University of Texas Southwestern Medical Center
Dallas, TX

Paul F. White, Ph.D., M.D.
Professor and McDermott Chair
Department of Anesthesiology and Pain Management
University of Texas Southwestern Medical Center
Dallas, TX

O.H.G. Wilder-Smith, M.D.
Division D'Anesthesiologie
Hospital Cantonal Universitaire De Geneve
CH-3646 Einigen Switzerland

Elizabeth J. Youngs, M.D.
Staff Anesthesiologist
Veterans Affairs Palo Alto Health Care System
Stanford University
Palo Alto, CA

Elemer K. Zsigmond, M.D.
Professor Emeritus
Department of Anesthesiology
University of Illinois
University of Illinois Hospital
Chicago, IL

CONTENTS

I INTRODUCTION

II PHARMACOKINETICS AND DYNAMICS OF SEDATIVE-HYPNOTICS

III PHARMACOKINETICS AND DYNAMICS OF OPIOID AND NONOPIOID ANALGESICS

IV PHARMACOKINETICS AND DYNAMICS OF MUSCLE RELAXANTS

V BASIC INTRAVENOUS ANESTHETIC TECHNIQUES

VI SPECIAL PATIENT POPULATIONS

VII CONTROVERSIES IN INTRAVENOUS ANESTHESIA

VIII CONCLUSIONS

I INTRODUCTION

1 History of Intravenous Anesthesia

Jan Van Hemelrijck and Igor Kissin

RISE OF INTRAVENOUS ANESTHESIA

In the mid-seventeenth century, soon after the description of the circulatory system by Harvey, Percival Christopher Wren and Daniel Johann Major conceived the idea of injecting medicinal compounds directly into the blood and performed the first experiments (1). Wren dissolved opium in water and injected the solution into the venous system of a dog by means of a quill fastened to a bladder. The injection "stupefied" the dog within a short time without killing it. In 1845, the hollow needle was invented by Francis Rynd, and a functional syringe was introduced by Charles Gabriel Pravaz in 1853. These tools were not initially designed for intravenous administration of drugs but for perineural and intra-arterial injections. Alexander Wood perfected the syringe and used it for injection of morphine into painful points (e.g., neuralgias) (2). Despite Wren's early discovery, the history of clinical intravenous anesthesia did not begin until the late nineteenth century.

One of the early pioneers in the field of intravenous anesthesia was Pierre-Cyprien Oré, who reported on the use of chloral hydrate as an intravenous anesthetic to the Société Chirurgicale de Paris in 1872 (3). In a monograph published in 1875, Oré described 36 cases involving the use of the intravenous chloral hydrate to provide anesthesia (4). Despite Oré's enthusiasm, a high incidence of mortality prevented further development of intravenous anesthesia until after the turn of the century (5).

The next stage in the development of intravenous anesthesia involved hedonal, a urethane derivative used for the treatment of insomnia. In 1909, Krawkow and Fedoroff administered this agent intravenously to provide general anesthesia (6). According to Adams (5), "hedonal was the first anesthetic agent for intravenous administration that produced fairly adequate surgical anesthesia with a moderate degree of safety." The drug did not have sufficient water solubility, acted too slowly, and had a long duration of effect. After the use of hedonal for intravenous anesthesia was reported, the search for other possible intravenous anesthetics continued. In 1913, Noel and Souttar (7) described the anesthetic effect of paraldehyde given intravenously. Three years later, Peck and Meltzer (8) reported the results of the intravenous administration of magnesium sulfate. Ethyl alcohol was also used intravenously by Naragawa (9) in 1921 and by Cardot and Laugier (10) in 1922.

The first barbiturates were used for intravenous anesthesia in 1921. A mixture of the diethylamines of diethyl- and diallyl-barbituric acid (Somnifen) was used by Bardet (11). Although the first barbiturate acid derivative with hypnotic activity, diethylbarbituric acid, was synthesized in 1903 by Fisher and von Mering (12), its low solubility in water and extremely prolonged duration of hypnotic effects delayed the search for intravenous barbiturate anesthetics. The sodium salt of sec-butyl-(2-bromoallyl)-barbiturate (Pernoston) had greater water solubility and, in 1927, it was the first barbiturate to gain widespread use as an intravenous anesthetic (13). The first short-acting barbiturate with a fast onset of action, hexobarbital (Evipan), was synthesized by Kropp and Taub and by Weese and Scharpff in 1932 (14). This drug had a high incidence of excitatory side effects. Another barbiturate, thiopental (Pentothal), a rapid-acting hypnotic devoid of excitatory side effects, was first administered in 1934 (15) by Lundy (16) and Waters (17). It was introduced in the United Kingdom by Jarman (18). Today, thiopental remains the reference (gold standard) intravenous hypnotic against which all newer compounds are compared. Despite thiopental's widespread clinical acceptance, the search for the ideal drug for intravenous anesthesia continues.

As soon as rapid-acting barbiturates became available, these drugs were used for the induction of anesthesia, a practice with considerable advantages over inhalation induction of anesthesia by ether or other volatile agents. Shortly afterward, infusions of thiopental were used alone to maintain anesthesia, not surprisingly with poor results. When infusions of barbiturates were administered without opioids or muscle relaxants, large doses were necessary to suppress movement, and these doses had considerable side effects and delayed awakening. The use of barbiturates as a monoanesthetic was the cause of a many deaths among the casualties at Pearl Harbor in 1941 and led to the statement that intravenous anesthesia was "an ideal method for euthanasia" (19).

HISTORY OF INTRAVENOUS ANESTHETIC AGENTS

Barbiturates

Since the introduction of thiopental, the search for the ideal intravenous hypnotic agent has led to the development of several other intravenous anesthetic drugs. Some of these drugs have not withstood the test of clinical safety or utility, where others have proved valuable additions to the practice of anesthesia (5). Thiamylal (Surital, Thioseconal) is as effective as thiopental, but it is used infrequently. Although the British anesthetic thialbarbitone (Kemithal) and the German compound Inaktin are thiobarbiturates with the same duration of action and spectrum of activity as thiopental but with a lower potency, these agents have not become popular. The introduction of a methyl-thioethyl group into the side chain of methitural (to accelerate breakdown of the drug and to protect the liver by the release of methionine) created a drug that enjoyed some popularity as Thiogenal in Germany and methitural (Neraval) in the United States. The quality of anesthesia was inferior to that achieved with thiopental. The same criticism was applied to buthalitone, a barbiturate that was popular briefly under the trade names of Transithal (UK), Ulbreval (US), and Baytinal (Germany). Other modifications of the side chains of thiobarbiturates included the spirobarbiturates and the spirothiobarbiturates (Rapital), but none of these compounds proved as acceptable as thiopental.

The rapid onset of anesthesia induced by an oxybarbiturate, hexobarbital, was attributed to the addition of a methyl group in the first position. Lilly Research Laboratories consequently produced another methyloxybarbiturate, methohexital which was introduced into clinical practice in 1957. Compared with thiopental, methohexital has a shorter duration of action and a shorter half-life. The drug can be used for continuous infusion without prolonging recovery times. Its use is associated with pain on injection and a relatively high incidence of involuntary muscle movements. Several other methylthiobarbiturates were studied, but all caused an unacceptably high incidence of excitatory side effects.

Benzodiazepines

The first benzodiazepine, chlordiazepoxide (Librium), was synthesized by Sternbach of Hoffman-LaRoche Laboratories in 1955 (20). The compound elicited a broad spectrum of anxiolytic, sedative, and anticonvulsive effects (21). The first anesthesiologists in the clinical evaluation of chlordiazepoxide first used the drug as preanesthetic medication to calm patients (22). Subsequently, Sternbach synthesized diazepam (Valium), for use in the treatment of psychiatric disorders. This drug was made available in a parenteral injectable form in 1960. Diazepam was used by anesthesiologists to decrease preoperative apprehension (23, 24). In 1965, Stovner and Andresen reported on the administration of diazepam as an intravenous anesthetic (25). Diazepam remains the standard and most widely used benzodiazepine despite its disadvantages, which include a slow onset and long duration of action, insolubility in water, and venous irritation. Diazepam has recently become available in an emulsion formulation (Diazemuls), which rarely causes pain or thrombophlebitis, but it has a slightly lower bioavailability.

Lorazepam (Ativan, Temesta) was developed in 1971 in an effort to find a more potent benzodiazepine. In 1976, Fryer and Walser synthesized midazolam (Versed, Dormicum) (26). Midazolam was the first water-soluble benzodiazepine and therefore produced minimal local irritation after either intravenous or intramuscular injection. Midazolam is short-acting and was the first benzodiazepine produced primarily for use in anesthesia (27, 28). Several other benzodiazepines with slightly different pharmacologic profiles have been synthesized and marketed for oral use. As a result of increased knowledge concerning the central nervous system (CNS) receptor mechanisms of action, the first specific benzodiazepine receptor antagonist, flumazenil (Romazicon, Anexate) was developed in 1987 (29). Currently, Hoffman LaRoche is initiating clinical trials with a water-soluble derivative of midazolam, Ro48–6791, which appears to have a shorter elimination half-life than the parent compound.

Steroids

In 1941, Hans Selye reported that the injection of progesterone into rodents produced sleep (30). In subsequent screening of 75 different steroids, he discovered that, (Brietal, Brevital), for a steroid compound to possess anesthetic properties, an oxygen atom at either end of the steroid molecule was necessary. This molecular construction was exemplified by pregnanedione, which proved to be the most potent of the various steroids tested (31). In 1955, a laboratory report on the anesthetic effect of hydroxydione, a water-soluble steroid, was published (32). After an initial clinical assessment (33, 34), this compound was used briefly under the trade names Viadril and Pressuren. However, the onset of hypnosis induced by this drug was delayed (3 to 5 minutes), the drug was long acting, and produced a high incidence of thrombophlebitis.

In the early 1970s, a mixture of two steroids, alphaxalone and alphadolone, was marketed in a Cremophor EL solution under the trade name Althesin (35). Whereas alphaxolone was the primary active hypnotic, alphadolone was added to increase its solubility. Althesin was a relatively short-acting drug that could easily be administered by continuous infusion to provide hypnosis or sedation (36). It became popular in the mid-1970s in the United Kingdom and in some European countries, but it was never marketed in the United States. Unfortunately, the use of Althesin was associated with a high incidence of hypersensitivity reactions, a factor that led to its withdrawal from clinical use in 1984. Efforts to find an alternative solvent or emulsion remained unsuccessful because of the instability of the solution. In 1979, minoxalone, a water-soluble, rapid-acting steroid, was developed. The drug was withdrawn after some 1200 administrations because of the high incidence of excitatory phenomena and prolonged recovery.

The search for an acceptable steroid hypnotic agent is ongoing. Pregnanolone (eltanolone), a naturally occurring metabolite of progesterone, is undergoing worldwide clinical investigation (Pharmacia). Eltanolone is a water-insoluble compound and is therefore formulated as a lipid emulsion similar to propofol (Diprivan). The hypnotic potency of eltanolone is three times greater than that of thiopental (37). Induction of anesthesia is rapid, but recovery appears to be slower than after propofol administration.* Several novel steroid anesthetics are being investigated by Organon and may be under active clinical investigation in the near future.

Phencyclidines (Ketamine)

Cyclohexylamine compounds produce a state of unconsciousness in which the patient appears to be in a cataleptic (dissociative) state and is able to undergo surgery without recall of intraoperative events. Several agents of this group including phencyclidine (Sernil, PCP) were used clinically (38). Unfortunately, an unacceptably high incidence of postanesthetic psychomimetic reactions and delirium precluded their widespread use. In veterinary anesthesia, phencyclidine (Sernyl) is still used successfully.

Only one drug of this group, ketamine, has gained clinical anesthetic utility. This agent was synthesized in 1962 by Stevens at the research laboratories of Parke-Davis and was first used clinically in 1965 by Corssen and Domino (39). Ketamine's properties of providing analgesia, as well as a unique form of unconsciousness, delineated a new concept of intravenous anesthesia characterized by the term dissociative anesthesia, in which the patient has the characteristic facial expression of being "disconnected" from the surroundings rather than being asleep. Ketamine was released for clinical use in 1970 and is still used in a variety of clinical settings, even though it produces psychomimetic activity and marked cardiovascular stimulation (40, 41).

The molecular structure of ketamine contains a chiral center producing two optical isomers. White and associates demonstrated that the S(+) isomer offered clinical advantages over the racemic mixture [or the R(−) isomer] because it is a more effective anesthetic and analgesic drug (42). S(+)-ketamine produces shorter emergence and recovery times and faster return of cognitive function (43). Although the incidence of dreaming is similar with S(+)-ketamine and the racemic mixture, subjective mood and acceptance in volunteers were better with the S(+) isomer (43). Clinical investigations with S(+)-ketamine are currently under way in Germany.

Propofol

The most important factor in the increasing popularity of intravenous anesthesia during the last decade has been the availability of propofol. Its rapid metabolism and high degree of lipophilicity are responsible for a pharmacokinetic profile that is more suitable for continuous intravenous administration than that of any other available intravenous hypnotic agent. Propofol, a substituted derivate of phenol, was synthesized in the early 1970s by Glen and colleagues at ICI in the United Kingdom. The drug is insoluble in water and was initially prepared with Cremophor EL solution. The first clinical trials involving this drug were performed in 1977 by Kay and Rolly (44). Because of concerns regarding anaphylactoid reactions with the Cremophor EL formulation, however, propofol was withdrawn from clinical investigation. In 1983, propofol became available in a lipid emulsion (Diprivan) and was first administered to human subjects by Nigel Kay in Oxford. The drug was officially released for clinical use in the late 1980s in Europe, and in 1989 it was approved by the Food and Drug Administration (FDA) of the United States. Since then, a multitude of studies have been conducted using propofol in combination with many other drugs for diverse anesthetic indications (45, 46, 47).

Etomidate

Etomidate is an imidazole derivate developed in 1964 at Janssen Pharmaceutica in Beerse, Belgium (48) and

*Q; J.

introduced into clinical practice in 1974 by Doenicke (49). Etomidate causes little hemodynamic depression and practically no histamine release. It is a short-acting hypnotic, and its pharmacokinetic profile prompted its use as a continuous infusion to maintain sedation and anesthesia. The pain on injection, which is due primarily to the propylene glycol solvent, myoclonic activity, and a high incidence of postoperative nausea and vomiting were the primary undesirable properties of the drug. The principal drawback to its use as an infusion, however, was the drug's inhibition of adrenal steroidogenesis (50). The increased mortality observed in patients who had multiple trauma and who had been sedated with etomidate infusions in the intensive care unit was attributed to the inhibition of cortisol production (51, 52). These observations were confirmed by several in vivo and in vitro studies (50, 53). The role of etomidate in modern anesthetic practice is therefore confined mainly to its use as an induction agent in patients who are at risk of hemodynamic instability or who suffer from polyallergic reactions. Nevertheless, an alternative formulation designed to decrease the problem of pain on injection has recently been introduced into clinical practice (54, 55).

Propanidid

The observation that eugenol, derived from oil of clover and cinnamon, exhibits anesthetic properties when given intravenously prompted Thuillier and Domenjoz in Basel, Switzerland to explore the suitability of some of the congeners of eugenol for use as intravenous anesthetics (56). The eugenol derivatives were the predecessors of propanidid, a phenoxyacetic acid derivate developed by Bayer Laboratories. Introduced in the 1960s, propanidid (Epontol, Fabontal) was the first acceptable nonbarbiturate hypnotic. The effects of propanidid were extremely short lasting as a result of its rapid metabolic breakdown by plasma pseudocholinesterase (57). The drug was popular for use during in short ambulatory procedures. To prolong the action of propanidid, large doses were administered, and these doses produced acute hemodynamic depression. Unfortunately, the compound was solubilized in Cremophor EL, which led to a high incidence of hypersensitivity reactions and its eventual withdrawal from clinical practice. Propanidid was never released for clinical use in the United States.

Opioids

Opium, obtained from the seeds of Papaver somniferum, had been used for analgesia and sedation for centuries. Opium is a complex mixture of alkaloids, containing the naturally occurring morphine and codeine. In 1803, Serturner isolated morphine from opium (58). In the second part of the nineteenth century, morphine was frequently used in the form of injections as a supplement during ether or chloroform anesthesia, and it was used postoperatively for analgesia. At the beginning of this century, large doses of morphine were used in combination with scopolamine for anesthesia (59). This technique rapidly fell into disfavor because of the increased mortality (60).

Meperidine (pethidine, Dolantin) was synthesized in 1939 and is still in clinical use (61). To achieve additional antinociceptive effect, Neff and colleagues introduced meperidine as a supplement during nitrous oxide anesthesia as part of a balanced anesthetic technique that rapidly achieved widespread popularity. Meperidine has many side effects and cannot be used in high doses because of cardiovascular depression and significant histamine release. Fentanyl was synthesized by Janssen in 1959 and was released for clinical use in the United States in 1967. At that time, it had the most rapid onset and shortest duration of action of the available opioid agents. Fentanyl is extremely potent and has relatively few side effects. This opioid analgesic has become the most common opioid supplement used during anesthesia.

Lowenstein and colleagues proposed high-dose morphine anesthesia for cardiac surgery in the 1960s (62). The efficacy and safety of fentanyl as a primary anesthesic was later shown to be superior (63). The extremely high doses of opioids necessary to obtain a hypnotic effect and to maintain unconsciousness have restricted this anesthetic technique to surgical interventions that benefit from intense analgesia and optimal suppression of the stress response and for which postoperative mechanical ventilation is necessary. Consequently, high-dose opioid anesthesia is almost exclusively used for cardiac anesthesia. Because unconsciousness is not guaranteed, anesthesiologists soon realized that high-dose opioid "anesthesia" necessitates the use of additional drugs to prevent intraoperative recall.

Newer phenylpiperidine derivates, sufentanil and alfentanil, were developed by Janssen Pharmaceuticals (64). Sufentanil (Sufenta), a thienyl derivate of fentanyl, was synthesized in 1974. It is highly lipophilic, potent opioid with a short onset time and an intermediate elimination half-life of 3 to 4 hours. Alfentanil (Alfenta, Rapifen) was synthesized in 1976, and it has an even more rapid onset and a shorter duration of action after a single-bolus administration than sufentanil. Alfentanil is less potent and less lipophilic than either fentanyl or sufentanil. Remifentanil, an ultrashort-acting opioid developed by Glaxo-Wellcome, is undergoing extensive clinical investigation (65). It has a rapid onset and is rapidly metabolized by nonspecific tissue esterases. Remifentanil may prove to be the most acceptable opioid for continuous intravenous administration. However, the speed with which its effect dissipates after terminating the infusion raises concern in circumstances where prolonged postoperative analgesia is desirable.

Other opioids have found only limited applications in anesthesia. Lofentanil, levorphanol, and buprenorphine are examples of long-acting opioids that are rarely used in anesthesia except for postoperative pain relief. The use of phenoperidine was curtailed by the advent of shorter-acting drugs. Pentazocine has become obsolete because of the high degree of σ-receptor agonism causing dysphoria and hallucinations, and its low efficacy at the μ-opioid receptors. Similarly, butorphanol, dezocine, and meptazinol all cause an unacceptably high incidence of side effects.

CHANGING CONCEPTS OF INTRAVENOUS ANESTHESIA

Balanced Anesthesia

The concept of balanced anesthesia, in which several drugs are used, each with a specific effect, dates back to the theory of "anociassociation" introduced by George Crile between 1900 and 1910 (66). Crile proposed to block psychic stimuli associated with surgery by light general anesthesia and noxious stimuli by local anesthesia. The term balanced anesthesia, as suggested by Lundy in 1926 (67), was used to indicate the balanced use of premedication, regional anesthesia, and general anesthesia. The meaning of balanced anesthesia changed with the introduction of new intravenous agents. In 1938, Organe and Broad (68) used a combination of thiopental with nitrous oxide and oxygen. In 1947, Neff, Meyer, and Perales (69) introduced a technique in which nitrous oxide anesthesia was supplemented with intravenous meperidine, d-tubocurarine, and sodium thiopental. Thus, the original concept of balanced anesthesia representing a combined use of regional and general anesthesia was transformed into a term for the combined use of general anesthetics, opioids, and muscle relaxants.

Components of General Anesthesia

When combinations of various intravenous agents including opioids, barbiturates, and neuromuscular blocking agents began to be widely used for induction and maintenance of anesthesia, the concept of anesthetic components was introduced. Woodbridge (70) divided anesthesia into four components: sensory block; motor block; blockade of reflexes; and mental block. This concept was based on the findings that different intravenous drugs have their predominant effects on different components of anesthesia. The concept that the state of general anesthesia consisted of a spectrum of effects represented by separate pharmacologic actions (optimally produced by different pharmacologic agents) found general acceptance (71). Unconsciousness, analgesia, muscle paralysis, suppression of the stress response, and amnesia are different aspects of general anesthesia. Each of these components of the anesthetic state may have a different priority, depending on the clinical situation.

Neuroleptanalgesia

In 1954, Laborit and Huguenard (72) introduced a technique that produced the state of artificial hibernation (or "neuroplegia"). This state was achieved by the combined use of neuroleptics (e.g., chlorpromazine and promethazine) and opioids (e.g., meperidine). The aim of neuroplegia was to block endocrine and autonomic mechanisms usually activated by surgical stimulation. DeCastro and associates (73) combined an opioid phenoperidine (a meperidine derivative) with a neuroleptic agent (haloperidol) in the first demonstration of neuroleptanalgesia, a detached, pain-free state. Later, neuroleptanalgesia was produced by the combination of fentanyl and droperidol (Innovar). Neuroleptanalgesia eventually became neuroleptanesthesia through the use of larger doses of the intravenous drugs or by the addition of an inhaled agent.

HISTORY OF PHARMACOKINETIC CONCEPTS AND INFUSION TECHNIQUES

The effects of intravenous drugs depend on their pharmacokinetic and pharmacodynamic properties. Pharmacokinetic concepts were first introduced into anesthesia in the 1950s by Brodie and associates of New York and by Kety of Philadelphia, who studied the uptake and distribution of inhaled anesthetics and the metabolism of thiopental (74). In 1960, Price and colleagues described a physiologic model for the distribution of thiopental in the body (75). These investigators were the first to suggest that the lean tissues were more important than fat for the redistribution of thiopental from the CNS. Saidman and Eger demonstrated in 1966 that the hepatic metabolism of thiopental was also important in the termination of its central effects (76). In 1968, Bischoff and Dedrick further elaborated on the pharmacokinetic model with inclusion of the influence of hepatic metabolism, tissue blood flows, and tissue and plasma protein binding (77). Gillis and associates presented a plausible physiologic model to explain the actions of thiopental and methohexital (78). Yamaoka and colleagues developed the concept of noncompartmental modeling in 1978 (79). According to their model, the disposition of drugs is considered in terms of area under concentration-time curve and mean "residence" time (i.e., the time necessary to eliminate 62.3% of an injected dose from the body). From these two parameters, the clearance and the volume of distribution at steady-state can be derived (80). The concept of an "effect compartment" (i.e., the biophase in which the drug concentration determines its predominant effect) was suggested by Hull and associates in 1978 (81). In 1985, Scott and colleagues described the delay between the change in plasma concentration of fentanyl and alfentanil and their CNS effects ("hysteresis") as measured using the electroencephalographic (EEG) spectral edge (82).

The design of an appropriate infusion regimen depends on the knowledge of the concentrations necessary to obtain a given effect and of the pharmacokinetic parameters of the drug (83). If the drug is given as a fixed-rate infusion, a steady-state plasma and effect-site concentration will eventually be reached after a time delay dependent on the drug's terminal half-life and volume of distribution, an approach that is obviously impractical in clinical practice. The solution proposed by Boyes and associates (84) and by Mitenko and Olgivie (85) in the early 1970's was to administer a loading dose followed by a zero-order infusion. This solution was not optimal because the bolus dose resulted in a transient plasma concentration that was either too high or too low, depending on the distribution volume used for the calculation. In 1974, Wagner proposed a double-infusion regimen to achieve a therapeutic blood concentration more rapidly (86, 87). Instead of a bolus dose, a rapid infusion was administered, followed by a slow infusion calculated to achieve and maintain the target steady-state concentration more rapidly. The magnitude of the "overshoot" of the loading dose could be minimized by extending the duration of the loading infusion. The combination of a single bolus dose with two or more constant-rate infusions was originally proposed in 1969 by Kruger-Thiemer (88), and it was subsequently refined by Vaughan and Tucker (89), Rigg and Wong (90), and Schwilden and associates (91). The infusion technique was characterized by the letters BET because it consisted of a bolus dose (B) to achieve the target concentration, a maintenance infusion rate to replace the drug eliminated (E) from the body, and an exponentially declining infusion rate to compensate for drug transfer (T) to the peripheral compartments. Although this infusion scheme is most easily used with computer-driven pumps, manual techniques can closely approximate the BET model (91).

Clinical techniques learned from the common practice of titrating volatile anesthetics shows that the concentration of intravenous drugs has to be adapted to the individual needs of the patient and the variations in the magnitude of the stress of surgery. This approach was demonstrated in a quantitative fashion for alfentanil by Ausems and colleagues in an elegant series of clinical studies in the 1980's (92–94). Consequently, the use of variable-rate instead of fixed-rate infusions was investigated by White and associates (95, 96), Doze and colleagues (97), Shafer and colleagues (98), Sear and associates (99), and other investigators in more recent studies.

Computer technology has permitted the development of sophisticated pharmacokinetic model-driven continuous infusion devices. The first practical example was developed in 1981 by Schwilden (100), who demonstrated that it was possible to maintain the desired plasma concentration by means of an infusion pump controlled by a computer using pharmacokinetic parameters obtained from the anesthesia literature. This was the origin of the concept of target-controlled infusion (TCI) or drug delivery, also referred to as computer-assisted continuous infusion (CACI) (101). Instead of deciding on an infusion regimen, the anesthesiologist chooses a plasma concentration according to the status of the patient and the degree of surgical stimulation anticipated, and the computer-driven infusion pump then controls the drug's infusion rate to obtain the theoretical plasma concentration as predicted by pharmacokinetic information derived from a similar population of patients.

Computer-simulation programs of continuous intravenous administration of anesthetic drugs have increased our understanding of clinical pharmacokinetics (102). The terminal half-life of an agent does not reliably predict the rate of decrease of the plasma concentration after discontinuation of drug administration. In 1991, Shafer and Varvel were the first to examine the dependency of the rate of decline in effect-site concentration of fentanyl, alfentanil, and sufentanil on the duration of the infusion and to translate this information into a series of recovery curves (103). Concurrently, Hughes and associates proposed the concept of "context-sensitive" half-time (i.e., the time to decrease the plasma concentration of a drug by 50% after discontinuing an infusion) (104). The concept was further extended from opioids to intravenous hypnotics. Anesthesiologists can now suggest qualitative guidelines for pharmacokinetic properties desirable in anesthetic drugs (105).

The ultimate development of a computer-based drug infusion technique is the closed-loop administration of intravenous agents. The most promising development in this regard is a feedback control system for administering neuromuscular blocking drugs during anesthesia. A system for automatic maintenance of neuromuscular block was described for infusion of pancuronium (106). Another system was used to induce and to maintain neuromuscular block with succinylcholine. The feedback signal of the system was based on the evoked, rectified, and integrated electromyographic recording (107). The development of closed-loop systems for control of other components of anesthesia is complicated by the absence of an adequate feedback signal. Although devices using EEG-derived parameters and brain stem evoked potential signals as feedback information have been demonstrated to be clinically applicable in certain situations (108), the greatest challenge for further progress in automating intravenous anesthetic delivery remains the identification of an adequate measure of anesthetic depth (109).

REFERENCES

1. Major DJ. Chirurgia infusoria placidis CL: vivorium dubiis impugnata, cun modesta, ad Eadem, Responsione. Kiloni, 1667.
2. Wood A. A new method of treating neuralgia by the direct application of opiates to the painful points. Edinburgh Med Surg J 1855;82:265–281.
3. Sykes WS. Essays on the first hundred years of anaesthesia. Edinburgh: Churchill Livingstone, 1960 (vol I), 1960 (vol II), 1982 (vol III).
4. Oré PC. Etudes, cliniques sur l'anesthésie chirurgicale par la methode des injection de choral dans les veines. Paris: JB Balliere et Fils, 1875.
5. Adams RC. Intravenous anesthesia. New York: Paul B. Hoeber, 1944.
6. Kissin I, Wright AG. The introduction of hedonal: a Russian contribution to intravenous anesthesia. Anesthesiology 1988; 69:242–245.
7. Noel H, Souttar HS. The anesthetic effects of the intravenous injection of paraldehyde. Ann Surg 1913;57:64–67.
8. Peck CH, Meltzer, SJ. Anesthesia in human beings by intravenous injection of magnesium sulphate. JAMA 1916;67:1131–1133.
9. Naragawa K. Experimentelle studien uber die intravenose infusionsnarkose mittels alkohols. J Exp Med 1921;2:81–126.
10. Cardot H, Laugier H. Anesthésie par injection intrareineuse d'un melange alcool-chloroform-solution physiologique chez le chien. C R Seances Soc Biol 1922;87:889–892.
11. Bardet D. Sur l'utilisation, comme anesthesique general, d'un produit nouveau, le diethyl-diallyl-barbiturate de diethylamine. Bull Gen Ther Med Chir Obstet Pharm 1921;172:27–33.
12. Fischer E, von Mering J. Ueber eine neue klasse von schlafmitteln. Ther Gengenwart 1903;44:97–101.
13. Bumm R. Intravenose narkosen mit barbitursaure-derivaten. Klin Wochenschr 1927;6:725–726.
14. Weese H, Scharpff W. Evipan, ein neuartiges einschlaffmittel. Dtsch Med Wochenschr 1932;58:1205–1207.
15. Dundee JW. Historical vignettes and classification of intravenous anesthetics. In: Aldrete JA, Stanley TH, eds. Trends in intravenous anesthesia. Chicago: Year Book, 1980:1.
16. Lundy JS, Tovell RM. Some of the newer local and general anesthetic agents: methods of their administration. Northwest Med (Seattle) 1934;33:308–311.
17. Platt TW, Tatum AL, Hathaway HR, Waters RM. Sodium ethyl (α-methyl butyl) thiobarbiturate: preliminary experimental and clinical study. Am J Surg 1936;31:464–466.
18. Jarman R, Abel AL. Intravenous anaesthesia with Pentothal sodium. Lancet 1936;1:422–424.
19. Halford HJ. A critique of intravenous anesthesia in war surgery. Anesthesiology 1943;4:67–69.
20. Sternbach LH. The benzodiazepine story. In: Jucker, E, ed. Drug research. Vol 22. Basel: Birkhauser, 1978.
21. Randall LO, Schallek W, Heise GA, et al. The psychosedative properties of methaminodiazepoxide. J Pharmacol Exp Ther 1960;129:163–166.
22. Brandt AL, Liu SCY, Briggs BD. Trial of chlordiazepoxide as a preanesthetic medication. Anesth Analg 1962;41:557.
23. DuCailar J, Rious J, Bellanger A, Grolleau D. Utilisation du diazepam (Valium) en premédication. Ann Anesth Fr 1964;5:706–710.
24. Campan L, Espagno M Th. Note sur le diazepam en anesthésiologie. Ann Anesth Fr 1964;5:711–717.
25. Stovner J, Andresen R. Diazepam in intravenous anesthesia. Lancet 1965;2:1298.
26. Walser A, Benjamin LE Sr, Flynn T, et al. Quinazolines and 1,4-benzodiazepines: synthesis and reactions of imidazo (1,5-a)(1,4)-benzodiazepines. J Org Chem 1978;43:936–940.
27. Reves JG, Corssen G, Holcome C. Comparison of two benzodiazepines for anaesthesia induction: midazolam and diazepam. Can Anaesth Soc J 1978;25:211–214.
28. Reves JG, Fragen RJ, Vinik HR, Greenblatt DJ. Midazolam: pharmacology and uses. Anesthesiology 1985;92:310–324.
29. Amrein R, Leishman B, Benmtzinger C, Roncari G. Flumazenil in diazepine antagonism: actions and clinical use in intoxications and anaesthesiology. Med Toxicol 1987;2:411–429.
30. Selye H. Anesthetic effect of steroid hormones. Poc Soc Exp Biol Med 1941;46:116.
31. Selye H. Studies concerning the correlation between anesthetic potency, hormonal activity and clinical structure among steroid compounds. Anesth Analg 1942;21:41–52.
32. P'An SY, Gardocki JE, Hutcheon DE, et al. General anesthetic and other pharmacological properties of a soluble steroid, 21-hydroxpregomedione sodium succinate. J Pharmacol Exp Ther 1955;115:432–437.
33. Murphy FJ, Guadagni N, DeBon FL. Use of steroid anesthesia in surgery. JAMA 1955;156,1412.
34. Gordon RA, Lunderville CWP, Scott JW. Clinical investigation of Viadril. Can Anaesth Soc J 1956;3:335–340.
35. Davis B, Pearce DR. An introduction to althesin (CT1341). In: Steroid anesthesia: proceedings of the conference of the Royal College of Physicians, London, 1972:40.
36. Savege TM, Ramsay MAE, Curran JPJ, et al. Intravenous anesthesia by infusion. Anaesthesia 1975;30:757–761.
37. Van Hemelrijck J, Muller P, Van Aken H, White PF. Relative potency of eltanolone, propofol, and thiopental for induction of anesthesia. Anesthesiology 1994;80:36–41.
38. Maddox VH. The historical development of phencyclidine. In: Domino, EF, ed. PCP (phencyclidine): historical and current perspectives. Ann Arbor, MI: NPP Books, 1981.
39. Corssen G, Domino EF. Dissociative anesthesia: further pharmacologic studies and first clinical experience with the phencyclidine derivate CI–581. Anesth Analg 1966;45:29–40.
40. White PF, Way WL, Trevor AJ. Ketamine: its pharmacology and therapeutic uses. Anesthesiology 1982;56:119–136.
41. White PF. Ketamine update: its clinical uses in anesthesia. Semin Anesth 1988;7:113–126.
42. White PF, Ham J, Way WL, Trevor AJ. Pharmacology of ketamine isomers in surgical patients. Anesthesiology 1980;52:231–239.
43. White PF, Schüttler J, Shafer A, et al. Comparative pharmacology of the ketamine isomers: studies in volunteers. Br J Anaesth 1985;57:197–203.
44. Kay B, Rolly G. ICI 35868, a new intravenous induction agent. Acta Anaesthesiol Belg 1977;28:303–316.
45. White PF. Propofol: pharmacokinetics and pharmacodynamics. Semin Anesth 1988;7:4–20.
46. Sebel PS, Lowdon JD. Propofol: a new intravenous anesthetic. Anesthesiology 1989;71:260–277.
47. Smith I, White PF, Nathanson M, Gouldson R. Propofol: An update on its clinical uses. Anesthesiology 1994;81:1005–1043.
48. Godefroi EF, Jansen PAJ, Van Der Eycken CAM, et al. Dl-1-(1-arylalkyl)imidazole–5 carboxylate ester. A novel type of hypnotic agent. J Med Chem 1965;8:222–228.
49. Doenicke A. Etomidate, a new intravenous hypnotic. Acta Anaesthesiol Belg 1974;25:307–315.

50. Wagner RL, White PF, Kan PB, et al. Inhibition of adrenal steroidogenesis by the anesthetic etomidate. N Engl J Med 1984; 310:1415–1421.
51. Ledingham IM, Watt I. Influence of sedation on mortality in critically ill multiple trauma patients. Lancet 1983;1:1270.
52. Ledingham IM, Finlay WEI, Watt I, McKee JI. Etomidate and adrenocortical function. Lancet 1983;1:1434.
53. Wagner RL, White PF. Etomidate inhibits adrenocortical function in surgical patients. Anesthesiology 1984;61:647–651.
54. Doenicke A, Kugler A, Vollmann N, et al. Etomidate with a new solubilizer: clinical and experimental investigations on venous tolerance and bioavailability. Anaesthesist 1990;39:475–480.
55. Kulka PJ, Bremer F, Schuttler J. Induction of anaesthesia with etomidate in lipid emulsion. Anaesthesist 1993;42:205–209.
56. Thuillier MJ, Domenjoz R. Zur pharmakologie der intravenoesen kurznarkose mit 2-metholxy-4-allylphenoxyessigsaeure-N, N-diathylamide (G 29, 505). Anaesthesist 1957;6:163–170.
57. Wynands JE, Burfoot MF. A clinical study of propanidid (F.B.A. 1420). Can Anaesth Soc J 1963;12:587–590.
58. Serturner FWA. Darstellung der reinen mohnsaure nebst einer chemischen untersuchung des opiums mit vorzuglicher hinsicht auf einen darin neu entdeckten stoff und die dahin gehorigen beherkungen. J Pharm Aerzte Apth Chem 1806;14:47–52.
59. Smith RR. Scopolamine-morphine anesthesia, with report of two hundred and twenty-nine cases. Surg Gynecol Obstet 1908; 7:414.
60. Sexton JC. Death following scopolamine-morphine injection. Lancet Clin 1905;55:582.
61. Eisleb O, Schaumann O. Dolantin, ein neuartiges spasmolytikum und analgeticum. Dtsch Med Wochenschr 1939;65:967–972.
62. Lowenstein E, Hallowell P, Levine FH, et al. Cardiovascular response to large doses of intravenous morphine in man. N Engl J Med 1969;281:1389–1393.
63. Stanley TH, Webster LR. Anesthetic requirements and cardiovascular effects of fentanyl-oxygen and fentanyl-diazepam-oxygen anesthesia in man. Anesth Analg 1978;57:411–416.
64. Janssen PAJ. Potent, new analgesics, tailor-made for different purposes. Acta Anaesthesiol Scand 1982;26:262–268.
65. Feldman PL, James MK, Brackeen MF, et al. Design, synthesis, and pharmacological evaluation of ultrashort- to long-acting opioid analgetics. J Med Chem 1991;34:2202–2208.
66. Crile GW, Lower WE. Surgical shock and the shockless operation through anoci-association. Philadelphia: WB Saunders, 1921.
67. Lundy JS. Balanced anaesthesia. Minn Med 1926;9:399.
68. Organe GSW, Broad RJB. Pentothal with nitrous oxide and oxygen. Lancet 1938;2:1170–1172.
69. Neff W, Mayer EC, Perales ML. Nitrous oxide and oxygen anesthesia with curare relaxation. Calif Med 1947;66:67.
70. Woodbridge PD. Changing concepts concerning depth of anesthesia. Anesthesiology 1957;18:536–550.
71. Kissin I. General anesthetic action: an obsolete notion? Anesth Analg 1993;76:215–218.
72. Laborit H, Huguenard P. Pratique de l'hibernotherapie en chirurgie et medicine. Paris: Masson, 1954:267.
73. DeCastro J, Mundeleer P, Bauduin T. Critical evaluation of ventilation and acid-base balance during neuroleptanalgesia. Ann Anaesthesiol Fr 1964;5:425–436.
74. Brodie BB, Mark L, Papper EM, et al. The fate of thiopental in man and a method for its estimation in biological material. J Pharmacol Exp Ther 1950;98:85–96.
75. Price HL, Kovnat PJ, Safer JN, et al. The uptake of thiopental by body tissues and its relations to duration of narcosis. Clin Pharmacol Ther 1960;1:16–22.
76. Saidman LJ, Eger EI II. The effect of thiopental metabolism on the duration of anesthesia. Anesthesiology 1966;27:118–126.
77. Bischoff KB, Dedrick RL. Thiopental pharmacokinetics. J Pharm Sci 1968;57:1346–1351.
78. Gillis PP, deAngelis RJ, Wynn RL. Non-linear pharmacokinetic model of intravenous anesthesia. J Pharm Sci 1976;65:1001–1006.
79. Yamaoka K, Nakagawa T, Uno T. Statistical moments in pharmacokinetics. J Pharmacokinet Biopharm 1978;6:547–558.
80. Chan KKH, Gibaldi M. Estimation of statistical moments and steady-state volume of distribution for a drug given by intravenous infusion. J Pharmacokinet Biopharm 1982;10:551–558.
81. Hull CJ, vanBeem HBH, McLeon K, Watson MJ. A pharmacodynamic model for pancuronium. Br J Anaesth 1978;50:1113–1123.
82. Scott JC, Ponganis KV, Stanski DR. EEG quantitation of narcotic effect: the comparative pharmacodynamics of fentanyl and alfentanil. Anesthesiology 1985;62:234–241.
83. White PF. Clinical uses of intravenous anesthetic and analgesic infusions. Anesth Analg 1989;68:161–171.
84. Boyes RN, Scott DB, Jebson PJ, et al. Pharmacokinetics of lidocaine in man. Clin Pharmacol Ther 1971;12:105–115.
85. Mitenko PA, Olgivie RI. Rapidly achieved plasma concentration plateaus with observations of theophylline kinetics. Clin Pharmacol Ther 1972;13:329–335.
86. Wagner JG. A safe method for rapidly achieving plasma concentration plateaus. Clin Pharmacol Ther 1974;16:691–700.
87. Wagner JG. Linear pharmacokinetic equations allowing direct calculation of many needed pharmacokinetic parameters from the coefficients and exponents of polyexponential equations which have been fitted to the data. J Pharmacokinet Biopharm 1976;4:443–467.
88. Kruger-Thiemer E. Continuous intravenous infusion and multicompartment accumulation. Eur J Pharmacol 1968;4:317–334.
89. Vaughan DP, Tucker GT. General theory for rapidly establishing steady-state drug concentrations using two consecutive constant rate intravenous infusion. Eur J Clin Pharmacol 1975; 9:235–238.
90. Rigg JRA, Wong TY. A method for achieving rapidly steady-state blood concentrations for i.v. drugs. Br J Anaesth 1981; 53:1247–1257.
91. Schwilden H, Stoeckel H, Schuttler J, Lauven PM. Pharmacological models and their use in clinical anaesthesia. Eur J Anaesthesiol 1986;3:175–208.
92. Ausems ME, Hug CC Jr. Plasma concentrations of alfentanil required to supplement nitrous oxide anaesthesia for lower abdominal surgery. Br J Anaesth 1983;55 (suppl 2):191s–197s.
93. Ausems ME, Hug CC Jr, deLange S. Variable rate infusion of alfentanil as a supplement to nitrous oxide anesthesia for general surgery. Anesth Analg 1983;62:982–986.
94. Ausems ME, Hug CC Jr, Stanski DR, Burm AGL. Plasma concentrations of alfentanil required to supplement nitrous oxide anesthesia for general surgery. Anesthesiology 1986;65:361–373.
95. White PF, Dworsky WA, Horai Y, Trevor AJ. Comparison of continuous infusion fentanyl or ketamine versus thiopental: determining the mean effective serum concentrations for outpatient surgery. Anesthesiology 1983;59:564–569.
96. White PF. Continuous infusions of thiopental, methohexital or etomidate as adjuvants to nitrous oxide for outpatient anesthesia. Anesth Analg 1984;63:282–287.
97. Doze VA, Westphal LM, White PF. Comparison of propofol with methohexital for outpatient anesthesia. Anesth Analg 1986;65:1189–1195.
98. Shafer A, Doze VA, White PF. Pharmacokinetics and pharmacodynamics of propofol infusions during general anesthesia. Anesthesiology 1988;69:348–356.

99. Sear JS, Shaw I, Wolf A, Kay NH. Infusion of propofol to supplement nitrous oxide for maintenance of anesthesia. Anaesthesia 1988;43 (suppl):18–22.
100. Schwilden H. A general method for calculating the dosage scheme in linear pharmacokinetics. Eur J Clin Pharmacol 1981; 20:379.
101. Jacobs JR, Reves JG, Glass PSA. Continuous infusions for maintaining anesthesia. Int Anesthesiol Clin 1991;29.
102. Shafer SL, Stanski DR. Improving the clinical utility of anesthetic drug pharmacokinetics [Editorial]. Anesthesiology 1992; 76:327–330.
103. Shafer SL, Varvel JR. Pharmacokinetics, pharmacodynamics, and rational opioid selection. Anesthesiology 1991;74:53–63.
104. Hughes MA, Glass PSA, Jacobs JR. Context-sensitive half-time in multicompartment pharmacokinetic models for intravenous anesthetic drugs. Anesthesiology 1992;76:334–341.
105. Youngs E, Shafer SL. Pharmacokinetic parameters relevant to recovery from opioids. Anesthesiology 1994;81:833–842.
106. Brown BH, Asbury J, Linkens DA, et al. Closed-loop control of muscle relaxation during surgery. Clin Phys Physiol Meas 1980; 1:203–210.
107. Ritchie G, Ebert JP, Jannett TC, et al. A microcomputer based controller for neuromuscular block during surgery. Ann Biomed Eng 1985;13:3–15.
108. Schwilden H, Schuttler J, Stoeckel H. Closed-loop feedback control of methohexital anesthesia by quantitative EEG analysis in humans. Anesthesiology 1987;67:341–347.
109. Stanski DR. Monitoring depth of anesthesia. In: Miller RD, ed. Anesthesia. 4th ed. New York: Churchill Livingstone, 1994:1127–1159.

2 Basic Pharmacokinetic and Pharmacodynamic Principles

Elizabeth J. Youngs and Steven L. Shafer

Providing anesthesia is the art of providing certain desired effects at appropriate times: quick induction, hypnosis, analgesia, and rapid emergence are some common goals. Most anesthesiologists are facile at titrating volatile agents to achieve these goals. Inhalational anesthesia is perceived to be "easier" than intravenous anesthesia because it is easier to deliver and easier to titrate and because one can measure the end-tidal concentration of volatile agents. Many anesthesiologists, however, prefer to give intravenous anesthetic agents because of specific effects that cannot be achieved with volatile agents, such as clear emergence from anesthesia with propofol or analgesia and suppression of the stress response with opioids. Admittedly, it is more difficult to use these agents, at least with current technology, but these drugs do permit the achievement of goals not regularly obtained with volatile agents.

To use intravenous agents optimally requires at least a basic understanding of pharmacokinetics and pharmacodynamics. Pharmacokinetics is the dose-concentration relationship (what the body does to the drug), and pharmacodynamics is the concentration-effect relationship (what the drug does to the body). One must use knowledge of both to choose a dosing scheme that will produce the desired effects.

This chapter introduces the basic pharmacokinetic and pharmacodynamic models used in the anesthesia literature today. Most of the examples given are of intravenous drugs that have short durations of action, but the principles apply to most drugs used in anesthesia, including volatile agents. These principles are then used to design several different dosing schemes for anesthetic practice. This chapter should allow the reader to gain further insight into the anesthesia literature, to better understand the behavior of anesthetic drugs, and to utilize intravenous anesthetics in a more optimal way.

PHARMACOKINETICS

The fundamental pharmacokinetic concepts are volume and clearance. When a given amount of drug is introduced into the body and the concentration is measured, the volume, or volume of distribution, is the proportionality constant that relates amount to concentration:

$$\textit{concentration} = \frac{\textit{dose}}{\textit{volume}}$$

The volume of distribution is not necessarily equal to the absolute volume of tissues in the body. It is the *apparent volume* into which a dose of drug would have to be mixed to obtain the concentration measured in the plasma. A drug such as digoxin, for example, has extensive tissue binding, which makes its volume of distribution about 500 L (1).

Clearance is the body's ability to remove drug from the blood or plasma. For the drugs discussed in this chapter, the rate of drug removal depends on the concentration of drug in the plasma. Clearance is the proportionality constant relating rate of drug removal to plasma concentration, and it has the units volume/time:

$$\textit{rate of drug removal} = \textit{clearance} \times \textit{concentration}$$

Clearance describes an intrinsic capability of the body, not an actual rate of drug removal. For example, if the body has a clearance of 1 L/min for a particular drug, the actual rate of drug removal will be 0 if no drug is present in the plasma, 1 mg/min if the plasma drug concentration is 1 mg/L, and 100 mg/min if the plasma drug concentration is 100 mg/L. For drugs with linear pharmacokinetics, the clearance is a constant.

One-Compartment Model

It is possible to combine one volume and one clearance to get the classic "one-compartment model." This model can be visualized as a tank of water with a pipe at the bottom, as in Figure 2-1. In this simple hydraulic model, the higher the level of water, the faster it runs out of the pipe, because of increasing water pressure. The pressure exerted by the column of water is analogous to the concentration of drug in the plasma. The size of the pipe corresponds to clearance, and the cross-sectional area of the tank corresponds to the volume of distribution. For a given amount of drug (amount of water), the larger the volume of distribution (cross-sectional area of tank), the lower the concentration (height of water).

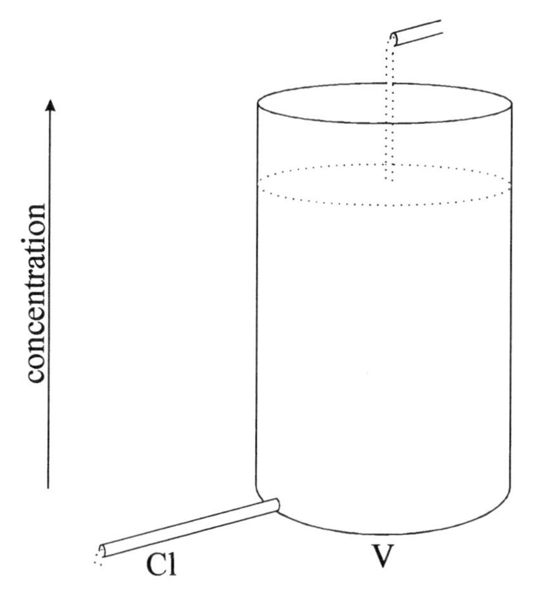

FIGURE 2-1. This hydraulic model is analogous to the one-compartment pharmacokinetic model. The cross-sectional area of the tank represents the volume of distribution (*V*), the cross-sectional area of the pipe leading out represents the clearance (*Cl*), and the height of fluid in the tank represents the concentration.

The process of clearing the drug from this compartment is a first-order process (i.e., directly proportional to concentration), so the concentration declines according to the following equation after a bolus:

$$C(t) = Ae^{-kt},$$

where A is the initial concentration, t is the time since the bolus, and k is the rate constant of elimination out of the body ($k = Cl/V$). The units of k are time^{-1}. The half-life of this process is simply $0.693/k$.

The concentration is usually plotted on a logarithmic scale to produce a straight line, as seen in Figure 2-2. The slope of this line is $-k$ and the y-intercept is A, the initial concentration. We can also visualize the decline using the hydraulic model in Figure 2-3, in which the concentrations are marked at different times after the bolus, as Eger originally described for inhalation anesthetics (2). Thus, the concentration decreases 50% after one half-life, 75% after two half-lives, and 87.5% after three half-lives.

During an infusion, the concentration is described by a more complicated expression:

$$C(t) = \frac{R}{Cl}(1 - e^{-kt}),$$

where R is the infusion rate. The concentration is not linear on a semilogarithmic graph, as in Figure 2-4.

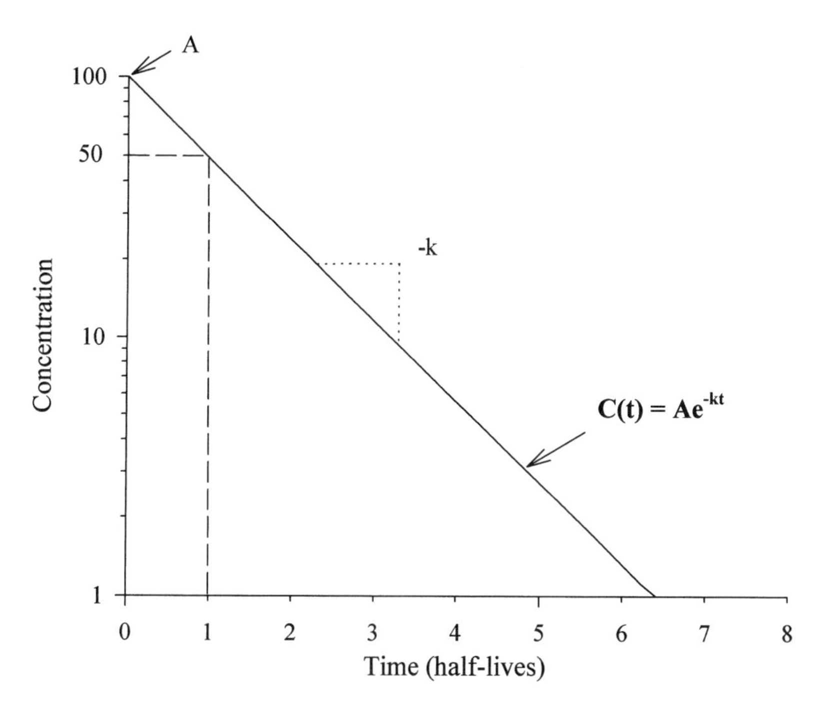

FIGURE 2-2. The solid line represents the concentration in a one-compartment model after a bolus. The y-intercept (A) is the initial concentration, and the slope is $-k$. It takes one half-life for the concentration to decrease by 50%. The concentration at time t is Ae^{-kt}.

However, the hydraulic model in Figure 2-5 can be used to show that the concentration reaches half of its eventual level after 1 half-life, 75% after 2 half-lives, and so on. Steady state is generally assumed to be reached after 4 or 5 half-lives (94% and 97% of steady-state concentration, respectively). Furthermore, from the foregoing equation, one can see that the steady-state concentration, C_{ss}, is equal to the infusion rate divided by the clearance. Therefore, at steady state, the volume of distribution has no effect on the concentration. The concentration at steady state is simply the level where the rate of flow out of the body is equal to the rate of flow into the body (i.e., the infusion rate).

If one wanted to achieve a constant target concentration (C_T) in a one-compartment model, one would simply give a bolus of C_T/V to achieve the concentration initially, then an infusion rate of $C_T \times Cl$, to maintain this concentration. This loading dose-maintenance rate scheme is traditionally used for many drugs in medicine.

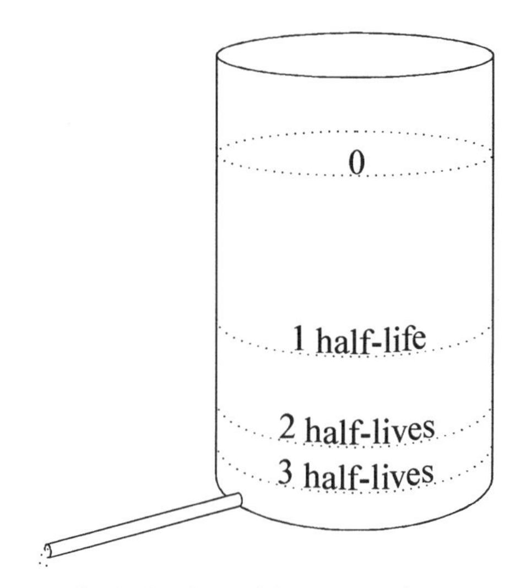

FIGURE 2-3. This hydraulic model represents the concentration in a one-compartment model after a bolus. It takes one half-life for the concentration to decrease by 50%, two half-lives for 75%, and three half-lives for 87.5%.

Three-Compartment Model

In contrast, most drugs used in anesthesia behave more like two- or three-compartment models. In Figure 2-6, an example of a three-compartment model is depicted. The tank receiving and eliminating the drug is the "central volume," and the other tanks are the "peripheral volumes." The drug initially is present only in the central volume. In time, it distributes into the peripheral volumes. V_2 is the compartment that equilibrates with plasma faster and is thus termed the "rapid peripheral volume;" and V_3 is the "slow peripheral volume." The sum of all the volumes is the volume of distribution at steady-state, or V_{ss}. The pipe leaving the central volume represents the "central clearance," also known as the metabolic or elimination clearance. The pipes connecting the peripheral volumes to the central volume are also clearances, the "intercompartmental clearances" or "distribution clearances." The pipe to V_2 is the "rapid intercompartmental clearance," and the pipe to V_3 is the "slow intercompartmental clearance." Each intercompartmental clearance is simply a proportionality constant relating net flow of drug between the compartments to the concentration gradient between the compartments.

The height of water in the tanks is now labeled "apparent concentration." Just as the volumes of distri-

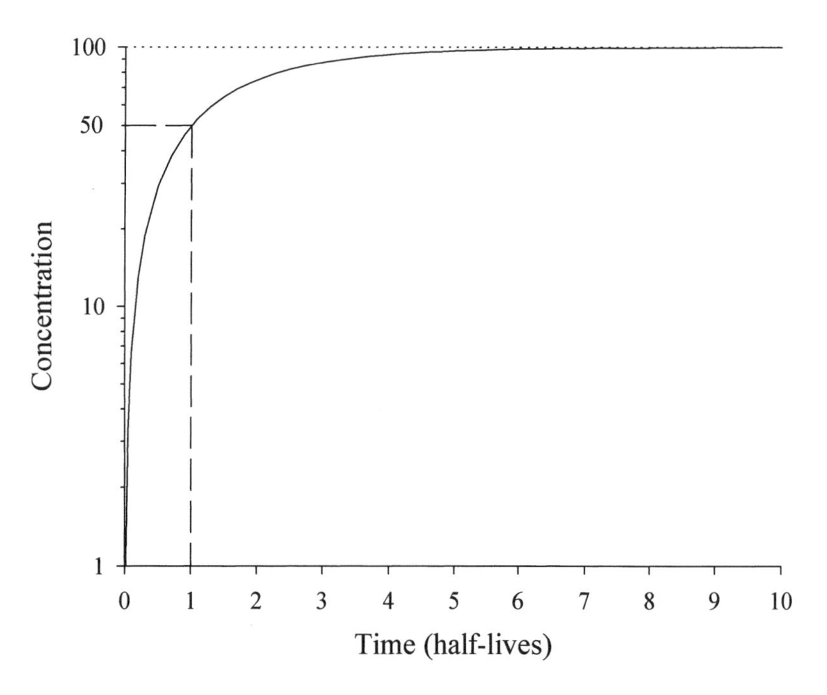

FIGURE 2-4. The solid line represents the concentration in a one-compartment model during a constant-rate infusion. It takes one half-life for the concentration to reach 50% of its final level.

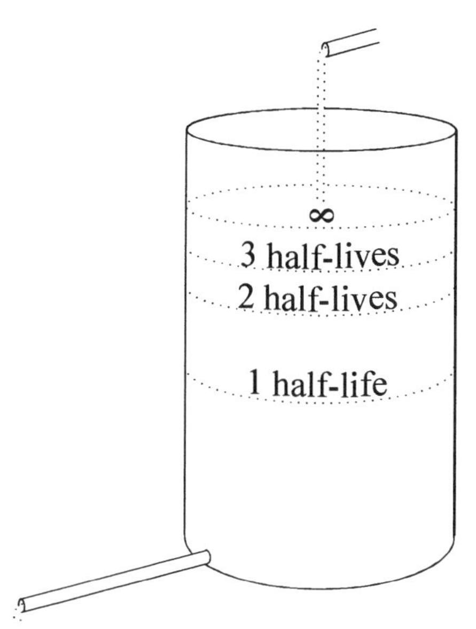

FIGURE 2-5. This hydraulic model represents the concentration in a one-compartment model during a constant-rate infusion. It takes one half-life for the concentration to reach 50% of its final level, two half-lives for 75%, and three half-lives for 87.5%.

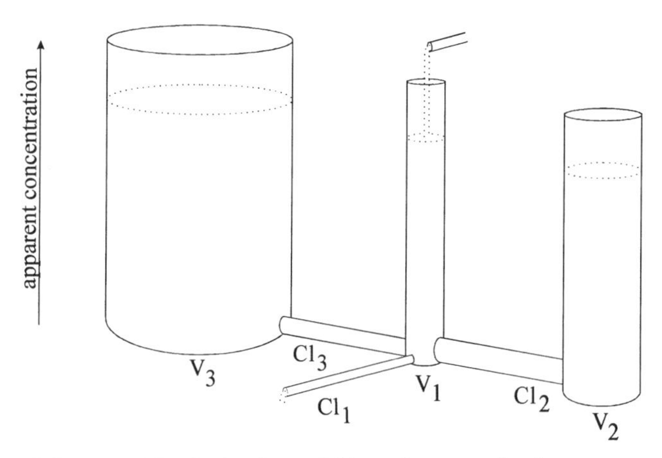

FIGURE 2-6. This hydraulic model is analogous to the three-compartment pharmacokinetic model. The tanks represent the three volumes of distribution (V_1, V_2, and V_3), and the three pipes represent the three clearances (Cl_1, Cl_2, and Cl_3). The height of fluid in the tanks represents the apparent concentration of drug.

bution are not actual volumes, the apparent concentration in the peripheral volumes is not necessarily equal to the true concentration of drug there. The peripheral volumes of distribution are determined such that, at steady-state, the *apparent* concentration in these compartments is equal to the concentration in the plasma. For example, a drug such as sufentanil has an extremely large V_3 (476 L) (3), presumably because it is highly lipophilic. At steady-state, the actual concentration in the tissues making up V_3 is much higher than the plasma concentration because sufentanil preferentially partitions into lipophilic tissues. Just as the apparent volume of distribution is much higher than the actual volume of slowly equilibrating tissues in the body, however, the apparent concentration is much lower than the actual concentration in those tissues.

What do the volumes and clearances estimated by pharmacokinetic modeling mean? The central volume of distribution represents the tissues into which the drug initially is dissolved. This includes the blood, along with tissues that have high blood flow. For three-compartment models, it is tempting to speculate that the rapidly equilibrating volume (V_2) corresponds to the vessel-rich group and the slowly equilibrating volume (V_3) corresponds to the fat- and vessel-poor group. This may provide some insight, particularly for highly lipophilic drugs, such as sufentanil in which a large V_3 may be explained by extensive distribution of the drug into fat. The peripheral volumes of drugs are not direct measures of discrete anatomic structures, however. In human patients, we cannot measure V_2 or V_3 because it would involve collecting multiple tissue specimens. The volumes reported for pharmacokinetic models are simply mathematical constants derived from equations that describe the plasma drug concentrations over time.

The central clearance is possible to measure with some accuracy. The central clearance, as in the one-compartment model, represents the sum of all processes clearing drug from the body: renal excretion, hepatic metabolism, metabolism by enzymes in the blood, or other mechanisms relevant for that drug. The intercompartmental clearances refer to flow of drug between compartments. These clearances are probably influenced by factors such as blood flow and capillary permeability. Like the peripheral volumes, however, the intercompartmental clearances are simply those values that mathematically explain the time course of the plasma concentration over time.

The time course of the drug's concentration in a three-compartment model can be described in three ways that are mathematically equivalent: 1) three volumes and three clearances, 2) five rate constants and a scaling factor, and 3) a triexponential equation. Each of these ways of examining the system has unique advantages, which is why pharmacokinetic studies frequently report all three sets of parameters.

The volume-clearance scheme is useful for visualizing how the drug moves throughout the body, as with the hydraulic models in Figure 2-7. Three distinct phases can be distinguished in the plasma concentration curve. The "rapid distribution phase" (solid line in Fig. 2-7) begins immediately after the bolus. This phase is characterized by rapid movement of the drug from the plasma to the rapidly equilibrating tissues. Then, a second "slow distribution phase" (dashed line in Fig. 2-7) is characterized by movement of drug into more slowly equilibrating tissues and out of the body, and by return of drug to the plasma from the most rapidly equilibrating tissues (i.e., those that reached equilibrium with the plasma at the end of phase 1). The

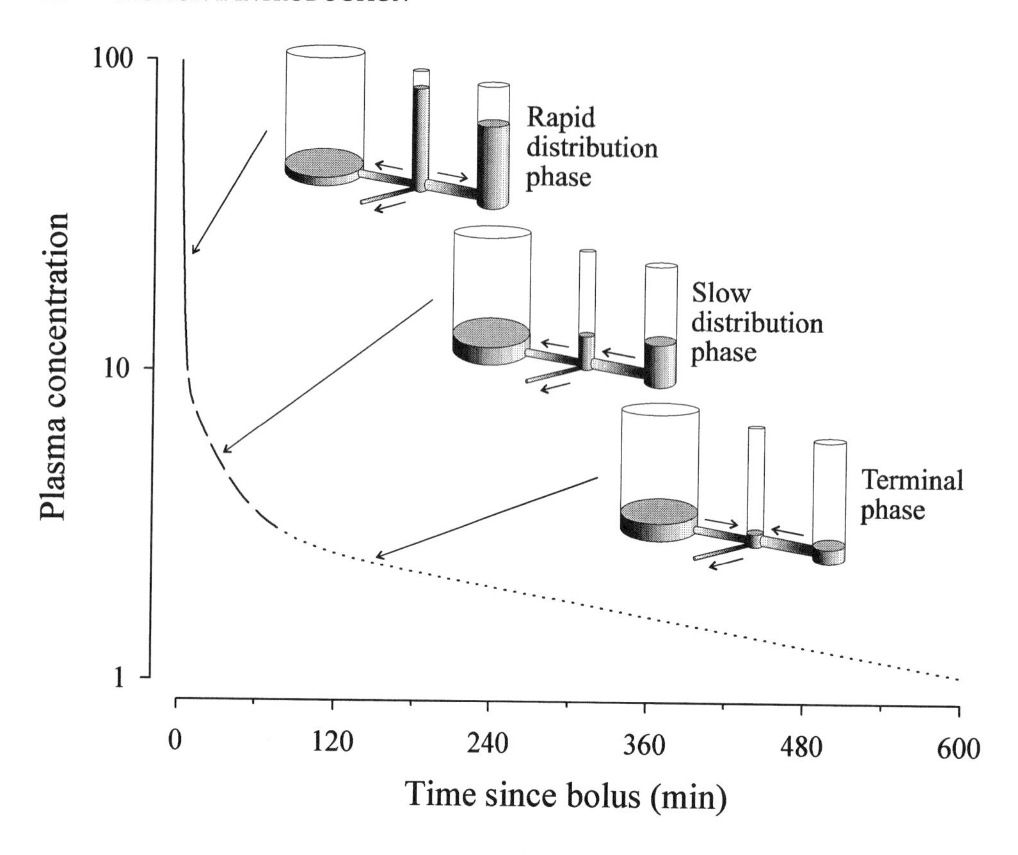

FIGURE 2-7. The graph represents the plasma concentration in a three-compartment model after a bolus. During the rapid distribution phase (solid line), drug is transferred from V_1 into V_2 and V_3 and out of the body. During the slow distribution phase (dashed line), drug is transferred from V_2 into V_1, and from V_1 into V_3 and out of the body. During the terminal phase (dotted line), drug is transferred from V_3 and V_2 into V_1, and from V_1 out of the body.

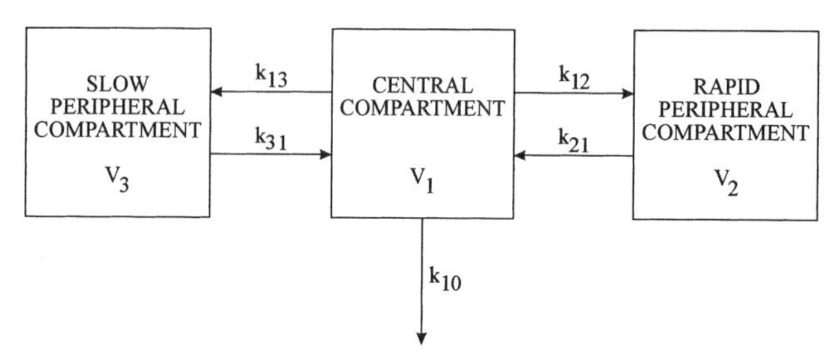

FIGURE 2-8. The boxes represent the three-compartment model in the rate-constant/scaling-factor parameterization. The arrows represent the rate constants for flow of drug.

"terminal phase" (dotted line in Fig. 2-7) approaches a straight line when plotted on semilog paper. The terminal phase is often called the "elimination phase" because the primary mechanism for decreasing drug concentration during the terminal phase is drug elimination from the body. During this phase, the drug also returns from the rapid and slow distribution volumes to the plasma, thereby slowing down the rate at which the plasma concentration decreases. Because elimination occurs during all three phases, "elimination phase" is a misnomer.

The rate constant-scaling factor scheme is depicted in Figure 2-8. Each "microrate constant," k_{ij}, defines the rate of drug transfer from compartment i to compartment j (Compartment 0 would be a compartment outside the model). This system is completely described by the five rate constants and V_1 as the scaling factor (V_2 and V_3 are also pictured, but are not independent parameters here). This scheme is useful for writing the differential equations that describe movement of drug in the body. The average anesthesiologist may not be particularly interested in differential equations, but these equations are useful for programming computers to simulate drug behavior (see the Appendix for these equations). The volume-clearance scheme and the rate constant-scaling factor scheme are simple to interconvert (see the Appendix).

Finally, the clearest way of describing the concentration data is with the third scheme, the triexponential equation:

$$C(t) = Ae^{-\alpha t} + Be^{-\beta t} + Ce^{-\gamma t},$$

where $C(t)$ is the drug concentration following a bolus dose, t is the time since the bolus, and A, α, B, β, C, and γ are parameters of a pharmacokinetic model. A, B, and C are called coefficients, whereas α, β, and γ are called exponents or hybrid rate constants. A, B, and C are occasionally called L_1, L_2, and L_3, and α, β, and γ are occasionally called λ_1, λ_2, and λ_3. After an infusion, there are still three coefficients, but they are different in value from the A, B, and C obtained after a bolus. The exponents remain the same after an infusion.

The triexponential equation really states that the concentrations over time are the algebraic sum of three separate functions, $Ae^{-\alpha t}$, $Be^{-\beta t}$, and $Ce^{-\gamma t}$. It is possible to graph each of these functions separately, as well as their algebraic sum at each point in time, as shown in Figure 2-9.

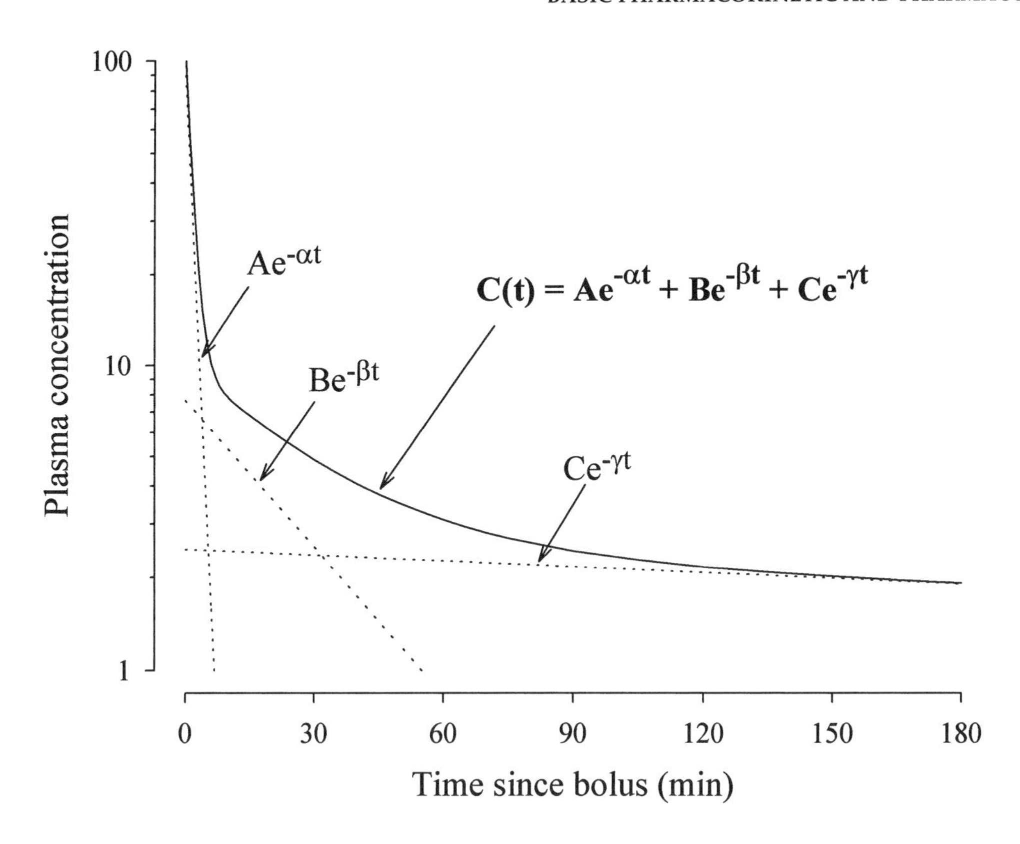

FIGURE 2-9 The solid line represents the plasma concentration in a three-compartment model after a bolus. The concentration is the sum of three monoexponential functions (dotted lines; $Ae^{-\alpha t}$, $Be^{-\beta t}$, $Ce^{-\gamma t}$).

At time 0, the previous equation reduces to:

$$C(0) = A + B + C$$

where $C(0)$ means concentration. Thus, the sum of the coefficients A, B, and C equals the concentration immediately following a bolus.

The exponents usually differ in size by about an order of magnitude. The exponential terms have several conventions. We prefer to order the exponentials as $\alpha > \beta > \gamma$. For historical reasons, however, some individuals always call the smallest exponent β. The context usually clarifies which exponent is the smallest.

The smallest exponent has a special significance. After sufficient time has passed, the values of $Ae^{-\alpha t}$ and $Be^{-\beta t}$ are so much smaller than $Ce^{-\gamma t}$ that the drug concentrations over time approach $Ce^{-\gamma t}$, which appears to be a straight line, with a slope of $-\gamma$, when plotted as log concentration versus time, as in Figure 2-9.

The three-compartment model has three half-lives: two distribution half-lives, calculated as $0.693/\alpha$ and $0.693/\beta$, and a terminal half-life (sometimes called the "elimination half-life"), calculated as $0.693/\gamma$. The literature often refers to the half-life of a drug. Unless stated otherwise, the half-life is the terminal half-life, i.e., 0.693/smallest exponent. The terminal half-life only refers to the third phase of the concentration-time curve. As pointed out by Shafer and Varvel (3) and by Hughes and associates (4), the terminal half-life for drugs with three exponential terms is not at all useful in predicting the decrease in concentration after a bolus or an infusion. The terminal half-life is always greater, often much greater, than the time it takes for drug concentrations to decrease by 50% after drug administration. The time for the concentration to decrease also depends on the duration of drug administration.

Mathematically, the coefficients and exponents are related to the volumes and clearances in an extremely complex way. Each phase of drug distribution, illustrated by volumes and clearances in Figure 2-7, is a sum of all three exponential terms, as seen in Figure 2-9. It is slightly easier to transform the rate constants and scaling factor into the triexponential equation, but each exponent is still a complex function of the rate constants.

In the literature, several sets of kinetic parameters are commonly published for a given drug. As our knowledge of pharmacokinetics has grown, pharmacokinetists have become more sophisticated at designing studies to obtain the most accurate results. For instance, the longer the sampling time, the better the third phase is defined for a three-compartment model. In addition, the sooner the first sample is drawn after administration of a bolus, the better the first phase is defined, unless, of course, the sample is drawn exactly at time 0, when the drug would still be en route from the venous injection site to the arterial sampling catheter. Arterial samples provide more accurate parameters than venous samples, because venous samples are affected by uptake into the tissues they directly drain

(5, 6). Moreover, a short infusion seems to give more precise parameters than a single bolus (5, 6).

Decline of Plasma Concentrations

In anesthesia, the offset of drug effect governs awakening from the hypnotic state. Thus, anesthesiologists are particularly concerned with the rate of decrease in the plasma concentration following drug administration. As described previously, the terminal half-life sets an upper limit on how long it will take the plasma concentrations to fall by 50%, but for drugs described by multicompartmental pharmacokinetics, the actual time for the plasma concentrations to fall by 50% is always faster than that and often much faster. The reasons for this discrepancy can be explained using volumes and clearances.

The bottom curve in Figure 2-10 shows the concentration of fentanyl after a bolus, in which most of the decrease in plasma concentration takes place in the first two phases. After a 1-hour infusion, however, the first and second phases are much less significant than after a bolus. This phenomenon can be explained by the finding that during that hour, the fentanyl was redistributing from the plasma into V_2 and V_3, and these compartments are partially filled by the end of the infusion. Therefore, when the infusion ends, less fentanyl can redistribute to these compartments, and the contribution of the distribution phases is smaller. After an infusion to steady-state, the first two phases still exist, although most of the decrease in plasma concentration takes place during the terminal phase. The dotted line in Figure 2-10 represents a 50% decrease in plasma concentration. This figure shows that infusion duration has an important influence on the time for a 50% decrease in concentration. The dot in Figure 2-10 represents the terminal half-life. Even after an infusion to steady-state, the time for a 50% decrease in plasma concentration is still less than the terminal half-life.

Because half-lives tell us almost nothing about the time required for the concentrations to fall by 50%, Hughes and associates (4) introduced the term "context-sensitive half-time" to describe the time required for a 50% decrease in plasma concentration following infusions of varying duration. The "context" is the duration of an infusion that maintains a steady drug concentration. In Figure 2-10, the points at which the concentration curves cross the dotted line represent the context-sensitive half-times for those infusion durations. Figure 2-11 shows the context-sensitive half-times for two opioids popular in anesthesia practice: alfentanil and sufentanil. The terminal half-lives for these drugs are 2 hours and 9 hours, respectively. Even though sufentanil has a longer terminal half-life, sufentanil concentrations fall much faster than the alfen-

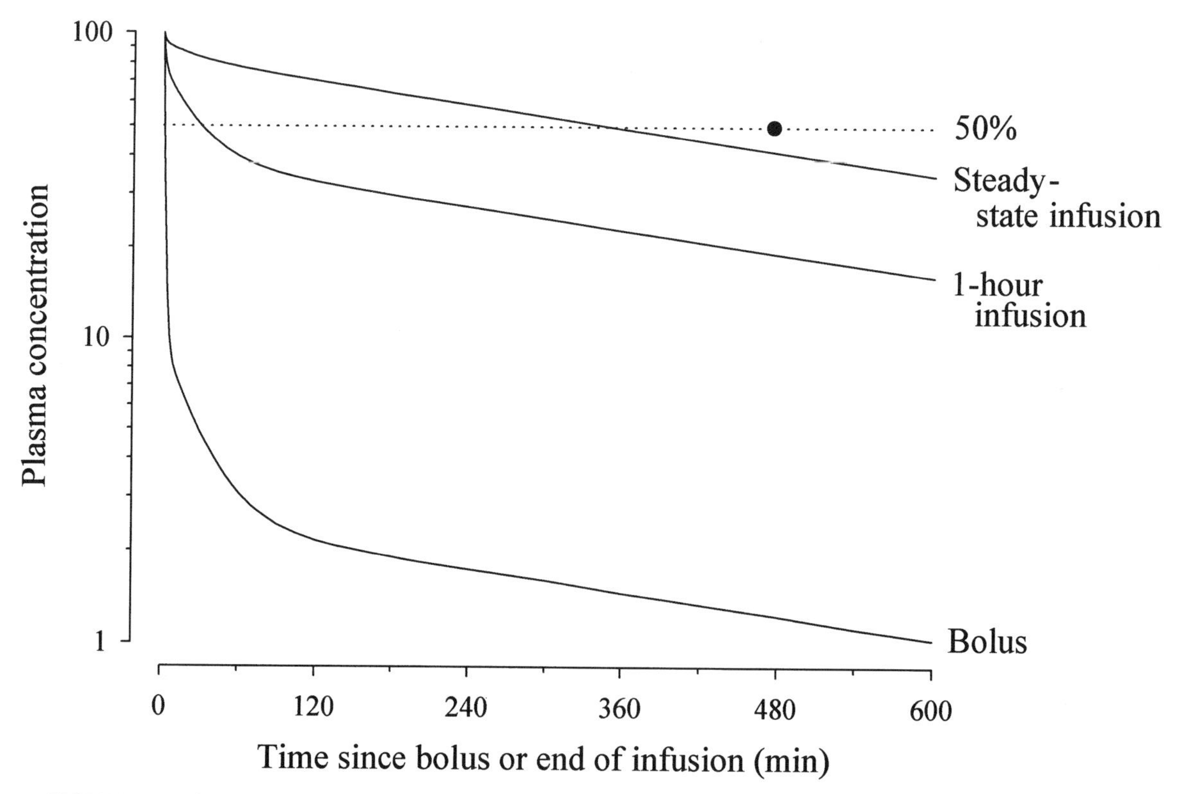

FIGURE 2-10. The solid lines represent the plasma concentration in a three-compartment model of fentanyl after either a bolus or an infusion that maintained a constant concentration. The dotted line represents 50% of the initial concentration, and the dot represents the terminal half-life.

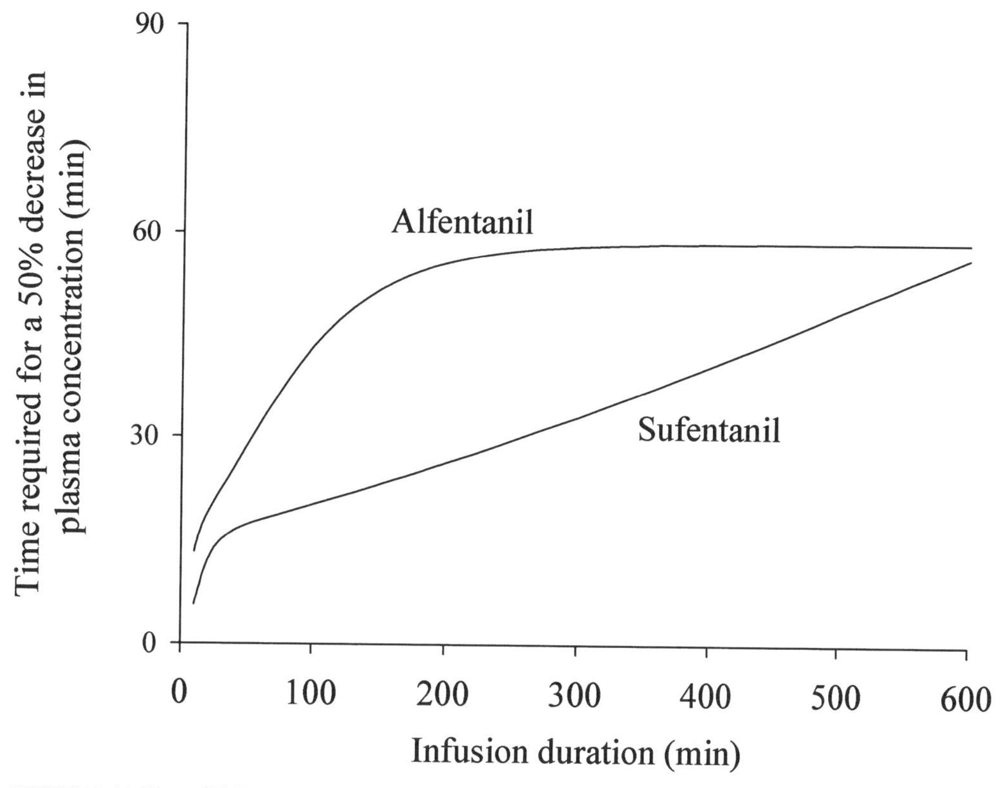

FIGURE 2-11. The solid lines represent the time required for a 50% decrease in plasma concentration after an infusion that maintained a constant concentration. After an infusion of any given duration, sufentanil takes less time than alfentanil to reach 50% of the initial concentration.

tanil concentrations for infusions of less than 10 hours' duration. This illustrates that terminal half-lives can be misleading because the 9-hour terminal half-life of sufentanil provides virtually no insight into how long it takes the plasma concentration to fall by 50% following drug administration.

PHARMACODYNAMICS

Pharmacodynamics is the relationship between drug concentration and drug effect. Most drug effects can be described by the so-called E_{max} model:

$$E = \frac{E_{max}C}{EC_{50} + C}$$

where E is effect, C is drug concentration, E_{max} is the maximum effect, and EC_{50} is the concentration that produces 50% of the maximum effect. The result is a sigmoidal curve, as illustrated in Figure 2-12.

A maximum effect, E_{max}, exists beyond which an increase in concentration has no further effect. In the case of simple receptor-mediated actions, this is when all the receptors are fully occupied. When the concentration is zero, no effect occurs, and when the concentration is equal to EC^{50}, the effect is half of E_{max}.

A more sophisticated model is the Hill equation:

$$E = \frac{E_{max}C^{\gamma}}{EC_{50}^{\gamma} + C^{\gamma}}$$

where γ is the Hill coefficient (not to be confused with the exponent γ from pharmacokinetic models). The symbol γ describes how steep the increasing portion of the curve is. A drug with a higher γ, such as the solid line in Figure 2-13, is difficult to titrate: this is a drug that either has no effect or the maximum effect, with a narrow range of concentrations in which an intermediate effect can take place. In contrast, a drug whose effect gradually increases with increasing concentration would have a smaller γ, as in the dashed line in Figure 2-13.

The EC_{50} is the index of drug potency; it is also referred to in the anesthesia literature as Cp_{50} and IC_{50}. Figure 2-14 shows the concentration *versus* effect relationship for three drugs of different potency. A drug with a lower potency simply needs a higher concentration to achieve a given effect. Although potency is often used to refer to the relationship between dose and effect, the dose-effect relationship is also influenced by pharmacokinetics. It is therefore more accurate to refer to the *concentration-effect* relationship.

Potency is not to be confused with efficacy. E_{max} is the measure of a drug's efficacy. The lower the E_{max},

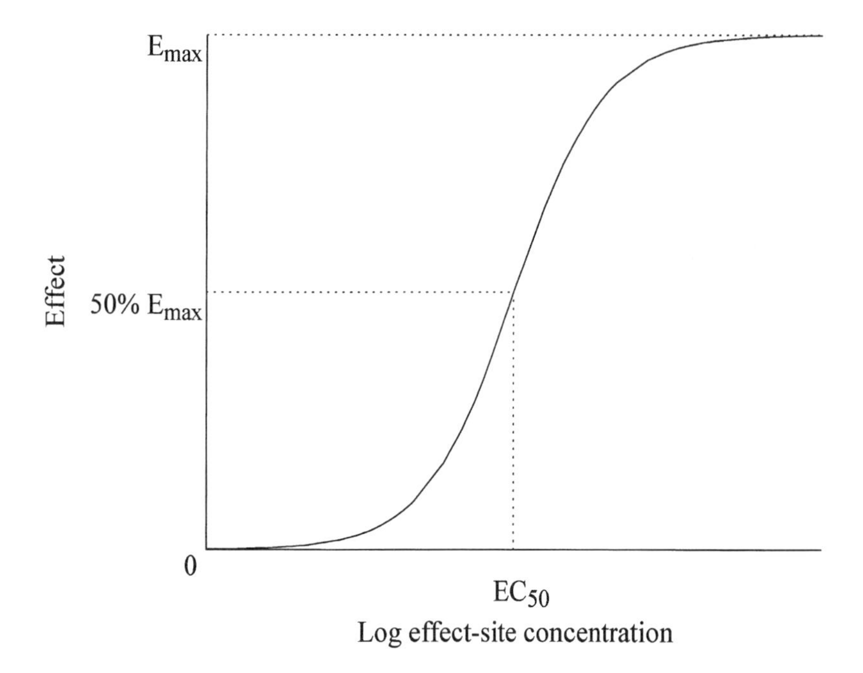

FIGURE 2-12. The solid line represents the effect at different effect site concentrations. EC_{50} is the concentration at which 50% of the maximum effect (E_{max}) is achieved.

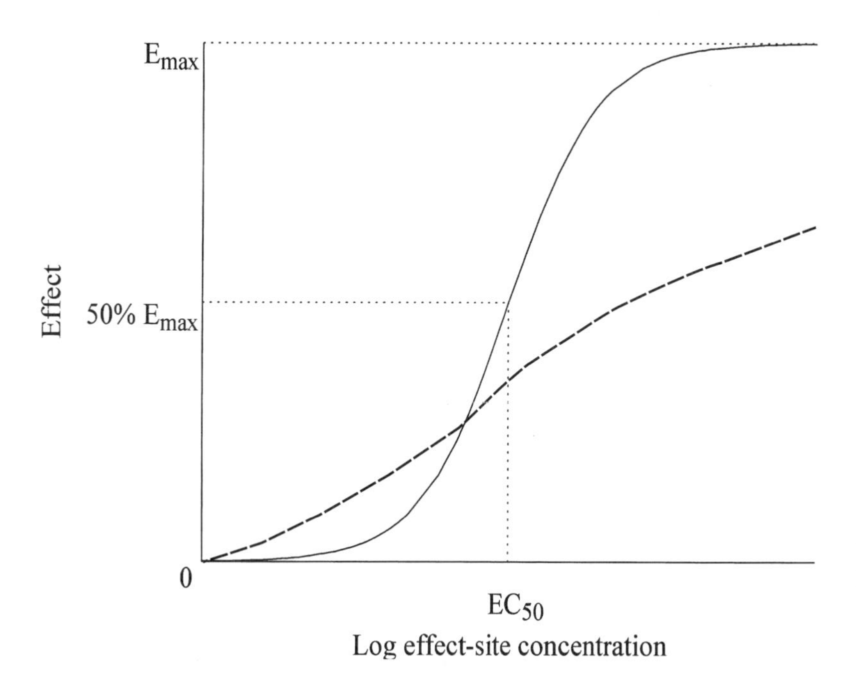

FIGURE 2-13. The solid line and the dashed line represent the concentration-effect relationship between two hypothetical drugs with different values of γ. The higher the γ, the steeper the ascending portion of the curve.

the less effective the drug at producing this particular effect, no matter how high the concentration.

The sigmoidal relationship as described earlier defines a continuous response to a drug in an average individual, such as change in heart rate in response to administration of a β-blocker. The sigmoidal relationship can also be used to characterize the probability of reaching a quantal (response-no response) effect in a population of patients. For example, Ausems and colleagues (7) examined the relationship between the opioid drug effect and the alfentanil concentrations in patients undergoing general anesthesia (Fig. 2-15). Using logistic regression, these investigators identified the probability of no response to three different noxious stimuli that patients receive in the operating room: intubation, skin incision, and skin closure. For a given concentration that falls within the steep portion area of the graph, some individuals respond and some do not.

With this type of quantal effect data, the steepness of the sigmoidal curve, γ, is related to the amount of variability in the study population. Drugs with little

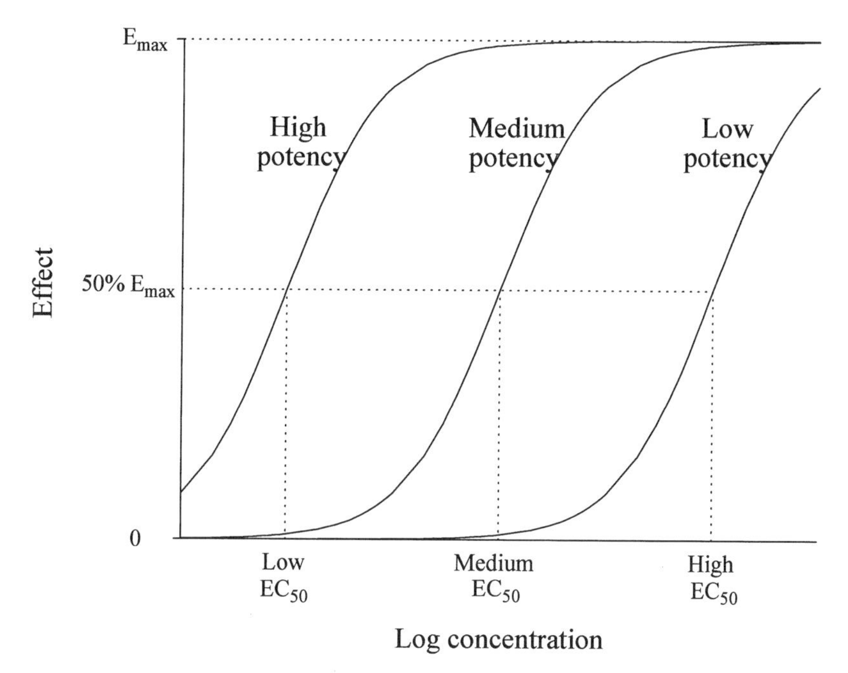

FIGURE 2-14. The curves represent the concentration-effect relationship between three hypothetical drugs with different values of EC_{50} (the concentration at which 50% of the maximum effect is achieved). The higher the EC_{50}, the lower the potency.

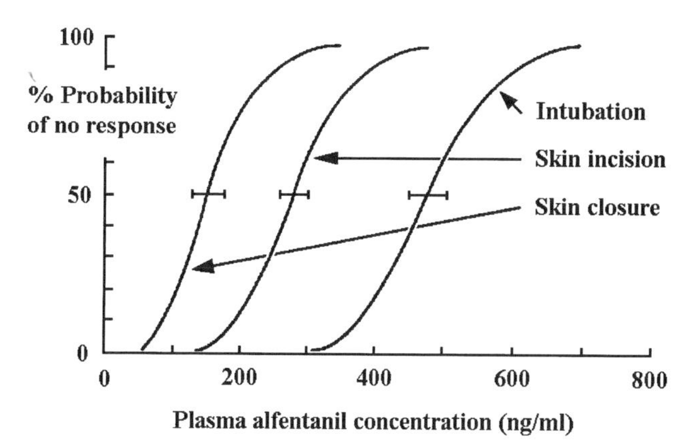

FIGURE 2-15. The curves represent the concentration-effect relationships for alfentanil. In this case, effect is the probability of no response to each of three stimuli. (From Ausems ME, Hug CC, Stanski DR, Burm AGL. Plasma concentrations of alfentanil required to supplement nitrous oxide anesthesia for general surgery. Anesthesiology 1986;65:362–373.)

variability between concentration and effect have steep curves and large γs. Drugs with more variability have more gently sloping curves and lower γs.

These pharmacodynamic relationships can be used to define a therapeutic window, as shown in Figure 2-16, to guide the initial choice of the optimal concentration. Just as we can construct models relating the therapeutic effect to the concentration, we can relate concentration to a toxic effect as well. The effect can be a continuous effect or a probability response, as long as information is available on how different individuals in the population will respond to a given concentration. In the case of propofol in Figure 2-16, sedation levels 2 and 3 were considered desirable levels of sedation. Level 4 was considered excessively deep, thereby exposing the patient to unnecessary risk. The therapeutic window for light propofol sedation was set between 0.5 and 1.0 μg/ml based on this analysis (Dyck et al, unpublished data).

By knowing the relationship among concentration, desired effect, and toxic effect, we can identify the therapeutic window at which most subjects will have the desired effect while few will show the toxic effect. Using the principles outlined in the next section, the practitioner can design a dosing scheme that has a high likelihood of achieving a concentration in the therapeutic window, which, in turn, has a high likelihood of producing the desired drug effect. Tables 2-1 and 2-2 list the therapeutic windows for fentanyl, alfentanil, sufentanil, and propofol. These therapeutic windows are based partly on analyses such as the foregoing one for propofol, and partly on simulations for those studies whose experimental design did not permit direct measurement. These simulations, which were based on current knowledge of each drug's pharmacokinetics and pharmacodynamics, are unpublished. With recent advances in experimental design, these therapeutic windows are expected to be formally validated or refined in the near future.

So far, the "concentration versus effect" relationship have been discussed without being specific about defining concentration. Although the plasma concentration following an intravenous bolus peaks nearly instantaneously, most anesthesiologist would not induce anesthesia with an intravenous bolus of a hypnotic and immediately intubate the patient's trachea. The reason, of course, is that although the plasma concentration peaks almost instantly, additional time is required for the drug concentration in the brain to rise and to induce unconsciousness, as shown in Figure 2-17. This

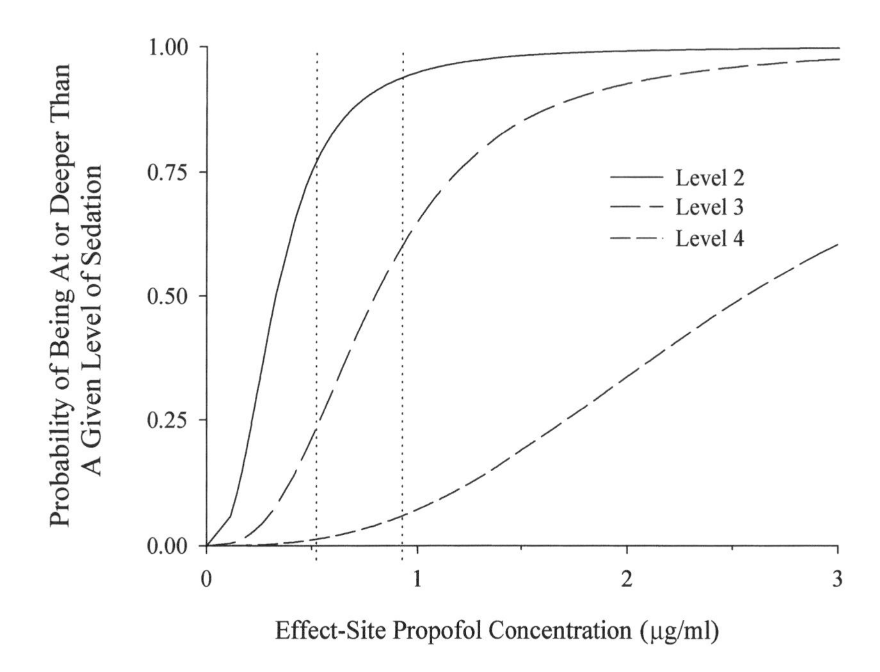

FIGURE 2-16. The curves represent the concentration-effect relationships for propofol. Effect is the probability of being at or deeper than one of three levels of sedation, with level 4 being the deepest. The dotted lines delineate the therapeutic window, where most patients should be at the desired levels of 2 or 3.

TABLE 2-1. Therapeutic Windows for Opioids*

Use	Fentanyl (ng/ml)	Alfentanil (ng/ml)	Sufentanil (ng/ml)
Induction and intubation			
With thiopental	3–5	250–400	0.4–0.6
With nitrous oxide (N_2O)	8–10	400–750	0.8–1.2
Maintenance			
With N_2O-volatile agent	1.5–4	100–300	0.25–0.5
With N_2O	1.5–10	100–750	0.25–1.0
With O_2 only	15–60	1000–4000	2–8, 10–60
Adequate ventilation on emergence	1.5	125	0.25

**Effect-site concentrations likely to achieve the desired effect during different stages of an anesthetic. (Adapted from Shafer SL, Varvel JR. Pharmacokinetics, pharmacodynamics, and rational opioid selection. Anesthesiology 1991;74:53–63.*

TABLE 2-2. Therapeutic Windows for Propofol*

Use	Therapeutic Window (µg/ml)
Induction and intubation	
Unpremedicated	6–9†
Premedicated	3–4.5†
Maintenance	
With nitrous oxide (N_2O)	2–5†,3–7‡
With opioid	2–4†,4–7‡
With O_2	6–9†,8–16‡
Adequate ventilation on emergence	1–2†
Sedation	0.5–1.5‡,1–2†

**Effect-site concentrations of propofol likely to achieve the desired effect during different stages of an anesthetic.*

†Data from Shafer SL, Kern DE, Stanski DR. The scientific basis of infusion techniques in anesthesia. North Reading, MA: Bard MedSystems Division, 1990.

‡Data from Diprivan package insert. Wilmington, DE: Stuart Pharmaceuticals, 1993.

delay reflects the fact that the plasma is usually not the site of the drug's action, only the mechanism of transport to that site. Drugs exert their biologic effect at the "biophase," or the "effect site," which is the precise location where the drug acts on the body, and may include membranes, receptors, or other molecular structures.

The concentration of drug in the biophase cannot be measured. First, it is usually inaccessible in human subjects. Second, even if we could take tissue samples, the drug concentration in the microscopic environment of the receptors would not necessarily be the same as the concentration grossly measured in brain tissue or cerebrospinal fluid. Although we cannot measure drug concentration in the biophase, using rapid measures of drug effect we can characterize the time course of the drug effect. Knowing the time course of the drug effect, one can characterize the rate of drug flow into and out of the biophase. Using these values to add to our model an effect compartment, is shown in Figure 2-18. The effect site is the hypothetical compartment whose concentration parallels the time course of drug effect.

The effect compartment, by definition, is so small that it has no influence on pharmacokinetics. The k_{e0} is the microrate constant out of the effect site compartment. In Figure 2-19, the k_{e0} refers to drug transfer from the effect site compartment to V_1 (in which case it should really be called k_{e1}). Mathematically, this figure is correct, although k_{e0} is occasionally represented as an arrow pointing out into empty space. This second version gives almost identical results in simulations because the amount of drug moving along that pathway does not significantly affect the plasma concentration.

If a constant plasma concentration is maintained, then the time required for the biophase concentration to reach 50% of the plasma concentration ($t½\ k_{e0}$) can be calculated as $0.693/k_{e0}$. Following a bolus dose, the time to achieve a peak effect site concentration is a function of *both* pharmacokinetics and k_{e0}. For drugs with an extremely rapid decline in plasma concentration following a bolus (e.g., adenosine, with a half-life of several seconds), the effect site concentration peaks within several seconds of the bolus, regardless of the k_{e0}. For drugs with a rapid k_{e0} and a slow decrease in concentration following bolus injection (e.g., pancuronium), the time to peak effect site concentration is determined more by the k_{e0} than by the plasma pharmacokinetics. The k_{e0} and $t½\ k_{e0}$ have been characterized for many drugs used in anesthesia. Equilibration between the plasma and the effect site is rapid for thiopental (9, 10), propofol (11), and alfentanil (12), intermediate for fentanyl (12) and sufentanil (13) and the nondepolarizing muscle relaxants (14), and slow for morphine (15) and ketorolac (Mandema and Stanski, unpublished data).

Using three hypothetical drugs with identical pharmacokinetics but different k_{e0}, values one can consider the influence of k_{e0} on the onset of drug effect. Figure 2-20 shows the plasma concentrations and apparent biophase concentrations after an intravenous bolus of these three drugs with these values for $t½\ k_{e0}$: 1, 2, and

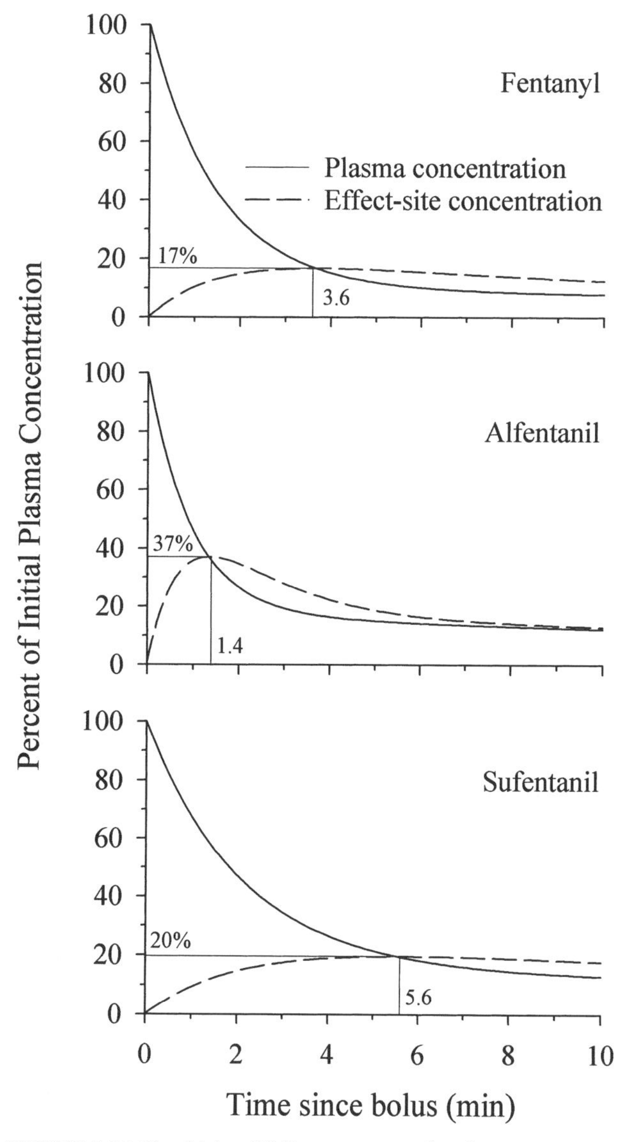

FIGURE 2-17. The thick solid lines represent the plasma concentrations after a bolus for fentanyl, alfentanil, and sufentanil. The dashed lines are the effect site concentrations. The thin solid lines identify the concentration and time at which the peak effect site concentration occurs. (From Shafer SL, Varvel JR. Pharmacokinetics, pharmacodynamics, and rational opioid selection. Anesthesiology 1991;74:53–63.)

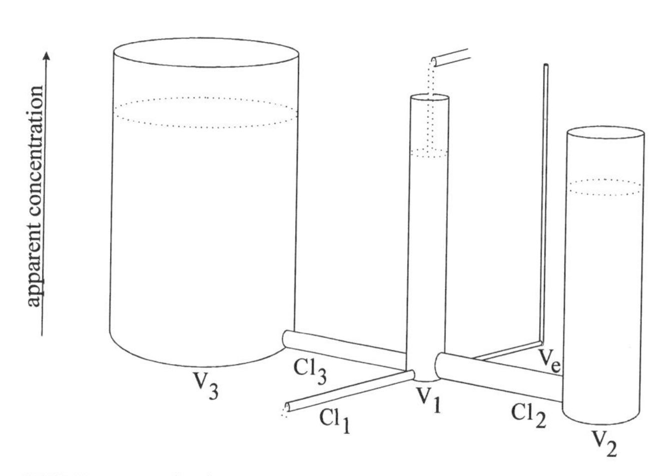

FIGURE 2-18. This hydraulic model represents the three-compartment model with a separate tank representing the effect site (V_e).

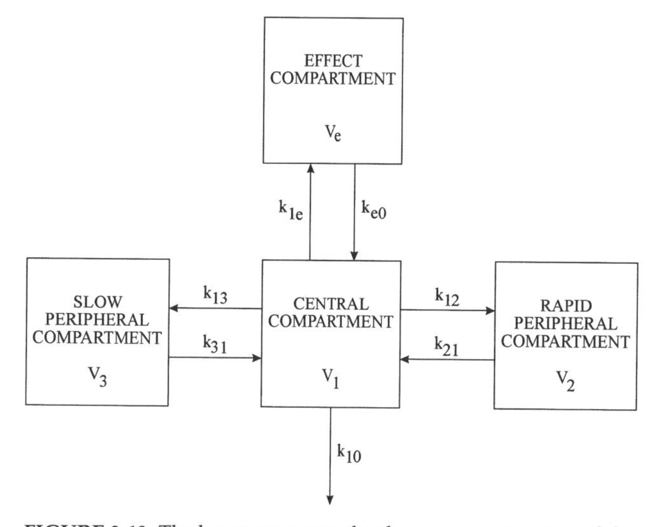

FIGURE 2-19. The boxes represent the three-compartment model with an effect site (V_e). The rate constant, k_{e0}, is commonly used to describe the time course of equilibration between the plasma and the effect site.

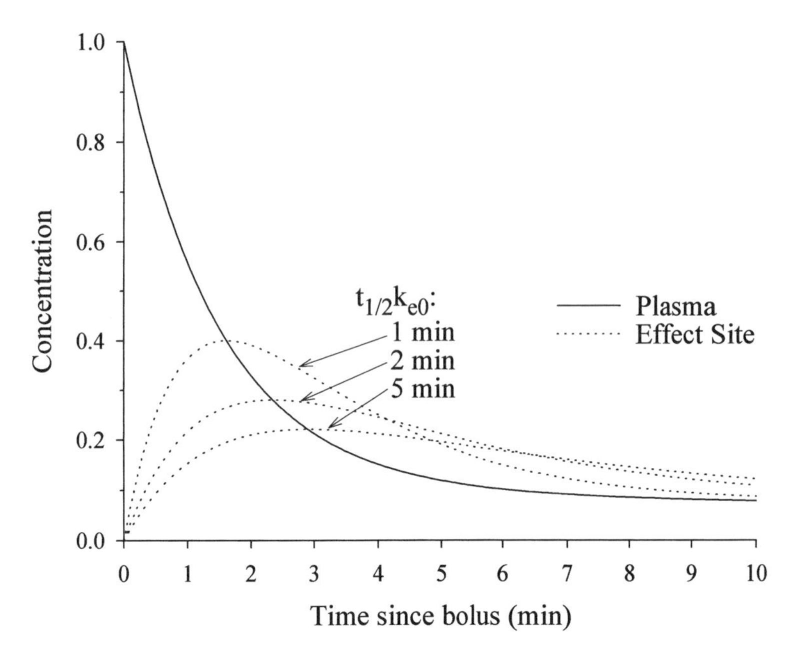

FIGURE 2-20. The solid line represents the plasma concentration after a bolus of a hypothetical drug. The dotted lines represent the effect site concentration of this drug, assuming different k_{e0}.

5 minutes. Regardless of the value of k_{e0}, the pattern remains the same. The plasma concentration peaks instantly and then steadily declines. The effect site concentration starts at 0 and increases over time until it equals the (descending) plasma concentration. The plasma concentration continues to fall, and after that moment of identical concentrations, the gradient between the plasma and the effect site favors drug removal from the effect site as the effect site concentrations decrease.

Examining the different values of $t½\ k_{e0}$ in Figure 2-20 shows that as $t½\ k_{e0}$ increases, the time to reach the peak apparent biophase concentration also increases. Concurrently, the magnitude of the peak effect site concentration relative to the initial plasma concentration decreases because slower equilibration between the plasma and biophase allows more drug to be distributed to other peripheral tissues.

Let us again turn to two newer opioids used in the practice of anesthesia: alfentanil and sufentanil. As shown in Figure 2-17, the rapid plasma-effect site equilibration (large k_{e0}, small $t½\ k_{e0}$) of alfentanil causes the effect site concentration to rise rapidly, producing a peak in about 90 seconds. At the time of the peak effect, about 60% of the alfentanil bolus will have been distributed into the peripheral tissues or eliminated from the body. For sufentanil, the effect site concentration rises much more slowly and peaks at 5 to 6 minutes following the bolus. At the time of the peak, over 80% of the initial bolus of sufentanil will have been distributed into the tissues or eliminated. To achieve an equivalent peak effect site concentration, relatively more sufentanil than alfentanil must be injected into the plasma, and the rate of drug offset from a sufentanil bolus is slower than that of an alfentanil bolus.

When one uses "a therapeutic window", the concept of the effect site is important in understanding the time course of drug effect. Figure 2-21 depicts the therapeutic window for fentanyl in supplementing induction with thiopental. If one gives a relatively low dose, the desired effect is achieved only for a moment. A relatively high dose not only achieves the desired effect for a longer period of time, but also results in a faster onset of this effect.

DESIGNING DOSING REGIMENS

After reviewing all the necessary concepts in pharmacokinetics and pharmacodynamics, one can use these principles to develop dosing regimens for different clinical situations. The practitioner can choose the bolus dose that has the greatest likelihood of achieving the desired effect in the desired time frame; and choose an infusion regimen to maintain a constant effect; and predict when to stop an infusion to achieve the desired clinical recovery.

Bolus Dosing Regimens

Unlike the dosing regimen described earlier for the one-compartment model, $dose = C_T \times V$, the three-compartment model with an effect site does not have a traditional volume of distribution to be used in this calculation. V_1 is too small (redistribution and elimination occur before the drug reaches the effect site, so the dose would be too low), and V_{ss} is too large (the drug is not expected to spread equally throughout the compartments for many hours, so the initial dose would be too high).

A simple method of calculating the bolus dose to achieve a desired peak concentration at the effect site

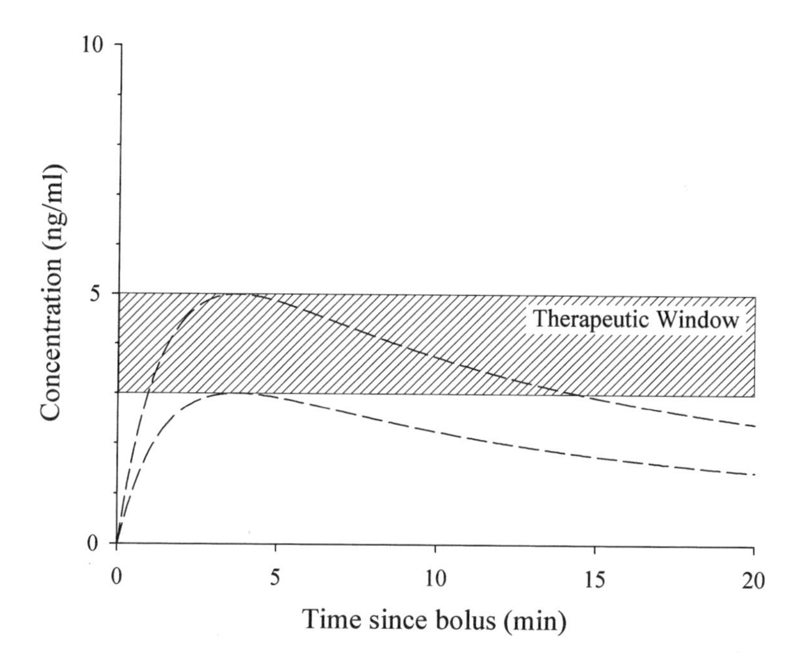

FIGURE 2-21. The hatched area represents the therapeutic window for fentanyl in supplementing induction with thiopental. If a small dose of fentanyl is given, the therapeutic level is achieved for a moment; if a larger dose of fentanyl is given, the therapeutic level is reached earlier and has a longer duration.

is available. As in Figure 2-17, for each drug the peak effect site concentration is a given percentage of the initial plasma concentration (17%, 37%, and 20% for fentanyl, alfentanil, and sufentanil, respectively). This number remains constant for all clinically relevant concentrations, because these drugs have linear pharmacokinetics. This peak effect site concentration is equivalent to the plasma concentration at the time of peak effect. If one thinks of the decline in plasma concentration after the bolus as a dilution into a larger and larger volume, one could calculate a volume of distribution for the bolus at the time of peak effect. Technically, this is not a true volume of distribution because elimination from the body also contributes to the decline in plasma concentration. The constant that describes this hypothetical volume has been called "V_d peak effect" (16); to be consistent with the nomenclature in this chapter, we call it "$V_{peak\ effect}$."

$V_{peak\ effect}$ can be easily calculated if one knows the ratio between the initial plasma concentration and the plasma concentration at the time of peak effect:

$$V_{peak\ effect} = V_1 \frac{C_{plasma,\ initial}}{C_{plasma,\ peak\ effect}},$$

where $C_{plasma,\ initial}$ is the initial concentration following a bolus and $C_{plasma,\ peak\ effect}$ is the concentration at the time of peak effect. Table 2-3 lists the $V_{peak\ effect}$ for several commonly used drugs in anesthesia, along with the time at which to expect that peak effect.

The next step is to calculate dose:

$$Dose = C_T \times V_{peak\ effect},$$

where C_T is the target effect site concentration. As an example, fentanyl has a $V_{peak\ effect}$ of 75 L, as listed in Table 2-3. To produce a peak fentanyl effect site concentration of 4.0 ng/ml (in the middle of the therapeutic window for supplementing induction with thiopental), the calculated dose is 300 μg, which should produce a peak effect in 3.6 minutes. This dose is useful and clinically relevant.

TABLE 2-3. $V_{peak\ effect}$* for Calculating Bolus Dose

Drug	$V_{peak\ effect}$ (L)	Time to peak effect (min)
Fentanyl	75	3.6
Alfentanil	5.9	1.4
Sufentanil	89	5.6
Propofol	24	2.0

*$V_{peak\ effect}$ is the proportionality constant which, when multiplied by the target concentration, should produce the desired peak effect in the number of minutes noted above. (Adapted from Shafer SL, Kern DE, Stanski DR. The scientific basis of infusion techniques in anesthesia. North Reading, MA: Bard MedSystems Division, 1990.)

Pharmacokinetic-pharmacodynamic modeling can also be used to choose the drug that would lead to the fastest clinical recovery. As mentioned earlier, because alfentanil equilibrates with the effect site faster than fentanyl or sufentanil, relatively less drug is needed to achieve a given peak effect, and recovery is more rapid. Therefore, alfentanil is a rational choice of opioid for a rapid recovery after a bolus.

Maintenance Dosing Regimens

To maintain a constant concentration at the effect site after the desired level is achieved, one needs to start an infusion exactly at the time of peak effect. At this time, no concentration gradient exists between the plasma and the effect site, and if $C_{plasma,\ peak\ effect}$ can be maintained, the effect site will also remain at this concentration. For the one-compartment model, as before,

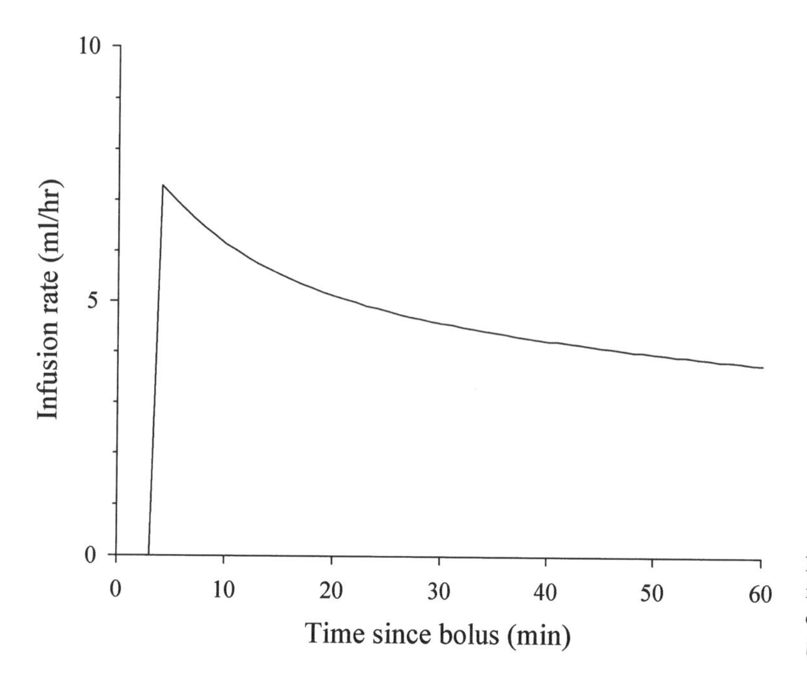

FIGURE 2-22. The curve represents the infusion rate of fentanyl necessary to achieve a constant effect site concentration of 1.5 ng/ml, after giving a bolus of 112.5 μg at time 0.

the infusion rate is simply $Cl \times C_T$, the rate at which the amount of drug entering the body equals the amount of drug leaving the body. For the three-compartment model, however, the infusion rate must match the rate of flow of drug out of V_1, both to V_2 and V_3, and out of the body.

To calculate these rates requires computer simulations. An example of this type of simulation is shown in Figure 2-22, which depicts the infusion rate of undiluted fentanyl (50 μg/ml) required to maintain an effect site concentration of 1.5 ng/ml. Immediately after the bolus based on the target concentration and $V_{peak\ effect}$ (112.5 μg, in this case), the infusion rate is 0, until the time of peak effect at around 4 minutes. At that point, the infusion begins at about 7 ml per hour, and then gradually decreases with time. At 30 minutes after the bolus, the infusion rate is about 4 ml per hour.

Figure 2-23 is a graph showing this type of curve for fentanyl, alfentanil, sufentanil, and propofol. As in Figure 2-22, each downward-sloping line represents a specific effect site concentration. The infusion rate can be adjusted either more or less frequently, depending on the degree of fluctuation one is willing to allow in effect site concentration. Of the four drugs depicted in Figure 2-23, sufentanil appears to require the fewest amount of rate changes, because the rates required after the bolus are fairly constant.

This approach has many variations, such as changing the effect site target according to the response of the patient, or achieving a high effect site concentration for intubation, then targeting a lower level for maintenance. These schemes can be approximated by using the infusion rates in Figure 2-23, but a more precise approach is to use a specialized computer program to take into account how much drug has been given already. Many such programs are currently available,

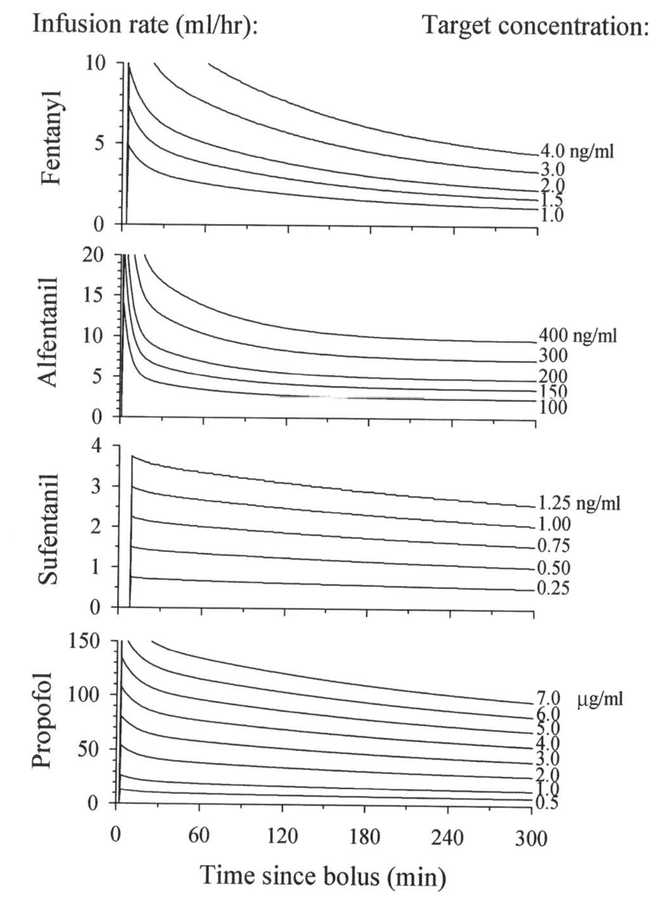

FIGURE 2-23. Each curve represents the infusion rate required to achieve a given constant effect site concentration after a bolus at time 0. The labels on the right denote the target concentrations.

including one written by one of the authors (SLS), called "Stanpump." Some of these programs, including Stanpump, have the ability to drive an infusion pump at the predicted rates. Several of these devices are currently being examined by the United States Food and Drug Administration, and they will likely be introduced into clinical practice over the next decade.

Planning for Recovery

Pharmacokinetic-pharmacodynamic modeling can be used to predict how long it will take for the effect site concentration to decrease from its desired intraoperative level to its desired level at extubation. Figure 2-24 depicts "recovery curves" for fentanyl, alfentanil, and sufentanil: the time required for the effect site concentration to decrease by a given amount after an infusion ends. For example, a sufentanil concentration of 0.5 ng/ml is in the therapeutic window for a balanced anesthetic, whereas a concentration of 0.25 ng/ml is desirable for adequate ventilation on emergence from anesthesia (a 50% decrease). Using the middle graph of Figure 2-24, if the maintenance infusion has been running for about 2 hours, it will need to be discontinued about 30 minutes before the end of the procedure to obtain the desired decrease in effect site concentration.

The fentanyl curve on the same graph demonstrates that it takes almost 2 hours to achieve the same percentage of decrease after an infusion is discontinued. This brings up another way to plan for recovery: choose an opioid that provides a reasonable recovery period. For extremely short procedures and when only a small decrease in effect site concentration is desired, any of these three opioids is a reasonable choice. For medium-length procedures, when a large decrease in concentration is required, sufentanil has the fastest recovery time. For extremely long procedures, alfentanil has the fastest recovery times.

Other Factors Influencing Dosing

The dosing schemes described in this chapter refer to the healthy adult of average size and age: the typical subject for a pharmacokinetic-pharmacodynamic study. Because patients who undergo surgery may vary in size or in physiology based age or disease processes, dosing must be tailored according to these individuals' needs. Current knowledge regarding scaling to weight or pathophysiologic features is imperfect. Therefore, one must use restraint and titrate to effect when applying these dosing regimens to different patient populations.

In conclusion, the basic principles of pharmacokinetics and pharmacodynamics have been discussed and used to derive dosing to derive dosing schemes for commonly used intravenous anesthetics. These dosing schemes suggest another way of providing anesthesia using intravenous drugs. Once computer-controlled infusion devices are available in the operating room, intravenous drugs will indeed be easier to deliver and easier to titrate, while achieving essential requirements for general anesthesia. In addition to the clinical applications, a more complete understanding of the principles of pharmacokinetics and pharmacodynamics should allow the reader to delve more deeply into this interesting field of study.

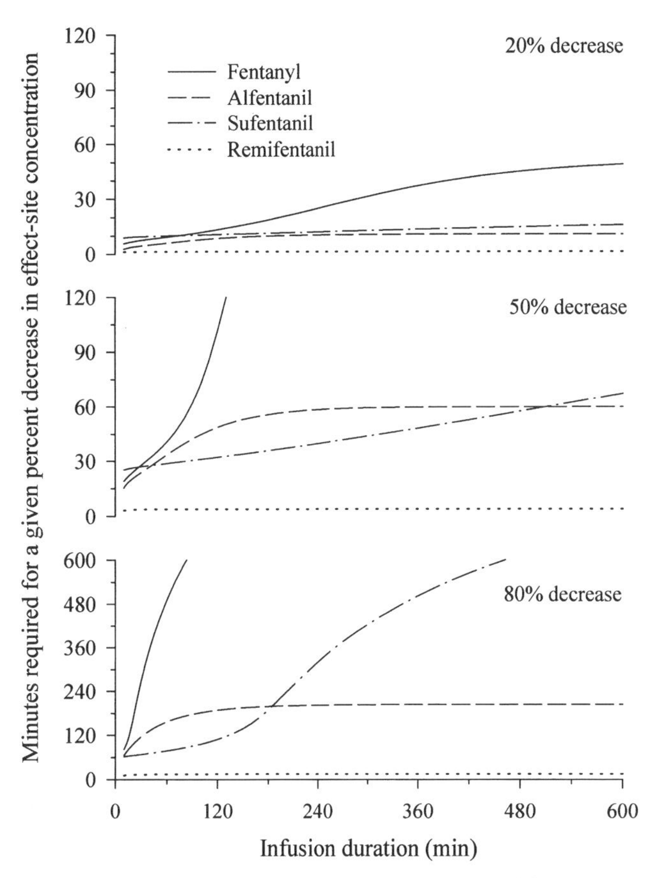

FIGURE 2-24. Each curve represents the time required for a given decrease in effect-site concentration after an infusion to a constant level for fentanyl, alfentanil, and sufentanil, and remifentanil (see Addendum). Adapted from Shafer and Varvel, with permission.

APPENDIX

Differential equations are used to describe the rate of change of a drug or physiologic process. In the case of pharmacokinetics, these equations describe the rate of change of the amount of drug. For the one-compartment model, if one gives a bolus, the amount of drug in the body will decline by a first-order process:

$$dX/dt = -kX,$$

where k is the rate constant for the one-compartment model, X is the amount of drug in the compartment, and dX/dt is the rate of change of X over time. In other words, the more drug in the body, the faster the elimination rate will be. To ensure an actual concentration of drug in the plasma at a given time, one needs to integrate the foregoing equation and divide by the volume of distribution, to obtain:

$$C(t) = Ae^{-kt},$$

where A is the concentration at time 0.

For the three-compartment model, the differential equation for the amount in compartment 1, which includes the plasma, has to incorporate all the rate constants for the processes going in and out of this compartment. These processes are depicted in Figure 2-8. The differential equation for a three-compartment model after a bolus is

$$dX_1/dt = -x_1k_{10} - x_1k_{12} + x_2k_{21} - x_1k_{13} + x_3k_{31},$$

where X_1, X_2, and X_3 are the amounts in compartments 1, 2, and 3, respectively. Because X_2 and X_3 need to be calculated to solve this equation, we need differential equations for them as well:

$$dX_2/dt = x_1k_{12} - x_2k_{21}$$

$$dX_3/dt = x_1k_{13} - x_3k_{31}$$

Now, to calculate the plasma concentration, we need to integrate the foregoing equation for dX_1/dt. This can be done exactly, using advanced procedures such as Laplace transforms, which are beyond the scope of this discussion. It is much easier to *approximate* the plasma concentration using a technique called Euler's numeric approximation. By substituting ΔX for dX and Δt for dt, one ends up with difference equations instead of differential equations. If one knows the amount at time 0 (the bolus dose) and the rate constants, one can calculate the amount at 1 second after the bolus dose, 2 seconds after, and so on. With a Δt of 1 second, the error from linearizing the differential equations is less than 1%. These difference equations are simple to incorporate into a computer program or spreadsheet. This technique is used in all the simulations presented in this chapter.

If one knows the volumes and clearances of a drug but not the rate constants, it is simple to interconvert these terms:

$$k_{10} = Cl_1 / V_1$$

$$k_{12} = Cl_2 / V_1$$

$$k_{13} = Cl_3 / V_1$$

$$k_{21} = Cl_2 / V_2$$

$$k_{31} = Cl_3 / V_3$$

Converting from either volumes and clearances or rate constants to coefficients and exponents, however, is complex.

Computer programs that simulate plasma concentrations and dosing regimens using the foregoing types of equations can be obtained free of charge from one of the authors (SLS) on request, or by anonymous ftp at pkpd.icon.palo-alto.med.va.gov.

REFERENCES

1. Rowland M, Tozer TN. Clinical pharmacokinetics: concepts and applications. Philadelphia: Lea & Febiger, 1989.
2. Eger EI. Mysterious models: uptake by intuition. In: Eger EI, ed. Anesthetic uptake and action. Baltimore: Williams & Wilkins, 1974:97–112.
3. Shafer SL, Varvel JR. Pharmacokinetics, pharmacodynamics, and rational opioid selection. Anesthesiology 1991;74:53–63.
4. Hughes MA, Glass PSA, Jacobs JR. Context-sensitive half-time in multicompartment pharmacokinetic models for intravenous anesthetic drugs. Anesthesiology 1992;76:334–341.
5. Chiou WL. The phenomenon and rationale of marked dependence of drug concentration on blood sampling site: implications in pharmacokinetics, pharmacodynamics, toxicology and therapeutics. Part I. Clin Pharmacokinet 1989;17:175–199.
6. Chiou WL. The phenomenon and rationale of marked dependence of drug concentration on blood sampling site: implications in pharmacokinetics, pharmacodynamics, toxicology and therapeutics. Part II. Clin Pharmacokinet 1989;17:275–290.
7. Ausems ME, Hug CC, Stanski DR, Burm AGL. Plasma concentrations of alfentanil required to supplement nitrous oxide anesthesia for general surgery. Anesthesiology 1986;65:362–373.
8. Shafer SL, Kern DE, Stanski DR. The scientific basis of infusion techniques in anesthesia. North Reading, MA: Bard Med-Systems Division, 1990.
9. Homer TD, Stanski DR. The effect of increasing age on thiopental distribution and anesthetic requirements. Anesthesiology 1985;62:714–724.
10. Stanski DR, Maitre PO. Population pharmacokinetics and pharmacodynamics of thiopental: the effect of age revisited. Anesthesiology 1990;72:412–422.
11. Dyck JB, Shafer SL. Effects of age on propofol pharmacokinetics. Semin Anesth;11:2–4, 1992.
12. Scott JC, Stanski DR. Decreased fentanyl and alfentanil dose requirements with age: a simultaneous pharmacokinetic and pharmacodynamic evaluation. J Pharmacol Exp Ther 1987; 240:159–166.
13. Scott JC, Cooke JE, Stanski DR. Electroencephalographic quantitation of opioid effect: comparative pharmacodynamics of fentanyl and sufentanil. Anesthesiology 1991;74:34–42.
14. Donati F. Onset of action of relaxants. Can J Anaesth 1988; 35:S52–S58.
15. Inturrisi CE, Colburn WA. Application of pharmacokinetic-pharmacodynamic modeling to analgesia. In: Foley KM, Inturrisi CE, eds. Advances in pain research and therapy. vol. 8. New York: Raven Press, 1986:441–452.
16. Shafer SL, Gregg KM. Algorithms to rapidly achieve and maintain stable drug concentrations at the site of drug effect with a computer-controlled infusion pump. J Pharmacokinet Biopharm 1992;20:147–169.

After this chapter went to press, the FDA approved a new opioid, remifentanil. This opioid is rapidly metabolized by esterases, which translates into an extremely high clearance and very short context-sensitive half-times (less than 4 minutes for cases less than 10 hours). This drug deserves special mention here because its short context-sensitive half-time has important pharmacokinetic implications: (1) its effects will terminate faster than those of any drug mentioned in this chapter, and (2) if continued opioid action is desired at the end of an anesthetic, remifentanil must not simply be turned off, but must be continued as an infusion or be replaced by a longer-acting opioid. See Chapter 11 for more information about remifentanil.

3A Mechanisms of Intravenous Anesthesia

James G. Bovill

The primary pharmacologic actions of the hypnotic and analgesic drugs used in intravenous anesthesia are the results of interactions at one of three types of central nervous system (CNS) receptors, the γ-aminobutyric acid $(GABA)_A$ receptor, the N-methyl-D-aspartate (NMDA) receptor, or the opioid receptor. In recent years, attention has also focused on the role of drugs acting on α_2-adrenoceptors in anesthesia. Receptors are specialized proteins containing stereospecific binding sites. Receptors incorporate two inherent properties, recognition and transduction. Recognition involves the ability of the receptor to bind specific ligands selectively. The interaction between the receptor and the ligand changes the functioning of the cell such that a molecular signal can be transduced into a cellular message.

RECEPTOR THEORY

At least four receptor superfamilies are recognized: 1) ligand-gated ion channel receptors that contain a transmitter binding site as part of the ion channel; 2) G-protein-coupled receptors, which are linked to their second messenger system by a guanine nucleotide protein; 3) ligand-regulated tyrosine kinases; and 4) nuclear receptors that alter DNA transcription. Only the first two classes of receptors, both of which span the entire cellular membrane, are directly relevant to the mechanisms of intravenous anesthetic actions. These receptors are formed by 7 hydrophobic domains spanning the lipid bilayer of the cell membrane and are connected by extra- and intracellular loops. The transmembrane domains are helices composed of 19 to 24 amino acids that have hydrophobic, nonpolar groups. The ends of the membrane-spanning regions and the joining loops are formed by polar amino acids exposed to the aqueous mileau outside and inside the cell.

The response of the receptor to ligand binding is a conformational change that triggers a transmembrane signal. The conformational change is caused by an agonist but not by an antagonist, which can bind to the receptor but does not activate the system. The initial signal generated by activation of a receptor by an agonist must be greatly amplified if it is to result in a cellular response. Activation of ligand-gated ion-channel receptors naturally results in amplification because the opening of even a single ion channel permits fluxes of about 10^6 ions per second, sufficient to change membrane potential. Receptors incorporating ion channels, such as acetylcholine (Ach) nicotinic receptors, are associated with rapid (1 millisecond) response times. These receptors are found when speed is essential to the signaling process. In contrast, receptors coupled to G proteins have intermediate response times of 10 to 100 milliseconds. This slower response is because the signal amplification requires an intracellular cascade of biochemical events involving second messenger molecules, such as cyclic adenosine monophosphate (cAMP) or calcium (Ca^{2+}), which, in turn, trigger reactions that result in cell activation.

DESENSITIZATION AND DOWNREGULATION

In some circumstances, receptor activity may be lost within minutes of receptor activation despite the continued presence of the agonist, a process called receptor desensitization, which results when the receptor assumes an altered conformation that precludes signal transduction. Desensitization results in a decrease in receptor efficacy and appears to be a built-in shutoff mechanism that prevents continuing receptor activation from interfering with the further processing of information. Desensitization may act to prevent the neuron from being overwhelmed with incoming signals because a typical neuron can receive information from a multitude of synapses.

Continuing exposure to an agonist can lead to a decrease in the number of binding sites, a process known as receptor downregulation. Receptor concentration on the cell surface is an important factor in signal processing even in the presence of "spare" receptor (i.e., more receptors than are necessary to give a maximum response). Receptor downregulation therefore reduces cell activity in the presence of an agonist and can be confused with receptor desensitization. The time frame and mechanism are different, however. Desensitization is a rapid process that occurs within minutes, whereas downregulation takes place over several hours (1). Downregulation is transmitter- or ligand-induced because it is blocked by receptor antagonists. Agonist-induced receptor downregulation is associated with changes in the cytoarchitecture of the cell and a reduction in the levels of receptor. For example, the expression of the c-fos protooncogene, a marker of neuronal activity, is dose-dependently suppressed by morphine (2).

EFFICACY

An important concept in receptor pharmacology is that of intrinsic activity or efficacy, a measure of the ability of a ligand to activate a specific receptor (Fig. 3A-1). If the binding of a ligand increases the cellular response (which may be either inhibitory or stimulatory), the ligand has positive intrinsic efficacy and is classified as an agonist. If the binding decreases the receptor-transducor association, the ligand possesses negative efficacy and is referred to as an inverse agonist. An antagonist is a ligand that binds to a specific receptor without affecting the receptor-transducor association (3). Agonists are further subclassified into full agonists and partial agonists. A full agonist is able to cause a maximum response, which, by definition, corresponds to an activity of unity, whereas partial agonists cannot produce the maximum response and therefore mani-

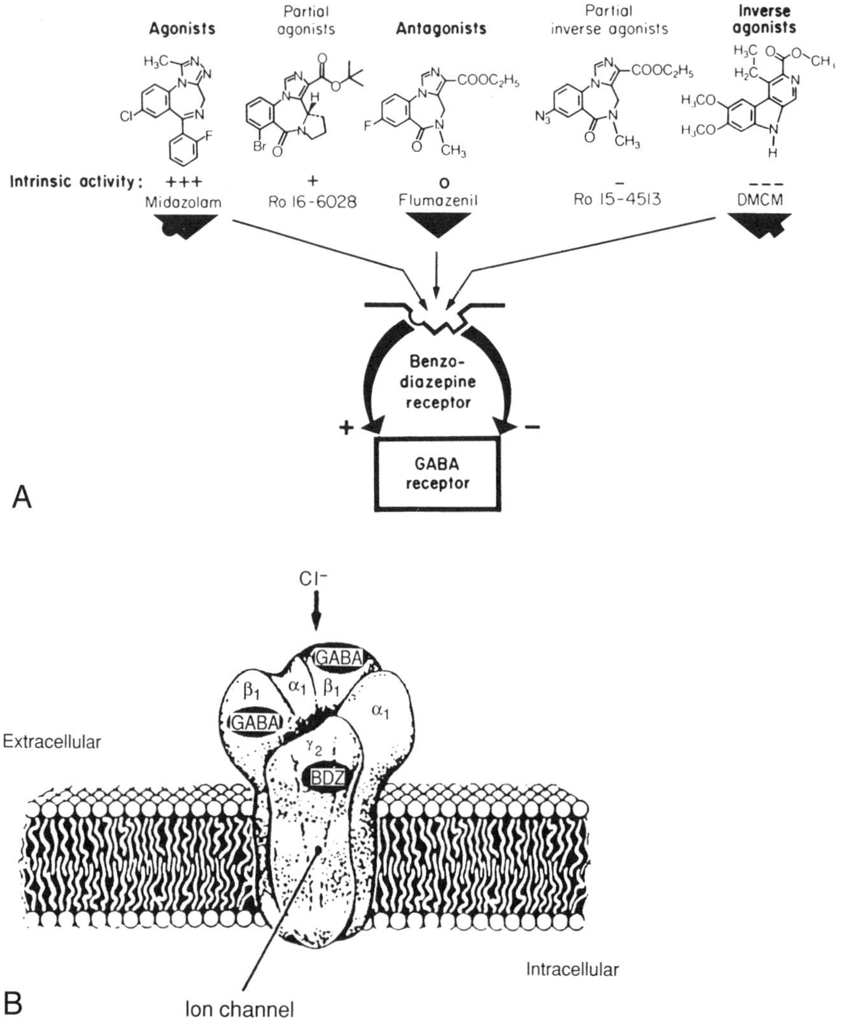

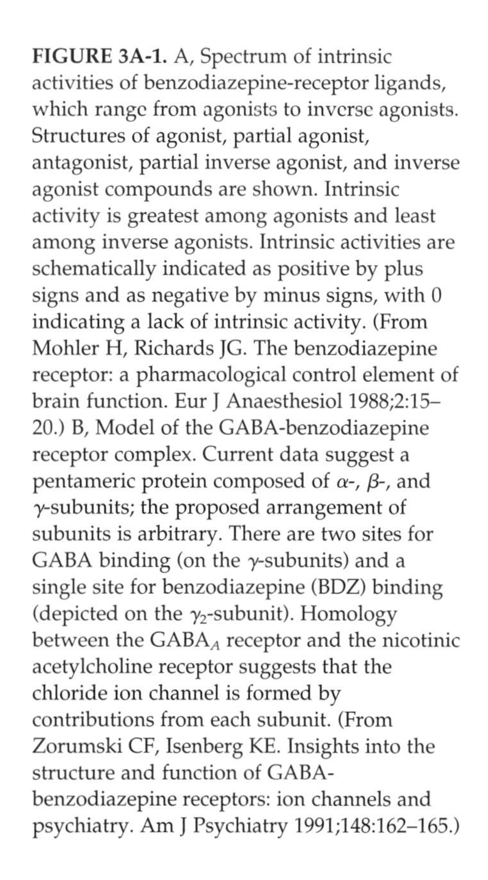

FIGURE 3A-1. A, Spectrum of intrinsic activities of benzodiazepine-receptor ligands, which range from agonists to inverse agonists. Structures of agonist, partial agonist, antagonist, partial inverse agonist, and inverse agonist compounds are shown. Intrinsic activity is greatest among agonists and least among inverse agonists. Intrinsic activities are schematically indicated as positive by plus signs and as negative by minus signs, with 0 indicating a lack of intrinsic activity. (From Mohler H, Richards JG. The benzodiazepine receptor: a pharmacological control element of brain function. Eur J Anaesthesiol 1988;2:15–20.) B, Model of the GABA-benzodiazepine receptor complex. Current data suggest a pentameric protein composed of α-, β-, and γ-subunits; the proposed arrangement of subunits is arbitrary. There are two sites for GABA binding (on the γ-subunits) and a single site for benzodiazepine (BDZ) binding (depicted on the γ_2-subunit). Homology between the $GABA_A$ receptor and the nicotinic acetylcholine receptor suggests that the chloride ion channel is formed by contributions from each subunit. (From Zorumski CF, Isenberg KE. Insights into the structure and function of GABA-benzodiazepine receptors: ion channels and psychiatry. Am J Psychiatry 1991;148:162–165.)

fest intrinsic activities less than unity. Not all full agonists have equal efficacy. For example, some may produce a maximum response when only 5% of the available receptors are occupied, whereas less efficient agonists may need to occupy 30% or more of the available receptors to obtain a full response.

The two types of antagonists are competitive and unsurmountable (noncompetitive). Competitive antagonism implies that the agonist and the antagonist bind at the same site on the receptor, so the binding is mutually exclusive. Provided the combination is freely reversible, then the blocked response caused by the presence of the antagonist can be fully overcome by sufficiently increasing the concentration of the agonist. In other words, the antagonism is *surmountable*. At equilibrium, the relative ratio of agonist and antagonist bound to the receptor is proportional to their respective effect-site concentrations and their affinities for the receptor. When the effect of an antagonist cannot be fully overcome by increasing the concentration of the agonist, then the antagonism is classified as *unsurmountable*. An example of unsurmountable antagonism is that produced by phenoxybenzamine at α-adrenoceptors.

AGONIST-RECEPTOR INTERACTIONS

Receptor identification and classification are based on ligand-binding specificity, whereas an important characteristic of ligands is their affinity for a receptor. This information is often obtained using radiolabeled ligands added to cellular (or subcellular) fractions of a tissue homogenate containing the receptor. The binding of an agonist to a receptor is a chemical process, involving chemical bonding and attractive forces between corresponding elements of the agonist and receptor. This interaction between agonist (A) and receptor (R) can be described by Equation 1:

$$A + R \underset{k_1}{\overset{k_2}{\rightleftarrows}} AR \tag{1}$$

where k_1 and k_2 are the association and dissociation constants, respectively. At equilibrium, the rates of association and dissociation are equal, and the law of mass action can be applied to determine the dissociation rate constant (Equation 2):

$$\frac{[A]\,[R]}{[AR]} = \frac{k_2}{k_1} = K_d \tag{2}$$

The square brackets denote concentration, and K_d is the equilibrium dissociation constant. K_d provides a measure of the affinity of the agonist for the receptor. High values of K_d denote a low affinity of the agonist for the receptor, whereas low values indicate a high affinity. The R in Equations 1 and 2 denotes the concentration of free receptor (i.e., not bound by the agonist). The fraction of the receptor that is occupied by the agonist is represented by $[AR]$. To eliminate R from Equation 2, the number of receptors in the specimen is assumed to be finite, R_T. Therefore,

$$[R_T] = [R] + [AR] \; or \; [R] = [AR] - [R_T]$$

substitution for $[R]$ in Equation 2 and rearranging gives Equation 3 for the fraction of occupied receptors $[AR]$:

$$[AR] = [R_T]\,\frac{[A]}{[A] + K_d} \tag{3}$$

Equation 3 reveals that when 50% of the receptors are occupied (i.e., $[AR]/[R_T] = 0.5$), K_d equals $[A]$. That is, K_d is numerically equal to the free ligand concentration when half the receptors are occupied.

Pharmacologists traditionally use the symbols B_{max} (maximum possible binding) for $[R_T]$, B for $[AR]$, the concentration of receptors bound to the agonist, and F for $[A]$, the concentration of free agonist. Equation 3 then becomes

$$\frac{B}{B_{max}} = \frac{F}{F + K_d} \tag{4}$$

The graph of B/B_{max} versus F is a rectangular hyperbole, and semilogarithmic plot yields a sigmoid relationship (Fig. 3A-2). Linear plots are often easier to evaluate than nonlinear curves. Various graphic methods are available to linearize the expression in Equation 4. One of the most popular methods is the Scatchard plot, which is derived by expressing Equation 4 as

$$B{\cdot}F + B{\cdot}K_d = B_{max}{\cdot}F$$

Dividing by $F{\cdot}K_d$ and rearranging yields Equation 5:

$$\frac{B}{F} = \frac{B_{max}}{K_d} - \frac{1}{K_d}B \tag{5}$$

which represents a linear relationship between B/F and B. A plot of B/F against B (i.e., the Scatchard plot), is a straight line with slope of $-1/K_D$ and an intercept on the B axis equal to B_{max} (Fig. 3A-3).

The primary advantage of the Scatchard plot is that it facilitates calculation of K_d and B_{max}. Several disadvantages are associated with its use, however. The Scatchard transformation contains a term for "B" on both axes, so errors in B are magnified in two directions. Further, marked compression of data often occurs at increasing value of F because evenly spaced data points on the hyperbolic curve become clustered in a Scatchard plot. A useful alternative to the Scatchard plot is the Hill plot (Fig. 3A-4), which relates logit Y_D (i.e., $\log[Y_D/(1\text{-}Y_D)]$) to $\log[A]$, where Y_D represents fractional receptor occupancy (i.e., $[AR]/R_T$). Although knowledge of R_T (e.g., from a preliminary

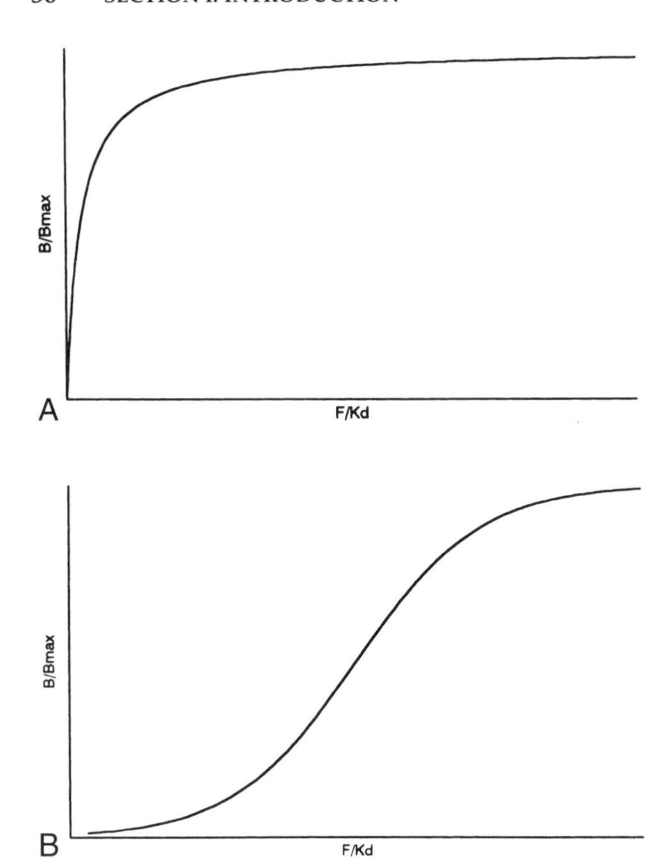

FIGURE 3A-2. A and B, The relationship between fraction of receptor occupied by a ligand (B) as a fraction of the total number of receptors (B_{max}), and the concentration of free ligand (F), normalized to multiples of K_d, plotted using linear (upper plot) and semilogarithmic (lower plot) axes.

semilogarithmic plot) is a prerequisite for the construction of the Hill plot, this method has the advantage of linearity.

Inhibition studies provide an alternative approach to measuring the affinity of a drug for a receptor binding site. In an inhibition experiment, the concentration of the radiolabeled drug is held constant, while the concentration of a nonlabeled competing ligand, $[I]$, is varied. The equilibrium dissociation constant, K_i, for the interaction of the competing ligand for the receptor can be determined by measuring the concentration of I that produces a 50% inhibition (IC_{50}) of the specific binding of the labeled drug. After determining the value of IC_{50}, K_i can then be calculated:

$$K_i = \frac{IC_{50}}{1 + [A]/K_d}$$

The foregoing discussion of drug-receptor binding does not consider the pharmacologic response elicited by the binding process. This follows logically, however, if one assumes that the magnitude of the pharmacologic response is linearly proportional to fractional receptor occupancy, as proposed by Clark (4) in his "occupation" theory of drug-receptor interaction. This relationship can be expressed as Equation 6:

$$\frac{E_A}{E_m} = \frac{[AR]}{[R_t]} = \frac{[A]}{[A] + K_d} \qquad (6)$$

where E_A is the observed response to agonist A and E_m is the maximum obtainable response. Note the similarity between the left-hand term in Equation 6 and the B/B_{max} term in Equation 4. An implicit assumption of this model is that 100% receptor occupancy is required to obtain a maximum response. Because this is not always the case, a more recent modification allows for the concept of reserve or "spare" receptors. Therefore, an agonist with high efficacy need only occupy a fraction of the total available receptors to produce a maximum response. This concept implies a nonlinear relationship between receptor occupancy and response (5). Stephenson (5) proposed that the response is a function of the stimulus (s) generated by the interaction between the agonist and the receptor. In Stephenson's model, the relationship between stimulus and response has been arbitrarily defined such as s = 1 when the response is 50% of the maximum response achieved by a full agonist. Thus,

$$\frac{E_A}{E_m} = f(s) = f\left(\frac{e[A]}{[A] + K_d}\right) \qquad (7)$$

where e is efficacy, the parameter that relates occupancy to stimulus, and therefore Equation 7 characterizes the capacity of a drug to induce a biologic response (6). The efficacy parameter can range from 0 to values greater than 1. When $e = 0$, the drug binds to the receptor but elicits no response (i.e., an antagonist). When $e > 1$, the drug has agonist activity, and for large values of e, the maximum response is obtained at low receptor occupancy.

COMPETITIVE ANTAGONISTS

When a competitive antagonist (I) is present concurrently with an agonist, the antagonist molecules compete with the agonist for binding sites on the receptor. Because an antagonist has no intrinsic efficacy, however, the pharmacologic response produced by the agonist is reduced. This interaction can be expressed by the following equation:

$$I + R \underset{k_3}{\overset{k_4}{\rightleftarrows}} IR$$

or, applying the law of mass action:

$$\frac{[I][R]}{[IR]} = K_I$$

In the presence of an antagonist, the occupancy in Equation 3 becomes

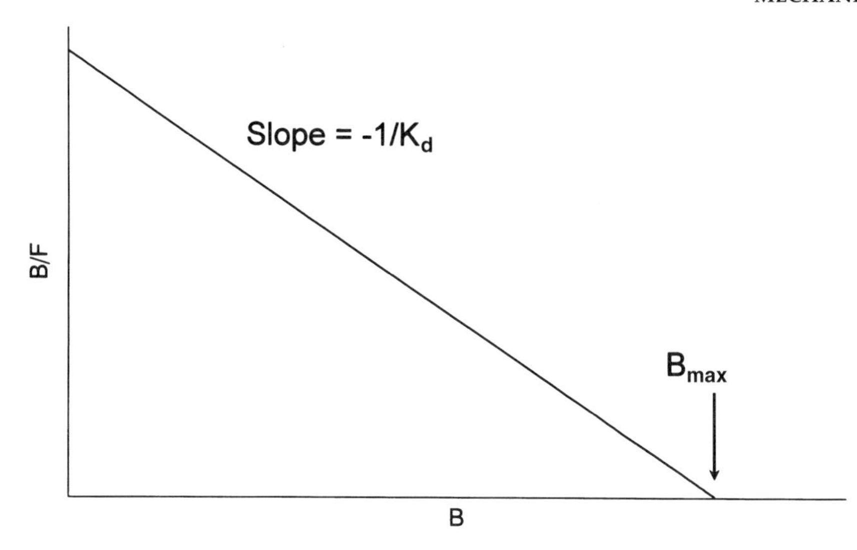

FIGURE 3A-3. The Scatchard plot, which represents the linear relationship between B/F and B given in Equation 5. The slope of the straight line is $-1/K_d$ and the x-axis intersect B_{max}.

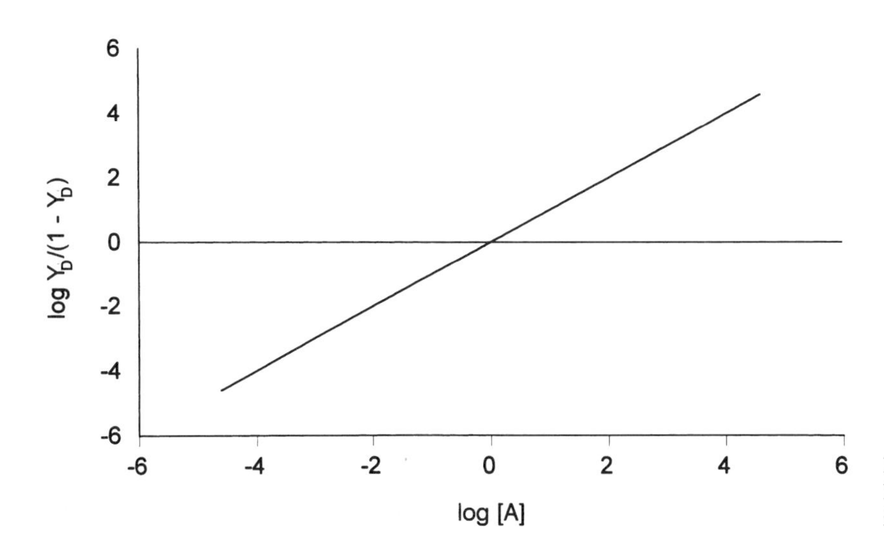

FIGURE 3A-4. The Hill plot, which relates $\log[Y_D/(1\text{-}Y_D)]$ to log[A] where Y_D represents fractional receptor occupancy, i.e., $[AR]/R_T$.

$$Y_D = \frac{[A]/K_d}{1 + [A]/K_d + [I]/K_I}$$

where $Y_D = [AR]/R_T$. When negligible antagonist is present, this equation reduces to Equation 3. As the concentration of the antagonist increases, the concentration of the agonist required to maintain the same occupancy increases (i.e., its value of K_d appears to increase). This phenomenon can be seen as a displacement of the agonist occupancy curves on the Hill plot to the right (Fig. 3A-5).

SPECIFIC RECEPTORS

The overall "activity" of the CNS is basically governed by two superior functions, excitation and inhibition. The major excitatory neurotransmitter in the mammalian nervous system is the amino acid L-glutamate, which depolarizes neurons through activation of many receptor subtypes. GABA is the major inhibitory transmitter in the CNS. GABA hyperpolarizes neurons through activation of multiple receptors (7). Because anesthesia represents a state of altered brain activity, involving either an inhibition of nervous system function or a suppression of excitatory functions, most anesthetic drugs modulate the functioning of GABA and glutamate receptors.

GABA Receptors

Several GABA receptor subtypes have been identified; $GABA_A$, $GABA_B$, and receptors that have been termed $GABA_C$ or "non-$GABA_A$, non-$GABA_B$ receptors" (7). The $GABA_B$ receptor is a G-protein-linked receptor coupled to Ca^{2+} or potassium ion (K^+) channels. It is of minor consequence for anesthetic mechanisms, compared with the $GABA_A$ receptor. $GABA_A$ receptors are members of a ligand-gated ion channel family of receptors, all of which possess a pentomeric structure, with the five subunits arranged perpendicular to the cell membrane around a central, relatively hydrophilic core, the ion channel (8). Investigators have suggested

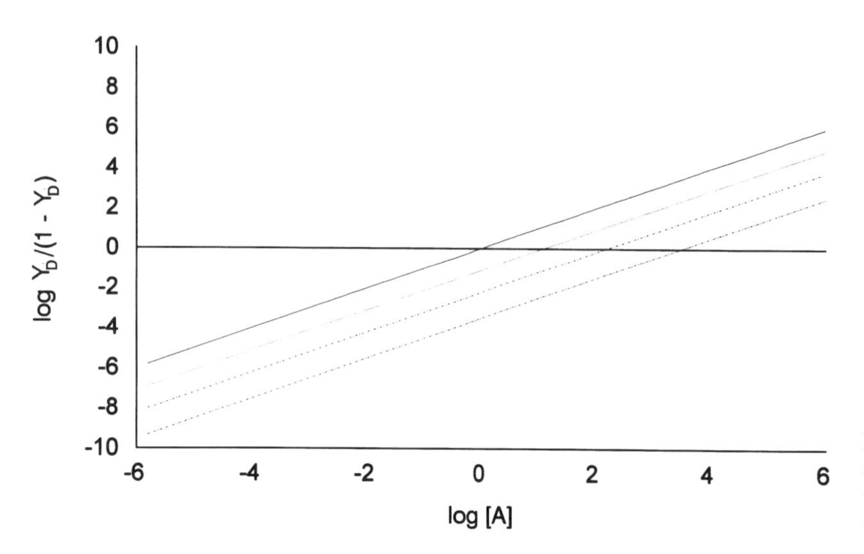

FIGURE 3A-5. A Hill plot showing the displacement of the agonist occupancy curves to the right with increasing concentrations of a competitive antagonist.

that at least two GABA molecules must bind to the receptor for full activation (9). Binding of GABA to the $GABA_A$ receptor increases membrane conductance for chloride (Cl^-), resulting in a Cl^- current into the cell, membrane hyperpolarization, and a reduction in neuronal excitability. GABA regulation of the Cl^- channel is not a simple gating between an open and closed state. Three open states, 10 closed states, and 1 "desensitized" state have been described (10). The average open duration increases with increasing GABA concentration because of a shift in the type of opening. Drugs may enhance $GABA_A$ current by increasing channel conductance, increase channel open and burst frequencies, or increase channel open and burst duration. Several anesthetic drugs, including barbiturates, benzodiazepines, steroids, etomidate, and propofol, bind to the $GABA_A$ receptor and augment $GABA_A$ mediated inhibition by allosteric modulation of receptor function (Fig. 3A-6).

NMDA Receptors

The amino acid L-glutamate is the most important excitatory neurotransmitter in the mammalian CNS. L-glutamate activates several amino acid receptors, which have been classified into three broad subtypes: 1) α-amino–3-hydroxy–5-methyl–4-isoxazole propionate (AMPA) receptors; 2) N-methyl-D-aspartate (NMDA) receptors; and 3) a non-NMDA receptor activated by kainite and quisqualate. These receptors are ligand-gated ion channels. A fourth family of glutamate receptors, the metabotropic glutamate or *trans*–1-aminocyclopentane–1,3-dicarboxylate (tACPD) receptors, which are G-protein-coupled receptors, has been identified (11). The NMDA receptor is the one most relevant to the mechanism of anesthesia. NMDA receptors are broadly distributed throughout the brain and spinal cord and have widespread physiologic functions (11, 12).

Activated NMDA receptors control ion channels that permit entry of monovalent (mainly sodium [Na^+]) and divalent (mainly Ca^{2+}) ions to enter the cell. Ca^{2+} flux is by far the most important and is some 70 times larger than comparable ionic currents mediated by activation of AMPA and kainate receptors. In addition to a binding site for L-glutamate, the NMDA receptor has recognition sites for the amino acid glycine, binding sites for magnesium (Mg^{2+}), and a separate divalent cation binding site with an affinity for zinc (Zn^{2+}). A recognition site for phenylcyclidine and ketamine lies in the opening of the ion channel (Fig. 3A-7).

The NMDA receptor is unique in that it is the only ligand-gated ion channel whose probability of opening depends strongly on the voltage across the membrane. The receptor is inoperative when the neuron is in the resting state, with a negative intracellular membrane potential. An important restriction is placed on Ca^{2+} flux through the ion channel by imposing a voltage-dependent Mg^{2+} block on the channel. Presynaptically released glutamate cannot activate ion flow through this channel unless the postsynaptic membrane is sufficiently depolarized to remove this Mg^{2+} block. Hence, generation of NMDA receptor-mediated responses requires both the binding of an agonist (e.g., L-glutamate), and a degree of membrane depolarization. As a result, NMDA receptor mechanisms contribute to synaptic responses only under certain conditions (e.g., high-frequency discharges). Glutamate dissociates relatively slowly from the NMDA receptor, with a decay time constant of 10 to 100 milliseconds, in contrast to the AMPA glutamate receptor, which has rapid kinetics (time constant of 1 to 3 milliseconds) (13).

The NMDA receptor is involved in important physiologic and cognitive functions relevant to anesthesia, including sensory information processing, memory and learning, locomotion, and regulation of vasomotor

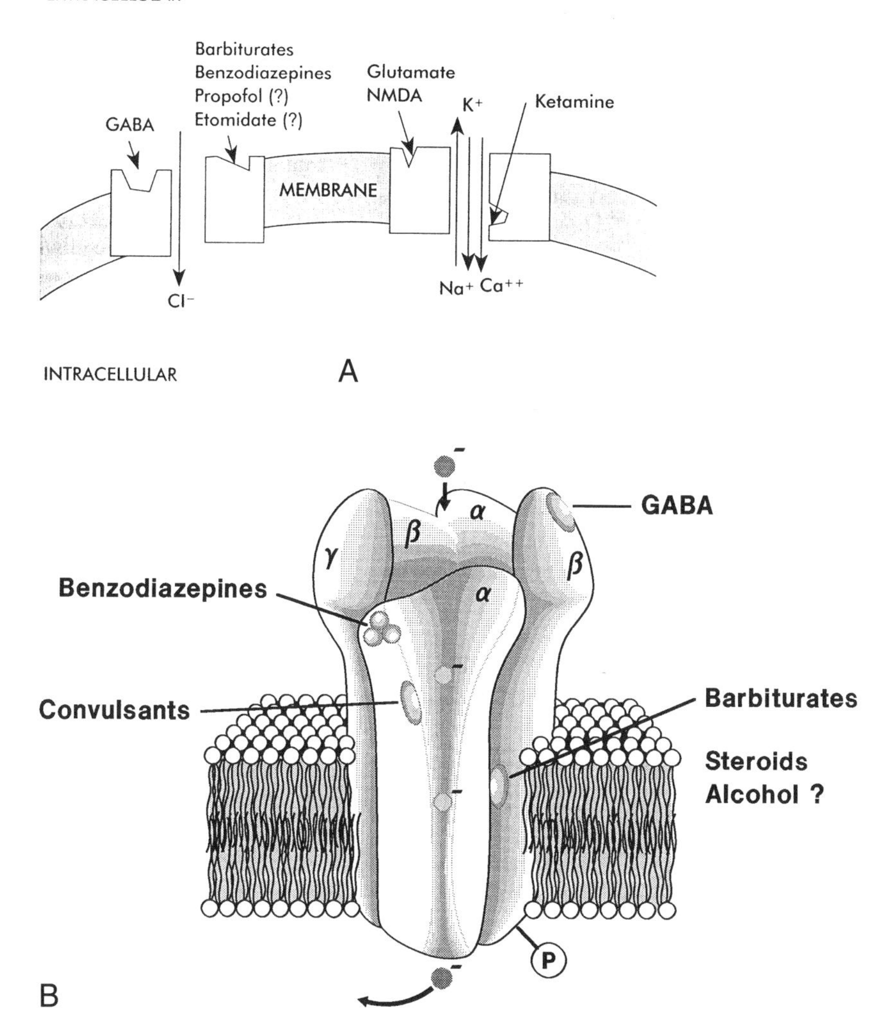

FIGURE 3A-6. A, This model depicts the postsynaptic site of action of GABA and glutamate within the central nervous system. GABA decreases the excitability of neurons by its action at the $GABA_A$ receptor complex. When GABA occupies the binding site of this complex, it allows inward flux of chloride ion, resulting in hyperpolarizing of the cell and therefore the subsequent resistance of the neuron to stimulation by excitatory transmitters. Barbiturates, benzodiazepines, and probably propofol and etomidate decrease neuronal excitability by enhancing the effect of GABA at this complex, facilitating this inhibitory effect in the postsynaptic cell. Glutamate (or its analog NMDA) is excitatory. When glutamate occupies the binding site on the NMDA subtype of glutamate receptor, the channel opens and allows Na^+, K^+, and Ca^{++} to enter or to leave the cell, as shown in the figure. Flux on these ions leads to depolarization of the postsynaptic neuron and initiation of an action potential and activation of other pathways. Ketamine blocks this open channel and prevents further ion flux, thus inhibiting the excitatory response to glutamate. This model does not attempt to represent any structural information pertaining to subunits or binding sites. (From Van Hemelrijck J, White PF. Use of intravenous sedative agents. In: Rogers MC, Tinker JH, Covino BG, Longnecker DE, eds. Principles and practice of anesthesiology St. Louis: CV Mosby, 1992:1131-1154.) B, Schematic model of the $GABA_A$ receptor complex illustrating recognition sites for many of the substances that bind to the receptor. The model is not meant to indicate subunit assembly or the exact location of recognition sites. (Courtesy of Rochelle D. Schwartz.)

tone and blood pressure. These receptors are also involved in the pathophysiology of cellular damage or death associated with ischemia, traumatic head injury, and strokes. The NMDA receptors also play an important role in nociception, in particular neuronal plasticity associated with chronic pain, tissue injury, and inflammatory states (14, 15). NMDA plays a pivotal role in multisynaptic local circuit nociceptive processing in the spinal cord. In situations of chronic pain with high-frequency or sustained afferent input producing a prolonged depolarization, the Mg^{2+} block on spinal NMDA receptors is removed, thereby allowing NMDA activation and an influx of Ca^{2+}.

In animals subjected to repeated peripheral nerve stimulation of sufficient intensity to activate *C* fibers, the responses of a proportion of neurons in the spinal dorsal horn increase with each subsequent stimulus. This phenomenon is referred to as "wind up" and is associated with facilitation of spinal nociceptive reflexes or hyperalgesia (16). It is related to a centrally mediated temporal summation and is closely related to the NMDA receptor (17, 18). Wind up of dorsal horn nociceptive neurons is selectively reduced by NMDA antagonists, including ketamine (17, 19). Temporal summation of secondary pain in humans appears to be selectively attenuated by an NMDA receptor antagonist (20).

Opioid Receptors

Extensive research during the last two decades has provided unequivocal evidence for the existence of three opioid receptor types, μ, δ and κ and substantial evidence for various subtypes of each of these receptors. The μ receptor has been subclassified into two subtypes, a high-affinity μ_1 receptor and a low-affinity μ_2 receptor (21). Subtypes of the δ and κ receptors also have been described (22, 23). The supraspinal mechanisms of analgesia produced by μ-opioid agonist drugs is thought to involve the μ_1 receptor, whereas spinal analgesia, respiratory depression, and the effects of opioids on gastrointestinal function have been associated with the μ_2 receptor (24, 25). The σ receptor, proposed by Martin and Eades (26) to explain the dys-

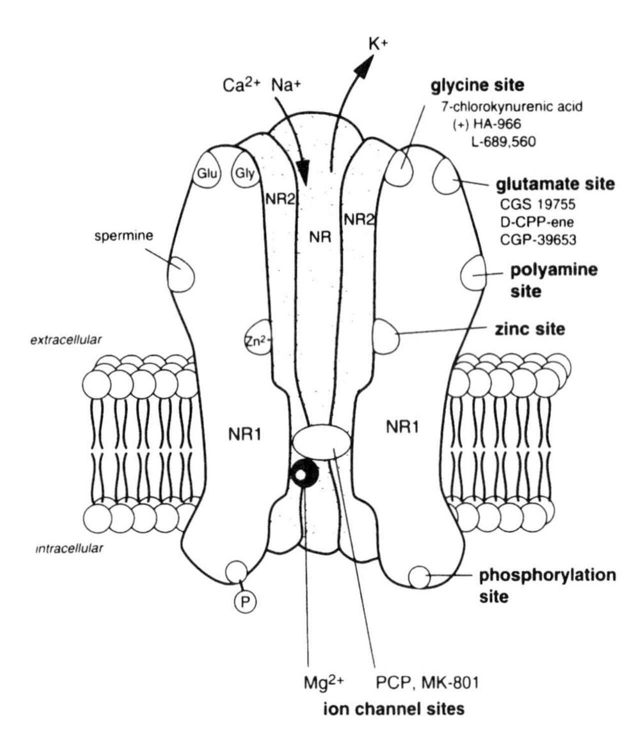

FIGURE 3A-7. Model of the NMDA receptor showing sites for antagonist action. Ketamine binds to the site labeled PCP (phencyclidine). The pentameric structure of the receptor, composed of a combination of the subunits NR 1 and NR 2, is illustrated. (From Leeson TD, Iversen LL. The glycine site on the NMDA receptor: structure-activity relationships and therapeutic potential. J Med Chem 1994;37:4053–4067.)

phoric effects of nalorphine, is not an opioid receptor because actions mediated by it are not reversed by naloxone, and it shows a preferential affinity for dextroisomers rather than levoisomers of some benzomorphans (27). Evidence indicates that the receptor is associated with the NMDA receptor and may be involved in nociceptive information processing in the spinal cord (28).

Opioid receptors are widely distributed within the CNS. The μ receptors are most dense in those regions of the CNS associated with the regulation of nociception and sensorimotor integration. The distribution of δ receptors is less extensive than μ receptors. Within the brain, κ receptors are located mainly in areas associated with nociception, such as the periaqueductal gray, and regulation of water balance and food intake. Opioid drugs produce analgesia by interacting with one or more of the opioid receptors and are thought to mimic the actions of the endogenous opioid peptides (29). These compounds are the natural ligands for the opioid receptors. All mammalian opioid peptides belong to one of three peptide families, the endorphin, the enkephalin, or the dynorphin group. β-endorphin binds primarily to μ opioid receptors, whereas met- and leu-enkephalin bind to both μ and δ receptors (although more so to δ receptors). The dynorphins appear to be the natural ligand for the κ opioid receptors.

The actions of opioids are primarily inhibitory as a result of alterations in the regulation of K^+ and Ca^{2+} ion channels. Activation of μ and δ receptors increases K^+ conductance by opening K^+ channels (30), whereas κ-opioid receptor agonists cause N-type Ca^{2+} channels to close, reducing Ca^{2+} conductance (31). Both result in hyperpolarization of the cell and a reduction in excitability of the postsynaptic neuron (or a shortening of the action potential) followed by a secondary decrease in Ca^{2+} conductance (32). Opioid-mediated inhibition of neurotransmitters such as substance P is probably regulated by changes in intracellular free calcium, $[Ca^{2+}]_i$ (33). δ-Receptor activation causes a transient increase in $[Ca^{2+}]$, the increase resulting from external Ca^{2+} influx due to opening of voltage-gated Ca^{2+} channels (34, 35).

Activation of an opioid receptor does not lead directly to changes in ion channels, but is mediated by G proteins. Activation of G proteins by opioids decreases adenyl cyclase activity, thereby decreasing the intracellular concentration of cAMP. Although opioid-induced alterations in cAMP can account for modulation of neurotransmitter release (e.g., substance P), the actions on K^+ and Ca^{2+} channels may be mediated by a direct coupling between G protein and the ion channels or by second messengers other than cAMP.

SPECIFIC DRUGS

Barbiturates

The primary mechanism for the hypnotic activity of barbiturates is through GABA receptors. Barbiturates bind to distinct sites on the $GABA_A$ receptor, enhancing the GABA response and also mimicking the actions of GABA by opening the Cl^- channel in the absence of GABA. The enhancement of GABA action is manifest by an increase in GABAergic inhibitory postsynaptic potentials (IPSPs) (36). By prolonging bursts of Cl^- channel openings, barbiturates increase the mean channel open time and slow the decay of inhibitory conductance changes (37). Although barbiturates do not alter the open duration time constants, they reduce the relative proportion of openings of a short duration (states 1 and 2) and increase the proportion with the longer duration (state 3) (38). The addition of pentobarbital and GABA together to dorsal horn neurons produced Cl^- currents that are three to four times greater than the algebraic sum of individual GABA and pentobarbital responses, both because of potentiation of GABA responses and because of the agonist action of pentobarbital (39).

Barbiturates allosterically inhibit the binding of picrotoxin, a convulsant that exerts a noncompetitive inhibition at a site distinct from the GABA receptor. Barbiturates also enhance the binding of GABA and benzodiazepines to their respective sites on the $GABA_A$ complex while inhibiting the binding of GABA antagonists and benzodiazepine inverse agonists (40). The enhancement of GABA and benzodiazepine affinity for the $GABA_A$ receptor by barbiturates is well correlated with their hypnotic and anesthetic potency (41).

In addition to an action at the GABA receptor, barbiturates have other important actions that contribute to their anesthetic and anticonvulsant effects. Barbiturates influence cAMP regulation, possibly through effects on G proteins. Pentobarbital enhances cAMP accumulation in cells by a mechanism dependent on G_s but independent of G_i (42). This effect is stereoselective, with the S-(−)-isomer of pentobarbital enhancing isoproterenol-stimulated cAMP accumulation more than the R-(+)-isomer. The properties of barbiturates responsible for the enhancement of cAMP accumulation may be responsible for producing sedation and anesthesia. Other possible mechanisms of barbiturate-induced hypnosis include an increase in depolarization-induced dopamine release in the striatum (42). Another potential site of action is the Ach receptor. De Armendi and colleagues (43) demonstrated that barbiturates inhibit the transient open-channel conformation of the nicotinic ACh receptor (nAChR) by binding to a discrete site. This site exhibits a different structure-activity relationship than an allosteric site established by equilibrium barbiturate binding on the resting conformation of the ACh receptor. Thus, barbiturate action depends on the nAChR's conformational state. Barbiturates have also been shown to inhibit the function of the excitatory amino acids AMPA and NMDA in a noncompetitive manner, and this may also be a mechanism whereby they produce anesthesia (44).

Etomidate and Steroids

Etomidate is even more potent than barbiturates in activating $GABA_A$ receptor channels, with a potency comparable to that of GABA (39). Etomidate has two optical isomers, the (+) isomer being the most active for the hypnotic and anticonvulsant actions (45). (+)-Etomidate also enhances the binding of benzodiazepines to the GABA receptor by increasing their binding affinity (46). Etomidate binds to the chloride-ionophore complex of the GABA-receptor complex to increase the efficacy of GABA-ergic neuronal inhibition (46, 47). Etomidate may also have presynaptic actions on the $GABA_A$ receptor-coupled Cl^- channel in the mammalian CNS, inhibiting the uptake of GABA, resulting in synaptic GABA accumulation, which contributes to etomidate's anesthetic activity (48).

Steroid anesthetics potentiate $GABA_A$ action similar to etomidate and the barbiturates (49). Despite similarities between barbiturates and steroid anesthetics, steroid activity at a cellular and molecular level is independent of the activity of these agents at the $GABA_A$ complex. The steroid binding site appears to lie on the extracellular surface of the receptor complex. Intracellular injection of a steroid failed to activate $GABA_A$ Cl^- conduction, whereas the same cells responded to extracellular application of the drug (50). Further research is required to understand the mechanism of steroid effects on the CNS fully.

Benzodiazepines

There are three pharmacologic classes of benzodiazepines, agonists, antagonists and inverse agonists (see Fig. 3A-1A). In this respect, the benzodiazepines are unique among anesthetic and analgesic compounds. The benzodiazepine agonists diazepam, lorazepam, and midazolam produce anxiolytic, anticonvulsant, and sedative-hypnotic effects. The benzodiazepine receptor antagonist, flumazenil, binds with a high affinity to the $GABA_A$ receptor while possessing minimal intrinsic activity and blocking the effects of both agonists and inverse agonists. Inverse agonists produce opposite pharmacologic effects to these of the agonists, namely, anxiogenic and proconvulsant activity. The first inverse agonists described were the β-carbolines 3-carboethoxy-β-carboline (β-CCB) and 3-carbobutoxy-β-carboline (β-CCE), which were extracted from human urine (51), and β-CCE was identified in pig brain (52). Subsequently, several benzodiazepine inverse agonists have been identified, although as yet no clear therapeutic role has been identified. Whereas benzodiazepine agonists increase the GABA response, inverse agonists decrease it.

Benzodiazepine agonists bind to distinct sites on the $GABA_A$ receptor complex, often referred to as the benzodiazepine receptor. The nature of the benzodiazepine binding site may be conferred only by specific subunit subtypes (10). For example, benzodiazepine sensitivity is conferred by the presence of the Y_2 subtype (53). Benzodiazepines alone have no effect on Cl^- currents in the absence of GABA or GABA agonists (54). When GABA molecules are present, benzodiazepines increase Cl^- ion flux in a concentration-dependent manner (55), and the increase is blocked by flumazenil. The binding of benzodiazepines is allosterically enhanced by GABA agonists, whereas inverse agonists and antagonists are unaffected (56). In contrast to the barbiturates, benzodiazepines increase channel current by increasing receptor open and burst frequency, but average open and burst durations are not altered (57). Benzodiazepines also enhance the probability of the $GABA_A$ channel remaining open in long-duration bursts (58). Inverse agonists reduce the Cl^- channel open and burst frequencies (10).

GABA is found in high concentrations in the dorsal horn of the spinal cord, in particular in the substance gelatinosa (59), and $GABA_A$ receptors may play an important role in spinal nociceptive processing. Intrathecally administered midazolam produces a modulation of these processes (60), and this effect is reversed by flumazenil (61), but not by naloxone (62). Intravenous midazolam suppresses noxiously evoked activity of spinal wide dynamic range neurons, an action that appears to be mediated by the $GABA_A$ receptor (62).

The presence of a specific binding site for benzodiazepines on the $GABA_A$ receptor and the finding that benzodiazepines also bind with high affinity to non-GABA sites on the outer mitochrondial membranes of brain and peripheral tissues (e.g., adrenal gland and testes) (63, 64) have led to speculation as to possible endogenous ligands. The discovery in human urine of the β-carboline, β-CCB, which has high affinity for the benzodiazepine binding site on $GABA_A$, raised expectations that this was an endogenous benzodiazepine (51). Unfortunately, investigators subsequently found that β-CCB was an artifact of the extraction process. Another potential candidate for this role is β-CCE, identified in pig brain (52); however, both β-CCB and β-CCE are inverse agonists. Several studies have provided evidence for the existence in the CNS of endogenous benzodiazepine ligands, including a diazepam binding inhibitor (DBI) (65) and a group of low-molecular-weight, nonpeptide substances referred to as endozepines (66). Endozepines have been purified and characterized in both animal and human brain tissue (67). DBI, an 11-kd polypeptide, has also been purified from the brains of animals and humans (68). DBI is concentrated in synaptic vesicles and released by depolarization, like classic neurotransmitters. High concentrations are found in cortical and limbic areas, the cerebellum, and brain stem, and preliminary data indicate that these compounds have a modulatory role in the human brain (69). The clinical syndrome of hepatic encephalopathy is associated with an increase in the brain content of endozepines (70), and flumazenil ameliorates the neurologic signs of this syndrome (67).

Propofol

Pharmacologic and electrophysiologic data suggest that at least some of the CNS actions of propofol are mediated by the $GABA_A$ receptor complex. Propofol reversibly and in a dose-dependent manner potentiates the amplitude of membrane currents evoked by locally applied GABA to bovine adrenomedullary chromaffin cells, which posses high concentrations of $GABA_A$ receptors (71). Propofol also augments GABA-induced neuronal inhibition cerebral cortex at clinically relevant concentrations (72, 73) or hippocampal CA1 pyramidal neurons (74, 75). At higher concentrations, the propofol-induced inward Cl^- current decreases considerably because of desensitization of the $GABA_A$ receptor (74). The action of propofol on the glycine receptor, which is also coupled to a Cl^- channel, is unclear. Glycine, along with GABA, is a major inhibitory transmitter, and glycine-induced chloride currents are enhanced by several CNS depressant drugs (76). Hales and Lambert (71) reported that propofol enhanced both GABA and glycine responses, whereas Hara and associates (75) found that the glycine response was not affected by propofol.

Propofol binding to the $GABA_A$ receptor is at a site distinct from those for barbiturates, benzodiazepines, or steroids. Propofol inhibits the binding of t-[^{35}S] butylbicyclophosphorothionate ([^{35}S] TBPS), a noncompetitive $GABA_A$ antagonist, to rat cerebral cortex membranes in a dose-dependent manner (73, 77). In the presence of pentobarbital or alphaxalone, propofol caused a supra-additive inhibition of [^{35}S] TBPS binding that was greater than that produced by either drug alone, a finding suggesting that barbiturates, steroids and propofol were acting at separate sites. Flumazenil did not affect the activation by propofol of $GABA_A$ receptor channels (74), and propofol did not displace flumazenil from the benzodiazepine binding site (73). Similarly, propofol did not displace [^3H] GABA from its binding site, indicating that the propofol binding site is different from that of GABA on the $GABA_A$ receptor complex (73).

Although numerous classes of anesthetic agents have been shown to enhance the effects mediated by the postsynaptic $GABA_A$ receptor-coupled Cl^- channel in the mammalian CNS, the presynaptic actions of anesthetics potentially relevant to clinical anesthesia remain to be clarified. Data suggest that inhibition of GABA uptake, which results in synaptic GABA accumulation, may contribute to both propofol- and etomidate-induced anesthesia (48).

The anesthetic effects of propofol are probably mediated by mechanisms other than those on the $GABA_A$ receptor. Propofol, in clinically relevant concentrations, induces changes in the concentrations of $[Ca^{2+}]_i$ and disrupts cellular communication by closing the gap junctions between non-neuronal astrocytes (78, 79). Like pentobarbital, propofol has a blocking effect on Na^+ channels in human brain cortex, leading to a voltage-independent reduction in the fractional channel open time (80). In contrast, midazolam and ketamine have produced similar changes only at supraphysiologic concentrations (10- to 50-fold higher) (81). Propofol also disrupts CNS function by nonspecific changes in the cytoskeletal organization of neurons and glial cells caused by increases in $[Ca^{2+}]_i$ (82).

Ketamine

NMDA antagonism is clearly an important mechanism for the anesthetic and analgesic effects of ketamine and other dissociative anesthetics (83). Phencyclidine and ketamine act as noncompetitive antagonists of the

NMDA receptor (84, 85). This action is selective for the NMDA receptor because the excitatory responses produced by kainate and quisqualate on dorsal horn interneurons are only minimally affected by ketamine (86). Other mechanisms may be involved in the pharmacologic actions of ketamine, however, including inhibition of Ca^{++} influx through voltage-gated Ca^{++} channels (87). The NMDA antagonistic actions of ketamine exhibit stereoselectivity that correlates with the anesthetic effects of its isomers. The S(+) isomer of ketamine, which produce more profound sedation and analgesia that the R(−) enantiomer, is three times as potent as R(−) ketamine as an NMDA antagonist (86). Blockade of the NMDA receptor by ketamine is voltage-dependent, with much greater blockade observed at hyperpolarized (versus depolarized) potentials. The degree of antagonism appears to be determined by the state of the NMDA receptor, and the agonist-activated form interacts most readily with the dissociative anesthetics (88). Observations by MacDonald and Nowcik (89) suggest that the NMDA channels must be gated open before the binding site for ketamine is exposed. These investigators concluded that the binding site for the dissociative anesthetics was in the vicinity of the extracellular mouth of the NMDA receptor channel pore. This extracellular region is associated with a large negative surface charge that enhances binding of these positively charged molecules.

The dissociation rate of ketamine from the NMDA receptor is much slower than the rates of channel gating. This phenomenon makes it possible for ketamine molecules to become trapped within the channel if closure occurs while they are still associated with the NMDA receptor. Not until the channel is reopened by depolarization does dissociation of ketamine from the receptor become possible. As a consequence, the number of blocked channels can accumulate as the channels are activated, contributing to the slow offset of the clinical effects of ketamine. In addition to a slow offset, the block of NMDA currents by ketamine is also slow, contributing to a slow onset (89). This slow onset means that the receptors must be exposed to the drug for relatively long periods before steady-state equilibration is achieved.

Like opioid analgesia, ketamine analgesia has both supraspinal and spinal components, resulting in analgesia after both systemic and spinal administration. Ketamine binds not only to NMDA receptors but also to opioid receptors, with a distinct preference for μ receptors (90, 91). The dose of naloxone required to reverse ketamine analgesia is considerably higher than the dose needed to reverse opioid-induced analgesia, however. Furthermore, injection of ketamine into the periaqueductal gray region of the brain did not elicit analgesia (92). Probably, therefore, most of the analgesic effects of ketamine are produced predominately by an antagonistic action at the NMDA receptor. The spinal analgesic action of ketamine may involve an interaction between several receptors involved in processing spinal nociception (93). Ketamine, because of its capacity to antagonize the NMDA receptor, may be useful for "preemptive analgesia" to decrease facilitation (wind up) of spinal neurons. The psychomimetic properties of ketamine are thought to result from an interaction with the nonopioid σ receptor.

Opioids

The primary pharmacologic action of opioids relevant to anesthesia is analgesia, and most of the other actions such as respiratory depression are considered side effects. Two anatomically distinct sites exist for opioid-receptor-mediated analgesia, supraspinal and spinal, and systemically administered opioids produce analgesia at both sites. The spinal dorsal horn is the primary site for nociceptive modulation. Supraspinal analgesia produced by opioids involves both a direct supraspinal action and activation of descending inhibition of dorsal horn cells. Opioid receptors are located presynaptically on the terminals of the primary afferents and on the dendrites of postsynaptic neurons, and descending inhibition of spinothalamic neurons is mediated in part by activation of these interneurons. Opioid peptides and opioid drugs are thought to regulate nociceptive transmission by a combination of presynaptic and postsynaptic actions. Presynaptically, opioids inhibit the release of substance P, glutamate, and other neurotransmitters from the sensory neurons (94). Opioids also act postsynaptically, decreasing the amplitude of the afferent evoked excitatory postsynaptic potentials (EPSP) and hyperpolarizing the cell (Fig. 3A-8). Substance P and opioid peptide-containing nerve terminals functionally interact in the dorsal horn as two opposing systems in the regulation of the nociceptive pathway and endogenous opioids regulate substance P receptor activity in the spinal cord (95).

The brain stem modulation of nociceptive neurons in the dorsal horn is mediated primarily by release of norepinephrine and serotonin (5-HT), as well as enkephalin and substance P. Enkephalin-containing interneurons in laminae I and II of the dorsal horn synapse with terminals of serotonergic neurons that most likely derive from the rostral ventral medulla (RVM). Synaptic connections also exist between 5-HT and GABAergic interneurons (96) and between enkephalin and GABA neurons. In addition to supraspinal effects, opioids also exert a direct analgesic action on the spinal cord. For example, morphine can inhibit the firing of dorsal horn nociceptive neurons in animals that have undergone spinal transection. The analgesic effectiveness produced by epidurally and intrathecally administered opioids to patients is further evidence of a direct spinal action by opioids.

Several studies investigating opioid-mediated su-

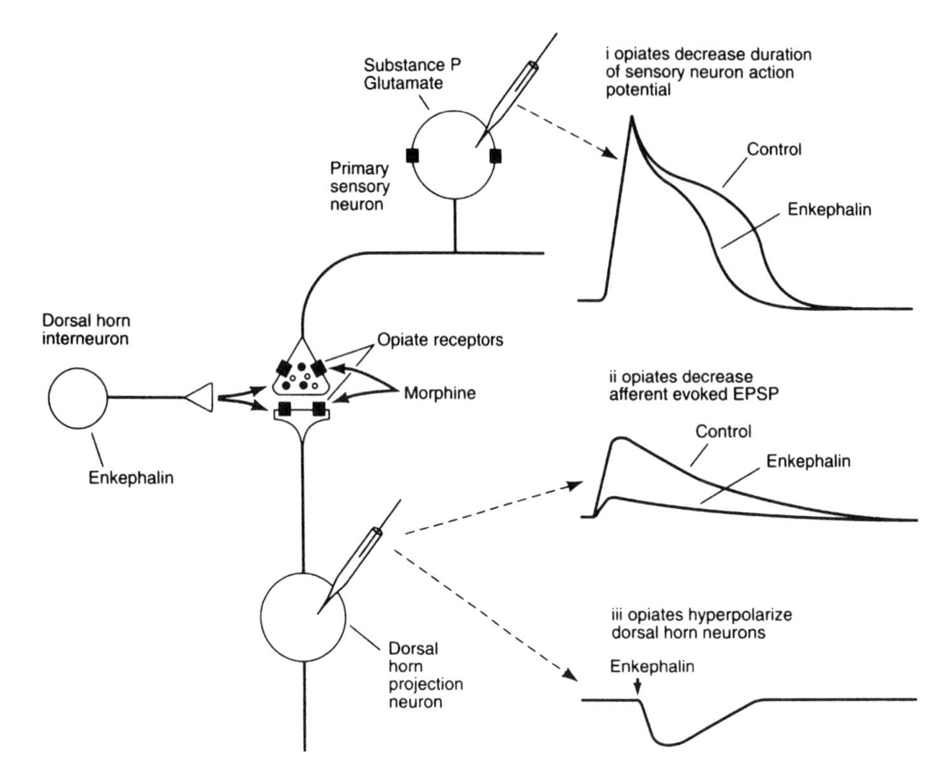

FIGURE 3A-8. Electrophysiologic analysis of the actions of opioids on sensory and dorsal horn neurons. A primary afferent neuron makes contact with a postsynaptic dorsal horn neuron. Opioids decrease the duration of the sensory neurons action potential, probably by decreased Ca^{2+} influx. Opioids may have a similar action at the terminals of the sensory neurons. Opioids hypolarize the membrane of dorsal horn neurons by activating a K^+ conductance. Stimulation of the sensory neurons normally produces a fast excitatory postsynaptic potential in the dorsal horn neurons; opioids decrease the amplitude of the postsynaptic potential. (From Jessel TM, Kelly JP. Pain and analgesia. In: Kandel ER, Schwartz JH, Jessel TM, eds. Principles of neural science. 3rd ed. New York: Elsevier, 1991).

praspinal analgesia have used the Fos protein product of the early immediate proto-oncogene, c-fos, as a marker of neuronal activity (2, 97, 98). Injection of a selective μ-opioid receptor agonist into the third ventricle also produced a dose-dependent inhibition of both pain behavior and Fos expression (98). When opioids are given systemically, they act concurrently at many sites in the CNS to produce analgesia, in addition to acting at more specific locations to produce undesirable side effects such as respiratory depression, nausea, and vomiting. In the RVM, opioids activate off-cells and inhibit on-cells, a likely mechanism of opioid analgesia. Off-cells and on-cells are classes of low-threshold neurons that are present in the RVM. On-cells show firing bursts during the hyperalgesia state just before a withdrawal reflex, and off-cells are neurons that shut off just before a behavioral response to a noxious stimulus and inhibit nociceptive reflexes. The activation of off-cells is an indirect action of opioids secondary to inhibition of an inhibitory input because off-cells are excited when opioids are directly applied. Opioid-induced disinhibition is thought to involve inhibition of GABAergic input to the off-cells (99–101).

α_2-Adrenoceptor Agonists

The α_2-adrenoceptor agonists, such as clonidine and dexmedetomidine, are a novel class of drugs that have been the subject of considerable attention in recent years because of their unique sedative-hypnotic and analgesic properties. These compounds reduce the anesthetic requirement and improve perioperative hemodynamic and sympathoadrenal stability (102). α_2-Adrenergic agonists are effective in blunting the perioperative stress response, and clonidine may have anti-ischemic effects related in part to a reduction in circulating plasma epinephrine and norepinephrine levels. Dexmedetomidine, which has a 10-fold greater α_2/α_1-receptor selectivity than clonidine (103), decreases circulating catecholamines in healthy volunteers by up to 90%, and in surgical patients it blunts the hemodynamic response to laryngoscopy and tracheal intubation (104–108). The various pharmacologic responses to these drugs are mediated by activation of α_2-adrenoceptors, although some of the hemodynamic effects may also involve the imidazoline receptor. α_2-Adrenoceptors are located both pre- and postjunctionally and are generally inhibitory, whereas α_1-adrenoceptors are excitatory. An exception is in vascular smooth muscle where α_2-adrenoceptor stimulation (analogous to α_1-activation) results in vasoconstriction.

Sedation is one the most consistent effects of α_2-adrenoceptor agonists and was a major limiting side effect for the clinical use of clonidine as an antihypertensive drug. This property can, however, be used to advantage in anesthesia, and both clonidine and dexmedetomidine have been used successfully as premedicants as well as adjuncts during balanced anesthesia (109). The CNS region where the sedative effects are mediated is the locus caeruleus (LC), the principal region for noradrenergic pathways in the mammalian CNS, which has a high density of α_2-adrenoceptors. The α_2-adrenoceptor agonists (and μ-opioid receptor agonists) hyperpolarize and silence LC neurons by inhibiting the cell membrane regulatory proteins that control inwardly rectifying K^+ channels (110). Microinjection of dexmedetomidine into the LC of rats produces a dose-dependent hypnotic effect (111). The cellular mechanism for this hypnotic-anesthetic effect involves inhibitory G proteins coupled to K^+ channels (112).

The mechanisms involved in the antinociceptive action of α_2-adrenoceptor agonists have attracted much interest following the publication of several articles describing the opioid-sparing effects of both systemic and spinally administered clonidine in the management of clinical pain syndromes. Although more recent evidence points to a spinal action for these drugs, they may also have a supraspinal component. The neurotransmitters primarily involved in descending antinociception in the dorsal horn are norepinephrine and 5-HT. The LC and the related subceruleus nuclei are the primary origins of fibers belonging to the noradrenergic descending inhibitory system. Analgesia produced by stimulation of the LC is mediated by release of norepinephrine activating α_2- adrenoceptors in the substantia gelatinosa in the spinal cord. Spinally adminstered α_2-adrenergic drugs such as clonidine probably produce their analgesia by mimicking the actions of norepinephrine in the dorsal horn. The depression of the evoked activity of nociceptive neurons in the dorsal horn by clonidine is blocked or reversed by α_2-receptor antagonists such as idazoxan or yohimbine (113). The supraspinal analgesic action of opioids is also mediated by descending inhibitory pathways. Like α_2-adrenoceptor agonists, opioids activate the adrenergic system in the LC and other medullary and pontine nuclei causing a reduction in the firing of nociceptive dorsal horn neurons, as well as inhibiting nociceptive spinal reflexes.

Because α_2-adrenergic drugs and opioids act through similar pathways but on different spinal receptors to produce analgesia, they can enhance each others' analgesic effects (114–116). Ossipov and associates, using isobolographic analysis, demonstrated a synergistic interaction between clonidine and medetomidine (a racemic mixture of which the d-enantiomer, dexmedetomidine, is the active ingredient) and a variety of μ-, δ-, and κ-opioid receptor agonists (117–119). Synergism was observed only with the tail-flick test, a spinally mediated response modulated at the spinal level, whereas an additive effect was seen after intravenous administration and in the supraspinally integrated hot plate response (119). These findings also support the hypothesis that the site of interaction between opioids and α_2-adrenoceptor agonists is at the spinal level and that the spinal cord is the principal site for the antinociceptive effects of α_2-adrenoceptor agonists. Spinal transection of mice reduces the antinociceptive potency of morphine, which acts both supraspinally and spinally, but not of clonidine (120). Destruction of descending noradrenergic neurons in the LC result in spinal supersensitivity to the antinociceptive effects of clonidine (121).

The interactions between α_2-adrenoceptor agonists and opioids may be attributable to their sharing common cellular effector mechanisms for antinociception. Both types of receptors belong to the G-protein family of cell membrane receptors. Like μ-opioid receptor agonists, α_2-adrenoceptor agonists produce membrane hyperpolarization through G proteins by altering K^+ channel conductance. Opening of K^+ channels effectively clamps the cell in a state that is unresponsive to excitatory input. Thus, in the presence of an opioid or an α_2-adrenergic agonist, the neuron is unable to depolarize, and the affected pathway is effectively severed (122).

Opioid and α_2 adrenoceptors are expressed in similar regions of the CNS and, in some cases, even on the same neurons. This makes possible an allosteric interaction between the receptors. Alternatively, activation of both receptors may elicit an enhanced effect by independently altering intracellular mechanisms coupled to G-protein activation, yielding a net effect greater than the sum of each independent effect (119). Attributing the synergistic interactions directly to a shared common second messenger system may be misleading, however, because it is likely that the combination could not enhance antinociceptive efficacy beyond that for the drug with the highest efficacy (123).

The G proteins involved in the signal transduction of α_2 adrenoceptor and opioids are sensitive to pertussis. The toxin from the bacterium Bordetella pertussis (PTX) covalently modifies these G proteins by the addition of an adenosine diphosphate (ADP)-ribose group to the subunit of the protein. Although PTX-sensitive G proteins are involved in both the hypnotic and analgesic effects of α_2-adrenergic agonists, these effects are mediated at different sites within the CNS. Intracerebroventricular pretreatment of rats with PTX significantly attenuates the hypnotic, but not the analgesic, effects of systemically administered dexmedetomidine, whereas intrathecal PTX pretreatment attenuates the analgesic, but not the hypnotic, effects (124). The hypnotic response is relatively inefficient, requiring activation of more than 80% of membrane receptors, whereas the analgesic response requires only 50% receptor occupancy (125). The anesthetic-sparing properties of dexmedetomidine appear not to involve PTX-sensitive G proteins (124). Although inhibition of adenyl cyclase and decreased formation of cAMP are important consequences of α_2-adrenoceptor activation, compelling evidence indicates that not all the physiologic consequences of this activation can be ascribed to this mechanism. Indeed, data suggest that the α_2 adrenoceptors involved in antinociception do not mediate their effects by reducing the cAMP content of cells (126). The antinociceptive effects of α_2 agonists may be due to a direct coupling between G proteins and K^+ channels, causing them to open or by inhibition of voltage-dependent Ca^{2+} channels by interacting with G proteins in a cAMP-independent fashion (127, 128). The LC-mediated hypnotic effect of these compounds does appear to be dependent on cAMP, however, because stable cAMP analogs were able to counteract dexmedetomidine-induced hypnosis (129).

Clonidine was initially introduced as a centrally active antihypertensive drug. Although α_2-adrenoceptor agonists lower blood pressure by reducing sympathetic outflow and vasomotor tone, only α_2 agonists with an imidazoline structure such as clonidine cause a decrease in blood pressure when they are injected into the RVM. The RVM area, which is rich in adrenergic neurons, is an important processing center for the control of arterial blood pressure and is considered to be the primary site of action for α_2-adrenoceptor agonist activity on sympathetic outflow (130, 131). Clonidine and other related imidazolines were originally considered to act only on the central α_2 adrenoceptor (132–134). Investigators now know, however, that certain drugs that were traditionally thought to act at α_2 adrenoceptors also act at nonadrenergic imidazoline-preferring sites, designated imidazoline receptors (135).

The physiologic role of the imidazoline receptor is still not well defined, but in the RVM it has a function in regulating blood pressure (101, 136–138). Good evidence indicates that the hypotensive activity of clonidine and other imidazolines is mediated by these imidazoline receptors (135–137, 139). A close correlation exists between the degree of hypotension induced by clonidine and the degree of occupancy of imidazoline receptors, but not α_2 receptors (101).

A low-molecular-weight noncatecholamine, nonpeptidergic agent, designated the clonidine-displacing substance (CDS), has been isolated and purified from bovine brain and has been characterized in various cells (101, 140, 141). CDS specifically displaces clonidine from rat brain membranes without affecting α_1- or β-adrenergic receptors (142). Injection of CDS into the RVM causes an increase in blood pressure. CDS may be the endogenous ligand for the imidazoline receptor (101, 141–143). Current opinion is that clonidine acts centrally at two receptors, the α_2 adrenoceptor and the imidazoline receptor, with the hypotensive effect of clonidine predominantly related to activity at the imidazoline receptor. Clonidine may be an antagonist at the imidazoline receptor, and its hypotensive effects may result from displacement of CDS (140).

Local Anesthetics

A long history relates to the administration of local anesthetic by the intravenous route for producing analgesia. Procaine has been given intravenously to ease the pruritus of jaundice, for dressing burns, and to produce obstetric and postoperative pain relief (144). Intravenous lidocaine has been used to relieve cancer pain (145), pain due to adiposis dolorosa (146, 147), and postoperative pain (148, 149). Intravenous lidocaine has also been used to provide analgesia during surgical operations in combination with thiopental and nitrous oxide-oxygen anesthesia (148). The alleged advantages of this technique include prolonged postoperative analgesia, no respiratory depression, and a low incidence of postoperative nausea and vomiting. More recently, Cassuto and colleagues (150) described the use of a continuous low-dose infusion of lidocaine for postoperative analgesia after cholecystectomy. The lidocaine infusion regimen consisted of a loading dose of 100 mg followed by 2 mg min^{-1} started 30 minutes before skin incision and continued for 24 hours after surgery. The lidocaine-treated patients had significantly lower pain scores and required significantly less meperidine during the first and second postoperative days. The use of lidocaine was devoid of postoperative side effects. Although intravenous local anesthetics for intraoperative analgesia have been largely replaced by other drugs, this technique remains popular in many South American and Asian countries. Local anesthetics are also widely used for intravenous regional blocks, peripheral nerve blocks, tissue infiltration and instillation, and for the treatment of cardiac arrhythmias.

The pharmacologic actions of local anesthetics are the result of blocking the generation and propagation of action potentials in excitable tissues, which include nerve cells and the pacemaker cells in the sinoatrial (SA) and atrioventricular nodes of the heart. Nerve cells respond to stimuli by undergoing a rapid but transient change in their electrical (action) potential. This action potential is then propagated as an impulse along the nerve axon to trigger the release of neurotransmitters or stimulate other excitable cells (e.g., skeletal muscle). Local anesthetics block these impulses by inhibiting the inward Na^+ current and preventing depolarization of the neuron. The Na^+, K^+, and Ca^{++} channels are each important for initiation and propagation of neuronal action potentials; however, the Na^+ channel is the most important and best understood. At rest, the inside of the neural cell is maintained at a voltage of -60 to -70 mV relative to the outside of the membrane (as a consequence of the relative impermeability of the neural membrane to Na^+ ions and a selective permeability to K^+ ions). This potential difference is maintained by an energy dependent mechanism, the Na^+-K^+ pump, which extrudes Na^+ ions from within the cell in exchange for K^+ ions. The result is an intracellular-to-extracellular K^+ ratio of 35:1. The potential across the membrane is thus largely determined by the K^+ gradient, according to the Nernst equation:

$$E = -61 \log \frac{[K^+]_i}{[K^+]_o}$$

where E *is membrane potential and* $[K^+]$ is the K^+ concentration inside (i) and outside (o) the cell. The Nernst potential for K^+ is −94 mV, but because Na^+ and Cl^- ions also make a contribution, the resting potential is lower and averages −60 to −70 mV. Although K^+ ions are primarily responsible for the resting potential, movement of Na^+ ions makes the initial contribution to the development of the action potential. The Na^+ channels are voltage-gated channels that can exist in one of three states; closed (or resting), open, and inactivated. During an action potential the Na^+ channels open allowing extracellular Na^+ ions to flow into the cell. The trigger for this opening is an increase in the intracellular potential toward a threshold potential of approximately −55 mV. This change in the resting potential causes a voltage-dependent change in the conformation of the Na^+ channel whereby the marked increase in the permeability of the membrane for Na^+ depolarizes the neurons. The opening of the Na^+ channel is transient (lasting less than 1 millisecond), and it spontaneously closes and enters the inactivated state. It can only return to its resting state when the membrane potential returns to near the resting potential. The same potential changes that lead to the opening of Na^+ channels also open K^+ channels. The K^+ channel opens more slowly than the Na^+ channels and becomes fully open when the Na^+ channel has almost returned to the inactivated state (Fig. 3A-9). The outward flow of K^+ ions is responsible for the repolarization of the neurons. Although an action potential is associated with large changes in membrane potential, the number of Na^+ ions entering and K^+ ions leaving the cell is small, and ionic equilibrium is rapidly restored by the Na^+-K^+ pump. During each action potential, 3 to 4 × 10^{-12} mol of Na^+ ions enter the cell through each cm^2 of surface area. When a squid axon has been poisoned with cyanide so that Na^+-K^+ ion pumping mechanism is abolished, the axon can fire nearly 100,000 action potentials before failing.

Because the Na^+ channel is sensitive to changes in transmembrane voltage (it is voltage gated), part of the channel must act as a voltage sensor. Current evidence suggests the fourth transmembrane helix (S4) segment of the channel protein is the likely site of this sensor (151). This segment of protein is unusual in that it contains an excess of arginine and lysine, the most positively charged of the amino acids, arranged in every third position among otherwise neutral amino acids. Investigators believe that the rotational and longitudinal movement of this segment in response to a change in transmembrane potential causes the ion pore to open and allow Na^+ ions to flow toward the inside of the cell, down their concentration gradient. Inactivation of the Na^+ channel involves a region of the channel exposed to the inside of the cell. The mechanism has been likened to a "ball and chain," with the ball being a globular part of the protein that can plug the inside mouth of the pore and the chain being a flexible part that can allow the ball to flop in and out of the mouth, depending on the voltage across the membrane.

Local anesthetics have different affinities for the different states in the Na^+ channel. They bind tightly to the inactivated state, thereby stabilizing this form of the channel (152). The closed or resting state has the

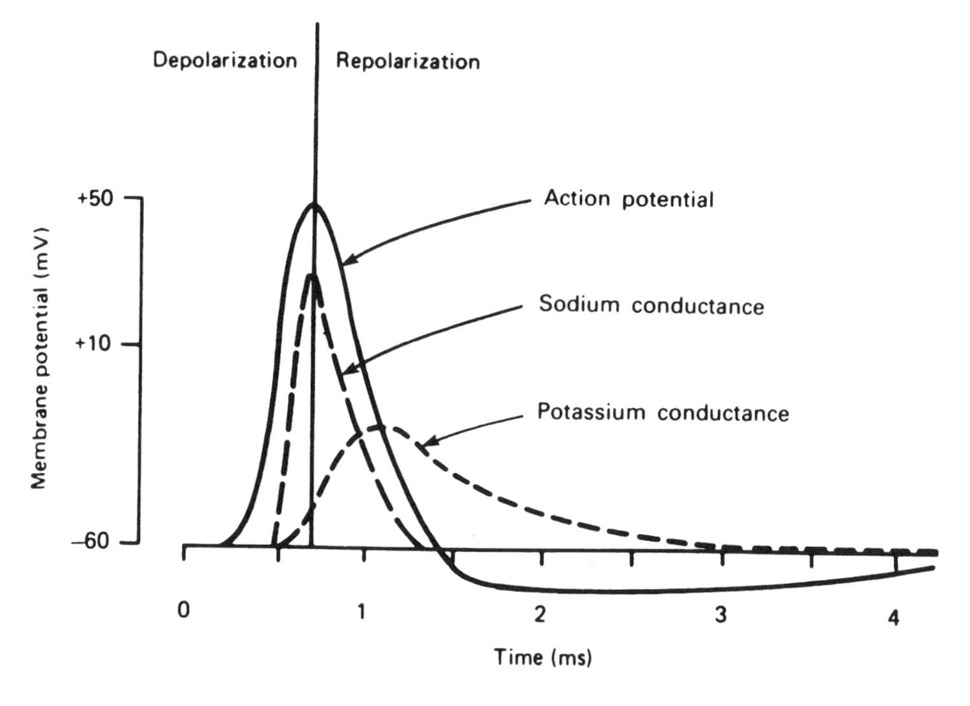

FIGURE 3A-9. Relationship between depolarization and repolarization phases of nerve action potential and sodium and potassiuim currents. (From Covino BG, Strichartz GR. Local anaesthetics. In: Feldman SA, Paton W, Scurr C, eds. Mechanisms of drugs in anaesthesia. 2nd ed. London: Edward Arnold, 1993.)

least affinity for local anesthetics. This differential affinity explains the phasic or frequency-dependent neuronal block produced by local anesthetics (153). The location of the local anesthetic receptors of the Na^+ channel are uncertain, and they appear to have at least three binding sites. The charged forms of amino esters and amino amides act at the axoplasmic surface of the Na^+ channel. The base form of local anesthetics binds to a lesser extent at the intramembrane portion of the channel, at the interface between the channel and the surrounding membrane lipid. Various toxins such as tetrodotoxin specifically bind to the outer aspects of the channel to block Na^+ conductance (154, 155).

An important mechanism of the antiarrhythmic action of local anesthetic (class I of antiarrhythmic drugs, Vaughan Williams classification) is inhibition of the fast inward depolarizing currents carried by Na^+ ions. Lidocaine is the standard drug for the treatment of ventricular arrhythmias. Lidocaine, a class I B drug, acts during phase 0 of the cardiac action potential to suppress the entry of Na^+ responsible for conduction in cardiac muscle and the His-Purkinje system. More important for its antiarrhythmic action, however, is the reduction in Na^+ current during phase 4 diastolic depolarization of the Purkinje fibers, thereby suppressing automaticity. Lidocaine only interferes with SA nodal activity when there is preexisting SA node disease. Because the Na^+ block produced by lidocaine dissociates rapidly, it has little effect on conduction at normal heart rates, but it may slow conduction during rapid tachyarrhythmias. Conduction velocity is also significantly decreased in regions of myocardial ischemia. Several factors may be responsible for this effect, including reduced regional perfusion in ischemic regions preventing drug washout. An alternative explanation may be potentiation of the local anesthetic action by the lowered pH in ischemic tissues as a result of "ion trapping." As the charged form of lidocaine gains access to the Na^+ channel from inside the cell membrane, an increase in intracellular drug concentration increases the degree of block of Na^+ channels.

In summary, several different theories have been advanced to explain the mechanism of action of centrally active intravenous anesthetic drugs. The concept of a common "nonspecific" mechanism has been abandoned with the identification and classification of specific receptor binding sites for sedative-hypnotics, opioid analgesics, α_2 agonists, and local anesthetics. The availability of more specific information on mechanism of action of these compounds should result in the synthesis and clinical development of safer and more efficacious intravenous anesthetics in the future.

REFERENCES

1. Law PY, Hom DS, Loh HH. Opiate receptors down-regulation and desensitization in neuroblastoma X glioma NG108–15 hybrid cells are two separate cellular adaptation processes. Mol Pharmacol 1983;24:413–424.
2. Presley RW, Menétrey D, Levine JD, Basbaum AI. Systemic morphine suppresses noxious stimulus-evoked Fos protein-like immunoreactivity in the rat spinal cord. J Neurosci 1990;10:323–335.
3. Kenakin T, Morgan P, Lutz M. Commentary on the importance of the "antagonist assumption" to how receptors express themselves. Biochem Pharmacol 1995;50:17–26.
4. Clark AJ. General pharmacology. In: Handbook of experimental physiology. Berlin: Springer-Verlag; 1937:64.
5. Stephenson RP. A modification of receptor theory. Br J Pharmacol 1956;11:379–393.
6. Leslie FM. Methods used for the study of opioid receptors. Pharmacol Rev 1987;39:197–249.
7. Krogsgaard-Larsen P, Frølund B, Jorgensen FS, Schousboe A. $GABA_A$ receptor agonists, partial agonists, and antagonists: design and therapeutic prospects. J Med Chem 1994;37:2489–2505.
8. Verdoorn TA, Draguhn A, Ymer S, et al. Functional properties of recombinant rat $GABA_A$ receptors depend upon subunit composition. Neuron 1990;4:919–928.
9. Sakmann B, Hamill OP, Bormann J. Patch-clamp measurements of elementary chloride currents activated by the putative inhibitory transmitters GABA and glycine in mammalian spinal neurons. J Neural Transm Suppl 1983;18:83–95.
10. Macdonald RL, Olsen RW. $GABA_A$ receptor channels. Annu Rev Neurosci 1994;17:569–602.
11. Monaghan DT, Bridges RJ, Cotman CW. The excitatory amino acid receptors: their classes, pharmacology and distinct properties in the function of the central nervous System. Annu Rev Pharmacol Toxicol 1989;29:365–402.
12. Daw NW, Stein PSG, Fox K. The role of the NMDA receptors in information processing. Annu Rev Neurosci 1993;16:207–222.
13. Seeburg PH. The molecular biology of mammalian glutamate receptor channels. Trends Pharmacol Sci 1993;14:297–303.
14. Dubner R, Ruda MA. Activity-dependent neuronal plasticity following tissue injury and inflammation. Trends Neurosci 1992;15:96–103.
15. Collingridge GL, Singer W. Excitatory amino acid receptors and synaptic plasticity. Trends Pharmacol Sci 1990;11:290–296.
16. Ghorpade A, Advokat C. Evidence of a role for N-methyl-D-aspartate (NMDA) receptors in the facilitation of tail withdrawal after spinal transection. Pharmacol Biochem Behav 1994;48:175–181.
17. Davies SN, Lodge D. Evidence for involvement of N-methylaspartate receptors in "wind-up" of class 2 neurons in the dorsal horn of the rat. Brain Res 1987;424:402–406.
18. Dickenson AH. A cure for wind up: NMDA receptor antagonists as potential analgesics. Trends Pharmacol Sci 1990;11:307–309.
19. Dickenson AH, Sullivan AF. Evidence for a role of the NMDA receptor in the frequency dependent potentiation of deep rat dorsal horn nociceptive neurons following C fibre stimulation. Neuropharmacology 1987;26:1235–1238.
20. Price DD, Mao J, Frenk H, Mayer DJ. The N-methyl-D-aspartate receptor antagonist dextromethorphan selectively reduces temporal summation of second pain in man. Pain 1994;59:165–174.
21. Pasternak GW, Wood PL. Multiple mu opiate receptors. Life Sci 1986;38:1889–1898.
22. Jiang Q, Takemori AE, Sultana M, et al. Differential antagonism of opioid delta antinociception by [D-Ala^2, Leu^5, Cys^6] enkephalin and naltrindole 5-isothiocynate: evidence for delta receptor subtypes. J Pharmacol Exp Ther 1991;257:1069–1075.
23. Clark AJ, Liu L, Price M, et al. Kappa-opiate receptor multiplicity: evidence for two U–50, 488 sensitive κ_1 subtypes and a novel κ_3 subtype. J Pharmacol Exp Ther 1989;251:461–468.
24. Heymans JS, Williams CL, Burks TF, et al. Dissociation of opi-

oid antinociception and central gastrointestinal propulsion in the mouse: studies with naloxonazine. J Pharmacol Exp Ther 1988;245:238–243.
25. Paul D, Bodnar RJ, Pasternak GW. Different mu receptor subtypes mediate spinal and supraspinal analgesia. Neurosci Abstr 1988;14:465.
26. Martin WR, Eades CG. The effects of morphine-and nalorphine-like drugs in the nondependent and morphine-dependent chronic spinal dog. J Pharmacol Exp Ther 1976;197:517–532.
27. Largent BL, Gundlach AL, Snyder SH. Pharmacological and autoradiographic discrimination of sigma and phencyclidine receptor binding sites in brain with (+)-[3H]SKF 10, 047, (+)-[3H]-3-PPP and [3H]TCP. J Pharmacol Exp Ther 1986;238:739–748.
28. Flagg GE, Foster AC, Ganong AH. Excitatory amino acid synaptic mechanisms and neurological function. Trends Pharmacol Sci 1986;7:357–363.
29. Zhang AZ, Pasternak GW. Opiates and enkephalins: a common binding mediates their analgesia actions in rats. Life Sci 1981; 29:843–851.
30. North RA. Opioid receptor types and membranes on ion channels. Trends Neurosci 1986;9:174–176.
31. Gross RA, Macdonald RL. Dynorphin A selectivity reduces a large transient (N-type) calcium current of mouse dorsal root ganglion neurons in cell culture. Proc Natl Acad Sci U S A 1987; 84:5469–5473.
32. McFadzean DF. The ionic mechanisms underlying opioid actions. Neuropeptides 1988;11:173–180.
33. Xu H, Gintzler AR. Opioid enhancement of evoked [Met5] enkephalin release requires activation of cholinergic receptors: possible involvement of intracellular calcium. Proc Natl Acad Sci U S A 1992;89:1978–1982.
34. Tang T, Kiang JG, Cox BM. Opioids acting through delta receptors elicit a transient increase in the intracellular free calcium concentration in dorsal root ganglion-neuroblastoma hybrid ND8–47 cells. J Pharmacol Exp Ther 1994;270:40–46.
35. Jin W, Lee NM, Loh HH, Thayer SA. Dual excitatory and inhibitory effects of opioids in the neuronal cell line NG108–15. Mol Pharmacol 1992;42:1083–1089.
36. Albertson TE, Walby WF, Joy RM. Modification of GABA-mediated inhibition by various injectable anesthetics. Anesthesiology 1992;77:488–499.
37. Gage PW, Robertson B. Prolongation of inhibitory postsynaptic currents by pentobarbitone, halothane and ketamine in CA1 pyramid cells in rat hippocampus. Br J Pharmacol 1985;85:675–681.
38. Macdonald RL, Rogers CJ, Twyman RE. Barbiturate modulation of kinetic properties of $GABA_A$ receptor channels in mouse spinal neurons in culture. J Physiol 1989;417:483–500.
39. Robertson B. Actions of anaesthetics and avermectin on $GABA_A$ chloride channels in mammalian dorsal root ganglion neurons. Br J Pharmacol 1989;98:167–176.
40. Olsen RW, Yang J, King RG. Barbiturate and benzodiazepine modulation of GABA receptor binding and function. Life Sci 1986;39:1969–1976.
41. Sieghart W. $GABA_A$ receptors: ligand-gated Cl^- ion channels modulated by multiple drug-binding sites. Trends Pharmacol Sci 1992;13:446–450.
42. Mantz J, Varlet C, Lecharny JB, et al. Effects of volatile anesthetics, thiopental, and ketamine on spontaneous and depolarization-evoked dopamine release from striatal synaptosomes in the rat. Anesthesiology 1994;80:352–363.
43. De Armendi AJ, Tonner PH, Bugge B, Miller KW. Barbiturate action is dependent on the conformational state of the acetylcholine receptor. Anesthesiology 1993;79:1033–1041.
44. Carla V, Moroni F. General anaesthetics inhibit the responses induced by glutamate receptor agonists in the mouse cortex. Neurosci Lett 1992;146:21–24.
45. Ashton D, Fransen J, Wauquier A. In vivo interactions between agonists and antagonists of the GABA-benzodiazepine-chloride ionophore receptor complex in a model of hypoxic hypoxia. In: Wauquier A, Borgers M, Amery WK, eds. Protection of tissues against hypoxia. Amsterdam: Elsevier Biomedical Press, 1982:115–119.
46. Ashton D, Geerts R, Waterkeyn C, Leysen JE. Etomidate stereospecifically stimulates forebrain but not cerebellar ^{3}H-diazepam binding. Life Sci 1981;29:2631–2636.
47. Thyagaran R, Ramanjaneyulu YMK. Enhancement of diazepam, and GABA binding by (+) etomidate and pentobarbital. J Neurochem 1983;41:578–585.
48. Mantz J, Lecharny JB, Laudenbach V, et al. Anesthetics affect the uptake but not the depolarization-evoked release of GABA in rat striatal synaptosomes. Anesthesiology 1995;82:502–511.
49. Harrison NL, Majewska MD, Harrington JW, Barker JL. Structure-activity relationships for steroid interaction with the γ-aminobutyric $acid_A$ receptor complex. J Pharmacol Exp Ther 1987;241:346–353.
50. Lambert JJ, Peters JA, Sturgess NC, Hales TG. Steroid modulation of the $GABA_A$ receptor complex: electro-physiological studies. In: Simmonds MA, ed. Steroids and neural activity. Chichester: Wiley, 1990:56–71.
51. Braestrup C, Nielsen M, Olsen C. Urinary and brain β-carboline–3-carboxylates as potent inhibitors of brain benzodiazepine receptors. Proc Natl Acad Sci U S A 1980;77:2288–2292.
52. Pena C, Medina J, Noval M, et al. Isolation and identification in bovine cerebral cortex of n-butyl-carboline–3-carboxylate, a potent endogenous benzodiazepine binding inhibitor. Proc Natl Acad Sci U S A 1986;83:4952–4956.
53. Prichett DB, Sontheimer H, Shivers BD, et al. Importance of a novel $GABA_A$ receptor subunit for benzodiazepine pharmacology. Nature 1989;338:582–585.
54. Schwartz R, Skolnick P, Seale T, Paul S. Demonstration of GABA/barbiturate-receptor mediated chloride transport in rat brain synaptoneurosomes: a functional assay of GABA receptor-effector coupling. Adv Biochem Psychopharmacol 1986; 41:33–49.
55. Morrow LA, Suzdak PD, Paul SM. Benzodiazepine, barbiturate, ethanol and hypnotic steroid hormone modulation of GABA-mediated chloride ion transport in rat brain synaptoneurosomes. Adv Biochem Psychopharmacol 1988;45:247–261.
56. Richards JG, Schoch P, Haefely W. Benzodiazepine receptors: new vistas. Semin Neurosci 1991;3:191–203.
57. Macdonald RL, Twyman RE. Kinetic properties and regulation of $GABA_A$ receptor channels. In: Narahashi T, ed. Ion channels. 4th ed. New York: Plenum, 1992:315–343.
58. Mathers DA. The $GABA_A$ rceptor: new insights from single channel recording. Synapse 1987;1:96–101.
59. Faull RL, Villiger JW. Benzodiazepine receptors in the human spinal cord: a detailed anatomical and pharmacological study. Neuroscience 1986;17:791–802.
60. Serrao JM, Goodchild CS, Gent JP. Intrathecal midazolam and fentanyl in the rat: evidence for different spinal antinociceptive effects. Anesthesiology 1989;70:780–786.
61. Edwards M, Serrao JM, Gent JP, Goodchild CS. GABA involvement in spinal analgesia with midazolam. Br J Anaesth 1989; 62:233P.
62. Sumida T, Tagami M, Ide Y, et al. Intravenous midazolam suppresses noxiously evoked activity of spinal wide dynamic range neurons in cats. Anesth Analg 1995;80:58–63.
63. Mukhin A, Papadopoulos V, Costa E, Krueger KE. Mitochondrial receptors regulate steroid biosynthesis. Proc Natl Acad Sci U S A 1989;86:9813–9816.
64. Yanagibashi K, Ohno Y, Nakmichi N, et al. Peripheral-type benzodiazepine receptors are involved in the regulation of cholesterol side chain cleavage in adrenocortical mitochondria. J Biochem (Tokyo) 1989;106:1026–1029.
65. Costa E, Guidotti A. Neuropeptides as cotransmitters: modulatory effects of GABAergic synapses. In: Meltzer HY, ed. Psy-

chopharmacology: the third generation process. New York: Raven Press, 1987:425–435.
66. Rothstein JD, Garland W, Puia G, et al. The role of endogenous benzodiazepines in physiology and pathology. In: Barnard EA, Costa E, eds. Transmitter amino acid receptors: structures, transductions and models for drug development. New York: Raven Press, 1991:325–340.
67. Rothstein JD, Garland W, Puia G, et al. Purification and characterization of neurally occurring benzodiazepine receptor ligands in rat and human brain. J Neurochem 1992;6:2102–2115.
68. Ferrero P, Costa E, Conti-Tronconi B, Guidotti A. A diazepam binding inhibitor (DBI)-like neuropeptide is detected in human brain. Brain Res 1986;399:136–142.
69. Ferrarese C, Appollonio I, Frigo M, et al. Distribution of a putative endogenous modulator of the GABAergic system in human brain. Neurology 1989;39:443–445.
70. Olasmaa M, Guidotti A, Costa E, et al. Endogenous benzodiazepines in hepatic encephalopathy. Lancet 1989;1:491–492.
71. Hales TG, Lambert JJ. The actions of propofol on inhibitory amino acid receptors of bovine adrenomedullary chromaffin cells and rodent central neurons. Br J Pharmacol 1991;104:619–628.
72. Collins GGS. Effects of the anaesthetic 2,6-diisopropylphenol on synaptic transmission in the rat olfactory cortex slice. Br J Pharmacol 1988;95:939–949.
73. Peduto VA, Concas A, Santoro G, et al. Biochemical and electrophysiologic evidence that propofol enhances GABAergic transmission in the rat brain. Anesthesiology 1991;75:1000–1009.
74. Hara M, Kai Y, Ikemoto Y. Propofol activates the $GABA_A$ receptor-ionophore complex in dissociated hippocampal neurons of the rat. Anesthesiology 1993;79:781–788.
75. Hara M, Kai Y, Ikemoto Y. Enhancement by propofol of the γ-aminobutyric $acid_A$ response in dissociated hippocampal pyramidal neurons of the rat. Anesthesiology 1994;81:988–994.
76. Wakamori M, Ikemoto Y, Akaike N. Effects of two volatile anesthetics and a volatile convulsant on the excitatory and inhibitory amino acid responses in dissociated CNS neurons of the rat. J Neurophysiol 1991;66:2014–2021.
77. Concas A, Santoro G, Mascia MP, et al. The action of the general anesthetic propofol on $GABA_A$ receptors. In: Biggio G, Concas A, Costa E, eds. GABAergic synaptic transmission. New York: Raven Press, 1992:349–363.
78. Mantz J, Delumeau JC, Cordier J, Petitet F. Differential effects of propofol and ketamine on cytosolic calcium concentrations of astrocytes in primary culture. Br J Anaesth 1994;72:351–353.
79. Mantz J, Cordier J, Giaume C. Effects of general anesthetics on intercellular communications mediated by gap junctions between astrocytes in primary culture. Anesthesiology 1993;78:892–901.
80. Frenkel C, Urban BW. Human brain sodium channels as one of the molecular target sites for the new intravenous anaesthetic propofol (2,6-diisopropylphenol). Eur J Pharmacol 1991;208:75–79.
81. Frenkel C, Urban BW. Interactions of intravenous anesthetics with human CNS ion channels: electrophysiologic studies with a new type of voltage clamp technique. Anaesthetist 1994;43:229–234.
82. Jensen AF, Lindroth M, Sjölander A, Eintrei C. Propofol induces changes in the cytosolic free calcium concentration and the cytoskeletal organization of cultured human glial cells and primary embryonic rat brain cells. Anesthesiology 1994;81:1220–1229.
83. Yamamura T, Harada K, Okamura A, Kemmotsu O. Is the site of action of ketamine anesthesia the N-methyl-D-aspartate receptor? Anesthesiology 1990;72:704–710.
84. Lodge D, Anis NA. Effects of phencyclidine on excitatory amino acid activation of spinal interneurons in the cat. Eur J Pharmacol 1982;77:203–204.
85. Lodge D, Anis NA. Effects of ketamine and three other anaesthetics on spinal reflexes and inhibition in the cat. Br J Anaesth 1984;56:1143–1147.
86. Lodge D, Anis NA. Effects of optical isomers of ketamine on excitation of cat and rat spinal neurons by amino acids and acetylcholine. Neurosci Lett 1982;29:281–286.
87. Wong BS, Martin CD. Ketamine inhibition of cytoplasmic calcium signalling in rat pheochromocytoma (PC–12) cells. Life Sci 1993;53:PL359-PL364.
88. MacDonald JF, Bartlett MC, Mody I, et al. Actions of ketamine, phencyclidine and MK–801 on NMDA receptor currents in cultured mouse hippocampal neurons. J Physiol 1991;432:483–508.
89. MacDonald JF, Nowcik LM. Mechanisms of blockade of excitatory amino acid receptor channels. Trends Pharmacol Sci 1990;11:161–172.
90. Finck AD, Ngai SH. Opiate receptor mediation of ketamine analgesia. Anesthesiology 1982;56:291–297.
91. Smith DJ, Bouchal RL, DeSanctis CA, et al. Properties of the interaction between ketamine and opiate binding sites in vivo and in vitro. Neuropharmacology 1987;26:1253–1260.
92. Smith DJ, Perrotti JM, Mansell AL, Monroe PJ. Ketamine analgesia is not related to an opiate action in the periaquaductal grey region of the rat brain. Pain 1985;21:253–265.
93. Song XJ, Zhao ZQ. Interaction between substance P and excitatory amino acid receptors in modulation of nociceptive responses of cat spinal dorsal horn neurons. Neurosci Lett 1994;168:49–52.
94. Chang HM, Berde CB, Holz GG4, et al. Sufentanil, morphine, met-enkephalin, and kappa-agonists (U–50,488H) inhibit substance P release from primary sensory neurons: a model for presynaptic spinal opioid actions. Anesthesiology 1989;70:672–677.
95. Igwe OJ. Modulation of substance P-ergic system in the rat spinal cord by an opioid antagonist. Brain Res Mol Brain Res 1994;21:263–273.
96. Alhaider AA, Lei SZ, Wilcox GL. Spinal 5-HT_3 receptor-mediated antinociception: possible release of GABA. J Neurosci 1991;11:1881–1888.
97. Tölle TR, Castro LJ, Coimbra A, Zieglgènsberger W. Opiates modify induction of c-fos proto-oncogene in the spinal cord of the rat following noxious stimulation. Neurosci Lett 1990;111:46 51.
98. Gogas KR, Presley RW, Levine JD, Basbaum AI. The antinociceptive action of supraspinal opioids results from an increase in descending inhibitory control: correlation of nociceptive behavior and c-fos expression. Neuroscience 1991;42:617–628.
99. Heinricher MM, Barbaro NM, Fields HL. Putative nociceptive modulating neurons in the rostral ventromedial medulla of the rat: firing of on-and off-cells is related to nociceptive responsiveness. Somatosens Mot Res 1989;6:427–439.
100. Heinricher MM, Haws CM, Fields HL. Evidence for GABA-mediated control of putative nociceptive modulating neurons in the rostral ventromedial medulla: iontophoresis of bicuculline eliminates the off-cell pause. Somatosens Mot Res 1991;8:215–225.
101. Heinricher MM, Morgan MM, Fields HL. Direction and indirect actions of morphine on medullary neurons that modulate nociception. Neuroscience 1992;48:533–543.
102. Maze M, Tranquilli W. Aplha–2 adrenoceptor agonists: defining the role in clinical anesthesia. Anesthesiology 1991;74:581–605.
103. Virtanen R, Savola JM, Saano V, Nyman L. Characterization of the selectivity, specificity and potency of medetomidine as an alpha 2-adrenoceptor agonist. Eur J Pharmacol 1988;150:9–14.
104. Aho M, Lehtinen A, Erkola O, et al. The effect of intravenously administered dexmedetomidine on perioperative hemodynamics and isoflurane requirements in patients undergoing abdominal hysterectomy. Anesthesiology 1991;74:997–1002.
105. Aantaa RE, Kanto JH, Scheinen M, et al. Dexmedetomidine, an

α_2 adrenergic agonist, reduces anesthetic requirements for patients undergoing minor gynecological surgery. Anesthesiology 1990;73:230–235.
106. Aho M, Scheinin M, Lehtinen AM, et al. Intramuscularly administered dexmedetomidine attenuates hemodynamic and stress hormone responses to gynecologic laparoscopy. Anesth Analg 1992;75:932–939.
107. Morgan MM, Heinricher MM, Fields HL. Circuitary linking opioid-sensitive nociceptive modulatory systems in periaqueductal gray and spinal cord with rostral ventromedial medulla. Neuroscience 1992;47:863–871.
108. Belleville JP, Ward DS, Bloor BC, Maze M. Effects of intravenous dexmedetomidine in humans. I. Sedation, ventilation, and metabolic rate. Anesthesiology 1992;77:1125–1133.
109. Flacke JW, Flacke WE. The use of α_2-adrenergic agonists during general anaesthesia. Anaesth Pharmacol Rev 1993;1:268–283.
110. North RA. Drug receptors and the inhibition of nerve cells. Br J Pharmacol 1989;98:13–28.
111. Correa-Sales C, Rabin B, Maze M. A hypnotic response to dexmedetomidine, an α_2 agonist, is mediated in the locus coeruleus in rats. Anesthesiology 1992;76:948–952.
112. Doze VA, Chen B, Tinklenberg JA, et al. Pertussis toxin and 4-aminopyridine differentially affect the hypnotic-anesthetic action of dexmedetomidine and pentobarbital. Anesthesiology 1990;73:304–307.
113. Tjolsen A, Lund A, Hole K. The role of descending noradrenergic systems in regulation of nociception: the effects of intrathecally administered α-adrenoceptor antagonists and clonidine. Pain 1990;43:113–120.
114. Rostaing S, Bonnet F, Levron JC, et al. Effect of epidural clonidine on analgesia and pharmacokinetics of epidural fentanyl in postoperative patients. Anesthesiology 1991;75:420–425.
115. Vercauteren M, Lauwers E, Meert T, et al. Comparison of epidural sufentanil plus clonidine with sufentanil alone for postoperative pain relief. Anaesthesia 1990;45:531–534.
116. Motsch J, Graber E, Ludwig K. Addition of clonidine enhances postoperative analgesia from epidural morphine: a double-blind study. Anesthesiology 1990;73:1067–1073.
117. Ossipov MH, Harris S, Lloyd P, Messineo E. An isobolographic analysis of the antinociceptive effect of systemically and intrathecally administered combinations of clonidine and opiates. J Pharmacol Exp Ther 1990;255:1107–1116.
118. Ossipov MH, Lozito R, Messineo E, et al. Spinal antinociceptive synergy between clonidine and morphine, U69593, and DPDPE: isobolographic analysis. Life Sci 1990;47:PL71-PL76.
119. Ossipov MH, Harris S, Lloyd P, et al. Antinociceptive interaction between opioids and medetomidine: systemic additivity and spinal synergy. Anesthesiology 1990;73:1227–1235.
120. Spaulding TC, Venafro JJ, Ma MG, Fielding S. Dissociation of the antinociceptive effect of clonidine from supraspinal structures. Neuropharmacology 1979;18:103–105.
121. Ossipov MH, Chaterjee TK, Gebhart GF. Locus coeruleus lesions in the rat enhance the antinociceptive potency of centrally administered clonidine but not morphine. Brain Res 1985;341: 320–330.
122. Bloor BC. General pharmacology of α_2-adrenoceptors. Anaesth Pharmacol Rev 1993;1:221–232.
123. Andrade RA, Aghajanian GK. Opiate and α_2-adrenergic-induced hyperpolarizations of locus coeruleus neurons in brain slices: reversal by cyclic-AMP analogs. J Neurosci 1985;5:2359–2364.
124. Hayashi Y, Rabin BC, Guo T, Maze M. Role of pertussis toxin-sensitive G-proteins in the analgesic and anesthetic actions of α_2-adrenergic agonists in the rat. Anesthesiology 1995;83:816–822.
125. Hayashi Y, Guo T, Maze M. Desensitization of the behavioral effects of α_2-adrenergic agonists in rats. Anesthesiology 1995; 82:954–962.
126. Uhlén S, Persson M, Alari L, et al. Antinociceptive actions of α_2-adrenoceptor agonists in the rat spinal cord: evidence for antinociceptive α_2-adrenoceptor subtypes and dissociation of antinociceptive α_2-adrenoceptors from cyclic AMP. J Neurochem 1990;55:1905–1914.
127. Hescheler J, Rosenthal W, Trautwein W, Schultz G. The GTP-binding protein, G_o, regulates neuronal calcium channels. Nature 1987;325:445–447.
128. Iyengar R, Birnbaumer L. Signal transduction by G-proteins. ISI Atlas Sci Pharmacol 1987;1:213–221.
129. Correa-Sales C, Nacif-Coelho C, Reid K, Maze M. Inhibition of adenylate cyclase in the locus coeruleus mediates the hypnotic response to an alpha-2 agonist in the rat. J Pharmacol Exp Ther 1992;263:1046–1049.
130. Reis DJ, Morrison S, Ruggiero DA. The C1 area of the brain stem in tonic and reflex control of blood pressure. State of the art lecture. Hypertension 1988;11:18–33.
131. Unnerstall JR, Kopajtic TA, Kuhar MJ. Distribution of alpha–2 agonist binding sites in the rat and human central nervous system: analysis of some functional, anatomic correlates of the pharmacologic effects of clonidine and related adrenergic agents. Brain Res 1984;319:69–101.
132. Isaac L. Clonidine in the central nervous system: site and mechanism of hypotensive action. J Cardiovasc Pharmacol 1980;2: S5–S19.
133. Brest AN. Hemodynamic and cardiac effects of clonidine. J Cardiovasc Pharmacol 1980;2:S39-S46.
134. Timmermans PBMWM, Schoop AMC, Kwa HY, van Zwieten PA. Characterization of alpha-adrenoceptors participating in the central hypotensive and sedative effects of clonidine using yohimbine, rauwolscine and corynanthine. Eur J Pharmacol 1981;70:7–15.
135. Hamilton CA. Adrenergic and nonadrenergic effects of imidazoline and related antihypertensive drugs in the brain and periphery. Am J Hypertens 1992;5:58S–63S.
136. Bousquet P, Feldman J, Tibirica E, et al. Imidazoline receptors, a new concept in central regulation of the arterial blood pressure. Am J Hypertens 1992;5:47S–50S.
137. Laragh JH. Imidazoline receptors: a new regulatory concept in blood pressure control. Am J Hypertens 1992;5:45S–46S.
138. van Zwieten PA. Different types of centrally acting antihypertensive drugs. Eur Heart J 1992;13:18–21.
139. Reis DJ, Regunathan S, Meeley MP. Imidazole receptors and clonidine-displacing substance in relationship to control of blood pressure, neuroprotection, and adrenomedullary secretion. Am J Hypertens 1992;5:51S–57S.
140. Atlas D, Diamant D, Zonnenschein R. Is imidazoline site a unique receptor? A correlation with clonidine-displacing substance activity. Am J Hypertens 1992;5:83S–90S.
141. Regunathan S, Meeley MP, Reis DJ. Clonidine-displacing substance from bovine brain binds to imidazoline receptors and releases catecholamines in adrenal chromaffin cells. Mol Pharmacol 1991;40:884–888.
142. Atlas D. Clonidine-displacing substance (CDS) and its putative imidazoline receptor: new leads for further divergence of alpha 2-adrenergic receptor activity. Biochem Pharmacol 1991; 41:1541–1549.
143. Fields HL, Basbaum AL. Central nervous system mechanisms of pain modulation. In: Wall PD, Melzack R, eds. Textbook of pain. 3rd ed. Edinburgh: Churchill Livingstone, 1994:243–257.
144. Morris DDB. Local analgesic drugs. In: Wylie WD, Churchill-Davidson HC, eds. A practice of anaesthesia. 2nd ed. London: Lloyd-Luke, 1966:1007–1029.
145. Gilbert CRA, Hanson IR, Brown AB, Hingson RA. Intravenous use of xylocaine. Anesth Analg 1951;30:301–313.
146. Iwane T, Maruyama M, Matsuki M, et al. Management of intractable pain in adiposis dolorosa with intravenous administration of lidocaine. Anesth Analg 1976;55:257–259.
147. Atkinson RL. Intravenous lidocaine for the treatment of intractable pain of adiposis dolorosa. Int J Obes 1982;56:351–357.

148. De Clive-Lowe SG, Desmond J, North J. Intravenous lignocaine anaesthesia. Anaesthesia 1958;13:138–146.
149. Bartlett EE, Hutaserani O. Xylocaine for the relief of postoperative pain. Anesth Analg 1961;40:296–304.
150. Cassuto J, Wallin G, Högström S, et al. Inhibition of postoperative pain by continuous low-dose intravenous infusion of lidocaine. Anesth Analg 1985;64:971–974.
151. Catterall WA. Structure and function of voltage-sensitive ion channels. Science 1988;242:50–61.
152. Chernoff DM. Kinetic analysis of phasic inhibition on neuronal sodium currents by lidocaine and bupivacaine. Biophys J 1990; 58:53–68.
153. Veering BT. Local anaesthetics: an update. Anaesth Pharmacol Rev 1993;2:159–167.
154. Ritchie JM, Rogart RB. The binding of saxitoxin and tetrodotoxin to excitable tissue. Rev Physiol Biochem Pharmacol 1977; 79:1–50.
155. Cohen CJ, Bean BP, Colatsky TJ. Tetrodotoxin block of sodium channels in rabbit Purkinje fibers: interactions between toxin binding and channel gating. J Gen Physiol 1981;78:383–411.

3B Central Analgetic Mechanisms: Opioid Receptor Physiopharmacology and Related Antinociceptive Systems

John M. Murkin, Scott Bowersox, Dawn McGuire, Nancy Tich, Jere Fellmann, and Robert Luther

The exponential growth of knowledge attending the identification of endogenous opioid receptors and their ligands, as well as the recognition and molecular characterization of neuronal calcium (Ca^{2+}) channels, has greatly increased the understanding of both the function and the complexity of mammalian antinociceptive systems. This advance has led to the development of increasingly varied and sophisticated approaches to opioid administration. Since the first reported use of epidural (1) or intrathecal (2) narcotics in 1979, numerous reports have noted the successful use of transmucosal (3), inhalational (4), and transdermal (5) routes of opioid administration. This greater insight into the mechanisms of antinociception has also fostered the selective investigation and utilization of nontraditional analgesic supplements such as subselective α-adrenergic agonists (6), serotinergics (7), and subselective neuronal Ca^{2+} channel blockers.

OPIOID RECEPTORS

The existence of endogenous receptor sites for the binding of opioids had long been postulated (8); however, stereospecific opioid receptors, demonstrating preferential binding of levo- (−) over dextro- (+) isomers, were first identified in mammalian brain homogenate in the early 1970s (9-11). This advance was followed by the isolation of two brain peptides with specific opioid receptor bioactivity in 1975 (12). Opioid receptors were subsequently localized to areas of the central nervous system (CNS) responsible for nociception and affect, as well as being distributed more diffusely in the smooth muscle of gut, bladder, and certain vascular beds.

Investigators now recognize that stereoselectivity for levorotatory isomers (13) and specific binding of the opioid antagonist naloxone (14) are characteristics uniquely defining the family of opioid receptors and enabling them to be distinguished from other receptor families (15).

Receptor types

Characterization of opioid receptors into specific types, each capable of producing distinct responses, was first established by Martin and associates (16). They described three different physiologic syndromes in nonopioid-dependent animals and attributed them to the action of prototypical agonists on distinguishable receptors. They identified three discrete, complementary, opioid receptors that could be selectively activated or blocked in vivo.

Morphine was shown to be acting on one distinct receptor type, designated as μ receptor, to produce miosis, bradycardia, hypothermia, suppression of nociceptive responses, and indifference to environmental stimuli. Ketocyclazocine administration produced differing responses consisting of sedation and miosis, with little effect on heart rate or skin twitch reflex. Administration of ketocyclazocine precipitated only a limited abstinence syndrome in morphine-dependent dogs, a finding indicating that its effects are due to selective action on a distinctive receptor, termed κ. The action of N-allylnormetazocine (SKF 10,047), caused mydriasis, tachypnea, tachycardia, and mania, through activation of a third receptor type defined as

σ receptor (16). Use of the dextrorotatory isomer of SKF, which is selective for σ-receptors, does not produce antinociception (17), indicating that σ-receptors are unlikely to have a significant role in analgesia. By the definition outlined previously, some investigators now believe that σ-receptors should not be considered true opioid receptors (14, 15), The σ receptor is believed to be an active site for phencyclidines (e.g., ketamine).

Two further putative opioid receptors were later isolated and designated as δ receptor (18) and ϵ receptor (19). Evidence for the occurrence of the ϵ receptor has been challenged based on refined receptor-ligand data, leading to skepticism regarding its existence (20); μ, κ, and δ receptors are all believed to be classic opioid receptors and are of primary importance in mediating analgesia.

The various opioid receptor types mediate responses to different nociceptive stimuli. μ Receptors fulfill an undisputed central role in the modulation of antinociception, and μ-receptor agonists are effective against all modes of stimuli, including thermal, pressure, or chemical stimuli (21). δ-Receptor agonists produce antinociception primarily against thermal stimuli, whereas κ-receptor agonists are active against nothermal stresses (21). Opioid receptor sites appear to be synthesized within neuronal cell bodies and are transported to the periphery (22). Sectioning of the vagus nerve decreases receptor density along its axonal membrane (23).

μ, κ Receptor Subtypes

The use of increasingly selective agonist and antagonist ligands has permitted the identification of additional subpopulations of receptors within the main opioid receptor types. Pasternak and Wood (24) have theorized that μ receptors may be further subdivided into two populations, correlating opiate analgesia with activation of a subpopulation of high-affinity μ_1 receptors, whereas low-affinity μ_2 receptors apparently mediate other opioid effects, such as respiratory depression. This concept was supported by autoradiographic studies demonstrating two distinct populations of μ receptors in mouse brain (25) and by work demonstrating reversal of the analgesic effects of morphine with naloxonazine (a noncompetitive selective μ_1 antagonist) without significant reversal of the degree of respiratory depression in treated animals (26).

Putative clinical evidence of the successful separation of pain threshold (analgesia) from respiratory depression has been demonstrated by Bailey and associates (27). These investigators were able to show that the magnitude and duration of respiratory depression produced by up to 4 μg/kg fentanyl were significantly greater than that occurring after 0.4 μg/kg sufentanil. However, elevations of the pain threshold were significantly greater and longer lasting after sufentanil, compared with fentanyl. The chosen dosage ratio of fentanyl to sufentanil was 10:1, whereas some evidence suggests that ratios of 7:1 or 5:1 are more nearly equipotent (28). These results likely reflect greater stereospecific binding of sufentanil compared with fentanyl to μ_1 receptors versus μ_2 receptors. Sufentanil has an overall affinity for μ receptors that is 12 to 27 times greater than that of fentanyl (29).

Based on data obtained from selective ligand binding assays, the existence of two subpopulations of κ receptors, one a high-affinity κ_1 receptor, the other a low-affinity κ_2 receptor, has also been reported (30). Subpopulations of κ receptors have also been inferred from studies of cerebral arteries wherein one population appears to mediate constriction, whereas the other produces dilatation (31). Some uncertainty remains as to the interpretation of these observations, and the issue of κ-receptor subpopulations is currently unresolved (32). Because agonists acting at κ receptors cause less respiratory depression and euphoria than μ-receptor agonists, but they have undesirable side effects including sedative (16) emetic and psychomimetic (33) actions, verification of the existence of μ-receptor subtypes could allow development of agents without the side effects.

Mechanisms of Action

Mechanistically, a receptor site can be viewed as a recognition site for determining ligand binding, coupled to an effector mechanism for producing effect. In vitro, receptor binding of opiate agonists becomes 12 to 60 times weaker in the presence of sodium, whereas antagonist binding is enhanced (23). Based on these observations, investigators have hypothesized that opiate receptor sites exist in 2 states, with localized sodium concentrations determining whether the recognition site is configured for agonist or antagonist binding. This agonist or antagonist binding determines whether the occupied recognition site subsequently activates the effector mechanism to ultimately produce its effect or whether the receptor-effector coupling is inhibited. Localized control of transcellular sodium concentrations may thus play a role in vivo, in modulating receptor activity (23).

Activation of either μ or δ receptors appears to evoke hyperpolarization of neuronal membranes. This is secondary to an increase in potassium (K+) conductance that is mediated by receptor-bound pertussis-sensitive guanine nucleotide regulatory protein (G-protein) (34). Increasing K+ conductance has the net effect of rendering the membrane more difficult to depolarize, thus decreasing synaptic transmission. The G-protein is activated in the presence of guanosine triphosphate (GTP), and activated G-protein dissociates from the receptor (35) to inhibit adenylate cyclase, resulting in decreased levels of cyclic adenosine monophosphate (cAMP) (36). Decreases in cAMP, in turn, open phosphorylation-dependent gated K+ channels, resulting in increased K+ conductance and membrane hyperpolarization (37). The same pool of K+ channels may be affected by either δ or μ opioid receptors, or α-adrenergic or muscarinic receptors, indicating G-protein to be a final common pathway. The neuromodulatory effects of opioid, monoaminergic, and muscarinic agonists on primary afferent networks in the spinal cord thus all appear to be mediated through binding to neuronal receptors that are negatively coupled by G-protein to a commmon pool of adenylate cyclase, which regulates conductance through specific ion channels (34). K+-induced membrane hyperpolarization decreases synaptic transmission.

κ receptors similarly appear to have G-protein as the effector mechanism, but they seem to function by a different mechanism of action because κ ligands appear to act by blocking voltage-sensitive Ca^{2+} currents (38). The net result of decreased Ca^{2+} influx is a decrease in neurotransmitter mobilization and release of substance P (a pain modulator) from afferent nerves sensitive to noxious stimuli. This may represent a mechanism, mediated by κ receptors, for presynaptic control of the processing of afferent nociceptive stimuli at the spinal level (39).

Two anatomically distinct sites appear to exist for analgesia mediated by opiate receptors. At the spinal level, multiple receptor subtypes (μ_1, δ, and κ) are involved, whereas only μ receptors appear to be significant supraspinally (40). Despite the distribution of several types of opioid receptors within the brain, the μ receptor is primarily active in mediating supraspinal analgesia (41). A primary characteristic of μ receptor-mediated analgesia is the ability to modify the concious appreciation of pain and to alleviate concomitant fear, anxiety, and emotional distress, the "suffering" component (42, 43). At the spinal segmental level, μ receptors also dominate antinociception, although intrathecal administration of selective δ agonists has produced analgesia in humans, indicating a separate role for δ receptors in spinal analgesia (44).

The role of segmental κ receptors, which are found in high densities in the substantia gelatinosa of the spinal cord along with μ receptors (45), is unclear. Spinal κ receptors have been shown to have a pivotal role in the suppression of the reflex hyperalgesia (46, 47). Thus, spinal κ receptors appear to have a specific role that is expressed at the segmental level for the modulation of chronic pain syndromes (21).

Dual Receptor Complex

In addition to exogenous opioids, μ receptors can be activated by β-endorphin, met-enkephalin, or enkephalin analogs with μ-receptor activity, and these agonists have produced marked antinociceptive effects clinically and in animal models (21). Moreover, evidence indicates cross reactivity in vivo between μ- and δ-receptor agonism, possibly reflecting an allosteric coupling (48) that does not appear to be due to noselectivity of ligand binding (49). Receptor proteins with mixed μ and δ properties have also been observed in in vitro systems, suggesting an anatomic as well as a functional linkage between the two receptor types (50).

The main role of δ receptors appears to be that of modulating μ-receptor activity. Allosteric coupling between separate μ and δ receptors is suggested by the potentiation of morphine analgesia by δ-selective ligands (49), giving rise to the concept of the dual-receptor complex whereby μ and δ receptors exist as a unit in which activation of the μ receptor produces coupling with an effector and an antinociceptive effect. The role of the δ receptor is not primarily to produce analgesia, but rather to modulate the activity of the μ receptor-effector coupling mechanism (49). A δ-receptor agonist is thus believed to interact with a δ receptor, facilitating coupling of the μ receptor with its effector, producing enhanced analgesia. Conversely, prolonged agonist occupation of one receptor site, either μ or δ, has been reported to reduce ligand binding allosterically at the associated site (51). In this system, μ agonists appear nocompetitively to decrease δ-agonist binding, intrepreted as further evidence of an allosteric linkage between these receptor types.

Tolerance

The demonstration of a decreased receptor response to a given concentration of agonist implies tolerance. A given degree of receptor response can be regained, at least temporarily, by increasing the agonist concentration. Although no evidence suggests cross tolerance among narcotic receptors, tolerance to a given agonist is confined to those receptor subtypes to which they specifically bind (52).

Tolerance is proportional to the exposure concentration of agonist and is reversible over time. In cell systems maintained in tissue culture, complete resistance to opioids can be demonstrated after 1 to 5 hours exposure to morphine (53). Proposed mechanisms include reduced affinity of receptor sites, a decreased number of receptor sites (downregulation), and uncoupling of the receptor from the intracellular messenger (G-protein). Increasingly, it appears as though tolerance initially reflects an initial receptor desensitization followed by receptor downregulation (54, 55). Receptor desensitization appears to reflect functional uncoupling of μ or δ receptors from their associated G-proteins. This is apparently the result of prolonged agonist occupation of the receptor, lowering G-protein affinity for GTP and inducing uncoupling of the unactivated receptor-G-protein complex (53). In addition to receptor desensitization, investigators have estimated that about 30 to 40% downregulation of opioid receptors occurs. Tolerance developing in one opioid receptor type does not influence agonists acting at other receptor types (56). Receptor-effector uncoupling appears to be the primary mechanism in opioid tolerance.

The observation that the degree of tolerance is related to the extent of receptor occupancy predicts that the magnitude of the tolerance produced after exposure to a drug with high intrinsic activity will be less than that seen after exposure to a less potent agonist (57). Thus, less tolerance would be expected to be produced by equianalgesic doses of sufentanil than fentanyl. This may have significance for the management of patients receiving maintenance opioid analgesia (e.g., patients with chronic pain from cancer) (58).

OPIOID RECEPTOR DISTRIBUTION

Radioligand binding and autoradiographic studies employing highly selective ligands for the various receptor types, together with functional studies, have suggested the presence of μ, δ, σ, and κ receptors within the CNS (21). The large regional variation in the types of opioid receptors distributed to various sites in the CNS demonstrates a differential distribution that presumably subserves a functional role in the processing of nonciceptive stimuli. Moreover, within certain tissues, including the dorsal horn of the spinal cord, particular neuronal tracts or even single neurons may carry multiple types of opioid receptors (59, 60).

Nociceptive stimuli are potentially modified by opioid systems at several sites. At peripheral nerve endings, opioid receptors are accessible to endogenous opioid peptides present in the systemic circulation or generated in situ. The dorsal horn of the spinal cord provides a second site for the processing and modulation of primary afferent nociceptive information. Relay sites within the midbrain, brain stem, and hypothalamus comprise a third locus for regulation of nociceptive traffic, interacting with inhibitory pathways descending to the dorsal spinal cord or facilitating the relay of nociceptive information to higher brain centers. Within the limbic system and cortex are sites that appear to be involved in the affective dimensions of pain perception and that are heavily vested with opioid receptors (21).

Spinal Cord

The human spinal cord in humans contains high concentrations of both μ and κ receptors, with κ sites predominant in some areas, and demonstrates a relative paucity of δ receptors (45). Within the spinal cord, the opioid receptors are located in a dense band in the subsantia gelatinosa (laminae II and III) and in the dorsal horns, a site for primary integration of afferent sensory nociceptive information from unmyelinated C fibers and small myelinated Aδ pain fibers (40). Opioid-induced blockade of transmission in ascending axons evoked by Aδ- and C-fiber afferent stimulation has been observed (61, 62). A high ratio of μ_1- to μ_2-receptor binding is found in the spinal cord, a finding suggesting that specific μ_1 agonists should have desired analgesic effects without undesirable side effects (40).

Brain Stem

In the brain stem and neocortex, μ sites predominate, although κ receptors are found in the hypothalamus, periaqueductal gray, substantia nigra, and deep laminae of the neocortex. Opioid receptors concentrated in the periaqueductal gray matter and in the floor of the fourth ventricle represent some of the few regions where microinjections of morphine, or direct electrical stimulation, elicit analgesia that can be blocked by naloxone (63) and in which prolonged stimulation can produce tolerance. Direct injection of morphine into the fourth ventricle also produces rapid onset of respiratory depression (64) because of the proximity of the respiratory center in the ventral pons.

The solitary nuclei receive visceral sensory input through the vagus and glossopharyngeal nerves and also contain high concentrations of opioid receptors. They are at least partly responsible for opiate-induced depression of the cough reflex, intestinal hypomotility, and the production of orthostatic hypotension. The area postrema, also in the brain stem and containing the chemoceptor trigger zone (CTZ), has clusters of opioid receptors that can sensitize the CTZ to vestibular stimulation, to produce opioid-induced nausea and vomiting. In high concentrations, opioids appear to act to depress the vomiting center, and this effect outweighs the CTZ stimulation.

Brain

In the brain, the highest concentrations of opioid receptors are found in the limbic system, most particularly the amygdala, but also in the frontal and temporal cortex and the hippocampus. These areas are primarily involved with affect, rather than with analgesia, and mediate some of the dissociative states that accompany narcotic administration. Medial thalamic nuclei receive inputs from the spinothalamic tract and trigeminal nuclei, relaying poorly localized and emotionally influenced deep pain; they also contain large numbers of opiate receptors.

Blood Vessels

The presence or absence of opioid receptors on vascular smooth muscle in various tissue beds appears to be, in part, a species-dependent phenomenon. Precontracted isolated feline middle cerebral arteries evidence dose-dependent relaxation during morphine application (65), whereas contraction occurs in isolated rat portal vein (66). Evidence demonstrating μ- and δ-opioid receptor activity in the mediation of cerebral microcirculatory dynamics in the cat has been reported (67), and the demonstration of morphine-induced hyperpolarization of feline middle cerebral artery smooth muscle cells has also supported the role of opioid-mediated systems in cerebral vascular control (68). In the dog, κ receptors (31, 69) and σ receptors (70) have been demonstrated to mediate relaxation and contraction of basilar and middle cerebral arteries. Whether such opioid-related mechanisms are operative in humans is unclear, but in vivo studies of the cerebrovascular effects of indermediate-dose (sufentanil 0.5 μg/kg) (71) or high-dose (sufentanil 10 μg/kg) (72) opioid administration in humans have demonstrated either no change (71) or increases in cerebrovascular resistance and decreases in cerebral blood flow (72) appropriate for the decreased cerebral metabolic rate associated with opioid administration.

Miscellaneous Distribution

Systemic opioids are known to alter gastrointestinal (GI) motility. Specific opioid receptors are located on neuronal, smooth muscle, and mucosal cells throughout the GI tract (73). Opioids increase the tone of the intestinal wall while decreasing propulsive peristalsis that can result in constipation or ileus.

The existence of a central opioid mechanism involving μ and δ receptors, and mediated by stimulation of the sympathetic nervous system to increase water and electrolyte absorption, has been postulated (73). The administration of intrathecal or epidural opioids results in urinary retention in 22 to 39% of patients (61). Opioid-induced urinary retention is a complex phenomenon that appears to be mediated both by an increase in external sphincter tone (74) and by inhibition of the volume-evoked micturation reflex (75).

ENDOGENOUS OPIOID PEPTIDES

Endogenous opioid peptide receptor agonists were isolated by purification and separation of brain extracts according to their ability to inhibit electrically induced contractions of guinea pig ileum, or mouse vas defrens, by two standardized opioid bioassays. This led to the isolation of two intrinsic opioid pentapeptides, leucine and methionine enkephalin, by Hughes and colleagues in 1975 (12).

Biosynthetic studies of pituitary opioid peptides have identified 3 separate precursors for the 3 related families of opioid peptides, giving rise to more than 20 distinct opioid peptides with biologic activity (76). All known opioid peptides have tyrosine as the amino terminus, and differences in the opposite, carboxy terminal, extensions underlie the marked differences in the actions of individual endogenous opiate peptide. Pro-opiomelanocortin is a presursor to β-endorphin, as well as corticotropin and melanocyte-stimulating hormone. Proenkephalin A is the prohormone yielding 1 leu-enkephalin and 4 met-enkephalin and is found both in brain and in adrenal tissue. Prodynorphin is a precursor for α-neoendorphin and dynorphin A as well as leu-enkephalin (21).

β-Endorphin

β-Endorphin is found primarily in the anterior pituitary and hypothalamus, from which it can be secreted into the systemic circulation (21). Evidence also indicates that, in humans, β-endorphin is generated and secreted by the adrenal medulla along with catecholamines (77). Hypothalamic perikarya synthesizing β-endorphin project to many brain regions involved in nociceptive processing including the periaqueductal gray and thalamus (78). No evidence of β-endorphin is detectable within the mature spinal cord, so it is unlikely to play a role in vivo in spinal antinociception (21). β-Endorphin is a relatively long-acting species, such that it is considered to be a neurohormone and is detectable within the systemic circulation. Oyama and associates (79) have produced 74 hours of analgesia in some patients with disseminated cancer after intrathecal administration of 4 mg β-endorphin. β-Endorphin appears to be the primary endogenous agonist interacting with μ and δ receptors (80). The identification of a substance chemically indistinguishable from morphine in human milk has, however, raised the suggestion that exogenous morphine-like compounds derived from commom dietary sources may also act as endogenous μ-receptor agonists (81).

Pituitary opioid peptides including β-endorphin appear to be involved in the regulation of pituitary function and hormone secretion. Morphine releases antidiuretic hormone (ADH) from the posterior pituitary, where most opiate receptor binding is located, and it also facilitates the release of ACTH and follicle-stimulating hormone (FSH) (23). Systemically administered opioid agonists also depress plasma thyroid-stimulating hormone (TSH) levels.

Enkephalins

The enkephalins are located more diffusely in interneurons and their processes than β-endorphin, and met-enkephalin somata are in close correspondence to the location of L-receptors within the periaqueductal gray, thalamus, amygdala (82), and, in particular abundance, in the superficial layers of the dorsal horn of the spinal cord, particularly those receiving primary afferent nociceptive information (83). The adrenal medulla is a primary site for the secretion of plasma met-enkephalin, from which it is secreted along with catecholamines (84). Enkephalins are short-lived species and are believed to function as neurotransmitters or modulators of synaptic function. Enkephalins appear to act as neurotransmitters within specific neuronal systems in the brain, to modulate integration of sensory information pertaining to pain and emotional behaviour, and they appear to be particularly active at the spinal level.

Endogenous μ-receptor activity, as produced by β-endorphin, appears to be modulated by the enkephalins. Binding of enkephalins at the δ receptor enhances or inhibits μ-receptor activity, depending on whether leu-enkephalin or met-enkephalin predominates. Leu-enkephalin appears to potentiate, whereas met-enkephalin depresses, μ activity. The clinical analgesic efficacy of the administration of δ-selective ligands has been reported (44), whereas the potential role of combined antinociceptive therapy with μ and δ agonists remains to be investigated.

Dynorphin

Dynorphin is found in lower concentrations than met-enkephalin or β-endorphin in the brain, but it is widely distributed throughout the CNS in the periaqueductal gray, limbic system, and thalamus (85, 86). Dynorphin is found in particularly high concentrations in the dorsal horn of the spinal cord, where it is concentrated in laminae I and V, wherein the processing of nociceptive information is coordinated (87, 88).

A close association between dynorphin and κ receptors has been demonstrated in humans (89, 90). In addition, dynorphin has a pronounced preference for κ-receptor binding (80, 91) and has effects in vivo similar to those of synthetic κ-receptor agonists (92), indicating that dynorphin is most probably an endogenous ligand for κ receptors (21). Dynorphin is responsible for the mediation of the antinociceptive effects of spinal electroacupuncture (93).

In summary, evidence indicates that β-endorphin is primarily a μ-receptor and, to a lesser extent, a δ-receptor agonist. Enkephalins are primarily δ-receptor agonists, but they also have some μ- and κ-receptor activity. Dynorphins have predominantly κ-receptor activity (94). These preferential binding affinities probably reflect the in vivo endogenous ligand status of the endogenous opiate peptides, although this is only clearly established for dynorphin and κ receptors (21).

RELATED ANTINOCICEPTIVE SYSTEMS

Despite the central role of opioid receptors and endogenous opioid peptides in the modulation of afferent nociceptive activity at the spinal level, increasing evidence suggests the involvement of other neural systems. These operate in part at the spinal level, but they have a major role as descending pathways modulating the processing and inhibition of nociceptive stimuli. Intracerebral microinjections of morphine into the periaqueductal gray, or focal electrical stimulation, inhibit spinal nociceptive reflex function (63). Mounting evidence indicates that at least some of these effects are mediated by descending noradrenergic and serotinergic systems (95). The common effector mechanism for all these systems appears to be an adenosine-receptor interaction functioning as the potential final common pathway (96).

α-Adrenergic Systems

The involvement of spinal adrenergic systems in the processing of nociceptive stimuli was demonstrated in 1904 (97, 98). Evidence of noradrenergic inhibition of transmitter release (substance P) from primary afferent terminals in spinal dorsal horn (99) demonstrates a role for noradrenergic receptors in the initial processing of nociceptive traffic. Subsequent investigations have demonstrated that supraspinally mediated analgesia, whether produced by focal administration of morphine or by electrical stimuli, inhibits nociceptive spinal function by the activation of descending noradrenergic pathways (95, 100). These descending pathways terminate in the substantia gelatinosa of the dorsal horn, as well as in the vicinity of motor nuclei in the ventral gray areas (101). Microinjection of norepinephrine into the dorsal gray of cat spinal cord was shown to depress nociceptive reflexes (102), as was the α_2-adrenergic agonist clonidine (103). Selective α_2-receptor antagonist administration produces dose-dependent suppression of agonist-induced antinociception (104), supporting the role of α_2-adrenergic systems in mediating analgesia.

Selective application of norepinephrine to spinal motor units results in significant depression of their activity associated with hyperpolarization (105). Evidence indicates that α_1 receptors may mediate an increase in ventral horn motor activity, whereas α_2 receptors produce hyperpolarization and decreased motor unit activity (97). These mechanisms appear to be of clinical significance in the etiology, treatment, and prevention of narcotic-induced muscle rigidity. The hyperpolarization and resultant depression of function of both dorsal and ventral horn neurons are thus primarily mediated by α_2 receptors (97). Although it is not clear that these descending adrenergic systems constitute a separate antinociceptive system, they do mediate some of the effects of brain stem morphine on spinal function. Other central adrenergic mechanisms mediate arousal, and the subselective α_2-adrenoceptor agonist dexmedetomidine has been demonstrated clinically to produce sedation and anxiolysis (106).

Clinical interest in the role of adrenergic systems in the production of opioid-induced truncal rigidity has increased. The association of high-dose opioid administration and the production of rigidity is unquestioned, and various strategies, including pretreatment with small doses of nondepolarizing muscle relaxants (107), midazolam (108), or concomitant administration of muscle relaxants (109), have been advocated. The mechanism responsible for the production of rigidity is unclear, but evidence implicates activation of μ receptors on the caudate nucleus of the basal ganglia (110). Other studies have suggested the involvement of central adrenergic (111) and serotinergic (112) mechanisms, and the close association among opioid, serotinergic, and adrenergic pathways in dorsal raphe regions of the brain stem provides a possible anatomic locus for these interactions (113). The demonstrated inhibition of alfentanil-induced rigidity in rats by the selective α_2 agonist dexmedetomidine (114) is further support for the role of α_2 receptors in the amelioration of rigidity and may reflect supression of ventral horn motor neurons. Dexmedetomidine is of clinical interest because it has a desirable physiologic profile that includes sedation and anxiolysis (106), as well as an ability to produce anesthesia (115).

Other evidence of the clinical importance of adrenergic pathways in the production of antinociception has been steadily accumulating. In clinical studies, intrathecal epinephrine has potentiated the duration of postoperative analgesia when coadministered with fentanyl (116). The α_2 agonist clonidine has decreased volatile anesthetic requirements (106), and intrathecal clonidine administration has been reported to produce powerful analgesia in patients with terminal cancer who were rendered refractory to spinal morphine (97). Dexmedetomidine has been decreased thiopental dosage required for induction of anesthesia in patients undergoing minor surgery (6).

Serotinergic Systems

In addition to noradreneric neurons, descending serotinergic pathways mediate antinociception at a spinal level as demonstrated by the inhibition of nociceptive dorsal horn neurons by electrical stimulation of dorsal raphe nuclei, a source of descending serotinergic inhibition (117). Considerable evidence also indicates interactions between descending serotinergic and noradrenergic systems (118, 119), and it appears as though serotonin-induced suppression of nociceptive activity in dorsal horn neurons may be mediated by a common pathway that involves release of norepinephrine and interaction with α_2 receptors (119).

Adenosine

Intrathecal opioids elicit analgesia by actions on the spinal cord, and actions at both pre- and postsynaptic sites have been implicated in the production of spinal opioid analgesia (120). Investigators have also proposed that by acting both on descending antinociceptive pathways (121) and directly at sites on the spinal cord, morphine may release adenosine to activate methylxanthine-sensitive adenosine receptors and to produce antinociception (122, 123). Direct application of adenosine has inhibited the release of substance P, a nociceptive neurotransmitter, from spinal nociceptive pathways (124). Neurally mediated antinociception may turn out to involve adenosine receptors, whether the initial stimulus is inititated by opioid, α_2-adrenergic, or serotinergic systems.

Both A_1 and A_2 subtypes of adenosine receptors have been identified (125) and subsequently localized to areas within the substantia gelatinosa (126). Evidence involving both A_1 (127) and A_2 receptors (128) in the mediation of antinociception has been presented, and whether one subtype predominates in the production of antinociception is unclear. Use of selective A_1-receptor agonists has been reported to produce A_2-mediated motor impairment and to confirm A_1-mediated antinociception (129).

Voltage-sensitive Calcium Channels

Voltage-sensitive Ca^{2+} channels (VSCCs) are found throughout the mammalian nervous system where they influence, both directly and indirectly, various cellular processes including neuronal excitability, transmitter release, intracellular metabolism, neurosecretory activity, and gene expression (130-132). The functional diversity of neuronal VSCCs, together with the availability of antagonists that block specific VSCC subtypes, has opened the way for the development of new therapeutic agents for the treatment of various neuropathologic conditions. These include a host of acute and chronic pain syndromes ranging from localized nociceptive pain induced by transient noxious stimuli to chronic, complex polyneuropathies. Although significant progress has already been made toward identifying highly potent and efficacious analgesic agents that target specific VSCC subtypes, an increased understanding of the structural and functional diversity of neuronal VSCCs is expected to provide ever greater opportunities for the development of novel analgesics possessing improved safety and efficacy profiles.

Structural and Functional Diversity of Neuronal VSCCs

At least six types of VSCC have been described in mammalian neural tissues to date; however, the molecular diversity of VSCC subunits and the fact that transcripts of these subunits are subject to alternative splicing (133, 134) suggest even greater heterogeneity. The molecular complex comprising neuronal VSCCs consists of a central α_2 subunit containing the Ca^{2+}-conducting pore and voltage sensing elements, an α_2/δ subunit, a β subunit, and a 95-kd subunit, possibly corresponding to the δ subunit found in VSCCs of skeletal muscle (Fig. 3B-1) (135-137). The α_1 subunit consists of a single, long-chained protein with homologous repeating regions, each containing six membrane-spanning domains. Molecular genetic studies have defined genes coding for α_1 subunits, designated A, B, C, D, and E. These correspond to P/Q- (α_{1a}), N- (α_{1b}), L- (α_{1c}, α_{1d}), and R-type (α_{1E}) VSCCs as defined by electrophysiologic criteria. The α_1 subunit copurifies with α_2/δ, β, and the 95-kd subunit of unknown function. The α_2/δ subunit consists of a membrane-spanning element (δ) linked covalently to an extracellular component (α_2); α_2 and δ are derived from the same gene by posttranslational proteolytic processing (135, 136). The β subunit, a long-chain polypeptide-containing repeat structure characteristic of cytoskeletal proteins, is located on the cytoplasmic side of the plasma membrane in close approximation to the α_1 and α_2/δ subunits. At least four distinct genes coding for β subunit protein (β_1, β_2, β_3, β_4) and six splice variants (β_1a, β_1b, β_1c, β_2a, β_2b, β_2c) have been described (138-141).

Six classes of neuronal VSCCs (L, N, T, P, Q, R) have been recognized, primarily on the basis of their electrophysiologic properties. Low-threshold channels mediating transient Ca^{2+} currents have been designated T-type. In contrast to the other VSCCs, the T-type channel has not yet been matched to a known α_1 subunit. It is nonspecifically blocked by octanol, amiloride, and certain polyamines (142-144). L- N-, P-, Q-, and R-type VSCCs are activated by large membrane depolarizations and have varied inactivation kinetics and unitary conductances (145, 146). Two α_1 subunit genes coding for functionally expressed L-type VSCCs have been cloned from mammalian brains (147, 148); splice variants of one of these (α_{1C}) have been identified, although their individual functional characteristics have not been well defined (149). L-type VSCCs are found in both central (150, 151) and peripheral (152) neurons and are blocked by compounds of several chemical classes including dihydropyridines, phenylalkylamines, benzothiazepines, and polypeptides (153, 154). N-type VSCCs are also found in both central and peripheral neural tissues and are particularly abundant in areas rich in synaptic endings (155). They are potently blocked by polypeptides, notably ω-conopeptides isolated from the venoms of predatory marine snails belonging to the genus *Conus* (156) and

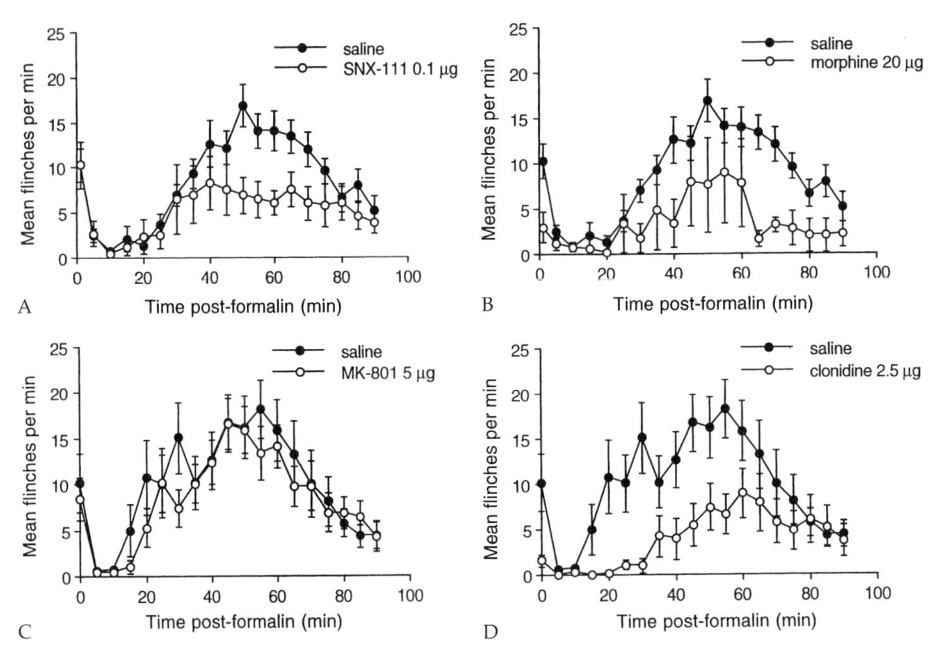

FIGURE 3B-1. Comparative effects of spinal N-type voltage-sensitive calcium channel (VSCC) blockade (A) opiate receptor activation (B) N-methyl-D-aspartate (NMDA) receptor blockade (C) and α-2 adrenoceptor activation (D) on nociceptive responses in the rat hindpaw formalin test. Animals of each group were given a single bolus injection of either SNX-111, morphine sulfate, MK-801, or clonidine 10 minutes before injection of dilute (5%) formalin subcutaneously into the dorsal hindpaw. Test articles were administered through indwelling spinal (intrathecal) catheters terminating at the lumbar enlargement. Pain behavior was quantified by counting paw flexions at regular intervals throughout a 90-minute observation period beginning immediately after formalin injection. The nociceptive response pattern depicted is typical of this test and consists of acute (phase 1: 0 to 9 minutes) and tonic (phase 2: 10 to 90 minutes) phases. Because nociceptive responses are elevated during the tonic phase and are disproportionate to the level of primary afferent discharge, they are thought to reflect a state of facilitated nociceptive processing. Plotted are means ± SEM. Group sizes ranged from 5 to 21 rats per group.

by certain synthetic ω-conopeptide analogs. P-type VSCCs are found in both central and peripheral neurons, but they exist in highest density in cerebellar Purkinje neuron cell bodies (157). They are blocked potently by the spider venom peptide ω-Aga IVA (158) and less potently by ω-conopeptide MVIIC (159). Neuronal Q- and R-type VSCCs are not as well characterized as other Ca^{2+} channels, because they are not subject to selective blockade by existing pharmacologic reagents. Current findings suggest, however, that Q-type VSCCs are colocalized with P-type channels (160). Immunocytochemical staining studies indicate that the R-type VSCC (α_{1E} subunit) is found widely throughout the brain, most prominently in deep midline structures (e.g., caudate putamen, thalamus, hypothalamus, amygdala, and cerebellum) and in nuclei of the ventral midbrain and brain stem (161).

Perhaps no other function of VSCCs in the nervous system is more important than the control of the Ca^{2+}-dependent secretion of neurotransmitters from presynaptic terminals to initiate synaptic transmission. This task is apparently handled by N- and P/Q-type VSCCs, whereas T-, L-, and R-types make little direct contribution to this process (162-165). Through the use of subtype-specific VSCC blockers, investigators now know that N- and P/Q-type VSCCs support the release of distinct but overlapping pools of neurotransmitters. This differential regulation of transmitter release and localization of transmitter classes within the nervous system forms one basis for the development of safe and effective analgesic agents directed against VSCC subtypes.

Neuronal VSCC Blockade and Analgesia

The analgesic properties of L-, P/Q-, and N-type VSCC blockers, administered alone or in combination with other pharmacologic agents, have been extensively studied. L-type VSCC blockers have been reported both to potentiate and to prolong the analgesic actions of opioids (166-171). Although several investigators have reported that parenterally administered L-type VSCC antagonists of the dihydropyridine, phenylalkylamine, and benzothiazepine classes block evoked nociceptive responses (168, 172), these observations have not been consistently confirmed (167, 173, 174). When administered spinally by intrathecal injection, L-type VSCC blockers suppress persistent pain produced by subcutaneous formalin injection (175, 176), but they fail to relieve acute nociceptive pain (177, 178) or mechanical allodynia induced by experimental nerve injury (179) (Fig. 3B-2). Like L-type VSCCs, P-type channels appear to be involved in the spinal processing of certain subtypes of nociceptive input, but they do not play a significant role in the pathophysiology of neuropathic pain. The selective P-type VSCC antagonist, ω-agatoxin IVA, produces a potent dose-dependent inhibition of both acute and persistent formalin-induced nociceptive responses in rats when it is administered intrathecally (180). Spinally administered ω-agatoxin IVA does not, however, suppress escape responses elicited by high-threshold thermal stimuli (hot-plate test), nor does it relieve mechanical allodynia induced by experimental nerve injury (179, 180). In marked contrast to L- and P-type VSCC blockade, selective blockade of N-type VSCCs produces powerful antinociceptive effects in animal models of acute, persistent, and neuropathic pain (179-181).

Acute and Persistent Pain

The synthetic version of the selective N-type VSCC blocker, ω-conopeptide MVIIA (SNX-111), suppresses evoked pain behavior in rodents when it is administered spinally by either intrathecal bolus injection or continuous infusion. A single bolus injection of SNX-111 delivered intrathecally through an indwelling spinal (lumbar) catheter significantly attenuates formalin-induced nociceptive behavior (see Fig. 3B-2). In rats, doses ranging from 10 to 100 ng decrease tonic (phase

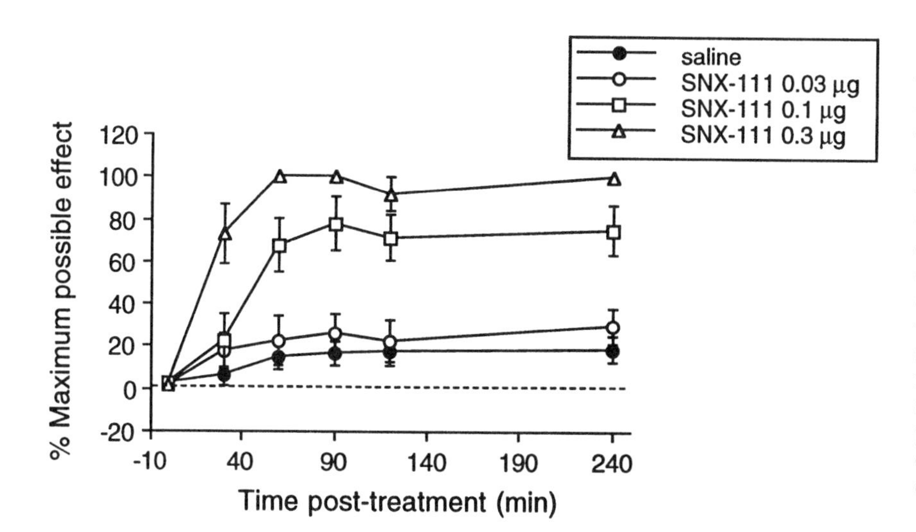

FIGURE 3B-2. Effects of spinal (intrathecal) bolus injections of the selective N-type voltage-sensitive calcium channel (VSCC) blocker, 0.03 μg SNX-111 0.1 μg SNX-111, and 0.3 μg SNX-111, on tactile allodynia in rats with painful peripheral neuropathy induced experimentally by unilateral ligation of the L5 and L6 spinal nerves using procedures described by Kim and Chung (63). Tactile allodynia was assessed by measuring the paw withdrawal response to mechanical stimulation of the plantar surface using nylon filaments of varying stiffness. Analgesic effects are expressed as a percentage of maximum possible effect, where scores of 0 and 100 correspond, respectively, to the presence and absence of tactile allodynia. Shown are means ± SEM. There were 8 to 24 rats in each group.

2) responses by 50% of control values (180-182). When administered spinally by intrathecal bolus injection, the selective P-type VSCC blocker, ω-Aga IVA, also potently suppresses formalin-induced pain behavior, as do the nonselective VSCC blockers lanthanum and neodymium (180). Although L-type VSCC antagonists (e.g., nifedipine, verapamil, and diltiazem) significantly attenuate tonic nociceptive behavior in the rat paw formalin test, high doses are required, and the analgesic effects are comparatively modest (175, 180).

The effect of N-type VSCC blockers on acute (phase 1) nociceptive responses in the rat paw formalin test varies. Although it has been reported that a single bolus injection of SNX-111 administered spinally significantly attenuates acute pain behavior with a median effective dose (ED_{50}) of 0.01 μg (180), this finding has not been consistently replicated. Both acute (phase 1) and tonic (phase 2) formalin-induced nociceptive responses are, however, powerfully attenuated when low doses of SNX-111 are administered for 72 hours by continuous spinal infusion (phase 1, ED_{50} = 14 ng/h; phase 2, ED_{50} = 0.8 ng/h).

Neuronal VSCC blockers have variable effects on acute pain responses elicited in rats by thermal activation of cutaneous nociceptors (i.e., hot-plate test). Doses of VSCC blockers that strongly suppress acute nociceptive responses in the rat formalin test are moderately analgesic in the hot-plate test when they are administered by spinal bolus injection. The latency of the hot-plate-induced nociceptive response (hindpaw lick or jump) is significantly increased 15 minutes after administering a single bolus injection of either the nonselective Ca^{2+} channel blocker, lanthanum, or the N-type VSCC blocker SNX-111, the response latency returns to normal within 30 minutes of treatment (180). Continuous, spinal infusion of SNX-111, however, produces a more favorable analgesic profile; within 2 days of initiating treatment with low doses (10 ng/h), response latencies are markedly elevated and remain so for as long as SNX-111 is administered (176).

Unlike μ- and δ-opioid antagonists, N-type VSCC blockers can be administered on a long-term basis to produce analgesia without leading to the development of tolerance. When opioids are administered to rats by continuous spinal infusion, a progressive, time-dependent diminution of their analgesic effects is observed (183). For example, formalin-evoked nociceptive responses are significantly decreased in Sprague-Dawley rats infused with 20 nmol/h morphine for 2 days before testing; after 7 days of morphine infusion, nociceptive responses are no different from those measured in saline-infused animals, indicating complete tolerance or desensitization (176). Comparable results are obtained in the hot-plate test, in which response latencies are significantly increased after 2 days of morphine infusion (20 nmol/h), but not after 7 days of treatment (176). Strikingly different outcomes are observed with N-type VSCC blockers; analgesic potency is not lost in either rat paw formalin or hot-plate test when low doses of SNX-111 (either 0.03 nmol/h or 0.003 nmol/h) are administered by continuous spinal infusion acutely or chronically (176, 184). Nociceptive responses return to control levels within 2 days of terminating long-term SNX-111 infusion, indicating that chronic N-type VSCC blockade does not permanently alter spinal sensory processing. In keeping with these observations, morphine-tolerant rats show no cross tolerance to the analgesic effects of SNX-111. Taken together, these findings indicate that long-term administration of certain opioid agonists and of N-type VSCC blockers has qualitatively different effects on experimentally evoked nociceptive behavior.

Painful Peripheral Neuropathy

Subtype-specific neuronal VSCC blockers are potently antinociceptive in rodent models of painful peripheral neuropathy. For example, N-type VSCC blockers prevent pain behavior elicited by tactile stimulation in animals with permanent peripheral nerve injuries when these agents are administered spinally by either intrathecal bolus injection or continuous infusion. Bolus injections of as little as 0.3 μg of SNX-111 acutely block tactile allodynia in rats with peripheral nerve injuries induced by the unilateral ligation of the L5 and L6 spinal nerves just distal to the dorsal root ganglia (179) (see Fig. 3B-2). A longer-lasting, reversible blockade of tactile allodynia is achieved when the compound is administered for 7 days by continuous, spinal infusion. Spinally administered L- and P-type VSCC blockers are without effect in this model (179). N-type VSCC blockers also produce analgesia when they are administered perineurally to the site of nerve injury through chronically implanted cuffs in rats with an experimental painful peripheral neuropathy induced by loose ligation of the common sciatic nerve (i.e., chronic constriction injury model of Bennett and Xie) (185). Investigators believe that this analgesic effect is due to the suppression of VSCC-mediated spontaneous ectopic discharge in injured primary afferent axons at or near the site of nerve damage (181).

N-type VSCC Blockers: Sites of Action

Findings indicate that N-type VSCC blockers interfere with nociceptive processing at both brain and spinal levels. Specific brain sites mediating the analgesic effects of N-type VSCC blockers have not yet been identified. Nonetheless, these blockers act at supraspinal levels, because SNX-111 decreases formalin-induced nociceptive responses in mice when it is administered intracerebroventricularly in doses several orders of magnitude lower than those necessary to produce analgesia by the spinal route (Hynansky, A, personal communication). A spinal site of action is indicated by the finding that N-type VSCCs are highly localized to the superficial layers (Rexed laminae I and II) of the dorsal horn (160), sites that receive dense innervation from Aδ and C nociceptive afferents (186) (Figs. 3B-3 and 3B-4). This would indicate that the analgesic effects of spinally administered N-type VSCC antagonists are mediated by local blockade of nociceptive input. Moreover, the fact that analgesic properties of N-type blockers in animal models correlate well with the rank order of affinities for N-type VSCC binding in rat brain synaptic membranes (176, 180) confirms that the molecular mechanism of action is specifically related to N-type VSCC blockade.

Clinical Investigations of the N-type VSCC Blocker: SNX-111

Phase I studies of the safety and tolerability of intravenously administered SNX-111 have been completed in over 100 patients with daily doses ranging from 0.0003 to 1.00 mg/kg. The main side effect is related to the sympatholytic activity of the drug causing a dose-dependent peripheral blockade of the sympathetic nervous system. At intravenous daily doses

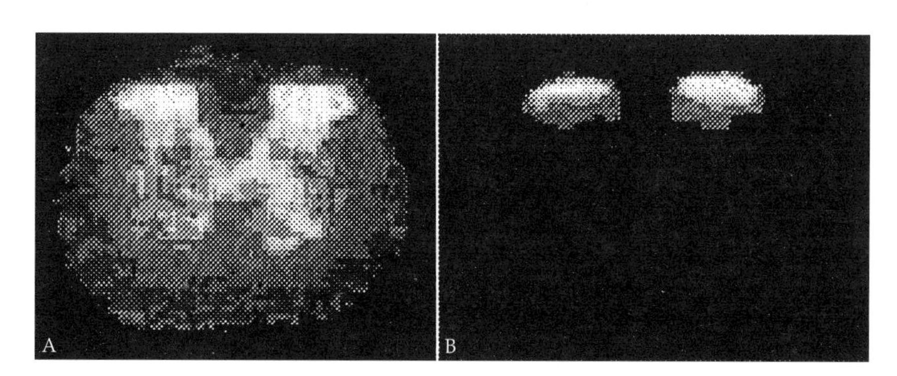

FIGURE 3B-3. Autoradiogram showing the distributions of radioiodinated ω-conopeptide MVIIA (^{125}I-SNX-111) (A) and ω-conopeptide MVIIC (^{125}I-SNX-230) (B) binding sites in the adult rat cervical cord. Lighter shades depict higher density binding. Putative N-type voltage-sensitive calcium channels (VSCCs) labeled by ^{125}I-SNX-111 are localized to superficial layers (Rexed laminae I and II) of the dorsal horn. These sites receive the majority of their inputs from primary nociceptive afferents. Blockade of transmitter release from these sites is a proposed mechanism for the analgesic actions of spinally administered N-type VSCC blockers.

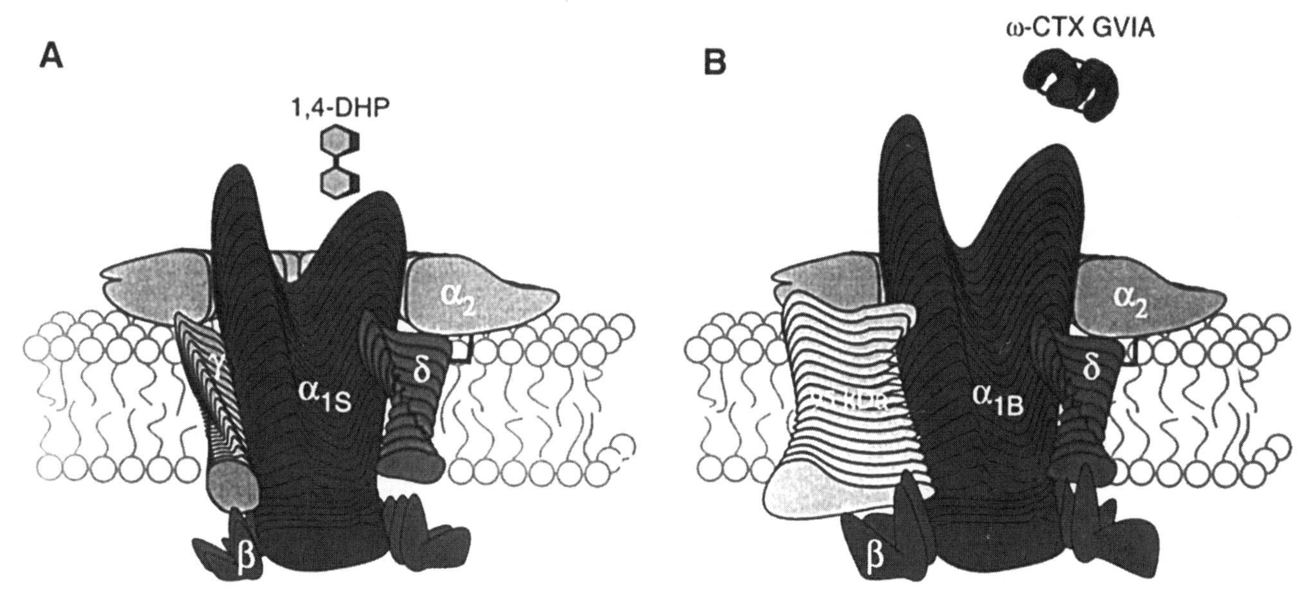

FIGURE 3B-4. Schematic diagrams showing the multisubunit complexes of calcium channels. A, The dihydropyridine-sensitive calcium channel purified from skeletal muscle. B, The ω-conotoxin (ω-CTX) GVIA-sensitive calcium channel purified from rabbit brain. The α_1 subunits form the ion pore and provide for voltage-dependent gating.The precise functions of the other subunits are unknown. Genes have been cloned for all except the 95-kd protein associated with the brain channel complex. The α_2 and δ subunits are encoded by a single gene and are linked by a disulfide bond. Although the positioning of the subunits in these diagrams takes into account published information about the biochemical properties of the subunits, this cartoon is speculative. It is meant only to provide a comparision of the general properties of skeletal muscle and brain calcium channels and, as such, should not be overinterpreted. (From Dunlop K, Luebke JI, Turner TJ. Exocytotic Ca^{2+} channels in mammalian central neurons. Trends Neurosci 1995;18:89–98.)

higher than 0.01 mg/kg, orthostatic hypotension without reflex tachycardia was seen in all volunteers. Apart from dose-related orthostatic hypotension, with associated symptoms of dizziness, the drug was well tolerated (187-189).

A phase I/II open-label rising dose safety, tolerability, and analgesic efficacy study of intrathecal administration of SNX-111 in patients with severe, intractable cancer and neuropathic pain has been completed at six investigative centers in the United States. Enrollment was restricted to patients with chronic, intractable pain in whom intrathecal opioid administration had failed. The study consisted of an in-hospital period of up to 7 days during which SNX-111 was titrated every 24 to 48 hours beginning at 0.3 ng/kg/h, increasing the dose at half-log increments (i.e., 0.3, 1.0, 3.0, 10.0, 30.0, 100.0, 300.0 ng/kg/h) up to 300.0 ng/kg/h. Patients who experienced a favorable response in terms of pain relief were enrolled in a long-term extension in which they could elect to continue to receive intrathecal SNX-111.

Of 31 patients enrolled in the phase I/II study, 25 were considered evaluable as defined by the length of time on study drug and adherence to the protocol. Sixteen patients were terminally ill with either cancer or AIDS, and 15 patients were enrolled with nonmalignant pain syndromes. Patients had various pain syndromes, such as spinal nerve root metastases, AIDS polyneuropathy, phantom limb pain, poststroke thalamic pain, spinal cord injury, and postherpetic neuralgia. With rare exceptions, all patients had failed intrathecal opioid administration; in all, systemic therapy with opioids and adjuvants had failed. Efficacy response was assessed every 4 hours during the in-hospital phase by the visual analog scale of pain intensity (VASPI), the visual analog scale of pain relief (VASPR), and a global patient satisfaction-dissatisfaction scale. Safety assessments consisted of an assessment of adverse events and routine laboratory evaluations. Twenty-one of the 25 evaluable patients reported partial to complete pain relief or, in 2 patients, an improvement in the quality or distribution of pain. The most commonly reported side effects were lateral gaze nystagmus, dose-related gait imbalance, and, in 2 patients, word-finding difficulty. Several patients with terminal cancer had episodes of mental confusion that were generally attributed to concomitant medications, to opiate withdrawal, or to their underlying disease; however, in 2 cases, confusion and aphasia were attributed to SNX-111. Orthostatic hypotension was observed in only 2 patients, 1 of whom had a history of orthostasis. In general, there was no evidence of sympatholysis as a side effect of the intrathecal route of administration. Ten patients continued receiving SNX-111 for up to 9 months with excellent pain control and without requiring an increase in dose, a finding supporting the nonclinical studies that indicate that, unlike opiates, SNX-111 does not induce tolerance to its analgesic effects (190, 191).

ACKNOWLEDGMENT

Parts of text exerpted with permission from Murin JM. Central Analgesic Mechanisms: A Review of Opioid Receptor Physiopharmacology and Related Antinociceptive Systems. J Cardiothorac Vasc Anesth 1991; 5:268–77.

REFERENCES

1. Wang JK, Nauss LE, Thomas JE. Pain relief by intrathecally applied morphine in man. Anesthesiology 1979;50:149–151.
2. Cousins MJ, Mather LE, Glynn CJ, et al. Selective spinal analgesia. Lancet 1979;1:1141–1142.
3. Streisand JB, Ashburn MA, LeMaire L, et al. Bioavailability and absorption of oral transmucosal fentanyl citrate. Anesthesiology 1989;71:A229.
4. Port JD, Stanley TH. Narcotic inhalational anesthesia. Anesthesiology 1982;57:A344.
5. Chauvin M, Strumza P, Levron JC, et al. Plasma fentanyl concentrations during transdermal delivery. Anesthesiology 1989; 71:A717.
6. Aantaa R, Kanto J, Scheinin M, et al. Dexmedetomidine, an O_2-adrenoceptor agonist, reduces anesthetic requirements for patients undergoing minor gynecologic surgery. Anesthesiology 1990;73:230.
7. Archer T, Jonsson G, Minor BG, Post C. Noradrenergic-serotinergic interactions and nociception in the rat. Eur J Pharmacol 1986;120:295–307.
8. Leimbach DG, Eddy NB. Synthetic analgesics. III. Methadols, isomethadols and their acyl derivatives. J Pharmacol Exp Ther 1954;110:135–147.
9. Pert CB, Snyder SH. Properties of opiate-receptor binding in rat brain. Proc Natl Acad Sci U S A 1973;70:2243–2247.
10. Terenius L. Stereospecific interaction between narcotic analgesics and a synaptic plasma membrane fraction of rat cerebral cortex. Acta Pharmacol Toxicol 1973;32:317–320.
11. Pert CB, Pasternak GW, Snyder SH. Opiate agonists and antagonists discriminated by receptor binding in brain. Science 1973; 182:1359–1361.
12. Hughes J, Smith TW, Kosterlitz HW, et al. Identification of two related pentapeptides from the brain with potent opiate receptor agonist activity. Nature 1975;258:577.
13. Teal JJ, Holtzman SG. Stereoselectivity of the stimulus effects of morphine and cyclazocine in the squirrel monkey. J Pharmacol Exp Ther 215:369–376.
14. Martin WR, Eades CG, Gilbert PE, et al. Tolerance to and physical dependence on N-allylnormetazocine (NANM) in chronic spinal dogs. Subst Alcohol Actions Misuse 1980;1:269–270.
15. Pfeiffer A, Brantl V, Herz A, et al. Psychotomimesis mediated by κ opiate receptors. Science 1986;233:774–776.
16. Martin WR, Eades CG, Thompson JA, et al. The effects of morphine- and nalorphine-like drugs in the nondependent and morphine-dependent chronic spinal dog. J Pharmacol Exp Ther 1976;197:517–532.
17. Aceto MD, May EL. Antinociceptive studies of the optical isomers of N-allylnormetazocine (SKF 10,047). Eur J Pharmacol 1983;91:267–272.
18. Lord JAH, Waterfield AA, Hughes AA, et al. Endogenous opi-

oid peptides: multiple agonists and receptors. Nature 1977; 267:495–499.

19. Schulz R, Wuster M, Herz A. Pharmacological characterization of the epsilon opiate receptor. J Pharmacol Exp Ther 1981; 216:604–606.
20. Sheehan MJ, Hayes AG, Tyers MB. Lack of evidence for ϵ-opioid receptors in the rat vas deferens. Eur J Pharmacol 1988; 154:237–245.
21. Millan MJ. Multiple opioid systems and pain. Pain 1986;27:303–347.
22. Laduron PM. Axonal transport of opiate receptors in capsaicin-sensitive neurons. Brain Res 1984;294:157–160.
23. Snyder SH. Opiate receptors in the brain. N Engl J Med 1977; 296:266–271.
24. Pasternak GW, Wood PJ. Minireview: multiple μ opiate receptors. Life Sci 1986;38:1889.
25. Moskowitz AS, Goodman RR. Autoradiographic distribution of μ1 and μ2 opioid binding in the mouse central nervous system. Brain Res 1985;360:117–129.
26. Ling GSF, Spiegel K, Lockhart SH, et al. Separation of opioid analgesia from respiratory depression: evidence for different receptor mechanisms. J Pharmacol Exp Ther 1985;232:149–155.
27. Bailey PL, Streisand JB, East KA, et al. Differences in magnitude and duration of opioid-induced respiratory depression and analgesia with fentanyl and sufentanil. Anesth Analg 1990;70:8–15.
28. Hall RI, Murphy MR, Hug CC Jr. The enflurane sparing effect of sufentanil in dogs. Anesthesiology 1987;67:518–525.
29. Stahl KD, VanBever W, Janssen P. Receptor affinity and pharmacological potency of a series of narcotic analgesic, anti-diarrheal and neuroleptic drugs. Eur J Pharmacol 1977;46:199–205.
30. Zukin, RS, Eghbali M, Olive D, et al. Characterization and visualization of rat and guinea pig brain k opioid receptors: evidence for κ1 and κ2 opioid receptors. Proc Natl Acad Sci U S A 1988;85:4061–4065.
31. Altura BT, Altura B, Quirion R. Identification of benzomorphan-kappa opiate receptors in cerebral arteries which subserve relaxation. Br J Pharmacol 1984;82:459–466.
32. Traynor J. Subtypes of the κ-opioid receptor: fact or fiction? Trends Pharmacol Sci 1989;10:52–53.
33. Pfeiffer A, Brantl V, Herz A, et al. Psychotomimesis mediated by κ opiate receptors. Science 1986;233:744–776.
34. Crain SM, Crain B, Makman M. Pertussis toxin blocks depressant effects of opioid, monoaminergic and muscarinic agonists on dorsal-horn network responses in spinal cord-ganglion cultures. Brain Res 1987;400:185–190.
35. Neer EJ, Claphan DE. Roles of G protein subunits in transmembrane signalling. Nature 1988;333:129–134.
36. Bogoch GM, Katada T, Northup JK, et al. Purification and properties of the inhibitory guanine nucleotide-binding regulatory component of adenylate cyclase. J Biol Chem 1984;259:3560–3567.
37. Siegelbaum S, Camardo JS, Kandel ER. Serotonin and cAMP close single K+ channels in aplysia sensory neurons. Nature 1982;299:413–417.
38. Gross RA, MacDonald RL. Dynorphin A selectively reduces a large transient (N-type) calcium current of mouse dorsal root ganglion neurons in cell culture. Proc Natl Acad Sci U S A 1987; 84:5469.
39. Werz MA, Macdonald RL. Dynorphin and neoendorphin peptides decrease dorsal root ganglion neuron calcium-dependent action potential duration. J Pharmacol Exp Ther 1985;234:49–54.
40. Blumenkopf B. Neurochemistry of the dorsal horn. Appl Neurophysiol 1988;51:89–103.
41. Fang FG, Fields HL, Lee NM. Action at the μ receptor is sufficient to explain the supraspinal analgesic effect of opiates. J Pharmacol Exp Ther 1986;238:1039–1044.
42. Millan MJ. Endorphins and nociception: an overview. Methods Find Exp Clin Pharmacol 1982;4:445–462.
43. Millan MJ, Duka T. Anxiolytic properties of opiates and endogenous opioid peptides and their relationship to the actions of benzodiazepines. Mod Probl Pharmacopsychiatry 1981; 17:123–141.
44. Onofrio BM, Yaksh TL. Intrathecal δ-receptor ligand produces analgesia in man. Lancet 1983;1:1386–1387.
45. Czlonkowski A, Costa T, Przewlocki R, et al. Opiate receptor binding sites in human spinal cord. Brain Res 1983;267:392–396.
46. Millan MJ, Millan MH, Czlonkowski A, et al. Functional response of multiple opioid systems to chronic arthritic pain in the rat. Ann N Y Acad Sci 1986;467:182–193.
47. Millan MJ, Millan MH, Pilcher CWT, et al. Spinal cord dynorphin may modulate nociception via a κ-opioid receptor in chronic arthritic rats. Brain Res 1985;340:156–159.
48. Rothman RB, Westfall TC. Allosteric coupling between morphine and enkephalin receptors in vitro. Mol Pharmacol 1982; 21:548–557.
49. Vaught JL, Rothman RB, Westfall TC. μ and δ receptors: their role in analgesia and in the differential effects of opioid peptides on analgesia. Life Sci 1982;30:1443–1455.
50. Haynes L. Opioid receptors and signal transduction. Trends Pharmacol Sci 1988;9:309–311.
51. Rothman RB, Bykov V, Long JB, et al. Chronic administration of morphine and naltrexone up-regulate μ-opioid binding sites labeled by [3H][D-Ala2, MePhe4, Gly-ol5]enkephalin: further evidence for two μ-binding sites. Eur J Pharmacol 1989;160:71–82.
52. Christie MJ, Williams JT, North RA. Cellular mechanisms of opioid tolerance: studies in single brain neurons. Mol Pharmacol 1987;32:633–638.
53. Puttfarcken PS, Werling LL, Cox BM. Effects of chronic morphine exposure on opioid inhibition of adenylyl cyclase in 7315c cell membranes: a useful model for the study of tolerance at μ opioid receptors. Mol Pharmacol 1988;33:520–527.
54. Law PY, Hom DS, Loh HH. Opiate receptor down-regulation and desensitization in neuroblastoma X glioma NG 108-15 hybrid cells are two separate adaptation processes. Mol Pharmacol 1983;24:413–424.
55. Yu VC, Sadee W. Efficacy and tolerance of narcotic analgesics at the μ opioid receptor in differentiated human neuroblastoma cells. J Pharmacol Exp Ther 1988;245:350–355.
56. Werling LL, McMahon PN, Cox BM. Selective tolerance at μ and κ opioid receptors modulating norepinephrine release in guinea pig cortex. J Pharmacol Exp Ther 1988;247:1103–1106.
57. Tung AS, Yaksh TL. The antinociceptive effects of epidural opiates in the cat: studies on the pharmacology and the effects of lipophilicity in spinal analgesia. Pain 1982;12:343–356.
58. Cousins MJ, Mather LE. Intrathecal and epidural administration of opioids. Anesthesiology 1984;61:276–310.
59. Fields HL, Emson PC, Leigh BK, et al. Multiple opiate receptor sites on primary afferent fibres. Nature 1980;284:351–353.
60. Zieglgansberger W, French ED, Mercuri N, et al. Multiple opiate receptors on neurones of the mammalian nervous system: in vivo and in vitro studies. Life Sci 1982;31:2343–2346.
61. Zieglgansberger W. Opioid actions on mammalian spinal neurons. Int Rev Neurobiol 1984;25:243–275.
62. Doi T, Jurna I. Analgesic effect of intrathecal morphine demonstrated in ascending nociceptive activity in the rat spinal cord and ineffectiveness of caerulein and cholecystokinin octapeptide. Brain Res 1982;234:399–407.
63. Yaksh TL, Rudy TA. Narcotic analgesics: CNS sites and mechanisms of action as revealed by intracerebral injection techniques. Pain 1978;4:299–359.
64. Florez J, McCarty LE, Borison HL. A comparative study in the cat of the respiratory effects of morphine injected intravenously and into the cerebrospinal fluid. J Pharmacol Exp Ther 1968; 163:448–455.

65. Hanko JH, Hardebo JE. Enkephalin-induced dilatation of pial arteries in vitro probably mediated by opiate receptors. Eur J Pharmacol 1979;51:295–297.
66. Yamamoto Y, Hotta K, Matsuda T. Effect of methionine-enkephalin on the spontaneous electrical and mechanical activity of the smooth muscle of the rat portal vein. Life Sci 1984;34:993–999.
67. Wahl M. Effects of enkephalins, morphine, and naloxone on pial arteries during perivascular microapplication. J Cereb Blood Flow Metab 1985;5:451–457.
68. Harder DR, Madden JA. Cellular mechanisms of opiate receptor stimulation in cat middle cerebral artery. Eur J Pharmacol 1984;102:411–416.
69. Altura BT, Altura BM, Quirion R. Identification of benzomorphan κ-opiate receptors in cerebral arteries which subserve relaxation. Br J Pharmacol 1984;82:459–466.
70. Altura BT, Quirion R, Pert CB, et al. Phencyclidine ("angel dust") analogs and σ-opiate benzomorphans cause cerebral arterial spasm. Proc Natl Acad Sci U S A 1983;80:865–869.
71. Mayer N, Weinstabl C, Podreka I, Spiss CK. Sufentanil does not increase cerebral blood flow in healthy human volunteers. Anesthesiology 1990;73:240–243.
72. Murkin JM, Farar JK, Tweed WA. Sufentanil anesthesia reduces cerebral blood flow and cerebral oxygen consumption. Can J Anaesth 1988;35:S131.
73. Kromer W. Endogenous and exogenous opioids in the control of gastrointestinal motility and secretion. Pharmacol Rev 1988; 40:121–162.
74. Aoki M, Watanabe H, Namiki A, et al. Mechanism of urinary retention following intrathecal administration of morphine. Masui 1982;31:939–943.
75. Reiz S, Westberg M. Side effects of epidural morphine. Lancet 1980;2:203–204.
76. Hokfelt T, Johansson O, Ljungdahl A, et al. Peptidergic neurons. Nature 1980;284:515–521.
77. Evans CJ, Erdelyi E, Weber E, et al. Identification of pro-opiomelanocortin-derived peptides in the human adrenal medulla. Science 1984;221:957–960.
78. Millan MJ, Herz A. The endocrinology of the opioids. Int Rev Neurobiol 1985;26:1–84.
79. Oyama T, Jin T, Yamaya R, et al. Profound analgesic effects of β-endorphin in man. Lancet 1980;1:122–124.
80. Garzon J, Sanchez-Blaquez P, Hollt, et al. Endogenous opioid peptides: comparative evaluation of their receptor affinities in the mouse brain. Life Sci 1983;33 (suppl 1):291–294.
81. Hazum E, Sabatka JJ, Chang K-J, et al. Morphine in cow and human milk: could dietary morphine constitute a ligand for specific morphine (μ) receptors? Science 1981;213:1010–1012.
82. Khachaturian H, Lewis ME, Watson SJ. Immunocytochemical studies with antisera against leu-enkephalin and an enkephalin-precursor fragment (BAM-22P) in the rat brain. Life Sci 1982; 31:1879–1882.
83. Cruz L, Basbaum A. Multiple opioid peptides and the modulation of pain: immunohistochemical analysis of dynorphin and enkephalin in the trigeminal nucleus caudalis and spinal cord of the rat. J Comp Neurol 1985;240:331–348.
84. Yang HYT, Hexum T, Costa E. Opioid peptides in the adrenal gland. Life Sci 1980;27:1119–1125.
85. Khachaturian H, Watson SJ, Lweis ME, et al. Dynorphin immunocytochemistry in the rat central nervous system. Peptides 1983;3:941–954.
86. Watson SJ, Akil H, Fischli W, et al. Dynorphin and vasopressin: common localization in magnocellular neurones. Science 1982; 218:1134–1136.
87. Basbaum AI, Cruz L, Weber E. Immunoreactive dynorphin B in sacral primary afferent fibres of the cat. J Neurosci 1986; 7:127–133.
88. Millan MJ, Millan MH, Czlonkowski A, et al. Vasopressin and oxytocin in the rat spinal cord: distributions and origins in comparison to met-enkephalin, dynorphin and related opioids and their irresponsiveness to stimuli modulating neurohypophyseal secretion. Neuroscience 1984;13:179–187.
89. Gramsch C, Hollt V, Pasi A, et al. Immunoreactive dynorphin in human brain and pituitary. Brain Res 1982;223:65–74.
90. Pfeiffer A, Pasi A, Mehraein P, et al. Opiate receptor binding sites in human brain. Brain Res 1982;248:87–96.
91. James IF, Fischli W, Goldstein A. Opioid receptor selectivity of dynorphin gene products. J Pharmacol Exp Ther 1984;228:88–93.
92. Han JS, Xie GX, Goldstein A. Analgesia induced by intrathecal injection of dynorphin B in the rat. Life Sci 1984;34:1573–1579.
93. Han JS, Xie GX. Dynorphin: important mediator for electroacupuncture in the spinal cord of the rabbit. Pain 1984;18:367–376.
94. Morley JS. Peptides in nociceptive pathways. In: Lipton S, et al, eds. Persistent pain: modern methods of treatment. vol 5. Orlando, FL: Grune & Stratton, 1985:65–91.
95. Yaksh TL. Direct evidence that spinal serotonin and noradrenaline terminals mediate the spinal antinociceptive effects of morphine in the periaqueductal grey. Brain Res 1979;160:180–185.
96. Sweeney MI, White TD, Sawynok J. Involvement of adenosine in the spinal antinociceptive effects of morphine and noradrenaline. J Pharmacol Exp Ther 1987;243:657–665.
97. Yaksh TL. Pharmacology of spinal adrenergic systems which modulate spinal nociceptive processing. Pharmacol Biochem Behavior 1985;22:845–858.
98. Weber H. Uber anasthesie durch adrenalin. Verh Dtsch Ges Inn Med 1904;21:616–619.
99. Kuraishi Y, Hirota N, Sato Y, et al. Noradrenergic inhibition of the release of substance P from the primary afferents in the rabbit spinal dorsal horn. Brain Res 1985;359:177–182.
100. Hammond DL, Tyce GM, Yaksh TL. Efflux of 5-hydroxytryptamine and noradrenaline into spinal cord superfusates during stimulation of the rat medulla. J Physiol 1985;359:151–162.
101. Westlund K, Bowker RM, Ziegler MG, et al. Descending noradrenergic projections and their spinal terminations. Prog Brain Res 1982;57:219–238.
102. Bell JA, Matsumiya T. Inhibitory effects of dorsal horn and excitant effects of ventral horn intraspinal microinjections of norephinephrine and serotonin in the cat. Life Sci 1981;29:1507–1514.
103. Kawasaki K, Takesue H, Matsushita A. Modulation of spinal reflex activities inacute spinal rats with alpha-adrenergic agonists and antagonists. Jpn J Pharmacol 1978;28:165–168.
104. Howe JR, Wang JY, Yaksh TL. Selective antagonism of the antinociceptive effects of intrathecally applied alpha adrenergic agonists by intrathecal prazocin and intrathecal yohimbine. J Pharmacol Exp Ther 1983;224:552–558.
105. Engberg I, Ryall RW. The inhibitory action of noradrenaline and other monoamines on spinal neurons. J Physiol 1966; 185:298–322.
106. Scheinin M, Kallio A, Koulu M, et al. Sedative and cardiovascular effects of medetomidine, a novel selective alpha-2-adrenoceptor agonist, in healthy volunteers. Br J Clin Pharmacol 1987;24:443–451.
107. Stanley TH, de Lange S. The effect of population habits on side effects and narcotic requirements during high-dose fentanyl anaesthesia. Can Anaesth Soc J 1984;31:368–376.
108. Sanford TJ, Smith NT, Weinger MB, et al. The effect of midazolam pretreatment on alfentanil-induced muscle rigidity. Anesthesiology 1988;69:A556.
109. Hill AP, Nahrwald ML, de Rosayro AM, et al. Prevention of rigidity during fentanyl-oxygen induction of anesthesia. Anesthesiology 1981;55:452–454.
110. Havemann U, Kuschinsky K. Further characterization of opioid

receptors in striatum mediating muscular rigidity in rats. Naunyn Schmiedebergs Arch Pharmacol 1981;317:321–325.
111. Jerussi TP, Capacchione JF, Benvenga MJ. Reversal of opioid-induced muscular rigidity in rats: evidence for alpha-2 adrenergic involvement. Pharmacol Biochem Behav 1987;28:283–289.
112. Weinger MB, Cline EB, Blasco TA. Ketanserin pretreatment prevents alfentanil-induced muscle rigidity in the rat. Anesthesiology 1987;67:348–355.
113. Weinger MB, Cline EJ, Smith NT, et al. Localization of brain stem sites which mediate alfentanil-induced rigidity in the rat. Pharmacol Biochem Behav 1988;29:573–580.
114. Weinger MB, Segal IS, Maze M. Dexmedetomidine, acting through central alpha-2 adrenoceptors, prevents opiate-induced muscle rigidity in the rat. Anesthesiology 1989;71:242–249.
115. Vickery RG, Sheridan BC, Segal BC, et al. Anesthetic and hemodynamic effects of the stereoisomers of medetomidine, an alpha-2-adrenergic agonist, in halothane-anesthetized dogs. Anesth Analg 1988;67:611–615.
116. Malinow AM, Mokriski BLK, Nomura MK, et al. Effect of epinephrine on intrathecal fentanyl analgesia in patients undergoing postpartum tubal ligation. Anesthesiology 1990;73:381–385.
117. Hammond DL, Yaksh TL. Antagonism of stimulation-produced antinociception by intrathecal administration of methysergide or phentolamine. Brain Res 1984;298:329–337.
118. Minor BG, Post C, Archer T. Blockade of intrathecal 5-hydroxyryptamine-induced antinociception in rats by noradrenaline depletion. Neurosci Lett 1985;54:39–44.
119. Nakagawa I, Omote K, Kitahata LM, et al. Serotonergic mediation of spinal analgesia and its interaction with noradrenergic systems. Anesthesiology 1990;73:474–478.
120. Yaksh TL, Noueihed R. The physiology and pharmacology of spinal opiates. Annu Rev Pharmacol Toxicol 1985;25:433–462.
121. DeLander GE, Hopkins CJ. Spinal adenosine modulates descending antinociceptive pathways stimulated by morphine. J Pharmacol Exp Ther 1986;239:88–93.
122. Sweeney MI, White TD, Sawynok J. Involvement of adenosine in the spinal antinociceptive effects of morphine and noradrenaline. J Pharmacol Exp Ther 1987;243:657–665.
123. Sawynok J, Sweeney MI, White TD. Adenosine release may mediate spinal analgesia by morphine. Trends Pharmacol Sci 1989; 10:186–189.
124. Delander GE, Wahl JJ. Behavior induced by putative nociceptive neurotransmitters is inhibited by adenosine or adenosine analogs coadministered intrathecally. J Pharmacol Exp Ther 1988;246:565–570.
125. Choca JI, Proudfit HK, Green RD. Identification of A1 and A2 adenosine receptors in the rat spinal cord. J Pharmacol Exp Ther 1987;242:905–910.
126. Choca JI, Green RD, Proudfit HK. Adenosine A1 and A2 receptors of the substantia gelatinosa are located predominantly on intrinsic neurons: an autoradiography study. J Pharmacol Exp Ther 1988;247:757–764.
127. Sawynok J, Sweeney MI, White TD. Classification of adenosine receptors mediating antinociception in the rat spinal cord. Br J Pharmacol 1986;88:923–930.
128. Delander GE, Hopkins CJ. Involvement of A2 adenosine receptors in spinal mechanisms of antinociception. Eur J Pharmacol 1987;139:215–223.
129. Karlsten R, Gordh T, Hartvig P, et al. Effects of intrathecal injection of the adenosine receptor agonists R-phenylisopropyladenosine and N-ethylcarboxamide-adenosine on nociception and motor function in the rat. Anesth Analg 1990;71:60–64.
130. Tsien RW, Lipscombe D, Madison DV, Bley KR, Fox AP. Multiple types of neuronal calcium channels and their selective modulation. Trends Neurosci 1988;11:431–438.
131. Miller RJ, Fox AP. Voltage sensitive calcium channels. In: Bronner LF, ed. Intracellular calcium regulation. New York: Wiley-Liss, 1990:97–138.
132. Olivera BM, Miljanich GP, Ramachandran J, Adams ME. Calcium channel diversity and neurotransmitter release: The ω-conotoxins and ω-agatoxins. Annu Rev Biochem 1994;63:823–867.
133. Tsien RW, Ellinor PT, Horn WA. Molecular diversity of voltage-dependent Ca^{2+} channels. Trends Pharmacol Sci 1991;12:349–354.
134. Snutch TP, Reiner PB. Ca^{2+} channels: diversity of form and function. Curr Opin Neurobiol 1992;2:247–253.
135. Campbell KP, Leung AT, Sharp AH. The biochemistry and molecular biology of dyhydropyridine-sensitive calcium channel. Trends Neurosci 1988;11:425–430.
136. Catterall WA. Structure and function of voltage-sensitive ion channels. Science 1988;242:50–61.
137. Dunlop K, Luebke JI, Turner TJ. Exocytotic Ca^{2+} channels in mammalian central neurons. Trends Neurosci 1995;18:89–98.
138. Pragnell M, Sakamato J, Jay SD, Campbell KP. Cloning and tissue-specific expression of the brain calcium channel beta-subunit. FEBS Lett 1991;291:253–258.
139. Hullin R, Singer-Lahat D, Freichel M, et al. Calcium channel β subunit heterogeneity: functional expression of the cloned cDNA from heart, aorta, and brain. EMBO J 1992;11: 885–890.
140. Castellano A, Wei X-Y, Birnbaumer L, Perez-Reyes E. Cloning and expression of a third β-subunit. J Biol Chem 1993;268:3450–3455.
141. Castellano A, Wei X-Y, Birnbaumer L, Prez-Reyes E. Cloning and expression of a neuronal calcium-channel β-subunit. J Biol Chem 1993;268:12359–12366.
142. Yaari Y, Hamon B, Lux HD. Development of two types of calcium channels in cultured mammalian hippocampal neurons. Science 1987;235:680–682.
143. Llinas R, Yarom Y. Specific blockade of the low threshold calcium channel by high molecular weight alcohols [Abstract]. Soc Neurosci 1986; 12:174.
144. Scott RH, Sweeney MI, Kobrinsky EM, et al. Actions of arginine polyamine on voltage-and ligand-activated whole cell currents recorded from cultured neurons. Br J Pharmacol 1992;106:199–207.
145. Bean BP. Classes of calcium channels in vertebrate cells. Annu Rev Physiol 1989;51:367–384.
146. Sather WA, Tanabe T, Zhang J-F, et al. Distinctive biophysical and pharmacological properties of class A (BI) calcium channel alpha 1 subunits. Neuron 1993;11:1–20.
147. Snutch TP, Leonard JP, Gilbert MM, et al. Rat brain expresses a heterogenous family of calcium channels. Proc Natl Acad Sci U S A 1990;87:3391–3395.
148. Williams ME, Feldman DH, McCue AF, et al. Structure and function of alpha 1, alpha 2, and beta subunits of a novel human neuronal calcium channel subtype. Neuron 1992;8:71–84.
149. Snutch TP, Tomlinson WJ, Leonard JP, Gilbert MM. Distinct calcium channels are generated by alternative splicing and are differentially expressed in the mammalian CNS. Neuron 1991; 7:45–57.
150. Supervilai P, Cortes R, Palacios JM, Karobath M. Calcium entry blockers: Autoradiographic mapping of their binding sites in rat brain. Prog Brain Res 1985;63:89–95.
151. Thayer SA, Murphy SN, Miller RJ. Widespread distribution of dihydropyridine-sensitive calcium channels in the central nervous system. Mol Pharmacol 1986;30:505.
152. Plummer MR, Logothetis DE, Hess P. Elementary properties and modulation of calcium channels in mammalian peripheral neurons. Neuron 1989;2:1453–1463.
153. Triggle DJ, Janis RA. Calcium channel ligands. Annu Rev Pharmacol Toxicol 1987;27:346–369.
154. Mintz IM, Venema VJ, Adams ME, Bean BP. Inhibition of N-

and L-type Ca^{2+} channels by the spider venom toxin omega-Aga-IIIA. Proc Natl Acad Sci U S A 1991;88:6628–6631.
155. Kerr LM, Filloux F, Olivera BM, et al. Autoradiographic localization of calcium channels with [^{125}I]omega-conotoxin in rat brain. Eur J Pharmacol 1988;146:181–183.
156. Olivera BM, Gray WR, Zeikus R, et al. Peptide toxins from fish-hunting cone snails. Science 1985;230:1338–1343.
157. Westenbroek RE, Sakurai T, Elliott EM, et al. Immunochemical identification and subcellular distribution of the α_{1A} subunits of brain calcium channels. J Neurosci 1995;15:6403–6418.
158. Mintz IM, Adams ME, Bean BP. P-type calcium channels in rat central and peripheral neurons. Neuron 1992;9:85–95.
159. Hillyard DR, Monje VD, Mintz IM, et al. A new *Conus* peptide ligand for mammalian presynaptic Ca^{2+} channels. Neuron 1992;9:69–77.
160. Gohil K, Bell JR, Ramachandran J, Miljanich GP. Neuroanatomical distribution of receptors for a novel voltage-sensitive calcium channel antagonist, SNX-230 (ω-conopeptide MVIIC). Brain Res 1994;653:258–266.
161. Yokoyama CT, Westenbroek RE, Hell JW, et al. Biochemical properties and subcellular distribution of the neuronal class E calcium channel α_1 subunit. J. Neurosci 1995;15:6419–6432.
162. Augustine GJ, Charlton MP, Smith SJ. Calcium action in synaptic transmitter release. Annu Rev Neurosci 1987;10:633–693.
163. Dooley D, Lupp A, Herting G. Inhibition of central neurotransmitter release by omega-conotoxin GVIA, a peptide modulator of N-type voltage-sensitive calcium channels. Naunyn Schmiedebergs Arch Pharamacol 1987;336:467–470.
164. Uchitel OD, Protti DA, Sanchez V, et al. P-type voltage-dependent calcium channel mediates presynaptic calcium influx and transmitter release in mammalian synapses. Proc Natl Acad Sci U S A 1992;89:3330–3333.
165. Bowersox SS, Miljanich GP, Sugiura Y, et al. Differential blockade of voltage-sensitive calcium channels at the mouse neuromuscular junction by novel ω-conopeptides and ω-agatoxin-IVA. J Pharmacol Exp Ther 1995;273:248–256.
166. Benedek G, Szikszay M. Potentiation of thermoregulatory and analgesic effects of morphine by calcium antagonists. Pharmacol Res Commun 1984;16:1009–1018.
167. Hoffmeister F, Tettenborn D. Calcium agonists and antagonists of the dihydropyridine type: antinociceptive effects, interference with opiate-μ-receptor agonists and neuropharmacological actions in rodents. Psychopharmacology (Berl) 1986;90:299–307.
168. Del Pozo E, Caro G, Baeyens JM. Analgesic effects of several calcium channel blockers in mice. Eur J Pharmacol 1987;137:155–160.
169. Kavaliers M. Stimulatory influences of calcium channel antagonists on stress-induced opioid analgesia and locomotor activity. Brain Res 1987;408:403–407.
170. Santillan R, Maestre JM, Hurle HA, Florez J. Enhancement of opiate analgesia by nimodipine in cancer patients chronically treated with morphine: a preliminary report. Pain 1994;58:129–132.
171. Carta F, Bianchi M, Argentron S, et al. Effect of nifedipine on morphine-induced analgesia. Anesth Analg 1990;70:493–498.
172. Miranda HF, Bustamante D, Kramer V, et al. Antinociceptive effects of Ca^{2+} channel blockers. Eur J Pharmacol 1992;217:137–141.
173. Contreras E, Tamayo L, Amigo M. Calcium channel antagonists increase morphine-induced analgesia and antagonize morphine tolerance. Eur J Pharmacol 1988;148:463–466.
174. Mecke E, Kauppila T, Carlson S, Pertovaara A. Differential effects of verapamil, a calcium channel antagonist, on morphine and cocaine-induced analgesia and locomotor behavior in rats. Neurosci Res Commun 1991;9:137–142.
175. Coderre TJ, Melzack R. The role of NMDA receptor-operated calcium channels in persistent nociception after formalin-induced tissue injury. J Neurosci 1992;12:3671–3675.
176. Malmberg AB, Yaksh TL. Effect of continuous intrathecal infusion of ω-conopeptides, N-type calcium-channel blockers, on behavior and antinociception in the formalin and hot-plate tests in rats. Pain 1995;60:83–90.
177. Omote K, Sonoda H, Kawamata M, et al. A potentiation of antinociceptive effects of morphine by calcium channel blockers at the level of the spinal cord. Anesthesiology 1993;79:746–752.
178. Omote K, Iwaksaki H, Kawamata M, et al. Effects of verapamil on spinal anesthesia with local anesthetics. Anesth Analg 1995;80:444–448.
179. Chaplan SR, Pogrel JW, Yaksh TL. Role of voltage-dependent calcium channel subtypes in experimental tactile allodynia. J Pharmacol Exp Ther 1994;269:1117–1123.
180. Malmberg AB, Yaksh TL. Voltage-sensitive calcium channels in spinal nociceptive processing: blockade of N- and P-type channels inhibits formalin-induced nociception. J Neurosci 1994;14:4820–4890.
181. Xiao W-H, Bennett GJ. Calcium channel blockade with synthetic omega-conopeptides applied to the site of nerve injury suppresses neuropathic pains in rats. J Pharmacol Exp Ther 1995;274:666–672.
182. Gohil K, Bowersox S, Singh T, Ramachandran J, Miljanich G. SNX-111, a selective inhibitor of N-type voltage-sensitive calcium channels, is antinociceptive in the rat hindpaw formalin test [Abstract]. Soc Neurosci 1993;19:235.
183. Stevens CW, Yaksh TL. Magnitude of opioid dependence after continuous intrathecal infusion of mu and delta selective opioids in the rat. Eur J Pharmacol 1989;166:467–472.
184. Bowersox S, Gadbois T, Singh T, et al. Selective N-type neuronal voltage-sensitive calcium channel blocker, SNX-111, produce spinal antinociception in rat models of acute, persistent and neuropathic pain. J Pharmac. Exp Ther (in press).
185. Bennett GJ, Xie Y-K. A peripheral mononeuropathy in rat that produces disorders of pain sensation like those seen in man. Pain 1988;33:87–107.
186. Cervero F, Iggo A. The substantia gelatinosa of the spinal cord. Brain 1980;103:717–772.
187. Luther R, Tich N, Sperzel WD, Cohen A. A double-blind, placebo controlled, safety and tolerability study of SNX-111 [Presentation]. The 24th Annual Meeting of the American College of Clinical Pharmacology, October, 1995.
188. McGuire D, Kugler A, Bowersox S, Luther R. The first N-type voltage-sensitive calcium channel antagonist administered to humans: pharmacokinetics and evidence of drug effect [Presentation]. The 48th Annual Meeting of the American Academy of Neurology, March, 1996.
189. McGuire D, Bowersox S, Fellmann J, Luther R. Sympatholysis after neuron-specific, N-type, voltage sensitive calcium channel blockade: first demonstration of N-channel function in humans. (Submitted for publication.)
190. Wermeling D, Pfeifer B, Berger J, et al. Successful use of SNX-111, a novel n-type neuronal calcium channel blocker, in the treatment of severe AIDS neuropathic pain [Abstract]. J Neurovirol 1996;2:52.
191. Brose W, Pfeifer B, Hassenbusch S, et al. SNX-111 produces analgesia in patients with intractable pain: phase I/II results. In: Proceedings of the 11th World Congress of Anesthesiologists. Sydney, Australia, April 1996.

II PHARMACOKINETICS AND DYNAMICS OF SEDATIVE-HYPNOTICS

4 Barbiturates

W. Brooks Gentry and Thomas K. Henthorn

Thiopental and methohexital are the most commonly used barbiturates in clinical anesthesia. These drugs are classified as ultrashort-acting barbiturates because the hypnotic effect of small doses of these drugs dissipates after only a few minutes, despite an elimination half-life of several hours. Thiopental was first introduced as an induction agent for surgical anesthesia in 1934 (1). The lessons learned from its long and storied history are invaluable to the modern anesthesiologist. An understanding of the pharmacology of thiopental is important because it is still the most commonly used intravenous induction agent, and the effect of thiopental wanes as a result of distribution of the drug away from the effect site before significant metabolism occurs. The elucidation of the mechanism of thiopental's biodisposition by Brodie and its subsequent refinement by Price were important milestones in anesthesia research (2, 3).

PHYSICOCHEMICAL PROPERTIES

Thiopental and methohexital are derivatives of the pharmacologically inert barbituric acid (Fig. 4-1). Barbiturates may be classified according to chemical structure, based on substitutions at positions 1 and 2 of the barbituric acid molecule. Both thiopental and methohexital have hydrogen atom substitutions at position 1 of the molecule. Thiopental is a thiobarbiturate with a sulfur substitution at position 2 of the barbituric acid molecule. Methohexital is an oxybarbiturate with an oxygen substitution on position 2 of the molecule.

Both thiopental and methohexital are useful for induction of general anesthesia because of their rapid onsets of action. Because they are highly lipid soluble and have slightly alkaline pKa values, these agents are able to cross the brain-capillary endothelial barrier rapidly. The pKa values of these two agents (7.6 for thiopental and 7.9 for methohexital) are such that at physiologic pH, thiopental (pKa 7.6) and methohexital (pKa 7.9) are predominantly un-ionized (61% for thiopental and 75% for methohexital) (4). Both agents are weak acids and are manufactured for clinical use as sodium salts to maintain water solubility, because their free acid forms are virtually insoluble in water (4). Aqueous solutions of the two drugs are strongly alkaline ($pH > 10$), and this high pH causes significant tissue damage if these agents are injected subcutaneously or intra-arterially. Admixture with most other agents, including succinylcholine, may result in precipitation and occlusion of intravenous tubing. The high pH is bacteriostatic and results in the drug's stability in solution for up to 2 weeks. However, the same care in the handling and storage is necessary with other anesthetic agents after storage to ensure sterility (4).

PROTEIN BINDING

Thiopental and methohexital are highly protein bound to plasma albumin. Morgan and associates reported that thiopental binds in a dose-dependent fashion, with the percentage bound varying between 60 and 97% for plasma thiopental concentrations of 15.0 to 0.2 μg/ml (5). Subsequently, Burch and Stanski reported that thiopental serum protein binding is not significantly concentration dependent over the range of plasma concentrations seen in patients given an induction dose of thiopental (6). Thiopental clearance is directly related to unbound thiopental concentration and thus can be altered by albumin levels and by drugs that displace the drug from albumin (7). However, when the drug is given for induction of anesthesia, changes in thiopental elimination clearance (Cl_e) rarely are clinically relevant. The hypnotic effect of thiopental is likely related to its unbound fraction, as evidenced by the return of unconsciousness caused by a rapid decrease in bound drug produced when intravenous

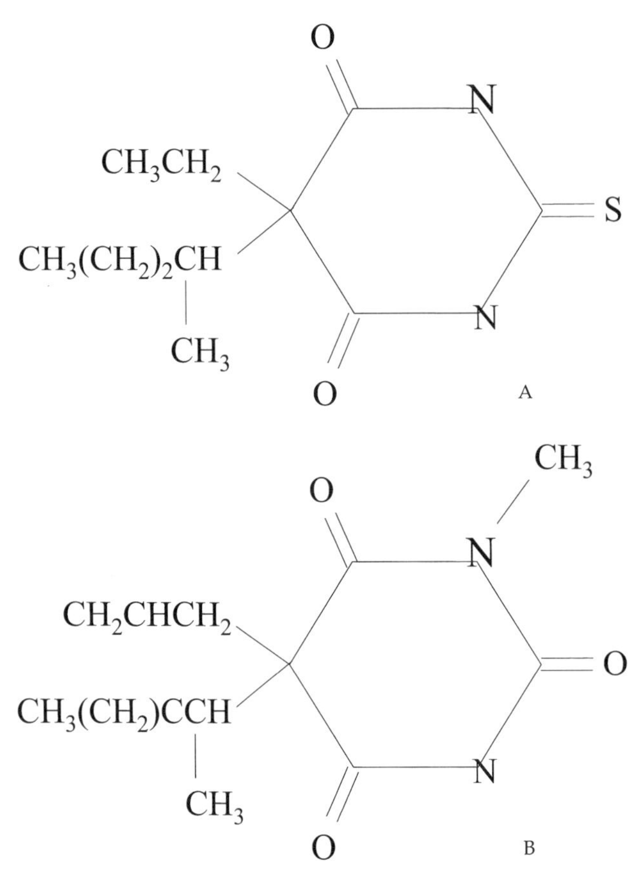

FIGURE 4-1. Chemical structures of thiopental (A) and methohexital (B). (From Dundee JW, Wyant GM. Intravenous anesthesia. Edinburgh: Churchill Livingstone 1988.)

aspirin is administered at the time of return of an eyelash reflex following an induction dose of thiopental (8).

MECHANISM OF ACTION

Many neurotransmitter systems are affected by barbiturates, but the anesthetic properties of these drugs are most likely due to effects on the γ-aminobutyric $acid_A$ ($GABA_A$) receptor (9) and its effects on voltage-sensitive sodium channels (10, 11). Barbiturate actions at the $GABA_A$ receptor correlate with anesthetic potency and are stereospecific, suggesting that these $GABA_A$ effects may in large part cause the hypnotic action of barbiturates. GABA is the major inhibitory neurotransmitter in the mammalian brain; virtually every neuron of the mammalian brain is responsive to GABA. $GABA_A$ receptors are pentameric transmembrane chloride channels that are ligand-gated chloride ion channels. Numerous anesthetic agents including volatile agents, barbiturates, benzodiazepines, and steroids enhance $GABA_A$-mediated inhibition in the mammalian central nervous system (CNS) (9).

Barbiturates have many effects on the $GABA_A$ receptor. Pentobarbital binding to the barbiturate receptor increases chloride ion flux into the cell even in the absence of GABA. In the presence of chloride ions, barbiturates increase the affinity of GABA for the $GABA_A$ receptor. The binding of benzodiazepines to their receptor on the $GABA_A$ receptor is enhanced by barbiturates in a chloride-dependent manner (9).

Sodium channels are common membrane proteins that are important in cellular communication because of their role in the generation of fast propagated action potentials. Barbiturates result in voltage-independent reduction of sodium channel open time and voltage-dependent depression of steady-state activation. These actions occur at clinically relevant concentrations and in a dose-dependent manner. The sodium channel may contribute to overall anesthetic depression, supporting the hypothesis that anesthesia results from superposition and integration of several different actions at the molecular level (11).

ONSET AND OFFSET OF BARBITURATE EFFECTS: A PHYSIOLOGIC MODEL OF DISTRIBUTION

Immediately after administration of an intravenous dose of thiopental or methohexital, the drug mixes within the central blood volume. During and after this process, the dose distributes throughout the body according to tissue perfusion, tissue affinity for the drug, and the thiopental concentration gradients between the various tissues and the blood. The rapid onset of effect of thiopental occurs in part because it rapidly traverses lipid capillary membranes in the brain because of its relatively high lipid solubility and low ionization at physiologic pH. It also achieves rapid equilibration between the blood and the effect site. The rate of tissue equilibration is determined by tissue perfusion and the apparent volume of the tissue. The apparent volume of a tissue or organ is the product of its mass and the tissue-to-blood partition ratio. The onset of effect occurs during the intravascular mixing and early distribution phases. The brain is exposed to high concentrations of the drug soon after administration because it is a highly perfused tissue of relatively low apparent volume and thus rapidly equilibrates with the concentration of thiopental in the blood.

Drug delivery to tissues other than the brain is also rapid. However, because the apparent volume of distribution of these tissues is much larger than that of the brain, equilibration of thiopental between these tissues and the blood takes a longer time. Therefore, thiopental reaches pseudoequilibrium initially with highly perfused tissues of relatively low apparent volume and only later with less well perfused tissues of higher apparent volume. The early rapid decline in thiopental

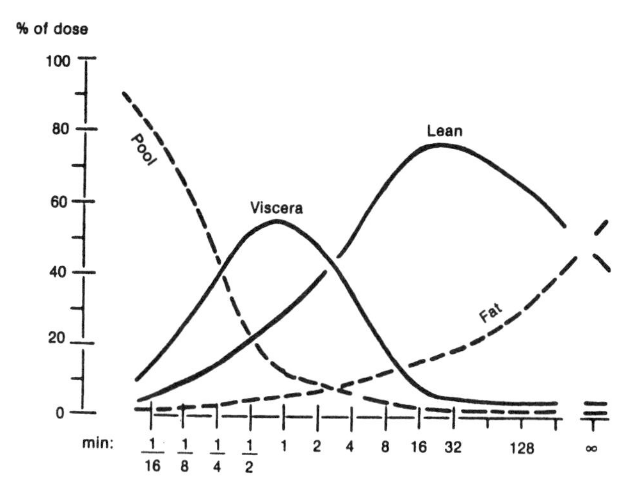

FIGURE 4-2. Percentage of thiopental dose in the central blood pool, viscera, lean tissue, and fat following bolus intravenous administration. (From Price HL. A dynamic concept of the distribution of thiopental in the human body. Anesthesiology 1960; 21:40.).

concentration in the blood, as tissue distribution progresses, results in the rapid wane in brain concentrations and cessation of effect after an induction dose of thiopental.

The theory that thiopental's central effects wane not as a result of metabolism, but rather from distribution to non-neural tissues, was reported as early as 1948 (12). In 1950, Brodie and colleagues reported that fat uptake of thiopental removed enough of the drug to end the sedative-hypnotic effects after an induction dose (2). A decade later, Price and colleagues used computer simulations to demonstrate that, because of low blood flow, uptake by fat is too slow to result in adequate removal of thiopental from the blood to explain the observed effects (Fig 4-2). These investigators suggested instead that uptake by more highly perfused tissues results in cessation of thiopental effects. These tissues include the relatively lower volume viscera and the relatively higher volume lean (muscle) tissues (3).

Metabolism of thiopental doses contributes significantly to the termination of effect when extremely large doses (30 mg/lb in dogs) are given (13). The contribution of metabolism of thiopental to the termination of effect of an induction dose, however, is small. In an average adult, the fraction of a 4 to 6-mg/kg dose of thiopental administered intravenously removed from the central compartment by metabolism is 0.14 at 1 minute and only 0.18 at 15 minutes after administration (6).

PHARMACOKINETICS

Early studies reported that methohexital had a much smaller volume of distribution at steady state (V_{dss}) than thiopental (14). However, more complete studies by Hudson and associates with longer sampling times (12 hours) provided a more accurate characterization of the late distribution and elimination phases and found that thiopental and methohexital distribute into a V_{dss} of 2.5 and 2.2 L/kg, respectively (15) (Table 4-1). The volume of distribution of the central compartment (V_c) for thiopental has been reported to range from 8.3L (16) to 26.1 L (15) for adults. Estimates for V_c depend on experimental conditions related to the speed of injection and the timing, location, and frequency of blood sampling, with small central distribution volumes associated with bolus injections and frequent, early arterial blood sampling. The rapid onset of effect of thiopental suggests that the brain is a part of a small volume that rapidly equilibrates with thiopental in the central compartment blood. Henthorn and associates reported a smaller V_c of 3.2 L determined by concomitant modeling of thiopental and the intravascular marker indocyanine green (ICG). Simultaneous analysis of thiopental and ICG allows characterization of late intravascular mixing and better approximation of early drug distribution (17, 18). Better definition of early kinetic events may provide an explanation for the interindividual differences in response to these drugs, as well as allow for more precise control of thiopental's concentrations by computer-controlled infusion devices.

The elimination of thiopental and methohexital is predominantly through the liver, with little involvement of the kidneys. Thiopental is oxidized primarily by the hepatic P450 system to a carboxylic acid derivative (19). Although the V_{dss} of the two drugs is similar, the Cl_e of the two differs. For single-bolus induction doses given to healthy patients, Hudson and colleagues found the Cl_e for thiopental to be 3.4 ± 0.5 ml/

TABLE 4-1. Thiopental and Methohexital Pharmacokinetic and Pharmacodynamic Values

Variable	Thiopental	Methohexital
V1 (L)	6	7
V3 (L)	36	25
V3 (L)	165	90
V_{ss} (L/kg)	2.5	2.2
C12 (L/min)	2.9	4.7
C13 (L/min)	0.6	0.6
Cl_e(ml/min)	250	690
k_{e0} (min^{-1})*	0.29	0.6
t_{max} (min)*	1.6	1.6
V_{pe} (L)	20	20
EC (μg/ml)†	10–15	3–5

**Estimated following a simulated intravenous bolus dose.*

†Effective concentration range for hypnosis when other agents are used for analgesia.

V_{ss}, Volume of distribution at steady state; Cl_e, elimination clearance; k_{e0}, effect site rate constant; t_{max}, time to maximal effect; V_{pe}, volume of distribution at pseudoequilibrium; EC, effect site concentration

(Data for thiopental from references 18, 77, and 78, data for methohexital from references 14 and 15.)

min/kg (15). Because the hepatic extraction of thiopental is only 10 to 20% (5), whereas that for methohexital is 50 to 87% (20, 21), methohexital's rate of elimination depends more on hepatic blood flow than does that of thiopental.

The elimination half-life for methohexital (3.9 hours) is less than half that of thiopental (11.6 hours). This difference in the barbiturates half-lives is due to the more rapid hepatic Cl_e of methohexital than of thiopental. Hudson and colleagues reported that more variability exists in the Cl_e of methohexital than with thiopental because of its greater dependence on hepatic blood flow for elimination. The metabolism of methohexital contributes to the termination of its effect. At 1 minute, approximately 29% of an induction dose of methohexital has been removed from the central compartment by metabolic processes; at 30 minutes, 38% has been lost. However, the major cause of dissipation of the clinical effects of methohexital is still redistribution, as is the case with thiopental (15), because at 30 minutes, 56% of the dose has been removed from the central compartment by redistribution.

The elimination of thiopental becomes zero-order at high blood concentrations (22, 23), and it exhibits Michaelis-Menten elimination kinetics (Fig. 4-3). The Michaelis-Menten equation states that

$$\text{elimination rate} = V_{max} \cdot C/(K_m + C)$$

where V_{max} is the maximum elimination rate, C is the drug concentration, and K_m is the concentration at which the elimination rate is half the maximum (the Michaelis constant). As concentration approaches and exceeds K_m, the elimination rate becomes less dependent on the concentration of thiopental and more dependent on the capacity of the hepatic P450 system. The K_m may be exceeded with either large bolus doses or prolonged infusions, or when bolus doses higher than 800 mg are given to healthy adults, the distribution of thiopental is unaffected and the concentration drops as rapidly as with normal induction doses (24). At extremely high sustained concentrations produced by continuous infusions of thiopental for barbiturate coma (electroencephalographic [EEG] silence), the elimination rate becomes constant. At lower concentrations associated with hypnosis (below the K_m), ordinary first-order processes are in effect (i.e., the elimination rate is proportional to the plasma concentration of thiopental). Stanski and colleagues found that the K_m varied from 8.1 to 67.5 μg/ml during a prolonged infusion of thiopental for cerebral resuscitation (22). In most patients, the K_m was found to be approximately 50 μg/ml, a concentration that results in EEG burst suppression (25).

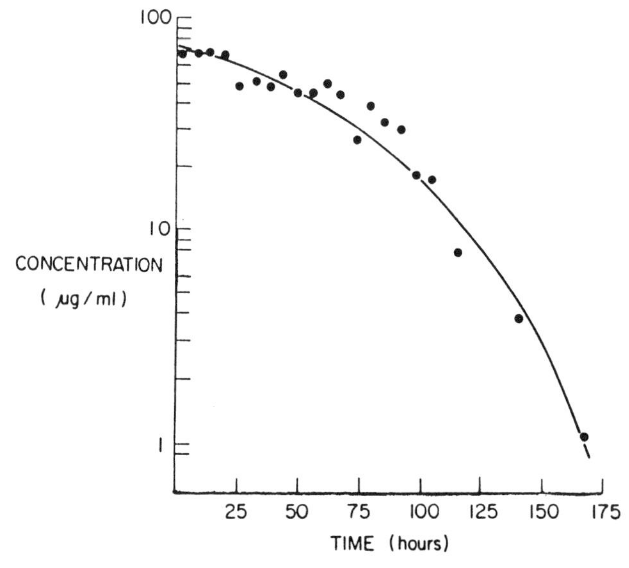

FIGURE 4-3. Decline in the plasma concentrations following a 42-hour infusion of 40.2 g of thiopental administered for cerebral resuscitation. This graph illustrates nonlinear (Michaelis-Menten) elimination kinetics. (From Stanski DR, Mihm FG, Rosenthal MH, Kalman SM. Pharmacokinetics of high-dose thiopental used in cerebral resuscitation. Anesthesiology 1980;53:169.)

Because thiopental exhibits zero-order kinetics at high concentrations, this agent is not a good choice for prolonged infusion when high concentrations are desired for reduced cerebral activity. Examination of simulations of the times required for a 25%, 50%, and 75% decrease in plasma concentrations after termination of a constant plasma concentration infusion shows that, with an infusion of 2 hours, the time for a 25% drop in concentration is only slightly more than 15 minutes, whereas the time required for a 50% drop exceeds an hour (Fig. 4-4A). The time for a 75% fall in the blood concentration almost always exceeds twice that necessary for a 50% fall suggesting that, even with prolonged infusions, the decay is multiexponential (i.e., due to distributional as well as elimination processes). The more rapid hepatic elimination of methohexital makes it a more logical choice for prolonged infusions than thiopental because the times required for both 25 and 50% decreases in concentrations remain 20 minutes or less for infusion durations commonly used in clinical anesthesia (Fig. 4-4B).

Organ System Effects

Induction doses of thiopental and methohexital result in a predictably rapid onset of sedation, hypnosis, and amnesia. In addition to these effects on the CNS, induction doses of these agents also have profound effects on other organ systems.

Central Nervous System Effects

After an initial activation at low concentrations, the barbiturates cause depression of cerebral electrical activity and dose-dependent depression of cerebral me-

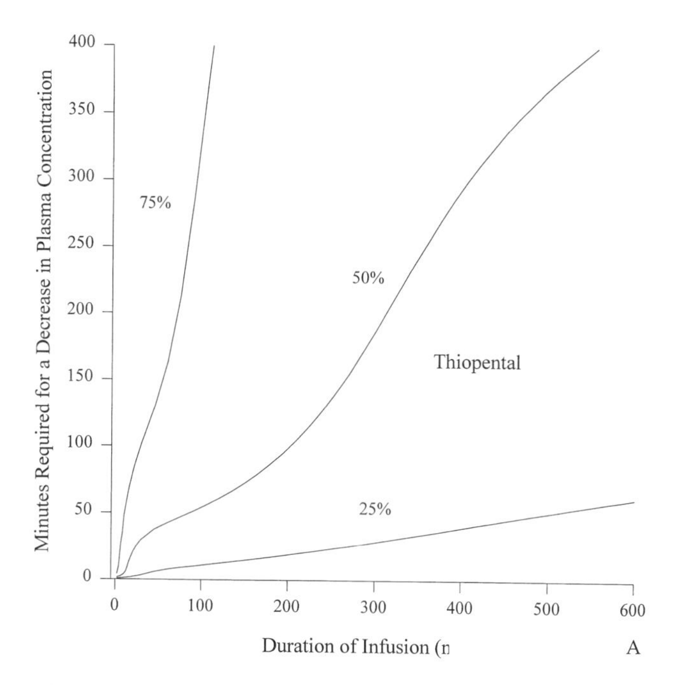

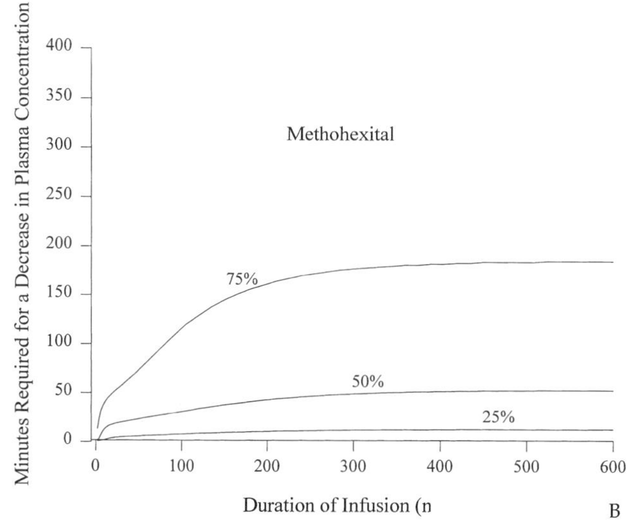

FIGURE 4-4. Recovery curves for thiopental (A) and methohexital (B) showing the time required for decreases in plasma concentrations of 25%, 50%, and 75% from the plasma concentration following termination of the infusion maintained by a computer-controlled infusion device.

tabolism (26). Thiopental results in a dose-dependent depression of cerebral metabolic rate for oxygen ($CMRO_2$). The depression of cerebral metabolism reaches a plateau at about 55% of control values (27). Thiopental reduces cerebral blood flow by reducing $CMRO_2$, which results in cerebral vasoconstriction and reduction in cerebral blood volume, reducing intracranial pressure (ICP) (28). Reduction in cerebral blood flow does not decrease cerebral perfusion pressure (CPP) because ICP is reduced more than mean arterial pressure. In fact, the decrease in ICP is often associated with an increase in CPP (29).

The reduction in cerebral metabolism caused by thiopental primarily reflects a reduction in neuronal activity. This results in a dose-dependent depression of the EEG, with the EEG amplitude increasing and frequency decreasing until a burst suppression pattern results. As the doses of thiopental increase, EEG isoelectricity is achieved (30), reflecting the maximum decrease in $CMRO_2$. The only way to decrease brain oxygen requirements further is with hypothermia (31). Although thiopental is an effective anticonvulsant, methohexital has been reported to have proconvulsant effects (32). Methohexital has been reported to cause seizures when given in high doses (33) to healthy patients and at lower doses in patients with undiagnosed epilepsy (34).

Cardiovascular Effects

The barbiturates have direct effects on the peripheral vasculature and the myocardium. The predominant effect of thiopental is venodilation resulting in blood pooling in the periphery (35). With normal induction doses, systemic vascular resistance and arterial blood pressure remain unchanged in healthy patients (36). At high doses, thiopental is a direct myocardial depressant and results in decreased myocardial contractility (37).

Thiopental and methohexital both increase heart rate by activating the barostatic reflex (38). Methohexital causes a greater increase in heart rate (40%) than thiopental (25%) in healthy patients (36). The net result of changes in heart rate and contractility is that cardiac index is decreased (36, 39). High doses of methohexital given for neurosurgery similarly result in modest reductions in stroke volume, arterial pressure, systemic vascular resistance, and total body oxygen consumption. Cardiac index is well maintained by the increase in heart rate (33).

The dose of thiopental should be decreased and administered more slowly in patients relying on high sympathetic tone to maintain cardiovascular function (i.e., hypovolemic shock and heart failure) (38). Price and colleagues suggested that hypovolemic patients have a greater percentage of their cardiac output going to the brain and myocardium because of peripheral redistribution of blood flow to core tissues (3). These patients have a higher percentage of an administered dose of thiopental in the central circulation and thus experience greater CNS depressant effects from a given dose. Likewise, thiopental has been shown to cause marked hemodynamic changes (e.g., decreased afterload, left ventricular stroke work index, coronary blood flow, and myocardial oxygen consumption) in patients with chronic, stable ischemic heart disease. However, the decreased coronary blood flow did not cause global or regional hypoxia in any of the patients studied (40).

Respiratory Effects

Thiopental and methohexital depress ventilation in a dose-dependent fashion depending on the rate of administration and the presence of other ventilatory depressant drugs. Apnea occurs in most patients given an induction dose of thiopental or methohexital. Barbiturates depress ventilatory responses to hypoxemia and hypercapnia even after normal minute ventilation resumes following anesthetic induction doses (41). Thiopental also suppresses airway protective reflexes against aspiration of stomach contents, but it does not usually obliterate laryngeal and tracheal reflexes to the degree that tracheal intubation can be accomplished without muscle relaxants unless extremely large doses are used (42). Thiopental is not as effective as propofol in blunting these reflexes (43); therefore, propofol is a better choice for induction when insertion of a laryngeal mask airway is planned. Thiopental depresses lung mucociliary clearance of foreign material to the same degree as halothane (44).

Renal and Hepatic Effects

Although large doses of thiopental and methohexital may cause transient decrements in liver function, doses used for induction of anesthesia cause no significant changes in liver function either in healthy patients or in patients with preexisting liver disease (45). Thiopental may decrease urine output because of decreased renal blood flow and renal artery constriction (46). However, proper fluid management and treatment of hypotension prevent clinically significant decreases in urine output during thiopental administration.

Protein binding decreases significantly in patients who are receiving long-term dialysis and who are cirrhotic and uremic. Ghoneim and Pandya showed that the free fraction of thiopental almost doubles in the plasma of these patients at plasma thiopental concentrations near the hypnotic threshold of 10 μg/ml (47). Induction doses should be administered more slowly in these patients, to prevent excessively high "free" thiopental levels. In the presence of normal liver function, the effects of a given dose of thiopental in a patient receiving dialysis may decrease quickly because of the greater availability of free drug to the liver for metabolism by decreased plasma protein binding.

Metabolic and Endocrine Effects

Thiobarbiturates can cause a dose-dependent release of histamine. However, oxybarbiturates have not been associated with this effect (48). Unless massive doses of thiopental are administered rapidly, this release of histamine rarely causes clinically significant hemodynamic or pulmonary changes. Thiopental does not prevent the adrenocortical stress response to surgery, but it does decrease plasma cortisol concentrations (49). Finally, clinically insignificant increases in blood glucose levels occur with thiopental induction, but serum insulin levels do not change (50).

Adverse Effects During Induction

Pain on injection occurs in 1 to 2% of patients given thiopental and in 5% of patients who receive methohexital, particularly when the drug is injected into small veins of the hand or wrist (51). Extravasation into subcutaneous tissues or accidental intra-arterial injection of methohexital results in minimal discomfort and almost no sequelae. Extravasation of thiopental causes pain, edema, erythema, and reactions ranging from slight soreness to tissue necrosis, depending on the amount and the concentration injected (4, 52). Intra-arterial injection of thiopental results in immediate pain and burning, which radiate into the hand and fingers. Anesthesia, hyperesthesia, and motor weakness may follow. Sequelae range from mild discomfort to gangrene. Treatment includes papaverine or lidocaine injection into the artery and sympathetic blockade through the stellate ganglion or brachial plexus (52).

Mild excitatory muscular movements and respiratory effects such as cough or hiccups can occur with induction doses of thiopental or methohexital. The incidence and severity of these effects are greater with equivalent doses of methohexital than with thiopental (53). Atropine or opioids given before induction minimize these effects, whereas phenothiazines or scopolamine may exacerbate them (31).

Anaphylactoid reactions (e.g., facial edema or urticarial rash of the chest, neck, and face) can occur with thiopental induction. These reactions are usually mild and last only a few minutes (54). Rarely, shock and bronchospasm occur with thiobarbiturate induction and require treatment with epinephrine. Barbiturates induce the production of δ-aminolevulinic acid synthetase, which catalyzes the rate-limiting step in the synthesis of porphyrins (55). Because of this phenomenon, barbiturate administration can precipitate attacks of acute intermittent porphyria or variegate porphyria in patients with this disease. Symptoms include nervous system dysfunction including paralysis, abdominal pain, and photosensitivity.

Drug Interactions

Patients taking CNS depressant drugs, including antihistamines, isoniazide, methylphenidate, and monoamine oxidase inhibitors, are more sensitive to the depressant effects of thiopental (31). Clonidine and dexmedetomidine, α_2-adrenergic agonists used as adjuvants in general and regional anesthesia, also reduce thiopental induction dose requirements (56, 57). Patients with long-term, extremely high ethanol intake and normal liver function were reported to require larger doses of thiopental for induction of anesthesia and to have prolonged Cl_e of the drug (58). However, Swerdlow and associates subsequently reported that alcoholic patients given an infusion of thiopental at 100 mg/min to a burst suppression EEG end point do not have increased requirements or altered pharmacokinetics of thiopental (59). Aminophylline administered concomitantly with thiopental reduces both the resultant depth and the duration of sedation (60). Thiopental may be displaced from albumin by high concentrations of nonsteriodal anti-inflammatory drugs (e.g., naproxen, indomethacin, mefenamic acid, and aspirin [61].) The antibiotic sulfizoxazole has also been reported to displace thiopental from albumin-binding sites (62).

Considerations for Use During Pregnancy and With Neonates

Thiopental crosses the placenta and enters the fetus, but umbilical arterial concentrations are less than half those seen in the maternal plasma at delivery when induction doses lower than 6 mg/kg are used. The explanation for the lower fetal levels relates to the following: 1) thiopental transit from the placental intervillous space to the fetal circulation is delayed; 2) extraction of drug by the fetal liver occurs before it reaches the brain; 3) thiopental is diluted by admixture with various components of the fetal circulation; and finally, 4) extensive right-to-left shunting of fetal blood occurs. Reports document that prompt delivery of the fetus by cesarean section following thiopental induction (4 to 8 mg/kg) is associated with minimal depression; however, lower Apgar scores may be seen with longer delivery times requiring repeat maintenance doses (63). The reasons for the lower Apgar scores may be the high thiopental dosage and factors associated with longer cesarean delivery times. Thiopental is as safe for the fetus as ketamine (64) when it is used for cesarean section, and it is safer than midazolam (65). Thiopental also has been used for induction of anesthesia for nonobstetrical surgery during pregnancy. Thiopental has little effect on the smooth muscle of the pregnant uterus, neither increasing nor decreasing its tone (4). Thiopental is not associated with an increase in preterm labor, nor has it been shown to be teratogenic in human patients (66).

Term, normal-weight neonates younger than 14 days of age require a significantly decreased dose of thiopental for induction of anesthesia when compared with infants 1 to 6 months old (3.4 mg/kg for neonates versus 6.3 mg/kg for infants) (67). Neonatal serum protein binding of thiopental is approximately 10% less than that of adults (68); increased free thiopental in the neonate may be partly responsible for the decreased dose requirement. Children aged 5 months to 13 years were found to have significantly increased Cl_e for thiopental over that of 11 healthy adults (6.6 $ml \cdot kg^{-1} \cdot min^{-1}$ versus 3.1 $ml \cdot kg^{-1} \cdot min^{-1}$) the V_{dss} and serum protein binding were not different between the two groups (69).

PHARMACODYNAMICS

Pharmacodynamics may be viewed as the relation of drug concentration to drug effect (73). Safe administration of anesthetic drugs relies on the integration of knowledge of concentration-time profiles (pharmacokinetics) with knowledge of concentration-effect relationships.

Early studies with thiopental found that venous plasma concentrations associated with loss of consciousness differ from those observed at emergence. In addition, these reports have demonstrated a strong positive correlation between the induction dose of thiopental and peripheral venous plasma thiopental concentration on emergence (70-72); that is, the larger the thiopental dose required for induction, the higher the plasma concentrations at emergence. This phenomenon was interpreted as evidence of the development of "acute" tolerance to the effects of thiopental. Acute tolerance implies that exposure of the brain to a dose of a centrally active drug renders it less sensitive to subsequent exposure to the same doses. Later studies of the transition from light to moderate depths of anesthesia with three different infusion rates of thiopental administered over the course of 1 hour found no differences in the peripheral venous plasma concentrations at which the EEG end point was attained with each of the three infusions. These results suggested that acute tolerance to thiopental doses not develop over the course of a 1-hour infusion (73).

Barratt and associates explained the discrepancies in venous concentrations at induction and emergence among these studies by pointing out that peripheral venous concentrations poorly reflect jugular venous concentrations, which may more accurately reflect thiopental concentrations in the brain (74, 75). The earlier studies involving a rapid infusion of thiopental measured effects before equilibration of concentrations in the brain and venous blood (70-72). The later study measured effects after equilibration of brain and venous plasma concentrations, such that concentrations in the venous plasma were the same as those in the brain at the onset and offset of clinical effects, and concluded that acute tolerance is not clinically relevant (73).

Concentration-Effect Hysteresis

Studies of thiopental pharmacodynamics in which arterial concentrations are related to CNS effects have shown that peak effect (and concentration) in the brain, as assessed by the EEG, lags behind peak arterial plasma concentrations because equilibration of thiopental across the brain-capillary membrane barrier is not instantaneous (76-78). On induction, plasma levels rise before the effect is seen, and on emergence, residual effects remain even after arterial concentrations decrease below those seen on induction. This phenomenon, called effect hysteresis, is defined as a situation in which a clinical effect lags behind the cause of that effect.

Several factors, the effects of which are additive, contribute to pharmacologic hysteresis. Before a tissue responds to a drug administered intravenously, time is required for four events: 1) for the drug to travel from the vein of administration to the target capillary bed; 2) for the drug to diffuse across the capillary membrane to the target organ; 3) for the drug to bind to its receptor; and 4) for the drug-receptor interaction to exert its pharmacodynamic effect (4).

Effect hysteresis is accounted for in pharmacokinetic models with the addition of an effect site or "biophase" compartment, which is related to the drug disposition model using an effect site rate constant, or k_{e0}. The k_{e0} is a first-order rate constant that characterizes the disequilibrium between plasma concentration and concentration at the effect site (e.g., brain). For a given pharmacokinetic model, a larger k_{e0} implies a more rapid equilibration (i.e., less temporal dissociation) between the plasma concentrations and the apparent effect site concentrations, whereas smaller k_{e0} values imply slower equilibration (i.e., more temporal dissociation). The k_{e0} may be incorporated into a pharmacokinetic-effect model to relate changes in the observed effect to concurrent plasma pharmacokinetics (79) during periods of rapidly changing plasma concentrations, such as those that occur during induction of anesthesia with thiopental. Stanski and associates added an effect compartment to their pharmacokinetic-pharmacodynamic model for thiopental to derive consistent, sigmoid relationships between plasma concentrations and effect (76-78).

Plasma Concentrations at Anesthetic End Points

Knowledge of the principles of thiopental pharmacokinetics and of the processes responsible for its distribution throughout the body is useful clinically only when it is combined with the appropriate pharmacodynamic information. Several studies have used various techniques to estimate thiopental plasma or effect site concentrations necessary to produce responses relevant to clinical anesthesia (Table 4-2). For loss of skeletal muscle power, an index of loss of consciousness, a concentration of 11.3 μg/ml is required. For EEG burst suppression, a concentration of 33.9 μg/ml is needed (80). This is a lower concentration than that required to prevent movement to a standard stimulus, such as trapezius squeeze, at 39.8 μg/ml. Still higher concentrations are required to blunt the response to laryngoscopy and endotracheal intubation (81). The higher concentrations required to blunt responses beyond (EEG) burst suppression suggest that these responses are mediated by central structures deeper than the cerebral cortex, and they are less sensitive to the effects of thiopental than the cortex (82).

TABLE 4-2. Concentration-Effect Relationships for Thiopental and Methohexital

Clinical End Point	Thiopental EC_{50} (μg/ml)	Methohexital EC_{50} (μg/ml)
Hypnosis (syringe drop)	11.3	3.4
Verbal command	13.6	—
Spectral edge	17.9–19.4	—
Electroencephalographic burst suppression	33.9	10.7
Laryngoscopy	50.7	—
Intubation	78.8	—

EC_{50}, Median effective concentration.

The ratio of methohexital effect site concentrations required for loss of consciousness and EEG burst suppression is the same as for thiopental; however, the methohexital concentrations required for loss of consciousness and EEG burst suppression are about 30% of those of thiopental, at 3.4 μg/ml and 10.7 μg/ml, respectively (83). These values are consistent with the estimates of the relative potency of the two barbiturates. Reports vary, but most sources agree that methohexital is approximately three times more potent that thiopental. Intravenous bolus doses resulting in unconsciousness are 3 to 5 mg/kg for thiopental and 1 to 3 mg/kg for methohexital (4).

Altered Dose Requirements

Neonates (67), females (84, 85), older patients (77, 84, 85), hypovolemic patients (86), and patients in renal failure (87) all exhibit increased sensitivity to the effects of thiopental. Changes in the total volume of distribution, Cl_e, and thus elimination half-life do not significantly affect the concentration-time relationship of an induction dose when that dose is exerting its clinical effect or when its effects are waning. Altered clinical responses to thiopental are primarily due to changes in pharmacodynamics or early distribution pharmacokinetics (31). Neonates and patients in renal failure have decreased protein binding of thiopental, resulting in an increased free fraction available to enter the brain. In hypovolemic patients, redistribution of blood flow from peripheral tissues to the central blood pool reduces distribution of drug to peripheral tissues, increasing the fraction of a given dose of drug to peripheral tissues and increasing the fraction of a given dose of drug in the central compartment and, thus, the dose entering the brain (3). Wulfsohn and Joshi have postulated that calculation of induction dose based on lean body mass results in similar reponses in obese patients and in those of average weight (88).

The reason for the increased response of aged patients has been extensively studied, but a consensus has not yet been reached. Thiopental infusion studies using EEG to evaluate thiopental brain effects demonstrated no increased sensitivity of the elderly brain to the drug (77). Homer and Stanski concluded that increased sensitivity to thiopental is due to a decreased initial volume of distribution. Subsequent studies by Stanski and Maitre suggested that this phenomenon could be the cause of the increased sensitivity of elderly patients to thiopental (78). Avram and colleagues concluded that this change alone would not affect peak-effect site concentrations following an intravenous bolus dose (89).

Changes in early distribution of thiopental caused by medications administered before the induction of anesthesia have also been reported to increase patient sensitivity to thiopental. Pharmacokinetic parameters for thiopental determined after treatment with the α_2-adrenergic agonist dexmedetomidine administered to healthy patients resulted in decreased fast and slow distribution volumes and decreased clearance to these volumes. The authors reported that a decrease in the movement of thiopental out of the central compartment decreased the dose necessary for induction (57).

Dose requirements to reach a given end point are also affected by the rate of administration of the drug (90-92). Cumulative dose versus infusion rate is not a simple linear relationship. In a study involving a 30-fold range of infusion rates administered to healthy men, the dose required to result in a loss of consciousness was not different at infusion rates of 40 to 150 mg/min (92) (Fig. 4-5). The dose required at these infusion rates was approximately 300 mg. As administration rates increased above 150 mg/min, the delivered dose at the end point increased significantly. Higher infusion rates increase the amount of drug in the vascular tree between the site of administration and the brain at the time the end point is attained, thus increasing the administered dose (92).

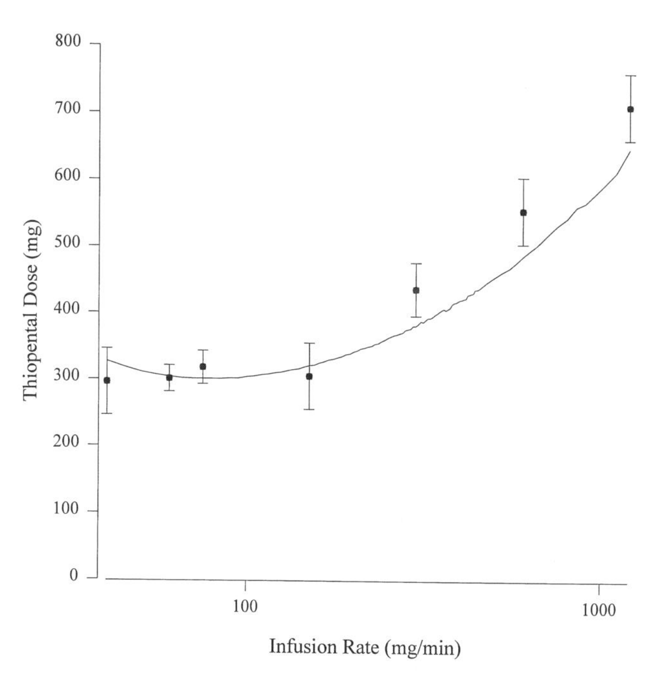

FIGURE 4-5. Simulations of thiopental infusion rates and thiopental doses required to produce an EC_{50} of 11.3 mg/L (four-compartment pharmacokinetic model), k_{e0}=0.29 min^{-1}, and three different doses are from a clinical study involving seven different infusion rates (filled circles). These values are shown with their 95% confidence intervals (From Gentry WB, Krejcie TC, Henthorn TK, et al. Effect of infusion rate on thiopental dose-response relationships. Anesthesiology 1994;81:316–324.)

Prediction of Induction Dose

Selection of the appropriate induction dose of an anesthetic agent that results in the desired end point without excessive side effects is a major goal in the overall perioperative care of the patient. Current knowledge of pharmacology of anesthetic drugs allows anesthesiologists to make reasonable predictions of dose requirements in most cases. However, interpatient variability in response to thiopental is difficult to predict and results in occasional underdoses and overdoses. Much of this interpatient variability in dose required to result in loss of consciousness with thiopental may be accounted for with a simple equation:

$$Dose\ (mg) = 350\ (300\ if\ female) + weight - 2 \times age - 50 \quad (89)$$

Combined pharmacokinetic-pharmacodynamic models are useful for predicting the influence of administration, disposition, and effect variables (e.g., target effect site concentration or pharmacodynamic end point) on dose-response relationships (92). These models, which characterize the time required for equilibration between plasma and effect sites, may be used to calculate the optimal (instantaneous) dose required to produce the desired concentration as rapidly as possible without "overshooting" the desired end point. Plasma and effect compartment concentrations reach pseudoequilibrium at the time of maximal effect of an induction dose. Using Niazi's concept of a time-dependent distribution volume (93), the volume of distribution at the time of maximal effect may be determined by dividing the amount of drug remaining in the body by the plasma concentration. The time of maximal effect may be determined by either of two methods (94). The first is by observation of the maximal drug effect, and the second is by examining the time of maximal effect site concentration using a simulation including plasma kinetics, an instantaneous central volume input, and the effect site rate constant, k_{e0} (94). The distribution volume at the time of maximal effect is the volume of distribution at pseudoequilibrium of blood and effects site (V_{dpe}). The optimal instantaneous dose may be determined by multiplying the V_{dpe} by the desired concentration. Dose determinations using the V_c or V_{dss} result in inappropriately low and high doses, respectively. For instance, calculation of an induction dose of thiopental based on a V_c of 7 L and a hypnotic concentration of 15 mg/L results in a dose of 105 mg. Likewise, calculation of an induction dose based on a V_{dss} of 200 L with the same target concentration results in a dose of 3000 mg. However, using the V_{dpe} for thiopental of 20 L, the calculated induction dose would be 300 mg, a clinically appropriate dose.

Dose predictions using combined pharmacokinetic-pharmacodynamic models depend on the rate of administration, the pharmacokinetic model describing the concentration history, k_{e0}, and the target effect site concentration (e.g., EC_{50}) (92). A complex relationship exists among the k_{e0}, target concentration, pharmacokinetic model, and infusion regimen. Changes in any one of these variables can change the predicted doses of thiopental (92). For instance, the combined models of Stanski and Maitre (78) and of Shanks and associates (80) make reasonable predictions of the thiopental dose required to result in a loss of consciousness when administered over many infusion rates to healthy patients. However, combining the k_{e0} of Stanski and Maitre with the pharmacokinetic model of Shanks and colleagues results in marked underpredictions of the doses required to achieve this end point (Fig. 4-6). Avoidance of similar mispredictions requires application of the variables used to construct the combined models with knowledge of the pharmacokinetics and pharmacodynamics used in their derivation (92).

The k_{e0} value is derived using pharmacokinetic and pharmacodynamic data and is frequently used to compare the onset time of clinical effects of different hypnotic drugs. However, the increase and decrease of the effect site concentration, and thus the degree of dissociation between the central compartment concentration and the effect site concentration, is the convolution of the drug concentration history of the central compartment (pharmacokinetic model) and the effect site unit disposition function. As stated earlier, combinations of pharmacokinetic models with k_{e0} values derived from different pharmacokinetic models may result in mispredictions of onset of effects (Fig. 4-7). A better way to compare onset of effects for different drugs may be with the time to maximal effect, or t_{max}. The t_{max} value can be determined by observation of a continuous end point such as EEG, and does not depend on a pharmacokinetic model for its determination, in contrast to the k_{e0} does.

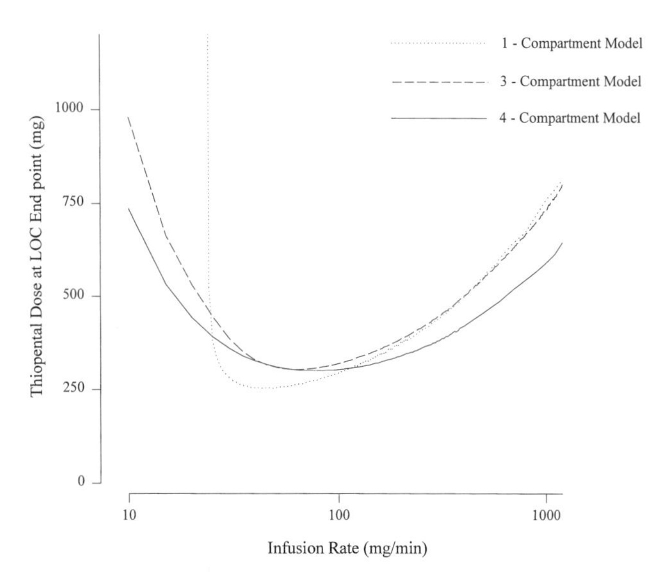

FIGURE 4-6. Simulations of infusion rates and thiopental doses calculated to result in an EC_{50} of 11.3 mg/L using a k_{e0} of 0.29 min^{-1} and three different pharmacokinetic models: a one-compartment model (dotted line) (78); a three-compartment model (dashed line) (78); and a four-compartment model (solid line) (92).

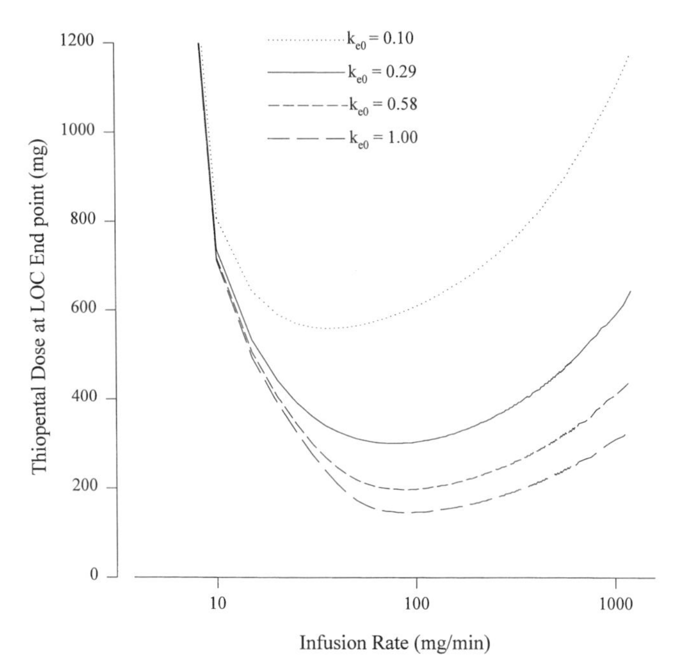

FIGURE 4-7. Simulations of infusion rates and thiopental doses calculated to result in an EC_{50} of 11.3 mg/L using a four-compartment model and four k_{e0}s: k_{e0} 0.10 min^{-1} (dotted line); k_{e0} 0.29 min^{-1} (solid line); k_{e0} 0.29 min^{-1} (solid line); k_{e0} 0.58 min^{-1} (dashed line); and k_{e0} 1.00 min^{-1} (long dashes). (From Gentry WB, Krejcie TC, Henthorn TK, et al. Effect of infusion rate on thiopental dose-response relationships. Anesthesiology 1994;81:316–324.)

REFERENCES

1. Dundee JW. Fifty Years of Thiopentone. Br J Anaesthesia. 56:211–213, 1984.
2. Brodie BB, Mark LC, Papper EM, Lief PA, Bernstein E, and Rovenstein EA. The fate of thiopental in man and a method for its estimation in biological material. J Pharmacol Exp Ther 98:85–96, 1950.

3. Price HL. A dynamic concept of the distribution of thiopental in the human body. Anesthesiology 1960;21:40.
4. Dundee JW, Wyant GM. Intravenous anesthesia. Edinburgh: Churchill Livingstone 1988.
5. Morgan DJ, Blackmann GL, Paull JD, Wolf LJ. Pharmacokinetics and plasma binding of thiopental. I. Studies in surgical patients. Anesthesiology 1983;54:468.
6. Burch PG, Stanski DR. The role of metabolism and protein binding in thiopental anesthesia. Anesthesiology 1983;58:146–152.
7. Pandele G, Chaux F, Salvadori C, et al. Thiopental pharmacokinetics in patients with cirrhosis. Anesthesiology 1983;59:123.
8. Hu OY-P, Chu KM, Liu HS, et al. Reinduction of the hypnotic effects of thiopental with NSAIDs by decreasing thiopental plasma protein binding in humans. Acta Anaesthesiol Scand 1993;37:258.
9. Tanelian DL, Kosek P, Mody I, Baclver B. The role of the $GABA_A$ receptor/chloride channel complex in anesthesia. Anesthesiology 78:757–776, 1993.
10. Frenkel C, Duch DS, Urban BW. Molecular actions of pentobarbital isomers on sodium channels from human brain cortex. Anesthesiology 1990;72:640–649.
11. Frenkel C, Duch DS, Urban BW. Effect of IV anaesthetics on human brain sodium channels. Br J Anaesth 1993;71:15–24.
12. Brooks LM, Bollman JL, Flock EV, Lundy JS. Tissue distribution with time following single intravenous administration of sodium pentothal (sodium ethyl (-methylbutly thiobarbiturate) [Abstract]. Am J Physiol 1948;155:429.
13. Saidman LJ, Eger EI. The effect of thiopental metabolism on duration of anesthesia. Anesthesiology 1966;27:118–126.
14. Breimer DD. Pharmacokinetics of methohexitone following intravenous infusion in humans. Br J Anaesth 1976;48:643–649.
15. Hudson RJ, Stanski DR, Burch PG. Pharmacokinetics of methohexital and thiopental in surgical patients. Anesthesiology 1983;59:215–219.
16. Christensen JH, Andreasen F, Jansen JA. Pharmacokinetics of thiopentone in a group of young women and a group of young men. Br J Anaesth 1980;52:913.
17. Henthorn TK, Avram MJ, Krejcie TC. Intravascular mixing and drug distribution: the concurrent disposition of thiopental and indocyanine green. Clin Pharmacol Ther 1989;45:56.
18. Avram Mj, Krejcie TC, Henthorn TK. The relationship of age to the pharmacokinetics of early drug distribution: the concurrent disposition of thiopental and indocyanine green. Anesthesiology 1990;72:403–411.
19. Mark LC, Brand L, Kamyyssi S, et al. Thiopental metabolism by human liver in vivo and in vitro. Nature 1965;206:1117.
20. Duvaldestin P, Charvin M, Lebrault C, et al. Effect of upper abdominal surgery and cirrhosis upon the pharmacokinetics of methohexital. Acta Anaesthesiol Scand 1991;35:159.
21. Lange H, Staphan H, Brand C, et al. Hepatic disposition of methohexitone in patients undergoing coronary bypass surgery. Br J Anaesth 1992;69:478.
22. Stanski DR, Mihm FG, Rosenthal MH, Kalman SM. Pharmacokinetics of high-dose thiopental used in cerebral resuscitation. Anesthesiology 1980;53:169.
23. Turcant A, Delhumeau A, Premel-Cavic A, et al. Thiopental pharmacokinetics under conditions of long-term infusion. Anesthesiology 1985;63:50–54.
24. Hull, CJ. Pharmacokinetics for anaesthesia. London: Butterworth-Heinemann, 1991.
25. Campbell GA, Morgan DJ, Kumar K, Crankshaw DP. Extended blood collection period required to define distribution and elimination kinetics of propofol. Br J Clin Pharmacol 1988; 26:187.
26. Michenfelder JD. the interdependency of cerebral functional and metabolic effects following massive doses of thiopental in the dog. Anesthesiology 1974;41:231.
27. Stullken EH, Milde JH, Michenfelder JD, Tinker JH. The nonlinear responses of cerebral metabolism to low concentrations of halothane, enflurane, isoflurane, and thiopental. Anesthesiology 1977;46:28–34.
28. Pierce EC, Lambertsen CJ, Deutsch S, et al. Cerebral circulation and metabolism during thiopental anesthesia and hyperventilation in man. J Clin Invest 1962;41:1664.
29. Rockoff MA, Marshall LF, Shapiro HM. High-dose barbiturate therapy in humans: a clinical review of 60 patients. Ann Neurol 1979;6:194.
30. Kiersey DK, Bickford RG, Faulkner A. electroencephalographic patterns produced by thiopental sodium during surgical operations: description and classification. Br J Anaesth 1951; 23:141.
31. Fragen RJ, Avram MJ. Barbiturates. In Miller RD, ed. Anesthesia. 4th ed. New York: Churchill Livingstone, 1994.
32. Rockoff MA, Goudsouzian NG. Seizures induced by methohexital. Anesthesiology 1981;54:333–335.
33. Todd MM, Drummond JC, U HS. The hemodynamic consequences of high-dose methohexital anesthesia in humans. Anesthesiology 1984;61:495–501.
34. Male CG, Allen EM. Methohexitone induced convulsions in epileptics. Anaesth Intensive Care 1977;5:226–230.
35. Eckstein JW, Hamilton WK, McCammond JM. The effect of thiopental on peripheral venous tone. Anesthesiology 1961; 22:525–528.
36. Allen GD, Kennedy WF, Everett G, Tolas AG. A comparison of the cardiorespiratory effects of methohexital and thiopental supplementation for outpatient dental anesthesia. Anesth Analg 1969;48:730–737.
37. Chamberlain JH, Seed RGFL, Chung DCW. Effect of thiopentone on myocardial function. Br J Anaesth 1977;49:865–870.
38. Skovsted P, Price ML, Price HL. The effects of short-acting barbiturates on arterial pressure, preganglionic sympathetic activity, and barostatic reflexes. Anesthesiology 1970;33:10–18.
39. Flickinger H, Fraimow W, Cathcart RT, Nealon TF. Effect of thiopental induction on cardiac output in man. Anesth Analg 1961;40:693–700.
40. Reiz S, Balfors E, Friedman A, et al. Effects of thiopental on cardiac performance, coronary hemodynamics and myocardial oxygen consumption in chronic ischemic heart disease. Acta Anaesthesiol Scand 1981;25:103–110.
41. Hirshman CA, McCullough RE, Cohen PJ, Weil JV. Hypoxic ventilatory drive in dogs during thiopental, ketamine or pentobarbital anesthesia. Anesthesiology 1975;43:628–634.
42. Harrison GA. The influence of different anaesthetic agents on the response to respiratory tract irritation. Br J Anaesth 1962; 34:804–811.
43. Barker P, Langton JA, Wilson IG, Smith G. Movements of the vocal cords on induction of anaesthesia with thiopentone or propofol. Br J Anaesth 1992;69:23–25.
44. Forbes AR, Gamsu G. Depression of lung mucociliary clearance by thiopental and halothane. Anesth Analg 1979;58:387–389.
45. Bittrich NM, Kane AV'R, Mosher RE. Methohexital and its effect on liver function tests: a comparative study. Anesthesiology 1963;24:81–90.
46. Guerra F. Thiopental forever after. In Aldrete JA, Stanley TH, eds. Trends in intravenous anesthesia. Chicago: Year Book, 1980:143.
47. Ghoneim MM, Pandya H. Plasma protein binding of thiopental in patients with impaired renal or hepatic function. Anesthesiology 1975;42:545–549.
48. Hirshman CA, Edelstein RA, Ebertz JM, Hanifin JM. Thiobarbiturate-induced histamine release in human mast cells. Anesthesiology 1985;63:353.
49. Fragen RJ, Shanks CA, Molteni A, Avram MJ. Effects of etomidate on hormonal responses to surgical stress. Anesthesiology 1984;61:652–656.

50. Kaniaris P, Katsilambros N, Castanas E, et al. Relation between glucose tolerance and serum insulin levels in man before and after thiopental intravenous administration. Anesth Analg 1975;54:718.
51. Whitwam JG, Methohexitone. Br J Anaesth 1976;48:641.
52. Stone HH, Donnelly CC. The accidental intra-arterial injection of thiopental. Anesthesiology 1961;22:995.
53. Clark RSJ. Adverse effects of intravenously administered drugs used in anaesthetic practice. Drugs 1981;22:26.
54. Thompson DS, Eason CN, Flacke JW. Thiamylal anaphylaxis. Anesthesiology 1973;39:556.
55. Remmer H. The role of the liver in drug metabolism. Am J Med 1970;49:617.
56. Wright PMC, Carabine UA, McClune S, et al. Preanaesthetic medication with clonidine: A dose-response study. Br J Anaesth 1990;65:628–632.
57. Buhrer M, Mappes A, Lauber R, et al. Dexmedetomidine decreases thiopental dose requirement and alters distribution pharmacokinetics. Anesthesiology 1994;80:1216–1227.
58. Couderc E, Ferrier C, Haberer JP, et al. Thiopentone pharmacokinetics in patients with chronic alcoholism. Br J Anaesth 1984;56:1393–1397.
59. Swerdlow BN, Holler FO, Maitre PO, Stanski DR. Chronic alcohol intake does not change thiopental anesthetic requirement, pharmacokinetics or pharmacodynamics. Anesthesiology 1990;72:455–461.
60. Krintel JJ, Wegmann F. Aminophylline reduces the depth and duration of sedation with barbiturates. Acta Anaesthesiol Scand 1987;31:352.
61. Chaplin MD, Roszkowski AP, Richards PK. Displacement of thiopental from plasma proteins by nonsteroidal anti-inflammatory agents. Proc Soc Exp Biol Med 1973;143:667–671.
62. Csogor SI, Kerek SF. Enhancement of thiopentone anaesthesia by sulphafurazole. Br J Anaesth 1970;42:988–990.
63. Kosaka Y, Takahashi T, Mark LC. Intravenous thiobarbiturate anesthesia for cesarean section. Anesthesiology 1969;31:489–506.
64. Bernstein K, Gisselsson L, Jacobsson L, Ohrlander S. Influence of two different anaesthetic agents on the new born and the correlation between foetal oxygenation and induction-delivery time in elective cesarean section. Acta Anaesthesiol Scand 1985; 29:157–160.
65. Bland BAR, Lawes EG, Duncan PW, et al. Comparison of midazolam and thiopental for rapid sequence anesthetic induction for elective cesarean section. Anesth Analg 1987;66:1165–1168.
66. Shnider SM, Levinson G. Anesthesia for obstetrics. 2nd ed. Baltimore: Williams & Wilkins, 1987.
67. Westrin Pl Jonmarker C, Werner O. Thiopental requirements for induction of anesthesia in neonates and in infants one to six months of age. Anesthesiology 1989;71:344–346.
68. Kingston HGG, Kendrick A, Sommer KM, et al. Binding of thiopental in neonatal serum. Anesthesiology 1990;72:428–431.
69. Sorbo S, Hudson RJ, Loomis JC. The pharmacokinetics of thiopental in pediatric surgical patients. Anesthesiology 1984; 61:666–670.
70. Brodie BB, Marc LC, Lief PA, et al. Acute tolerance to thiopentone in man. J Pharmacol Exp Ther 1951;102:215.
71. Dundee JW, Price HI, Dripps Rd. Acute tolerance to thiopentone in man. Br J Anaesth 1956;28:344.
72. Toner W, Howard PJ, McGowan WAW, Dundee JW. Another look at acute tolerance to thiopentone. Br J Anaesth 1980; 52:1005.
73. Hudson RJ, Stanski DR, Saidman LJ, Meathe E. A model for studying depth of anesthesia and acute tolerance to thiopental. Anesthesiology 1983;59:301–307.
74. Barratt R, Graham GG, Torda TA. The influence of sampling site upon the distribution phase kinetics of thiopentone. Anaesth Intensive Care 1984;12:5.
75. Barratt R, Graham GG, Torda TA. Kinetics of thiopentone on relation to the site of sampling. Br J Anaesth 1984;56:1385–1391.
76. Stanski DR, Hudson RJ, Homer TD, et al. Pharmacodynamics modeling of thiopental anesthesia. J Pharmacokinet Biopharm 1984;12;223–240.
77. Homer TD, Stanski DR. The effect of increasing age on thiopental disposition and anesthetic requirement. Anesthesiology 1985;62:714–724.
78. Stanski DR, Maitre PO. Population pharmacokinetics and pharmcodynamics of thiopental: the effect of age revisited. Anesthesiology 1990;72:412–422.
79. Sheiner LB, Stanski DR, Vozeh S, et al. Simultaneous modeling of pharmacokinetics and pharmacodynamics: application to d-tubocurarine. Clin Pharmacol Ther 1979;25;358–371.
80. Shanks CA, Avram MJ, Krejcie TC, et al. A pharmacokinetic-pharmacodynamic model for quantal responses with thiopental. J Pharmacokinet Biopharm 1993;21:309–321.
81. Hung OR, Varvel JR, Shafer SL, Stanski DR. Thiopental pharmacodynamics. II. Quantitation of clincial and electroencephalic depth of anesthesia. Anesthesiology 1992;77:237–244.
82. Henthorn TK. Pharmacokinetics of intravenous induction agents. In: Bowdle TA, Horita A, Kharasch ED, eds. The Pharmacologic Basis of Anesthesiology. New York: Churchill Livingstone, 1994.
83. Lauven PM, Schwilden H, Stoekel H. Threshold hypnotic concentration of methohexitone. Eur J Clin Pharmacol 1987;33:261.
84. Christensen JH, Andreasen F. Individual variation in response to thiopental. Acta Anaesthesiol Scand 1978;22:203–213.
85. Dundee JW, Hassard TH, McGowan WAW, Henshaw J. The "induction" dose of thiopentone: a method of study and preliminary illustrative results. Anaesthesia 1982;37:1176–1184.
86. Halford FJ. A critique of intravenous anesthesia in war surgery. Anesthesiology 1943;4:67.
87. Dundee JW, Richards RK. Effect of azotemia upon the action of intravenous barbiturate anesthesia. Anesthesiology 1954; 15:333–346.
88. Wulfsohn NL, Joshi CW. Thiopentone dosage based on lean body mass. Br J Anaesth 1969;41:516–521.
89. Avram MJ, Sanghvi R, Henthorn TK, et al. Determinants of thiopental induction dose requirements. Anesth Analg 1993; 76:10–17.
90. Danhof M, Levy G. Kinetics of drug action in disease states. I. Effect of infusion rate on phenobarbital concentrations in serum, brain and cerbrospinal fluid of normal rates at onset of loss of righting reflex. J Pharmacol Exp Ther 1984;229:44–50.
91. Klockowski PM, Levy G. Kinetics of drug action in disease states. XXI. Relationship between drug infusion rate and dose required to produce a pharmacologic effect. J Pharm Sci 1987; 76:516–520.
92. Gentry WB, Krejcie TC, Henthorn TK, et al. Effect of infusion rate on thiopental dose-response relationships. Anesthesiology 1994;81:316–324.
93. Niazi S. Volume of distribution as a function of time. J Pharm Sci 1976;65:452–454.
94. Henthorn TK, Krejcie TC, Shanks CA, Avram MJ. Time-dependent distribution volume and kinetics of the pharmacodynamic effector site. J Pharm Sci 1992;81:1136–1138.

5 Benzodiazepines

Robert Litz Coleman and Jim Temo

The nearly coincidental discovery and subsequent commercial development of benzodiazepines offered a class of drugs that arguably has been one of the most intensely evaluated and widely used drug groups in modern medicine (1) (Table 5-1). The reasons for the acceptance of benzodiazepines include their broad spectrum of central nervous system (CNS) activity, proven efficacy in reducing anxiety and treating sleep irregularities, relative therapeutic safety, and aggressive product marketing. Over 15 benzodiazepine compounds are available for clinical use in the United States, several of which are commonly administered during the perioperative period (Fig. 5-1).

In 1957, Dr. Leo Sternbach submitted the first benzodiazepine (Ro 5-0690 or chlordiazepoxide) for pharmacologic testing by Dr. Lowell O. Randall, who described the drug's sedative and muscle relaxant properties in animals. These features were especially notable because they were unlike the properties of the convulsant compounds that were previously submitted by Dr. Sternbach for laboratory evaluation. The first reported use of benzodiazepines in conjunction with anesthesia was by Brandt and associates, who used chlordiazepoxide as a component of preanesthetic medication (5). With additional study, analogs of the original sedative compound were evaluated and were found to possess less desirable qualities than the parent compound. Nonetheless, the repeated screening of newer analogs demonstrated that the benzodiazepine molecule exhibited multiple traits consisting of anticonvulsant properties, "taming" (calming) effects, and appetite stimulation (2).

In 1959, Sternbach and Reeder initiated studies with one of the chlordiazepoxide analogs and found it to be 3 to 10 times more potent than the original compound. The superior potency of the substance, coupled with its impressive pharmacologic and toxicologic data (3), led to the introduction of diazepam (4).

In 1964, DuCailar and associates and Campan and Espagno of France successfully used diazepam for relief of preoperative anxiety. Shortly thereafter, the drug's utility was also demonstrated in the United States as a component of neuroleptanalgesic techniques (3). About this same time, the use of diazepam as an anesthetic induction agent was investigated in several countries outside the United States (6). Subsequent studies also evaluated the efficacy of diazepam in relieving maternal anxiety during labor and in managing eclampsia, status epilepticus, and tetanus (7-12).

In 1971, lorazepam was discovered in the search for a more potent benzodiazepine. This exploration was encouraged by the synthesis of an active metabolite of diazepam, oxazepam, in 1961 (1). In 1976, investigators at the Roche Laboratories in Basel, Switzerland, synthesized midazolam, the first water-soluble benzodiazepine. Midazolam had a shortened half-life ($t_{1/2}$), it possessed more profound amnestic qualities, and it lacked the irritant effects of diazepam following parenteral administration (13-17). Midazolam has become one of the most widely used intravenous drugs in anesthesiology.

Finally, the isolation and discovery of a γ-aminobutyric acid (GABA)-benzodiazepine receptor complex in 1977 (Fig. 5-2) gave research chemists an avenue for synthesizing and testing many new benzodiazepine agonist and antagonist compounds (1). This receptor discovery also led to the synthesis of the first specific benzodiazepine antagonist, flumazenil. The history of benzodiazepines continues to evolve and will possibly lead to even more clinically useful compounds in the future (e.g., Ro 48-6791).

MECHANISMS OF ACTION

The benzodiazepines exert their general effects by occupying the benzodiazepine receptor, facilitating the inhibitory action of GABA on neuronal transmission. The benzodiazepine receptors are found in highest

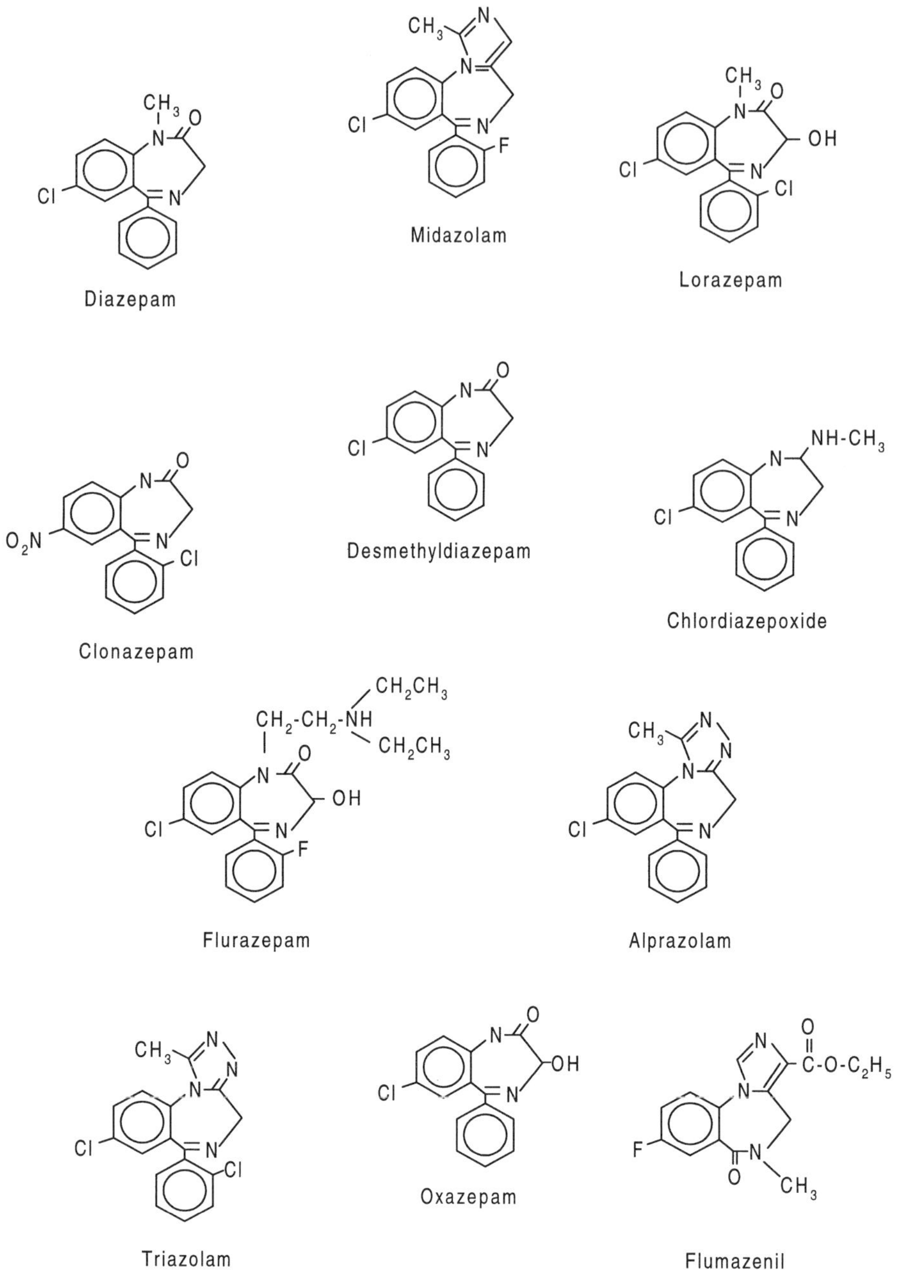

Diazepam

Midazolam

Lorazepam

Clonazepam

Desmethyldiazepam

Chlordiazepoxide

Flurazepam

Alprazolam

Triazolam

Oxazepam

Flumazenil

FIGURE 5-1. Structures of the benzodiazepines.

density in the olfactory bulb, cerebral cortex, cerebellum, hippocampus, substantia nigra, and inferior colliculus. However, high receptor densities are also found in the striatum, lower brain stem, and spinal cord (18-24). The anxiolytic, anticonvulsant, and muscle relaxation effects of benzodiazepines are mediated at the GABA receptor, whereas the hypnotic effects appear to be mediated elsewhere (25). The binding of benzodiazepines to the receptor is stereospecific and saturable, with the potency depending on receptor affinity. Plasma concentration influences the drug effect because 20% receptor occupancy is sufficient to produce anxiolysis, 30 to 50% occupancy produces sedation, and 60% or greater occupancy is necessary to produce hypnosis or unconsciousness (26, 27).

Two GABA receptors have been identified, and the benzodiazepine receptor is part of the $GABA_A$ receptor complex on the subsynaptic membrane of the effector neuron. This complex is made up of three protein subunits, α, β, and γ, arranged in a five-member complex (25, 28, 29). The benzodiazepine receptor is located on the γ subunit, and the GABA appears to bind on each on the two β subunits (25, 29). Activation of the receptor results in hyperpolarization of the cell from opening of the chloride ion channel, which is formed by contributions of each subunit (25, 28, 30-32). Hyperpolarized neurons are resistant to excitation. Investigators have postulated that the hypnotic effects are mediated by alterations in a potential-dependent calcium ion flux (25). Long-term administration of ben-

TABLE 5-1. Benzodiazepines Used Clinically in the United States

Generic Name	Trade Name	Half-life (h)	Clinical Applications
Alprazolam	Xanax	12–15	Anxiolysis
Chlordiazepoxide	Librium	8–18	Alcohol withdrawal, etc.
Clonazepam	Klonopin	18.7–39	Treatment of epilepsy
Clorazepate	Tranxene	2.4	Treatment of epilepsy and alcohol withdrawal
Desmethyldiazepam	Nordiazepam and Nadar	20–200	
Diazepam	Valium		Sedation, induction and maintenance of anesthesia
Estazolam	ProSom	14	Treatment of insomnia
Flumazenil	Mazicon	0.7–1.3	Reversal of benzodiazepine agonists
Flurazepam	Dalmane	2–3	Treatment of insomnia
Lorazepam	Ativan	10–22	Anxiolysis and sedation
Midazolam	Versed	1.7–2.6	Sedation, induction and maintenance of anesthesia
Oxazepam	Serax	3–21	Anxiolysis
Prazepam	Centrax	63–70	Anxiolysis
Quazepam	Doral	25–41	Treatment of insomnia
Temazepam	Restoril	10–21	Treatment of insomnia
Triazolam	Halcion	2–3	Treatment of insomnia

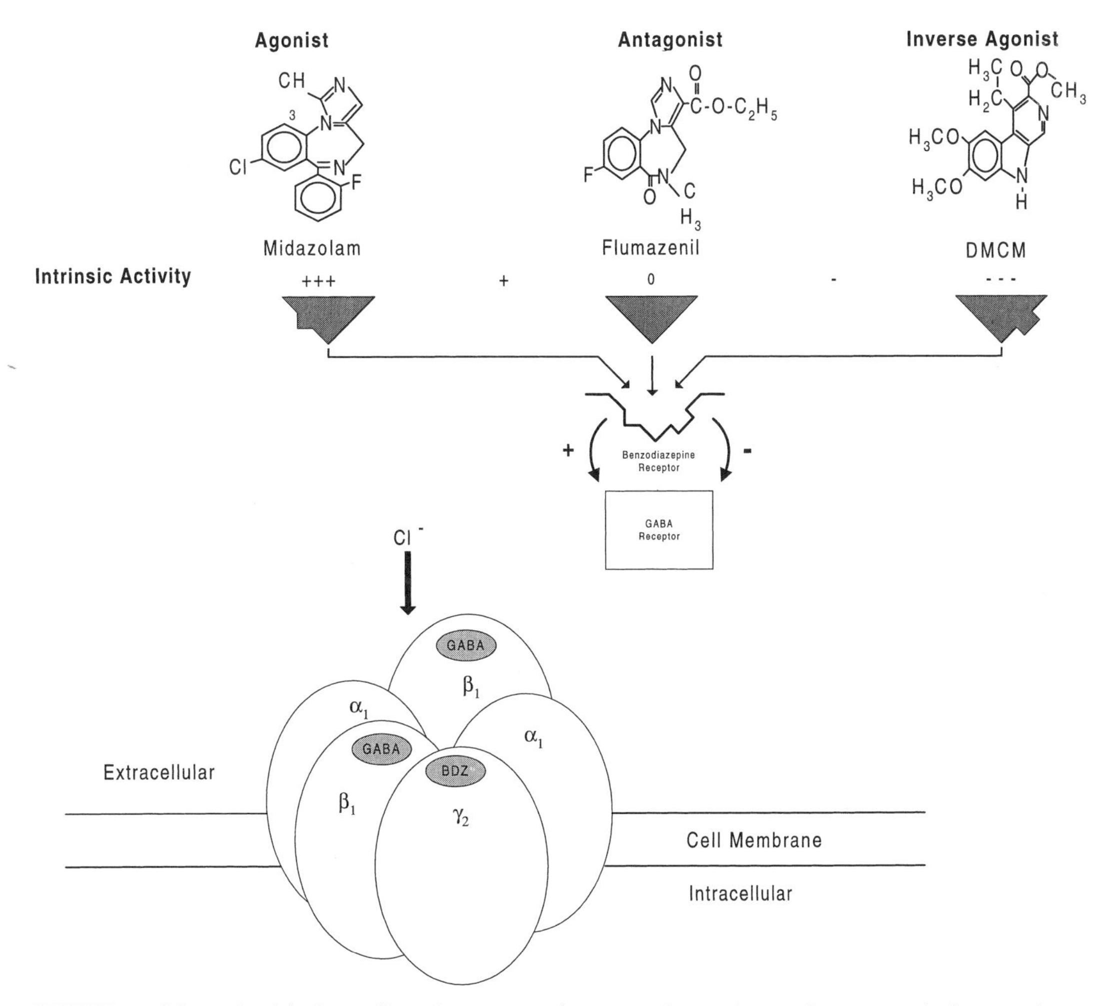

FIGURE 5-2. Schematic of the benzodiazepine receptor. A pentameric protein complex composed of α, β, and γ subunits. The site of the benzodiazepine receptor is on the β subunit, and γ-aminobutyric acid (GABA) receptors are located on each of the two β subunits. Benzodiazepine receptor ligands range in activity from agonists to inverse agonists. Agonists have the greatest inverse activity, and inverse agonists have the least. (Data from references 23 and 28.)

zodiazepines (e.g., continuous infusions in the intensive care unit [ICU]) produces downregulation of the CNS receptor, resulting in tolerance to the drug (33).

Three different type of ligands for the GABA receptor have been identified (23). Agonists alter the affinity for the receptor complex so binding affinity of GABA is increased. Antagonists occupy the receptor, but they produce no intrinsic activity, thereby blocking GABA action. Inverse agonists reduce the efficiency of GABA-adrenergic synaptic transmission, resulting in CNS stimulation (26, 34) (Fig. 5-2).

MIDAZOLAM

Midazolam is a water-soluble, short-acting benzodiazepine with potency that is two to three times greater than diazepam. It has a distribution $t_{1/2}$ ($t_{1/2\alpha}$) value of 5 to 10 minutes and an elimination $t_{1/2}$ ($t_{1/2\beta}$) value of 2 to 4 hours (14, 17). Its imidazole ring structure contributes to its rapid metabolism and stability in aqueous solution. Midazolam has been most effective as an antianxiety medication in the immediate preanesthetic and preprocedure period and also as an anesthetic induction agent in selected clinical situations. Like other benzodiazepines, midazolam has been used to provide sedation and amnesia, as well as to treat convulsions, with anticonvulsant properties comparable to those of diazepam (35). Routes of administration for this compound have included intravenous, intramuscular, oral, intranasal, and rectal (36).

Chemistry and Physical Properties

Midazolam (8-chloro-6(2-fluorophenyl-1-methyl)-4H-imidazo [1,5a][1,4] benzodiazepine) is a water-soluble agent with a pKa of 6.15. Therefore, it requires no potentially harmful or irritating solvents as carrier solutions, and it does not breakdown into strongly active metabolites, unlike other members of the benzodiazepine group (37, 38). In solution, midazolam is buffered to a pH of 3.5, which allows the imidazole ring to remain open and maintain water solubility. Following parenteral injection, the imidazole ring closes, allowing midazolam to become highly lipid soluble and leading to a rapid onset of its central effects. In clinical use, midazolam preparations are compatible with crystalloid solutions, opioids, and anticholinergic drugs.

Pharmacokinetics and Pharmacodynamics

Midazolam is highly protein bound, with approximately 96% of an injected dose bound to albumin (15, 39-41). This binding does not appear to depend on its plasma concentration (42). However, in the presence of extreme hypoalbuminemia, rapid and profound CNS effects may result because of the increased concentration of free drug (15, 39, 43, 44). In normal physiologic states, the highly lipophilic compound is still notable for its rapid CNS effects and a large volume of distribution (4). The disappearance of its CNS effects is primarily a result of redistribution, although after extensive and prolonged infusion of midazolam, increased dosage is required because of progressively greater hepatic clearance (41). The usual clearance rate of midazolam ranges from 6 to 11 ml/kg/min, compared with 0.2 to 0.5 ml/kg/min for diazepam and 0.8 to 1.8 ml/kg/min for lorazepam.

Metabolism and biotransformation of midazolam are similar to those of other benzodiazepines and involve oxidative hepatic microsomal pathways or glucuronide conjugation. The total body clearance is high and exceeds that of other benzodiazepine drugs (39, 45). When given orally, midazolam is absorbed from the gastrointestinal tract, with approximately 50% of the administered dose reaching the circulation (42), indicating a sizable "first-pass" hepatic effect. Midazolam is broken down into at least four relatively inactive metabolites, with only small amounts of the parent compound excreted unchanged in the urine. The principal metabolite is α-hydroxymidazolam, which is partially active; however, the contribution of this metabolite is negligible because of its rapid conjugation and subsequent elimination. Two other notable metabolites are 4-hydroxymidazolam and α,4-hydroxymidazolam, which are also excreted in the urine as glucuronide conjugates (46).

Central Nervous System Effects

Midazolam is associated with dose-related effects on cerebral metabolism and blood flow and has been used for induction of anesthesia in patients with intracranial disorders or decreased intracranial compliance (47). Midazolam may also protect the brain against cerebral hypoxic events, although its effect was less than those produced by pentobarbital (48). The time for induction of anesthesia appears to be dose related, partly because of extensive protein binding (42, 49). Midazolam is not associated with protection against the acute hemodynamic response to laryngoscopy and intubation. Midazolam, like diazepam and lorazepam, increases the seizure threshold and lowers mortality rates in animals exposed to toxic levels of local anesthetics (48).

Cardiovascular Effects

When used for induction of anesthesia, midazolam causes a greater decrease in arterial blood pressure than related benzodiazepine compounds, but the hypotensive effect is similar to that of thiopental 3 to 4 mg/kg (50). This transient hypotensive effect has not prevented the successful use of midazolam at doses up to 0.2 mg/kg in patients with severe aortic stenosis

(51). In the presence of severe hypovolemia, midazolam exerts the same hypotensive effects expected with other intravenous induction agents (52).

The hemodynamic effects of midazolam are dose related, but apparently a plasma level (ceiling) exists above which additional administration does not result in increasingly profound consequences (53). In patients who have increased left ventricular filling pressures, midazolam can lower filling pressures and increase cardiac output, mimicking the effects found with nitroglycerin administration (54-56). Studies show that the combination of midazolam with nitrous oxide results in minimal hemodynamic changes. The combined administration of opioids and midazolam, however, may produce a supra-additive hypotensive effect related to reduced sympathetic tone (57, 58) and decreased catecholamine release (59).

Respiratory Effects

Midazolam is associated with a depression of central respiratory drive that is related to both dose and rate of administration (60). Most investigators report that midazolam is similar to diazepam with respect to its effects on central respiratory drive. According to at least two clinical studies, the peak onset of ventilatory depression with intravenous midazolam, 0.13 to 0.2 mg/kg, occurs in 3 to 5 minutes and lasts 60 to 120 minutes (61, 62). In patients with chronic obstructive pulmonary disease, respiratory depression is more profound and lasts longer with midazolam compared with thiopental (26). Investigators have observed that midazolam and other benzodiazepines also have an additive or even synergistic respiratory depressant effect when they are given in combination with opioids because these drugs act at different receptors (26). Analogous to thiopental, transient apnea may be induced with midazolam; however, its occurrence is more frequent than with diazepam. This depressant effect is enhanced by increased dosage of the drug, coadministration with opioids, preexisting disease states, and administration to elderly patients (26). Reports have indicated synergism between the respiratory effects of midazolam and the respiratory effects of spinal anesthesia (63, 64). This association has led to the need for vigilant monitoring of respiratory and ventilatory function when midazolam is administered during central neuraxis blockade (26).

Clinical Use

A positive correlation becomes evident between plasma concentrations of midazolam and its sedative and psychomotor effects (40, 43, 44). Individual differences in drug-response relationships appear to be less with midazolam than with diazepam (65). Midazolam can be used for premedication, induction of anesthesia, supplementation of regional and local anesthesia, and in the relief of postoperative anxiety states.

As preanesthetic medication, midazolam meets the primary criterion of providing anxiolysis (17) in many clinical situations (66-70). It has been administered orally, rectally, nasally, intramuscularly, and intravenously, with the first three routes of administration displaying differing efficacy in pediatric patients. Intravenous administration of midazolam is associated with a rapid onset of action (2 to 3 minutes), but it has an initial recovery time similar to that of diazepam because of redistribution effects (71). Following intravenous administration for sedation, midazolam produces profound anterograde amnesia lasting approximately 20 to 30 minutes (71). The residual amnestic effects of midazolam in the immediate postpartum period have contributed to a lack of maternal recall of interactions with her newborn.

Midazolam is considered the benzodiazepine of choice for intravenous induction of anesthesia (26). When administered to premedicated patients in doses of 0.15 to 0.3 mg/kg over 5 to 15 seconds, it induces anesthesia within 30 seconds (72). In unpremedicated patients, White reported that 0.2 to 0.3 mg/kg of midazolam given over 30 to 60 seconds induced loss of consciousness in 110 seconds (73). Anesthesia induction dosages and times can be altered by several factors including the patient's age, physical status, and rate of administration, as well as the presence of other centrally active drugs (Fig. 5-3) (16, 74). Advanced age,

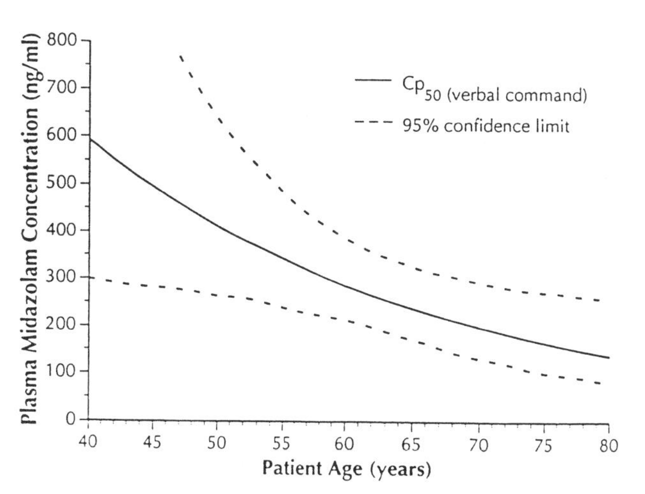

FIGURE 5-3. Midazolam $Cp_{50\ (verbal\ command)}$ as a function of age computed from Equation 4. Confidence limits are included to indicate the effect of the net uncertainty in the mean model parameters estimated on the Cp_{50} calculation. The increasing width of the confidence limits on the calculated Cp_{50} values associated with patient age less than approximately 55 years is presumed to be due to the relatively small number of subjects less than 50 years of age included in the study. (From Jacobs JR, Reves JG, Marty J, et al. Aging increases pharmacodynamic sensitivity to hypnotic effects of midazolam. Anesth Analg 1995;80:143–148.)

preexisting diseases, and rapid bolus injection lead to a reduction of the dose recommended in otherwise healthy individuals (75). Induction of anesthesia is considered complete when the patient experiences loss of responsiveness to verbal commands (26).

Midazolam has also been recommended for use as a continuous infusion in balanced anesthesia because of its desirable hemodynamic stability and amnestic qualities (14, 76). Infusions have also been used to ensure an adequate depth of anesthesia (77, 78). Midazolam produces up to a 30% reduction in the minimum alveolar concentration (MAC) of halothane and presumably of other inhalation agents (77). Maintenance of midazolam infusions also appears to reduce adjuvant drug requirements (26). Continuous infusion regimens of midazolam, in conjunction with opioid analgesics, have been demonstrated to keep patients adequately anesthetized while providing for a prompt emergence from anesthesia at the end of the procedure (79, 80). Midazolam infusions have also proved useful for sedation in the ICU (81, 82). However, marked individual pharmacokinetic variability exists among critically ill patients receiving midazolam infusions (83). Midazolam, like diazepam and lorazepam, can accumulate after repeated bolus dosages or infusions. With midazolam, this accumulation seems to be less problematic because of its high clearance and rapid redistribution properties (26). Additionally, as a result of the current development and use of the benzodiazepine antagonist, flumazenil, reservations about benzodiazepine accumulation seem to be of less concern.

DIAZEPAM

Diazepam is an intravenous and orally active benzodiazepine used as an anxiolytic and an anesthetic induction drug, and it is the drug of first choice in the treatment of status epilepticus.

Chemical and Physical Properties

Diazepam (7-chloro-1,3-dihydro-1-methyl-5-phenyl-2H-1,4-benzodiazepine-2-one) is highly lipid soluble and is virtually insoluble in water (with an octanol-water partition coefficient of 840) (84, 85). The most commonly available parenteral preparation of diazepam is formulated in propylene glycol (40%) and ethyl alcohol (10%), in addition to containing sodium benzoate and benzoic acid as buffers and benzyl alcohol as a preservative. Intravenous use of diazepam is associated with a high incidence of venous thrombosis, phlebitis, and local irritation (86). A lipid emulsified formulation (Dizac) has become available in the United States. The emulsion consists of fractionated soybean oil, factionated egg yolk phospholipids, glycerin, and water (87). The pharmacokinetic and pharmacodynamic effects of diazepam in the lipid emulsion are reported to be comparable to those of other diazepam formulations (88, 89).

Pharmacodynamics

Diazepam is metabolized by hepatic microsomal enzymes to N-desmethyldiazepam and 3-hydroxydiazepam. Both metabolites are then converted to oxazepam, which is then conjugated before its elimination. All the metabolites have some pharmacologic activity (26, 90-93). Diazepam has a relatively long $t_{1/2}\alpha$ of 30 to 60 minutes. The elimination $t_{1/2}$ ($t_{1/2}\beta$) of diazepam is 20 to 50 hours, and its clearance is 0.24 to 0.53 ml/kg/min. The steady-state volume of distribution is 0.7 to 1.7 L/kg. Diazepam is extensively protein bound (96 to 99%), and its metabolites also have long $t_{1/2}\beta$ values (e.g., desmethyldiazepam, 20 to 200 hours; 3-hydroxydiazepam, 10 to 21 hours; and oxazepam, 3 to 21 hours) (90, 91, 94-100).

The $t_{1/2}\beta$ of diazepam is prolonged in elderly patients, in neonates, and in patients with liver disease. Age increases the $t_{1/2}\beta$ of diazepam in a linear fashion. The $t_{1/2}\beta$ in a 20-year-old patient is approximately 20 hours and in an 80-year-old patient it is approximately 90 hours. Metabolism is also affected by genetic, traits, preexisting disease, endocrine status, nutritional status, smoking, sex, and concurrent drug therapy. Diazepam and its metabolites readily cross the blood-brain barrier and the placental barrier and are excreted in breast milk (7, 85, 90, 101-110). Following oral administration, diazepam is rapidly absorbed from the gastrointestinal tract. Peak plasma concentrations occur within 30 to 90 minutes. Absorption following intramuscular administration is erratic. Peak plasma concentration may be lower following intramuscular injection than following oral administration, possibly because of precipitation of diazepam at the site of injection (85, 111-114). Minimal clinical effects are seen at blood levels below 400 μg/L. Sleep occurs at a blood level of approximately 1000 μg/L. Individual responses widely vary (41).

Clinical Pharmacology

The pharmacologic effects of diazepam on the CNS are dose related. The effects of chronic administration of diazepam are cumulative because of the long $t_{1/2}\beta$ of the parent compound and its metabolites (41, 115, 116). Diazepam, like all other benzodiazepines, causes CNS depression ranging from mild sedation to deep coma (18, 41). The response varies widely, especially when diazepam is combined with other CNS depressants (e.g., barbiturate, propofol, opioids) (41). Diazepam has neither analgetic nor antianalgetic effects (117). Tolerance to the CNS depressant effects may develop with long-term therapy or during continuous infusions for sedation (111, 118). Diazepam administration also results in antegrade, but not retrograde, amnesia (119-121). Diazepam reduces both the cerebral metabolic rate for oxygen and cerebral blood flow in a dose-dependent manner (47). Electroencephalographic (EEG) changes associated with diazepam administration resemble those of light sleep, with the appearance of rhythmic β activity (122). Like the other benzodiazepines, diazepam raises the seizure threshold.

Diazepam has minimal cardiovascular depressant effects in humans. Systemic vascular resistance is slightly reduced, resulting in a corresponding slight drop in blood pressure. Although homeostatic mechanisms are preserved, some evidence indicates that diazepam may impair the baroreceptor reflex (123, 124). One study has reported a dose-related "nitroglycerin-like" effect on coronary blood vessels, with preservation of coronary blood flow and cardiac index despite the reduced systemic blood pressure (53, 54).

Intravenous diazepam causes modest respiratory depression, with decreases in tidal volume of 20 to 30%. However, the resultant increase in respiratory rate minimizes the decrease in minute ventilation (125). Opioid analgesics and sedative-hypnotics potentiate its respiratory depressant properties (126-128). Diazepam also produces skeletal muscle relaxation. Increased presynaptic inhibition at the spinal level and a direct peripheral action on the contractile process of the muscle are possible sites of this effect (129). It does not increase the action of neuromuscular blocking agents (125, 130).

Clinical Uses

Because diazepam is a highly effective anxiolytic, sedative, and amnestic, it has widespread clinical applications during the perioperative period. Diazepam has been used for the induction and maintenance of intravenous anesthesia (72, 127, 131-148). Diazepam is effective in the symptomatic relief of anxiety and tension associated with anxiety disorders and acute situational disturbances (86, 149-152). Intravenous diazepam is the drug of choice for initial control of grand mal seizures (10, 153-155). Diazepam is also effective in treating muscle rigidity and spasm caused by low back pain or neurologic disorders (95, 156-159). In one study, diazepam was reported to be effective in reducing postoperative muscle pain (myalgias) following the use of succinylcholine (160).

Toxicity and Side Effects

The most common side effects of intravenous diazepam are pain on injection and venous irritation resulting from the solvents (namely, propylene glycol, ethyl alcohol, and benzyl alcohol) used in the intravenous preparation. The resultant venous irritation may result in thrombosis, phlebitis, and sclerosis. Because of concerns regarding teratogenicity in animals, use in pregnant patients is not advised (41, 86, 87).

LORAZEPAM

Chemistry and Physical Properties

Lorazepam is 7-chloro-5-(*o*-chlorophenyl)1,3-dihydro-3-hydroxy-2H-1,4-benzodiazepin-2-one. Lorazepam is insoluble in water, and this lipid- soluble compound has an octanol-water partition coefficient of 240 (compared with 840 for diazepam) (84).

Pharmacokinetics

Over 90% of an oral dose of lorazepam is absorbed, with peak plasma levels occurring within 2.5 hours (161, 162). Unlike diazepam and chlordiazepoxide, lorazepam is dependably and rapidly absorbed after intramuscular injection, with plasma concentrations peaking within 60 minutes. Intramuscular injection causes minimal discomfort (163). When given intravenously, lorazepam has a rapid $t_{1/2}\alpha$ of 15 to 20 minutes (164) and a $t_{1/2}\beta$ that ranges from 10 to 22 hours. However, the elimination of lorazepam is prolonged by liver disease (41, 164, 165). Lorazepam's volume of distribution ranges from 0.8 to 1.3 L/kg, and its protein binding of 80 to 92% is lower than that of most of other benzodiazepines (165). At equipotent sedative doses, lorazepam provides significantly longer amnestic activity than diazepam despite is shorter $t_{1/2}\beta$ (166, 167). Lorazepam is primarily metabolized to a glucuronide, which is pharmacologically inactive (162, 168).

Clinical Uses

Lorazepam is one of the most potent benzodiazepines. It produces anxiolytic, sedative, and amnestic effects in a dose-related fashion (41). As a result of its profound sedative properties, lorazepam has been widely used for premedication (163, 169-171). The usual premedicant doses do not cause significant changes in cardiorespiratory function (172). Lorazepam's sedative properties also make it useful as an adjunct to local and regional anesthesia (41).

Toxicity and Side Effects

Sedation, dizziness, vertigo, weakness, and unsteadiness are the most frequent side effects. Less frequent side effects of lorazepam include disorientation, depression, headache, confusion, agitation, and delirium (173-175). As a result of its potential for producing prolonged drowsiness following standard premedicant dosages, lorazepam should be used with caution in patients whose neurologic status requires careful monitoring in the postoperative period (176).

CHLORDIAZEPOXIDE

Chlordiazepoxide (7-chloro-2-methylamino-5-phenyl-3H-1,4-benzodiazepine-4-oxide) was the first psychotropic agent in the benzodiazepine class. Unlike most benzodiazepines, chlordiazepoxide is soluble in water (95). When given orally, chlordiazepoxide is rapidly and completely absorbed; pharmacologic effects are detectable within 10 minutes (177-179). Intramuscular absorption is slow and unpredictable (179). Plasma concentrations are maximal at approximately 8 hours (179). Absorption and disposition of the drug are slower in elderly persons and in patients with parenchymal liver disease (180, 181). Chlordizepoxide has a short $t_{1/2}\alpha$ (10 minutes) (177, 178) and a $t_{1/2}\beta$ of 8 to 18 hours, but the drug has two long-acting metabolites (namely, demoxepan and desmethyldiazepam). The volume of distribution of chlordiazepoxide is small (0.3 to 0.6 L/kg), with total clearance values ranging from 0.21 to 0.56 ml/kg/min, and the degree of protein binding is relatively high (94 to 97%) (182).

Chlordiazepoxide can be used for preanesthetic medication because of its anxiolytic and sedative properties (5). The drug is also used to treat withdrawal symptoms of acute alcoholism (183). In patients with proven drug (alcohol) addiction, the use of chlordiazepoxide is not recommended because development of physical and psychologic dependence and withdrawal symptoms can occur after discontinuation of this drug (41, 184).

ALPRAZOLAM

Alprazolam (8-chloro-1-methly-6-phenly-4H-5-triazolo [4,3α] 1,4-benzodiazepine) is useful in the management of anxiety disorders, panic disorders, and depression (185, 186). The drug achieves its peak plasma concentration within 1 to 2 hours after oral administration. Its metabolites are α-hydroxyalprazolam and a benzophenone derivative of alprazolam, and its $t_{1/2}\beta$ is 12 to 15 hours. Safe and effective doses for the short-term relief of anxiety and depression range from 0.25 to 0.5 mg given orally three times daily, with a maximum total daily dose of 4 mg. Use of alprazolam is contraindicated in pregnant women and in patients with acute narrow-angle glaucoma (187, 188).

CLONAZEPAM

Clonazepam (5-(2-chlorophenyl)-1,3-dihydro-7-nitro-2H-1,4-benzodiazepin-2-one) is a benzodiazepine derivative that is useful in the treatment of all forms of epilepsy (including absence seizures). Onset of activity is within 20 to 40 minutes of oral administration, the volume of distribution is 1.8 to 4.4 L/kg, and the $t_{1/2}\beta$ is 18.7 to 39 hours; clonazepam undergoes extensive hepatic metabolism (189, 190). It has been found to be 5 to 10 times more effective as an anticonvulsant than diazepam (191). Clinical uses of clonazepam include the treatment of trigeminal neuralgias, Gilles de la Tourette syndrome, and endogenous depression (192-195).

CLORAZEPATE

Clorazepate is primarily used for the treatment of anxiety and is occasionally used for the treatment of epilepsy and alcohol withdrawal. It can also be used to reduce the anxiety of patients undergoing surgical procedures (196-199). At higher doses, clorazepate may be associated with personality changes such as rage, depression, irratibility, and aggressive behavior (200-204). Clorazepate is rapidly converted in the liver to nordiazepam, which is responsible for most of its central pharmacologic activity. Clorazepate has a $t_{1/2}$ of 2.4 hours, and nordiazepam has a $t_{1/2}$ of 44 hours (205).

DESMETHYLDIAZEPAM

Desmethyldiazepam (7-chloro-1,3-dihydro-5-phenyl-2H-1,4-benzodiazepin-2-one) is a pharmacologically active metabolite of diazepam, chlordiazepoxide, and prazepam. The drug is slightly less potent than the parent compounds and has a long $t_{1/2}\beta$ of 20 to 200 hours (98). This long-acting metabolite of chlordiazepoxide and diazepam may contribute to prolonged postoperative drowsiness when these agents are used for premedication (98, 184).

ESTAZOLAM

Estazolam is a triazobenzodiazepine derivative that is used in the short-term treatment of insomnia. It is particularly useful in patients suffering from nocturnal awakenings. Estrazolam is extensively metabolized, with a $t_{1/2}\beta$ of approximately 14 hours, and its metabolites are primarily excreted in the liver (206, 207).

FLURAZEPAM

Flurazepam (7-chloro-1-diethylaminoethyl-5-[2-fluorphenyl]-2H-1,4-benzodiazepine) is a commonly used sedative and hypnotic drug. Despite its short $t_{1/2}\beta$ of 2 to 3 hours, flurazepam has a prolonged duration of clinical activity because of the long $t_{1/2}\beta$ of its primary active metabolite, desalkylflurazepam. In clinical practice, flurazepam is used primarily to control insomnia (208).

OXAZEPAM

Oxazepam (7-chloro-3-hydroxy-5-phenyl-2H-1,4-benzodiazepin-2-one) is another active metabolite of chlordiazepoxide and diazepam, with a $t_{1/2}\beta$ of 3 to 21 hours, and it has no known active metabolites. The drug is 87 to 97% protein bound (96, 97). Oxazepam is used as an oral anxiolytic agent during the preoperative period, as well as for treatment of acute alcohol withdrawal (94). Fewer side effects are associated with oxazepam than with diazepam or chlordiazepoxide (209).

PRAZEPAM

Prazepam (8-chloro-1-[cyclopropylmethyl]-1,3-dihydro-5-phenyl-2-1,4-benzodiazepin-2-one) is also used as an anxiolytic for preanesthetic medication. However, it is slowly absorbed over a prolonged period after oral administration. Its major metabolite, norprazepam, has a $t_{1/2}\beta$ of 63 to 70 hours. Before elimination from the body, most of the prazepam is metabolized to 3-hydroxyprazepam and oxyazepam (210).

QUAZEPAM

Quazepam (7-chloro-1[2,2,2-trifluroethyl]-5-[0-fluorophenyl]-1,3-dihydro-2H-1,4-benzodiazepin-2-thione) is a long-acting benzodiazepine use primarily for the treatment of insomnia. As a result of its long $t_{1/2}$, quazepam has minimal tendency to cause rebound insomnia even during withdrawal periods. However, it can impair performance on the day after its use as a nighttime hypnotic ("hangover effect") (211-215). The volume of distribution of quazepam is 5.0 L/kg, and it is metabolized to 2-oxoquazepam and N-desalkylflurazepam. The parent drug has a $t_{1/2}\beta$ is 25 to 41 hours, whereas 2-oxoquazepam and N-desalkylflurazepam have $t_{1/2}\beta$ values of 28 to 43 hours and 40 to 114 hours, respectively. In elderly patients, the elimination of N-desalkylflurazepam is approximately twice that in younger patients (216-218).

TEMAZEPAM

Temazepam or 3-hydroxydiazepam (7-chloro-1,3-dihydro-3-hydroxy-1-5-phenyl-2H-1,4-benzodiazepin-2-one) is another hypnotic agent that is absorbed within 20 to 40 minutes and achieves a peak concentration within 2 to 3 hours after oral administration. Temazepam has a $t_{1/2}\beta$ is 10 to 21 hours (95, 100), and no active metabolites have been identified (100). The drug is effective in the relief of insomnia by prolonging total sleeping time and by reducing the number of nocturnal awakenings with a minimum of residual (hangover) effects. Its use in pregnant women is contraindicated (41).

TRIAZOLAM

Triazolam (8-chloro-6-[*o*-chlorophenyl]-1-methyl-4H-5-triazolo-[4,3-α-1,4-benzodiazepine]) is a hypnotic agent that is rapidly absorbed orally; it has inactive metabolites (219) and a $t_{1/2}\beta$ of only 2 to 3 hours. As a result of its strong hypnotic action, the drug is used primarily in the short-term management of insomnia characterized by difficulty in falling asleep and frequent nocturnal awakenings. The most frequent adverse effects of triazolam include fatigue, ataxia, euphoria, incoordination, and drowsiness (220). Hallucinations have been reported after the administration of triazolam, and its use is contraindicated in pregnant patients (221). Analogous to other short-acting hypnotics, rebound insomnia has been reported with triazolam. Controversy surrounds the safety and efficacy of triazolam. Some investigators have reported a high incidence of excitement and violence, whereas others have stated that these side effects are not well documented (220, 222-228).

FLUMAZENIL

Chemistry and Physical Properties

Flumazenil interacts at the central benzodiazepine receptor to antagonize the behavioral, neurologic, and electrophysiologic effects of benzodiazepine agonists and inverse agonists (229). Flumazenil was first synthesized by Hunkeler and associates in 1979 and is the first benzodiazepine antagonist approved for clinical use in the United States (62, 230-238). Chemically, flumazenil is ethyl 8-fluro-5,6-dihydro-5-methyl-6-oxo-4H-imadazo[1,5a](1,4)benzodiazepine-3-carboxylate and is structurally similar to the other benzodiazepines except for the absence of the phenyl group, which is replaced by a carboxyl group [m84, rc2]. Flumazenil has an octanol:water partition coefficient of 14:1 at pH 7.4 and a pK of 1.7, and it is soluble in acidic aqueous solutions (230).

Pharmacokinetics

Flumazenil is rapidly cleared from the plasma secondary to hepatic metabolism (239), with less than 0.2% of an intravenous dose recovered unchanged in the urine (239). Metabolism is partially dependent on hepatic blood flow (239), and three metabolites have been identified, namely, N-desmethylflumazenil, N-desmethylflumazenil acid, and flumazenil acid (239). The activities of these metabolites of flumazenil and their glucuronide conjugates are unknown. Flumazenil's $t_{1/2}\beta$ is 0.7 to 1.3 hours, with a clearance rate of 5 to 20 ml/kg/min and a volume of distribution at steady state of 0.6 to 1.6 L/kg (239-241). Analogous to other benzodiazepines, flumazenil is partially protein bound (239).

Pharmacodynamics

Flumazenil doses of 0.1 to 0.2 mg (corresponding to plasma levels of 3 to 6 ng/ml) produce partial antagonism of benzodiazepine agonist effects. Doses of 0.4 to 1.0 mg (plasma level of 12 to 28 ng/ml) produce antagonism of benzodiazepine-induced sedative and amnestic effects in patients who have received standard premedicant or coinduction-sedation doses of benzodiazepines (e.g., midazolam 3 to 10 mg intravenously or intramuscularly).

Pharmacology

Central Nervous System Effects

Flumazenil has little intrinsic CNS activity in the recommended therapeutic doses and produces no clinically apparent CNS effects in the absence of benzodiazepine receptor agonists (21, 22, 31, 232, 233, 241-245). Although investigators have postulated that low doses may produce a stimulating effect and high doses may cause central depression, these effects are difficult to detect clinically (27). No consistent effect of flumazenil has been demonstrated on the EEG or in studies of cerebral metabolism (242-243). Flumazenil has no anticonvulsant properties, and it reverses the anticonvulsant effects of benzodiazepine receptor agonists in local anesthetic-induced seizures (246).

Clinical effects occur rapidly following intravenous administration (247, 248). Penetration into the brain and binding to the benzodiazepine receptors is rapid, as evidenced by positron emission tomography studies (249). The number of CNS binding sites and the topography of the sites appear to be identical to those of the other benzodiazepines (21, 22, 250). Flumazenil precipitates withdrawal in animals made dependent on benzodiazepines (234). However, flumazenil does not antagonize the effects of barbiturates, meprobamate, alcohol, GABA mimetics, or opioids (21).

Cardiovascular and Respiratory Effects

Flumazenil has little (if any) respiratory depressant effects. Even an overdose of flumazenil, 0.1 mg/kg, failed to produce respiratory depression in healthy volunteers (251). Flumazenil has no significant hemodynamic effect when given alone or to reverse agonists (27, 252-256). Rapid administration of doses of up to 3 mg has been reported to be safe in patients with ischemic heart disease; however, reversal of sedation with higher doses (5 to 10 mg) may precipitate acute anxiety-type reactions and may result in elevations of plasma catecholamine levels (252, 254, 255, 257-260).

Clinical Uses

Flumazenil is used for the therapeutic and diagnostic reversal of benzodiazepine receptor agonists. It improves the level of alertness in patients, and it may also be indicated in the treatment of benzodiazepine overdose (229). Flumazenil should be given in incremental doses of 0.2 to 1 mg up to a maximum dose of 3 mg; it can partially reverse the respiratory depression produced by the benzodiazepine agonists (261). The reversal of midazolam-induced respiratory depression only lasts 3 to 30 minutes (62).

Because flumazenil has a shorter $t_{1/2}\beta$ and a higher plasma clearance than the benzodiazepine receptor agonists, the possibility of resedation exists when a single dose of flumazenil is given to reverse the a benzodiazepine agonist (247, 248). Repeated doses or a continuous infusion of flumazenil, 0.5 to 1.0 mg/kg/min, can be used to minimize the risk of resedation (262).

Contraindications

Flumazenil is contraindicated in patients experiencing a tricyclic antidepressant overdose. Therefore, flumazenil should be used with extreme caution when a mixed overdose with tricyclic antidepressants is suspected because it may unmask tricyclic antidepressant-induced seizures by antagonizing the antiepileptic effect of the concomitantly ingested benzodiazepine (263, 264).

REFERENCES

1. Randall L. Discovery of benzodiazepines. In: Usdin E, Skolnik J, Tallman J, et al, eds. Pharmacology of benzodiazepines. 1982.
2. Tobin J, Bird I, Beyle D. Preliminary evaluation of Librium (Ro5-0690) in the treatment of anixety reactions. Dis Nerv Syst 1960;21 (suppl 3):11.
3. Randall L, Heise G, Schallek W, et al. Pharmacological and clinical studies on Valium, a new psychotherapeutic agent of the benzodiazepine class. Curr Ther Res 1961;3:405.
4. Sternbach L. The discovery of CNS active 1,4-benzodiazepine (chemistry). In: Usdin E, Skolnik J, Tallman J, et al, eds. Pharmacology of benzodiazepines. 1982.
5. Brandt A, Liu S, Briggs B. Trial of chlordiazepoxide as a preanesthetic medication. Anesth Analg 1962;41:557.
6. Blondeau P. Diazepam et anésthesie générale. Cah Anesthesiol 1965;13:207.

7. Bepko F, Lowe E, Waxman B. Relief of the emotional factor in labor with parenterally administered diazepam. Obstet Gynecol 1965;26:852.
8. Lean T, Ratnam S, Sivasamboo R. Use of benzodiazepines in the management of eclampsia. Br J Obstet Gynaecol 1965; 26:852.
9. Gastaut H, Naquet R, Pire R, Tassinari C. Treatment of status epilepticus with diazepam (Valium). Epilepsia 1965;6:167.
10. Lombroso C. Treatment of status epilepticus with diazepam. Neurology 1966;16:629.
11. Shershin P, Katz S. Diazepam in the treatment of tetanus: report of a case following tooth extraction. Clin Med 1964;71:362.
12. Weinberg W. Control of the neuromuscular and convulsive manifestations of severe systemic tetanus: case report with a new drug. Clin Pediatr 1964;3:226.
13. Walser A. Literature review of Ro 21-3981. Basel: Roche Laboratories, Hoffman-LaRoche, 1977 to 1978.
14. Reves JG. Midazolam compared with thiopentone as a hypnotic component in balanced anaesthesia: a randomized, double-blind study. Can Anaesth Soc J 1979;26:42.
15. Reves JG, Newfield P, Smith LR. Influence of serum protein, serum albumin concentrations, and dose on midazolam anesthesia induction times. Can Aneaesth Soc J 1981;28:556.
16. Reves JG, Fragen RJ, Vinik HR, Greenblatt DJ. Midazolam: pharmacology and uses. Anesthesiology 1985;62:310–324.
17. Khanderia U, Pandit SK. Use of midazolam hydrochloride in anesthesia. Clin Pharm 1987;6:533–547.
18. Richter J. Current theories about the mechanisms of benzodiazepines and neuroleptic drugs. Anesthesiology 1981;54:66.
19. Bertillson L. Mechanisms of action of benzodiazepines: GABA hypothesis. Acta Psychiatr Scand Suppl 1978;274:19.
20. Costa E, Giudotti A. Molecular mechanisms in the receptor actions of benzodiazepines. Annu Rev Pharmacol Toxicol 1979; 19:531.
21. Haefely W. The biological basis of benzodiazepine actions. J Psychoactive Drugs 1983;15:19.
22. Haefely W, Pieri L, Polc P, Schaffner R. General pharmacology and neuropharmacology of benzodiazepine derivatives. In: Hoffmeister F, Stille G, eds. Handbook of experimental pharmacology. vol 2. Berlin: Springer, 1981:55.
23. Moehler H, Richards J. The benzodiazepine receptor: a pharmacological control element of brain function. Eur J Anaesthesiol 1988;2:15.
24. Amrein R, Hetzel W. Pharmacology of Dormicum (midazolam) and Anexate (flumazenil). Acta Anaesthesiol Scand 1990; 92:6.
25. Mendelson WB. Neuropharmacology of sleep induction by benzodiazepines. Neurobiology 1992;16:221.
26. Reves JG, Glass PSA, Lubarsky DA. Nonbarbiturate intravenous anesthetics. In: Miller RD, ed. Anesthesia. New York: Churchill Livingstone, 1994.
27. Amrein R, Hetzel W, Harmann D, Lorscheid T. Clinical pharmacology of flumazenil. Eur J Anaesthesiol 1988;2:65.
28. Zorumski CF, Isenberg KE. Insights into the structure and function of GABA-benzodiazepine receptors: ion channels and psychiatry. Am J Psychiatry 1991;148:162.
29. Strange PG. D1/D2 dopamine receptor interaction at the biochemical level. Trends Pharmacol Sci 1991;12:48.
30. Richards J, Moehler H, Haefley W. Benzodiazepine binding sites: receptors or acceptors? Trends Pharmacol Sci 1982;3:233.
31. Young WS, Kuhar MJ. Autoradiographic localization of benzodiazepine receptors in rat brain. J Pharmacol Exp Ther 1980; 212:337.
32. Haefely W, Kulscar A, Moehler H, et al. Possible involvement of GABA in the central actions of benzodiazepines. In: Costa E, Greengard P, eds. Mechanism of action of the benzodiazepines. New York: Raven, 1975.
33. Miller LG. Chronic benzodiazepine administration: from the patient to the gene. J Clin Pharmacol 1991;31:492.
34. Haefely W. The preclinical pharmacology of flumazenil. Eur J Anaesthesiol 1988;2:25.
35. Stoelting RK. Benzodiazepines. In: Stoelting RK, ed. Pharmacology and physiology in anesthetic practice. 2nd ed. Philadelphia: JB Lippincott, 1991.
36. Crevoisier PC, Eckert M, Heizmann P. Relation entre l'effect clinique et pharmacocinetique du midazolam après administration i.v. et i.m. Arznemittelforschung 1981;31:2211.
37. Ziegler WH, Schalch E, Leishman B, Eckert M. Comparison of the effects of intravenously administered midazolam, triazolam and their hydroxymetabolites. Br J Clin Pharmacol 1983;16:63S.
38. Carrougher JG, Kadakia S, Shaffer RT, Barrilleaux C. Venous complications of midazolam versus diazepam. Gastrointest Endosc 1993;39:3.
39. Smith M, Eadie M, O'Rourke B. The pharmacokinetics of midazolam in man. Eur J Clin Pharmacol 1981;19:271–278.
40. Allonen H, Ziegler G, Klotz U. Midazolam kinetics. Clin Pharmacol Ther 1981;30:653–661.
41. Reves J. Benzodiazepines. In: Roberts C, Hug C, eds. Pharmacokinetics of anesthesia. Oxford: Blackwell, 1984:219–251.
42. Greenblatt D, Abernathy D, Morse D, et al. Effect of age, gender and obesity on midazolam kinetics. Anesthesiology 1984;61:27–35.
43. Crevoisier C, Ziegler W, Eckert M, et al. Relationship between plasma concentration and effect of midazolam after oral and intravenous administration. Br J Clin Pharmacol 1983;16 (suppl 1):51–61.
44. Godtilsben O, Jerko D, Gordeladze J. Residual effect of single and repeated doses of midazolam and nitrazepam in relation to their plasma concentrations. Eur J Clin Pharmacol 1986; 19:595–600.
45. Jochemsen R, Rijn PV, Hazelset T. Comparative pharmacokinetics of midazolam and lorazepam in healthy subjects after oral administration. Biopharm Drug Dispos 1986;7:53–61.
46. Heizmann P, Eckert M, Ziegler W. Pharmacokinetics and bioavailability of midazolam in man. Br J Clin Pharmacol 1983;16 (suppl 1):43–49.
47. Forster A, Juge O, Morel D. Effects of midazolam on cerebral blood flow in human volunteers. Anesthesiology 1980;53:494–499.
48. deJong R, Bonin J. Benzodiazepines protect mice from local anesthetics and deaths. Anesth Analg 1981;60:385.
49. Dundee J, Kawar P. Consistency of action of midazolam. Anesth Analg 1982;61.
50. Lebowitz P, Cote M, Daniels A, et al. Comparative cardiovascular effects of midazolam and thiopental in healthy patients. Anesth Analg 1982;61:771.
51. Croughwell N, Reves J, Hawkins E. Cardiovascular changes after midazolam in patients with aortic stenosis: effects of nitrous oxide. Anesth Analg 1988;67 (suppl 1).
52. Adams P, Gelman S, Reves J, et al. Midazolam pharmacodynamics and pharmacokinetics during acute hypovolemia. Anesthesiology 1985;63:140–146.
53. Sunzel M, Paalzow L, Berggren L, Eriksson I. Respiratory and cardiovascular effects in relation to plasma levels of midazolam and diazepam. Br J Clin Pharmacol 1988;25:561.
54. Cote P, Gueret P, Courassa M. Systemic and coronary hemodynamic effects of diazepam in patients with mormal and diseased coronary arteries. Circulation 1974;50:1210.
55. Reves J, Samuelson P, Lewis S. Midazolam maleate induction in patients with ischemic heart disease: haemodynamic observations. Can J Anaesth 1979;26:402.
56. Reves J, Samuelson P, Linnan M. Effects of midazolam maleate in patients with elevated pulmonary artery occluded pressure.

In: Aldrete J, Stanley T, eds. Trends in intravenous anesthesia. Chicago: Year Book, 1980.
57. Tomichek R, Rosow C, Schneider R. Cardiovascular effects of diazepam-fentanyl anesthesia in patients with coronary artery disease. Anesth Analg 1982;61:217.
58. Reves J, Croughwell N. Valium-fentanyl interaction. P356. In: Reves J, Hall K, eds. Common problems in cardiac anesthesia. Chicago: Year Book, 1987.
59. Ruff R, Reves J. Hemodynamic effects of a lorazepam-fentanyl anesthetic induction for coronary artery bypass surgery. J Cardiothorac Anesth 1990;4:314.
60. Alexander C, Teller L, Gross J. Slow injection does not preclude midazolam induced ventilatory depression. Anesth Analg 1992;74:260.
61. Gross J, Zebrowski M, Carel W, et al. Time course of ventilatory depression after thiopental and midazolam in normal subjects and in patients with chronic obstructive pulmonary disease. Anesthesiology 1983;58:540.
62. Brogden R, Goa K. Flumazenil. Drugs 1991;42:1061.
63. Gauthier R, Dyck B, Chung F. Respiratory interaction after spinal anesthesia and sedation with midazolam. Anesthesiology 1992;77:909.
64. Ben-David B, Vaida S, Gaitini L. The influence of high spinal on sensitivity to midazolam sedation. Anesth Analg 1995; 81:525–528.
65. Dundee J, Samuel I, Howard P. Midazolam: a water soluble benzodiazepine. Anaesthesia 1980;35:454.
66. Rosenberg M, Raymond C, Bridge P. Comparison of midazolam/ketamine with methohexital for sedation during peribulbar block. Anesth Analg 1995;81:173–174.
67. Feld LH, Negus JB, White PF. Oral midazolam preanesthetic medication in pediatric outpatients. Anesthesiology 1990; 73:831–834.
68. Milgrom P, et al. The safety and efficacy of outpatient midazolam intravenous sedation for oral surgery with and without fentanyl. Anesth Prog 1993;40:57–62.
69. Orman R. Nasal midazolam in children. Anesthesiology 1995; 82:1535–1536.
70. Lyons B, Cregg N, et al. Premedication for ambulatory surgery in school children: a comparison of oral midazolam and rectal thiopentone. Can J Anaesth 1995;42:473–478.
71. Cole S, Brozinsky S, Isenbert J. Midazolam, a new more potent benzodiazepine compared with diazepam: a randomized double blind study of preendoscopic sedatives. Gastrointest Endosc 1983;29:219.
72. Samuelson P, Reves J, Kouchoukos N, et al. Hemodynamic responses to anesthetic induction with midazolam or diazepam in patients with ischemic heart disease. Anesth Analg 1981; 60:802.
73. White PF. Comparative evaluation of intravenous agents for rapid sequence induction-thiopental, ketamine, and midazolam. Anesthesiology 1982;57:279–284.
74. Kanto J, Sjovall S, Vuori A. Effect of different kinds of premedication on the induction properties of midazolam. Br J Anaesth 1982;54:507.
75. Gamble J, Kawar P, Dundee J, et al. Evaluation of midazolam as an intravenous induction agent. Anaesthesia 1981;36:868–873.
76. Crawford M, Carl P, Andersen R, Mikkelsen B. Comparison between midazolam and thiopentone-based balanced anesthesia for day care surgery. Br J Anaesth 1984;56:165.
77. Melvin M, Johnson B, Quasha A, Eger E. Induction of anesthesia with midazolam decreases halothane MAC in humans. Anesthesiology 1982;57:238.
78. Reves J, Sladen R. Anesthesia and sedation by continuous infusion. In: Reves J, Sladen R, eds. Proceedings of a symposium. Princeton, NJ: Excerpta Medica, 1991.
79. Reves J, Jacobs J, Croughwell N, Smith L. Continuous infusions of midazolam and fentanyl for anesthesia during cardiac surgery. In: Vinik R, ed. Midazolam infusion for anesthesia and intensive care. Princeton, NJ: Excerpta Medica, 1989.
80. Theil D, Stanley T, White W, et al. Continuous intravenous anesthesia for cardiac surgery: a comparison of two infusion systems. J Thorac Cardiovasc Anesth 1993;7:300.
81. Shapiro J, Westphal LM, White PF, et al. Midazolam infusion for sedation in the intensive care unit: effect on adrenal function. Anesthesiology 1986;64:394–398.
82. Westphal LM, Cheng E, White PF, et al. Use of midazolam infusion for sedation following cardiac surgery. Anesthesiology 1987;67:257–262.
83. Shafer A, Doze VA, White PF. Pharmacokinetic variability of midazolam infusions in critically ill patients. Crit Care Med 1990;18:1039–1041.
84. Ritschel W, Hammer G. Prediction of the volume of distribution from in vitro data and use for estimating the absolute extent of aborption. Int J Clin Pharmacol Res 1980;18:298.
85. Mandelli M, Tognoni G, Garattini S. Clinical pharmacokinetics of diazepam. Clin Pharmacokinet 1978;3:72–91.
86. Valium product information. In: Physician's desk reference. Montvale, NJ: Medical Economics Data Production, 1995:2077–2079.
87. Dizac product information. 1994.
88. Thorn-Alquist AM. Parenteral use of diazepam in an emulsion formulation: a clinical study. Acta Anaesthesiol Scand 1977; 21:400–404.
89. Naylor HC, Burlingham AN. Pharmacokinetics of diazepam emulsion. Lancet 1985;1:518–519.
90. Greenblatt DJ, Allen MD, Harmatz JS, Shade R. Diazepam disposition determinants. Clin Pharmacol Ther 1980;27:301.
91. Yamamoto K, Kuze S, Muradmai S, Tsuji A. Pentazocine-diazepam-N_2O anesthesia: influence of pentazocine on protein binding and distribution of diazepam. In: Aldrete JA, Stanley TH, eds. Trends of intravenous anesthesia. Miami: Symposia Specialists, 1980.
92. DeSilva JAF, Koechlin BA, Bader G. Blood level distribution patterns of diazepam and its major metabolite in man. J Pharm Sci 1966;55:692–702.
93. Schwartz MA, Koechlin BA, Postma E, et al. Metabolism of diazepam in rat, dog, and man. J Pharmacol Exp Ther 1965; 149:423–435.
94. British National Formulary. London: British Medical Association and Pharmaceutical Society of Great Britain, 1983:123.
95. Drug information 86. Bethesda, MD: American Society of Hospital Pharmacists, American Hospital Formulary Service, 1986.
96. Alvan G, Siwers B, Vessman J. Pharmacokinetics of oxazepam in healthy volunteers. Acta Pharmacol Toxicol 1977;40:40.
97. Alvan G, Cederlof O. The pharmacokinetics profile of oxazepam. Acta Psychiatr Scand 1978;274:47.
98. Randall L, Scheckel C, Banzinger R. Pharmacology of the metabolites of chlordiazepoxide and diazepam. Curr Ther Res 1965;7:590.
99. Curry SH, Whelpton R. Pharmacokinetics of closely related benzodiazepines. Br J Clin Pharmacol 1979;8:15S.
100. Heel R, Brogden R, Speight T, Avery G. Temazepam: a review of pharmacological properties and therapeutic efficacy as a hypnotic. Drugs 1981;21:321.
101. Gilman AG, Goodman LS, Rall TW, et al. The pharmacologic basis of therapeutics. 7th ed. New York: Macmillan, 1985.
102. Caccia S, Garattini S. Formation of active metabolites of psychoactive drugs: an updated review of their significance. Clin Pharmacokinet 1990;18:434–459.
103. Klotz U, Avant GR, Hoyumpa A, et al. The effects of age and liver disease on disposition and elimination of diazepam in adult man. J Clin Invest 1975;55:347.

104. Kerkkola R, Kangas L. The transfer of diazepam across the placenta during labor. Acta Obstet Gynecol Scand 1973; 52:167.
105. Cavanagh D, Condo C. Diazepam: a pilot study of drug concentrations in maternal blood, amniotic fluid, and cord blood. Curr Ther Res 1964;6:122.
106. DeSilva JAF, D'Arconte L, Kaplan L. The determination of blood levels and the placental transfer of diazepam in humans. Curr Ther Res 1964;6:115.
107. Idanpaan HJE, Jouppila PI, Poulakka JO, Vorne MD. Placental transfer and fetal metabolism of diazepam in early human pregnancy. Am J Obstet Gynecol 1971;109:1011.
108. MacLeod SM, Giles HG, Bengert B, et al. Age- and gender-related differences in diazepam pharmacokinetics. J Clin Pharmacol 1979;19:15.
109. Ghoneim MM, Korttila K, Chiang CK. Diazepam effects and kinetics in Caucasians and Orientals. Clin Pharmacol Ther 1981; 29:749.
110. Klotz U, Reaming I. Delayed clearance of diazepam due to cimetidine. N Engl J Med 1980;302:1012.
111. Hillestad L, Hansen T, Melsom H. Diazepam metabolism in normal man. I. Serum concentrations and clinical effects after intravenous, intramuscular, and oral administration. Clin Pharmacol Ther 1974;16:479.
112. Stanski D, Watkins W. Drug disposition in anesthesia. New York: Grune and Stratton, 1982.
113. Greenblatt DJ, Kock-Weser J. Intramuscular injection of drugs. N Engl J Med 1976;295:542.
114. Korttila K, Linnoila M. Absorption and sedative effects of diazepam after oral administration and intramuscular administration into the vastus lateralis muscle and the deltoid muscle. Br J Anaesth 1975;47:857.
115. Kaplan SA, Jack ML, Alexander K, Weinfeld RE. Pharmacokinetic profile of diazepam in man following single intravenous and oral and chronic oral administrations. J Pharm Sci 1973; 62:1789.
116. Gamble JAS, Dundee JW, Gray RC. Plasma diazepam concentrations following prolonged administration. Br J Anaesth 1976; 48:1087.
117. Brown SS, Dundee JW. Clinical studies of induction agents. XXXV. Diazepam. Br J Anaesth 1968;40:108.
118. Greenblatt DJ, Shader RI. Dependence, tolerance and addiction to benzodiazepines: clinical and pharmacokinetic considerations. Drug Metab Rev 1978;8:13.
119. Clarke PRF, Eccersley PS, Frisby JP, Thornton JA. The amnesic effect of diazepam (Valium). Br J Anaesth 1970;42:690.
120. Dundee JW, Pandit SK. Anterograde amnesic effects of pethidine, hyoscine, and diazepam in adults. Br J Pharmacol 1972; 44:140.
121. Pandit SK, Dundee JW, Keilty SR. Amnesia studies with intravenous premedication. Anaesthesia 1971;26:421.
122. Brown CR, Sarnquist FH, Canup CA, Pedley TA. Clinical and electroencephalographic and pharmacokinetic studies of water-soluble benzodiazepine, midazolam maleate. Anesthesiology 1979;50:467.
123. Reves JG, Gelman S. Cardiovascular effects of intravenous anesthetic drugs. In: Covino BG, Fozzard HA, Rehder K, Strichartz G, eds. Effects of anesthesia. Bethesda, MD: American Physiological Society, 1985.
124. Marty J, Gauzit R, Lefevre P, et al. Effects of diazepam and midazolam on barofeflex control of heart rate and on sympathetic activity in humans. Anesth Analg 1986;65:113.
125. Stovner J, Andresen R. Diazepam in intravenous anesthesia. Lancet 1966;1:1042.
126. Stanley TH. Pharmacology of intravenous narcotic anesthetics. In: Miller RD, ed. Anesthesia. New York: Churchill Livingstone, 1981.
127. Dundee JW, Haslett WHK, Keilty SR, Pandit SK. Studies of drugs given before anaesthesia. XX. Diazepam-containing mixtures. Br J Anaesth 1970;42:143.
128. Prensky AL, Raff MC, Moore MJ, Schwab RS. Intravenous diazepam in the treatment of prolonged seizure activity. N Engl J Med 1967;276:770.
129. Haefely W. Synaptic pharmacology of barbiturates and benzodiazepines. Agents Action 1977;7:353–359.
130. Hunter AR. Diazepam (Valium) as a muscle relaxant during general anaesthesia: a pilot study. Br J Anaesth 1967;39:633.
131. Eryasa Y. The use of diazepam in surgery. South Med J 1971; 64:27–29.
132. Dowell T. Diazepam in intravenous anesthesia. Lancet 1966; 1:369.
133. Brandt AL, Oakes FD. Preanesthesia medication: double blind study of a new drug, diazepam. Anesth Analg 1965;44:125.
134. Brown PRH, Main DMG, Lawson JIM. Diazepam in dentistry. Br Dent J 1968;125:498.
135. Rogers WK, Waterman DH, Domm SE, Sunay A. Efficacy of a new psychotropic drug in bronchoscopy. Dis Chest 1965; 13:562.
136. McClish A. Diazepam as an intravenous induction agent for general anesthesia. Can Anaesth Soc J 1966;13:562.
137. Samuelson PN, Lell WA, Kouchoukos NT, Strong SD, Dole KM. Hemodynamics during diazepam induction of anesthesia for coronary artery bypass grafting. South Med J 1980;73:332.
138. Davidau A. La premédication pur les malades difficiles: ou sur les séances de soir trés longues. Rev Stomatol Chir Macillofac 1966;67:589.
139. Aldrete JA, Tan ST, Carron DJ, Watts MK. Pentazepam (pentazocine and diazepam) supplementing local analgesia for laparoscopic sterilisation. Anesth Analg 1976;55:177.
140. Baird ES, Curson I. Orally administered diazepam in conservative dentistry. Br Dent J 1970;128:26.
141. Healy T, Robinson J, Vickers M. Physiological responses to intravenous diazepam as a sedative for conservative denistry. Br Med J 1970;3:10.
142. Healy TEJ, Hamilton M. Intravenous diazepam in the apprehensive child. Br Dent J 1972;130:25.
143. Healy TEJ, Edmondson HD, Hall N. The use of intravenous diazepam during dental surgery in the mentally handicapped patient. Br Dent J 1970;128:22.
144. Vinge LN, Wyant GM, Lopez JF. Diazepam in cardioversion. Can Anaesth Soc J 1971;18:166.
145. Orko R. Anaesthesia for cardioversion. Br J Anaesth 1976; 48:257.
146. Nutter DO, Massumi RA. Diazepam in cardioversion. N Engl J Med 1965;273:650.
147. McClish A, Andres D, Tetreault L. Intravenous diazepam for psychiatric reactions following open heart surgery. Can Anaesth Soc J 1968;15:63.
148. Conner JT, Katz RL, Pagano RR, Graham CW. Ro 21-3981 for intravenous surgical premedication and induction of anesthesia. Anesth Analg 1978;57.
149. Uhlenhuth EH, Turner DA, Purchatzke G, et al. Intensive design in evaluating anxiolytic agents. Psychopharmacology 1977;52:79–85.
150. Jacobs MA, Heim E, Chassau JB. Intensive design in the study of differential therapeutic effects. Comp Psychiatry 1966;7:278–289.
151. Kellner R, Kelly AV, Sheffield BF. The assessment of changes in anxiety in a drug trial: a comparison of methods. Br J Psychiatry 1968;114:863–869.
152. Hesbacher PT, Rickels K, Hutchinson J, et al. Setting, patient, and doctor effects on drug response in neurotic patients. II. Differential improvement. Psychopharmacologia 1970;18:209–226.
153. Browne TR. Drug therapy reviews: drug therapy of status epilepticus. Am J Hosp Pharm 1978;35:915–921.

154. Josephson DA. Status epilepticus. Am Fam Phys 1974;10:168–173.
155. Drugs for epilepsy. Med Lett Drugs Ther 1989;31:1–4.
156. Olafson RA, Mulder DW, Howard FH. "Stiffman" syndrome: a review of the literature, report of three additional cases, and discussion of pathophysiology and therapy. Mayo Clin Proc 1964;39:131.
157. Nathan PW. The action of diazepam in neurologic disorders with excessive motor activity. J Neurol Sci 1970;10:33.
158. DeLee JC, Rockwood CA. Skeletal muscle spasm and a review of muscle relaxants. Curr Ther Res 1980;27:64–74.
159. Young RR, Delwaide PJ. Spasticity (second of two parts). N Engl J Med 1981;304:96–99.
160. Davies AO. Oral diazepam premedication reduces the incidence of post-succinylcholine muscle pains. Can Anaesth Soc J 1983;30:603–606.
161. Greenblatt D, Comer W, Elliott H, et al. Clinical pharmacokinetics of lorazepam. III. Intravenous injecion: preliminary results. J Clin Pharmacol 1977;17:490.
162. Greenblatt D, Shader R, Franke K, et al. Pharmacokinetics and bioavailability of intravenous, intramuscular and oral lorazepam in humans. J Pharm Sci 1979;68:57.
163. Verschraegen R, Rolly G. Intra-muscular premedication with lorazepam (Temesta). Acta Anaesthesiol Belg 1974;25:68.
164. Greenblatt D, Knowles J, Comer W, et al. Clinical pharmacokinetics of lorazepam. IV. Long-term oral administration. J Clin Pharmacol 1977;17:495.
165. Kraus J, Desmond P, Marshall J, et al. Effects of aging and liver disease on disposition of lorazepam. Clin Pharmacol Ther 1978; 24:411.
166. George K, Dundee J. Relative amnesic actions of diazepam, flunitrazepam and lorazepam in man. Br J Clin Pharmacol 1977; 4:45.
167. Dundee J, McGowan W, Lilburu J, et al. Comparison of the actions of diazepam and lorazepam. Br J Anaesth 1979; 51:439.
168. Elliott H. Metabolism of lorazepam. Br J Anaesth 1976;48:1017.
169. Seitz W, Hempelmann G, Piepenbrock S. Zur kardiovaskulaeren Wirkung von Flunitrazepam (Rohypnol, RO 5-4200). Anaesthesist 1977;26:249.
170. Hedges A, Turner P, Harry T. Preliminary studies on the central effects of lorazepam: a new benzodiazepine. J Clin Pharmacol 1971;11:243.
171. Aleniewkis M, Bulas B, Maderazo L, Mendoza C. Intramuscular lorazepam vs. pentobarbital premeditation: a comparison of patient sedation, aniolysis and recall. Anesth Analg 1977; 56:498.
172. Knapp R, Fierro L. Evaluation of the cardiopulmonary safety and effects of lorazepam as a premedicant. Anesth Analg 1974; 53:122.
173. Olgiati S. Clinical assessment of lorazepam in anxiety: a double-blind study. Curr Ther Res 1975;17:13.
174. Krueger G. Use of lorazepam in treating patients with neurotic and somatized psychovegetative symptoms. Ther Res 1973; 15:907.
175. Blitt C, Petty W. Reversal of lorazepam delirium by physostigmine. Anesth Analg 1975;54:607.
176. Korttila K, Tarkkanen L, et al. Unpredictable central nervous system effects after lorazepam premedication for neurosurgery. Acta Anaesth Scand 1982;26:213–216.
177. Schwartz M, Postma E, Gaut Z. Biological half-life of chlordiazepoxide and its metabolit, demoxepam, in man. J Pharm Sci 1971;60:1500.
178. Boxenbaum H, Geitner K, Jack M, et al. Pharmacokinetic and biopharmaceutic profile of chlordiazepoxide HCl in healthy subjects: single-dose studies by the intravenous, intramuscular, and oral routes. J Pharmacokinet Biopharm 1977;5:3.
179. Greenblatt D, Shader R, MacLeod S, et al. Absorption of oral and intramuscular chlordiazepoxide. Eur J Pharmacol 1978; 13:267.
180. Shader R, Greenblatt D, Harmatz J, et al. Absorption and disposition of chlodiazepoxide in young and elderly male volunteers. J Clin Pharmacol 1977;17:709.
181. Roberts R, Wilkinson G, Branch R, Schenker S. Effects of age and parenchylmal liver disease on the disposition and elimination of chlordiazepoxide (Librium). Gastroenterology 1978; 75:479.
182. Greenblatt D, Shader R, MacLeod S. Clinical pharmacokinetics of chlordiazepoxide. Clin Pharmacokinet 1978;3:381.
183. Kissen M. Comparative study of chlorpromazine and chlordiazepoxide in the prevention and treatment of alcohol withdrawal symptoms. Cin Med 1960;72:59.
184. Holister L, Motzebecker P, Degan R. Withdrawal reactions from chlordiazepoxide ("Librium"). Psychopharmacologia 1961;2:63.
185. Moschitto L, Greenblatt D, Divoll M. Alprazolam kinetics in the elderly: relation to antipyrine disposition. Clin Pharmacol Ther 1981;29:267.
186. Study C-NCP. Drug treatment of panic disorder. Br J Psychiatry 1992;160:191–202.
187. Greenblatt D, Divoll M, Abernethy D, et al. Clinical pharmacokinetics of the newer benzodiazepines. Clin Pharmacokinet 1983;8:233–252.
188. Fawcett J, Kravitz H. Alprazolam: pharmacokinetics, clinical efficacy, and mechanism of action. Pharmacotherapy 1982; 2:243–254.
189. Kaplan S, et al. Pharmacokinetic profiles of clonazepam in dog and humans and of flunitrazepam in dog. J Pharm Sci 1974; 63:527.
190. Berlin A, Dahlstrom H. Pharmacokinetics of the anticonvulsant evaluated from single oral and intravenous doses and by repeated oral administration. Eur J Clin Pharmacol 1975;9:155.
191. Gastaut H. Exceptional antiepileptic properties of a new benzodiazepine (RO5-4023). Vie Med 1970;51:1575.
192. Diener H-C, Pfaffenrath V, Soyka D, et al. Therapie und Prophylaxe der Gesichtsneuralgien and anderer Gesichtsschmerzen: Empfehlungen der Deutschen Migraene- und Kopfschmerz-Gesellschaft. Arzneimitteltherapie 1994;11:349–353.
193. Jones B, Chouinard G. Clonazepam in the treatment of recurrent symptoms of depression and anxiety in a patient with systemic lupus erythematosus. Am J Psychiatry 1985;142:345–355.
194. Kaim B. A case of Gilles de la Tourette's syndrome treated with clonazepam. Brain Res Bull 1983;11:213–214.
195. Court J, Kase C. Treatment of tic douloureux with a new anticonvulsant (clonazepam). J Neurol Neurosurg Psychiatr 1976; 39:297.
196. Greco F, Menthonnex P, Micoud M, et al. Action of a tranquilizing agent on preoperative anixety. Anesth Analg 1973;30:289–312.
197. Granger J, et al. Anxiety and anesthesia. Study of injectable Tranxene: 1161 observations. Anesth Analg 1973;30:459.
198. Eydan R, Moussa O. Post operative sedation and analgesia by the association of dipotassic chlorazepate and pentazocine. Anesth Analg 1973;30:559.
199. Troupin A, Friel P, Wilensky A, et al. Evaluation of clorazepate (Tranxene) as an anticonvulsant: a pilot study. Neurology 1979; 29:488–566.
200. Lion J, Azcarate C, Koepke H. "Paradoxical rage reactions" during psychotropic medication. Dis Nerv Syst 1975;36:557–558.
201. Livingston S, Pauli L, Pruce L. Clorazepate in epilepsy. JAMA 1977;237:1561.
202. Feldman R. Clorazepate in temporal lobe epilepsy. JAMA 1979; 236:2603.
203. Karch F. Rage reaction associated with clorazepate dipotassium. Ann Intern Med 1979;91:61–62.

204. Idman R. Clorazepate in temporal lobe epilepsy. JAMA 1976; 236:2603.
205. Bertler A, Lindgren S, Malmgren H. Pharmacokinetics of dipotassium chlorazepate in patients after repeated 50 mg oral doses. Psychopharmacology 1980;71:165–167.
206. Pierce MW, Shu VS. Safety of estazolam: the United States clinical experience. Am J Med 1990;88 (suppl 3A):6–17.
207. Gustavson LE, Carrigan PJ. The clinical pharmacokinetics of single dose of estazolam. Am J Med 1990;88 (suppl 3A):2–5.
208. Kales J, Kales A, Bixler E, Slye E. Effects of placebo and flurazepam on sleep patterns in insomniac subjects. Clin Pharmacol Ther 1971;12:691.
209. Dundee J, Haslett W. The benzodiazepines: a review of their actions and uses relative to anesthetic practice. Br J Anaesth 1970;42:217.
210. Allen M, Greenblatt D, Harmatz J, Shader R. Desmethyl-diazepam kinetics in the elderly after oral prazepam. Clin Pharmacol Ther 1980;28:196.
211. Hahn EF, Battista D, Arnold J. Recent developments in hypnotic benzodiazepines: clinical implications. Drugs Today 1990; 25:41–48.
212. Kales A, Scharf MB, Soldatos CR, et al. Quazepam, a new benzodiazepine hypnotic: intermediate-term sleep laboratory evaluation. J Clin Pharmacol 1980;20:184–192.
213. Kales A, Bixler EO, Scharf M, et al. Sleep laboratory studies of flurazepam: a model for evaluating hypnotic drugs. Clin Pharmacol Ther 1976;19:576–583.
214. Dement WC, Carskadon MA, Mitler MM, et al. Prolonged use of flurazepam: a sleep laboratory study. Behav Med 1978;5:25–31.
215. Dement WC. Objective measurements of daytime sleepiness and performance comparing quazepam with flurazepam in two adult populations using the multiple sleep latency test. J Clin Psychiatry 1991;52 (suppl):31–37.
216. Chung M, Hilbert JM, Gural RPE, et al. Multiple-dose quazepam kinetics. Clin Pharmacol Ther 1984;35:520–524.
217. Hilbert JM, Chung M, Radwanski E, et al. Quazepam kinetics in the elderly. Clin Pharmacol Ther 1984;36:566–569.
218. Jochemsen R, Breimer DD. Pharmacokinetics of benzodiazepines: metabolic pathways and plasma level profiles. Curr Med Res Opin 1984;8 (suppl 4):60–79.
219. Eberts F, Philopoulos Y, Reineke L, Vliek R. Triazolam disposition. Clin Pharmacol Ther 1981;29:81.
220. Vogel G, Thurmond A, Gibbons P, et al. The effect of triazolam on the sleep of insomniacs. Psychopharmacologia 1975;41:65–69.
221. Einarson T, Moschitto L, Greenblatt D, et al. Hallucinations from triazolam. Drug Intell Clin Pharm 1980;14:714.
222. Kales A, Bixler E, Vgontzas A. Triazolam safety. Lancet 1993; 341:1602.
223. Vela-Bueno A. Triazolam safety. Lancet 1993;341:1602.
224. Jonas J. Adverse events after triazolam substitution. Lancet 1993;341:1150–1151.
225. Jonas J, Coleman B, Sheridan A, et al. Comparative clinical profiles of trizolam versus other shorter-acting hypnotics. J Clin Psychiatry 1992;19–31.
226. Jonas J. Triazolam. Br Med J 1993;307.
227. Wang R. Determining optimum dose and acute tolerance of triazolam. J Int Med Res 1977;5:184–190.
228. Kripke D, Grant I. A double-blind study of triazolam. Sleep Res 1974;3:57.
229. Hoffman E, Warren E. Flumazenil: a benzodiazepine antagonist. Clin Pharm 1993;12:641–656.
230. Hunkeler W. Preclinical research findings with flumazenil (Ro15-1788, Anexate) chemistry. Eur J Anaesthesiol 1988;2:37.
231. Hunkeler W, Moehler H, Pieri L, et al. Selective antagonists of benzodiazepines. Nature 1981;290:514.
232. Polc P, Laurent J, Scherschlicht R, Haefely W. Electrophysiological studies on the specific benzodiazepine antagonist (RO 15-1788). Naunyn Schmiedebergs Arch Pharmacol 1981; 316:317.
233. Bonetti E, Pieri L, Cumin R, et al. Benzodiazepine antagonist Ro 15-1788: neurological and behavioural effects. Psychopharmacology (Berl) 1982;78:8.
234. Cumin R, Bonetti E, Scherschlidht R, Haefely W. Use of the specific benzodiazepine antagonist, Ro 15-1788, in studies of physiological dependence on benzodiazepines. Experientia 1982;38:833.
235. Lauven P, Stoeckel H, Schwilden R, et al. Application of a benzodiazepine antagonist (Ro 15-1788) under steady state conditions of midazolam. Anesthesiology 1982;57:A325.
236. Darragh A, Lambe R, Kenny M, et al. Ro 15-1788 antagonizes the central effect of diazepam in man without altering diazepam bioavailability. Br J Clin Pharmacol 1982;14:677.
237. Ziegler W, Schalch E. Antagonism of benzodiazepine-induced sedation in man. In: Koella W, ed. Basel: Karger, 1983.
238. Scollo-Lavizzari G. First clinical investigation of the benzodiazepine antagonist Ro 15-1788 in comatose patients. Eur Neurol 1983;22:7.
239. Klotz U. Drug interactions and clinical pharmacokinetics of flumazenil. J Anaesthesiol Suppl 1988;2:103–108.
240. Klotz U, Kanto J. Pharmacokinetics and clinical use of flumazenil (Ro 15-1788). Clin Pharmacokinet 1988;20:491.
241. Breimer L, Hennis P, Burm A. Pharmacokinetics and EEG effects of flumazenil in volunteers. Clin Pharmacokinet 1991; 20:491.
242. Knudsen L, Cold G, Holdgard H, et al. Effects of flumazenil on cerebral blood flow and oxygen consumption after midazolam anesthesia for craniotomy. Br J Anaesth 1991;67:277.
243. Wolf J, Fribert L, Jensen J, et al. The effect of the benzodiazepine antagonist flumazenil on regional cerebral blood flow in human volunteers. Acta Anaesthesiol 1990;34:628.
244. Haefely W. Alleviation of anxiety: the benzodiazepine saga. In: Barnham M, Bruinvels J, eds. Discoveries in pharmacology. vol 1. Amsterdam: Elsevier, 1983.
245. Moehler H, Burkard W, Keller H, et al. Benzodiazepine antagonist Ro 15-1788: binding characteristics and interaction with drug-induced changes in dopamine turnover and cerebellar GMP levels. J Neurochem 1981;37:714.
246. Yokoyama M, Benson K, Arakawa K, Goto H. Effects of flumazenil on intravenous lidocain-induced convulsions and anticonvulsant property of diazepam in rats. Anesth Analg 1992; 75:87.
247. Lauven P, Schwilden H, Stoeckel H, Greenblatt D. The effect of a benzodiazepine antagonist RO 15-1788 in the presence of stable concentrations of midazolam. Anesthesiology 1985;63:61–64.
248. Ghouri AF, Ramirez Ruiz MA, White PF. Effect of flumazenil on recovery after midazolam and propofol sedation. Anesthesiology 1994;81:333–339.
249. Samson Y, Hantraye P, Baron J, et al. Kinetics and displacement of [C11] Ro 15-1788, a benzodiazepine receptor antagonist, studied in human brain in vivo by positron tomography. Eur J Pharmacol 1985;110:247–251.
250. Schoemaker H, Bliss M, Yamamura H. Specific high-affinity saturable binding of [3H] Ro 5-4864 to benzodiazepine binding sites in the rat cerebral cortex. Eur J Pharmacol 1984;71:713.
251. Forster A, Crettenand G, Morel D. Absence of ventilatory agonist or inverse agonist effects of an overdose of Ro 15-1788: a specific benzodiazepine antagonist. Anesthesiology 1987; 67:A144.
252. Duka T, Achenheil M, Noderer J, et al. Changes in noradrenaline plasma levels and behavioral responses induced by benzodiazepine agonists with the benzodiazepine antagonist Ro 15-1788 in cardiac patients. Pharmacology 1986;90:351.
253. Geller E, Chernilas J, Halpern P, et al. Haemodynamics follow-

ing reversal of benzodiazepine sedation with Ro 15-1788 in cardiac patients. Anesthesiology 1986;65:A49.

254. Geller E, Halpern P, Chernilas J, et al. Cardiorespiratory effects of antagonism of diazepam sedation with flumazenil in patients with cardiac disease. Anesth Analg 1991;72:207.
255. Nilsson A. Autonomic and hormonal responses after the use of midazolam and flumazenil. Acta Anaesthesiol Scand 1990; 92:51.
256. Ritter J, Flacke W, Hoshizaki G. Flumazenil reversal of midazolam lacks adrenergic, hemodynamic, and anixiogenic response. Anesth Analg 1991;68:S1–S321.
257. Marty J, Joyon D. Haemodynamic reponses following reversal of benzodiazepine-induced anaesthesia or sedation with flumazenil. Eur J Anaesthesiol 1988;2:167.
258. White P, Shafer A, Boyle W, Doze V. Stress response following reversal of benzodiazepine-induced sedation. Eur J Anaesthesiol 1988;2:173.
259. White P, Shafer A, Boyle W, et al. Benzodiazepine antagonism does not provoke a stress response. Anesthesiology 1989; 70:636.
260. Croughwell N, Reves J, Will C, et al. Safety of rapid administration of flumazenil in patients with ischemic heart disease. Acta Anaesthesiol Scand 1990;34 (suppl 92):55–58.
261. Rouiller M, Forster A, Gemperle M. Evaluation de l'efficacité et de la tolerance d'un antagoniste des benzodiazepines (Ro 15-1788). Ann Fr Anesth Reanim 1987;6:1.
262. Kleinberger G, Grimm G, Laggner A, et al. Weaning patients from mechanical ventilation by benzodiazepine antagonist Ro 15-1788. Lancet 1986;2:268.
263. McDuffee A, Tobias J. Seizure after flumazenil administration in a pediatric patient. Pediatr Emerg Care 1995;11:186–187.
264. Haverkos G, DiSalvo R, Imhoff T. Fatal seizures after administration in a patient with mixed overdose. Ann Pharmacother 1994;28:1347–1349.

6 Etomidate

Alfred Doenicke and P. Ostwald

Etomidate (R (+)-ethyl-1-(1-phenylethyl)-1H-imidazole-5-carboxylate), is a potent and short-acting intravenous hypnotic, with a simple molecular structure (1) (Fig. 6-1). Etomidate exists as two isomers, but only the (+) isomer is active as a hypnotic. It is water insoluble and is unstable in a neutral solution. Etomidate is supplied as the sulfate (molecular weight 342.36) dissolved in a phosphate buffered solution (1.8 mg $Na_2HPO_4{\cdot}12\ H_2O$ and 2.2 mg $NaH_2PO_4{\cdot}1\ H_2O$ and 4.2% glucose) in a concentration of 1.5 mg etomidate base per milliliter (pH about 3.4, osmolality 270 mOsm/L). Since 1977, etomidate has been solubilized in 35% propylene glycol (pH 5.6, osmolality 4600 mOsm/L) and is marketed as Amidate (Abbott Laboratories) or Hypnomidate (Janssen Pharmaceutica or Etomidate Lipuro (Braun)).

Following rapid (2 seconds) intravenous injection, etomidate (median effective dose [ED_{50}] of 0.57 mg/kg) is about 6 times more potent than methohexital (ED_{50} of 3.51 mg/kg) and about 25 times more potent than thiopental (ED_{50} of 13.4 mg/kg) (1). The margin of safety (LD_{50}/ED_{50}) of etomidate is higher (26.0) than those of methohexital (9.5), propanidid (6.7), and thiopental (4.6) in rats (1). The potency and toxicity of etomidate increase slightly with increasing speed of injection without affecting the drug's safety margin (1).

Thus, the effects of opioids and benzodiazepines in reducing myoclonic activity appear to be additive. In addition, clinical observations showed that a priming dose of 2–3 mg etomidate administered 1–2 min before induction of general anesthesia can completely attenuate myocloni. To exert its full effect it is important that the priming dose of etomidate is high enough to show clinical effects like sleepiness of the patient. A premedication with opioids or benzodiazepines is not necessary. The use of a priming dose of etomidate has been used successful clinically and may be especially useful in anesthesia for outpatients.

Etomidate was initially investigated in humans in 1972. At a dosage of 0.2 mg/kg, etomidate produced no significant effects on the cardiovascular or respiratory system (Doenicke, unpublished results). However, myoclonic activity, as well as an increase in heart rate during the surgical procedure (and other signs of insufficient analgesia), suggested that etomidate should not be used as a single anesthetic in subsequent clinical trials. After 2 years of clinical experience, an acceptable regimen for induction of general anesthesia using etomidate has been developed consisting of benzodizepine premedication (e.g., midazolam 2 to 5 mg intravenously) and administration of fentanyl 100 to 200 μg, 1 to 2 minutes before induction of anesthesia, followed by etomidate, 0.2 to 0.3 mg/kg, slowly injected (2). Induction of anesthesia using etomidate as described previously was free of major hemodynamic changes and led to its widespread clinical use in Europe until 1983. In a letter to the *Lancet,* two surgical colleagues, Ledingham and Watt, reported an increased mortality in patients in the intensive care unit who were sedated with etomidate; this complication allegedly was due to adrenocortical suppression, a newly described side effect of etomidate (3). Following these reports, etomidate has been used cautiously because of concerns regarding the well-characterized effects of etomidate on adrenocortical function during the perioperative period.

The problem of pain on injection of etomidate became an issue in 1977 when the solvent of etomidate was changed to propylene glycol (4, 5). However, this problem has been solved with the introduction of etomidate dissolved in lipofundin (Etomidate Lipuro) (6). This preparation of etomidate is approved and available in several European countries. With the change of the solvent from propylene glycol (7-11) to lipofundin, a lipid emulsion (6), the side effects related to the unphysiologic high osmolality of etomidate have disappeared (12, 13). As a result of the lack of further reports regarding the negative effects of adrenal suppression and its beneficial physiologic profile, etomidates has increased in the last several years. With

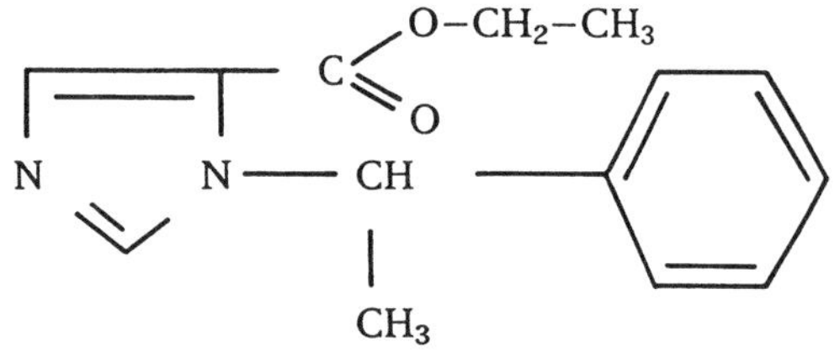

FIGURE 6-1. Chemical structure of etomidate.

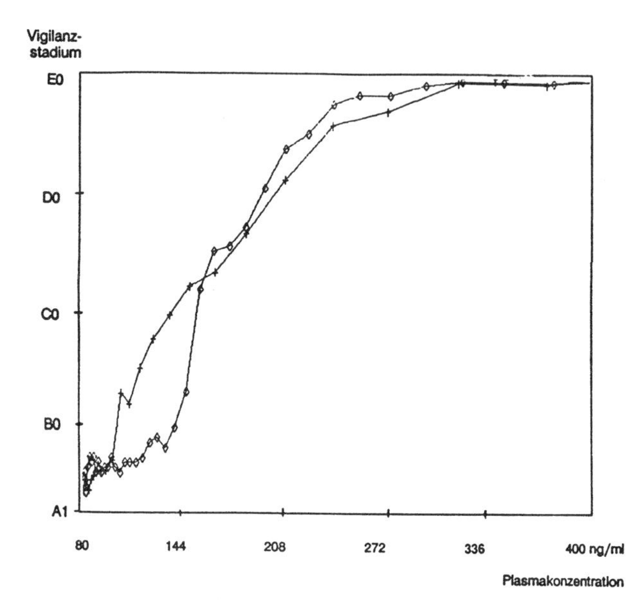

FIGURE 6-2. Hypnotic effects of etomidate. Concentration-response relationship after etomidate (0.3 mg/kg within 60 seconds). Etomidate in propylene glycol (n = 8;plus signs) versus etomidate in lipofundin (n = 8;circles). Deep anesthesia occurred in both groups when serum concentration of etomidate exceeded 170 ng/ml. (From Doenicke A, Kugler A, Vollmann N, et al. Etomidate with a new solubilizer: clinical and experimental investigations on venous tolerance and bioavailability. Anaesthesist 1990;39:475–480.

the availability of etomidate in lipofundin, this intravenous anesthetic may eventually become more popular than it was in the 1970s.

PHARMACOKINETICS

Etomidate is highly bound to plasma proteins (93.7%) (14), predominantly to albumin (643.7% at a pH of 7.4) (15). The volume of distribution has been determined at steady state to be 2.5 to 4.5 L/kg (16-20). The initial distribution half-life is approximately 2.8 minutes, and the redistribution half-life is about 28.7 minutes (15-18, 20). The elimination half-life (the terminal β-phase) varies from 2.9 to 5.3 hours (18). Pharmacokinetic properties of etomidate were not altered by the use of lipofundin as a solvent (6) (Fig. 6-2).

DISTRIBUTION AND METABOLISM

During the first 30 minutes after administration of an induction dose of etomidate to humans, the plasma level of unchanged etomidate decreases rapidly and then more slowly, with an elimination half-life of 75 minutes (21). Following intravenous injection, etomidate is extensively bound to plasma proteins (14). Etomidate penetrates the blood-brain barrier rapidly, and peak levels are reached within 1 minute of administration (22), corresponding to the fast onset of the hypnotic effect. Elimination of etomidate from the brain is also rapid (22). Rapid uptake of etomidate also occurs in lung, kidney, muscle, heart, and spleen. In these tissues, maximum etomidate levels are reached within 2 minutes after injection (20). A significantly slower uptake of etomidate is seen in fat, with maximal levels achieved between 7 and 28 minutes after intravenous administration (22). These observations may be explained by the limited solubility of etomidate in an acidic medium (stomach) and by the highly lipophilic properties of the unionized drug (22). Etomidate is rapidly metabolized in the liver by ester hydrolysis to its major metabolite, the carboxylic acid of etomidate. This metabolite is pharmacologically inactive (22). In humans, 75% of the intravenously injected dose is excreted as its primary metabolite in the urine during the first 24 hours after intravenous administration (21). Over this period, about 13% of the administered dose is found in the feces (20). Because the breakdown of etomidate occurs primarily in the liver, the hepatic concentration of the etomidate is higher than plasma etomidate concentrations even 3 minutes after intravenous administration.

The distribution of the optical isomers of etomidate, R (+) and S (−), do not differ substantially in blood, brain, and liver (22). In spite of almost equal brain concentrations for both isomers, the S (+) form has considerably less hypnotic activity, suggesting the presence of a stereospecific receptor for etomidate in the brain (22).

TOXICOLOGY AND TERATOLOGY

The electrocardiogram (ECG), urinalysis, and histopathologic examination fail to reveal any drug-related adverse effects after the daily intravenous injection of etomidate for 3 weeks to rats (highest dose 5.0 mg/kg) and 2 weeks to dogs (highest dose 1.5 mg/kg) (23). Etomidate is devoid of any teratogenic effect in rats (Sprague-Dawley strain) (24) or rabbits (23). The highest dose of etomidate given to rats was 5.0 mg/kg intravenously daily from day 6 through day 15 of pregnancy and to rabbits 4.5 mg/kg intravenously daily from day 6 through day 18 of pregnancy (23).

Etomidate has been safely used in humans during pregnancy without reports of adverse effects.

PHARMACODYNAMICS

Central Nervous System (CNS)

The electroencephalographic (EEG) changes provoked by etomidate are similar to the EEG stages produced by the barbiturates thiopental and methohexital (25). Effects of etomidate depend on the administered dose, the injection rate, and the individual's initial state of consciousness. The EEG changes represent the hypnotic effects of etomidate and indicate the impairment of integrative performance capacity of the neocortex structures of the brain. Analogous to the experimental findings in animals receiving barbiturates, transient activation of cortical neuronal activity occurs. However, EEG changes recorded using surface electrodes cannot detect effects of etomidate on subcortical structures. The hypnotic effect of etomidate, with its corresponding EEG changes and lack of analgesic activity, suggests that etomidate does not alter pain conduction in the thalamus or the brain stem. The primary site of etomidate action seems to be located in the neocortex, whereas diencephalic or mesencephalic structures are less affected (25). Primary actions of etomidate in the CNS appear to be inhibition of the formatio reticularis. However, etomidate seems to have additional activating or uninhibiting effects on spinal centers (26). Evans and Hill (27) showed in vitro and in vivo that etomidate exerts its central inhibiting effects by γ-aminobutyric acid (GABA)-adrenergic actions.

Myoclonic Activity

The induction of anesthesia with etomidate is characterized by a high incidence of myoclonia, especially when etomidate is used without premedication (25, 26). The occurrence of myoclonia and dyskinesia can be explained by disinhibition of subcortical structures. Regulation of involuntary movements is located in the extrapyramidal system, which is controlled by the neocortex. During the transition from consciousness to "deep" anesthesia, the inhibiting cortical influences are absent, and myoclonic activity is enhanced. This theory is supported by the finding that disappearance of myoclonic activity may be absent when etomidate is administered in combination with benzodiazepines and fentanyl, drugs known to have inhibiting effects on subcortical structures (2, 16, 25). Investigators have suggested that fentanyl stimulates GABAergic neurons in the basal ganglia by μ receptors and thereby either reduces GABA release or alters the function of the GABA receptors (28). Thus, the effects of opioids and benzodiazepines in reducing myoclonic activity appear to be additive.

Epileptogenic Activity

The use of etomidate has been associated with an increase in seizure activity (29). However, myoclonic activity must not be equated with generalized tonic-clonic seizures. Myoclonia can occur under the physiologic conditions of a reduction in cortical activity during physiologic sleep as a result of disinhibition of subcortical structures. To date, no definite paroxysmal or recruited epileptic discharges or clinical signs of generalized epileptic seizures have been observed in the EEG of patients without a history of epileptic disease after etomidate (25). Even in epileptic patients, no activation of paroxysms has been observed under etomidate anesthesia. Kugler and associates monitored EEG during anesthesia after induction with etomidate in patients with a history of convulsive disorders (25). No seizures were observed during anesthesia in any of these cases, and only 1 patient developed an epileptic attack during the late postanesthetic phase. In addition, etomidate has demonstrated anticonvulsive properties in several experimental models. It has been shown to reduce seizure activity after D,L-allyglycine (30), after stimulation of the amygdala region (31), and after electric stimulation (32). Although etomidate appears to have no convulsant or epileptogenic action in nonepileptic patients, Ebrahim and colleagues (29) reported an increase in epileptiform activity after the injection of etomidate in 9 of 12 patients with known epilectic disease. Because the injection of etomidate followed an induction dose of thiopental, the barbiturate may have interfered with etomidate's activity and may have altered its EEG response. Concerns regarding etomidate's epileptogenic action based on case reports understandably led to the unproven opinion that etomidate is "epileptogenic." During etomidate anesthesia, epileptic attacks occur infrequently, and their incidence is far lower than would be expected if it possessed significant convulsant activity (25). Hence, etomidate can be used safely even in patients with a known epileptic disorder provided they are premedicated with a benzodiazepine.

Effects on the Electroencephalogram

The EEG stages following a 0.3 mg/kg bolus dose of etomidate resemble the classic stages of anesthesia as observed with barbiturates and other intravenous and inhaled anesthetics (25). The first noticeable EEG changes occur after a latency of 30 to 40 seconds (the latency period depends on the rate of injection) (16), consisting of diffuse and irregular fast-wave activity comparable to the "induction" stage with barbiturates. After a brief period, there is a transition to a mixed activity pattern, with slow 5- to 3-second waves superimposed by rapid activity and corresponding to the "light" stage of anesthesia (Fig. 6-3). Subsequently, slow activity develops, corresponding to an intermediate stage of anesthesia consisting of an hypnotic ac-

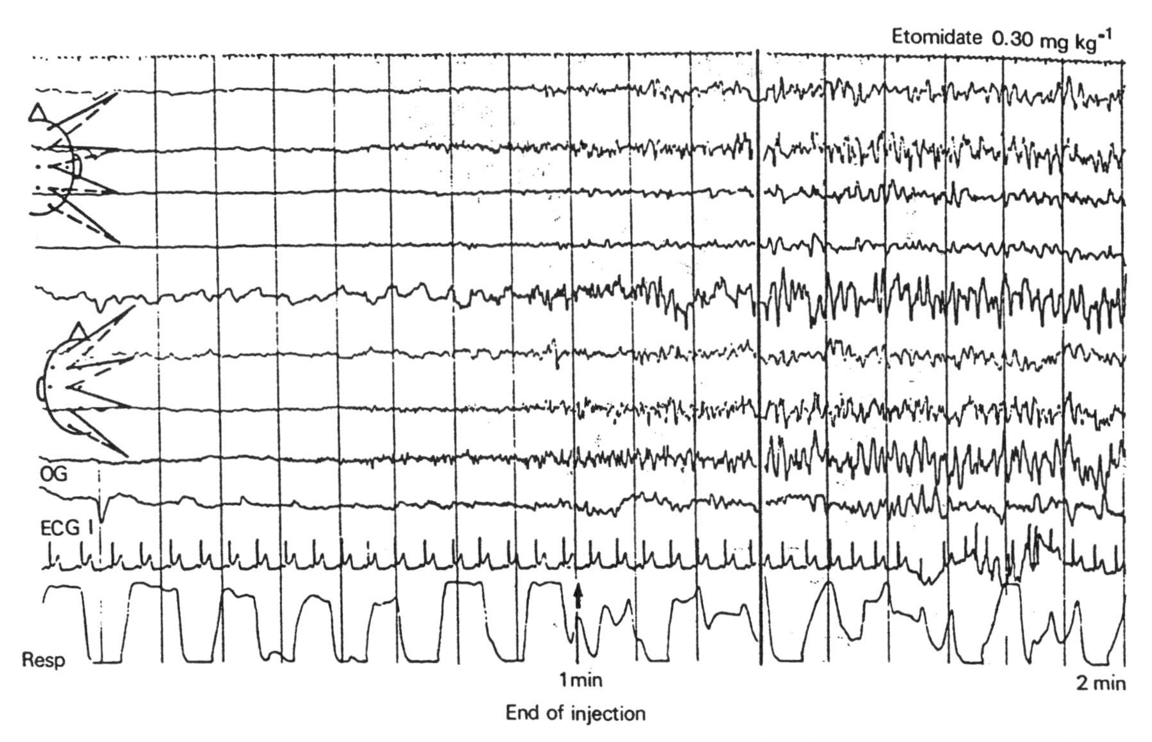

FIGURE 6-3. Etomidate-induced EEG changes (healthy volunteer): 10 seconds before the end of injection (0.3 mg/kg within 60 seconds), relatively fast irregular EEG activity occurred. At the end of the injection (1 minute), low-amplitude slow waves were noted. One minute later (2 minutes), high-amplitude slow-wave activity was seen, with superimposed waves. The oculogram (OG; right to left epicanthus) showed decreasing rapid eye movements of wakefulness. ECG (ECG I) showed increasing heart rate (up to 88 beats/min). Respiration was irregular and fast (22 breaths/min). (From Kugler J, Doenicke A, Laub M. The EEG after etomidate. In: Doenicke A, ed. Etomidate. Anaesthesiol Wiederbelebung 1977;106:31–48.)

tion that can already be utilized for surgical purposes (Fig. 6-3, right). The slow activity then increases, and the superimposed rapid activity becomes lower, corresponding to deep anesthesia and the so-called "burst-suppression" activity, that is, groups of irregular slow waves alternating with intervals of burst suppression ("electrocerebral inactivity"). This state is usually an expression of exceeding the tolerance limit and of an appreciable functional disturbance in synchronizing brain stem regions (16).

The EEG allows determination of the stages of anesthesia in arbitrarily chosen epochs, which are then entered into graphs to illustrate the time course of the changes (Fig. 6-4). After the injection of etomidate, these "hypnograms" show a rapid transition from the conscious state to deep anesthesia and subsequently a rapid subsidence of anesthesia with postanesthesia oscillations of vigilance (see Fig. 6-4). The hypnograms of all the subjects can be superimposed to give "mean-value curves" (16). With smaller doses (0.15 mg/kg) of etomidate, the standard deviations are larger than after larger (0.3 mg/kg) doses (see Fig. 6-4) (16).

After premedication with diazepam (10 mg), the EEG displays a transition from consciousness to states of reduced vigilance and increased sleepiness. After intravenous induction with etomidate (0.3 mg/kg), the transition to the medium and deep stages of anesthesia was faster in premedicated patients than after the injection of etomidate alone (Fig. 6-5). The hypnogram also showed a longer duration of the deep and medium stages than without premedication. The hypnogram showed that increasing doses of etomidate were followed by a deeper and longer-lasting hypnotic effect (Fig. 6-6). Plasma concentrations of etomidate correlated well with the observed changes in the hypnogram. With increasing the doses of etomidate, "acute tolerance" was observed analogous to the barbiturates (33-35).

EFFECTS DURING INDUCTION AND MAINTENANCE OF ANESTHESIA. In our studies, the rate of injection of etomidate (10 versus 60 seconds) did not significantly alter onset of the hypnotic effect or the onset of changes in the EEG (Fig. 6-7). The EEG changes and hypnosis correlated with plasma concentrations of etomidate, even after repeated bolus injections (Fig. 6-8). Maintenance of anesthesia with a continuous infusion of etomidate resulted in predictable changes in the EEG (Fig. 6-9) (16, 36).

SUMMARY OF EFFECTS

1. The doses of etomidate required for anesthesia in adults (0.3 mg/kg) lead to EEG changes comparable to the classic stages of barbiturate anesthesia.
2. The combination with benzodiazepines and fentanyl prolongs the anesthetic action of etomidate; a premedication with benzodiazepines and fen-

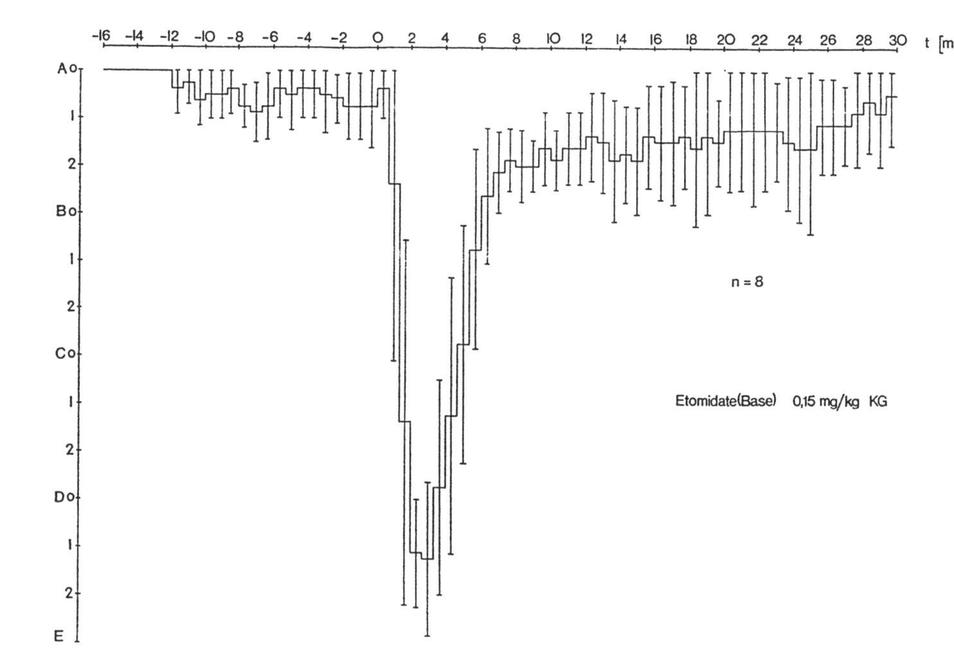

FIGURE 6-4. Hypnogram with EEG stages (A_0 = wakefulness, E = very deep sleep) of all succeeding 40-second epochs in eight healthy volunteers without premedication (mean values and standard deviations): at 0 begin, at 1 end of injection of 0.15 mg/kg etomidate (within 60 seconds). The hypnotic state lasted about 5 minutes. The state of vigilance was decreased. (From Doenicke A, Kugler J, Penzel G, et al. Cerebral function under etomidate, a new non-barbiturate iv hypnoticum. Anaesthesist 1973; 22:357–366.)

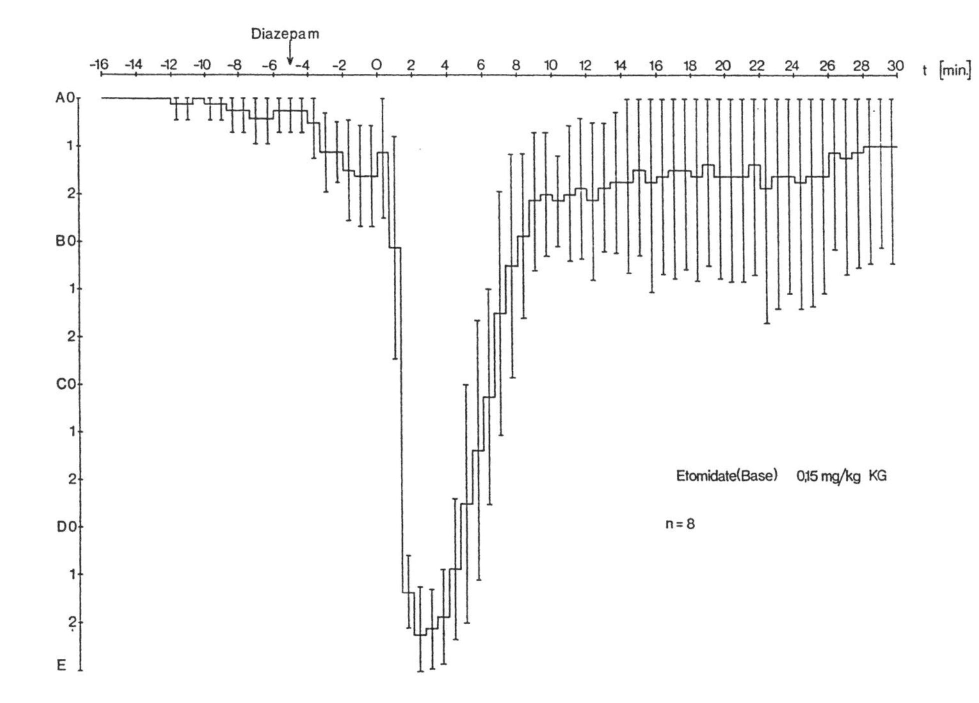

FIGURE 6-5. Hypnogram with EEG stages (A_0 = wakefulness, E = very deep sleep) of all succeeding 40-second epochs in eight healthy volunteers with a premedication of 0.1 mg/kg of intravenous diazepam (mean values and standard deviations): at 0 begin, at 1 end of injection of 0.15 mg/kg etomidate (within 60 seconds). The hypnotic state lasted about 7 minutes. Impairment of vigilance was increased and longer lasting. (From Doenicke A, Kugler J, Penzel G, et al. Cerebral function under etomidate, a new non-barbiturate iv hypnoticum. Anaesthesist 1973; 22:357–366.)

tanyl or a priming dose of etomidate suppresses the motor "excitatory" phenomena (e.g., myoclonic activity, dyskinesia) observed after administration of etomidate alone.

3. Etomidate has no specific pharmacodynamic epileptogenic or convulsant action.
4. Etomidate has a short plasma elimination half-life value. Plasma concentrations correlate well with the "depth of anesthesia" and changes in the EEG, respectively.

Effects on Intracranial Pressure

Etomidate can be used for induction of anesthesia in patients with increased intracranial pressure (ICP) values. Like thiopental (and methohexital), etomidate lowers cerebral blood flow (CBF) and ICP. The reduction in ICP does not necessarily correlate with cerebral perfusion pressure (37-39). The decrease in CBF (36%) is caused by a reduction in brain metabolism, with the cerebral metabolic rate of oxygen reduced by 45% (38).

Effects on the Respiratory System

Etomidate has minimal ventilatory depressant properties. In spontaneously breathing volunteers, the $PaCO_2$ value increased from 37.5 to 42 mm Hg, whereas PaO_2 values remained unchanged after 0.3 mg/kg of etomidate (40). In opioid-premedicated pa-

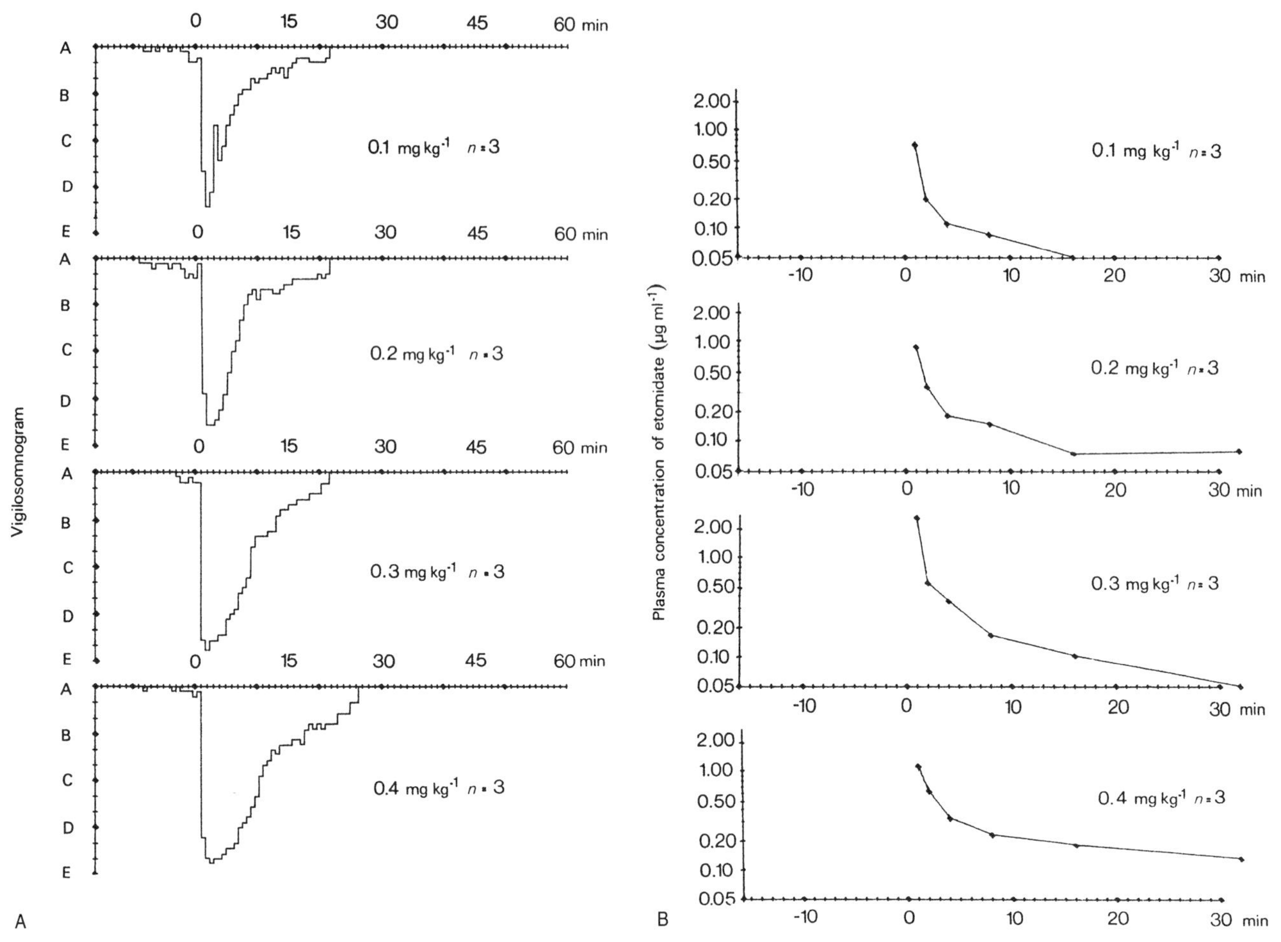

FIGURE 6-6. Hypnogram of increasing doses (A) corresponding with etomidate concentrations in the plasma (B). Premedication: 15 minutes, atropine 0.5 mg; 10 minutes, diazepam 0.05 mg/kg; 5 minutes, fentanyl 0.1 mg. (From Doenicke A, Löffler B, Kugler J, et al. Plasma concentration and EEG after various regimens of etomidate. Br J Anaesth 1982;54:393–400.)

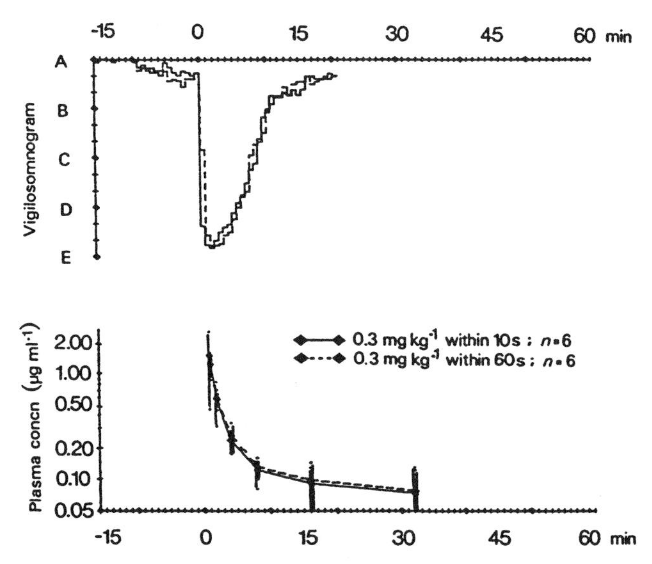

FIGURE 6-7. Hypnogram after a bolus injection of etomidate 0.3 mg/kg and corresponding etomidate concentration in the plasma. Premedication: 15 minutes, atropine 0.5 mg; 10 minutes, diazepam 0.05 mg/kg; 5 minutes, fentanyl 0.1 mg. (From Doenicke A, Löffler B, Kugler J, et al. Plasma concentration and EEG after various regimens of etomidate. Br J Anaesth 1982;54:393–400.)

tients suffering from congestive heart failure, the PaO_2 value decreased from 85 to 72 mm Hg after 0.3 mg/kg of etomidate (41). The incidence of apnea is lower after etomidate compared with thiopental (42) or methohexital (43), with an incidence between 12 and 30% (42, 44). In contrast to the barbituates, minute ventilation may actually increase after etomidate administration (42, 44).

Effects on the Cardiovascular System

Etomidate has only minimal effects on hemodynamic variables and myocardial function (45). Etomidate produces a 10% reduction in mean arterial blood pressure, a 12% reduction of peripheral vascular resistance, and a 10% increase of heart rate and cardiac index (45). However, stroke volume, left ventricular end diastolic pressure, and contractility (dP/dT) remain unchanged after an induction dose of etomidate (46). Even in cardiac patients, etomidate (0.3 mg/kg) results in only minor cardiovascular changes (47-49). Etomidate, in a dose of 0.3 mg/kg, resulted in a slight decrease of sys-

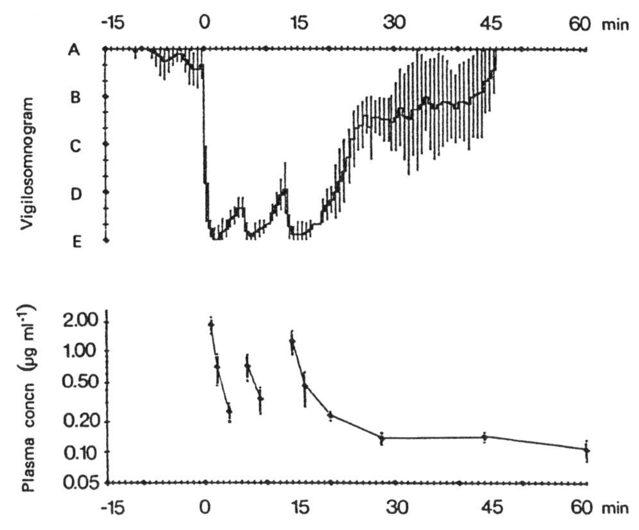

FIGURE 6-8. Hypnogram (mean values ± SD) of prolonged anesthesia: additional injections of etomidate 0.3 mg/kg (60 seconds at 0 minute), 0.15 mg/kg (60 seconds at 5 minutes), 0.15 mg/kg (60 seconds at 12 minutes), and corresponding etomidate concentrations in the plasma. Premedication: 15 minutes, atropine 0.5 mg; 10 minutes, diazepam, 0.05 mg/kg; 5 minutes, fentanyl 0.1 mg. (From Doenicke A, Löffler B, Kugler J, et al. Plasma concentration and EEG after various regimens of etomidate. Br J Anaesth 1982;54:393–400.)

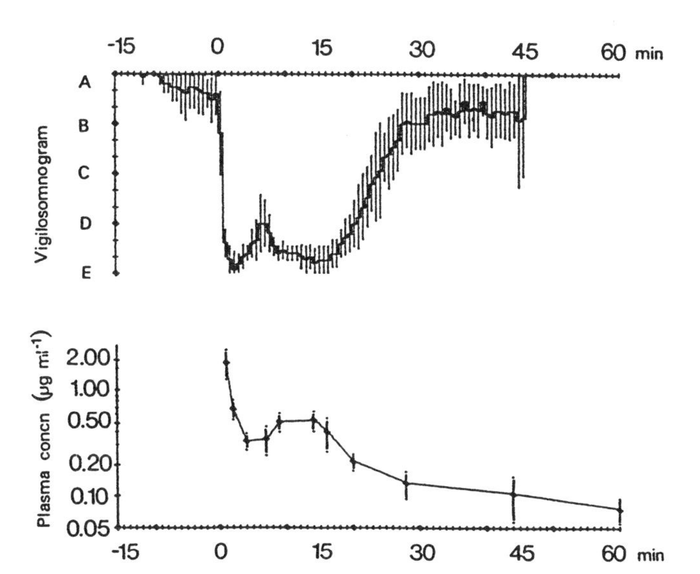

FIGURE 6-9. Hypnogram (mean values ± SD) with continuous infusion of etomidate 0.3 mg/kg in glucose 250 ml from 5 to 14 minutes (0.3 mg/kg given over 60 seconds at 0 minutes). Premedication: 15 minutes, atropine 0.5 mg; 10 minutes, diazepam 0.05 mg/kg; 5 minutes, fentanyl 0.1 mg. (From Doenicke A, Löffler B, Kugler J, et al. Plasma concentration and EEG after various regimens of etomidate. Br J Anaesth 1982;54:393–400.)

tolic blood pressure and only an 8% decrease of cardiac index in patients with myocardial disease (41). Cardiovascular changes in patients with ischemic heart disease were also modest (48, 50).

Etomidate can produce a slight increase of myocardial oxygen consumption as a result of an increase in heart rate. Because coronary perfusion pressure is unchanged, the 20% increase in coronary perfusion is a result of a decrease in coronary vascular resistance. Arteriovenous oxygen extraction is reduced by etomidate, leading to myocardial "luxury" perfusion, with the ratio of oxygen supply to demand well maintained (46, 51). Clinical and experimental data reveal that etomidate is well suited for induction of anesthesia even in patients with cardiovascular risk factors (50, 51). Compared with methohexital, thiopental, Althesin, propanidid, and propofol, etomidate is clearly the induction agent with the least cardiovascular effects. Etomidate's lack of negative inotropic effects is advantageous in patients with preexisting cardiovascular disease (52). After induction of anesthesia with etomidate, the heart rate remains almost unchanged (45, 53). To minimize the increase in heart rate during layngoscopy and intubation, etomidate should be administered in combination with fentanyl (1.5 to 5.0 µg/kg) (51, 54, 55).

Investigations using etomidate in higher dosages may reflect, in part, the adverse effects of high concentrations of propylene glycol (56). When etomidate was used for induction (18 mg) and maintenance of anesthesia (24 mg/min) (57), the reported side effects may have been related in part to the effects of propylene glycol and the high osmolality of the solution (7-13). Future investigations using etomidate in lipofundin formulation should answer this question (6). The hemodynamic stability seen with etomidate may in part be due to its unique lack of effect on the sympathetic nervous system and on baroreceptor function (58).

Effects on Other Organ Systems

Neither nephrotoxicity nor adverse effects of etomidate on hepatic function have been described, even after prolonged infusions of etomidate. Intraocular pressure is also reduced by 60% after an induction dose of etomidate (59).

SIDE EFFECTS

Inhibition of Cortisol Synthesis

The report of Ledingham and Watt (3) of an increased mortality in ICU patients who were sedated with etomidate has arguably had more impact on anesthesiologists than any other publication during the last two decades. In a retrospective analysis of their ICU patients, these investigators found that mortality was almost double in the subgroup of patients sedated with etomidate (3). The increased mortality in the etomidate-sedated group was attributed to low cortisol levels resulting from etomidate-induced suppression of cortisol synthesis. In this retrospective analysis, patients were not well characterized, and assignment to the sedation treatment groups was not randomized. In the benzodiazepine-treated group, 47 of 55 patients in the ICU were sedated, whereas in the etomidate-treated group, only 26 of 88 patients were sedated. Thus, it is possible that, during the period when etomidate was used for sedation in the ICU, only severely ill patients with the worst prognosis were sedated, suggesting that the increased mortality in the etomidate-treated group may have been caused by patient selection. Furthermore, patients in the etomidate-treated group received 75 to 120 mg of morphine as a continuous infusion, whereas the benzodiazepine-treated group received a maximum of 60 mg of morphine per day (personal communication).

In discussions of etomidate, the important role of opioid analgesics in regulating stress hormones has been almost completely ignored (60-62). Endorphins appear to play an important role in the regulation of the stress hormone response (63-66). Administration of corticotropin-releasing factor (CRF) leads to release of both adrenocorticotropic hormone (ACTH) and β-endorphin. Both centrally released hormones display a similar concentration pattern during the circadian variation over 24 hours and after surgical stress (67). In addition, negative feedback on CRF release has been demonstrated with both ACTH and β-endorphin. Thus, systemically administered opiates have a direct effect on the blood concentrations of ACTH and on cortisol levels (68-71). Even in the absence of painful stress, opiates can cause major changes in hormone levels (72).

Ledingham and Watt found that the etomidate-treated group had decreased cortisol levels, and they concluded that etomidate was associated with an increased mortality because of the suppressed cortisol synthesis. Etomidate directly inhibits 11-β-hydroxylase in the adrenal cortex (73-77). In vitro studies have shown that etomidate is the most effective adrenostatic agent on a molar basis (73). At higher dose levels, etomidate also inhibits β-desmolase (74, 78). Because opioids and etomidate are shown to reduce serum cortisol levels, it is difficult to differentiate the effects of these two drug groups. Hence, the conclusion of Ledingham and Watt that etomidate caused a higher mortality has to be viewed critically. To date, questions remain regarding the impact (if any) of low cortisol levels on patient outcome.

In light of these findings, etomidate was questioned as an induction agent (79). However, experimental results clearly demonstrate that suppression of cortisol synthesis after a single dose of 0.3 mg/kg of etomidate is short lasting. Time course of cortisol suppression after a single dose of etomidate has been investigated in several studies and suggests that cortisol function returns to normal within 6 to 8 hours of an induction dose of etomidate (73-80). Recovery of cortisol levels to normal is accompanied by increases of ACTH levels, suggesting a compensatory effect.

The time course of the cortisol response to stressful stimuli was investigated in healthy volunteers after a single dose of 0.3 mg/kg of etomidate (81). Ergometric exercise increased systolic blood pressure to 200 mm Hg, heart rate to 180 beats/min, and plasma ACTH levels to 250 pg/ml; however, plasma cortisol levels remained unchanged. When the cold stress was performed 4 hours after an induction dose of etomidate, however, a sharp rise in cortisol levels above 10 μg/dl was noted (Fig. 6-10) (81). Clinical investigations of the effect of a single dose of etomidate on cortisol levels during anesthesia are difficult to interpret because opioid analgesics can also influence cortisol levels (68-71). In volunteers, cortisol levels exceeded baseline values as early as 3 hours following etomidate (0.3 mg/kg) and increased from 5.8 to 6.3 μg/dl after 4 hours (Fig. 6-11) (75). After morphine, cortisol levels ranged be-

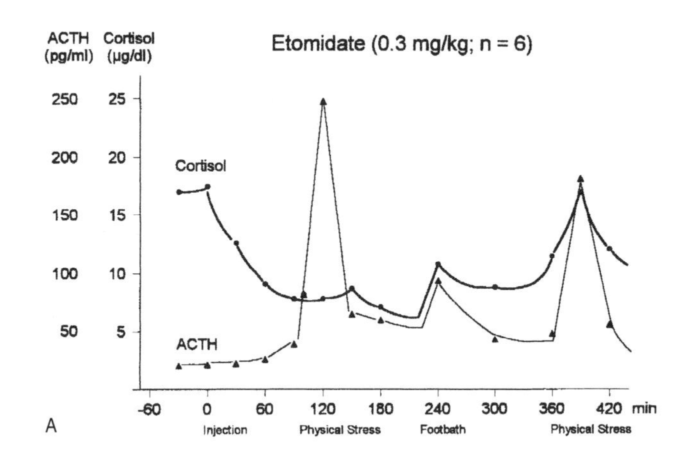

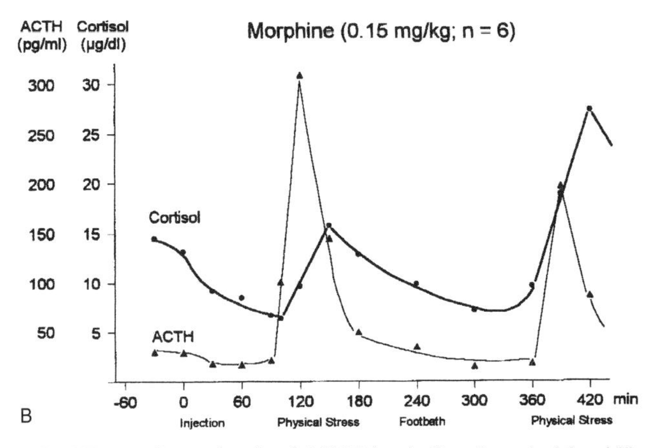

FIGURE 6-10. Serum levels of ACTH (pg/ml) and cortisol (μg/dl) after etomidate (n = 6;A) and morphine (n = 6;B). Both drugs cause a similar decrease in plasma cortisol concentration after injection. After etomidate, there was no increase of cortisol after ergometric stress. After morphine, ACTH and cortisol increased after ergometric stress. Cold stress (ice water foot bath) after 4 hours caused ACTH to rise from 60 to 90 pg/ml, with a cortisol response (from 7 to 11.2 μg/dl) with etomidate. With morphine, no ACTH and cortisol response occurred. Ergometric stress after 6 hours caused an increase of ACTH and cortisol in both groups. (From Doenicke A, Shay J, Mayer M, et al. Cortisol and ACTH increase 4 hr after etomidate. Anesthesiology 1992;77:A336.)

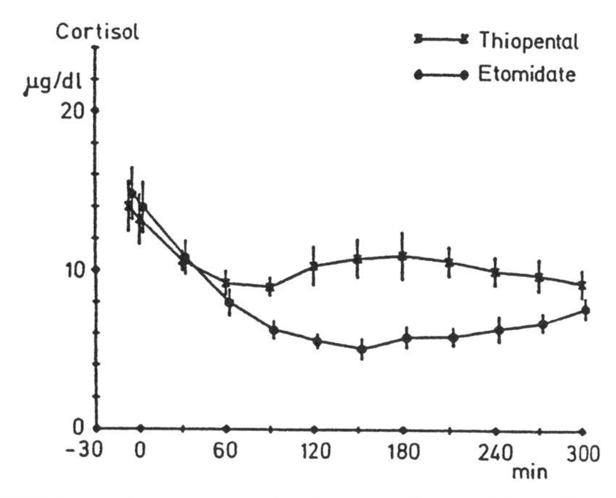

FIGURE 6-11. Cortisol serum levels (µg/ml) after 0.3 mg/kg etomidate or 4 mg/kg thiopental. Values are shown as mean and SEM at the 12 time points. Cortisol serum levels after etomidate are significantly reduced from 90 to 240 minutes, compared with thiopental. (From Engelhardt D, Doenicke A, Suttmann H, et al. The influence of etomidate and thiopentone on ACTH and cortisol levels in serum: a prospective controlled trial in healthy men. Anaesthesist 1984;33:583–587.)

tween 3.8 and 4 µg/dl at 3 and 6 hours, respectively (Fig. 6-12) (82), emphasizing the ACTH-suppressing effects of opioid analgesics.

Independent of the report by Ledingham and Watt (3), several prospective studies have been performed to investigate cortisol levels during general anesthesia (83). In patients receiving etomidate-lormetazepam-fentanyl anesthesia, cortisol levels decreased to 54% of baseline values. Increases in cortisol levels were only seen during anesthesia with a combination of thiopental, halothane, and enflurane (Table 6-1). The cortisol values 3 hours after anesthesia increased 100% above baseline values with a halothane-enflurane technique compared with a 52% increase after a etomidate-fentanyl-based technique. These increases are even more remarkable given that they were observed in the afternoon, when cortisol levels are usually lower than in the morning (83).

The question of whether etomidate can be safely administered to severely ill patients has been investigated in several clinical trials. Crozier and associates (84, 85) stated that it was inappropriate to assume that patients having transient low cortisol levels after etomidate anesthesia are in a life-threatening condition. In a study involving patients with burns who were subdivided into two groups according to their cortisol levels, the survival rate was considerable lower in the group with higher cortisol levels than in the group with low cortisol levels. These investigators also demonstrated (86) incomplete inhibition of cortisol levels in patients after induction with etomidate and subsequent etomidate infusion (total etomidate dose of 63 ± 6.4 mg). The inhibition of cortisol synthesis induced by etomidate was dose related. At plasma etomidate levels under 50 nmol/L, there was no significant inhibi-

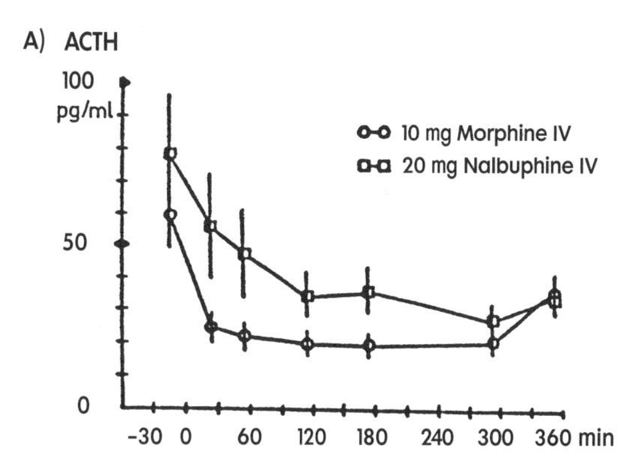

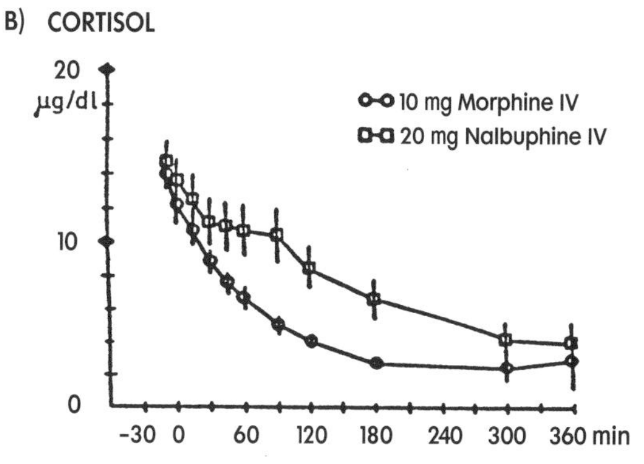

FIGURE 6-12. Plasma ACTH (A) and cortisol (B) levels after the intravenous administration of 10 mg of morphine or 20 mg of nalbuphine. Morphine reduces ACTH and cortisol levels significantly for more than 360 minutes. All values are given as mean ± SEM for n = 16. (From Suttmann H, Doenicke A, Lorenz W, et al. Is perioperative stress a real surgical phenomena or merely a drug induced effect? Theor Surg 1986;1:119–135.)

TABLE 6-1. Serum Cortisol Levels Before and After Anesthesia for Abdominal Surgery

	Cortisol (nmol/L)		
Anesthetic Group (n = 10)	**I**	**II**	**III**
A. Halothane Thiopental	603 ±235	746[†] ±242	1330[*] ±256
B. Enflurane Thiopental	578 ±170	764[†] ±211	1157[*] ±344
C. Neuroleptic anesthetic Droperidol-benzodiazepine-fentanyl	450 ±165	460[†] ±172	835[*] ±293
D. Electrostimulation lormetazepam etomidate	432 ±118	371 ±137	515 ±175
E. Lormetazepam fentanyl etomidate	515 ±168	327[†] ±55	691 ±347

*$p < 0.05$ I vs II and III

†$p < 0.05$ II vs III

Group A received anesthesia with thiopental and halothane; group B with thiopental and enflurane; group C with droperidol and fentanyl; group D with electrostimulation, etomidate, and lormetazepam; group E with lormetazepam, fentanyl, and etomidate (n = 10 in each group); values given as mean and standard deviation; cortisol levels were measured before anesthesia (I), after intraperitoneal preparation (II) and 3 hours after anesthesia (III). (Adapted from Dorow R, Doenicke A, Suttmann H, et al. Einfluss verschiedener Narkosemethoden auf hormonelle Parameter und auf das sympathonervale systems. In: Doenicke A, Koenig U, eds. Immunologie in Anaesthesie und Intensivmedizin. vol 3. Berlin: Springer-Verlag (Sertürner Workshop), 1983:97.)

tion of cortisol synthesis. Etomidate concentrations of 50 nmol/L are achieved approximately 4 hours after a normal induction dose. Similar results were obtained by Stuttmann and colleagues (87), suggesting that short-term cortisol suppression during anesthesia with etomidate had no adverse clinical consequences.

In addition, one study was performed to investigate whether prolonged use of etomidate as part of a total intravenous anesthesia (TIVA) technique had an adverse effect on clinical outcome. An etomidate-fentanyl-based TIVA technique was compared with midazolam-fentanyl for coronary artery surgery (86). Both anesthetic groups received the same dose of fentanyl, and the total drug doses were etomidate, 87 ± 3 mg, and midazolam, 46 ± 2 mg. Plasma cortisol concentrations decreased in the etomidate-treated group from 20 (10 to 31) to 10 (6 to 31) μg/dl (median and range) before extracorporeal circulation, but they returned to baseline values 1 hour after anesthesia and were significantly increased at 6 hours (29 μg/dl) and 20 hours (46 μg/dl) after anesthesia (Fig. 6-13). No difference was noted between the groups, except cortisol levels were higher in the etomidate-treated group at 20 hours after anesthesia. The stimulated increase in cortisol was markedly impaired in the etomidate-treated group, ACTH and β-endorphin were markedly increased in the etomidate-treated group, and ACTH concentrations were eight times higher than the corresponding postoperative values in the midazolam-treated group (ACTH 141 versus 18 pmol/L). Plasma catecholamine concentrations were increased significantly in both treatment groups; however, norepinephrine concentrations were greater in the etomidate-treated group at 6 hours after anesthesia. Two patients in the midazolam group and none in the etomidate group required circulatory support with exogenous catecholamines. Crozier and associates (86) concluded that the stress of cardiac surgery can overcome the block in cortisol synthesis caused by the administration of high-dose etomidate by substantially increasing ACTH secretion. The administration of high-dose etomidate was not associated with perioperative cardiovascular instability. Therefore, the use of etomidate as a component of TIVA should not be excluded simply because of transiently decreased cortisol secretion.

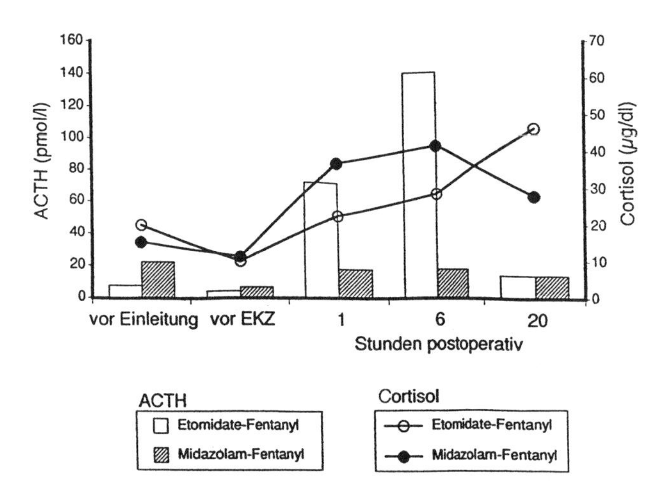

FIGURE 6-13. Serum concentrations of ACTH (pg/dl) and cortisol (μg/dl) during and after anesthesia for coronary artery surgery. In one group, anesthesia was induced with fentanyl 0.5 mg and etomidate 0.3 mg/kg and then maintained as total intravenous anesthesia (TIVA) with etomidate (0.36 mg/kg/h) and fentanyl 0.01 mg/kg/h. In the other group, anesthesia was induced with fentanyl 0.5 mg and midazolam 0.2 mg/kg and then maintained as TIVA with midazolam (0.16 mg/kg/h) and fentanyl 0.01 mg/kg/h. Cortisol levels had returned to baseline 1 hour after anesthesia and were significantly increased in both groups 6 and 20 hours after anesthesia. (From Crozier TA, Schlaeger M, Wuttke W, Kettler D. The stress of coronary artery surgery overcomes the inhibition of cortisol synthesis caused by etomidate-fentanyl anaesthesia. Anaesthesist 1994;43:605–613.)

Pain on Injection

The problem of pain on injection after etomidate was addressed as long ago as 1978, when it was suggested that any new anesthetic drug to be introduced has certain specific features that must become familiar to the anesthesiologist. Etomidate, a hypnotic generally recognized as preserving hemodynamic stability, was expected to gain further approval when its side effect of venous pain could be reduced. It was also suggested that the manufacturer works on this problem, to achieve a pleasant induction of anesthesia for the patient (4).

Sensations of pain after the intravenous injection of etomidate occur with a frequency of 18 to 81%, depending on the size of the vein and the solvent. Of 400 patients studied, 81% reported pain after the injection of etomidate into veins on the dorsum of the hand, 44% after injection into forearm veins, and 18% after injection into the cubital or brachial vein (88). A multinational study (5) intended to provide an objective measure of pain after injection of etomidate reported an incidence of 13% in 4452 patients. The pain on injection of etomidate depended not only on the dose and vein diameter, but also on the choice of premedication and the induction dose (increasing from 9% to around 22% when the etomidate dose was doubled). Injection pain was minimized by preadministration of fentanyl (88).

Polyethylene Glycol Solvent

Hendry and colleagues reported in 1977 (89) that etomidate formulated in polyethylene glycol caused pain on injection in only 4% of patients. Unfortunately, this formulation (with a normal osmolality) was not stable and therefore was not developed for commercial use.

Hydroxypropyl-β-Cyclodextrin Solvent

The combination of etomidate with hydroxypropyl-β-cyclodextrin demonstrated some advantages over the

TABLE 6-2. Venous Tolerance of Etomidate in Propylene Glycol (n = 50) and in Lipofundin (n = 50)

	Propylene Glycol		Lipid Emulsion	
Injection pain	n = 50	(%)	n = 50	(%)
None	32	64	50	100
Mild	7	14	0	0
Moderate	4	8	0	0
Severe	7	14	0	0
Vein reaction day 1	n = 47		n = 49	
None	35	74	49	100
Phlebitis	9	19	0	0
Thrombosis	3	6	0	0
Vein reaction day 7	n = 47		n = 48	
None	36	77	48	100
Phlebitis	2	4	0	0
Thrombosis	5	11	0	0
Thrombophlebitis				
< 4 cm	2	4	0	0
> 4 cm	2	4	0	0

(From Doeniche A, Kugler A, Vollmann N, et al. Etomidate with a new solubilizer: clinical and experimental investigations on venous tolerance and bioavailability. Anaesthesist 1990;39:475–480.)

commercial formulation of etomidate in propylene glycol in that irritation of the veins and the resultant thrombophlebitis were less common. However, pain during the injection of etomidate was not completely suppressed (13). Hydroxypropyl-β-cyclodextrin, when injected alone, did not cause significant pain (13). Because hydroxypropyl-β-cyclodextrin does not have the chemical ability to bind etomidate completely, pain on injection of etomidate is probably caused by etomidate itself.

Intralipid (Long-Chain Triglycerides) Solvent

In 1983 and 1984, the first results with etomidate dissolved in intralipid were reported (90, 91). In these comparative studies, the most remarkable finding, apart from the injection, on pain after administration of etomidate in propylene glycol was long-lasting thrombophlebitis, occurring a few days after the injection of etomidate. In contrast, no venous irritation occurred after etomidate administration when it was dissolved in an intralipid solution.

Lipofundin (Medium-Chain Triglycerides) Solvent

The question of venous irritation was again addressed in 1989 (92). In a prospective randomized study, etomidate was dissolved in either propylene glycol or lipofundin (6). Half the subjects given etomidate in propylene glycol complained of pain during the injection. At the final examination 1 week after the anesthetic injection, thrombophlebitis was noted in three patients given etomidate in the form of a painful hard vein over 10 to 15 cm proximal to the site of injection. The inflammation appeared 3 to 4 days after the administration of etomidate. No association was noted between the intensity of the pain on injection and subsequent thrombophlebitis. In no case did the subjects given etomidate in lipofundin experience pain during the injection. More important, no local venous irritation was observed during the 7-day study period. The bioavailability of etomidate in lipofundin was equivalent to that of etomidate in propylene glycol, with the mean plasma levels nearly identical in both groups (6). Blood pressure and heart rate were stable and similar in both treatment groups (6).

The experimental results in volunteers have been confirmed by a clinical study (6). Following administration etomidate in propylene glycol, 36% of the patients described the injection as painful. On the first postoperative day, 9 of the 47 patients studied had phlebitis (tenderness on palpation of the vein), and 3 others had evidence of thrombosis (hardness of the vein). On the seventh day after the operation, a venous reaction was evident in 22% of the patients receiving etomidate in propylene glycol. Two patients had phlebitis (4%), 5 patients (10%) had thrombosis with obvious hardening of the vein, and 4 patients (8%) had thrombophlebitis (tender and hard vein) (Table 6-2) (6). However, patients had no signs of local irritation after etomidate administration in lipofundin.

Therefore, two of the most unpleasant side effects of etomidate, namely, pain on injection and postoperative thrombophlebitis, can be abolished when etomidate is dissolved in lipofundin. This drug preparation is available for clinical use as Etomidate Lipuro (6). In a comparison of pain on injection with propofol, Etomidate Lipuro was associated with significantly less discomfort than propofol (Table 6-3) (94). Lipofundin is the preferable vehicle for clinical use (93). The incidence of myoclonic activity is also lower (10%) than in previous studies in which etomidate was dissolved in propylene glycol. Thus, the solvent lipofundin may possibly reduce the incidence of etomidate-induced myoclonic activity.

TABLE 6-3. Pain on Injection and Burning After Either Etomidate in Lipofundin (0.3 mg/kg) or Propofol (2 mg/kg) for Induction of Anesthesia (n = 50 in each group)

	Etomidate Lipuro	Propofol
Number	50	50
Burning	1 (2%)	19 (38%)
No discomfort	49 (98%)	31 (62%)
Pain on injection	3 (6%)	15 (30%)
No pain	47 (94%)	35 (70%)

(Adapted from Hepting L. Vergleichende Wirksamkeits-und Verträglichkeitsuntersuchung von Thiopental-Natrium: ein Vergleich mit Etomidat-Emulsion und Propofol [Thesis]. Munich: Ludwig-Maximilians University, 1995.

TABLE 6-4. Postoperative Nausea and Vomiting After Induction of Anesthesia With Either Etomidate in Lipofundin (0.3 mg/kg) or Propofol (2 mg/kg)

	Etomidate Lipofundin (n = 50)	Propofol (n = 50)
Nausea (n, %)	13 (26%)	12 (24%)
Vomiting (n, %)	11 (22%)	12 (24%)

(Adapted from Hepting L. Vergleichende Wirksamkeits-und Verträglichheitsuntersuchung von Thiopentae-Natrium: ein Vergleich mit Etomidat-Emulsion und Propofol [Thesis]. Munich: Ludwig-Maximilians University, 1995.

Nausea and Vomiting

The incidence of postoperative nausea and vomiting (PONV) after etomidate is reported to be as high as 30 to 40% (74, 95-99). This side effect is a major limiting factor in the use of etomidate for ambulatory (day-case) surgery (100). In contrast, the incidence of PONV after methohexital (97) or thiopental (96) is reported to be in the range of 10 to 20%. However, other studies showed no difference (101). When the incidence of PONV associated with etomidate in lipofundin was compared with that associated with propofol in a randomized, double-blind study, 25% of the patients in each group developed PONV (Table 6-4) (102). The solvent may possibly influence the incidence of PONV, compared with earlier studies in which etomidate in propylene glycol was used (94-99).

Histamine Release and Osmolality

Whenever a new anesthetic drug is introduced, the question of histamine release arises. In 1973, histamine release after etomidate was investigated. Etomidate was originally formulated as a sulfate in phosphate buffer (with a pH of 3.4 and an osmolality of 270 mOsm/L), a preparation that was not associated with histamine release (102). Unfortunately, phosphate-buffered etomidate was unstable for long-term storage, and in 1977, etomidate was reformulated in a 35% propylene glycol solution with an osmolality of 4900 mOsm/L (11, 13). The high osmolality of etomidate formulations in propylene glycol caused histamine release, pain on injection, and phlebitis (103). Histamine release and venous sequelae are not related because the mechanisms responsible for these events are different (103). In 1978, histamine release after etomidate was first reported (104). Later, several reports of anaphylactoid reactions occurred (105-107). In one report, a greater than eightfold increases in the plasma histamine concentration was observed in one volunteer without any associated hemodynamic compromise (103). The absence of hypotension may be explained by the transistory nature of the histamine in the circulation (108). The small amount of histamine released from destroyed blood and tissue cells is not sustained by the cascade mechanism of mediators and, therefore, does not produce untoward hemodynamic sequelae (108). Even though etomidate in propylene glycol can cause histamine release, etomidate is a safe hypnotic drug (108).

The hyperosmolality of the propylene glycol formulation may cause direct injury to vascular endothelium (109), resulting in local vessel damage. The pain and venous sequelae reported in previous studies (6, 90, 110-113) can be interpreted as symptoms of irritation of the intravascular tissue (109). Etomidate formulated in propylene glycol was associated with pain on injection, phlebitis, and histamine release, whereas etomidate formulated in lipofundin was not (Table 6-5). The hyperosmolar vehicle, propylene glycol, may be responsible for the pain and phlebitis by directly irritating the vascular endothelium of the veins (109). The lack of a direct association among histamine release, pain on injection, and venous sequelae implies that the mechanisms producing these effects may be different.

Hemolysis

Whereas the side effects of propylene glycol have been well described in the literature and include hypotension, lactic acidosis, pain, pulmonary hypertension, and cerebral edema, hemolysis had not been previously described (114-121). The first indication that etomidate in propylene glycol possibly caused hemolysis was as an accidental observation of the serum from volunteers participating in a pharmacokinetic study. A study was initiated to compare pain associated with etomidate in two different solvents. The serum from subjects treated with etomidate dissolved in propylene glycol were noted to be reddish, whereas the serum of subjects treated with etomidate in hydroxypropyl-β-cyclodextrin were normal (12). This ef-

TABLE 6-5. Osmolality and pH of Etomidate and of Propofol

	mOsm/L	pH
Etomidate in propylene glycol (35% vol, 362.6 mg/mL)*	4900	5.1
Etomidate in propylene glycol (diluted to 17.5 vol %, 181.3 mg/mL, 1:2 dilution with 0.9% NaCl)*	2450	5.5
Etomidate in 2-hydroxypropyl-β-cyclodextrin	307	6.4
Etomidate in lipid emulsion*	400	7.6
Propofol*	295	8.2
Propofol (1:4 dilution with glucose 5%)*	285	8.1

*Commercial preparation.

(From Doenicke A, Nebauer AE, Hoerneclee R, et al. Osmolalities of propylene glycol containing drug formulations for parenteral use: should propylene glycol be used as a solvent? Anesth Analg 1992;75:431–435.)

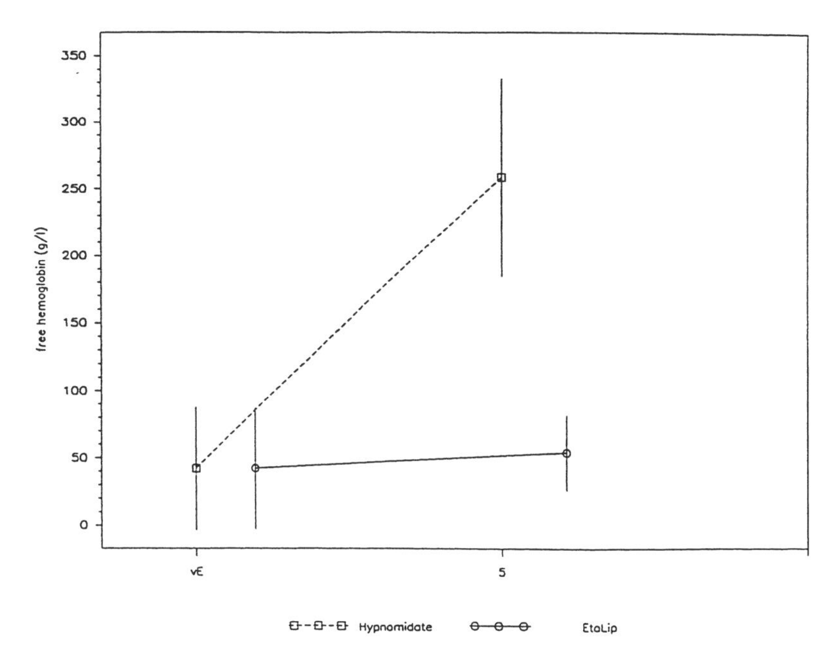

FIGURE 6-14. Serum free hemoglobin concentrations (g/L) 5 minutes after the induction of anesthesia with either etomidate in propylene glycol (circles) or etomidate in lipofundin (EtoLip;squares). Free hemoglobin increased significantly after etomidate in propylene glycol indicating hemolysis. (From Doenicke A, Roizen MF, Hoernecke R, et al. Hemolysis after etomidate: comparison of formulation with propylene glycol versus lipid emulsion. (submitted).)

fect was likely due to the solvent's different osmolality because etomidate in propylene glycol has an osmolality of 4965 mOsm, whereas etomidate in hydroxypropyl-β-cyclodextrin has an osmolality of 307 mOsm (10, 12). When serum from patients who received etomidate in lipofundin was examined, it was also found to be normal. Etomidate in lipofundin (like etomidate in hydroxypropyl-β-cyclodextrin) has a near physiologic osmolality of 400 mOsm/L. One clinical study (122) demonstrated that, in the first few minutes after administration of etomidate in propylene glycol, free hemoglobin increases to 259 mg/L, suggesting that intravascular hemolysis has occurred (Fig. 6-14). Free hemoglobin is not detectable at a later time, but the transient hemolysis caused by injecting etomidate in propylene glycol increases haptoglobin-hemoglobin complex and results in a 52% reduction in the serum haptoglobin concentration. The haptoglobin concentration in the serum of patients with etomidate in propylene glycol fell from a baseline value of 1.78 $\pm$ 0.15 g/L to a value of 0.89 $\pm$ 0.12 g/L after 360 minutes (Fig. 6-15) (122). After etomidate in lipofundin, only a slight reduction was noted in haptoglobin, from a baseline value of 1.79 $\pm$ 0.13 to 1.51 $\pm$ 0.14 g/L.

On careful inspection, serum from patients who received etomidate in propylene glycol may be red for up to 360 minutes because the haptoglobin-hemoglobin complex has a red color similar to that of free hemoglobin. Hemolysis and cell lysis associated with an induction dose of etomidate in propylene glycol are not sufficient in healthy patients to cause detectable renal injury. However, if etomidate in propylene gly-

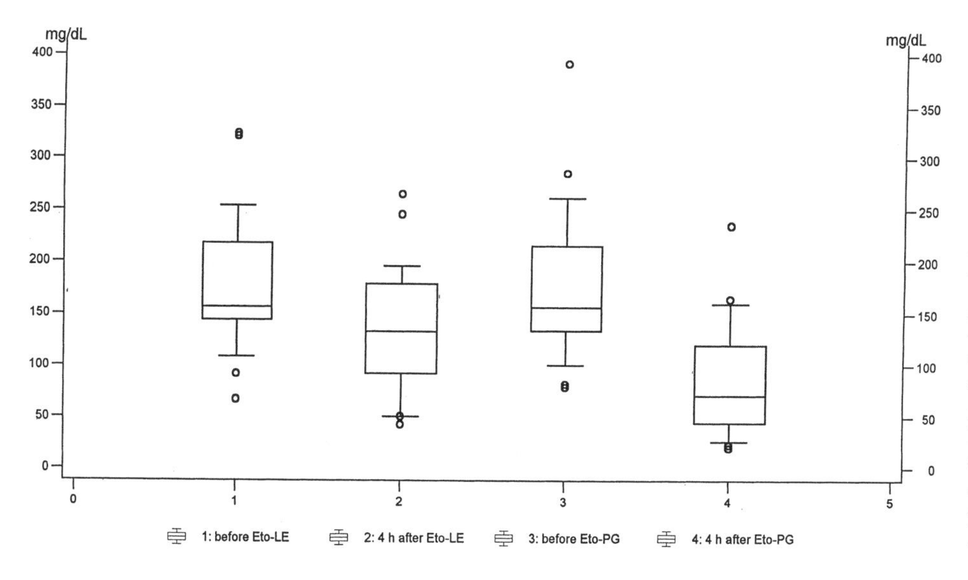

FIGURE 6-15. Serum haptoglobin concentrations (mg/dl) before and 4 hours after the induction of anesthesia with either etomidate in propylene glycol (Eto-PG) or etomidate in lipofundin (Eto-LE). Haptoglobin concentration decrease significantly more after etomidate in propylene glycol indicating hemolysis. (From Doenicke A, Roizen MF, Hoernecke R, et al. Hemolysis after etomidate: comparison of formulation with propylene glycol versus lipid emulsion. (submitted).)

col is injected repeatedly at short intervals, or if it is used as an anesthetic agent in combination with other drugs dissolved in propylene glycol such as diazepam, lorazepam, or nitroglycerin (13), significant hemolysis may occur leading to hemoglobinuria (117) and even acute renal failure, especially in patients with preexisting renal disease. In addition, use of intraoperative autotransfusion (IAT) poses another situation that can make hemolysis with etomidate in propylene glycol problematic. After an induction dose of etomidate in propylene glycol, haptoglobin fell from 1.78 ± 0.15 to 0.89 ± 0.12 g/L. A similar degree of haptoglobin depletion has been observed after IAT (123). Etomidate's cardiovascular stability makes it a desirable agent to use in older, sicker patients, who also may undergo procedures in which IAT is useful (e.g., total hip replacement, vascular surgery). The combination of etomidate in propylene glycol and IAT may lead to pronounced hemolysis, causing haptoglobin to become virtually undetectable.

These data suggest that it may be important to know the osmolalities of intravenous sedative-hypnotics. Etomidate in propylene glycol, with an osmolality of 4900 mOsm/L, is not the only hyperosmolar drug dissolved in propylene glycol. Lorazepam, with an osmolality of 12,800 mOsm/L, nitroglycerin (50 μg), with an osmolality of 4550 mOsm/L (13), and diazepam may have effects similar to those of etomidate in propylene glycol on intravascular cellular elements (e.g., erythrocytes and basophilis and endothelial cells). Moreover, propylene glycol-induced damage to basophils may cause histamine and other mediators to be released.

In conclusion, the intravenous anesthetic etomidate has experienced "ups and downs" during the 25 years since its introduction into clinical practice. The change of the solvent from a phosphate-buffered solution to propylene glycol and more recently to lipofundin has changed its side effect profile without altering its desirable clinical properties. The newer formulation of etomidate in lipofundin emulsion appears to reduce many of etomidate's unpleasant side effects. Hence, etomidate lipofundin may provide beneficial physiologic properties without the high incidence of untoward side effects which characterize the current propylene glycol formulation, thereby making etomidate a more attractive alternative to currently available intravenous hypnotic agents.

REFERENCES

1. Janssen PAJ, Niemegeers CJE, Schellekens KHL, Lemperts PM. Etomidate, R-(+)-ethyl-1 (-methyl-benzyl) imidazole-5-carboxylate (R 16 659), a potent, short-acting and relatively atoxic intravenous hypnotic agent in rats. Arzneimittelforschung 1971; 21:1234–1243.
2. Doenicke A, Kugler J, Penzel G, et al. Cerebral function under etomidate, a new non-barbiturate iv hypnoticum. Anaesthesist 1973;22:357–366.
3. Ledingham IM, Watt I. Influence of sedation on mortality in critically ill multiple trauma patients, letter. Lancet 1983;1:1270.
4. Doenicke A. Etomidate [Editorial]. Anaesthesist 1978;27:51.
5. Schuermans V, Dom J, Dony J, et al. Multinational evaluation of etomidate for anesthesia induction: conclusions and consequences. Anaesthesist 1978;27:52–59.
6. Doenicke A, Kugler A, Vollmann N, et al. Etomidate with a new solubilizer: clinical and experimental investigations on venous tolerance and bioavailability. Anaesthesist 1990;39:475–480.
7. Christopher MM, Eckfeldt JH, Eaton JW. Propylene glycol ingestion causes D-lactic acidosis. Lab Invest 1990;62:114–118.
8. Demey HE, Daelemans RA, Verpooten GA, et al. Propylene glycol-induced side effects during nitroglycerin therapy. Intensive Care Med 1988;14:221–226.
9. Martin G, Finberg L. Propylene glycol: a potentially toxic vehicle in liquid dosage form. Pediatrics 1970;77:877–878.
10. Fligner CL, Jack R, Twiggs GA, Raisys VA. Hyperosmolality induced by propylene glycol. JAMA 1985;253:1606–1609.
11. Bretschneider H. Osmolalities of commercially supplied drugs often used in anesthesia. Anesth Analg 1987;66:361–362.
12. Doenicke A, Roizen MF, Nebauer AE, et al. A comparison of two formulations for etomidate, 2-hydroxypropyl-β-cyclodectrin (HPCD) and propylene glycol. Anesth Analg 1994;79:933–939.
13. Doenicke A, Nebauer AE, Hoernecke R, et al. Osmolalities of propylene glycol containing drug formulations for parenteral use: should propylene glycol be used as a solvent? Anesth Analg 1992;75:431–435.
14. Meuldermans WEG, Heykants JJP. The plasma protein binding and distribution of etomidate in dog, rat and human blood. Arch Int Pharmacodyn Ther 1976;221:150.
15. Mannes GA, Doenicke A. Protein binding of etomidate. In: Doenicke A, ed. Etomidate. Anaesthesiol Wiederbelebung 1977; 106:6–8.
16. Doenicke A, Löffler B, Kugler J, et al. Plasma concentration and EEG after various regimens of etomidate. Br J Anaesth 1982; 54:393–400.
17. Ghoneim MM, Korttila K. Pharmacokinetics of intraveous anaesthetics: implications for clinical use. Clin Pharmacokinet 1977;2:344.
18. Hamme MJ van, Ghonheim MM, Ambre JJ. Pharmacokinetics of etomidate, a new intravenous anesthetic. Anesthesiology 1978;49:274.
19. Schüttler J, Wilms M, Lauven PM, et al. Pharmakokinetische Untersuchungen über Etomidat beim Menschen. Anaesthesist 1980;29:658.
20. Fragen RJ, Avram MJ, Henthorn TK, Caldwell NJ. Pharmakokinetically designed etomidate infusion regimen for hypnosis. Anaesth Analg 1983;62:654–660.
21. Heykants J, Brugmans J, Doenicke A. On the pharmacokinetics of etomidate (R 26490) in human volunteers: plasma levels, metabolism and excretion: clinical research report R 26 490/1. Beerse, Belgium: Janssen Pharmaceutica, 1973.
22. Heykants J. The distribution, metabolism and excretion of etomidate in the rat: biological research report R 26 490/5. Beerse, Belgium: Janssen Research Products Information Service, 1974.
23. Janssen PAJ, Niemegeers CJE Marsboom RPN. Etomidate, a potent non-barbiturate hypnotic: intravenous etomidate in mice, rats, guinea-pigs, rabbits and dogs. Arch Int Pharmacodyn Ther 1975;214:92–132.
24. Doenicke A, Haehl M. Teratogenicity of etomidate. In: Doenicke A, ed. Etomidate. Anaesthesiol Wiederbelebung 1977; 106:23–24.

25. Kugler J, Doenicke A, Laub M. The EEG after etomidate. In: Doenicke A, ed. Etomidate. Anaesthesiol Wiederbelebung 1977; 106:31–48.
26. Baiker-Heberlein M, Kenins P, Kikullus H, et al. Investigations on the site of the central nervous action of the short-acting hypnotic agent R-(+)-ethyl-1-(-methyl-benzyl) imidazole-5-carboxylate (etomidate) in cats. Anaesthesist 1979;28:78.
27. Evans RH, Hill RG. GABA-mimetic action of etomidate. Experientia 1978;34:1325.
28. Harvey SC. Hypnotics and sedatives. In: Goodman, Gilman, eds. The pharmacological basis of therapeutics. 7th ed. New York: Macmillan, 1985:339.
29. Ebrahim ZY, DeBoer GE, Luders H, et al. Effect of etomidate on the electroencaphologram of patients with epilepsy. Anesth Analg 1986;65:1004–1006.
30. Ashton D, Wauquier A. Effects of some antiepileptic, neuroleptic, and gabaminergic drugs on convulsions induced by D, L-allyglycine. Pharmacol Biochem Behav 1979;11:221.
31. Ashton D, Wauquier A. Behavioral analysis of the effects of 15 anticonvulsants on the amygdaloid kindeld rat. Psychopharmacology 1979;65:7.
32. Wauquier A, Ashton D, Clincke G, et al. Etomidat, ein barbituratfreies Hypnotikum: antikonvulsive, antianoxische und hirnprotektive Wirkung im Tierexperiment. In: Opitz A, Degen R, eds. Anästhesie bei zerebralen Krampfanfällen und Intensivtherapie des Status epilepticus. Erlangen, Verlagsgesellschaft, 1980:183.
33. Brodie BB, Mark CC, Lief PA, et al. Acute tolerance to thiopental. J Pharmacol Exp Ther 1951;102:215.
34. Dundee JW, Price HL, Dripps RD. Acute tolerance to thiopentone in man. Br J Anaesth 1956;28:344.
35. Maynert EW, Klingmann GI. Acute tolerance to intravenous anaesthetics in dogs. J Pharmacol Exp Ther 1960;128:192.
36. Schüttler J, Stoeckel M, Wilms M, et al. Ein pharmakokinetisch begründetes Infusionsmodell für Etomidate zur Aufrechterhaltung von Steady State Plasmaspiegeln. Anaesthesist 1980; 29:662.
37. Moss E, Powell D, Gibson RM, McDowall DG. Effect of etomidate on intracranial pressure and cerebral perfusion pressure. Br J Anaesth 1979;51:347.
38. Renou AM, Vernhiet J, Macrez P, et al. Cerebral blood flow and metabolism during etomidate anaesthesia in man. Br J Anaesth 1978;50:1047.
39. Kochs E, Thiel H. Neurochirurgie/Psychiatrie. In: Doenicke A, Kettler D, List WF, et al, eds. Anästhesiologie. Berlin: Springer-Verlag, 1995:540–590.
40. Doenicke A, Wagner E, Beetz KH. Arterial blood gas analysis following administration of three short-acting iv hypnotics (propanidid, etomidate, methohexital). Anaesthesist 1973; 22:353–356.
41. Hempelmann G, Hempelmann W, Oster W, et al. Die Beeinflussung der Blutgase und Hämodynamik durch Etomidate bei myokardial vorgeschädigten Patienten. Anaesthesist 1974; 23:423.
42. Ghoneim MM, Yamada T. Etomidate: a clinical and electroencephalographic comparison with thiopental. Anesth Analg 1977;56:479.
43. Choi SD, Spaulding BC, Gross JB, Apfelbaum JL. Comparison of the ventilatory effects of etomidate and methohexital. Anesthesiology 1985;62:442–447.
44. Morgan M, Lumley J, Whitwam JG. Respiratory effects of etomidate. Br J Anaesth 1977;49:233–236.
45. Doenicke A, Gabanyi D, Lemcke H, Schürk-Bulich M. Haemodynamics and Myocardial function after administration of three short-acting i.v. hypnotics, etomidate, propanidid, methohexital. Anaesthesist 1974;23:108–115.
46. Kettler D, Sonntag H, Donath U, et al. Hemodynamics, myocardial mechanics, oxygen requirements and oxygen consumption of the human heart during etomidate induction into anaesthesia. Anaesthesist 1974;23:116.
47. Hempelmann G, Oster W, Piepenbrock S, Karliczek G. Haemodynamic effects of etomidate—a new hypnotic—in patients with myocardial insufficiency. In: Doenicke A, ed. Etomidate. Anaesthesiol Wiederbelebung 1977;106:72.
48. Gooding JM, Weng J, Smith RA, et al. Cardiovascular and pulmonary responses following etomidate induction of anesthesia in patients with demonstrated cardiac disease. Anesth Analg 1979;58:40.
49. Gooding J, Corssen G. Effect of etomidate on the cardiovascular system. Anesth Analg 1977;56:717.
50. Lindeburg T, Spotoft H, Sorensen MB, Skovsted P. Cardiovascular effects of etomidate used for induction and in combination with fentanyl-pancuronium for maintenance of anaesthesia in patients with valvular heart disease. Acta Anaesthesiol Scand 1982;26:205.
51. Haessler R, Madler C, Klasing S, et al. Propofol/fentanyl versus etomidate/fentanyl for the induction of anesthesia in patients with aortic insuffiency and coronary artery disease. J Cardiothorac Vasc Anesth 1992;6:173.
52. Patschke D, Brückner JB, Eberlein HJ, et al. Effects of althesin, etomidate and fentanyl on haemodynamics and myocardial oxygen consumption in man. Can Anaesth Soc J 1977;24:57.
53. Kettler D, Sonntag H. Intravenous anesthetics: coronary blood flow and myocardial oxygen consumption (with special reference to Althesine). Acta Anaesthesiol Belg 1974;25:384.
54. Doenicke A. Etomidate, a new intravenous hypnotic. Acta Anaesthesiol Belg 1974;25:307.
55. DeBruijn NP, Hlatky MA, Jacobs JR, et al. General anesthesia during percutaneous transluminary coronary angioplasty for acute myocardial infarction: results of a randomised controlled clinical trial. Anesth Analg 1989;68:201.
56. Criado A, Maseda J, Navarro E, et al. Induction of anaesthesia with etomidate: haemodynamic study of 36 patients. Br J Anaesth 1980;52:803.
57. Larsen R, Rathgeber J, Bagdahn A, et al. Effects of propofol on cardiovascular dynamics and coronary blood flow in geriatric patients: a comparison with etomidate. Anaesthesia 1988; 435:25.
58. Ebert TJ, Muzi M, Berens R, et al. Sympathic responses to induction of anesthesia in humans with propofol or etomidate. Anesthesiology 1992;76:725.
59. Thompson MF, Brock-Utne JG, Bean P, et al. Anesthesia and intraocular pressure: a comparative of total intravenous anesthesia using etomidate with inhalational anesthesia. Anaesthesia 1982;37:758.
60. Doenicke A. Etomidate. Lancet 1983;2:168.
61. Doenicke A. Verunsichert eine Cortisolstory die Anaesthesisten? Anaesthesist 1984;33:391–394.
62. Kochs E, Schulte am Esch J. Hormone des Hypophysen-Nebennierenrindensystems bei Patienten unter Langzeitsedierung mit Etomidat und Fentanyl. Anaesthesist 1984;33:402.
63. Dubois M, Pickar D, Cohen MR, et al. Surgical stress in humans is accompanied by an increase in the plasma β-endorphin immunoreactivity. Life Sci 1981;29:1249.
64. Fragen R, Shanks CA, Molteni A, Avram MJ. Effect of etomidate on hormonal responses to surgical stress. Anesthesiology 1984;61:652–656.
65. Besser GM, Rees LH. Endocrine correlations of β-endorphin and metenkephalin in man. In: Müller EE, Agnoli A, eds. Neuroendocrine correlates in neurology and psychiatry. Amsterdam: Elsevier, 1979.
66. Govoni S, Pasenetti MR, Inzoli MR, et al. Correlation between β-endorphin/β-lipotropin-immunoreactivity and cortisol plasma concentrations. Life Sci 1984;35:2549.
67. Friaolo F, Moretti C, Paolucci D, et al. Physical exercise stimulates marked concomitant release of beta-endorphin and adre-

nocorticotropin hormone (ACTH) in peripheral blood in man. Experientia 1979;36:987.
68. George R, Way EL. Studies on the mechanism of pituitary-adrenal activation by morphine. Br J Pharmacol Chemother 1955; 10:260.
69. Munson P. Effects of morphine and related drugs on the corticotropin (ACTH)-stress reaction. In: Zimmermann E, ed. Drug effects on neuroendocrine regulation. Prog Brain Res 1973; 39:361.
70. Owen H, Spence AA. Etomidate [Editorial]. Br J Anaesth 1984; 56:557–558.
71. Hall GM, Young C, Holdcroft A, Alaghband-Zadeh J. Substrate mobilisation during surgery: a comparison between halothane and fentanyl and anaesthesia. Anaesthesia 1978;33:924.
72. Heybach JP, Vernikos J. Naloxone inhibits and morphine potentiates the adrenal steroidogenic response to ACTH. Eur J Pharmacol 1981;75:1.
73. Fry DE, Griffith H. The inhibition by etomidate of the 11 β-hydroxylation of cortisol. Clin Endocrinol 1984;20:625.
74. Wagner RL, White PF. Etomidate inhibits adrenocortical function in surgical patients. Anesthesiology 1984;61:647–651.
75. Engelhardt D, Doenicke A, Suttmann H, et al. The influence of etomidate and thiopentone on ACTH and cortisol levels in serum: a prospective controlled trial in healthy men. Anaesthesist 1984;33:583–587.
76. Wagner RL, White PF, Kan PB, et al. Inhibition of adrenal steroidogenesis by the anesthetic etomidate. N Engl J Med 1984; 310:1415–1421.
77. Fragen RJ, Molteni A. Effect on plasma cortisol concentration of a single induction dose of etomidate of thiopentone. Lancet 1983;2:625.
78. Duthie DJR, Fraser R, Nimmo WS. Effect of induction of anaesthesia with etomidate on corticosteroid synthesis in man. Br J Anaesth 1985;57:156–159.
79. Longnecker DE: Stress free: to be or not to be? [Editorial] Anesthesiology 1984;61:643–644.
80. Allolio B, Stuttmann R, Fischer H, et al. Adrenocortical suppression by a single induction dose of etomidate. Lancet 1983; 2:626.
81. Doenicke A, Shay J, Mayer M, et al. Cortisol and ACTH increase 4 hr after etomidate. Anesthesiology 1992;77:A336.
82. Suttmann H, Doenicke A, Lorenz W, et al. Is perioperative stress a real surgical phenomen or merely a drug induced effect? Theor Surg 1986;1:119–135.
83. Dorow R, Doenicke A, Suttmann H, et al. Einfluβ verschiedener Narkosemethoden auf hormonelle Parameter und auf das sympathonervale System. In: Doenicke A, Koenig U, eds. Immunologie in Anaesthesie und Intensivmedizin. vol 3. Berlin: Springer-Verlag (Sertürner Workshop), 1983:97.
84. Crozier TA, Beck D, Wuttke W, Kettler D. In vivo suppression of steroid synthesis by etomidate is concentration-dependant. Anaesthesist 1988;37:337–339.
85. Crozier TA. Endokrines System und perioperative Streβreaktionen. In: Doenicke A, Kettler D, List WF, et al, eds. Anästhesiologie. Berlin: Springer-Verlag, 1995:1186–1222.
86. Crozier TA, Schlaeger M, Wuttke W, Kettler D. The stress of coronary artery surgery overcomes the inhibition of cortisol synthesis caused by etomidate-fentanyl anaesthesia. Anaesthesist 1994;43:605–613.
87. Stuttmann R, Allolio B, Becker A, et al. Etomidate versus etomidate plus hydrocortisone in major abdominal surgery. Anaesthesist 1988;37:576–582.
88. Holdcroft A, Morgan M, Whitwam JG, Lumley J. Effect of dose and premedication on induction complications with etomidate. Br J Anaesth 1976;48:199–205.
89. Hendry JGB, Miller BM, Lees NW. Etomidate in a new solvent: a clinical evaluation. Anaesthesia 1977;32:996–999.
90. Gran L, Bleie H, Jeppson R, Maartmann-Moe H. Etomidate in intralipid. Anaesthesist 1983;32:475–477.
91. Doenicke A, Duka T, Suttmann H. Venous reactions following etomidate [Letter]. Br J Anaesth 1984;56:933.
92. Suttmann H, Doenicke A, Kugler J, Laub M. Eine neue Zubereitung von Etomidat in Lipidemulsion: Bioverfügbarkeit und Venenreizung. Anaesthesist 1989;38:421–423.
93. Doenicke A, Kugler A, Vollmann N. Venous tolerance to etomidate in lipid emulsion or propylene glycol (hypnomidate). Can J Anaesth 1990;37:823–824.
94. Hepting L. Vergleichende Wirksamkeits- und Verträglichkeitsuntersuchung von Thiopental-Natrium: ein Vergleich mit Etomidat-Emulsion und Propofol. [Thesis]. Munich: Ludwig-Maximilians University, 1995.
95. Fragen RJ, Caldwell N. Comparison of a new formulation of etomidate with thiopental:side effects and awakening times. Anesthesiology 1979;50:242.
96. Giese JL, Stockham RJ, Stanley T, et al. Etomidate versus thiopental for induction of anesthesia. Anesth Analg 1985;64:871.
97. Craig J, Cooper GM, Sear JW. Recovery from day-case anaesthesia: comparison between methohexitone, althesin and etomidate. Br J Anaesth 1982;54:447.
98. Wells JKG. Comparison of ICI 35868, etomidate and methohexitone for day-case anesthesia. Br J Anaesth 1985;57:732.
99. Zacharias M, Dundee JW, Clark RS, Hegarty JE. Effect of preanesthetic medication on etomidate. B J Anaesth 1979; 51:127.
100. Diez R. Labajo A, White PF: Pros and cons of intravenous versus inhaled anesthetics for ambulatory surgery. Anesth Analg (in press).
101. Carli F, Stribley GC, Clark MM. Forum: etomidate infusion in thoracic anesthesia. Anaesthesia 1983;38:784.
102. Doenicke A, Lorenz W, Beigl R, et al. Histamine release after intravenous applications of short acting hypnotics: a comparison of etomidate, althesin (CT 1341) and propanidid. Br J Anaesth 1973;45:1097–1104.
103. Doenicke A, Roizen MF, Hoernecke R, et al. The solvent for etomidate may cause pain and adverse effects. (submitted).
104. Doenicke A, Lorenz W, Hug P. Histamine et etomidate. Ann Anesth Fr 1978;19:207–213.
105. Krumholz W, Müller H, Gerlach H, et al. Ein Fall von anaphylaktoider Reaktion nach Gabe von Etomidat. Anaesthesist 1984; 33:161–162.
106. Sold M, Rothhammer A. Lebensbedrohliche anaphylaktische Reaktion nach Etomidat. Anaesthesist 1985;34:208–210.
107. Lorenz W, Doenicke A. Anaphylactoid reactions and histamine release by intravenous drugs used in surgery and anesthesia. In: Watkins J, Ward MA, eds. Adverse reactions to intravenous drugs. London: Academic Press, 1978:83–112.
108. Watkins J. Allergic and pseudoallergic mechanisms in anesthesia. In: Sage JD, ed. Anaphylactoid reactions in anesthesia. Int Anesthesiol Clin 1985;23:17–40.
109. Ruo W, Shay J, Attele A, et al. Propylene glycol damages vascular smooth muscle and endothelium. Anesthesiology 1992; 77S:A1096.
110. van Dijk B. Venous pain and involuntary muscular movements during and after administration of etomidate. Anaesthesist 1978;27:60–63.
111. Zacharias M, Clarke RSJ, Dundee JW, Johnson SB. Elevation of three preparations of etomidate. Br J Anaesth 1978;50:925–929.
112. Zacharias M, Clarke RSJ, Dundee JW, Johnson SB. Venous sequelae following etomidate. Br J Anaesth 1979;51:779–783.
113. Schou Olesen A, Hüttel MS, Hole P. Venous sequelae following the injection of etomidate or thiopentone i.v. Br J Anaesth 1984; 56:171–173.
114. Bedichek E, Kirschbaum B. A case of propylene glycol toxic

reaction associated with etomidate infusion. Arch Intern Med 1991;151:2297–2298.
115. Christopher MM, Eckfeldt JH, Eaton JW. Propylene glycol ingestion causes o-lactic acidosis. Lab Invest 1990;62:114–118.
116. Demey HE, Daelemars RA, Verpooten GA, et al. Propylene glycol-induced side effects during intravenous nitroglycerin therapy. Intensive Care Med 1988;14:221–216.
117. Potter PJ. Haemoglobinuria caused by propylene glycol in sheep. Br J Anaesth 1991;66:189–195.
118. Klement W, Arndt JO. Pain on iv injection of some anaesthetic agent is evoked by the unphysiological osmolality or pH of their formulations. Br J Anaesth 1991;66:189–195.
119. Martin G, Finberg L. Propylene glycol: a potentially toxic vehicle in liquid dosage form. Pediatrics 1970;77:877–878.
120. Pearl RG, Rice SA. Propylene-glycol-induced polmonary hypertension in sheep. Pharmacology 1989;39:383–389.
121. Levy ML, Aranda M, Zelma V, Glannotta SL. Propylene glycol toxicity following continuous etomidate infusion for the control of refractory cerebral edema. Neurosurgery 1995;37:363–369.
122. Doenicke A, Roizen MF, Hoernecke R, et al. Hemolysis after etomidate: comparison of formulation with propylene glycol versus lipid emulsion. (submitted).
123. Henn A, Hoffmann R, Müller HAG. Haptoglobin determination in patients serum after intraoperative autotransfusion with haemonetics cell-server. III. Hemolysis and intraoperative autotransfusion. Anaesthesist 1988;37:741–745.

7 Propofol

Paul F. White

Since the introduction of propofol into clinical practice in the late 1980s, over 1000 articles on the intravenous (IV) anesthetic have been published in the peer-reviewed anesthesia literature. Although propofol was initially approved for use as an induction and maintenance hypnotic agent (1), its clinical uses have expanded greatly to include indications for cardiac, neurosurgical, and pediatric anesthesia, as well as monitored anesthesia care and sedation in the intensive care unit (ICU). Propofol has rapidly become the drug of choice for induction of anesthesia in outpatients undergoing ambulatory procedures, and it is becoming increasingly popular for pediatric anesthesia. Propofol's unique antiemetic (2) and mood-altering (3) properties may lead to new clinical applications in the future. Although anecdotal reports suggest that propofol may possess euphorigenic (sense of well-being) properties, this finding has not been substantiated in controlled, double-blind studies (4). Yet subjects clearly "like" the effects of propofol, and it may have potential for abuse or diversion (5).

Information regarding propofol's pharmacokinetic and pharmacodynamic properties has facilitated the use of this drug in clinical practice (6). As expected, patients' responses to propofol during the perioperative period vary widely. Therefore, the dosage and rate of propofol administration should be titrated to the needs of the individual patient. Factors that influence propofol dosage requirements include age, weight, preexisting medical conditions, type of surgical procedure, and concomitant medical therapy. As part of a balanced or total intravenous anesthetic (TIVA) technique, infusion rates of 75 to 300 $\mu g \cdot kg^{-1} \cdot min^{-1}$ are usually required, whereas adequate sedation can be maintained with infusion rates of 25 to 100 $\mu g \cdot kg^{-1} \cdot min^{-1}$ (Fig. 7-1). Anesthesiologists can define "target" plasma concentrations for hypnosis (2 to 6 $\mu g \cdot ml^{-1}$) and sedation (0.5 to 1.5 $\mu g \cdot ml^{-1}$) during a variety of clinical conditions (Fig. 7-2). Pharmacokinetically based delivery systems can rapidly achieve targeted plasma concentrations of propofol (7). However, careful titration to the desired clinical effect is essential because of the inherent pharmacokinetic and pharmacodynamic variability of the drug among patients. In addition, the therapeutic propofol concentration depends on the surgical stimulus (8).

Studies on the molecular mechanism of propofol's effects on the central nervous system (CNS) suggest that, like other CNS depressants (e.g., barbiturates, etomidate), propofol activates the $GABA_A$ receptor-chloride ionophore complex (9). At clinically relevant concentrations, propofol increases chloride conductance. However, at high concentrations of propofol, desensitization of the $GABA_A$ receptor results in suppression of the inhibitory system.

In addition to discussing information regarding propofol's clinical pharmacologic and physiologic effects, the relevant literature relating to its use ambulatory, pediatric, cardiac anesthesia and for neuroanesthesia is reviewed in this chapter. Clinical applications of propofol infusions for sedation during local and regional anesthesia, as well as outside the operating room (e.g., ICU, radiologic suite), are discussed.

PHARMACOKINETICS

Several investigators have examined the pharmacokinetics of propofol in healthy adults and children, as well as in a variety of disease states. The pharmacokinetics and pharmacodynamics of propofol were initially reviewed in 1988 (10), and published studies are summarized in Table 7-1. The unique pharmacokinetic properties of propofol contribute to its favorable clinical characteristics. Of greatest importance is the rapid metabolic clearance of propofol, which is approximately 10 times faster than that of thiopental (6). The metabolic clearance of propofol exceeds hepatic blood flow, a finding that has led to the suggestion that pro-

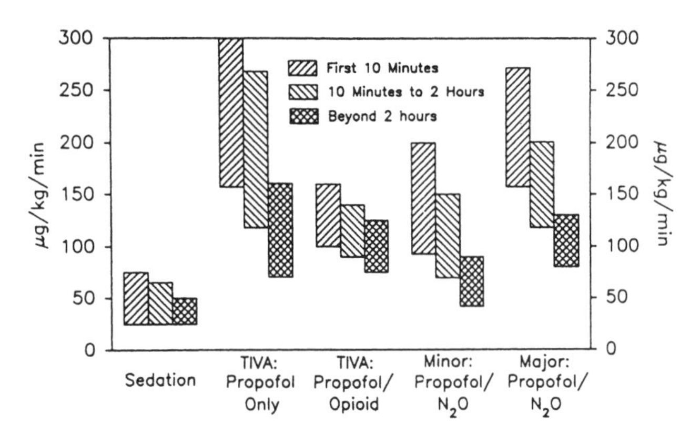

FIGURE 7-1. Recommended propofol infusion regimens to achieve satisfactory conditions for sedation, total intravenous anesthesia (TIVA) with and without supplemental opioid analgesics, and nitrous oxide-supplemented anesthesia for minor and major surgical procedures. (From Shafer SL. Advances in propofol pharmacokinetics and pharmacodynamics. J Clin Anesth 1993;5 (suppl 1):14S–21S.)

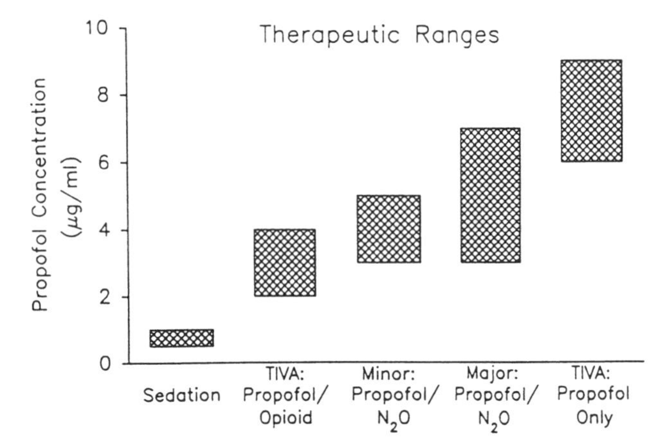

FIGURE 7-2. Therapeutic plasma propofol concentrations required for a variety of anesthetic applications. TIVA, Total intravenous anesthesia. (From Shafer SL. Advances in propofol pharmacokinetics and pharmacodynamics. J Clin Anesth 1993;5 (suppl 1):14S–21S.)

pofol is also metabolized in extrahepatic sites (6). Evidence for this hypothesis is provided by the detection of propofol metabolites following administration of propofol during the anhepatic phase of orthotopic liver transplantation (11).

Following an initial bolus of propofol, plasma levels decline rapidly, mainly because of redistribution of propofol from the brain and other highly perfused tissues into less well-perfused sites (e.g., muscle). In one study, the propofol dose for unconsciousness was 6.2 $mg \cdot kg^{-1} \cdot h^{-1}$ and the median effective concentration (EC_{50}) for unconsciousness was 2.3 $\mu g \cdot ml^{-1}$ (12). For adequate sedation using a target-controlled infusion system, a propofol concentration of 0.9 $\mu g \cdot ml^{-1}$ was required (13). The distribution clearance of propofol (3 to 4 $L \cdot kg^{-1} \cdot min^{-1}$) is similar to that of thiopental, and initially, plasma levels of thiopental and propofol decline at similar rates (6). Subsequently, the rate of decline of propofol is much more rapid than that of thiopental because of its high metabolic clearance rate. Propofol can impair its own clearance by decreasing hepatic blood flow, an effect enhanced in the presence of mild hypothermia (14). The pharmacokinetics of propofol is not altered by either an infusion of alfentanil or epidural analgesia (15). Given the similar pharmacokinetic profiles of propofol and alfentanil, Kay suggested mixing the two drugs together in the same syringe (16). These mixtures have been used for general surgery (17), gynecologic procedures (18), ambulatory surgery (19), and military (field) anesthesia (20).

The elimination half-life ($t_{1/2}\beta$) of propofol is long, yet recovery from its clinical effects is rapid, even after prolonged administration. The reason for this apparent discrepancy is that the long elimination half-life is related to slow elimination from the highly lipophilic tissue compartments (e.g., fat) and is largely irrelevant in clinical situations (21). Hughes and colleagues introduced the concept of "context-sensitive half-time" to describe recovery from anesthetic infusions of varying duration (22). The half-time is the time required for the drug concentration in the central compartment to decrease by 50% following discontinuation of the infusion. The context relates to the duration of drug infusion before its discontinuation. Propofol has a context-sensitive half-time of less than 25 minutes following infusions lasting up to 3 hours, and the half-time is still only 50 minutes following prolonged infusions. If the propofol infusion is titrated to effect, so the plasma propofol concentration has to decline by only 10 to 20% to permit awakening, recovery is extremely rapid. Adjunctive use of opioid analgesics (e.g., alfentanil) decreases the propofol concentration at which patients regain consciousness (23).

Hughes and associates provide a comprehensive description of the way in which the pharmacokinetic parameters of propofol interact to permit rapid recovery (22). Propofol has a large steady-state volume of distribution, indicating extensive redistribution of the drug into muscle, fat, and other poorly perfused tissues. The capacity of these sites is large. However, their rate of equilibration with the central compartment is slow. When an infusion of propofol is terminated, the concentration in the central compartment is much higher than in the peripheral compartments, and hence redistribution continues to occur. Thus, the concentration in the central compartment declines both from metabolism (elimination) and from continuing redistribution. Because the capacity of these peripheral compartments is so large, redistribution from the cen/tral compartment can still occur even after prolonged drug administration. The net result is a rapid decline in propofol concentration to levels below those re-

TABLE 7-1. Summary of Pharmacokinetic Variables in Adult and Pediatric Populations

Reference	Volume of Distribution (L • kg⁻¹)			Total Body Clearance	Half-life Values (min)		
	Compartment Central	Equilibrium	Steady State	(ml • kg⁻¹ • min⁻¹)	a	β	γ
Adults:							
Shafer et al, 1988[212]	0.12	—	3.4	28	1.3	30	232
Gepts et al, 1988[448]	0.27	9.76	3.81	25.9	2.7	23.6	281
Kirkpatrick et al, 1988[449]	0.42	27.1	11.9	27.7	2.04	52.4	674
Servin et al, 1990[450]	0.21	—	1.84	23.8	2.2	24	212
Morgan et al, 1990[292]	—	36.2	—	18.8	—	—	1795
Servin et al, 1993[27]	0.2	—	2.09	28.3	1.81	24.2	246
Adult subpopulations:							
Male[451]	0.55	9.23	4.29	23.6	2.4	56	262
Female[451]	0.58	12.9	5.06	29.1	2.2	44.9	309
Female[452]	0.72	12.6	5.31	32.9	2.85	45	284
Elderly[449]	0.31	28.4	12.4	23.2	1.84	69.3	834
Obese[27]	0.15	—	1.83	24.3	2.16	29.1	243
Uremic[453]	0.7	30.3	22.6	12.9	—	—	1638
Cirrhotic[450]	0.2	—	3.12	27.0	2.4	22	234
Pediatric:							
Saint-Maurice et al, 1989[454]	0.72	31.4	10.9	30.6	4.13	56.1	735.0
Valtonen et al, 1989[455]	0.53	7.15	2.16	32.0	1.5	9.3	214.6
Jones et al, 1990[456]	0.6	12.38	5.01	40.35	3.05	24.33	209.2
Kataria et al, 1994[457]	0.52	—	9.7	34.0	2.0	27.0	329.0

quired for hypnosis (or deep sedation), permitting rapid awakening. Eventually, the concentration in the central compartment becomes lower than that of the peripheral sites, and drug then begins to move back into the central compartment. However, the rate of this transfer is slow (resulting in a long terminal half-life value), such that the concentration of propofol in the central compartment may remain at subtherapeutic levels for a prolonged period. The complete elimination of propofol from the body may take many hours, or even days, but it has little effect on clinical recovery.

The effects of age and various disease states on propofol pharmacokinetics are summarized in Table 7-1. As with the barbiturates, elderly patients have a reduced dose requirement for propofol that appears to be related to pharmacokinetic rather than pharmacodynamic factors (24).

Four published pharmacokinetic studies have been performed in children. Variations among these four studies may be due to differing sampling intervals (which influence the size of the central compartment), small numbers of patients, the effects of adjunctive anesthetic drugs, and the use of different kinetic modeling techniques (25). In spite of these intrastudy differences, all four studies demonstrated that the volume of propofol's central compartment is larger in children than in adults on the basis of kilograms of body weight. The clearance rate of propofol is also higher in children. Therefore, children require a larger induction dose and an increased maintenance infusion rate than adults (26). As in adults, other factors (e.g., infusion duration) also influence the effect of propofol on recovery in children (25).

Although dosage adjustments are clearly indicated in severely debilitated patients, the clinical duration of effect of propofol does not appear to be greatly effected by obesity or by moderate hepatic or renal dysfunction (27). Although propofol metabolites accumulate in patients in renal failure, the lack of difference in emergence times suggests that these metabolities have no clinically significant effects (28). Because considerable interpatient variability exists in both healthy and sick patients, careful titration of the propofol dose to effect minimizes adverse effects such as hypotension, while permitting a rapid recovery from the drug's central effects. For patients weighing 60 to 90 kg, a "standard" dose infusion regimen is a useful starting point (29).

With improvements in computer technology, increasing interest has developed in automated IV delivery systems. Computer-assisted target-controlled infusions can facilitate the maintenance of anesthesia and sedation with propofol (7). Although the relationship between the targeted concentration and the actual measured blood concentration depends on the pharmacokinetic valuables used in programming the delivery system, the choice of the pharmacokinetic model does not appear to make any difference clinically (30, 31). Although a target-controlled delivery system was more convenient than using intermittent bolus injections, it offered no obvious advantages over a simple, variable-rate infusion system (32). For target-controlled infusion to gain widespread acceptance as a delivery system for propofol, the device will have to be user-friendly, easy to set up, and associated with a small incremental cost (33).

PHARMACODYNAMICS

General anesthesia

The ideal general anesthetic technique should provide for a rapid onset and stable operating conditions, while ensuring a rapid recovery of protective reflexes, as well as cognitive and psychomotor functions. In evaluating recovery from anesthesia in both inpatient and outpatient settings, the recovery process is commonly divided into three distinct phases. Early recovery is usually referred to as emergence, and it describes the time at which the patient awakens from anesthesia and obeys simple commands. Intermediate recovery (or simply "recovery") describes the return of cognitive and psychomotor function sufficient to permit discharge to a postanesthesia care unit (PACU). Late recovery describes a return to the preoperative state and resumption of normal activities. Although most comparative studies involving propofol have focused on "recovery times," other factors should be considered. For example, when a propofol infusion was used for maintenance of general anesthesia during endoscopic sinus surgery, less bleeding was noted, compared with an inhalation technique (34).

Anesthetic techniques used in the ambulatory setting should be associated with a low incidence of postoperative side effects because they can delay the patient's discharge and can result in unanticipated hospital admissions. Since its introduction into clinical practice, propofol has become an extremely popular IV anesthetic for ambulatory surgery procedures because of its predictable recovery and favorable side effect profile. Recovery is not only rapid following a single bolus dose, but also following repeated doses or a titrated continuous infusion, thereby allowing propofol to be effectively used for maintenance of anesthesia during short ambulatory procedures (35). Compared with the investigational IV anesthetic eltanolone (pregnanolone), propofol was associated with a shorter time to "home readiness" [37 minutes (32 to 100 minutes) versus 57 minutes (41 to 190 minutes)] (36).

Many of the early clinical trials involving propofol compared its use for induction and maintenance of anesthesia with "traditional" techniques involving thiopental for induction and a volatile anesthetic agent for maintenance of anesthesia. Despite considerable variation in patient populations, type and duration of operative procedures, use of adjuvant agents, and methods of titrating the anesthetics, the results were remarkably consistent (Table 7-2). Most investigators have reported a more rapid recovery from a propofol-based anesthetic than with a barbiturate-volatile anesthetic technique. For example, Millar and Jewkes (37)

TABLE 7-2. Comparison of Propofol For Induction and Maintenance of Outpatient Anesthesia With "Conventional" Intravenous and Inhalation Techniques

Reference	Population	Adjuvants	Propofol Administration	Comparative Group		Principal Findings†
				Induction	Maintenance*	
Ding et al, 1993[35‡]	44 laparoscopies	fentanyl	VRI	thiopental	enflurane	Faster emergence; later recovery equal
Millar and Jewkes, 1988[37]	130 outpatients	alfentanil	IB	thiopental	enflurane	Faster emergence and discharge
Price et al, 1988[83]	98 dilatation and curettage	fentanyl	VRI	thiopental	enflurane	Faster recovery at 15–30 minutes
Puttick and Rosen, 1988[263]	38 children	—	IB	thiopental	halothane	Faster emergence and discharge
Sear et al, 1988[458]	50 outpatients	papavaretum	VRI	thiopental	halothane	Faster emergence
Doze et al, 1988[84]	80 outpatients	meperidine	VRI	thiopental	isoflurane	Faster emergence and ambulation
Gold et al, 1989[459]	60 outpatients	morphine	FRI	thiopental	isoflurane, 1MAC	Earlier discharge from recovery room
Korttila et al, 1990[85]	41 outpatients	fentanyl	FRI	thiopental	isoflurane	Faster emergence and discharge
Lim and Low, 1992[460]	50 dental	—	FRI	thiopental	isoflurane, 0.5%	Faster emergence and ambulation
Marais et al, 1989[43]	100 outpatients	—	not reported	thiopental	isoflurane	Faster emergence and discharge
Sung et al, 1991[40]	99 females	fentanyl	VRI	thiopental	isoflurane	Faster recovery and discharge

VRI, Variable-rate infusion; FRI, fixed-rate infusion; IB, intermittent bolus doses.
**Volatile agent titrated to clinical end points, unless otherwise stated.*
†Findings are expressed with respect to the propofol group.
‡This study was a multiple-group comparison but has been subdivided for ease of interpretation.

studied 130 spontaneously breathing patients undergoing short (<30 minutes) outpatient procedures. Patients receiving propofol for induction and maintenance of anesthesia awakened and reached recovery milestones significantly faster than a control group receiving a thiopental-enflurane combination. As a result, patients receiving propofol were fit for discharge 40 to 50 minutes earlier than the thiopental-enflurane group. However, this difference was decreased when either technique was supplemented with alfentanil. Following discharge, propofol-treated patients were less likely to "feel unwell" during the journey home, they resumed normal alimentation sooner, and they reported significantly less drowsiness, dizziness, and weakness on the first postoperative day (37). Yet in patients undergoing middle ear surgery, no differences were noted between patients receiving propofol-N_2O combinations and those receiving thopental-enflurane-N_2O combinations with respect to recovery from anesthesia or psychometric testing (38). When propofol was used for induction of anesthesia before oral surgery (39), recovery times were similar irrespective of whether halothane or propofol was used for maintenance of anesthesia.

In a study involving 99 women undergoing breast biopsy procedures, Sung and colleagues (40) compared a propofol bolus followed by a variable-rate continuous infusion with a thiopental-isoflurane combination. All patients received fentanyl, 1 $\mu g \cdot kg^{-1}$ IV, and nitrous oxide (N_2O). In addition to a shortened recovery time and earlier discharge, propofol-treated patients were able to resume normal activities sooner and also reported returning to work half a day earlier (1.5 ± 0.1 versus 2.0 ± 0.1 days) than those in the thiopental-isoflurane group. Controversy exists regarding the effect of N_2O when administered in combination with propofol. Most investigators have found that the propofol-sparing effects of N_2O contribute to more rapid emergence from anesthesia without increasing side effects (e.g., postoperative nausea and vomiting [PONV]) (41). However, a study by Lindekaer and associates (42) suggested that the addition of N_2O to propofol-alfentanil-vecuronium anesthesia did not reduce the propofol dosage requirement or shorten the recovery period.

The "short" recovery times after propofol have led some authors to speculate on the potential cost savings resulting from the use of propofol-based anesthetic techniques. Sung and colleagues (40) suggested that extrapolating their results to a 4000 case-per-year outpatient facility would save 1000 nursing hours per year. Using the results of two separate comparisons of continuous propofol with thiopental-isoflurane, Marais and associates (43) suggested that widespread use of propofol-based techniques could reduce the requirement for recovery room nurses by as much as 25%. This evaluation was based on the shorter recovery time following propofol-based anesthetics, as well as the reduced workload imposed on recovery room nurses as a result of the lower incidence of side effects, in particular, nausea and vomiting. However, the authors comment that actual savings would vary, depending on site-specific factors such as case mix and volume, as well as decisions on minimum nursing staffing requirements in the PACU.

Induction of Anesthesia

The major criticism of the previous studies is that they compared propofol-based techniques with a combination technique involving a barbiturate and a volatile anesthetic. Such comparisons are usually justified on the grounds that they are comparing a new technique with a "standard practice." However, the substitution of propofol for other induction agents should be studied independently of its effects as a maintenance agent. In comparisons with thiopental, emergence from anesthesia induced with propofol has generally been faster, irrespective of the maintenance agent used (Table 7-3). However, Sanders and colleagues failed to detect a significant difference when halothane was employed for maintenance of anesthesia (44).

Several investigators have reported improved performance on postoperative psychomotor tests when patients received propofol for induction of anesthesia, compared with patients receiving thiopental (45-47). Although psychomotor tests are intended to assess the patient's ability to cope without supervision and to aid in determining the appropriate time for discharge following ambulatory surgery, investigators do not agree on the most useful measure of these important end points (48). Nevertheless, using traditional discharge criteria, the use of propofol (versus thiopental) for induction of anesthesia may allow for an earlier discharge from the ambulatory facility after brief outpatient procedures (49, 50).

When propofol was compared with induction agents other than thiopental for outpatient anesthesia, smaller differences were observed. In comparison with methohexital, propofol was reported to be associated with greater alertness, reduced ataxia, and improved choice reaction times during the first 20 minutes following isoflurane anesthesia (51). However, after 40 minutes these differences were no longer significant. In a comparison with etomidate, propofol induction resulted in only moderate improvements in psychomotor performance following 20 to 30 minutes of isoflurane-N_2O anesthesia (46). Compared with induction of anesthesia with midazolam followed by reversal with flumazenil at the end of anesthesia, induction with propofol was associated with significant improvement in performance on postoperative psychomotor testing when anesthesia was maintained with isoflurane (52). Similar findings were obtained when

TABLE 7-3. Comparison of Propofol With Alternative Induction Agents for Outpatient Anesthesia

Reference	Population	Adjuvants	Comparator	Maintenance	Principal Findings*
O'Toole et al, 1987[51]	50 females	—	methohexital	isoflurane	Faster emergence, improved test results at 20 min
Valanne and Korttila, 1985[461]	73 oral surgery	—	methohexital	enflurane	Similar times to orientation and ambulation
Chittleborough et al, 1992[49]	40 dental	fentanyl	thiopental	enflurane	Faster emergence and discharge
Ding et al, 1993[35]*	40 laparoscopies	fentanyl	thiopental	enflurane	Faster emergence, recovery times similar
Gupta et al, 1992[45]	30 arthroscopies	alfentanil	thiopental	isoflurane	Improved test results for first 90 min of recovery
Rolly and Versichelen, 1985[462]	30 females	fentanyl	thiopental	halothane-isoflurane	Faster emergence, later events not reported
Runcie et al, 1993[50]	102 children	—	thiopental	halothane-isoflurane	Faster emergence, earlier discharge in older children only
DeGrood et al, 1987[46†]	30 laparoscopies	fentanyl	thiopental	isoflurane	Faster emergence and improved test results
DeGrood et al, 1987[46†]	30 laparoscopies	fentanyl	etomidate	isoflurane	Not significantly faster recovery
Mackenzie and Grant, 1985[47†]	40 urology	—	thiopental	enflurane	Greatly improved psychomotor performance
Mackenzie and Grant, 1985[47†]	40 urology	—	methohexital	enflurane	Improved psychomotor performance
Sanders et al, 1989[44]	40 dental	—	thiopental	halothane	Similar emergence and recovery
Norton and Dundas, 1990[52†]	40 vasectomy	—	midazolam-flumazenil	isoflurane	Improved psychomotor performance

Findings are expressed with respect to the propofol group.

†This study was a multiple-group comparisons but has been subdivided for ease of interpretation.

comparing a propofol-based TIVA technique with a midazolam-isoflurane-flumazenil technique (53).

The effect of propofol on succinylcholine-induced myalgias is also controversial. McClymont (54) reported that induction with propofol was associated with a lower incidence of postoperative myalgias compared with thiopental (19% versus 63%) when succinylcholine was used to facilitate tracheal intubation. However, Smith and associates (55) found no difference in the effects of the two induction agents on the incidence of succinylcholine-induced myalgias when enflurane-N_2O was used for maintenance of anesthesia.

Maintenance of Anesthesia

Investigations in which anesthesia was induced with propofol and maintained with either propofol or a volatile anesthetic agent are summarized in Table 7-4. When propofol-N_2O was used to maintain outpatient anesthesia lasting approximately 3 hours, recovery and discharge occurred significantly earlier, compared with isoflurane-N_2O (56). However, use of propofol as part of a TIVA technique was no better than a balanced technique with isoflurane-alfentanil (57). Biro and colleagues (58) reported that for procedures lasting up to 2 hours, patients who received propofol (versus thiopental-enflurane) experienced "a faster and more pleasant recovery, leading to an earlier discharge from the recovery unit." Although propofol was 1.4 to 1.7 times more costly than thiopental-enflurane, the shorter recovery was a cost-reducing factor.

When comparing recovery from different anesthetic techniques, the investigator must ensure that all patients are maintained at a similar depth of anesthesia. Unfortunately, many of the previous investigations used fixed-dosage infusions or boluses of propofol and "standardized" concentrations of the volatile anesthetic (59-63). Because these rigid study designs do not allow for individual variations in the anesthetic requirements, one cannot be certain that patients were at comparable depths of anesthesia. In the absence of an objective monitor of anesthetic depth, common practice is to titrate the anesthetic drugs using clinical signs (e.g., hemodynamic and respiratory variables) (64) and to regard comparable cardiorespiratory stability as indicative of a similar depth of anesthesia. When propofol and isoflurane were administered using this clinical titration method, propofol was found to be associated with improved performance on psychomotor testing during the first hour of recovery (65). However, this difference was no longer apparent 2 hours after the operation.

In clinical comparisons with enflurane (35), desflurane (66, 67), and sevoflurane (68), maintenance of anesthesia with propofol did not improve recovery times (Fig. 7-3). Although the use of IV adjuvants such as fentanyl (35, 66, 67) and midazolam (35) may possibly have masked small differences among the study groups, these data suggest that the differences found

TABLE 7-4. Comparison of Propofol for Induction and Maintenance of Outpatient Anesthesia With a Propofol-Volatile Anesthetic Combination

Reference	Population	Adjuvants	Propofol Adminis-tration	Comparative Maintenance*	Principal Findings†
Herregods et al, 1988[59‡]	40 arthroscopies	—	FRI	isoflurane, 1%	Similar emergence and psychomotor performance
Larsen et al, 1992[60]	74 arthroscopies	alfentanil	FRI	isoflurane	Impaired psychomotor performance in first 30 min
Marshall et al, 1992[61]	114 females	± alfentanil	FRI	isoflurane, 1%	Similar emergence and psychomotor performance
Milligan et al, 1987[62]	60 D & Cs	—	IB	isoflurane, 1%	Faster emergence, recovery times similar
Nightingale and Lewis, 1992[65]	50 D & Cs	alfentanil	IB	isoflurane	Improved psychomotor performance
Valanne, 1992[56]	50 dental	—	VRI	isoflurane	Faster emergence, recovery, and discharge
Zuurmond et al, 1987[63]	40 arthroscopies	—	FRI	isoflurane, 0.9%	Similar emergence and psychomotor performance
Ding et al, 1993[35‡]	38 laparoscopies	fentanyl	VRI	enflurane	Similar emergence, recovery, and discharge
Rapp et al, 1992[66‡]	45 orthopedic	fentanyl	VRI	desflurane	Similar emergence and psychomotor performance
Van Hemelrijck et al, 1991[67‡]	46 females	fentanyl	VRI	desflurane	Similar emergence and psychomotor performance

D & Cs, Dilatation and curettage procedures; VRI, variable-rate infusion; FRI, fixed-rate infusion; IB, intermittent bolus doses.
**Volatile agent titrated to clinical end points, unless otherwise stated.*
†Findings are expressed with respect to the propofol group.
‡This study was a multiple-group comparisons but has been subdivided for ease of interpretation.

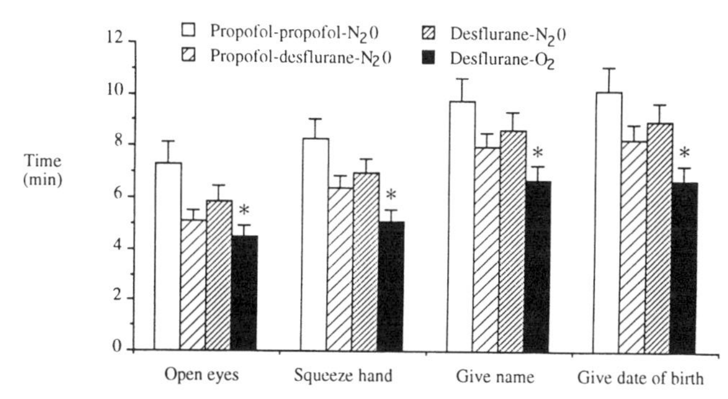

FIGURE 7-3. Emergence times after discontinuation of anesthesia with propofol-N_2O, propofol-desflurane-N_2O, desflurane-N_2O, and desflurane-O_2. *$p < 0.05$, from propofol-N_2O. (From Van Hemelrijck J, Smith I, White PF. Use of desflurane for outpatient anesthesia: a comparison with propofol and nitrous oxide. Anesthesiology 1991;75:197–203.)

in routine practice may indeed be of little clinical significance. A meta-analysis of recovery data following the use of propofol or the newer volatile anesthetics would suggest only minor differences with respect to time to following commands and time to discharge (69). Cost analysis would suggest that the combination of an IV induction agent followed by maintenance with a volatile agent is more cost-effective than using an IV technique for both induction and maintenance of anesthesia (58, 70). Finally, a large multicenter survey found that when isoflurane was used to supplement propofol-N_2O anesthesia, emergence times were only slightly prolonged compared with propofol-N_2O alone, and the incidence of side effects was unchanged (71). After major intra-abdominal surgery, early and later recovery were similar with propofol and isoflurane (72). However, patients anesthetized with propofol reported fewer "negative" symptoms and were more "socially oriented" during the postoperative period.

Propofol versus Inhaled Induction

When propofol induction and maintenance were compared with an inhalation induction using halothane followed by isoflurane for maintenance of pediatric anesthesia, recovery times were remarkably similar (73). However, the concomitant use of meperidine and diazepam premedication as well as intraoperative morphine, may well have masked differences between the two study groups. Although the use of propofol for induction of anesthesia was associated with pain on injection, it significantly decreased the incidence of upper airway obstruction, compared with halothane (73). Postoperative lung function was also less impaired after maintenance with propofol (versus isoflurane) anesthesia (74).

Induction of anesthesia with propofol was more rapid than inhalation induction in adults, even when newer volatile anesthetics with low blood gas partition coefficients were used (67, 75). Propofol induction was also associated with less airway irritation compared with desflurane (67), but not sevoflurane (75). Recovery times following use of propofol-N_2O for induction and maintenance were similar to those achieved with sevoflurane-N_2O (76) or desflurane-N_2O (67). Use of desflurane-O_2 resulted in a more rapid emergence than propofol-N_2O (see Fig. 7-3). However, late recovery times were similar (67).

Propofol versus Alternative Total Intravenous Anesthetic Techniques

During the last decade, TIVA (using a combination of hypnotic, analgesic, and muscle relaxant drugs) has gained increased popularity as an alternative to balanced anesthesia with volatile agents. Some investigators have compared recovery after TIVA with propofol with that obtained with other IV or volatile anesthetic agents (Table 7-5). Most comparisons have shown that propofol is associated with faster emergence and with improvements in the patient's assessment of their recovery or enhanced performance in psychomotor testing. Comparisons with methohexital have tended to yield smaller differences than with other commonly used IV agents (e.g., thiopental, midazolam, etomidate). For outpatients undergoing dental surgery, recovery was reported to be faster after methohexital than after propofol (77). However, this finding may have been related to the comparatively large propofol dose (3 mg•kg^{-1}) used for induction of anesthesia. Unfortunately, most of these studies have not reported discharge times, an important measure of the efficiency of an outpatient anesthetic technique. Two investigations reported similar discharge times following propofol and methohexital for extremely short operations (78, 79). Following lower abdominal surgery, TIVA with either propofol or methohexital was an acceptable alternative to balanced anesthesia with isoflurane-N_2O (80). For laparoscopic cholecystectomy, Blobner and associates (81) found that a propofol-based TIVA technique offered no advantages over balanced anesthesia with isoflurane. A further investigation found similar discharge times for propofol and thiopental, although the preoperative use of diazepam may have delayed discharge in both groups (82).

Several investigators have commented on the quality of anesthetic maintenance with propofol in comparison with other IV agents. For example, propofol-opioid techniques are generally considered superior to midazolam-opioid-flumazenil techniques (57). TIVA with propofol has generally been reported as "smooth" (46), with a reduced incidence of coughing and hiccuping, resulting in improved surgical conditions (79) compared with barbiturates or etomidate. A further common finding with propofol has been a reduced incidence of PONV. This finding has been reported when propofol is used both for induction and for maintenance (35-40, 43, 46, 56, 61, 66, 67, 73, 78, 83-87), as well as when it is used solely as an induction agent (46, 49). A TIVA technique involving propofol (1 mg/kg followed by 100 to 200 μg/kg/min) and ketamine (1 mg/kg followed by 17 to 34 μg/kg/min) was associated with a high incidence of side effects

TABLE 7-5. Comparison of Propofol With Alternative Intravenous Techniques for Outpatient Anesthesia (TIVA)

Reference	Population	Adjuvants	Administration	Comparator	Principal Findings*
DeGrood et al, 1987[46†]	31 laparoscopies	fentanyl	FRI	etomidate	Faster and more predictable recovery
Heath et al, 1988[463†]	40 TOPs	alfentanil	IB	etomidate	Faster emergence, smoother induction
Cade et al, 1991[78]	70 females	fentanyl	IB	methohexital	Faster recovery to ambulation
Cundy and Arunasalam, 1985[464]	60 TOPs	fentanyl	IB	methohexital	Improved quality of anesthesia, less drowsy
Doze et al, 1986[86]	60 females	meperidine	VRI	methohexital	Earlier orientation and ambulation
Heath et al, 1988[463†]	40 TOPs	alfentanil	IB	methohexital	Similar recovery times
Kay and Healy, 1985[465†]	60 cystoscopies	alfentanil	IB	methohexital	Faster emergence and psychomotor recovery
Logan et al, 1987[77]	40 dental	—	Single bolus	methohexital	Slower emergence, similar recovery times
Mackenzie and Grant, 1985[466]	40 orthopedic	papavaretum	VRI	methohexital	Faster emergence, smoother anesthetic
Noble and Ogg, 1985[467]	50 TOPs	alfentanil	IB	methohexital	Similar emergence and recovery times
Ræder and Misvær, 1988[79†]	50 D & Cs	alfentanil	IB	methohexital	Faster emergence, recovery times similar
Sampson et al, 1988[87]	40 TOPs	—	IB	thiamylal	Faster emergence, later events not reported
Edelist, 1987[468]	90 TOPs	—	IB	thiopental	Faster emergence and orientation
Heath et al, 1988[463†]	40 TOPs	alfentanil	IB	thiopental	Faster emergence, recovery times similar
Heath et al, 1990[469]	60 D & Cs	alfentanil	IB	thiopental	Reduced tiredness at 24 h postoperative
Henriksson et al, 1987[470]	120 D & Cs	—	IB	thiopental	Faster emergence, later events not reported
Johnston et al, 1987[471]	93 D & Cs	—	IB	thiopental	Faster emergence, later events not reported
Korttila et al, 1992[472]	12 volunteers	—	2 boluses	thiopental	Faster emergence and psychomotor recovery
Nielsen et al, 1991[82]	57 females	diazepam	FRI	thiopental	Similar emergence and recovery times
Ræder and Misvær, 1988[79†]	50 D & Cs	alfentanil	IB	thiopental	Faster emergence and psychomotor recovery
Ryom et al, 1992[473]	76 females	meperidine	IB	thiopental	Similar performance in postoperative testing
Sanders et al, 1991[474]	36 females	—	IB	thiopental	Faster emergence, improved performance at 24 h

D & Cs, Dilatation and curettage procedures; TOPs, termination of pregnancy procedures; VRI, variable-rate infusion; FRI, fixed-rate infusion; IB, intermittent bolus doses.
**Findings are expressed with respect to the propofol group.*
†This study was a multiple-group comparisons but has been subdivided for ease of interpretation.

(e.g., tachycardia, hypertension) (88). Other investigators have found that the use of a propofol-ketamine combination was not associated with an increased incidence of untoward cardiorespiratory side effects (89). To control hypertension during TIVA, larger amounts of propofol and alfentanil were required, contributing to a slower recovery (90). Use of coinduction technique consisting of a midazolam-propofol combination decreases the propofol and opioid dosage requirements during TIVA (91).

In summary, compared with traditional techniques involving barbiturate-volatile agent combinations, balanced or TIVA techniques with propofol may offer advantages in terms of a more rapid early recovery and reduced PONV. However, some of this benefit appears to result from the substitution of propofol for barbiturates during the induction period. Following short cases (<30 minutes), the maintenance anesthetic appears to have less impact on recovery time. When propofol is used for induction of anesthesia, followed by maintenance with a volatile agent, one sees only a small increase in direct costs with propofol. The suggested benefits of using propofol for maintenance of anesthesia include greater hemodynamic stability, a more pleasant recovery, and lack of operating room and environmental pollution (92). However, careful cost-to-benefit analysis is needed to determine whether the additional cost associated with the use of propofol for both induction and maintenance of anesthesia is justified.

Monitored Anesthesia Care

Monitored anesthesia care usually involves the administration of IV adjuvants to produce sedation, anxiolysis, and amnesia during minor diagnostic and therapeutic procedures and to supplement analgesia provided by local or regional anesthetic techniques. Monitored anesthesia care is perhaps the purest form of IV anesthesia varying from minimal sedation (e.g., patient-controlled sedation) to profound "deep" sedation (e.g., TIVA). During these procedures, patients are monitored to ensure their safety and comfort during the operation. The optimum sedative-analgesic technique uses a drug or combination of drugs with sedative-hypnotic, analgesic, anxiolytic, and amnestic properties, a low incidence of perioperative side effects (e.g., respiratory depression, nausea, and vomiting), and ease of titration to the desired level of sedation and analgesia, while providing for a rapid return to a "clearheaded" state on completion of the procedure. Compared with general anesthesia for laparoscopic sterilization (93), use of local anesthesia with sedation was associated with less time in the operating room and faster recovery, as well as decreased postoperative pain and fewer sore throats, contributing to an overall reduction in anesthesia and surgery costs.

Traditionally, benzodiazepines have been the most widely used drugs for sedation during monitored anesthesia care. However, even drugs such as midazolam and triazolam with relatively short elimination half-life values (2 to 4 hours) can produce prolonged residual sedation, and the resultant psychomotor impairment can delay recovery (94). Opioid analgesics (e.g., fentanyl and its newer analogs) are often administered in combination with sedative-hypnotics to reduce pain resulting from the injection of local anesthetic solutions and traction on deeper tissue structures. Although a combination of midazolam and fentanyl is the most popular regimen, this combination can produce profound respiratory depression (95). Compared with the nonsteroidal anti-inflammatory ketorolac, adjunctive use of fentanyl provided for improved intraoperative patient comfort during propofol sedation (96). However, when used alone, the potent opioid analgesics generally do not produce adequate sedation and appear to be associated with more undesirable side effects (e.g., itching, respiratory depression, nausea) (97, 98).

Because the use of low-dose propofol infusions is associated with rapid recovery when used as part of a balanced anesthetic technique (86), anesthesiologists displayed increased interest in using propofol to produce sedation during local and regional anesthesia. The use of propofol for sedation was initially described by Mackenzie and Grant in 1987 (99). These investigators utilized a variable-rate propofol infusion (mean dose 63 $\mu g \cdot kg^{-1} \cdot min^{-1}$) to provide sedation for patients undergoing lower limb surgery under spinal anesthesia. This low-dose propofol infusion resulted in a sleep-like state from which patients were arousable with verbal commands. More important, maintenance of the desired sedation level was easily achieved by varying the propofol infusion rate. Following completion of the operation, patients were completely awake within 4 minutes after terminating the propofol infusion, and they rapidly became clearheaded with "a strong desire for food." The investigators also commented on the ease with which the transition to general anesthesia could be made if the operation became more extensive than originally planned. In a follow-up study, these investigators compared infusions of propofol and midazolam used to supplement spinal anesthesia (100). Propofol, 62 $\mu g \cdot kg^{-1} \cdot min^{-1}$, provided sedation comparable to that provided by midazolam, 4.5 $\mu g \cdot kg^{-1} \cdot min^{-1}$, but propofol was associated with a significantly more rapid recovery. Following discontinuation of the sedative infusions, patients receiving propofol were wide awake in 2.1 $\pm$ 0.3 minutes, compared with 9.2 $\pm$ 1.5 minutes after midazolam. Patients receiving midazolam or methohexital for sedation during epidural analgesia also required more time to recall their date of birth, compared with those sedated with propofol (101).

When propofol and midazolam infusions were used during monitored anesthesia care (102), propofol was associated with decreased levels of residual sedation, drowsiness, confusion, clumsiness, and amnesia compared with midazolam (Fig. 7-4). Impairment of cognitive function in the early postoperative period was significantly greater in the midazolam-treated patients. Although midazolam produced more effective intraoperative amnesia, residual amnesia persisted for 60 minutes or longer into the postoperative period. Similarly, Fanard and associates also found that all patients had recovered to baseline levels within 15 minutes after discontinuing propofol, 44 $\mu g{\bullet}kg^{-1}{\bullet}min^{-1}$, whereas 24% of those receiving midazolam, 0.67 $\mu g{\bullet}kg^{-1}{\bullet}min^{-1}$, required more than 2 hours to achieve comparable recovery end points (103). In handicapped children receiving either propofol or midazolam infusions for sedation during dental procedures, propofol was preferred by the patients, their parents, and their care givers because of its rapid and smooth recovery profile (104). During regional anesthesia, propofol infusion rates of 2 to 5 $mg{\bullet}kg^{-1}{\bullet}h^{-1}$ are recommended in children (105).

Low-dose propofol infusions have also been used as an adjunct to local infiltration anesthesia in patients undergoing central venous catheter placement (106), oral surgery (107), ophthalmologic surgery (108), and superficial surgical procedures (e.g., breast biopsy and herniorrhaphy procedures) (102). Recovery was superior following propofol sedation compared with midazolam (102, 106) and diazepam (107, 108). Intraoperative motor agitation and postoperative fatigue were more common with the benzodiazepines. Even when the residual effects of midazolam were antagonized by flumazenil, recovery was no more rapid than following propofol infusion (109). Compared with methohexital, propofol was superior with respect to recovery of psychomotor performance (110). Ferrari and Donlon (111) compared bolus injections of propofol, 0.5 $mg{\bullet}kg^{-1}$, with midazolam, 0.02 $mg{\bullet}kg^{-1}$, and methohexital, 0.45 $mg{\bullet}kg^{-1}$, for sedation during retrobulbar or peribulbar blocks for ophthalmologic procedures. Propofol was associated with the lowest incidence of awareness during injection of the local anesthetic block and also resulted in more satisfactory sedation during the remainder of the surgical procedure. Additional advantages of propofol for this procedure include its ability to decrease intraocular pressure and to reduce postoperative nausea (111). Furthermore, sedative doses of propofol had no adverse effects on tidal volume, minute ventilation, end-expiratory carbon dioxide (CO_2), or arterial blood gas values (112). Because propofol can depress the ventilatory response to hypoxia (113), supplemental oxygen should be supplied, especially when propofol is administered in combination with an opioid analgesic. Use of ketamine in combination with propofol decreases the likelihood of ventilatory depression and may improve the operating conditions (114).

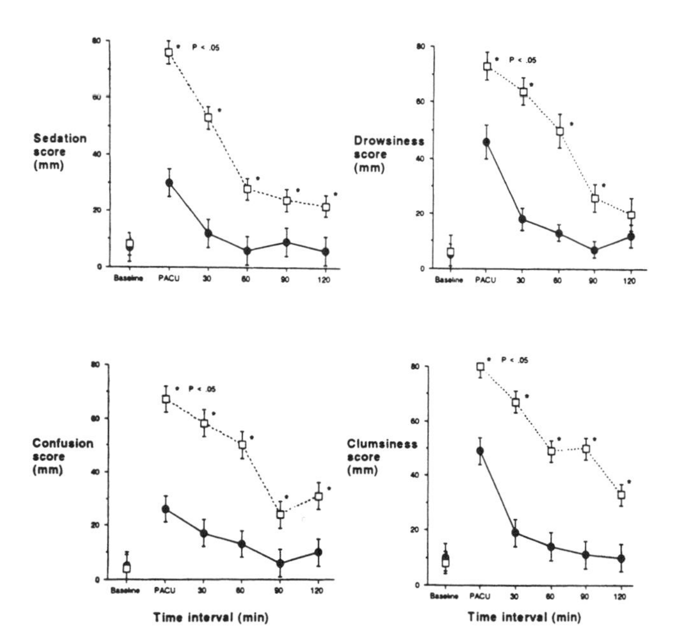

FIGURE 7-4. Perioperative sedation, drowsiness, confusion, and clumsiness visual analog scores for patients receiving either midazolam (open squares) or propofol (solid circles). Values represent median ± SEM. *$p < 0.05$, from propofol group. (From White PF, Negus JB. Sedative infusions during local and regional anesthesia: a comparison of midazolam and propofol. J Clin Anesth 1991;3:32–39.)

Propofol sedation has also been used to provide satisfactory conditions for upper gastrointestinal (GI) endoscopic procedures (115). Use of an infusion of propofol, 72 $\mu g{\bullet}kg^{-1}{\bullet}min^{-1}$, produced a cooperative patient with complete amnesia for the procedure, while providing for awakening and orientation in 4.8 ± 5.9 and 6.1 ± 5.7 minutes, respectively, after discontinuing the infusion. Patterson and colleagues (116) reported faster recovery and reduced hangover effects following propofol compared with midazolam when these drugs were administered for upper GI endoscopic procedures. However, the shorter duration of hypnosis following the bolus dose of propofol resulted in more recall of the end of the endoscopic procedure. The use of one or more supplemental doses of propofol would have extended the period of unconsciousness and reduced recall. Similar results were obtained in a comparison of propofol and midazolam for outpatient bronchoscopy (117, 118). Because of the potential for profound cardiovascular and respiratory depression, propofol should always be administered by personnel trained in the administration of general anesthesia, and not by gastroenterologists, radiologists, or surgeons (117). The usual dosages of propofol are 10- to 20-mg boluses for anxiolysis, 0.5 to 1.0 mg/kg/h for "light" sedation, and 2 to 4 $mg{\bullet}kg^{-1}{\bullet}h^{-1}$ for "deep" sedation (118).

Several investigators have commented on the minimal degree of amnesia produced by subhypnotic doses of propofol (100, 102, 106, 119, 120). Smith and associates administered four different bolus dose-infusion regimens to patients undergoing urologic procedures with regional anesthesia (119). Propofol infusion rates of 8, 17, 33, and 67 $\mu g \cdot kg^{-1} \cdot min^{-1}$ resulted in dose-related increases in the level of sedation (Fig. 7-5). Recall was assessed by showing the patients a picture 30 minutes after the start of the propofol infusion. Amnesia was not evident in the two low-dose propofol groups, with 88 and 86% of patients recalling the picture. However, at propofol infusion rates of 33 and 67 $\mu g \cdot kg^{-1} \cdot min^{-1}$, recall was reduced to 65 and 18%, respectively (119). At comparable levels of sedation, midazolam has a more profound amnesic effect than propofol (121). Analogous to the volatile agents, subanesthetic concentrations of propofol were able to suppress recall of emotionally charged information (122). Chortkoff and colleagues suggested that propofol may be a more potent amnestic agent than desflurane (123).

Sedation, amnesia, and anxiolysis are well-recognized pharmacologic features of benzodiazepines such as midazolam. However, the persistence of sedation and amnesia into the postoperative period is undesirable. The use of a midazolam and propofol combination takes advantage of the rapid recovery from propofol, whereas the benzodiazepine reduces intraoperative recall and anxiety. Taylor and associates (124) used a variable-rate propofol infusion (25 to 100 $\mu g \cdot kg^{-1} \cdot min^{-1}$) to provide sedation for outpatients undergoing operations with local anesthesia lasting 45 to 55 minutes. Before injection of the local anesthetic, patients received either midazolam, 2 mg IV, or a similar volume of saline according to a randomized, double-blind protocol. The addition of midazolam resulted in a significant increase in the level of sedation, decreased intraoperative anxiety, and reduced recall of painful intraoperative events (e.g., infiltration of the local anesthetic solution). When given at the outset, midazolam did not compromise the rapid recovery or favorable side effect profile following propofol sedation.

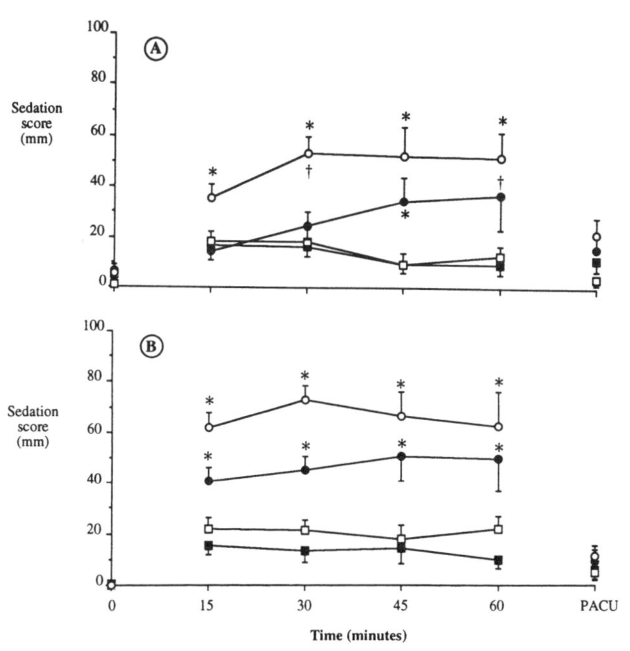

FIGURE 7-5. Sedation visual analog scores recorded by patients (A) and by a blinded observer (B) before (time 0), during, and after (PACU) sedation with propofol. Patients received propofol, 0.2 $mg \cdot kg^{-1}$ and 8 $\mu g \cdot kg^{-1} \cdot min^{-1}$ (group 1; solid squares); 0.4 $mg \cdot kg^{-1}$ and 17 $\mu g \cdot kg^{-1} \cdot min^{-1}$ (group 2; open squares); 0.5 $mg \cdot kg^{-1}$ and 33 $\mu g \cdot kg^{-1} \cdot min^{-1}$ (group 3; solid circles); and 0.7 $mg \cdot kg^{-1}$ and 67 $\mu g \cdot kg^{-1} \cdot min^{-1}$ (group 4; open circles). Values represent mean ± SEM. *$p < 0.05$, from group 1. $p < 0.05$, from 15-minute value in same group. (From Smith I, Monk TG, White PF, Ding Y. Propofol infusion during regional anesthesia: sedative, amnestic and anxiolytic properties. Anesth Analg 1994;79:313–319.)

Propofol sedation can also be supplemented by opioid analgesics to provide sedation and analgesia for uncomfortable procedures performed without local anesthesia. During extracorporeal shock wave lithotripsy, a combination of propofol and fentanyl produced comparable sedation and improved cardiorespiratory stability compared with an alfentanil-midazolam mixture, whereas both techniques decreased the anesthesia time and permitted a more rapid recovery than an epidural-based technique (120). Similarly, a mixture of alfentanil and propofol provided satisfactory conditions for transvaginal oocyte removal without clinically significant respiratory depression (18). In contrast, significant respiratory depression has been reported when midazolam-fentanyl and midazolam-alfentanil combinations are used (95, 120).

One of the advantages of propofol's pharmacologic profile relates to the ease with which the resultant level of sedation can be altered. A continuous propofol infusion, 2 to 4 mg/kg/h, provides for ease of titration of the level of sedation and a rapid recovery when used during loco-regional anesthesia (119-125). Several investigative groups have experimented with alternative methods for providing propofol sedation (13, 32, 126-130). The use of a computer-controlled infusion device (Diprafusor™) to achieve a target plasma propofol concentration derived from population pharmacokinetics resulted in satisfactory levels of sedation during 88% of the total infusion time (13). However, a comparative study failed to find any clinically significant advantages of the pharmacokinetic-based delivery system compared with conventional manual bolus-infusion schemes (32).

An alternative approach is to allow patients to self-administer sedative medications during monitored anesthesia care using a patient-controlled analgesia (PCA) device. Using bolus doses of propofol, 0.7 $mg \cdot kg^{-1}$, with a lockout interval of 3 minutes, satisfactory sedation and a high level of patient satisfaction was achieved during dental extractions (126) and during procedures performed with the patient under regional anesthesia (127). Using a crossover study design, Osborne and colleagues reported that patient-controlled sedation (PCS) with propofol was preferred over a continuous infusion of propofol by 66% of the patients (128). In a comparison of PCS by propofol and anesthesiologist-administered fentanyl-midazolam, the PCS group reported greater satisfaction and more rapid recovery of postoperative cognitive function (129). However, these differences were likely due to the use of propofol versus midazolam, rather than being specifically related to the use of the PCS technique. Ghouri and colleagues compared propofol, midazolam, and alfentanil when administered using a PCA device to supplement a basal infusion during operations performed under local anesthesia (130). Although all three drugs were associated with a high degree of patient satisfaction, propofol was associated with less postoperative nausea than alfentanil. Propofol produced more pain on injection, whereas midazolam was associated with decreased intraoperative recall. Discharge times were similar with propofol and midazolam, but discharge was delayed following alfentanil, probably secondary to the higher incidence of nausea. Although PCS with propofol may be an acceptable method of intraoperative drug delivery, no controlled trial has yet compared PCS with conventional bolus-infusion administration of propofol by an anesthesiologist.

In summary, propofol is capable of producing easily controllable levels of sedation during a variety of procedures performed with or without supplemental local or regional anesthesia. Its mood-altering (e.g., euphoriogenic) properties are believed to be "well-suited for conscious sedation procedures" (3). Low-dose infusions of propofol are associated with a predictably rapid recovery with few (if any) postoperative side effects. When amnesia and supplemental analgesia are needed, small doses of midazolam (2 to 3 mg) and fentanyl (50 to 75 μg) or alfentanil (0.5 to 1 mg) can be administered without affecting recovery times or increasing the incidence of perioperative side effects. Novel methods of propofol delivery (e.g., PCS) are associated with a high degree of patient acceptance. However, comparative trials are needed to determine whether these new modalities provide any additional benefit over conventional techniques for administering IV sedative medications during local anesthesia.

NEUROANESTHESIA

Considerable interest has been shown in the use of propofol for maintenance of neurosurgical anesthesia because a rapid recovery profile would facilitate an earlier postoperative assessment of CNS function. Propofol infusions can be used as an alternative to the volatile anesthetic agents, which all have the ability to cause cerebrovascular dilatation and thereby increase intracranial pressure (ICP). In contrast to the volatile anesthetics, propofol preserves cerebral autoregulation (131). Like the barbiturates, propofol can reduce ICP and intraocular pressure, can decrease cerebral metabolic requirements, and may provide "cerebral protection." In 1993, the United States Food and Drug Administration (FDA) approved the use of propofol for neurosurgical procedures.

Cerebrovascular Circulation

In clinical practice, use of propofol has been associated with cerebral vasoconstriction, decreased cerebral blood flow (CBF), and reduced cerebral metabolic requirement for oxygen ($CMRO_2$) (Table 7-6). Propofol also reduces the cerebral consumption of metabolic substrates (132). In contrast, in vitro studies have suggested that propofol has direct cerebral arterial and venous dilating properties (133, 134). In patients undergoing coronary artery bypass (CABG) surgery, induction with propofol, 2 mg•kg^{-1} IV, produced a 51% decrease in CBF, a 36% reduction of $CMRO_2$, and a 25% decrease in cerebral perfusion pressure (CPP) (135). However, the relationship between the cerebral effects and the systemic hypotensive effects following induction of anesthesia with propofol in neurosurgical patients is unclear.

In patients with brain tumors who were undergoing ventriculostomy for intracranial hypertension, induction of anesthesia with propofol, 2.5 mg•kg^{-1}, resulted in significant decreases in both mean arterial pressure (MAP) and CPP, whereas ICP remained unchanged (136). In patients with severe head injuries and normal ICP values, Pinaud and colleagues assessed regional CBF using a ^{133}xenon internal carotid artery injection technique (137). During a propofol-based anesthetic technique, these investigators found a 25% reduction in MAP, a 26% decrease in mean regional CBF, and a similar decrease in CPP.

Decreases in CBF have also been recorded when blood pressure was maintained at baseline values using vasopressor drugs (138, 139). Utilizing a canine model, Artu and associates found a significant reduction in CBF despite unchanged MAP values (140). These authors concluded that although the reductions in CBF and $CMRO_2$ (52 and 28%, respectively) were numerically different, they remained coupled. If propofol reduces CBF independent of changes in perfusion pressure, the mechanism for this action could be secondary to a reduction in cerebral metabolism. However, the decreases in CBF have not always been associated with equivalent reductions in $CMRO_2$ (138, 140, 141).

TABLE 7-6. Changes in Cerebral Hemodynamics, Cerebral Metabolic Rate for Oxygen, Intracranial Pressure, and Mean Arterial Pressure Following Induction of Anesthesia With Propofol

Reference	Population	Propofol Regimen	CBF (Ø)	CVR (_)	$CMRO_2$ (Ø)	ICP (Ø)	MAP (Ø)	CPP (Ø)	Comments
Stephan et al, 1987[135]	11 cardiac	2 mg•kg^{-1} 200 μg•kg^{-1}•min^{-1}	51%*	55%*	36%*	NR	NR	25%*	
Herregods et al, 1988[145]	6 head injury	2 mg•kg^{-1}	NR	NR	NR	56%*	34%*	46%*	Air-O_2 ICP > 25 mm Hg
Ravussin et al, 1988[146]	23 intracranial	1.5 mg•kg^{-1}	NR	NR	NR	32%* ‖	10%*	15%*	100% O_2 ICP > 15 mm Hg in 4/23
Vandesteene et al, 1988[138]	13 vertebral disk	100 μg•kg^{-1}•min^{-1} 100–350 μg•kg^{-1}•min^{-1}	27%*	51%†	18%	NR	a§	NR	0.5% enflurane, 65% N_2O; phenylephrine
Van Hemelrijck et al, 1989[136]	7 treated _ ICP		NR	NR	NR		45%†	49%†	100% O_2
Pinaud et al, 1990[137]	10 head injury	2.5 mg•kg^{-1} 2 mg•kg^{-1}	26%†	—	NR	16%§	26%‡	28%‡	Air-O_2
Van Hemelrijck et al, 1990[141]	7 baboons	150 μg•kg^{-1}•min^{-1}	39%*	NR	22%	NR	17%*	NR	Phencyclidine 70% N_2O
Artu et al, 1992[140]	6 dogs	200 μg•kg^{-1}•min^{-1}	52%*	155%*	28%*	28%*	4%§	3%	1% halothane, 66% N_2O
Muzzi et al, 1992[147]	10 mass lesions	400 μg•kg^{-1}•min^{-1} 1.7–3.5 mg•kg^{-1}	NR	NR	NR	45% ‖			Air-O_2; phenylephrine
Ramani et al, 1992[139]	9 rabbits	117–200 μg•kg^{-1}•min^{-1} 283–1100 μg•kg^{-1}•min^{-1}	38%¶	43%¶	NR	NR	10%§	NR	Opioid-70% N_2O; angiotensin II

*$p < 0.05$.
†$p < 0.01$.
‡$p < 0.001$.
§*Mean arterial pressure maintained at baseline values with vasopressors.*
‖ *ICP estimated from lumbar cerebrospinal fluid pressure.*
¶*p-value not recorded.*
CBF, Cerebral blood flow; CVR, cerebral vascular resistance; $CMRO_2$, cerebral metabolic rate for oxygen; ICP, intracranial pressure; MAP, mean arterial pressure; CPP, cerebral perfusion pressure; NR, not rated.

Ramani and associates administered a progressively increasing propofol infusion to rats during a "basal" opioid-N_2O anesthetic (139). While maintaining the MAP constant with an angiotensin II infusion, these investigators reported a close relationship between CBF and $CMRO_2$. As with the benzodiazepines (142), an increase in electroencephalogram (EEG) activity was noted at low propofol concentrations. However, at higher concentrations of propofol, the EEG showed progressive suppression (with an apparent correlation between EEG power and $CMRO_2$). To achieve EEG burst suppression during clinical neuroanesthesia, blood propofol concentrations of 6.3 ± 1.4 μg•ml^{-1} were required (143). Propofol also decreased the long latency cognitive P300 auditory evoked response (144).

Herregods and associates studied patients with raised ICP (>25 mm Hg) following severe head injury (145). They found that propofol, 2 mg•kg^{-1}, resulted in a 34% decrease in MAP and a 56% decline in ICP. However, the associated decrease in the CPP was 46%. Although most studies have found a reduction in ICP following induction of anesthesia with propofol, the associated decrease in MAP usually leads to a decreased CPP (137, 145, 146). Ravussin and colleagues studied patients undergoing craniotomy and found that an induction dose of propofol, 1.5 mg•kg^{-1}, followed by a maintenance infusion, 100 μg•kg^{-1}•min^{-1}, resulted in 32 and 10% decreases in cerebrospinal fluid (CSF) pressure and MAP values, respectively (146). Investigations have described reductions of ICP even when CPP was maintained during propofol anesthesia (140, 147). For example, in patients with supratentorial mass lesions without intracranial hypertension, TIVA with propofol led to a decrease in lumbar CSF pressure from 9.3 ± 3.9 (mean ± SD) to 5.1 ± 2.9 mm Hg when arterial blood pressure was maintained with vasopressor drugs (147).

The autoregulatory capacity of the cerebral circulation appears to remain intact during propofol anesthesia (Fig. 7-6) (140, 141, 148-150). In an animal model, Werner and colleagues demonstrated that cerebral autoregulation was preserved even after high doses of propofol (150). Several investigative groups have reported that the response of the cerebrovascular system to changes in CO_2 tension is also preserved during propofol anesthesia (Fig. 7-7) (151-156). Eng and associates studied CBF noninvasively using transcranial Doppler assessment of the velocity of middle cerebral artery blood flow during conditions of normocapnia, hypocapnia, and hypercapnia in both the awake state and during propofol anesthesia (156). Reactivity to CO_2 was preserved. However, the slope of the CO_2-response curve was decreased in the presence of propofol. Furthermore, no detectable difference was seen when N_2O was added, a finding since confirmed by Craen and colleagues (152).

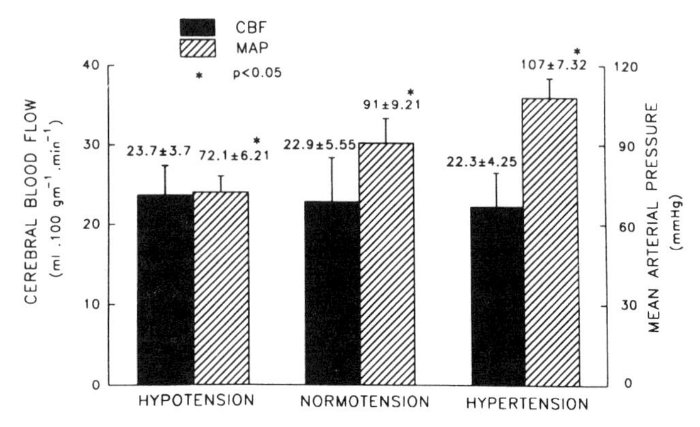

FIGURE 7-6. Autoregulation of cerebral blood flow (CBF, measured by ^{133}xenon technique) during manipulation of mean arterial blood pressure (MAP) with phenylephrine in humans anesthetized with a propofol infusion. (From Craen RA, Gelb AW, Murkin JM, Chong KY. Human cerebral autoregulation is maintained during propofol air/O_2 anesthesia [Abstract]. Anesthesiology 1992;77:A220.)

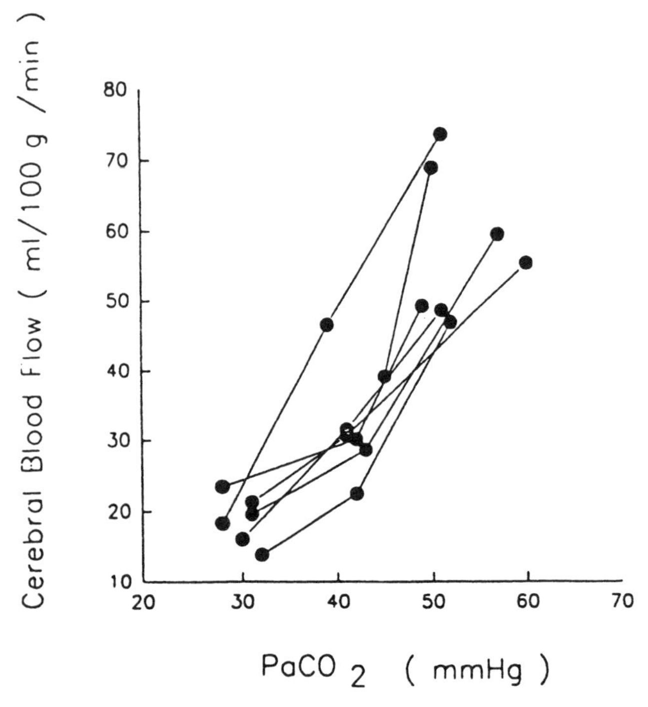

FIGURE 7-7. Autoregulation of cerebral blood flow (measured by ^{133}xenon technique) during changes in arterial CO_2 concentrations in humans anesthetized with a propofol infusion. (From Fox J, Gelb AW, Enns J, et al. The responsiveness of cerebral blood flow to changes in arterial carbon dioxide is maintained during propofol-nitrous oxide anesthesia in humans. Anesthesiology 1992; 77:453–456.)

Cerebral Protection

Investigators have suggested that propofol can reduce neuronal injury following incomplete ischemia by reducing cerebral oxygen requirements (157). In an hypoxic animal model, propofol was reported to improve tolerance of global cerebral ischemia (158). The improvement in survival was similar to that seen in a barbiturate control group. Using a hypotensive model of global ischemia, Weir and colleagues reported that the animals receiving an infusion of propofol showed higher postinsult CBF, improved electrolyte homeostasis, and a better recovery of EEG activity compared with control animals (159). However, histologic outcome was unchanged in the propofol-treated animals. Using positron emission tomography (PET), investigators have shown propofol to produce global metabolic depression of the CNS (160).

Following incomplete focal ischemia produced by temporary right common carotid artery ligation and hemorrhage-induced hypotension, neurologic outcome was improved and neuronal damage reduced in animals receiving propofol titrated to produce EEG burst suppression compared with a group receiving fentanyl-N_2O (157). However, in another study of focal ischemia following temporary middle cerebral artery occlusion, administration of propofol resulted in no significant difference in outcome or infarct size, compared with halothane anesthesia (161). The same model was able to demonstrate a reduction in infarct size when a barbiturate anesthetic was compared with halothane (162). In a different animal model of focal ischemia, Gelb and associates were also unable to demonstrate any significant reduction in the area of ischemia when propofol or thiopental was compared with halothane (163).

Ravussin and de Tribolet used a continuous infusion of propofol to provide anesthesia for cerebral aneurysm surgery (164). Following induction with propofol, 1.8 ± 0.1 $mg \cdot kg^{-1}$, anesthesia was maintained with a propofol infusion, 87 ± 3 $\mu g \cdot kg^{-1} \cdot min^{-1}$. EEG burst suppression was achieved during the temporary clipping of the vessel by increasing the propofol infusion to 500 $\mu g \cdot kg^{-1} \cdot min^{-1}$. During this treatment period, volume loading and dopamine infusions were used to avoid hypotension and to provide moderate hypertension (MAP of 100 mm Hg) in an attempt to improve collateral blood flow. None of the patients who required a temporary clip (three of whom had the temporary clip applied for more than 20 minutes) showed signs of neurologic deterioration. As might be expected, the use of propofol to achieve EEG burst suppression is associated with a reduction in cardiac output (CO) and MAP. Propofol, 1 $mg \cdot kg^{-1}$, followed by an infusion of 333 $\mu g \cdot kg^{-1} \cdot min^{-1}$ for 30 minutes and then 250 $\mu g \cdot kg^{-1} \cdot min^{-1}$, was used to produce burst suppression (165). While the cardiac filling pressure was maintained at baseline levels with supplemental fluids, MAP, CO and left ventricular stroke work index (LVSWI) decreased by 20%, 23%, and 26%, respectively. These cardiovascular changes are similar to those reported with thiopental (166).

Propofol Compared with Other Agents

Numerous studies have been published comparing different anesthetic techniques for neuroanesthesia. Todd and colleagues reported on the results of a randomized, prospective comparison of three neuroanesthetic regimens (167). All patients were undergoing elective craniotomy for supratentorial mass lesions and were randomized to receive one of the following regimens: (1) a propofol-fentanyl based anesthetic consisting of propofol, 1 to 2 $mg \cdot kg^{-1}$, followed by infusions of propofol, 50 to 300 $\mu g \cdot kg^{-1} \cdot min^{-1}$, and fentanyl, 0.03 to 0.05 $\mu g \cdot kg^{-1} \cdot min^{-1}$; (2) thiopental, 4 to 6 $mg \cdot kg^{-1}$, followed by isoflurane-N_2O anesthesia; or (3) thiopental followed by fentanyl-N_2O anesthesia with supplemental isoflurane as needed to maintain hemodynamic stability. The isoflurane-N_2O group recorded higher heart rate (HR) values during induction of anesthesia and a lower MAP during the maintenance period compared with the other anesthetic techniques. However, this treatment group had significantly more patients with an ICP greater than 24 mm Hg. Overall, the fentanyl-N_2O group had the most rapid emergence, whereas isoflurane-N_2O was associated with the slowest emergence. The fentanyl-N_2O group had a higher incidence (17%) of vomiting on emergence than the propofol-fentanyl group (2.5%) or the isoflurane-N_2O (5%) groups. No differences were noted among the three groups with respect to recovery milestones or neurologic outcome. These authors concluded that all three different anesthetic regimens were equally acceptable.

Ravussin and colleagues compared a thiopental-isoflurane technique with a propofol-based anesthetic technique in patients undergoing elective neurosurgical procedures (168). These investigators found that hemodynamic variables were similar in the two groups during induction. However, during application of the Mayfield head-holder, the propofol-based technique provided improved control of HR, MAP, and CSF pressure. During the early recovery period, the propofol-treated patients had shorter recovery times and higher Glasgow coma scale scores compared with the thiopental-isoflurane group. Yet the differences between the two groups were no longer significant after 30 minutes. Paillot and associates compared recovery after carotid endarterectomy surgery with either propofol or etomidate-isoflurane anesthesia (169). Although hemodynamic stability was similar with both techniques, subjective feelings and cognitive functioning, as assessed using sedation scores and psychometric testing, respectively, recovered more rapidly in the propofol group.

Given the length of many neurosurgical procedures, the issue of cost-effectiveness of drugs such as propofol has assumed greater importance (170). Todd and colleagues calculated the cost of the propofol-fentanyl anesthetic to be three times higher than the thiopental-isoflurane-N_2O combination and ten times more costly than thiopental-fentanyl-N_2O techniques (167). In addition, the use of IV anesthetic and analgesic infusions also requires specialized equipment for drug administration (e.g., infusion pump, IV tubing sets). Aitken and Farling estimated that an anesthetic regimen for aneurysm clipping using propofol is twice as expensive as an isoflurane-based technique (171). However, the relative costs of anesthetic and analgesic drugs change over time. More important, the cost of the anesthetic drugs is only a small fraction of the total hospital costs for a neurosurgical procedure.

Electroencephalogram

One of the primary concerns when using propofol for neuroanesthesia relates to the reports of alleged seizure-like activity following propofol anesthesia. Yet in animal models of status epilepticus, propofol suppressed seizures and possessed anticonvulsant properties similar to thiopental (172, 173). For example, propofol increases the lidocaine seizure threshold in rats (174). However, subanesthetic doses of propofol have been shown to augment the proconvulsant activity of the excitatory amino acids kainic acid and quisqualic acid (175).

Propofol, in common with other IV sedative-hypnotic drugs, induces dose-dependent changes in the EEG (176). When propofol is infused at a low rate to provide sedation, the most commonly observed EEG change is an increase in β activity (177). However, when given at a rate sufficient to produce unconsciousness, propofol produces an increase in δ activity (178). At even higher infusion rates, propofol can achieve EEG burst suppression (143, 179). No evidence suggests that propofol produces epileptiform activity in nonepileptic patients (178). Indeed, some reports indicate that propofol is successfully used to treat status epilepticus (180-182). Several research groups have investigated the relationship among propofol infusion rates, blood concentrations, and effects on the EEG. Kearse and associates (183) reported that the EEG bispectral index (BI) was a more useful predictor of patient movement in response to skin incision during propofol-N_2O anesthesia than other EEG variables or propofol blood concentrations. The EEG-BI decreases linearly as propofol blood concentrations increase.

During propofol administration, learning was suppressed when the EEG BI value was less than 90, and recall was decreased at values less than 90 (184, 185). In contrast to the EEG spectral edge frequency (186), the EEG BI appears to correlate with the depth of propofol anesthesia (187). An increase in the EEG δ power band ratio may be useful in predicting arousal after propofol anesthesia (188). Although pronounced EEG changes occur during emergence from propofol anesthesia, the EEG does not reliably predict eye opening (189).

Propofol decreases the duration of seizures in patients receiving electroconvulsive therapy (ECT) when induction doses are compared with methohexital (190). However, the use of propofol in patients with known epilepsy remains controversial. Hodkinson and colleagues described three patients who developed increased epileptiform activity on EEG recordings when these patients received propofol, 2 mg•kg^{-1}, as part of an anesthetic technique for seizure surgery (191). Areas of the brain that had not previously been shown to contain an epileptogenic focus displayed abnormal activity after propofol administration. The effect of propofol on the EEG activity of epileptic patients appears to be variable; some patients show increased spike activity, whereas others display decreased EEG activity (192).

Ebrahim and colleagues found that epileptiform activity increased in only 1 of 13 patients with temporal lobe epilepsy following a 2 mg•kg^{-1} bolus dose of propofol (193). The CNS depressant effects of propofol appear to be dose-dependent (194), because low doses may increase the activity of an epileptic focus, whereas higher doses (>1 mg•kg^{-1}) lead to suppression of EEG activity (195). In a study of 11 mentally retarded patients with pharmacologically controlled epilepsy, Oei-Lim and associates found that the use of a low-dose infusion of propofol to provide conscious sedation during dental surgery (92 ± 18 μg•kg^{-1}•min^{-1}, mean ± SD) did not increase interictal EEG activity (196).

Reports of adverse neurologic sequelae following propofol administration led the United Kingdom Committee on Safety of Medicines to report that "convulsions" and involuntary movements have been associated with the use of propofol (197). This committee subsequently advised that care should be taken when propofol is used in epileptic patients (198). The case reports include descriptions of convulsions (199, 200) and myoclonic movements with opisthotonos (hyperreflexia and arching of the back) (201, 202). These clinical signs can be associated with depressed levels of consciousness. Saunders and Harris reported four such cases and suggested that many of the reports of convulsions may actually represent opisthotonos and an associated depressed conscious level due to a drug-induced state of decerebrate rigidity (203). In three of the four cases, an EEG demonstrated a sleep-like EEG pattern consistent with cortical depression without any evidence of epileptiform activity. Other workers have confirmed the absence of seizure activity by EEG recording during involuntary movements with propofol (182) and have suggested that these events result from preferential depression of subcortical areas (204). Even in patients with complex partial epilepsy, propofol failed to produce seizure-like activity (205). Excitatory events (e.g., myoclonus, tremor, and dystonic posturing) during induction of anesthesia appear to be less prominent with propofol than with etomidate, thiopental, or methohexitone (206).

In summary, the use of propofol is associated with significant reductions in CBF, $CMRO_2$, and ICP. Propofol appears to have a cerebral protective action similar to that of the barbiturates. Because changes in blood pressure after induction doses of propofol are frequently reflected by changes in CPP, propofol should be administered with caution to avoid acute hemodynamic changes in patients with reduced intracranial compliance, as well as in patients receiving diuretic therapy. Propofol was approved by the FDA for use in neuroanesthesia, although the package insert cautions against its use in patients with raised ICP or abnormal cerebral circulation. The use of propofol in patients with seizure disorders remains controversial. However, increasing evidence would suggest that propofol possesses profound anticonvulsant activity (393).

CARDIAC ANESTHESIA

The optimal anesthetic technique for cardiac surgery should provide for (1) intraoperative hypnosis, amnesia, and analgesia, (2) hemodynamic stability with minimal direct myocardial depression, and (3) rapid recovery without the need for inotropic support. High-dose opioid techniques became popular because of the excellent hemodynamic stability associated with fentanyl and its newer analogs. However, opioid-based techniques may not provide an optimum degree of hemodynamic stability throughout the operation (207) and are more likely to be associated with intraoperative awareness (208). Supplementation of an opioid-based anesthetic with volatile agents reduces the incidence of intraoperative awareness and improves hemodynamic stability, but it may increase the potential for myocardial ischemia (209). The use of a high-dose opioid technique also prolongs the duration of postoperative mechanical ventilatory support (210). Prolonged stays in the ICU are expensive and may increase the risk of nosocomial infections (211).

Propofol's unique pharmacokinetic profile provides for a rapid recovery from its sedative and hypnotic effects (212). Although propofol appears to have an advantage over existing anesthetic techniques with respect to emergence times (213), its safety in patients with poor cardiac reserve has been the subject of considerable debate in the anesthesia literature (214-217). Most of the early clinical studies involving the use of propofol during cardiac surgery focused on its acute hemodynamic effects when used for induction of anesthesia in patients with good left ventricular function who were undergoing elective CABG surgery. More recently, investigators have evaluated the use of propofol-based maintenance anesthetic techniques in both healthy patients and in those with impaired left ventricular function (218). Compared with thiopental or etomidate, propofol appears to possess greater direct negative inotropic effects on papillary muscle (219). The decrease in systemic arterial blood pressure during propofol infusions is a result of its direct negative inotropic actions as well as its effects on arterial and venous vascular tone (220). Therefore, propofol should be used with caution in patients with preexisting cardiac disease.

Induction and the Prebypass Period

Use of propofol for induction of anesthesia in patients undergoing cardiac surgical procedures can produce significant hypotension before laryngoscopy and tracheal intubation. For example, in patients with good left ventricular function scheduled for elective CABG, induction with propofol, 1.5 mg•kg^{-1} IV, resulted in decreases in systolic and diastolic arterial pressures of 28 and 23%, respectively (221). However, these patients had received diazepam, 0.1 mg•kg^{-1}, and fentanyl, 8 μg•kg^{-1}, before propofol administration. Although HR, CO, and filling pressures were unchanged, decreases in systemic vascular resistance (SVR) and LVSWI of 25 and 32%, respectively, were reported. Anesthesia was maintained with a continuous propofol infusion adjusted to maintain hemodynamic stability (mean infusion rate of 86 μg•kg^{-1}•min^{-1}). Tracheal intubation was associated with a transient increase in MAP in 50% of patients. However, no MAP value exceeded the preoperative baseline value. Sternotomy resulted in a hypertensive reaction in only one patient.

A more recent study using a similar protocol design confirmed these hemodynamic changes but failed to find any adverse effects on myocardial blood flow or deleterious changes in cardiac metabolism during the prebypass period (222). Use of a smaller dose of propofol (0.5 mg•kg^{-1}) in combination with alfentanil, 50 μg•kg^{-1}, followed by infusions of propofol, 50 to 85 μg•kg^{-1}•min^{-1}, and alfentanil, 0.8 μg•kg^{-1}•min^{-1}, failed to prevent the initial decrease in arterial pressure following induction (223). Even without an opioid, induction with propofol, 2 mg•kg^{-1}, followed by an infusion of 200 μg•kg^{-1}•min^{-1}, produced a similar postinduction decrease in MAP (224). Although intubation was associated with an increase in MAP and HR, the addition of fentanyl, 10 μg•kg^{-1} IV, prevented the acute hemodynamic response to sternotomy. Another study involving patients undergoing cardiac surgery was prematurely terminated because two patients with three-vessel coronary artery disease became hypotensive after propofol, 1 mg•kg^{-1}, and fentanyl, 6 μg•kg^{-1} (225). The hypotensive responses were due to the vasodilator effects of propofol, enhanced by its interaction with fentanyl, in patients with low initial pulmonary capillary wedge pressure (PCWP) values. However, no electrocardiographic (ECG) evidence of myocardial ischemia was noted during the periods of hypotension. In comparison with alternative anesthetic induction agents, propofol produces a greater degree of hypotension as a result of decreased venous tone and reductions in total peripheral resistance. In addition, in common with other hypnotics, an interaction with opioid analgesics exacerbates these hypotensive effects.

The desire to avoid hypotension on induction, while maintaining hemodynamic stability during laryngoscopy, tracheal intubation, and sternotomy, led to the use of sedative-opioid combinations for induction of anesthesia followed by a propofol infusion for maintenance of anesthesia. In a recent study, Mora and colleagues compared anesthetic techniques involving the use of diazepam premedication followed by induction with fentanyl, 25 μg•kg^{-1} IV, and maintenance with either a propofol infusion, 50 to 500 μg•kg^{-1}•min^{-1}, or enflurane, 0.25 to 2% adjusted to maintain MAP within 15% of the postinduction values (213). These investigators found that both maintenance techniques resulted in comparable myocardial depression and control of hemodynamic variables. Russell and colleagues utilized a similar sedative-opioid induction (diazepam 0.1 mg•kg^{-1} and fentanyl 25 μg•kg^{-1}) followed by a two-stage propofol infusion, consisting of 167 μg•kg^{-1}•min^{-1} for 15 to 20 minutes and 50 μg•kg^{-1}•min^{-1} after sternotomy. A steady-state propofol concentration of 4.85 μg•ml^{-1} was achieved within 15 minutes and was not associated with untoward hemodynamic responses to either intubation or sternotomy (226). Analogous to the study by Mora and associates, Underwood and associates followed an opioid induction with either a two-stage propofol infusion or enflurane (227). Fewer patients in the propofol-treated group required vasodilator therapy in the propofol-treated group. However, one patient receiving enflurane developed increased myocardial lactate production and ECG evidence of ischemia, and one propofol-treated patient developed lactate production without any ECG changes. In comparing cardiac patients with normal versus impaired left ventricular function (ejection fraction $< 45\%$ and left ventricular end-diastolic pressure values > 16 mm Hg), Phillips and associates found no significant differences in hemodynamic variables when propofol was used for maintenance of anesthesia in the prebypass period (228).

In a prospective randomized trial, Hall and associates compared the safety of a propofol-based technique consisting of sufentanil, 0.2 $\mu g \cdot kg^{-1}$, and propofol, 1 to 2 $mg \cdot kg^{-1}$, and followed by a variable-rate propofol infusion (50 to 200 $\mu g \cdot kg^{-1} \cdot min^{-1}$), with an opioid-volatile technique consisting of sufentanil 5 $\mu g \cdot kg^{-1}$, supplemented with enflurane (229). Aside from an increased incidence of hypotension following induction in the propofol-treated group, these investigators found no significant differences between the anesthetic treatment groups with respect to hemodynamic stability, myocardial metabolic indices, or the incidence of adverse effects before the onset of cardiopulmonary bypass (CPB). In a more recent study, Hall and associates evaluated three anesthetic techniques in patients with decreased left ventricular function (218). In addition to the two treatment groups described previously, these investigators added a third study group consisting of an opioid induction (sufentanil 5 $\mu g \cdot kg^{-1}$) followed by a variable-rate propofol infusion (50 to 200 $\mu g \cdot kg^{-1} \cdot min^{-1}$) for maintenance of anesthesia. Although the overall control of hemodynamic variables was satisfactory in all three groups, propofol caused hypotension when used for induction with sufentanil, 0.2 $\mu g \cdot kg^{-1}$. Patients in the group receiving the opioid induction-propofol maintenance regimen tended to have decreased requirements for vasopressor medication and had less biochemical evidence of myocardial ischemia than the group receiving the opioid-volatile regimen.

Cardiopulmonary Bypass

Pharmacokinetic studies of propofol during CPB revealed the rapid onset of a transient decrease in propofol concentrations following the onset of CPB because of acute hemodilution, followed by a gradual rise in the blood concentration during the hypothermic phase (Fig. 7-8). These changes permitted the achievement of high propofol concentrations (5 $\mu g \cdot ml^{-1}$) during sternotomy while still maintaining hypnotic drug concentrations during CPB without changing the propofol infusion rate. Rewarming on CPB led to a decrease in propofol concentration to prebypass levels, suggesting that the hypothermic state was associated with changes in both hepatic enzyme activity and regional blood flow. However, hypnotic levels were maintained throughout the operation. Mora and colleagues also investigated propofol levels during CPB and observed that higher propofol infusion rates were required during CPB to achieve propofol levels similar to those measured during the prebypass period (230). However, Massey and colleagues failed to find a significant change in the propofol blood concentration during CPB when a zero order infusion of propofol, 67

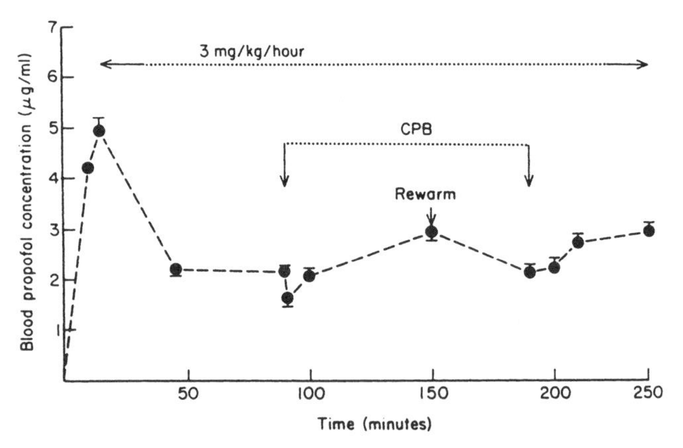

FIGURE 7-8. Changes in blood propofol concentrations during coronary artery surgery under propofol-fentanyl anesthesia. The time scale shows the mean time from induction of anesthesia to specific events. CPB, cardiopulmonary bypass period. (From Russell GN, Wright EL, Fox MA, et al. Propofol-fentanyl anaesthesia for coronary artery surgery and cardiopulmonary bypass. Anaesthesia 1989;44:205–208.)

$\mu g \cdot kg^{-1} \cdot min^{-1}$, was administered during cardiac surgery (231). Differences in the sampling site and timing of sample collections may explain the differences between these kinetic studies. The propofol concentrations remained above 1 $\mu g \cdot ml^{-1}$ throughout the operation, the concentration at which noncardiac patients awaken from propofol anesthesia (212). Not surprisingly, none of the patients recalled intraoperative events.

Propofol has been found to be a vasodilator during CPB (232), and high-dose infusion regimens (5 $mg \cdot kg^{-1}$ followed by 333 $\mu g \cdot kg^{-1} \cdot min^{-1}$) can further reduce oxygen consumption during hypothermic CPB (233). Propofol also inhibits thermoregulatory vasoconstriction (234), but only slightly alters the shivering threshold (235). When using propofol, the combination of vasodilation and decreased oxygen consumption may confer additional protection against the adverse effects of CPB. In comparative cardiac studies involving propofol-based techniques and standard opioid-volatile balanced anesthetic techniques, no differences have been found in the need for inotropic support on termination of CPB (218, 299).

Recovery Phase

Mora and associates reported that in cardiac surgical patients receiving fentanyl, 25 to 50 $\mu g \cdot kg^{-1}$, for induction of anesthesia, use of a propofol maintenance infusion (50 to 500 $\mu g \cdot kg^{-1} \cdot min^{-1}$) was associated with comparable intraoperative hemodynamic stability and a more rapid emergence from anesthesia than either fentanyl (0.15 to 0.45 $\mu g \cdot kg^{-1} \cdot min^{-1}$) or thiopental infusions (0.05 to 1.0 $mg \cdot kg^{-1} \cdot min^{-1}$) (236). Propofol also permitted earlier extubation compared with high-dose fentanyl and thus enhanced the ability to "fast track" cardiac surgery patients by reducing their stay in the ICU. Chong and colleagues studied 198 consecutive patients undergoing a variety of cardiac procedures using a standard anesthetic technique involving a propofol infusion (67 to 100 $\mu g \cdot kg^{-1} \cdot min^{-1}$) at the start of CPB (237). If patients were hemodynamically stable and bleeding was not excessive in the PACU, weaning from ventilatory support was attempted on return of patients to consciousness. The median time to extubation was 2 hours, and by 24 hours, only 2.5% of the patients required continuing ventilatory and inotropic support. Five patients in the propofol-treated group required reintubation, 4 of whom had undergone a repeat CABG procedure. A retrospective comparison with a comparable group of patients anesthetized with an opioid-based technique demonstrated a median time to extubation of 7 hours. However, these data conflict with the results of Mora and colleagues, who found no significant differences in the time to extubation between opioid-propofol and opioid-volatile anesthetic techniques. In the series by Hall and colleagues, a significantly longer time to extubation was noted in patients in whom an opioid induction was followed by a propofol infusion (218). However, these investigators suggested that the larger cumulative doses of morphine required for postoperative analgesia by the propofol induction-maintenance group contributed to prolonging their time to extubation.

In summary, induction of anesthesia with an opioid-benzodiazepine combination followed by a maintenance infusion of propofol, supplemented with an inhalational agent or opioid analgesic as needed to control blood pressure and HR, appears to provide highly acceptable anesthetic conditions for patients undergoing routine cardiac surgery and is associated with rapid emergence and early extubation. The use of a titrated infusion of propofol for maintenance of anesthesia is not associated with an increased requirement for inotropic support after cardiac surgery.

PEDIATRIC ANESTHESIA

The use of propofol in children was initially described in 1985 (238). Although IV induction techniques are generally considered less popular in infants and children because of difficulty in obtaining vascular access, the availability of EMLA cream (a eutectic mixture of local anesthetics) and propofol has renewed interest in the use of IV techniques in this patient population. With the increased use of the laryngeal mask airway (LMA), particularly for pediatric ambulatory surgery and for diagnostic procedures outside the operating room, propofol has advantages over other IV induction drugs. Compared with propofol (2.5 mg/kg), thiopental (4 mg/kg) produced less cardiovascular depression, and midazolam (0.5 mg/kg) caused greater psychomotor impairment on awakening (239). However, within 1 hour, all children were equally awake, cooperative, and coordinated. Runcie and colleagues (50) reported that propofol hastened early recovery in children undergoing day-case surgery, compared with thiopental. However, an earlier discharge was only found in the older children.

Dosage Requirements

The pharmacokinetics of propofol in children is optimally described by a standard three-compartment model, as summarized in Table 7-1. Marsh and associates maintained propofol anesthesia in children using a computer-controlled infusion device similar to the one described by White and Kenny (240) in adults. As expected, the pharmacokinetic-based infusion system systematically overpredicted the measured blood propofol concentrations when adult parameters were used for children aged 1 to 12 years (241). When pharmacokinetic data derived from children were used to program the kinetic-based infusion pump, the device more accurately achieved predicted plasma propofol concentrations. Compared with adults, the initial dose of propofol should be increased by 50% in children, and at equilibrium, the maintenance infusion should be increased by 25 to 50%. Browne and colleagues reported that the propofol infusion rate needed to suppress movement in children (ED_{95}) was 175 $\mu g \cdot kg^{-1} \cdot min^{-1}$ (242), twice the ED_{95} required for adults (223).

Early studies involving the use of propofol for induction of anesthesia in children have reported that the ED_{90} for loss of the eyelash reflex with propofol was 2.8 $mg \cdot kg^{-1}$ in unpremedicated children, and it was 2.0 $mg \cdot kg^{-1}$ in children premedicated with trimeprazine, 3.0 $mg \cdot kg^{-1}$ (243). A more recent study suggested that premedication with meperidine, 1 $mg \cdot kg^{-1}$ intramuscularly, or trimeprazine, 2 $mg \cdot kg^{-1}$ orally, had no effect on the propofol induction dose requirement (2.9 $mg \cdot kg^{-1}$) (244). In 90 unpremedicated children aged 3 to 12 years, Hannallah and associates found the ED_{95} for loss of the eyelash reflex to be 2.0 $mg \cdot kg^{-1}$, and the ED_{95} for subsequent acceptance of the face mask without disruptive movements was 2.3 $mg \cdot kg^{-1}$ (245).

When comparing a computerized, target-controlled propofol infusion with intermittent manual bolus dosing in 40 children aged 1 to 12 years, no difference was found in the induction dose requirement (246). The ED_{50} was found to be higher in infants aged 1 to 6 months than children aged 10 to 16 years (3.0 $mg \cdot kg^{-1}$ versus 2.4 $mg \cdot kg^{-1}$) (247). Using an incremental dosing technique, propofol, 2.5 $mg \cdot kg^{-1}$, produced loss of consciousness in 95% of children aged 3 to 15 years who had been pretreated with alfentanil, 5 $\mu g \cdot kg^{-1}$

(248). When using a smaller induction dose of propofol (1.5 mg•kg^{-1} IV), significantly more older children (10 to 15 year) lost consciousness than younger children.

Cardiorespiratory Effects

Several studies have suggested that induction of anesthesia with propofol decreases HR by 10 to 20% in children (238, 249). Irrespective of whether an induction dose of propofol is followed by an inhalation agent (249) or a propofol infusion (250), the HR response was similar. Propofol does not attenuate the transient increase in HR associated with the rapid introduction of desflurane (251). However, the HR decrease associated with propofol is significantly greater in toddlers than in older children (252). During strabismus surgery, the incidence of bradycardia secondary to the oculocardiac reflex has been found to be higher in children receiving propofol infusions, compared with an inhalation technique (253, 254). Furthermore, propofol does not alter sinoatrial or atrioventricular mode function in pediatric patients undergoing radiofrequency catheter ablation (255), and it has no direct effect on the accessory pathway in patients with Wolff-Parkinson-White syndrome (256).

In children, a 10 to 25% decrease in MAP usually occurs immediately following induction with propofol (249, 252). Hannallah and colleagues found that 48% of children had a 20% or greater decrease in MAP during the first 10 minutes following an induction dose of propofol (245). However, a majority of these "hypotensive" episodes occurred while patients were breathing 1 to 3% halothane, and all returned to within 20% of baseline MAP values after decreasing the inspired halothane concentration. Induction doses of propofol (1.6 to 2.6 mg•kg^{-1}), followed by a mixture of halothane, 0.5%, and 30% N_2O in oxygen in spontaneously breathing children, resulted in a 15% decrease in MAP at 1 minutes and a 30% decrease at 5 minutes following injection of propofol (249). These investigators reported that the magnitude of the hemodynamic change was not related to the size of the induction dose of propofol. In a study involving 40 children aged 1 to 13 years, Doyle and colleagues found no differences in intraoperative MAP values between children maintained with a computer-controlled propofol infusion (range of infusion rates 300 to 600 μg•kg^{-1}•min^{-1}) or halothane 0.5 to 2%, in combination with N_2O, 67%, in oxygen (246).

Use of propofol to produce "deep" sedation has facilitated outpatient transesophageal echocardiography (257) and cardiac catheterization (258). Using pulsed Doppler echocardiography, Aun and associates compared the hemodynamic effects of propofol, 2.5 mg•kg^{-1}, and thiopental, 5 mg•kg^{-1}, for induction of anesthesia in toddlers (younger than 2 years) and older children (2 to 12 years) (252). The decrease in MAP was greater after propofol (28 to 31%) than thiopental (14 to 21%) in both age groups. The decrease in SVR was similar (15%) in toddlers after thiopental or propofol, but in older children, the decrease in SVR was almost three times greater with propofol (19% versus 7%). Cardiac index decreased by 10 to 15% with both anesthetic agents. In preschool children ventilated with 60% N_2O in oxygen during a maintenance infusion of propofol, 400 μg•kg^{-1}•min^{-1}, investigators found a 25% decrease in MAP and a 23% decrease in stroke volume (250). Administration of atropine, 20 μg•kg^{-1} IV, increased HR and MAP but did not influence propofol's effect on stroke volume.

Propofol appears to suppress the pharyngeal and laryngeal reflexes more effectively than thiopental (259). Propofol has been used to facilitate tracheal intubation without muscle relaxants after inhalational induction in children undergoing outpatient surgery (260); it reportedly produces intubating conditions similar to those seen with succinylcholine. However, in children aged 2 to 7 years, Rodney and colleagues found intubating conditions to be poor when using propofol, 3.5 mg•kg^{-1}, as the sole agent for tracheal intubation (261). The addition of alfentanil, 20 μg•kg^{-1}, improved intubating conditions and effectively attenuated the pressor response to tracheal intubation compared with propofol alone or with a thiopental-succinylcholine combination. The 20% incidence of apnea (lasting more than 20 seconds) following induction with propofol, 2.5 mg•kg^{-1} (245, 248), is similar to that observed with thiopental (262). However, premedication with opioids or benzodiazepines increases the incidence of apnea (244, 262). Manschot and associates reported age- and dose-related increases in the incidence of apnea in children (namely, more than 12% at 3 to 5 years versus 38% at 10 to 15 years; and 3% with propofol, 2.0 mg•kg^{-1}, versus 28% with propofol, 2.5 mg•kg^{-1}) (248). Although Martin and colleagues (73) found a higher incidence of airway obstruction before tracheal intubation when anesthesia was induced in children with halothane (34%) than with propofol (10%), the ability to establish IV access and to administer muscle relaxant drugs more rapidly may have facilitated airway management in the propofol-treated group.

Recovery Profile

Mirakhur reported a significantly shorter time to awakening in children who received propofol for induction of general anesthesia (11 to 14 minutes) compared with thiopental (16 to 22 minutes) (244). These investigators also noted a significantly lower incidence of nausea with propofol. A more recent study comparing induction with propofol (3 mg•kg^{-1}) with thiopental (5 mg•kg^{-1}) reported that the time required for children over 5 years of age to give their name and to be discharged from the hospital was significantly shorter in the propofol group (50). In children aged 1 to 5 years, propofol only reduced the time to eye opening. Puttick and Rosen compared a propofol-N_2O technique with thiopental-N_2O-halothane in 38 children undergoing outpatient dental extractions and found that the times to spontaneous eye opening and discharge were significantly shorter with propofol (8 ± 3 and 36 ± 7 minutes, respectively) than with thiopental-halothane (11 ± 6 and 44 ± 13 minutes, respectively) (263). Times to extubation and discharge from the PACU were also significantly shorter in a study of 40 children aged 3 to 8 years who underwent minor otorhinolaryngologic operations when propofol was used for induction followed by a propofol maintenance infusion, 100 μg•kg^{-1}•min^{-1}, compared with a thiopental-halothane technique (264). However, Aun and colleagues (265) reported that recovery was slower after a target-controlled propofol infusion (compared with thiopental-halothane) in children undergoing superficial procedures. Although Hannallah and associates (266) reported no difference in awakening (extubation) times, children maintained with a propofol infusion (versus halothane) recovered faster, were discharged sooner, and had less postoperative vomiting. Using a more sensitive test of residual drug effect, Hiller and colleagues reported that propofol offered advantages over halothane (266a).

In a more recent study comparing inhalational induction and maintenance with halothane with IV induction and maintenance with propofol (3 mg•kg^{-1}, followed by 150 μg•kg^{-1}•min^{-1}) in infants aged 2 to 12 months, investigators reported significantly shorter times to spontaneous movement, extubation, and sucking response in the propofol-treated group (267). However, Aun and associates found that recovery was slower in children maintained with a propofol infusion compared with halothane. Watcha and colleagues found a significant decrease in times to ambulation and discharge, as well as a lower incidence of postoperative emesis, following strabismus surgery when anesthesia was maintained with a propofol infusion, 160 mg•kg^{-1}•min^{-1}, as part of a TIVA technique compared with either a balanced or inhalation technique (253). Similarly, Weir and colleagues found a significant decrease in the incidence of vomiting during the first 24 hours after strabismus surgery with propofol, 150 to 300 μg•kg^{-1}•min^{-1}, compared with halothane, 0.5 to 1% (41% versus 64%) (268). In a subgroup of children who did not require postoperative opioid analgesics, an even greater difference was found (24% versus 71%). Tramèr and associates failed to find any significant difference in the incidence of postoperative vomiting between propofol and isoflurane when N_2O was avoided (269). In patients with strabismus, the adjunctive use of ondansetron (5 mg•m^{-2}) was ineffective in reducing the incidence of nausea and vomiting after either propofol or isoflurane anesthesia (269).

In a study involving 40 children aged 1 to 12 years who underwent general surgical procedures while spontaneously breathing N_2O 67% in oxygen through an LMA (246), the investigators failed to find a significant difference in the time to spontaneous eye opening between a group maintained with a propofol infusion and a group maintained with halothane. The major difference between this investigation and earlier studies may relate to the shorter duration of anesthesia (263), the adjunctive use of N_2O (253), and the fact that these children were allowed to breath spontaneously (264). On the basis of recovery of postural stability, a balanced anesthetic technique consisting of propofol-alfentanil-N_2O offered no advantage over thiopental-halothane-N_2O for minor pediatric otolaryngologic procedures (265). In children undergoing cardiac catheterization, propofol infusions with fentanyl were associated with significantly shorter recovery times than midazolam-ketamine anesthesia (258). Finally, in pediatric patients undergoing brief diagnostic or therapeutic procedures outside the operating room, propofol was associated with less postanesthetic vomiting and agitation than ketamine or etomidate (270).

Magnetic Resonance Imaging

Magnetic resonance imaging (MRI) sequence images can be difficult to obtain in awake children because these images are extremely sensitive to motion artifacts. In the noisy environment of the MRI scanner, children are often unable to remain immobile long enough for a successful scan to be performed (271). Concerns about maintenance of airway patency have led some clinicians to secure the airway with a tracheal tube while maintaining anesthesia with a propofol infusion (272). Other investigators have used infusions of propofol for sedation of spontaneously breathing children (273) and found it to be a safe technique that provides scanning conditions superior to those seen with thiopental or methohexital (274), with no repeat scans required in children receiving propofol, compared with 75% of those children receiving barbiturates for sedation (275). Propofol also offers significant advantages over barbiturates with respect to recovery parameters (276). The peak CO_2 values measured at the oral or nasal cannulae can be used to monitor the respiratory rate and the pattern of ventilation (277), and these values have been shown to correlate with arterial CO_2 pressure measurements (278).

During computed tomography (CT) scanning, the minimum effective infusion rate following induction of anesthesia with propofol was 25 μg•kg^{-1}•min^{-1}.

However, higher infusion rates and supplemental boluses were required to prevent a motor response to subsequent head positioning (279). Tracheal intubation may also be avoided by maintaining a patent airway using an LMA device. When using an LMA in the CT scanner, the recommended doses of propofol are 2.5 mg•kg^{-1}, followed by an infusion of 83 μg•kg^{-1}•min^{-1} (280). Sedation with propofol also avoids the concerns associated with repeat exposures to halothane. With short-term administration, tolerance to propofol does not appear to develop in children following repeated exposures (281). However, the apparent safety of propofol infusion techniques for sedation in spontaneously breathing children is not a valid reason to dispense with the services of the anesthesiologist (282, 283).

In summary, propofol is used increasingly in children of all ages. On the basis of dosage per kilograms of body weight, the induction and maintenance dosage requirements for propofol are higher in neonates and children than in adults. Propofol's pharmacokinetic profile, recovery characteristics, and apparent antiemetic activity make it a particularly useful agent for pediatric outpatient anesthesia and for sedation during radiologic procedures.

INTENSIVE CARE UNIT

The primary objectives of sedation in the ICU are to enhance patient comfort, reduce anxiety, facilitate sleep, and minimize resistance to mechanical ventilation. The level of sedation should be rapidly adjustable depending on the patient's clinical condition. The ideal sedative agent for critically ill patients in the ICU would also have minimal depressant effects on the respiratory and cardiovascular systems, would not influence the biodegradation of other drugs, and would be eliminated by pathways independent of renal, hepatic, or pulmonary function, resulting in a short elimination half-life without active metabolites (284). The most commonly used sedative-analgesic agents (namely, midazolam and morphine) lack many of these properties. Although lacking some of the properties of an ideal sedative, propofol was approved by the FDA for ICU sedation in 1993. The advantages and disadvantages of using propofol for sedation in the ICU have been reviewed (285). However, caution is necessary until further information becomes available on the complications of propofol use in critically ill patients (286).

The first clinical report describing the use of propofol for sedation in the ICU was published in 1987 (287). Ten patients who required mechanical ventilation were sedated with an infusion of propofol for 8 hours at a mean infusion rate of 32 μg•kg^{-1}•min^{-1}. Patients were maintained at a level of sedation in which they appeared comfortable and were asleep when left undisturbed, but they were arousable with verbal or light tactile stimulation. Two of the 3 patients who received an initial bolus dose of propofol (1 mg•kg^{-1}) experienced 40 and 53% decreases in MAP, respectively. In addition, the mean and diastolic blood pressure values for the study group were significantly lower than baseline values throughout the study period. The range of blood propofol concentrations during the infusion was 0.1 to 1.9 μg•ml^{-1}. These blood levels are similar to the propofol concentrations reported by Barr and colleagues during light sedation of patients in the ICU (288). In the latter study, recovery was so rapid that 8 of the 10 ICU patients required "resedation" within 45 minutes of discontinuing the propofol infusion. In critically ill patients in septic shock and respiratory failure, propofol sedation did not adversely affect whole-body oxygen transport (289).

Pharmacokinetics

Early pharmacokinetic studies involving rapid bolus injections or short-term infusions suggested that propofol was rapidly eliminated from the body. Although of limited clinical significance, studies evaluating the pharmacokinetics of propofol after prolonged infusion in critically ill patients have suggested the presence of a long elimination half-life (290). Beller and colleagues performed an extensive pharmacokinetic study in 14 general surgical ICU patients who were sedated with propofol over a 4-day period (291). A constant-rate propofol infusion was discontinued every 24 hours for assessment of elimination kinetics and clinical recovery. The awakening times were similar after the 24-, 48-, 72-, and 96-hour study periods. Furthermore, propofol concentrations before the infusion was discontinued were similar, and the slopes of the plasma propofol decay curves did not change over the 4-day study period. The investigators found no evidence of a change in receptor sensitivity or drug accumulation despite the duration of the propofol infusion.

Albanese and colleagues also studied the pharmacokinetics of a constant rate infusion of propofol (50 μg•kg^{-1}•min^{-1}) in ICU patients (290). These investigators found a prolonged elimination half-life of 726 to 3000 minutes [1878 $\pm$ 672 minutes (mean $\pm$ SD)], a total body clearance of 0.95 to 2.58 L•min^{-1} (1.57 $\pm$ 0.56 L•min^{-1}), and a large volume of distribution of 415 to 2836 L (1666 $\pm$ 756 L), suggesting that propofol was extensively redistributed from the blood and other well-perfused tissues into the less well-perfused ("deep") tissue compartments. These variables are similar to those reported by Morgan and colleagues in their study involving propofol infusion during general anesthesia lasting up to 9 hours (292). Bailie and col-

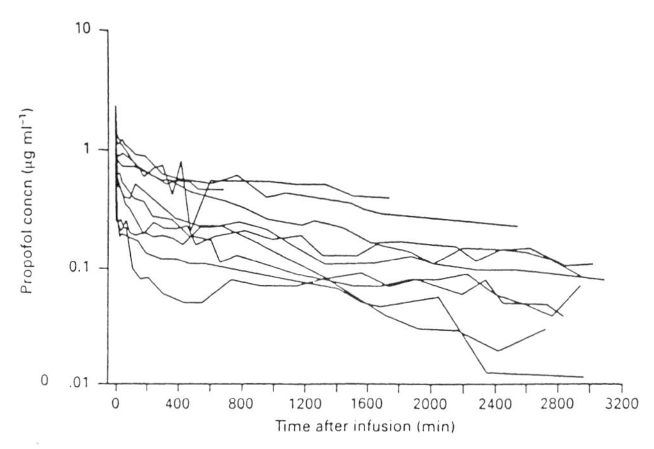

FIGURE 7-9. Decline in blood concentration of propofol after discontinuation of infusion in 12 patients in an intensive care unit. Mean duration of infusion was 85.6 hours, mean rate of infusion was 43 $\mu g \cdot kg^{-1} \cdot min^{-1}$, and mean elimination half-life was 23.5 hours. (From Bailie GR, Cockshott ID, Douglas EJ, Bowles BJM. Pharmacokinetics of propofol during and after long term continuous infusion for maintenance of sedation in ICU patients. Br J Anaesth 1992;68:486–491.)

leagues calculated clearance values ranging from 1.1 $L \cdot min^{-1}$ to 40.1 $L \cdot min^{-1}$, with a median total body clearance of 2.1 $L \cdot min^{-1}$ and a mean (± SD) elimination half-life value of 1411 ± 586 minutes (293). Surprisingly, blood concentrations of propofol decreased by 50% in the first 10 minutes after terminating the propofol infusion (Fig. 7-9). Because this decline was more rapid than would be predicted from the clearance rate, the authors concluded that redistribution of propofol between blood and the peripheral tissue compartments occurred even after the cessation of an 86-hour infusion. The long "terminal" elimination half-life of propofol after prolonged administration appears to represent drug elimination from a "shallow" tissue compartment, and the residual levels produce no clinically significant effects.

Weaning from Ventilatory Support

In comparing propofol with midazolam, propofol is typically associated with a faster recovery from its clinical and EEG effects (294-296). Carrasco and associates (294) studied 88 critically ill patients who were allocated to receive either propofol or midazolam for short-term (< 24 hours), medium-term (24 hours to 7 days), or long-term (> 7 days) sedation. The mean doses of propofol and midazolam were 38 $\mu g \cdot kg^{-1} \cdot min^{-1}$ and 2.8 $\mu g \cdot kg^{-1} \cdot min^{-1}$, respectively. Patients in the propofol treatment group were adequately sedated for a higher proportion of the study period than those receiving midazolam. Propofol was also associated with a significantly shorter time to tracheal extubation than midazolam after discontinuing short-, medium-, and long-term infusions. In each treatment group, the time to extubation correlated with the duration of the sedative infusion. On the basis of estimated costs (including drug costs and additional nursing care), the faster recovery from propofol sedation in the short-term subgroup was associated with significant cost savings compared with midazolam. However, this advantage was not evident in the medium- or long-term subgroups. These data suggest that propofol is more cost-effective than midazolam for short-term sedation in the ICU.

In a large multicenter study, Aitkenhead and colleagues (297) compared propofol and midazolam infusions in 101 critically ill patients. Patients received either propofol (30 $\mu g \cdot kg^{-1} \cdot min^{-1}$) or midazolam (1.7 $\mu g \cdot kg^{-1} \cdot min^{-1}$) for 24 hours. The infusion rates were adjusted to maintain a "light" level of sedation, and most patients in both treatment groups were able to obey simple commands immediately after discontinuing the sedative infusions. Of the patients not responding immediately after discontinuing the propofol infusion, all but 1 of the propofol-treated patients responded within 20 minutes. However, only 6 of the remaining 15 midazolam-treated patients responded within 20 minutes. In a subgroup of 39 patients who were judged to be fit for weaning from ventilatory support, this was achieved in a mean of 5 minutes (range 0 to 13 minutes) in the patients receiving propofol, compared with 148 minutes (range 17 to 555 minutes) in the midazolam-treated group ($p < 0.001$). Compared with flunitrazepam, weaning from ventilatory support was also achieved more rapidly with propofol (< 15 minutes versus < 264 minutes) (298).

Combinations of opioids and benzodiazepines are most commonly used for sedation. Comparisons between opioid-benzodiazepine and opioid-propofol combinations have revealed similar clinical conditions in the ICU (299, 300). Carrasco and colleagues also confirmed that recovery was more rapid after propofol alone than after either midazolam or an opioid-benzodiazepine combination. Interest in speed of recovery has led to investigations of the use of volatile agents for sedation in the ICU. Isoflurane has been shown to be superior to midazolam for short-term sedation in patients who require mechanical ventilation, with a faster recovery and a better quality of sedation (301). Millane and associates studied the quality of sedation and the time to recovery between isoflurane (median inspired concentration of 0.35%) and propofol (median infusion rate of 23 $\mu g \cdot kg^{-1} \cdot min^{-1}$) in 24 patients requiring mechanical ventilation (302). No significant differences were noted with respect to cardiovascular variables, analgesic requirements, sedation scores, or the quality of sedation as assessed by the ICU nurses. Although the results suggested a more rapid recovery after long-term sedation with isoflurane, analysis of the results is difficult because only 7 of the 24 patients actually completed the entire study.

Sedation after Head Injury

The use of propofol was studied in 10 patients with severe head injuries who required sedation during controlled mechanical ventilation (303). The rate of propofol infusion was adjusted to maintain the ICP below 10 mm Hg and the CPP above 60 mm Hg. After 24 hours, the propofol was stopped, and the patients were allowed to recover from the sedative medication. The mean rate of propofol infusion was 48 $\mu g \cdot kg^{-1} \cdot min^{-1}$ (range 30 to 83). No significant changes were seen in MAP. However, mean CPP tended to increase during the study. The quality of sedation was judged to be "good" in 9 of the 10 patients. In a comparison of propofol with a combination of morphine and pentobarbital, Pearson and associates found no significant difference in cardiovascular stability, ICP, or outcome between these groups (304).

Sedation after Cardiac Surgery

Several publications in the anesthesia literature have described the use of propofol infusions for sedation in the ICU following cardiac surgery. Many of these studies have demonstrated faster recovery following the use of propofol compared with midazolam (Table 7-7). However, Higgins and colleagues (305) found no difference between the two drugs with respect to extubation or ICU discharge times. Grounds and associates randomized patients to receive either an infusion of propofol or intermittent bolus doses of midazolam to maintain a stable level of sedation (306). Sedation was discontinued when predetermined criteria were met, and patients were then weaned from ventilatory support. The average doses of the sedative drugs were propofol, 13 $\mu g \cdot kg^{-1} \cdot min^{-1}$, and midazolam, 0.27 $\mu g \cdot kg^{-1} \cdot min^{-1}$. Propofol permitted patients to be maintained at the desired sedation level for a significantly higher percentage of time (90 to 96%) compared with midazolam (80 to 89%). In this study, and in a similar one by McMurray and associates, the requirements for analgesic medications were greater in the midazolam-sedated patients, suggesting that less ideal sedative conditions existed in the latter group (306, 307). To maintain a more profound level of sedation, higher mean infusion rates of propofol (45 $\mu g \cdot kg^{-1} \cdot min^{-1}$) and midazolam (1.5 $\mu g \cdot kg^{-1} \cdot min^{-1}$) were required (308). Use of propofol for sedation in the ICU decreases the requirement for both antihypertensive agents and opioid drugs (309).

For cardiac surgical patients who require sedation and mechanical ventilation for a short period followed by rapid weaning from the ventilator, propofol appears to be a more suitable agent. However, concerns regarding cardiovascular stability may limit the usefulness of propofol in this setting (310). A 15 to 20% decrease in MAP has been reported after a loading dose of propofol ranging from 0.24 to 1.0 $mg \cdot kg^{-1}$ in patients who have undergone cardiac surgery (308, 311, 312). Roekaerts and colleagues reported that the pressure started to return toward presedation values approximately 15 minutes after the start of the propofol infusion. Although MAP values remained below baseline levels throughout the 10-hour study period, these values were believed to be clinically acceptable in these patients with an ejection fraction of less than 40%. McMurray and associates reported that MAP values were "significantly lower" than awake values during propofol infusions lasting 9 to 12 hours at a mean infusion rate of 12.7 $\mu g \cdot kg^{-1} \cdot min^{-1}$ (307). No increased use of inotropes or sign of myocardial ischemia during the propofol infusion was reported. Roekaerts and colleagues found that the use of propofol infusions for sedation was associated with lower heart rates than the

TABLE 7-7. Comparative Recovery Times Following Sedation With Propofol or Midazolam After Coronary Artery Bypass Surgery

Reference	Number of Patients	Infusion Regimen $\mu g \cdot kg^{-1} \cdot min^{-1}$)	Time to Responsiveness (min)	Time to Spontaneous Ventilation (min)	Time to Tracheal Extubation (min)
Grounds et al, 1987[306]	60	propofol (13)	NR	13.6 (2.68)*	24.9 (2.97)*
		midazolam (0.27†)	NR	198 (22.5)*	226 (22.8)*
McMurray et al, 1990[307]	100	propofol (19.2)	NR	NR	11.9 (2.5)*
		midazolam (0.57†)	NR	NR*	127.9 (9.9)*
Snellen et al, 1990[311]	40	propofol (15.2)	NR	24 (7)‡	154 (33)
		midazolam (0.63)	NR	66 (16)‡	243 (44)
Roekaerts et al, 1993[308]	30	propofol (45.2)	11 (8)*	52 (32)*	250 (135)
		midazolam (1.5)	72 (70)*	195 (119)*	391 (128)

Times are means (± SEM), except Roekaerts et al means (± SD), recorded from the cessation of the study drug; NR, not recorded.
**$p < 0.001$.*
†Bolus dose administration, figure given is the calculated rate over the study period.
‡$p < 0.05$.

use of midazolam (308). This difference may be have been due to the effects of propofol on the baroreflex response, resulting in lower heart rate values despite decreased MAP values (313). In patients at risk of developing myocardial ischemia, the lower heart rate values may be of benefit (314). However, the effect of propofol on baroreflex activity during long-term infusions has not been studied. Furthermore, a propofol infusion of 50 $\mu g \cdot kg^{-1} \cdot min^{-1}$ altered the inotropic state of the right ventricle (315).

Sedation of Children

Propofol has been successfully used for pediatric sedation in the ICU (316). However, the use of propofol for sedation of young children in the ICU has resulted in reports of neurologic sequelae following withdrawal of propofol and the occurrence of metabolic acidosis during propofol infusions in the presence of upper respiratory tract infections. Thus, controversy surrounds the use of propofol for sedating neonates and young children in the ICU.

In 1992, Trotter and Serpell described neurologic sequelae in two children (aged 2½ and 4 years) sedated with propofol infusions following tracheal intubation for stridor secondary to presumed viral infections (317). The children were sedated with high doses of propofol (up to 300 $\mu g \cdot kg^{-1} \cdot min^{-1}$), and both developed abnormal movements, particularly fine twitching movements of the extremities after the propofol was stopped. However, both children made a full recovery. Lanigan and colleagues described a case of a 23-month-old child requiring sedation after tracheal intubation for stridor. Although the child had received various different sedative regimens including high-dose propofol (318), jerky, twitchy movements and functional blindness occurred following the withdrawal of propofol. Imray and Hay described similar clinical signs in an 18-month-old girl who received propofol for sedation for 2 weeks after severe burn injury (319).

Parke and colleagues reported five children (ages 4 weeks to 6 years) who required propofol infusions following intubation for upper respiratory tract infections (320). The average rate of infusion of propofol was high (125 to 167 $\mu g \cdot kg^{-1} \cdot min^{-1}$), and all five children developed lipemic serum, an increasing metabolic acidosis, bradyarrhythmias, and fatal myocardial failure. In view of the lack of evidence of another cause of death, as well as the presence of lipemic serum, the authors believed that the propofol emulsion (containing Intralipid 10%) may have been a contributing factor.

A review of a large database of preterm infants who had received high doses of IV lipids as part of parenteral nutrition found that those infants who required ventilation for respiratory disease were not at risk of developing metabolic acidosis (321). Other possible causes of the reported metabolic disturbances included adrenocortical suppression and an unexplained association between viral infections, high-dose propofol infusions, and metabolic acidosis (322, 323). The manufacturers of propofol have emphasized that the drug is not licensed for sedation of critically ill children (Diprivan package insert, Zeneca Pharmaceuticals, Macclesfield, England).

Hyperlipidemia during Propofol Sedation

Gottardis and colleagues studied changes in serum lipid concentrations in 10 patients receiving propofol (approximately 33 $\mu g \cdot kg^{-1} \cdot min^{-1}$) over a 3-day period (324). In this study, no significant rise in triglyceride or cholesterol levels was seen. In contrast, in another report, 10 of 22 patients sedated with a propofol infusion (mean infusion rate of 39 $\mu g \cdot kg^{-1} \cdot min^{-1}$) experienced a doubling of their triglyceride levels after 3 days (294). Cook and Palma also found a progressive rise in lipid levels in patients sedated with propofol for 2 to 3 days at a mean infusion rate of 38.5 $\mu g \cdot kg^{-1} \cdot min^{-1}$ (325). After a week, the triglyceride levels were more than 3 times normal. The patients with elevated lipid levels appeared to have a slower return of higher mental functions. This finding is consistent with the effects of hypertriglyceridemia on cerebral function (326). Boyle and associates studied lipid levels in 22 patients receiving propofol sedation for up to 14 days (327). The maintenance infusion rates of propofol ranged from 10 to 230 $\mu g \cdot kg^{-1} \cdot min^{-1}$. Lipid levels were not altered in those patients receiving low rates of infusion of propofol (< 33 $\mu g \cdot kg^{-1} \cdot min^{-1}$). However, serum triglyceride levels were increased in the 2 patients who received infusion rates in excess of 100 $\mu g \cdot kg^{-1} \cdot min^{-1}$ (6 $mg \cdot kg^{-1} \cdot h^{-1}$) over a 2-week period (Fig. 7-10). One case report described the occurrence of endobronchial lipid deposits in a patient with adult respiratory distress syndrome who had received propofol sedation for 16 days in the ICU (328).

Other Pharmacologic Actions

Adrenal Cortex

The potency of etomidate in inhibiting adrenal steroidogenesis is 1500 times greater than that of propofol (329). Two studies have looked at cortisol secretion during propofol sedation in ICU patients, and both concluded that although cortisol levels tend to decrease during the infusion period, no evidence of a clinically significant impairment of steroidogenesis was present (287, 297). Van Hemelrijck and associates (330) reported that propofol anesthesia did not inhibit stimulation of cortisol synthesis.

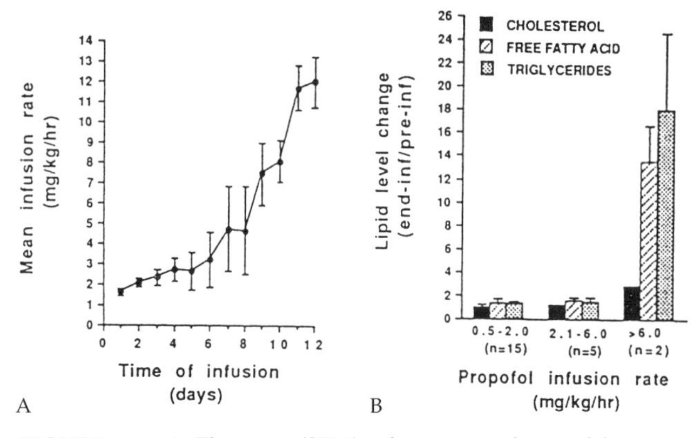

FIGURE 7-10. A, The mean (SEM) infusion rate of propofol necessary to maintain a constant level of sedation in 22 ventilator-dependent patients in an intensive care unit (ICU) who were sedated for up to 14 days. B, Mean (SEM) increase in serum lipid levels before discontinuation of propofol, relative to preinfusion levels during sedation at three rates of infusion in 22 patients in an ICU. (From Boyle WA, Shear JM, White PF, Schuller D. Tolerance and hyperlipemia during long-term sedation with propofol [Abstract]. Anesthesiology 1990;73:A245.)

Infection and Contamination

With prolonged infusions of propofol in the ICU, concerns have been raised regarding the risk of infections because of the well-known ability of the propofol (Intralipid) emulsion to support microbial growth. For example, Sosis and colleagues (331) found that propofol supported the rapid growth of *Candida albicans* after a latent period of 6 to 16 hours. Furthermore, small glass fragments from the exterior of a propofol ampule can contaminate its contents when the ampule is opened. Farrington and colleagues (332) compared the incidence of contamination when continuous infusions of propofol or midazolam were used for sedation of critically ill patients. These investigators found no evidence to suggest that the use of propofol infusions in the ICU increases the incidence of infections when the drug is prepared using conventional aseptic precautions. The new EDTA-containing formulation of propofol may decrease the risk of infectious contamination.

Tetanus

Borgeat and associates demonstrated reduced electrical muscular activity as measured by an electromyographic (EMG) device in a patient with tetanus who was given propofol (333). Although the site of action was not determined, a central site appears likely.

Bronchodilatation

Pedersen reported two patients who developed severe bronchospasm following aortic valve replacement and whose wheezing decreased after the administration of propofol (334). A reduction in peak inspiratory pressure and airway resistance and an increase in dynamic compliance in patients with chronic obstructive pulmonary disease who underwent mechanical ventilation have also been reported following a 2 mg•kg^{-1} bolus dose of propofol (335). The mechanism of the apparent bronchodilating action is not known, but it may be related to a direct effect of propofol on the bronchial smooth muscle (analogous to propofol's relaxant effects on vascular smooth muscle). Alternatively, the sedative effects of propofol may have simply decreased the stimulation from the tracheal tube. Compared with induction with the barbiturates, propofol was associated with less wheezing after tracheal intubation in both asthmatic and nonasthmatic patients (336).

Discoloration

Propofol has been reported to cause green discoloration of the hair and urine (337, 338). In addition, long-term sedation with propofol has been reported to produce reversible green discoloration of the liver (339). These phenomena are apparently due to metabolism of propofol that leads to a phenolic green chromophore. However, the appearance of white urine during prolonged propofol anesthesia (340) may be related to lipiduria.

Antioxidant Activity

Propofol has been demonstrated to possess antioxidant properties similar to those of vitamin E (341). These properties make propofol a free radical scavenger and suggest that the drug may be useful in conditions such as multiorgan failure and adult respiratory distress syndrome.

Status Epilepticus

Propofol has been successfully used in the ICU for the management of status epilepticus (180), severe generalized myoclonus (342), and severe delirium tremens (343). Propofol appears to modify the EEG pattern of patients in status epilepticus in a positive manner (344). However, propofol has also been implicated as the cause of agitation and "grand mal" convulsions following the withdrawal of sedative infusions (345). One patient experienced a generalized tonic-clonic seizure 6 days after propofol withdrawal (346). This phenomenon may be similar to the "withdrawal syndrome" reported earlier in children.

In summary, propofol provides a quality of sedation comparable to that provided by other sedative-hypnotic drugs in the ICU (347). With respect to its ability to produce short-term changes in the level of sedation, propofol offers advantages over all currently available benzodiazepines (348). Compared with the benzodiazepines and the barbiturates, recovery is faster following sedation with propofol, and this effect leads to a more rapid recovery of patient responsiveness, spontaneous ventilation, and tracheal extubation. A comparative study has also suggested that patients tolerate the ICU environment better with propofol than with midazolam (347). As a result of its favorable recovery profile, propofol may reduce overall costs when used for short-term sedation. However, the use of propofol for long-term sedation in the ICU is expensive and may result in hyperlipidemia and abnormal motor activity. Although some investigators have suggested that propofol has higher clinical effectiveness and a better cost-to-benefit ratio than midazolam in the ICU (294), others have suggested that the higher cost, development of tolerance, immunosuppression, and hyperlipidemia after long-term infusion administration may be more problematic (285, 348). Therefore, improvements in recovery may not offset the increased cost and complications associated with propofol compared with other available sedative agents in the ICU.

SPECIALIZED USES

Obstetric Anesthesia

The first reports describing the use of propofol for induction of general anesthesia in patients undergoing elective cesarean section were published in 1989. In a randomized comparison, anesthesia was induced with thiopental, 4.5 ± 0.3 mg•kg^{-1}, or propofol, 2.2 ± 0.3 mg•kg^{-1}, and subsequently maintained with isoflurane-N_2O (349). Because similar Apgar scores were recorded in both groups, propofol does not appear to affect fetal outcome adversely. Furthermore, the drug had no adverse effects on uterine contraction or intraoperative blood loss. In this study, maternal recovery was not significantly modified by the use of propofol. However, other investigators reported more rapid recovery when propofol was used in a similar protocol (350). In the latter investigation, patients received either propofol, 2.5 mg•kg^{-1}, or thiopental, 5 mg•kg^{-1}, followed by isoflurane-N_2O for the remainder of the operation, which lasted approximately 45 minutes. Propofol was associated with a significantly shorter time to orientation than thiopental (1.0 ± 0.9 versus 2.3 ± 1.0 minutes) and improved performance on the Maddox wing test (a test of extraocular muscle balance) during the first hour of recovery (350). However, when propofol was administered by infusion to maintain anesthesia, maternal recovery was not significantly faster compared with patients receiving thiopental-enflurane-N_2O (351, 352).

Following induction of anesthesia with propofol, maternal blood pressure values were found to be significantly lower than when thiopental was used (349). Compared with thiopental, propofol has also been reported more effective in attenuating the hypertensive response (353), and the associated catecholamine rise (354), following tracheal intubation. Like other IV anesthetic agents, propofol readily crosses the placenta and reaches the fetal circulation (355, 356). Compared with the use of thiopental (5 mg•kg^{-1}), neonates of parturients whose anesthesia was induced with propofol (2.4 mg•kg^{-1}) had lower Apgar and neurobehavioral scores (357). Neonatal depression may occur when propofol is infused for a prolonged period before delivery (352, 355) or when higher rates of propofol infusion (e.g., > 150 μg•kg^{-1}•min^{-1}) are used for maintenance of anesthesia (351). Propofol is also present in the breast milk of the mothers who received propofol for induction of anesthesia before cesarean delivery (358). However, the propofol concentrations are low when compared with the transplacental transfer of propofol.

In summary, propofol can reduce the response to tracheal intubation in obstetric patients, in whom the use of opioid analgesics may be undesirable. Propofol readily crosses the placenta, but the usual induction doses do not appear to depress the neonate. Despite its rapid clearance in pregnant women (359), propofol does not appear to produce a clinically significant advantage with respect to maternal recovery. However, propofol represents an acceptable alternative for obstetric patients in whom barbiturates are contraindicated (360).

Laryngeal Mask Airway

The LMA has become available in the United States and is increasing in popularity. Preliminary experience suggested that the use of propofol for induction of anesthesia produces more acceptable conditions for LMA insertion than other IV agents (e.g., thiopental) (361). An early, noncomparative clinical trial demonstrated that LMA insertion was possible within 20 seconds of a bolus dose of propofol, 2.5 mg•kg^{-1} (362). Of the 100 patients studied, 6 coughed, and 2 demonstrated a mild "laryngeal reaction" to insertion of the LMA. In a dose-ranging study, LMA insertion was equally successful following propofol, 2.0, 2.5, or 2.8 mg•kg^{-1}, but it was unsatisfactory following 1.5 mg•kg^{-1} (363). In young children undergoing MRI scanning (280), insertion of a laryngeal mask was found to be successful on the first attempt in 84% of cases following propofol, 2.5 mg•kg^{-1}.

Brown and associates compared propofol and thiopental for LMA insertion (364). Eighty patients received equihypnotic doses of propofol, 2.5 mg•kg^{-1}, or thiopental, 4 mg•kg^{-1}, for induction of anesthesia, and the incidence of gagging was found to be significantly higher with thiopental compared with propofol. However, this effect could be overcome by the use of larger doses of thiopental. Deepening anesthesia with a volatile agent before LMA insertion has also been recommended when thiopental is used for anesthetic induction (361).

During maintenance of anesthesia with the LMA, many anesthetic techniques are available. Supplementation of a propofol infusion with N_2O has been demonstrated to provide satisfactory conditions for the use of the LMA during both spontaneous (365) and controlled ventilation (366). TIVA with infusions of propofol and alfentanil have also been administered using the LMA to maintain the airway (367).

Antiemetic and Antipruritic Properties

An increasing body of literature suggests that propofol possesses antiemetic activity (368). Antagonism of the dopamine D_2 receptor by propofol has been suggested as a possible mechanism for this effect (369). Compared with volatile agents, the use of propofol for general anesthesia was associated with less PONV and decreased requirements for antiemetic medication (36-40, 43, 56, 61, 66, 67, 73, 83-85, 253, 264, 370-372). Similar findings have been found when using propofol as an alternative to other IV induction (45, 49) or maintenance agents (46, 78, 86, 87). More recently, propofol has been administered in subhypnotic doses to treat nausea and vomiting, a use suggesting that propofol possesses direct antiemetic properties (2). When PONV occurred in the recovery room, propofol (10 to 20 mg IV) was successful in 81% of patients, compared with 35% of those given a lipid emulsion. However, 6 of the 21 patients in the propofol-treated group experienced a relapse within 30 minutes after receiving the propofol. The antiemetic effect of propofol appears not to be due to the lipid emulsion (10% Intralipid) used to solubilize the drug (373). Unfortunately, the rapid clearance of IV propofol limits its clinical usefulness as a therapeutic antiemetic drug, unless a continuous infusion technique is utilized.

Propofol infusions have also been used successfully to treat refractory nausea and vomiting after surgery (374) and in patients receiving cytotoxic chemotherapy (375, 376). Borgeat and associates used a subhypnotic infusion of propofol (16.7 $\mu g \cdot kg^{-1} \cdot min^{-1}$ or 1 $mg \cdot kg^{-1} \cdot h^{-1}$) in 14 patients with emetic symptoms refractory to ondansetron and dexamethasone (376). All patients experienced complete resolution of their symptoms during the infusion period, and 12 reported improved appetite. These patients also manifested slight euphoric effects, with little evidence of sedation. Nonsedating doses of propofol had little effect on apomorphine-induced vomiting in volunteers (377).

Subhypnotic doses of propofol appear to protect against itching after intrathecal morphine (378). Propofol has subsequently been compared with naloxone for the treatment of pruritus produced by spinally administered opioid analgesics (379). Propofol, 10 mg, and naloxone, 2 $\mu g/kg$, were equally effective in treating opioid-induced pruritus. However, use of propofol was associated with less postoperative pain compared with naloxone.

Cardioversion

Cardioversion is often performed as a day-case procedure, and anesthetic agents with a short recovery profile and good cardiorespiratory stability are useful. Propofol has been compared with other available IV anesthetics, including etomidate, methohexital, thiopental, and midazolam. Propofol produced a greater depression of blood pressure than etomidate, but recovery times were similar (380-382). Pain on injection and myoclonus are frequently seen during induction of anesthesia with etomidate, and the myoclonus may be severe enough to interfere with the ECG interpretation (381). Methohexital and propofol produce similar conditions for cardioversion, although use of propofol may be associated with faster emergence from the hypnotic state (383, 384). Two studies report similar 16 to 29% decreases in systolic blood pressure during cardioversion with thiopental, 3.0 to 3.5 $mg \cdot kg^{-1}$, or propofol, 1.5 to 2.1 $mg \cdot kg^{-1}$ (382, 385). However, Gupta and colleagues used larger mean doses (± SD) of both thiopental (5.2 ± 1.0 $mg \cdot kg^{-1}$) and propofol (2.2 ± 0.3 $mg \cdot kg^{-1}$) and found that a decrease in blood pressure was only seen in the propofol-treated group (386).

Data on recovery when thiopental or propofol were used for cardioversion are conflicting (385, 387). However, the results differ because different adjuvant drugs and clinical end points were studied. Valtonen and colleagues (387) and Jan and associates (387a) reported a more rapid recovery following propofol using psychometric tests for assessment, whereas Sternlo and Hägerdal (385) found a prolongation of the time to awakening after propofol. Although midazolam remains a popular drug for providing sedation during cardioversion, recovery after midazolam is significantly longer than when propofol is used for cardioversion (382, 386, 388) Although the overall success rate for cardioversion is similar with all IV anesthetic agents, propofol may increase the energy required for successful cardioversion (387).

Electroconvulsive Therapy (ECT)

In the published comparisons of propofol and methohexital for ECT, propofol is consistently associated with a shortened duration of seizure activity (190, 389-391). Propofol also decreases the duration of seizures compared with thiopental (392). The effect of propofol on seizure duration is dose-related, and the minimally effective dose (0.75 to 1.25 $mg \cdot kg^{-1}$) should be used for ECT (194, 393). Although investigators have suggested that the efficacy of ECT is related to the duration of the motor seizure (e.g., > 30 seconds) (394), Malsch and colleagues have found that the efficacy of ECT was similar in patients anesthetized with either propofol or methohexital, despite shortened seizure duration in the propofol-treated group (395). In addition, propofol was more effective than methohexital in attenuating the rise in blood pressure and HR immediately after ECT (190, 194, 390, 391, 396). The incidence of myocardial infarction following ECT is surprisingly high (397). Thus, the ability of propofol to attenuate the sympathetic response to ECT may offer additional protection against this potentially serious complication of the treatment. Recovery following ECT appears to be more dependent on the duration of the seizure than on the type of hypnotic agent administered. Compared with methohexital and etomidate, propofol was associated with less confusion in the immediate post-ECT treatment period (393). Overall, recovery from ECT appears to be similar after the use of either propofol or methohexital (190, 194, 398, 399).

Malignant Hyperthermia

Propofol-based anesthetics have been used for providing anesthesia to patients susceptible to malignant hyperthermia (MH) (400). Propofol does not stimulate MH-susceptible ryanodine receptors (401). Furthermore, animal studies using the MH-susceptible swine model have found no evidence of the disorder during propofol anesthesia (402, 403). Propofol infusions have also been used to provide anesthesia for muscle biopsy procedures in patients being tested for susceptibility to MH (400, 404). McKenzie and colleagues have shown that not only can propofol be used successfully in susceptible patients, but also that propofol does not affect the sensitivity of in vitro contracture testing (404). Propofol does not simulate MH-susceptible or normal ryanodine receptor channel activity (401). Hence, propofol appears "safe" in patients susceptible to MH and can be used during muscle biopsy procedures in patients whose susceptibility has not yet been established.

Miscellaneous Indications

Propofol has also been used successfully in two patients with a history of acute intermittent porphyria. However, further work is required before declaring propofol safe in this patient population (405, 406). Propofol was administered for termination of pregnancy in a patient experiencing an exacerbation of acute intermittent porphyria, and her neurologic symptoms resolved, suggesting that propofol is a safe drug to use in the presence of this disease (406a).

In summary, propofol can be used successfully for both ECT and cardioversion. However, a minimally effective dose should be used to avoid the need to increase the energy requirements for successful treatments. Propofol also appears to be a useful agent in patients who are susceptible to MH and in those with acute intermittent porphyria. Finally, propofol has a distinctive antiemetic action, and its use during surgery can decrease emetic sequelae after general anesthesia.

Pain on Intravenous Injection

Pain following injection of propofol occurs in 28 to 90% of patients (244, 407, 408). Even when low-dose propofol infusions are administered for sedation, the incidence of pain can vary from 33 to 50% (102, 409). Although the mechanism responsible for the propofol-induced venous pain is unknown, it may be due to activation of the kinin cascade system (410). The original diluent, Cremophor EL, was initially thought to be the causative agent. However, no measurable reduction in pain occurred following the change to the current lipid emulsion formulation (411). Klement and Arndt have demonstrated that the pain is a function of the drug itself, rather than of the formulation (412).

The use of small veins on the dorsum of the hand is associated with a greater incidence of pain compared with the use of large veins in the antecubital fossa (245, 247, 407, 410, 411). Scott and colleagues found that decreasing the speed of injection or injecting propofol into a fast-flowing IV infusion in the dorsum of the hand was of little benefit in reducing the incidence of pain (410). However, dilution of propofol with either 5% glucose solution or 10% Intralipid resulted in a significant reduction in the incidence of pain (412, 413).

The use of local anesthetics (e.g., lidocaine 1 to 2%) reduces the pain resulting from propofol injection. King and associates found that the reduction in pain from the addition of lidocaine to the propofol formulation was dose-related (414). However, 6% of patients still reported severe pain when lidocaine, 20 mg, was mixed with 190 mg (19 ml) of propofol. Lin and colleagues reported a reduced incidence of pain and discomfort when lidocaine, 40 mg, was added to propofol, 200 mg (415). Gehan and colleagues found that lidocaine, 0.1 $mg{\cdot}kg^{-1}$, significantly reduced the incidence of pain, and no additional benefit occurred from increasing the dose to 0.4 $mg{\cdot}kg^{-1}$ (416). In children, lidocaine, 0.2 $mg{\cdot}kg^{-1}$, was reported to prevent pain from propofol injection (417). However, other investigators have reported pain in 6% (263) and 27% (243) of children receiving as much as 0.5 $mg{\cdot}kg^{-1}$ lidocaine. Johnson and colleagues found 40 mg of lidocaine to be highly effective, and better than 20 mg (418). This dose of lidocaine was equally effective when mixed with the propofol or when given as a "pretreatment" dose with simultaneous occlusion of the venous drainage of the forearm 20 seconds before the injection of propofol. Some investigators have suggested that venous occlusion with a tourniquet increases the effectiveness of lidocaine pretreatment (408). However, the addition of lidocaine to propofol was more effective than pretreatment without venous occlusion (410, 419). When a mixture is used, the lidocaine and propofol should be freshly mixed and used within 30 minutes; otherwise, a significant fraction of the lidocaine will have entered the lipid phase and resulted in a decline in the effective "free" concentration.

Manschot and colleagues reported a 4% incidence of pain when alfentanil, 5 $\mu g \cdot kg^{-1}$, was administered to children 30 seconds before an induction dose of propofol through a vein on the dorsum of the hand (248). However, in another investigation, alfentanil, 15 $\mu g \cdot kg^{-1}$ IV, failed to prevent propofol injection pain in 55% of the children studied (254). In adults, several investigators have demonstrated that alfentanil, 10 to 30 $\mu g \cdot kg^{-1}$, administered 1 to 2 minutes before infusing propofol, significantly reduced pain on injection (420-422). Fentanyl, 100 μg, may be equally effective (423). Finally, cooling propofol to 4°C or the injection of cold saline at 4°C into the IV cannula immediately before administering propofol is apparently as effective as the addition of lidocaine, 10 mg, to the propofol emulsion (424, 425).

In summary, in reviewing the numerous studies published over the past few years, propofol has obviously become an extremely valuable adjuvant for many diagnostic and therapeutic procedures (71, 426, 427). Although propofol was initially viewed as an "outpatient" (day-case) anesthetic, it is becoming more widely used during pediatric, neurosurgical, and cardiovascular anesthesia, as well as for sedation in the ICU. Although the cardiovascular depressant effects of propofol are well tolerated in healthy outpatients, these effects may be more problematic in high-risk patients with intrinsic cardiac disease, as well as those with multiorgan system disease. In hypovolemic patients and in those with limited cardiac reserve, even small induction doses of propofol (0.75 to 1.5 $mg \cdot kg^{-1}$) can produce profound hypotension. Therefore, use of a carefully titrated loading (priming) infusion minimizes the cardiovascular depression commonly associated with bolus (loading) doses of propofol in the operating room and ICU.

In high-risk patients, a two-stage infusion (i.e., rapid "loading" infusion followed by a slower "maintenance" infusion) improves hemodynamic stability. In premedicated patients receiving an opioid-propofol combination for induction of anesthesia, an initial propofol dose of 0.5 to 1 $mg \cdot kg^{-1}$ may be adequate. When smaller induction doses of propofol are administered, a higher initial maintenance infusion rate is required. To avoid untoward cardiovascular depression, a variable-rate maintenance infusion should be employed as part of a balanced or TIVA technique, as well as for sedation during the perioperative period. Propofol's cardiovascular effects during induction of anesthesia were not significantly different from the new steroid anesthetic eltanolone (pregnenolone) (428).

The use of propofol for maintenance of general anesthesia has not been widely accepted in the United States. Although propofol has proved to be a valuable adjuvant during short ambulatory procedures, its use for more prolonged operations (e.g., > 2 hours) has been questioned because of the increased cost and marginal differences in recovery times compared with standard inhalation or balanced anesthetic techniques (84). When propofol is used for maintenance of anesthesia in combination with an opioid infusion, the practitioner is confronted with the dilemma of whether to vary the hypnotic (propofol) or the opioid analgesic. Preliminary studies (429) suggest that the outcome is similar in either case. The availability of computer-controlled IV drug delivery systems may improve the ability of anesthesiologists to titrate drugs such as propofol and, therefore, to utilize IV anesthetic techniques more widely in their clinical practices.

Judging the depth of anesthesia remains a challenge when utilizing IV anesthetic techniques. The use of the EMG, EEG (e.g., EEG BI), and lower esophageal contractility (LEC) devices to monitor depth of anesthesia during surgery has proved disappointing. The correlation between the changes in EEG and LEC variables and hemodynamic responsiveness during propofol anesthesia is poor (186, 430). Studies involving newer approaches to cerebral function monitoring (e.g., EEG BI) (431), as well as brain stem evoked potentials, may prove to be of greater clinical benefit in the future. A good correlation appears to exist between the level of sedation and the EEG-BI (431). A EEG-BI less than 75 is associated with a significant decrease in intraoperative recall (475). The P300 long latency component of the auditory evoked potential is decreased in a dose-related manner (432). The correlation between changes in the P300 amplitude and memory performance suggests that it may be a useful indicator for amnesia. A simple, reliable, and noninvasive monitor of anesthetic depth would clearly enhance the ability of practitioners to titrate centrally active drugs such as propofol. Until a reliable cerebral function monitor is available, adjunctive use of midazolam and N_2O with propofol will decrease the likelihood of intraoperative recall.

With the increasing popularity of low-dose propofol infusions (e.g., 25 to 100 $\mu g \cdot kg^{-1} \cdot min^{-1}$) for sedation, questions have been raised regarding the appropriateness of nonanesthesiologists' using propofol infusions outside the operating room (e.g., radiology suites, radiation therapy, ICU). According to the package insert (Zeneca Pharmaceuticals), when propofol is used for general anesthesia or sedation in monitored anesthesia care, it should be administered only by persons trained in the administration of general anesthesia and not involved in the conduct of the surgical or diagnostic procedure. Patients should be continuously monitored, and facilities for maintenance of a patent airway, artificial ventilation, and oxygen enrichment and circulatory resuscitation must be immediately available. For sedation of intubated, mechanically ventilated adult patients in the ICU, propofol should be administered only by persons skilled in the management of critically ill patients and trained in cardiovascular resuscitation and airway management. It is extremely dangerous for nonanesthesiologists to administer propofol infusions for diagnostic and therapeutic procedures outside the operating room.

To minimize the well-known side effects associated with propofol, the following are recommended: (1) patients should be adequately hydrated before receiving a bolus dose or a rapid infusion of propofol; (2) when propofol is infused into small veins, prior administration of 1% lidocaine, 1 to 2 ml IV, decreases the pain on injection; (3) use of a rapid loading infusion over 30 to 60 seconds (versus bolus injection over 10 to 15 seconds) for induction and a variable-rate infusion for maintenance of hypnosis or sedation decreases propofol's acute cardiovascular and respiratory depressant effects; (4) when propofol is administered in combination with benzodiazepines as part of a coinduction technique or opioid analgesics as part of a balanced technique, the propofol induction dose requirement should be decreased in both adults and children; (5) in elderly and debilitated patients, both the induction and maintenance dose requirements should be reduced by 25 to 50%; (6) the dose of propofol should always be carefully titrated against the needs and responses of the individual patient, because of the considerable interpatient variability in anesthetic requirements; (7) adjunctive use of local anesthetics, nonsteroidal anti-inflammatory drugs, and opioids to provide postoperative analgesia improves the quality of emergence following propofol anesthesia and sedation; and (8) strict aseptic techniques must always be maintained during the handling of propofol, because the lipid emulsion contains no antimicrobial preservatives and is capable of supporting rapid growth of microorganisms (433).

Controversy surrounds the appropriate handling of propofol. The manufacturer has recommended that the solution be prepared for use "just prior to initiation of each individual procedure." Based on an in vitro study of questionable clinical relevance (434), "the ampule neck surface or vial rubber stopper should be disinfected using 70% isopropyl alcohol. Administration should commence promptly and be completed within 6 hours after the ampules or vials have been opened." According to the manufacturers, any unused portions of propofol must be discarded at the end of the anesthetic (or sedative) procedure or at 6 hours (whichever occurs sooner). In the ICU setting, the tubing and any unused portion of propofol must be discarded after 12 hours. Studies have also suggested that clinically relevant concentrations of propofol adversely affect the functional activity of white blood cells in vitro (435, 436, 436a, 436b). However, Davidson and colleagues (437) found that propofol had minimal effects on leukocyte phagocytosis and free radical production. Given the cost of the drug, many practitioners have questioned the appropriateness of discarding all unused drug at the end of every case. This practice is cost-ineffective and results in wastage of up to one-third of the propofol drawn up for a case (438), and it may lead to reluctance to use this otherwise excellent drug. The incidence of clinical infection secondary to bacterial contamination of propofol is extremely low (439-441). Most of these cases involved propofol that had been drawn up the day before its administration. However, one report suggested that when propofol is aseptically drawn into an uncapped syringe, it remains sterile at room temperature for several days (442). Further studies are clearly needed to determine the most cost-effective manner to utilize propofol in clinical practice (443).

In conclusion, propofol has become a widely used IV anesthetic for induction and maintenance of general anesthesia and sedation. In patients with asthma, propofol offers significant advantages over the barbiturates for induction of anesthesia (336). The favorable recovery profile associated with propofol offers advantages over traditional anesthetic and sedative medications in clinical situations where rapid recovery is important. However, faster recovery will only reduce overall costs if it permits a reduction in manpower or equipment utilization. Controversy exists regarding the cost-effectiveness of propofol-based (versus inhalation) anesthetic techniques (58, 443-445). In the future, outcome studies involving propofol should address specific patient populations and should also include an assessment of patient well-being. Although propofol would appear to be an ideal anesthetic for outpatient laparoscopic pronuclear stage transfer (PROST) procedures because of its excellent recovery profile and low incidence of PONV, its use was allegedly associated with lower clinical and ongoing pregnancy rates compared with isoflurane (446). Further studies are needed in this patient population, as well as in other clinical situations where controversy exists regarding the use of this agent. Although many questions still remain regarding this unique sedative-hypnotic drug, propofol has indeed provided a "new awakening" in anesthesia (447).

REFERENCES

1. Sebel PS, Lowdon JD. Propofol: a new intravenous anesthetic. Anesthesiology 1989;71:260–277.
2. Borgeat A, Wilder-Smith OHG, Saiah M, Rifat K. Subhypnotic doses of propofol possess direct antiemetic properties. Anesth Analg 1992;74:539–541.
3. Zacny JP, Lichtor JL, Coalson DW, et al. Subjective and psychomotor effects of subanesthetic doses of propofol in healthy volunteers. Anesthesiology 1992;76:696–702.

4. Whitehead C, Sanders LD, Oldroyd G, et al. The subjective effects of low-dose propofol: a double-blind study to evaluate dimensions of sedation and consciousness with low-dose propofol. Anaesthesia 1994;49:490–496.
5. Zacny JP, Lichtor JL, Zarogoza JG. Assessing the behavioral effects and abuse potential of propofol bolus injections in healthy volunteers. Drug Alcohol Depend 1993;32:45–57.
6. Shafer SL. Advances in propofol pharmacokinetics and pharmacodynamics. J Clin Anesth 1993;5 (suppl 1):14S–21S.
7. Kenny GNC. Practical experience with computer-controlled propofol infusion. Semin Anesth 1992;11 (suppl 1):12–13.
8. Glass PSA, Markham K, Ginsberg B, Hawkins ED. Propofol concentrations required for surgery [Abstract]. Anesthesiology 1989;71:A273.
9. Hara M, Kai Y, Ikemoto Y. Propofol activates $GABA_A$ receptor-chloride inophore complex in dissociated hippocampal pyramidal neurons of the rat. Anesthesiology 1993;79:781–788.
10. White PF. Propofol: pharmacokinetics and pharmacodynamics. Semin Anesth 1988;7:4–20.
11. Veroli P, O'Kelly B, Bertrand F, et al. Extrahepatic metabolism of propofol in man during the anhepatic phase of orthotopic liver transplantation. Br J Anaesth 1992;68:183–186.
12. Forrest FC, Tooley MA, Saunders PR, Prys-Roberts C. Propofol infusion and the suppression of consciousness: the EEG and dose requirements. Br J Anaesth 1994;72:35–41.
13. Skipsey IG, Colvin JR, Mackenzie N, Kenny GN. Sedation with propofol during surgery under local blockade: assessment of a target-controlled infusion system. Anaesthesia 1993;48:210–213.
14. Leslie K, Daniel IS, Bjorksten AR, Moayeri A. Mild hypothermia alters propofol pharmacokinetics and increases the duration of action of atracurium. Anesth Analg 1995;80:1007–1014.
15. Wessen A, Persson PM, Nilsson A, Hartvig P. Clinical pharmacokinetics of propofol given as a constant-rate infusion and in combination with epidural blockade. J Clin Anesth 1994; 6:193–198.
16. Kay B. Propofol and alfentanil infusion: a comparison with methohexitone and alfentanil for major surgery. Anaesthesia 1986; 41:589–595.
17. Sandin R, Norstrom O. Awareness during total i.v. anaesthesia. Br J Anaesth 1993;71:782–787.
18. Sherry E. Admixture of propofol and alfentanil: use of intravenous sedation and analgesia during transvaginal oocyte retrieval. Anaesthesia 1992;47:477–479.
19. Naurer WG, Kalhan SB. Propofol and alfentanil mixture for outpatient surgery [Letter]. J Clin Anesth 1994;6:166–167.
20. Wilson RJ, Ridley SA. The use of propofol and alfentanil by infusion in military anaesthesia. Anaesthesia 1992;47:231–233.
21. Shafer SL, Stanski DR. Improving the clinical utility of anesthetic drug pharmacokinetics [Editorial]. Anesthesiology 1992; 76:327–330.
22. Hughes MA, Glass PSA, Jacobs JR. Context-sensitive half-time in multicompartment pharmacokinetic models for intravenous anesthetic drugs. Anesthesiology 1992;76:334–341.
23. Vuyk J, Lim T, Engbers FH, et al. The pharmacodynamic interaction of propofol and alfentanil during lower abdominal surgery in women. Anesthesiology 1995;83:8–22.
24. Dyck JB, Shafer SL. Effects of age on propofol pharmacokinetics. Semin Anesth 1992;11 (suppl 1):2–4.
25. Fisher DM. Propofol in pediatrics: lessons in pharmacokinetic modeling [Editorial]. Anesthesiology 1994;80:2–5.
26. Hannallah RS. Induction dose of propofol in unpremedicated children. Semin Anesth 1992;11 (suppl 1):48–49.
27. Servin F, Farinotti R, Haberer JP, Desmonts JM. Propofol infusion for maintenance of anesthesia in morbidly obese patients receiving nitrous oxide. Anesthesiology 1993;78:657–665.
28. Nathan N, Debord J, Narcisse F, et al. Pharmacokinetics of propofol and its conjugates after continuous infusion in normal and in renal failure patients: a preliminary study. Acta Anaesthesiol Belg 1993;44:77–85.
29. Sear JW, Glen JB. Propofol administered by a manual infusion regimen. Br J Anaesth 1995;74:362–367.
30. Coetzee JF, Glen JB, Wium CA, Boshoff L. Pharmacokinetic model selection for target controlled infusions of propofol: assessment of three parameter sets. Anesthesiology 1995;82:1328–1345.
31. Vuyk J, Engbers FHM, Burm AGL, et al. Peformance of computer-controlled infusion of propofol: an evaluation of five pharmacokinetic parameter sets. Anesth Analg 1995;81:1275–1282.
32. Newson C, Joshi GP, Victory R, White PF. Comparison of propofol administration techniques for sedation during monitored anesthesia care. Anesth Analg 1995;81:486–491.
33. White PF. Intravenous anesthesia and analgesia: what is the role of target-controlled infusion (TCI)? J Clin Anesth 1996; 8:26S–28S.
34. Blackwell KE, Ross DA, Kapur P, Calcaterra TC. Propofol for maintenance of general anesthesia: a technique to limit blood loss during endoscopic sinus surgery. Am J Otolaryngol 1993; 14:262–266.
35. Ding Y, Fredman B, White PF. Recovery following outpatient anesthesia: use of enflurane versus propofol. J Clin Anesth 1993;5:447–450.
36. Kallela H, Haasio J, Korttila K. Comparison of eltanolone and propofol in anesthesia for termination of pregnancy. Anesth Analg 1994;79:512–516.
37. Millar JM, Jewkes CF. Recovery and morbidity after daycase anaesthesia: a comparison of propofol with thiopentone-enflurane with and without alfentanil. Anaesthesia 1988;43: 738–743.
38. Bembridge JL, Moss E, Grummitt RM, Noble J. Comparison of propofol with enflurane during hypotensive anaesthesia for middle ear surgery. Br J Anaesth 1993;71:895–897.
39. Pollard BJ, Bryan A, Bennett D, et al. Recovery after oral surgery with halothane, enflurane, isoflurane or propofol anaesthesia. Br J Anaesth 1994;72:559–566.
40. Sung YF, Reiss N, Tillette T. The differential cost of anesthesia and recovery with propofol-nitrous oxide anesthesia versus thiopental sodium-nitrous oxide anesthesia. J Clin Anesth 1991; 3:391–394.
41. Sukhani R, Lurie J, Jabamoni R. Propofol for ambulatory gynecologic laparoscopy: does omission of nitrous oxide alter postoperative emetic sequelae and recovery? Anesth Analg 1994;78:831–835.
42. Lindekaer AL, Skielboe M, Guldager H, Jensen EW. The influence of nitrous oxide on propofol dosage and recovery after total intravenous anaesthesia for day-case surgery. Anaesthesia 1995;50:397–399.
43. Marais ML, Maher MW, Wetchler BV, et al. Reduced demands on recovery room resources with propofol (Diprivan) compared to thiopental-isoflurane. Anesth Rev 1989;16:29–40.
44. Sanders LD, Isaac PA, Yeomans WA, et al. Propofol-induced anaesthesia: double-blind comparison of recovery after anaesthesia induced by propofol or thiopentone. Anaesthesia 1989; 44:200–204.
45. Gupta A, Larsen LE, Sjöberg F, et al. Thiopentone or propofol for induction of isoflurane-based anaesthesia for ambulatory surgery? Acta Anaesthesiol Scand 1992;36:670–674.
46. DeGrood PMRM, Harbers JBM, Van Egmond J, Crul JF. Anaesthesia for laparoscopy: a comparison of five techniques including propofol, etomidate, thiopentone and isoflurane. Anaesthesia 1987;42:815–823.
47. Mackenzie N, Grant IS. Comparison of the new emulsion formulation of propofol with methohexitone and thiopentone for induction of anaesthesia in day cases. Br J Anaesth 1985;57:725–731.

48. Korttila K. Recovery period and discharge. In: White PF, ed. Outpatient Anesthesia. New York: Churchill Livingstone, 1990:369–395.
49. Chittleborough MC, Osborne GA, Rudkin GE, et al. Double-blind comparison of patient recovery after induction with propofol or thiopentone for day-case general anaesthesia. Anaesth Intensive Care 1992;20:169–173.
50. Runcie CJ, Mackenzie SJ, Arthur DS, Morton NS. Comparison of recovery from anaesthesia induced in children with either propofol or thiopentone. Br J Anaesth 1993;70:192–195.
51. O'Toole DP, Milligan KR, Howe JP, et al. A comparison of propofol and methohexitone as induction agents for day case isoflurane anaesthesia. Anaesthesia 1987;42:373–376.
52. Norton AC, Dundas CR. Induction agents for day-case anaesthesia: a double-blind comparison of propofol and midazolam antagonised by flumazenil. Anaesthesia 1990;45:198–203.
53. Forrest P, Galletly DC. Comparison of propofol and antagonised midazolam anaesthesia for day-case surgery. Anaesth Intensive Care 1987;15:394–401.
54. McClymont C. A comparison of the effect of propofol or thiopentone on the incidence and severity of suxamethonium-induced myalgia. Anesth Intensive Care 1994;22:147–149.
55. Smith I, Ding Y, White, PF. Muscle pain following outpatient laparoscopy: influence of propofol versus thiopental and enflurane. Anesth Analg 1993;76:1181–1184.
56. Valanne J. Recovery and discharge of patients after long propofol infusion vs isoflurane anaesthesia for ambulatory surgery. Acta Anaesthesiol Scand 1992;36:530–533.
57. Monedero P, Carracosa F, Garcia-Pedrajas F, et al. Does propofol have advantages over midazolam and isoflurane? Comparative study of 2 total intravenous anesthesia techniques using midazolam and propofol, versus balanced anesthesia with isoflurane. Rev Esp Anesthesiol Reanim 1994;41:156–164.
58. Biro P, Suter G, Alon E. Intravenous anesthesia with propofol versus thiopental-enflurane anesthesia: a consumption and cost analysis. Anaesthesist 1995;4:163–170.
59. Herregods L, Capiau P, Rolly G, et al. Propofol for arthroscopy in outpatients: comparison of three anaesthetic techniques. Br J Anaesth 1988;60:565–569.
60. Larsen LE, Gupta A, Ledin T, et al. Psychomotor recovery following propofol or isoflurane anaesthesia for day-care surgery. Acta Anaesthesiol Scand 1992;36:276–282.
61. Marshall CA, Jones RM, Bajorek PK, Cashman JN. Recovery characteristics using isoflurane or propofol for maintenance of anaesthesia: a double-blind controlled trial. Anaesthesia 1992; 47:461–466.
62. Milligan KR, O'Toole DP, Howe JP, et al. Recovery from outpatient anaesthesia: a comparison of incremental propofol and propofol-isoflurane. Br J Anaesth 1987;59:1111–1114.
63. Zuurmond WA, Van Leeuwen L, Helmers JH. Recovery from propofol infusion as the main agent for outpatient arthroscopy: a comparison with isoflurane. Anaesthesia 1987;42:356–359.
64. Stanski DR. Monitoring depth of anesthesia. In: Miller RD, ed. Anesthesia. New York: Churchill Livingstone, 1990:1001–1029.
65. Nightingale JJ, Lewis IH. Recovery from day-case anaesthesia: comparison of total i.v. anaesthesia using propofol with an inhalation technique. Br J Anaesth 1992;68:356–359.
66. Rapp SE, Conahan TJ, Pavlin DJ, et al. Comparison of desflurane with propofol in outpatients undergoing peripheral orthopedic surgery. Anesth Analg 1992;75:572–579.
67. Van Hemelrijck J, Smith I, White PF. Use of desflurane for outpatient anesthesia: a comparison with propofol and nitrous oxide. Anesthesiology 1991;75:197–203.
68. Fredman B, Nathanson MH, Smith I, et al. Sevoflurane for outpatient anesthesia: a comparison with propofol. Anesth Analg 1995;81:823–828.
69. Dexter F, Tinker JH. Comparisons between desflurane and isoflurane or propofol on time to following commands and time to discharge. Anesthesiology 1995;83:77–82.
70. Rosenberg ML, Bridge P, Brown M. Cost comparison: a desflurane-versus a propofol-based general anesthetic technique. Anesth Analg 1994;79:852–855.
71. White PF, Stanley TH, Apfelbaum JL, et al. Effects on recovery when isoflurane is used to supplement propofol-nitrous oxide anesthesia. Anesth Analg 1993;77:s15–s20.
72. Kalman SH, Jensen AG, Ekberg K, Eintrei C. Early and late recovery after major abdominal surgery: comparison between propofol anaesthesia with and without nitrous oxide and isoflurane anaesthesia. Acta Anaesthesiol Scand 1993;37:730–736.
73. Martin TM, Nicolson SC, Bargas MS. Propofol anesthesia reduces emesis and airway obstruction in pediatric outpatients. Anesth Analg 1993;76:144–148.
74. Speicher A, Jessberger J, Braun R, et al. Postoperative pulmonary function after lung surgery: total intravenous anesthesia with propofol in comparison to balanced anesthesia with isoflurane. Anaesthesist 1995;44:265–273.
75. Smith I, Ding Y, White PF. Comparison of induction, maintenance and recovery characteristics of sevoflurane-N_2O and propofol-sevoflurane-N_2O with propofol-isoflurane-N_2O. Anesth Analg 1992;74:253–259.
76. Fredman B, Nathanson MH, Wang J, et al. Use of sevoflurane vs propofol for outpatient anesthesia: recovery profiles. Anesth Analg 1994;78:s121.
77. Logan MR, Duggan JE, Levack ID, Spence AA. Single-shot i.v. anaesthesia for outpatient dental surgery. Br J Anaesth 1987; 59:179–183.
78. Cade L, Morley PT, Ross AW. Is propofol cost-effective for day-surgery patients? Anaesth Intensive Care 1991;19:201–204.
79. Ræder JC, Misvær G. Comparison of propofol induction with thiopentone or methohexitone in short outpatient general anaesthesia. Acta Anaesthesiol Scand 1988;32:607–613.
80. Crozier TA, Muller JE, Quittkat D, et al. Total intravenous anesthesia with methohexital-alfentanil or propofol-alfentanil in hypogastric laparotomy: clinical aspects and the effects of stress reaction. Anaesthesist 1994;43:594–604.
81. Blobner M, Schneck HJ, Felber AR, et al. Comparative study of the recovery phase: laparoscopic cholecystectomy following isoflurane, methohexital and propofol anesthesia. Anaesthesist 1994;43:573–581.
82. Nielsen J, Jenstrup M, Gerdes NU, et al. Awakening and recovery of simple cognitive and psychomotor functions 2 h after anaesthesia for day-case surgery: total intravenous anaesthesia with propofol-alfentanil versus thiopentone-alfentanil. Eur J Anaesthesiol 1991;8:219–227.
83. Price ML, Walmsley A, Swaine C, Ponte J. Comparison of a total intravenous anaesthetic technique using a propofol infusion, with an inhalational technique using enflurane for day case surgery. Anaesthesia 1988;43 (suppl):84–87.
84. Doze VA, Shafer A, White PF. Propofol-nitrous oxide versus thiopental-isoflurane-nitrous oxide for general anesthesia. Anesthesiology 1988;69:63–71.
85. Korttila K, Östman P, Faure E, et al. Randomized comparison of recovery after propofol-nitrous oxide versus thiopentone-isoflurane-nitrous oxide anaesthesia in patients undergoing ambulatory surgery. Acta Anaesthesiol Scand 1990;34:400–403.
86. Doze VA, Westphal LM, White PF. Comparison of propofol with methohexital for outpatient anesthesia. Anesth Analg 1986;65:1189–1195.
87. Sampson IH, Plosker H, Cohen M, Kaplan JA. Comparison of propofol and thiamylal for induction and maintenance of anaesthesia for outpatient surgery. Br J Anaesth 1988;61:707–711.
88. Dunnihoo M, Wuest A, Meyer M, Robinson M. The effects of total intravenous anesthesia using propofol, ketamine, and vecuronium on cardiovascular response and wake up time. Am Assoc Nurse Anesth J 1994;62:261–266.

89. Hui TW, Short TG, Hong W, et al. Additive interactions between propofol and ketamine when used for anesthesia induction in female patients. Anesthesiology 1995;82:641–648.
90. Kirvela M, Yli-Hankala A, Lindgren L. Comparison of propofol/alfentanil anaesthesia with isoflurane/N_2O/fentanyl anaesthesia for renal transplantation. Acta Anaesthesiol Scand 1994;38:662–666.
91. Gonzalez-Arrieta ML, Juarez Melendez J, Silva Hernandez J, et al. Total intravenous anesthesia with propofol vs propofol/midazolam in oncology patients. Arch Med Res 1995;26:75–78.
92. Viviand X, Guidon-Attali C, Granthil C, et al. Computer-assisted intravenous anesthesia: value, method and use. Ann Fr Anesth Reanim 12:38–47, 1993
93. Bordahl PE, Raeder JC, Nordentoft J, et al. Laparoscopic sterilization under local or general anesthesia? A randomized study. Obstet Gynecol 1993;81:137–141.
94. Urquhart ML, White PF. Comparison of sedative infusions during regional anesthesia: methohexital, etomidate and midazolam. Anesth Analg 1989;68:249–254.
95. Bailey PL, Pace NL, Ashburn MA, et al. Frequent hypoxemia and apnea after sedation with midazolam and fentanyl. Anesthesiology 1990;73:826–830.
96. Ramirez-Ruiz M, Smith I, White PF. Use of analgesics during propofol sedation: a comparison of ketorolac, dezocine and fentanyl. J Clin Anesth 1995;7:481–485.
97. Bosek V, Smith DB, Cox C. Ketorolac or fentanyl to supplement local anesthesia? J Clin Anesth 1992;4:480–483.
98. Avramov MN, Smith I, White PF. Use of remifentanil and midazolam during monitored anesthesia care. Anesthesiology (in press).
99. Mackenzie N, Grant IS: Propofol for intravenous sedation. Anaesthesia 1987;42:3–6.
100. Wilson E, Mackenzie N, Grant IS. A comparison of propofol and midazolam by infusion to provide sedation in patients who receive spinal anaesthesia. Anaesthesia 1988;43 (suppl):91–94.
101. Atanassoff PG, Alon E, Pasch T. Recovery after propofol, midazolam, and methohexitone as an adjunct to epidural anaesthesia for lower abdominal surgery. Eur J Anaesth 1993;10:313–318.
102. White PF, Negus JB. Sedative infusions during local and regional anesthesia: a comparison of midazolam and propofol. J Clin Anesth 1991;3:32 39.
103. Fanard L, Van Steenberge A, Demeire X, van der Puyl F. Comparison between propofol and midazolam as sedative agents for surgery under regional anaesthesia. Anaesthesia 1988;43 (suppl):87–89.
104. Stephens AJ, Sapsford DJ, Curzon ME. Intravenous sedation for handicapped dental patients: a clinical trial of midazolam and propofol. Br Dent J 1993;175:20–25.
105. Dalen B, Mansoor O. Practical methods of using propofol as a complement to locoregional anesthesia in children. Cah Anesthesiol 1993;41:245–249.
106. Pratila MG, Fischer ME, Alagesan R, et al. Propofol versus midazolam for monitored sedation: a comparison of intraoperative and recovery parameters. J Clin Anesth 1993;5:268–274.
107. Valtonen M, Salonen M, Forssell H, et al. Propofol infusion for sedation in outpatient oral surgery: a comparison with diazepam. Anaesthesia 1989;44:730–734.
108. Holas A, Faulborn J. Propofol versus diazepam: sedation in ophthalmologic surgery under local anesthesia. Anaesthesist 1993;42:766–772.
109. Ghouri AF, Ramirez-Ruiz M, White PF. Midazolam-flumazenil versus propofol for routine outpatient sedation [Abstract]. Anesthesiology 1992;77:A33.
110. Meyers CJ, Eisig SB, Kraaut RA. Comparison of propofol and methohexital for deep sedation. J Oral Maxillofac Surg 1994; 52:897.
111. Ferrari LR, Donlon JV. A comparison of propofol, midazolam, and methohexital for sedation during retrobulbar and peribulbar block. J Clin Anesth 1992;4:93–96.
112. Rosa G, Conti G, Orsi O, et al. Effects of low-dose propofol administration on central respiratory drive, gas exchanges and respiratory pattern. Acta Anaesthesiol Scand 1992;36:128–131.
113. Blouin RT, Seifert HA, Babenco HD, et al. Propofol depresses the hypoxic ventilatory response during conscious sedation and isohypercapnia. Anesthesiology 1993;79:1177–1182.
114. Senn P Johr M, Kaufman S, et al. Brief narcosis with propofol/ketamine for administering retrobulbar anesthesia. Klin Monatsbl Augenheilkd 1993;202:528–532.
115. Dubois A, Balatoni E, Peeters JP, Baudoux M. Use of propofol for sedation during gastrointestinal endoscopies. Anaesthesia 1988;43 (suppl):75–80.
116. Patterson KW, Casey PB, Murray JP, et al. Propofol sedation for outpatient upper gastrointestinal endoscopy: comparison with midazolam. Br J Anaesth 1991;67:108–111.
117. Crawford M, Pollock J, Anderson K, et al. Comparison of midazolam with propofol for sedation in outpatient bronchoscopy. Br J Anaesth 1993;70:419–422.
118. Janvier G. Use of Diprivan in radiology. Ann Fr Anesth Reamin 1994;13:589–592.
119. Smith I, Monk TG, White PF, Ding Y. Propofol infusion during regional anesthesia: sedative, amnestic and anxiolytic properties. Anesth Analg 1994;79:313–319.
120. Monk TG, Bouré B, White PF, et al. Comparison of intravenous sedative-analgesic techniques for outpatient immersion lithotripsy. Anesth Analg 1991;72:616–621.
121. Polster MR, Gray PA, O'Sullivan G, et al. Comparison of the sedative and amnesic effects of midazolam and propofol. Br J Anaesth 1993;70:612–616.
122. Chortkoff BS, Gonsowski CT, Bennett HL, et al. Subanesthetic concentrations of desflurane and propofol suppress recall of emotionally charged information. Anesth Analg 1995;81:728–736.
123. Chortkoff BS, Eger EI II, Crankshaw DP, et al. Concenterations of desflurane and propofol that suppress response to command in humans. Anesth Analg 1995;81:737–743.
124. Taylor E, Ghouri AF, White PF. Midazolam in combination with propofol for sedation during local anesthesia. J Clin Anesth 1992;4:213–216.
125. Eledjam JJ. Use of Diprivan in addition to locoregional anesthesia. Ann Fr Anesth Reanim 1994;13:593–597.
126. Rudkin GE, Osborne GA, Curtis NJ. Intra-operative patient-controlled sedation. Anaesthesia 1991;46:90–92.
127. Grattidge P. Patient-controlled sedation using propofol in day surgery. Anaesthesia 1992;47:683–685.
128. Osborne GA, Rudkin GE, Jarvis DA, et al. Intra-operative patient-controlled sedation and patient attitude to control: a crossover comparison of patient preference for patient-controlled propofol and propofol by continuous infusion. Anaesthesia 1994;49:287–292.
129. Osborne GA, Rudkin GE, Curtis NJ, et al. Intra-operative patient-controlled sedation: comparison of patient-controlled propofol with anaesthetist-administered midazolam and fentanyl. Anaesthesia 1991;46:553–556.
130. Ghouri AF, Taylor E, White PF. Patient-controlled drug administration during local anesthesia: a comparison of midazolam, propofol, and alfentanil. J Clin Anesth 1992;4:476–479.
131. Strebel S, Lam AM, Matta B, et al. Dynamic and static cerebral autoregulation during isoflurane, desflurane and propofol anesthesia. Anesthesiology 1995;83:66–76.
132. Cavazzuti M, Porro CA, Barbieri A, Galetti A. Brain and spinal cord metabolic activity during propofol anaesthesia. Br J Anaesth 1991;66:490–495.
133. Gelb AW, Zhang C, Hamilton JT. The in vitro cerebrovascular

effects of propofol are due to calcium channel blockade [Abstract]. Anesthesiology 1992;77:A774.
134. Gelb AW, Hamilton JT, Zhang C, Henderson S. Propofol dilates human cerebral veins [Abstract]. Anesthesiology 1993;79:A208.
135. Stephan S, Sonntag H, Schenk HD, Kohlhausen S. Effect of Disoprivan (propofol) on the circulation and oxygen consumption of the brain and CO_2 reactivity of brain vessels in the human. Anaesthetist 1987;36:60–65.
136. Van Hemelrijck J, Van Aken H, Plets C, et al. The effects of propofol on intracranial pressure and cerebral perfusion pressure in patients with brain tumours. Acta Anaesthesiol Belg 1989;40:95–100.
137. Pinaud M, Lelausque JN, Chetanneau A, et al. Effects of propofol on cerebral hemodynamics and metabolism in patients with brain trauma. Anesthesiology 1990;73:404–409.
138. Vandesteene A, Trempont V, Engelman E, et al. Effect of propofol on cerebral blood flow and metabolism in man. Anaesthesia 1988;43 (suppl):42–43.
139. Ramani R, Todd MM, Warner DS. A dose-response study of the influence of propofol on cerebral blood flow, metabolism and the electroencephalogram in the rabbit. J Neurosurg Anesth 1992;4:110–119.
140. Artu AA, Shapira Y, Bowdle TA. Electroencephalogram, cerebral metabolic, and vascular responses to propofol anesthesia in dogs. J Neurosurg Anesth 1992;4:99–109.
141. Van Hemelrijck J, Fitch W, Mattheussen M, et al. Effect of propofol on cerebral circulation and autoregulation in the baboon. Anesth Analg 1990;71:49–54.
142. Seifert HA, Blouin RT, Conard PF, Gross JB. Sedative doses of propofol increase beta activity of the processed electroencephalogram. Anesth Analg 1993;76:976–978.
143. Van Hemelrijck J, Tempelhoff R, White PF, Jellish WS. EEG-assisted titration of propofol infusion during neuroanesthesia: effect of nitrous oxide. Anesthesiology 1996;84:64–69.
144. Davidson B, Kishimoto T, Kadoya C, Domino EF. Electrophysiologic effects of propofol sedation. Anesth Analg 1994;79:1151–1158.
145. Herregods L, Verbeke J, Rolly G, Colardyn F. Effect of propofol on elevated intracranial pressure: preliminary results. Anaesthesia 1988;43 (suppl):107–109.
146. Ravussin P, Guinard JP, Ralley F, Thorin D. Effect of propofol on cerebrospinal fluid pressure and cerebral perfusion pressure in patients undergoing craniotomy. Anaesthesia 1988;43 (suppl):37–41.
147. Muzzi D, Losasso T, Weglinski M, Milde L. The effect of propofol on cerebrospinal fluid pressure in patients with supratentorial mass lesions [Abstract]. Anesthesiology 1992;77:A216.
148. Craen RA, Gelb AW, Murkin JM, Chong KY. Human cerebral autoregulation is maintained during propofol air/O_2 anesthesia [Abstract]. Anesthesiology 1992;77:A220.
149. Enns J, Gelb AW, Manninen PH, et al. Cerebral autoregulation is maintained during propofol-nitrous oxide anaesthesia in humans [Abstract]. Can J Anaesth 1992;39:A43.
150. Werner C, Hoffman WE, Kochs E, et al. The effects of propofol on cerebral and spinal cord blood flow in rats. Anesth Analg 1993;76:971–975.
151. Craen RA, Gelb AW, Murkin JW, Chong KY. CO_2 reponsiveness of cerebral blood flow is maintained during propofol anaesthesia. Can J Anaesth 1992;39:A7.
152. Craen RA, Gelb AW, Brodkin I, et al. CO_2 reactivity and the rate of change of cerebral blood flow velocity during propofol anaesthesia with and without N_2O in humans. Can J Anaesth 1993;40:A59.
153. Jansen GFA, Kagenaar D, Kedaria MB, Bosch DA. Effects of propofol on the relation between CO_2 and cerebral blood flow velocity [Abstract]. Anesth Analg 1993;76:S163.
154. Schramm W, Czech T, Illevich U, et al. The impact of high-dose propofol on blood flow velocity and CO_2-reactivity in man [Abstract]. Anesthesiology 1992;77:A214.
155. Fox J, Gelb AW, Enns J, et al. The responsiveness of cerebral blood flow to changes in arterial carbon dioxide is maintained during propofol-nitrous oxide anesthesia in humans. Anesthesiology 1992;77:453–456.
156. Eng C, Lam AM, Mayberg TS, et al. The influence of propofol with and without nitrous oxide on cerebral blood flow velocity and CO_2 reactivity in humans. Anesthesiology 1992;77:872–879.
157. Kochs E, Hoffman WE, Werner C, et al. The effects of propofol on brain electrical activity: neurological outcome and neuronal damage following incomplete ischemia in rats. Anesthesiology 1992;76:245–252.
158. Varner PD, Vinik HR, Funderburg C. Survival during severe hypoxia and propofol or ketamine anesthesia in mice [Abstract]. Anesthesiology 1988;69:A571.
159. Weir DL, Goodchild CS, Graham DI. Propofol: effects on indices of cerebral ischemia. J Neurosurg Anesth 1989;1:284–289.
160. Alkire MT, Haier RJ, Barker SJ, et al. Cerebral metabolism during propofol anesthesia in humans studied with positron emission tomography. Anesthesiology 1995;82:393–403.
161. Ridenour TR, Warner DS, Todd MM, Gionet TX. Comparative effects of propofol and halothane on outcome from temporary middle cerebral artery occlusion in the rat. Anesthesiology 1992;76:807–812.
162. Warner D, Zhou J, Ramani R, Todd MM. Reversible focal ischemia in the rat: effects of halothane, isoflurane and methohexital anesthesia. J Cereb Blood Flow Metab 1991;11:794–802.
163. Gelb AW, Zhang C, Henderson SM. A comparison of the cerebral protective effects of propofol, thiopental, and halothane in temporary feline focal cerebral ischemia [Abstract]. Anesth Analg 1993;76:S115.
164. Ravussin P, de Tribolet N. Total intravenous anesthesia with propofol for burst suppression in cerebral aneurysm surgery: preliminary report of 42 patients. Neurosurgery 1993;32:236–240.
165. Illievich UM, Petricek W, Schramm W, et al. Electroencephalographic burst suppression by propofol infusion in humans: hemodynamic consequences. Anesth Analg 1993;77:155–160.
166. Todd MM, Drummond JC, Hoi SU. The hemodynamic consequences of high-dose thiopental anesthesia. Anesth Analg 1985; 64:681–687.
167. Todd MM, Warner DS, Sokoll MD, et al. A prospective, comparative trial of three anesthetics for elective supratentorial craniotomy. Anesthesiology 1993;78:1005–1020.
168. Ravussin P, Templehoff R, Modica PA, Bayer-Berger MM. Propofol vs thiopental-isoflurane for neurosurgical anesthesia: comparison of hemodynamics, CSF pressure, and recovery. J Neurosurg Anesth 1991;3:85–95.
169. Paillot V, Van Hemelrijck J, Van Aken H. Anesthesia for carotid endarterectomy: Propofol vs etomidate-isoflurane [Abstract]. Anesthesiology 1991;75:A180.
170. White PF, Watcha MF. Are new drugs cost-effective for patients undergoing ambulatory surgery? [Editorial]. Anesthesiology 1993;78:2–5.
171. Aitken HA, Farling PA. The cost of propofol infusion in neurosurgery [Letter]. Anaesthesia 1991;41:329.
172. De Riu PL, Petruzzi V, Testa C, et al. Propofol anticonvulsant activity in experimental epileptic status. Br J Anaesth 1992; 69:177–181.
173. Lowson S, Gent JP, Goodchild CS. Anticonvulsant properties of propofol and thiopentone: comparison using two tests in laboratory mice. Br J Anaesth 1990;64:59–63.
174. Hartung J, Ying H, Weinberger JM, Cottrell JE. Propofol forestalls or prevents lidocaine-induced seizures in rats [Abstract]. Anesthesiology 1993;79:A431.
175. Bansinath M, Shukla VK, Turndorf H. Proconvulsant effect of

propofol on the excitatory amino acid agonists induced convulsions [Abstract]. Anesthesiology 1992;77:A211.
176. Bendriss P, Stoiber HP, Bendriss-Brusset AC, et al. Propofol effects on EEG and relationship with plasma concentration during neurosurgery [Abstract]. Anesthesiology 1990;73:A203.
177. Seifert HA, Blouin RT, Conrad PF, Gross JB. Sedative doses of propofol increase beta activity of the processed electroencephalogram. Anesth Analg 1993;76:976–978.
178. Mahla ME, Grundy BL, Schmidt RP, et al. Propofol does not cause epileptiform electrographic activity [Abstract]. Anesthesiology 1991;75:A183.
179. Bendriss P, Stoiber HP, Bendriss-Brusset AC, et al. Propofol effects on EEG and relationship with plasma concentration during neurosurgery [Abstract]. Anesthesiology 1990;73:A203.
180. Wood PR, Browne GPR, Pugh S. Propofol infusion for the treatment of status epilepticus [Letter]. Lancet 1988;1:480–481.
181. Mackenzie SJ, Kapadia F, Grant IS. Propofol infusion for control of status epilepticus. Anaesthesia 1990;45:1043–1045.
182. Borgeat A, Wilder-Smith OHG, Jallon P, Suter PM. Propofol in the management of refractory status epilepticus: a case report. Intensive Care Med 1994;20:148–149.
183. Kearse LA, Manaberg P, Chamoun N, et al. Bispectral analysis of the electroencephalogram correlates with patient movement to skin incision during propofol/nitrous oxide anesthesia. Anesthesiology 1994;81:1365–1370.
184. Leslie K, Sessler DI, Schroeder M, Walters K. Propofol blood concentration and the bispectral index predict suppression of learning during propofol/epidural anesthesia in volunteers. Anesth Analg 1995;81:1269–1274.
185. Liu J, Singh H, White PF. EEG bispectral index predicts intraoperative recall and depth of propofol-induced sedation. Anesthesiology (in press).
186. White PF, Boyle WA: Relationship between hemodynamic and electroencephalographic changes during anesthesia. Anesth Analg 1989;68:177–181.
187. Vernon JM, Lang E, Sebel PS, Manberg P. Prediction of movement using bispectral electroencephalographic analysis during propofol/alfentanil or isoflurane/alfentanil anesthesia. Anesth Analg 1995;80:780–785.
188. Chen CL, Liu CC, Chen TL, et al. Recovery from propofol anesthesia: a quantitative electroencephalographic analysis. Acta Anaesthesiol Sin 1994;32:77–82.
189. Traast HS, Kalkman CJ. Electroencephalographic characteristics of emergence from propofol/sufentanil total intravenous anesthesia. Anesth Analg 1995;81:366–371.
190. Rampton AJ, Griffin RM, Stuart CS, et al. Comparison of methohexital and propofol for electroconvulsive therapy: effects on hemodynamic responses and seizure duration. Anesthesiology 1989;70:412–417.
191. Hodkinson BP, Frith RW, Mee EW. Propofol and the electroencephalogram [Letter]. Lancet 1987;2:1518.
192. Samra SK, Sneyd JR, Ross DA, Henry TR. Effect of propofol on electroencephalogram of epileptic patients [Abstract]. Anesthesiology 1993;79:A172.
193. Ebrahim ZY, Schubert A, Van Ness P, et al. The effect of propofol on the electroencephalogram of patients with epilepsy [Abstract]. Anesthesiology 1992;77:A217.
194. Fredman B, Husain MM, White PF. Anaesthesia for electroconvulsive therapy: use of propofol revisited. Eur J Anaesthesiol 1994;11:423–425.
195. Nadstawek J, Hufnagel A, Elger CE, Stoeckel H. Does propofol activate the seizure focus of epileptic patients? [Abstract]. Anesthesiology 1993;79:A171.
196. Oei-Lim VLB, Kalkman CJ, Bouvy-Berends ECM, et al. A comparison of the effects of propofol and nitrous oxide on the electroencephalogram in epileptic patients during conscious sedation for dental procedures. Anesth Analg 1992;75:708–714.
197. Committee on Safety of Medicines. Propofol. Curr Probl 1987; 20:5.
198. Committee on Safety of Medicines. Propofol: convulsions, anaphylaxis and delayed recovery from anaesthesia. Curr Probl 1989;26:3.
199. Collier C, Kelly K. Propofol and convulsions: the evidence mounts. Anaesth Intensive Care 1991;19:573–575.
200. Victory RAP, Magee D. A case of convulsion after propofol anaesthesia [Letter]. Anaesthesia 1988;43:904.
201. DeFriez CB, Wong HC. Seizures and opisthotonos after propofol anesthesia. Anesth Analg 1992;75:630–632.
202. Hopkins CS. Recurrent opisthotonus associated with anaesthesia [Letter]. Anaesthesia 1988;43:904.
203. Saunders PRI, Harris MNE. Opisthotonus and other unusual neurological sequelae after outpatient anaesthesia. Anaesthesia 1990;45:552–557.
204. Borgeat A, Wilder-Smith OHG, Tassonyi E, Suter PM. Propofol and epilepsy: Time to clarify! [Letter]. Anesth Analg 1994; 78:198–199.
205. Samra SK, Sneyd JR, Ross DA, Henry TR. Effects of propofol sedation on seizures and intracranially recorded epileptiform activity in patients with partial epilespy. Anesthesiology 1995; 82:843–851.
206. Reddy RV, Moorthy SS, Dierdorf SF, et al. Excitatory effects and electroencephalographic correlation of etomidate, thiopental, methohexital, and propofol. Anesth Analg 1993;77:1008–1011.
207. Hug C Jr. Does opioid "anesthesia" exist? Anesthesiology 1990; 73:1–4.
208. Goldman L, Shah MV, Hebden MW. Memory of cardiac anaesthesia. Anaesthesia 1987;42:596–603.
209. Reiz S, Balfors E, Sorenson MB, et al. Isoflurane: a powerful coronary vasodilator in patients with coronary artery disease. Anesthesiology 1983;59:91–97.
210. Mora CT, Dudek C, Epstein R, et al. Comparison of fentanyl to thiopental and propofol for maintenance of anesthesia during cardiac surgery [Abstract]. Anesthesiology 1988;69:A59.
211. Cross AS, Rorep B. Role of respiratory assistance devices in endemic nosocomial pneumonia. Am J Med 1981;70:681–685.
212. Shafer A, Doze VA, Shafer SL, White PF. Pharmacokinetics and pharmacodynamics of propofol infusions during general anesthesia. Anesthesiology 1988;69:348–356.
213. Mora CT, Dudek C, Epstein R, et al. Cardiac anesthesia techniques. fentanyl alone or in combination with enflurane or propofol [Abstract]. Anesth Analg 1989;68:S202.
214. Sebel PS, Lowdon JD. Propofol causes cardiovascular depression: reply [Letter]. Anesthesiology 1990;72:396.
215. Van Aken H, Brussel T. Propofol causes cardiovascular depression. II. Anesthesiology 1990;72:394–395.
216. Merin RG. Propofol causes cardiovascular depression. I. Anesthesiology 1990;72:393–394.
217. Lippman M, Mok MS. Propofol causes cardiovascular depression. III. Anesthesiology 1990;72:395.
218. Hall RI, Murphy JT, Landymore R, et al. Myocardial metabolic changes during propofol anesthesia for cardiac surgery in patients with reduced ventricular function. Anesth Analg 1993; 77:680–689.
219. Boyle WA, White PF, Rendig SV. Negative inotropic effects of propofol versus etomidate and thiopental on rabbit papillary muscle [Abstract]. Anesth Analg 1989;68:S35.
220. Pagel PS, Warltier DC. Negative inotropic effects of propofol as evaluated by the regional preload recruitable stroke work relationship in chronically instrumented dogs. Anesthesiology 1993;78:100–108.
221. Vermeyen KM, Erpels FA, Janssen LA, et al. Propofol-fentanyl anaesthesia for coronary bypass surgery in patients with good left ventricular function. Br J Anaesth 1987;59:1115–1120.
222. Vermeyen KM, De Hert SG, Erpels FA, Adriaensen HF. Myo-

cardial metabolism during anesthesia with propofol-low dose fentanyl for coronary artery bypass surgery. Br J Anaesth 1991; 66:504–508.
223. Roberts FL, Dixon J, Lewis GTR, et al. Induction and maintenance of propofol anaesthesia: a manual infusion scheme. Anaesthesia 1988;43 (suppl):14–17.
224. Stephan H, Sonntag H, Schenk HD, et al. Effects of propofol on cardiovascular dynamics, myocardial blood flow and myocardial metabolism in patients with coronary artery disease. Br J Anaesth 1986;58:969–975.
225. Haessler R, Madler C, Klasing S, et al. Propofol/fentanyl versus etomidate fentanyl for the induction of anesthesia in patients with aortic insufficiency and coronary artery disease. J Cardiothorac Vasc Anesth 1992;6:173–180.
226. Russell GN, Wright EL, Fox MA, et al. Propofol-fentanyl anaesthesia for coronary artery surgery and cardiopulmonary bypass. Anaesthesia 1989;44:205–208.
227. Underwood SM, Davies SW, Feneck RO, Walesby RK. Anaesthesia for myocardial revascularisation: a comparison of fentanyl/propofol with fentanyl/enflurane. Anaesthesia 1992; 47:939–945.
228. Phillips AS, McMurray TJ, Mirakhur RK, et al. Propofol-fentanyl anaesthesia in cardiac surgery: a comparison in patients with good and impaired ventricular function. Anaesthesia 1993;48:661–663.
229. Hall RI, Murphy JT, Moffitt EA, et al. A comparison of the myocardial and metabolic and haemodynamic changes produced by propofol-sufentanil and enflurane-sufentanil anaesthesia for patients having coronary artery bypass graft surgery. Can J Anaesth 1991;38:996–1004.
230. Mora CT, Torjman M, White PF. Use of propofol during cardiac anesthesia: maintenance infusion rates and therapeutic blood levels [Abstract]. Anesth Analg 1990;70:S276.
231. Massey NJA, Sherry KM, Oldroyd S, Peacock JE. Pharmacokinetics of an infusion of propofol during cardiac surgery. Br J Anaesth 1990;65:475–479.
232. Pensado A, Molins N, Alvarez J. Effects of propofol on mean arterial pressure and systemic vascular resistance during cardiopulmonary bypass. Acta Anaesthesiol Scand 1993;37:498–501.
233. Laycock GJA, Alston RP. Propofol and hypothermic cardiopulmonary bypass: vasodilation and enhanced protection? Anaesthesia 1992;382–387.
234. Lin CS, Lin IS, Liu CH, et al. The thermoregulatory threshold during surgery with propofol-nitrous oxide anaesthesia. Acta Anaesthesiol Sin 1995;33:15–20.
235. Matsukawa T, Kurz A, Sessler D, et al. Propofol linearly reduces the vasoconstriction and shivering thresholds. Anesthesiology 1995;82:1169–1180.
236. Mora CT, Dudek C, Torjman MC, White PF. The effects of anesthetic technique on the hemodynamic response and recovery profile in coronary revascularization patients. Anesth Analg 1995;81:90–10.
237. Chong JL, Grebenik C, Sinclair M, et al. The effect of a cardiac surgical recovery area on the timing of extubation. J Cardiothorac Vasc Anesth 1993;7:137–141.
238. Purcell-Jones G, James IG. The characteristics of propofol (Diprivan) for induction of general anaesthesia for paediatric surgery. Postgrad Med J 1985;61 (suppl 3):115.
239. Jones RD, Visram AR, Chan MM, et al. A comparison of three induction agents in paediatric anaesthesia: cardiovascular effects and recovery. Anaesth Intensive Care 1994;22:545–555.
240. White M, Kenny GNC. Intravenous propofol anaesthesia using a computerised infusion system. Anaesthesia 1990;45:204–209.
241. Marsh B, White M, Morton N, Kenny GNC. Pharmacokinetic model driven infusion of propofol in children. Br J Anaesth 1991;67:41–48.
242. Browne BL, Prys-Roberts C, Wolf AR. Propofol and alfentanil in children: infusion technique and dose requirement for total i.v. anaesthesia. Br J Anaesth 1992;69:570–576.
243. Patel DK, Keeling PA, Newman GB, Radford P. Induction dose of propofol in children. Anaesthesia 1988;43:949–952.
244. Mirakhur RK. Induction characteristics of propofol in children: comparison with thiopentone. Anaesthesia 1988;43:593–598.
245. Hannallah RS, Baker SB, Casey W, et al. Propofol: effective dose and induction characteristics in unpremedicated children. Anesthesiology 1991;74:217–219.
246. Doyle E, McFadzean W, Morton NS. I.V. anaesthesia with propofol using a target-controlled infusion system: comparison with inhalational anaesthesia for general surgical procedures in children. Br J Anaesth 1993;70:542–545.
247. Westrin P. The induction dose of propofol in infants 1–6 months of age and in children 10–16 years of age. Anesthesiology 1991;74:455–458.
248. Manschot HJ, Meursing AEE, Axt P, et al. Propofol requirements for induction of anesthesia in children of different age groups. Anesth Analg 1992;75:876–879.
249. Short SM, Aun CST. Haemodynamic effects of propofol in children. Anaesthesia 1991;46:783–785.
250. Murray T, Oyos TL, Forbes RB, et al. Hemodynamic depression during propofol infusions in children [Abstract]. Anesthesiology 1993;79:A1157.
251. Daniel M, Eger EI II, Weiskopf RB, Noorani M. Propofol fails to attenuate the cardiovascular response to rapid increase in desflurane concentration. Anesthesiology 1996;84:75–80.
252. Aun CST, Sung RYT, O'Meara ME, et al. Cardiovascular effects of i.v. induction in children: comparison between propofol and thiopentone. Br J Anaesth 1993;70:647–653.
253. Watcha MF, Simeon RM, White PF, Stevens JL. Effect of propofol on the incidence of postoperative vomiting after strabismus surgery in pediatric outpatients. Anesthesiology 1991; 75:204–209.
254. Snellen FT, Vanacker B, Van Aken H. Propofol-nitrous oxide versus thiopental sodium-isoflurane-nitrous oxide for strabismus surgery in children. J Clin Anesth 1993;5:37–41.
255. Lavoie J, Walsh EP, Burrows FA, et al. Effects of propofol or isoflurane anesthesia on cardiac conduction in children undergoing radiofrequency catheter ablation for tachydysrhythmias. Anesthesiology 1995;82:884–887.
256. Sharpe MD, Dobkowski WB, Murkin JM, et al. Propofol has no direct effect on sinoatrial node function or on normal atrioventricular and accessory pathway conduction in Wolff-Parkinson-White syndrome during alfentanil/midazolam anesthesia. Anesthesiology 1995;82:888–895.
257. Marcus B, Steward DJ, Khan, NR, et al. Outpatient transesophageal echocardiography with intravenous propofol anesthesia in children and adolescents. J Am Soc Echocardiocardiogr 1993; 6:205–209.
258. Lebovic S, Reich DL, Steinberg LG, et al. Comparison of propofol versus ketamine for anesthesia in pediatric patients undergoing cardiac catheterization. Anesth Analg 1992;74:490–494.
259. McKeating K, Bali IM, Dundee JW. The effects of thiopentone and propofol on upper airway integrity. Anaesthesia 1988; 43:638–640.
260. Montasser AM. Propofol for tracheal intubation in paediatric outpatient anaesthesia [Abstract]. Br J Anaesth 1993;70:A161.
261. Rodney GE, Reichert CC, O'Regan DN, Blackstock D. Propofol or propofol/alfentanil compared to thiopentone/succinylcholine for intubation of healthy children [Abstract]. Can J Anaesth 1992;39 (suppl II):A129.
262. Valtonen M, Iiaslo E, Kanto J, Tikkanen J. Comparison between propofol and thiopentone for induction of anaesthesia in children. Anaesthesia 1988;43:696–699.

263. Puttick N, Rosen M. Propofol induction and maintenance with nitrous oxide in paediatric outpatient dental anaesthesia. Anaesthesia 1988;43:646–649.
264. Borgeat A, Popovic V, Meier D, Schwander D. Comparison of propofol and thiopentone/halothane for short-duration ENT surgical procedures in children. Anesth Analg 1990;71:511–515.
265. Aun CST, Short TG, O'Meara ME, et al. Recovery after propofol infusion anaesthesia in children: comparison with propofol, thiopentone or halothane induction followed by halothane maintenance. Br J Anaesth 1994;72:554–558.
266. Hannallah RS, Britton JT, Schafer PG, et al. Propofol anaesthesia in paediatric ambulatory patients: a comparison with thiopentone and halothane. Can J Anaesth 1994;41:12–18.
266a. Hiller A, Pyykko I, Saarnivaara L. Evaluation of postural stability by computerised posturography following outpatient paediatric anaesthesia: comparison of propofol/alfentanil/N_2O anaesthesia with thiopentone/halothane/N_2O anaesthesia. Acta Anaesthesiol Scand 1993;37:556–561.
267. Tsai S, Lee L, Sheen J, et al. Outpatient surgery in infants: comparative recovery times from propofol and halothane anesthesia [Abstract]. Anesth Analg 1993;76:S437.
268. Weir PM, Munro HM, Reynolds PI, et al. Propofol infusion and the incidence of emesis in pediatric outpatient strabismus surgery. Anesth Analg 1993;76:760–764.
269. Tramèr M, Borgeat A, Rifat K. Postoperative nausea and vomiting after strabismus surgery in children-effects of propofol, ondansetron and lidocaine [Abstract]. Anesthesiology 1993; 79:A1193.
270. McDowall RH, Scher CS, Barst SM. Total intravenous anesthesia for children undergoing brief diagnostic or therapeutic procedures. J Clin Anesth 1995;7:273–280.
271. Patteson SK, Chesney JT. Anesthetic management for magnetic resonance imaging: problems and solutions. Anesth Analg 1992;74:121–128.
272. Martin L, Pasternak LR, Pudimat MA. Total intravenous anesthesia with propofol in pediatric patients outside the operating room. Anesth Analg 1992;74:609–612.
273. Lefever EB, Poter PS, Seeley NR. Propofol sedation for pediatric MRI [Letter]. Anesth Analg 1993;76:919–920.
274. Valtonen M. Anaesthesia for computerised tomography of the brain in children: a comparison of propofol and thiopentone. Acta Anaesthiol Scand 1989;33:170–173.
275. Kain ZV, Gaal DJ, Tatiana SK, et al. A first-pass cost analysis of propofol versus barbiturates for children undergoing magnetic resonance imaging. Anesth Analg 1994;79:1102–1106.
276. Bloomfield EL, Masaryk TJ, Caplin A, et al. Intravenous sedation for MR imaging of the brain and spine in children: pentobarbital versus propofol. Radiology 1993;186:93–97.
277. Vangerven M, Van Hemelrijck J, Wouters P, et al. Light anaesthesia with propofol for paediatric MRI. Anaesthesia 1992; 47:706–707.
278. Flanagan J, Wheeler T, Burney C, Tobias JD. Non-invasive monitoring of end-tidal CO_2 in spontaneously breathing children [Abstract]. Anesthesiology 1993;79:A1159.
279. Bready R, Spear R, Fisher B, et al. Propofol infusion; dose-response for CT scans in children [Abstract]. Anesth Analg 1992; 74:S36.
280. Van Obbergh LJ, Muller G, Zeippen B, Dooms G. Propofol infusion and laryngeal mask insertion for magnetic resonance imaging in children [Abstract]. Anesthesiology 1992;77:A1177.
281. Setlock MA, Palmisano BW. Tolerance does not develop to propofol used repeatedly for radiation therapy in children [Abstract]. Anesth Analg 1992;74:S278.
282. Cauldwell CB, Fisher DM. Sedating pediatric patients: is propofol a panacea? Radiology 1993;186:9–10.
283. Bloomfield EL. Propofol for sedation of pediatric patients. Radiology 1993;186:580–581.
284. Anonymous. Sedation in the intensive-care unit [Editorial]. Lancet 1984;1:1388–1389.
285. Mirenda J, Broyles G. Propofol as used for sedation in the ICU. Chest 1995;108:539–548.
286. Wiebalck A, Van Aken H. Propofol: the ideal long-term sedative? Anaesthesist 1995;44:178–185.
287. Newman LH, McDonald JC, Walace PGM, Ledingham IM. Propofol infusion for sedation in intensive care. Anaesthesia 1987; 42:929–937.
288. Barr J, Egan T, Feeley T, Shafer S. Depth of sedation vs. propofol concentration in mechanically ventilated ICU patients [Abstract]. Anesthesiology 1992;77:A313.
289. Nimmo GT, Mackenzie SJ, Grant IS. Haemodynamic and oxygen transport effects of propofol infusion in critically ill adults. Anaesthesia 49:485–489.
290. Albanese J, Martin C, Lacarelle B, et al. Pharmacokinetics of long-term propofol infusion used for sedation in ICU patients. Anesthesiology 1990;73:214–217.
291. Beller JP, Pottecher T, Lugnier A, et al. Prolonged sedation with propofol in ICU patients: recovery and blood concentration changes during periodic interruptions in infusion. Br J Anaesth 1988;61:583–588.
292. Morgan DJ, Campbell GA, Crankshaw DP. Pharmacokinetics of propofol when given by intravenous infusion. Br J Clin Pharmacol 1990;30:144–148.
293. Bailie GR, Cockshott ID, Douglas EJ, Bowles BJM. Pharmacokinetics of propofol during and after long term continuous infusion for maintenance of sedation in ICU patients. Br J Anaesth 1992;68:486–491.
294. Carrasco G, Molina R, Costa J, et al. Propofol vs midazolam in short-, medium-, and long-term sedation of critically ill patients. Chest 1993;103:557–564.
295. Ronan K, Gallagher J, George B, Hamby B. Comparison of propofol and midazolam for sedation in the intensive care unit (ICU) [Abstract]. Crit Care Med 1992;20:S36.
296. Gravino E, Leone D, Caruso C, et al. EEG variations following prolonged sedation with propofol and midazolam [Abstract]. Intensive Care Med 1992;18 (suppl 2):S157.
297. Aitkenhead AR, Pepperman ML, Willatts SM, et al. Comparison of propofol and midazolam for sedation in critically ill patients. Lancet 1989;2:704–709.
298. Moritz F, Petit J, Kaeffer N, et al. Metabolic effects of propofol and flunitrazepam given for sedation after aortic surgery. Br J Anaesth 1993;70:451–453.
299. Harris CE, Grounds RM, Murray AM, et al. Propofol infusion for long-term sedation in the intensive care unit: a comparison with papavaretum and midazolam. Anaesthesia 1990;45:366–372.
300. Carrasco G, Molina R, Costa J, et al. Usefulness of sedation scales in ICU: a comparative-randomized study in patients sedated with propofol, midazolam or opiates plus benzodiazepines [Abstract]. Intensive Care Med 1992;18 (suppl): S157.
301. Kong KL, Willatts SM, Prys-Roberts C. Isoflurane compared with midazolam for sedation in the intensive care unit. Br Med J 1989;298:1277–1280.
302. Millane TA, Bennett ED, Grounds RM. Isoflurane and propofol for long-term sedation in the intensive care unit. Anaesthesia 1992;47:768–774.
303. Farling PA, Johnston JR, Coppel DL. Propofol infusion for sedation of patients with head injury in intensive care: a preliminary report. Anaesthesia 1989;44:222–226.
304. Pearson K, Kruse G, Demetrion E. Sedation of patients with severe head injury: a randomized, prospective comparison of propofol versus morphine and barbiturates [Abstract]. Anesthesiology 1991;75:A248.
305. Higgins TL, Yared JP, Estafanous FG, et al. Propofol versus

midazolam for intensive care unit sedation after coronary artery bypass grafting. Crit Care Med 1994;22:1415–1423.
306. Grounds RM, Lalor JM, Lumley J, et al. Propofol infusion for sedation in the intensive care unit: preliminary report. Br Med J 1987;294:397–400.
307. McMurray TJ, Collier PS, Carson IW, et al. Propofol sedation after open heart surgery: a clinical and pharmacokinetic study. Anaesthesia 1990;45:322–326.
308. Roekaerts PMHJ, Huygen FJPM, de Lange S. Infusion of propofol versus midazolam for sedation in the intensive care unit following coronary artery surgery. J Cardiothorac Vasc Anesth 1993;7:142–147.
309. Higgins TL, Yared JP, Estafanous FG, et al. Propofol versus midazolam for intensive care unit sedation after coronary artery bypass grafting. Crit Care Med 1994;22:1415–1423.
310. Searle NR, Sahab P. Propofol in patients with cardiac disease. Can J Anaesth 1993;40:730–747.
311. Snellen F, Lauwers P, Demeyere R, et al. The use of midazolam versus propofol for short-term sedation following coronary artery bypass grafting. Intensive Care Med 1990;16:312–316.
312. Higgins TL, Yared JP, Estafanous FG, et al. ICU sedation following CABG: propofol vs. midazolam [Abstract]. Anesthesiology 1991;75:A278.
313. Cullen PM, Turtle M, Prys-Roberts C, Way WL, Dye J. Effect of propofol anesthesia on baroreflex activity in humans. Anesth Analg 1987;66:1115–1120.
314. Smith RC, Leung JM, Mangano DT. SPI Research Group: postoperative myocardial ischemia in patients undergoing coronary artery bypass graft surgery. Anesthesiology 1991;74:464–473.
315. Martin C, Perrin G, Saux P, et al. Right ventricular end-systolic pressure-volume relation during propofol infusion. Acta Anaesth Scand 1994;38:223–228.
316. Norreslet J, Wahlgreen C. Propofol infusion for sedation of children. Crit Car Med 1990;18:890–892.
317. Trotter C, Serpell MG. Neurological sequelae in children after prolonged propofol infusion. Anaesthesia 1992;47:340–342.
318. Lanigan C, Sury M, Bingham R, et al. Neurological sequelae in children after prolonged propofol infusion [Letter]. Anaesthesia 1992;47:810–811.
319. Imray JM, Hay A. Withdrawal syndrome after propofol [Letter]. Anaesthesia 1991;46:704.
320. Parke TJ, Stevens JE, Rice ASC, et al. Metabolic acidosis and fatal myocardial failure after propofol infusion in children: five case reports. Br Med J 1992;305:613–616.
321. Lucas A. Propofol infusion in children [Letter]. Br Med J 1992; 305:1501.
322. O'Flaherty D, Adams AP. Propofol infusion in children [Letter]. Br Med J 1992;305:952–953.
323. Macrae D, James I. Propofol infusions in children [Letter]. Br Med J 1992;305:953.
324. Gottardis M, Khünl-Brady KS, Koller W, et al. Effect of prolonged sedation with propofol on serum triglyceride and cholesterol concentrations. Br J Anaesth 1989;62:393–396.
325. Cook S, Palma O. Propofol as a sole agent for prolonged infusion in intensive care. J Drug Dev 1989;2 (suppl):65–67.
326. Durrington PN, Millar JP. Clinical aspects of hyperlipidaemia. Br J Hosp Med 1984;32:28–34.
327. Boyle WA, Shear JM, White PF, Schuller D. Tolerance and hyperlipemia during long-term sedation with propofol [Abstract]. Anesthesiology 1990;73:A245.
328. Brown E (in press).
329. Robertson WR, Reader SCJ, Davison B, et al. On the biopotency and site of action of drugs affecting endocrine tissue with special reference to the anti-steroidogenic effect of anaesthesic agents. Postgrad Med J 1985;61 (suppl 3):145–151.
330. Van Hemelrijck JV, Weekers F, Van Aken H, et al. Propofol anesthesia does not inhibit stimulation of cortisol synthesis. Anesth Analg 1995;80:573–576.
331. Sosis MB, Braverman B, Villaflor E. Propofol, but not thiopental, supports the growth of Candida albicans. Anesth Analg 1995;81:132–134.
332. Farrington M, McGinnes J, Matthews I, Park GR. Do infusions of midazolam and propofol pose an infection risk to critically ill patients? Br J Anaesth 1994;72:415–417.
333. Borgeat A, Dessibourg C, Rochani M, Suter PM. Sedation by propofol in tetanus: is it a muscular relaxant? Intensive Care Med 1991;17:427–429.
334. Pedersen CM. The effect of sedation with propofol on postoperative bronchoconstriction in patients with hyperreactive airway disease. Intensive Care Med 1992;18:45–46.
335. Conti G, Dell'Urti D, Vilardi V, et al. Propofol induces bronchodilation in mechanically ventilated chronic obstructive pulmonary disease (COPD) patients. Acta Anaesthesiol Scand 1993;37:105–109.
336. Pizov R, Brown RH, Weiss YS, et al. Wheezing during induction of general anesthesia in patients with and without asthma. Anesthesiology 1995;82:1111–1116.
337. Bowling P, Belliveau RR, Butler TJ. Intravenous medications and green urine [letter]. JAMA 1981;246:216.
338. Bodenham A, Culank LS, Park GR. Propofol infusion and green urine [Letter]. Lancet 1987;2:740.
339. Motsch J, Schmidt H, Bach A, et al. Long-term sedation with propofol and green discoloration of the liver. Eur J Anaesthesiol 1994;11:499–502.
340. Nates J, Avidan A, Gozal Y, Gertel M. Appearance of white urine during propofol anesthesia. Anesth Analg 1995;81:210.
341. Murphy PG, Myers DS, Davies MJ, et al. The antioxidant potential of propofol (2,6-diisopropylphenol). Br J Anaesth 1992; 68:613–618.
342. O'Connor R, Cranfield K. Use of propofol to terminate generalised myoclonus [Letter]. Anaesthesia 1992;47:443.
343. Ermakov S, Crippen D. Continuous propofol infusion for sedation in delirium tremens [Abstract]. Crit Care Med 1992; 20:S37.
344. Mazzarino A, DeMaria G, Candiani A. Effects of propofol in patients in status epilepticus of various origins: electroencephalographic analysis. Minerva Anestesiol 1994;60:A681–A685.
345. Au J, Walker WS, Scott DHT. Withdrawal syndrome after propofol infusion. Anaesthesia 1990;45:741–742.
346. Valente JF, Anderson GL, Branson RD, et al. Disadvantages of prolonged propofol sedation in the critical care unit. Crit Care Med 1994;22:710–712.
347. Ronan KP, Gallagher TJ, George B, Hamby B. Comparison of propofol and midazolam for sedation in intensive care unit patients Crit Care Med 1995;23:286–293.
348. Boyd O, Mackay CJ, Rushmer F, et al. Propofol or midazolam for short-term alernatives in sedation. Can J Anaesth 1993; 40:1142–1147.
349. Moore J, Bill KM, Flynn RJ, et al. A comparison between propofol and thiopentone as induction agents in obstetric anaesthesia. Anaesthesia 1989;44:753–757.
350. Valtonen M, Kanto J, Rosenberg P. Comparison of propofol and thiopentone for induction of anaesthesia for elective caesarean section. Anaesthesia 1989;44:758–762.
351. Gregory MA, Gin T, Yau G, et al. Propofol infusion anaesthesia for Caesarean section. Can J Anaesth 1990;37:514–520.
352. Yau G, Gin T, Ewart MC, et al. Propofol for induction and maintenance of anaesthesia at caesarean section. Anaesthesia 1991; 46:20–23.
353. Gin T, Gregory MA, Oh TE. The haemodynamic effects of propofol and thiopentone for induction of caesarean section. Anaesth Intensive Care 1990;18:175–179.
354. Gin T, O'Meara ME, Kan AF, et al. Plasma catecholamines and

neonatal condition after induction of anaesthesia with thiopentone at caesarean section. Br J Anaesth 1993;70:311–316.
355. Gin T, Yau G, Chan K, et al. Disposition of propofol infusions for caesarean section. Can J Anaesth 1991;38:31–36.
356. Gin T, Yau G, Jong W, et al. Disposition of propofol at caesarean section and in the postpartum period. Br J Anaesth 1991;67: 49–53.
357. Costantino P, Sebastiani M. Which induction drug for cesarean section? A comparison of thiopental sodium, propofol, and midazolam. J Clin Anesth 1993;5:284–288.
358. Dailland P, Cockshott ID, Lirzin JD, et al. Intravenous propofol during Caesarean section: placental transfer, concentrations in breast milk, and neonatal effects. A preliminary study. Anesthesiology 1989;71:827–834.
359. Gin T, Gregory MA, Chan K, et al. Pharmacokinetics of propofol in women undergoing elective caesarean section. Br J Anaesth 1990;64:148–153.
360. Holdcroft A, Morgan M. Intravenous induction agents for caesarean section [Editorial]. Anaesthesia 1989;44:719–720.
361. Brain AIJ. Further developments of the laryngeal mask [Letter]. Anaesthesia 1989;44:530.
362. Brain AIJ. The development of the laryngeal mask: a brief history of the invention, early clinical studies and experimental work from which the laryngeal mask evolved. Eur J Anaesthesiol Suppl 1991;4:5–17.
363. Blake DW, Donnan G, Bjorksten AR, Dawson P. Propofol induction for laryngeal mask insertion: dose requirement and cardiorespiratory effects [Abstract]. Anaesth Intensive Care 1992; 20:108.
364. Brown GW, Patel N, Ellis FR. Comparison of propofol and thiopentone for laryngeal mask insertion. Anaesthesia 1991;46:771–772.
365. Smith I, White PF. Use of the laryngeal mask airway as an alternative to a face mask during outpatient arthroscopy. Anesthesiology 1992;77:850–855.
366. Akhtar TM, McMurray P, Kerr WJ, Kenny GNC. A comparison of laryngeal mask airway with tracheal tube for intra-ocular ophthalmic surgery. Anaesthesia 1992;47:668–671.
367. Goodwin APL, Rowe WL, Ogg TW. Day case laparoscopy: a comparison of two anaesthetic techniques using the laryngeal mask during spontaneous breathing. Anaesthesia 1992;47:892–895.
368. Borgeat A, Wilder-Smith OHG, Suter PM. The nonhypnotic therapeutic applications of propofol. Anesthesiology 1994; 80:642–656.
369. DiFlorio T. Is propofol a dopamine antagonist? [Letter]. Anesth Analg 1993;77:200–201.
370. Gunawardene RD, White DC. Propofol and emesis. Anaesthesia 1988;43 (suppl):65–67.
371. Korttila K, Östman PL, Apfelbaum JL, et al. Randomized comparison of outcome after propofol-nitrous oxide or enflurane-nitrous oxide anaesthesia in operations of long duration. Can J Anaesth 1989;36:651–657.
372. Raftery S, Sherry E. Total intravenous anaesthesia with propofol and alfentanil protects against postoperative nausea and vomiting. Can J Anaesth 1992;39:37–40.
373. Östman PL, Faure E, Glosten B, et al. Is the antiemetic effect of the emulsion formulation of propofol due to the lipid emulsion? Anesth Analg 1990;71:536–540.
374. Schulman SR, Rockett CB, Canada AT, Glass PSA. Long-term propofol infusion for refractory postoperative nausea: a case report with quantitative propofol analysis. Anesth Analg 1995; 80:636–637.
375. Scher CS, Amar D, McDowall RH, Barst SM. Use of propofol for the prevention of chemotherapy-induced nausea and emesis in oncology patients. Can J Anaesth 1992;39:170–172.
376. Borgeat A, Wilder-Smith OHG, Forni M, Suter PM. Adjuvant propofol enables better control of nausea and emesis secondary to chemotherapy for breast cancer. Can J Anaesth 1994;41:1117–1119.
377. Hvarfner A, Hammas B, Thorn SE, Wattwil M. The influence of propofol on vomiting induced by apomorphine. Anesth Analg 1995;80:967–969.
378. Torn K, Tuominen M, Tarkkila P, Lindgren L. Effects of subhypnotic doses of propofol on the side effects of intrathecal morphine. Br J Anaesth 1994;73:411–412.
379. Saiah M, Borgeat A, Wilder-Smith OH, et al. Epidural-morphone-induced pruritus: propofol versus naloxone. Anesth Analg 1994;78:1110–1113.
380. Kick O, Kessler J, Conradi R, et al. Anesthesia for outpatient cardioversion: etomidate versus propofol [Abstract]. Anesthesiology 1993;79:A5.
381. Hullander RM, Leivers D, Wingler K. A comparison of propofol and etomidate for cardioversion. Anesth Analg 1993;77:690–694.
382. Canessa R, Lema G, Urzúa J, et al. Anesthesia for elective cardioversion: a comparison of four anesthetic agents. J Cardiothorac Vasc Anesth 1991;5:566–568.
383. Brown M. Comparison of methohexital and propofol for elective cardioversion [Abstract]. Anesthesiology 1993;79:A2.
384. Gale D, Grissom TE, Mirenda JV. Titration of intravenous anesthetics for elective cardioversion: a comparison of propofol, methohexital and midazolam [Abstract]. Anesthesiology 1992; 77:A316.
385. Sternlo JE, Hägerdal M. Anaesthesia for cardioversion: clinical experiences with propofol and thiopentone. Acta Anaesthesiol Scand 1991;35:606–608.
386. Gupta A, Lennmarken C, Vegfors M, Tydén H. Anaesthesia for cardioversion: a comparison between propofol, thiopentone and midazolam. Anaesthesia 1990;45:872–875.
387. Valtonen M, Kanto J, Klossner J. Anaesthesia for cardioversion: a comparison of propofol and thiopentone. Can J Anaesth 1988; 35:479–483.
387a. Jan KT, Wang KY, Lo Y, et al. Anesthesia for elective cardioversion: a comparison of thiopentone and propofol. Acta Anaesthesiol Sin 1995;33:35–39.
388. Gale DW, Grissom TE, Mirenda JV. Titration of intravenous anesthetics for cardioversion: a comparison of propofol, methohexital, and midazolam, Crit Care Med 1993;21:1509–1513.
389. Simpson KH, Halsall PJ, Carr CME, Stewart KG. Propofol reduces seizure duration in patients having anaesthesia for electroconvulsive therapy. Br J Anaesth 1988;61:343–344.
390. Rouse EC. Propofol for electroconvulsive therapy: a comparison with methohexitone. Preliminary report. Anaesthesia 1988; 43 (suppl):61–64.
391. Dwyer R, McCaughey W, Lavery J, et al. Comparison of propofol and methohexitone as anaesthetic agents for electroconvulsive therapy. Anaesthesia 1988;43:459–462.
392. Boey WK, Lai FO. Comparison of propofol and thiopentone as anaesthetic agents for electroconvulsive therapy. Anaesthesia 1990;45:623–628.
393. Avramov M, White PF. Comparative effects of methohexital, propofol and etomidate for electroconvulsive therapy. Anesth Analg 1995;81:596–602.
394. Maletzky BM. Seizure duration and clinical effect in electroconvulsive therapy. Compr Psychiatry 1978;19:541–550.
395. Malsch E, Gratz I, Mani S. Efficacy of electroconvulsive therapy (ECT) after propofol (P) or methohexital (M) anesthesia [Abstract]. Anesth Analg 1992;74:S192.
396. Malsch E, Mani S, Gratz I. The effect of anti-hypertensive medication on the cardiovascular (CV) response to electroconvulsive therapy (ECT) after methohexital (M) or propofol (P) anesthesia [Abstract]. Anesthesiology 1992;77:A76.
397. Selvin BL. Electroconvulsive therapy: 1987. Anesthesiology 1987;67:367–385.
398. Bone ME, Wilkins CJ, Lew JK. A comparison of propofol and

methohexitone as anesthetic agents for electroconvulsive therapy. Eur J Anaesthesiol 1988;5:279–286.
399. Martensson B, Bartfai A, Hallen B, et al. A comparison of propofol and methohexital as anesthetic agents for ECT: effects on seizure duration, therapeutic outcome, and memory. Biol Psychiatry 1994;35:179–189.
400. Harrison GG. Propofol in malignant hyperthermia [Letter]. Lancet 1991;337:503.
401. Fruen BR, Mickelson JR, Roghair TJ, et al. Effects of propofol on calcium regulation by malignant hyperthermia-susceptible muscle membranes. Anesthesiology 1995;82:1274–1282.
402. Krivosic-Horber R, Reyfort H, Becq MC, Adnet P. Effect of propofol on the malignant hyperthermia susceptible pig mode. Br J Anaesth 1989;62:691–693.
403. Raff M, Harrison GG. The screening of propofol in MHS swine. Anesth Analg 1989;68:750–751.
404. McKenzie AJ, Couchman KG, Pollock N. Propofol is a "safe" anaesthetic agent in malignant hyperthermia susceptible patients. Anaesth Intensive Care 1992;20:165–168.
405. Mitterschiffthaler G, Theiner A, Hetzel H, Fuith LC. Safe use of propofol in a patient with acute intermittent porphyria. Br J Anaesth 1988;60:109–111.
406. Tidmarsh MA, Baigent DF. Propofol in acute intermittent porphyria [Letter]. Br J Anaesth 1992;68:230.
406a. Kroh UF, Frank M, Schwerk C, Doss MO. Anesthesia with propofol during an exacerbated course of acute intermittent porphyria. Anasthesiol Intensivmed Notfallmed Schmerzther 1993;28:531–533.
407. Stark RD, Binks SM, Dukta VN, et al. A review of the safety and tolerence of propofol (Diprivan). Postgrad Med J 1985;61 (suppl 3):152–156.
408. Mangar D, Holak EJ. Tourniquet at 50 mm Hg followed by intravenous lidocaine diminishes hand pain associated with propofol injection. Anesth Analg 1992;74:250–252.
409. Ghouri AF, Ramirez Ruiz MA, White PF. Effect of flumazenil on recovery after midazolam and propofol sedation. Anesthesiology 1994.
410. Scott RPF, Saunders DA, Norman J. Propofol: clinical strategies for preventing the pain on injection. Anaesthesia 1988;43:492–494.
411. McCulloch MJ, Lees NW. Assessment and modification of pain on induction with propofol (Diprivan). Anaesthesia 1985; 40:1117–1120.
412. Klement W, Arndt JO. Pain on injection of propofol: effects of concentration and diluent. Br J Anaesth 1991;67:281–284.
413. Stokes DN, Robson N, Hutton P. Effect of diluting propofol on the incidence of pain on injection and venous sequelae. Br J Anaesth 1989;62:202–203.
414. King SY, Davis FM, Wells JE, et al. Lidocaine for the prevention of pain due to injection of propofol. Anesth Analg 1992;74:246–249.
415. Lin SS, Chen GT, Lin JC, et al. Pain on injection of propofol. Acta Anaesthesiol Sin 1994;32:773–776.
416. Gehan G, Karoubi P, Quinet F, et al. Optimal dose of lignocaine for preventing pain on injection of propofol. Br J Anaesth 1991; 66:324–326.
417. Cameron E, Johnston G, Crofts S, Morton NS. The minimum effective dose of lignocaine to prevent injection pain due to propofol in children. Anaesthesia 1992;47:604–606.
418. Johnson RA, Harper NJN, Chadwick S, Vohra A. Pain on injection of propofol: methods of alleviation. Anaesthesia 1990; 45:439–442.
419. Brooker J, Hull CJ, Stafford M. Effect of lignocaine on pain caused by propofol injection [Letter]. Anaesthesia 1985;40: 91–92.
420. Wall RJ, Zacharais M. Effects of alfentanil on induction and recovery from propofol anaesthesia in day surgery. Anaesth Intensive Care 1990;18:214–218.
421. Saarnivaara L, Klemola U-M. Injection pain, intubating conditions and cardiovascular changes following induction of anaesthesia with propofol alone or in combination with alfentanil. Acta Anaesthesiol Scand 1991;35:19–23.
422. Fletcher JE, Seavell CR, Bowen DJ. Pretreatment with alfentanil reduces pain caused by propofol. Br J Anaesth 1994;72:342–344.
423. Helmers JHJH, Kraaijenhagen RJ, Leeuwen LV, Zuurmond WWA. Reduction of pain on injection caused by propofol [Letter]. Can J Anaesth 1990;37:267–268.
424. McCrirrick A, Hunter S. Pain on injection of propofol: the effect of injectate temperature. Anaesthesia 1990;45:443–444.
425. Barker P, Langton JA, Murphy P, Rowbotham DJ. Effect of prior administration of cold saline on pain during propofol injection: a comparison with cold propofol and propofol with lignocaine. Anaesthesia 1991;46:1069–1070.
426. Nahrwold ML, Roizen MF, Stanely TH, et al. Phase IV study of propofol: validation of the data set. Anesth Analg 1993;77:S34–S43.
427. Apfelbaum JL, Grasela TH, Hug CC Jr, et al. The initial clinical experience of 1819 physicians in maintaining anesthesia with propofol: characteristics associated with prolonged time to awakening. Anesth Analg 1993;77:S10–S14.
428. Sear JW, Jewkes C, Wanigasekera V. Hemodynamic effects during induction, laryngoscopy, and intubation with eltanolone (5 beta-pregnanolone) or propofol: a study in ASA I and II patients. J Clin Anesth 1995;7:126–131.
429. Monk TG, Ding Y, White PF. Total intravenous anesthesia: effects of opioid versus hypnotic supplementation on autonomic responses and recovery. Anesth Analg 1992;75:798–804.
430. Ghouri AF, Monk TG, White PF. Electroencephalogram spectral edge frequency, lower esophageal contractility, and autonomic responsiveness during general anesthesia. J Clin Monit 1993;9:176–185.
431. Liu J, Singh H, White PF. EEG bispectral analysis predicts the depth of midazolam-induced sedation. Anesthesiology (in press).
432. Reinsel RA, Veselis RA, Wronski M, Marino P. The P300 event-related potential during propofol sedation: a possible marker for amnesia? Br J Anaesth 1995;74:674–680.
433. Thomas DV. Propofol supports bacterial growth [Letter]. Br J Anaesth 1991;66:274.
434. Zacher AN, Zornow MH, Evans G. Drug contamination from opening glass ampules. Anesthesiology 1991;75:893–895.
435. Jensen AG, Dahlgren C, Eintrei C. Propofol decreases random and chemotactic stimulated locomotion of human neutrophils in vitro. Br J Anaesth 1993;70:99–100.
436. Krumholz W, Endrass J, Hempelmann G. Propofol inhibits phagocytosis and killing of Staphylococcus aureus and Escherichia coli by polymorphonuclear leukocytes in vitro. Can J Anaesth 1994;41:446–449.
436a. Krumholz W, Endrass J, Hempelmann G. Propofol inhibits phagocytosis and killing of Staphylococcus aureus and Escherichia coli by polymorphonuclear leukocytes in vitro. Can J Anaesth 1994;41:446–449.
436b. Pirttikangas CO, Perttila J, Salo M. Propofol emulsion reduces proliferative responses of lymphocytes from intensive care patients. Intensive Care Med 1993;19:299.
437. Davidson JA, Boom SJ, Pearsall FJ, et al. Comparison of the effects of four iv anaesthetic agents on polymorphonuclear leucocyte function. Br J Anaesth 1995;74:315–318.
438. Song D, Sun R, White PF. In preparation.
439. Smith I, White PF. Drug contamination from opening glass ampules [Letter]. Anesthesiology 1992;76:486.
440. Veber B, Gachot B, Bedos JP, Wolff M. Severe sepsis after intravenous injection of contaminated propofol [Letter]. Anesthesiology 1994;80:712.
441. Carr S, Waterman S, Rutherford G, et al. Postsurgical infections associated with an extrinsically contaminated intravenous an-

esthetic agent: California, Illinois, Maine, and Michigan. MMWR Morbid Mortal Wkly Rep 1990;39:426–427, 433.
442. Warwick JP, Blake D. Drawing up propofol [Letter]. Anaesthesia 1994;49:172.
443. White PF, Watcha MF. The practice of anesthesiology and the package insert: decision-making regarding drug use in anesthesiology. Anesth Analg 1993;76:928–930.
444. Johans TG. The cost of propofol. Anesth Analg 1995;80:1252.
445. Joshi GP. Cost comparison: a desflurane-versus a propofol-based general anesthetic technique. Anesth Analg 1995; 80:1251–1252.
446. Vincent RD, Syrop CH, Van Voorhis BJ, et al. An evaluation of the effect of anesthetic technique on reproductive success after laparoscopic pronuclear stage transfer: propofol/nitrous oxide versus isoflurane/nitrous oxide. Anesthesiology 1995;82:352–358.
447. Anonomous. New awakening in anesthesia: at a price. Lancet 1987;1:1469–1470.
448. Gepts E, Jonckheer K, Maes V, et al. Disposition kinetics of propofol during alfentanil anesthesia. Anaesthesia 1988;43 (suppl):8–13.
449. Kirkpatrick T, Cockshott ID, Douglas EJ, Nimmo WS. Pharmacokinetics of propofol (Diprivan) in elderly patients. Br J Anaesth 1988;60:146–150.
450. Servin F, Cockshott ID, Farinotti R, et al. Pharmacokinetics of propofol infusions in patients with cirrhosis. Br J Anaesth 1990; 65:177–183.
451. Kay NH, Sear JW, Uppington J, et al. Disposition of propofol in patients undergoing surgery. Br J Anaesth 1986;58:1075–1079.
452. Cockshott ID, Briggs LP, Douglas EJ, White M. Pharmacokinetics of propofol in female patients. Br J Anaesth 1987;59:1103–1110.
453. Kirvelä M, Olkkola KT, Rosenberg PH, et al. Pharmacokinetics of propofol and haemodynamic changes during induction of anaesthesia in uraemic patients. Br J Anaesth 1992;68:178–182.
454. Saint-Maurice C, Cockshott ID, Douglas EJ, et al. Pharmacokinetics of propofol in young children after a single dose. Br J Anaesth 1989;63:667–670.
455. Valtonen M, Iisalo E, Kanto J, Rosenberg P. Propofol as an induction agent in children: pain on injection and pharmacokinetics. Acta Anaesthesiol Scand 1989;33:152–155.
456. Jones RDM, Chan K, Andrew LJ. Pharmacokinetics of propofol in children. Br J Anaesth 1990;65:661–667.
457. Kataria BK, Ved SA, Nicodemus HF, et al. The pharmacokinetics of propofol in children using three different data analysis approaches. Anesthesiology 1994;80:104–122.
458. Sear JW, Shaw I, Wolf A, Kay NH. Infusions of propofol to supplement nitrous oxide-oxygen for the maintenance of anaesthesia. Anaesthesia 1988;43 (suppl):18–22.
459. Gold MI, Sacks DJ, Grosnoff DB, Herrington CA. Comparison of propofol with thiopental and isoflurane for induction and maintenance of general anesthesia. J Clin Anesth 1989;1:272–276.
460. Lim BL, Low TC. Total intravenous anaesthesia versus inhalational anaesthesia for dental day surgery. Anaesth Intensive Care 1992;20:475–478.
461. Valanne J, Korttila K. Comparison of methohexitone and propofol (Diprivan) for induction of enflurane anaesthesia in outpatients. Postgrad Med J 1985;61 (suppl 3):138–143.
462. Rolly G, Versichelen L. Comparison of propofol and thiopentone for induction of anaesthesia in premedicated patients. Anaesthesia 1985;40:945–948.
463. Heath PJ, Kennedy DJ, Ogg TW, et al. Which intravenous induction agent for day surgery? A comparison of propofol, thiopentone, methohexitone and etomidate. Anaesthesia 1988; 43:365–368.
464. Cundy JM, Arunasalam K. Use of an emulsion formulation of propofol (Diprivan) in intravenous anaesthesia for termination of pregnancy: a comparison with methohexitone. Postgrad Med J 1985;61 (suppl 3):129–131.
465. Kay B, Healy TEJ. Propofol (Diprivan) for outpatient cystoscopy: efficacy and recovery compared with Althesin and methohexitone. Postgrad Med J 1985;61 (suppl 3):108–114.
466. Mackenzie N, Grant IS. Propofol (Diprivan) for continuous intravenous anaesthesia: a comparison with methohexitone. Postgrad Med J 1985;61 (suppl 3):70–75.
467. Noble J, Ogg TW. The effect of propofol (Diprivan) and methohexitone on memory after day case anaesthesia. Postgrad Med J 1985;61 (suppl 3):103–104.
468. Edelist G. A comparison of propofol and thiopentone as induction agents in outpatient surgery. Can J Anaesth 1987;34:110–116.
469. Heath PJ, Ogg TW, Gilks WR. Recovery after day-case anaesthesia: a 24-hour comparison of recovery after thiopentone or propofol anaesthesia. Anaesthesia 1990;45:911–915.
470. Henriksson B-À, Carlsson P, Hallén B, et al. Propofol vs thiopentone as anaesthetic agents for short operative procedures. Acta Anaesthesiol Scand 1987;31:63–66.
471. Johnston R, Noseworthy T, Anderson B, et al. Propofol vs thiopental for outpatient anesthesia. Anesthesiology 1987;67:431–433.
472. Korttila K, Nuotto EJ, Lichtor JL, et al. Clinical recovery and psychomotor function after brief anesthesia with propofol or thiopental. Anesthesiology 1992;76:676–681.
473. Ryom C, Flarup M, Suadicani P, et al. Recovery following thiopentone or propofol anaesthesia assessed by computerized coordination measurements. Acta Anaesthesiol Scand 1992; 36:540–545.
474. Sanders LD, Clyburn PA, Rosen M, Robinson JO. Propofol in short gynaecological procedures: comparison of recovery over 2 days after anaesthesia with propofol or thiopentone as sole anaesthetic agents. Anaesthesia 1991;46:451–455.

8 Steroids

John W. Sear

Interest in the pharmacology and clinical use of intravenous steroid hypnotic agents for both induction and maintenance of anesthesia has been renewed. These drugs have two major advantages over the traditional intravenous barbiturates: greater therapeutic (safety) indices and faster removal from the body by hepatic (and perhaps pulmonary) metabolism and elimination.

This chapter considers historical, currently available, and developmental steroid induction agents and their role in current anesthetic practice.

STRUCTURE-ACTIVITY RELATIONSHIPS FOR STEROID MOLECULES

In 1927, Cashin and Moravek induced anesthesia in cats following the administration of a colloidal suspension of cholesterol (1). However, the first systematic review of the hypnotic properties of steroids belonging to the pregnane and androstane groups was conducted by Selye (2). Of the screened steroids, no apparent relationship was noted between hypnotic (anesthetic) and hormonal properties; the most potent anesthetic steroid, pregnane-3,20-dione (pregnanedione) was virtually devoid of endocrinologic activity. The potency of all the active agents was increased by partial hepatectomy.

CHEMISTRY OF HYPNOTIC STEROIDS

All steroids have at least six asymmetric carbon atoms, resulting in optical isomers with varying degrees of hypnotic activity. However, for the naturally occurring steroids, isomerism only occurs around the AB ring junction (*cis-trans*; "chair" and "boat" forms); the BC and CD rings are in the *trans* arrangement. This compares with the *cis* arrangement of the CD rings in most plant sterols. Both 5α- and 5β-steroids are found to occur naturally, but the 5β-isomers are more predominant.

The various steroid anesthetic agents are divided into two main classes:

1. Naturally occurring: progesterone, pregnanedione, pregnenolone, allopregnenolone, and 11-keto pregnenolone.
2. Synthetic: hydroxydione, GR 2/146, Althesin (alphaxalone-alphadolone acetate), minaxolone citrate, and the aminosteroids (ORG 20599 and ORG 21465) (Fig. 8-1).

Pregnanedione and most of the synthetic steroids described by Selye were water insoluble, and little further work was conducted until Laubach and associates synthesized hydroxydione (3).

Hydroxydione

This 21-hydroxy derivative of pregnanedione was made water soluble by esterification at the C21 position as the sodium hemisuccinate. Hydroxydione had a high therapeutic index and few adverse effects in animals (4). In clinical practice, hydroxydione produced minimal changes in cardiorespiratory function, good muscle relaxation, a low incidence of coughing and pleasant recovery, with an extremely low incidence of vomiting (5, 6). Although induction was slow, there was early obtundation of the pharyngeal and laryngeal reflexes. The respiratory rate increased with an accompanying decrease in tidal volume, resulting in an increased minute volume. Although marked respiratory depression and apnea were not usually observed, cardiac output and arterial blood pressure decreased. Other side effects included pain on injection and a high incidence of venous postanesthetic irritation at the injection site and along the associated vein.

The recommended induction dose of hydroxydione was between 250 and 500 mg, with some patients receiving up to 2000 mg when incremental doses of the

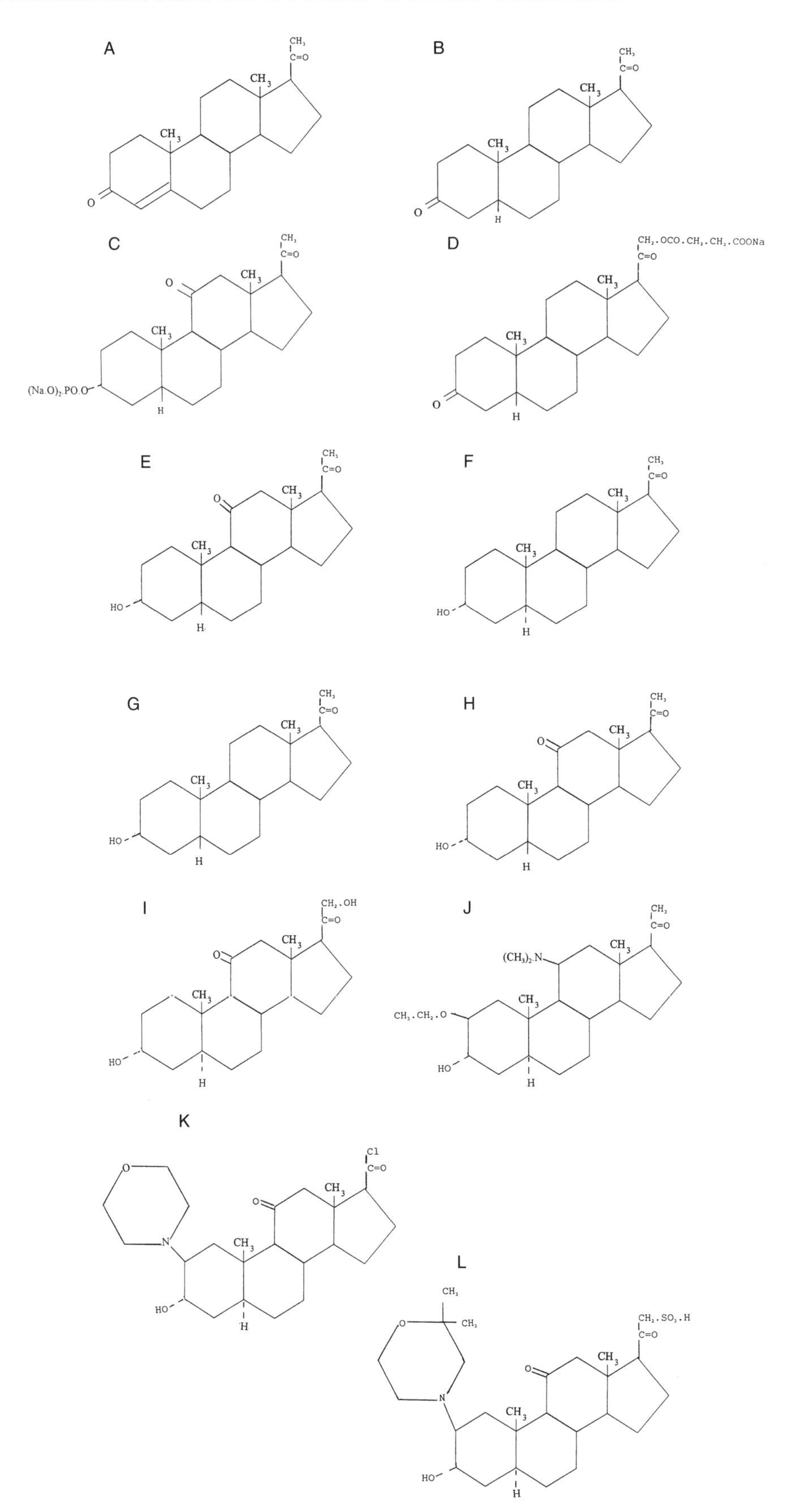

FIGURE 8-1. Structures of steroid anesthetic agents: A, progesterone; B, pregnanedione; C, GR 2/146 (3α-OH, 5β-pregnan-11-dione, 3-disodium phosphate); D, hydroxydione; E, 11-keto pregnanolone; F, 5α-pregnanolone; G, 5β-pregnanolone; H, alphaxalone; I, alphadolone; J, minaxolone; K, ORG 20599; L, ORG 21465.

drug were given to supplement 70% nitrous oxide (N_2O). Recovery from hydroxydione anesthesia was due to its hepatic metabolism and then urinary excretion of glucuronide conjugates. Because of side effects, chemists and pharmacologists at Glaxo-Wellcome began to look for other steroids having the clinical advantages of hydroxydione but without the tendency to cause pain on injection and thrombophlebitis. They noted a number of important structure-activity features:

- Anesthetic activity requires the presence of an oxygen function (either hydroxy or ketone) at each end of the steroid molecule (in the C3 position and in the C20 position of pregnanes or the C17 position of androstanes).
- Substitutions into the steroid structure, such as hydroxy groups, reduced anesthetic activity and occasionally introduced convulsant properties (e.g., 11β-hydroxy).
- Highly active compounds were found among both 5α- and 5β-series.
- The C3 hydroxyl group could be either in the α or β position. In general, 3α-hydroxy-5α- and 3α-hydroxy-5β- were molecules with the greatest anesthetic activity, followed by 3β-hydroxy-5β- and 3β-hydroxy-5α- compounds. 3-keto substituents have little or no anesthetic activity.
- Esters of hydroxy compounds are in general less active and slower than the parent alcohols (7).
- A single double bond in the A or B ring does not significantly affect anesthetic activity, but two or more double bonds in these rings or a single double bond in the D ring is associated with non-activity.
- The presence of C_5 hydrogen atom, which is *cis* to the C_{10} methyl group, is associated with high anesthetic potency.

Because of the difficulties in forming active agents with minimal side effects, Atkinson and associates set out to develop water-soluble steroid anesthetics. These investigators synthesized and evaluated 5β-pregnane-3α-ol, 11,20-dione-3-phosphate disodium [GR 2/146] (8). This was a promising hypnotic compound in several animal species, but when given to human patients, it resulted in a delayed onset of anesthesia and caused paresthesia in the arm and neck following intravenous administration (9). Although paresthesia ceased before loss of consciousness and did not recur when a second dose of the steroid was given during the induction sequence, the drug was not developed further.

Gyermek and associates also continued the search for suitable steroid anesthetics and reevaluated some of the pregnanes described by earlier authors (10). These agents were administered either as aqueous suspensions or were dissolved in water-miscible ketones or alcohols. The main results of their studies were as follows:

- Solutions of the native steroid were more potent than the water-soluble ester salts.
- High therapeutic indices were characteristic of all steroid agents.
- Onset of effect following administration of both suspensions and solutions was rapid.

The metabolites of progesterone (shown by Selye to be effective hypnotic agents) were found to be more potent than the hormone itself (as assessed by studies with both pregnanolone and pregnanedione). The 11-keto analogs of pregnanolone (11-keto pregnenolone and alphaxalone) were also active as hypnotics. On the other hand, the 17-hydroxy derivatives of hydrocortisone were found on evaluation to be convulsive, although some hormonal steroids and synthetic aminosteroids had both anticonvulsant and antianxiety properties. Other central nervous system (CNS) effects of these active steroids included potentiation of brain potentials evoked by adrenocortical steroids (11) and depression of the hypothalamic neuronal activity (12-14).

Althesin Steroids

Although hydroxydione was used for over 10 years after its introduction in 1955, the most important steroid anesthetic to date has been Althesin, a mixture of two steroids (alphaxalone 9 mg/ml) and alphadolone acetate (3 mg/ml). Because of their hydrophobicity, the two steroids were formulated in Cremophor EL.

Alphaxalone (3α-hydroxy, 5α-pregnane 11,20-dione) is an odorless, white crystalline powder with a melting point of 165 to 171°C; it is virtually insoluble in water, but freely soluble in chloroform and acetone. Its 11β-isomer, betaxalone, and the analog Δ 16-alphaxalone (3α-hydroxy, 5α-pregnan-16-ene-11,20-dione) are pharmacologically inactive (7). The other steroid, alphadolone acetate (21-acetoxy, 3α-hydroxy, 5α-pregnane 11,20-dione), is a similar crystalline powder with a higher melting point (175 to 181°C). It is wholly insoluble in water. Both these steroids possess anesthetic activity in animals, but the potency of alphaxalone is approximately twice that of the alphadolone acetate, the latter being present solely to increase the solubility of alphaxalone in Cremophor EL. The anesthetic effects of alphaxalone and alphadolone acetate appear additive.

Althesin remains an effective induction agent for many animal species (marketed as Saffan), except in dogs, in which the Cremophor EL solvent often causes marked hypotension because of histamine release.

MECHANISM OF ACTION

In neurophysiologic studies, all anesthetic steroids depress ascending extralemniscal pathways of the reticular formation, as well as descending tracts between the thalamus and the rostral reticular formation (15). At a cellular level, Makriyannis and Fesik showed that steroid agents perturb the organizational structure of biologic membranes; alphaxalone (in concentrations of 4 mmol/L) increases the fluidity and mobility of phospholipid bilayers to a greater extent than the inactive $_{\Delta}$16-alphaxalone (16).

Evidence now indicates that steroids may act to produce hypnosis through interaction at specific sites on the γ-aminobutyric acid$_A$ ($GABA_A$) receptor-chloride channel complex (17). Thus, at concentrations between 30 and 300 nmol/L, alphaxalone (and 3α-hydroxy, 5α- or 5β-pregnan-20-one, androsterone, and deoxycorticosterone metabolites) causes an increase in chloride conductance in GABA-stimulated receptors (18-22). At alphaxalone concentrations greater than 1 μmol/L (which were associated with clinical anesthesia in human patients), Cottrell and colleagues demonstrated a *direct* effect of alphaxalone in "opening" unstimulated chloride channels. This effect could, in turn, be blocked by 3 μmol/L bicuculline (18). Further experiments by Peters and associates have shown that the steroid anesthetics increase both the frequency of chloride channel opening (a benzodiazepine-like effect) and the duration of opening (as is seen with the barbiturates) (23). Other researchers have shown steroids to increase GABA-stimulated chloride uptake into brain synaptosomes and to increase the binding of the GABA agonist muscimol. This latter effect is the result of either an increase in binding affinity or an increase in the number of available binding sites (24).

Thus, the anesthetic steroids appear to have two effects on the $GABA_A$ receptor. The exact site of action of these steroids on the receptor protein subunits is uncertain, but it appears to be at an extracellular site, because intracellularly applied steroids have no pharmacologic effects. A possible mechanism for the steroid-receptor interaction has been proposed by Im and associates (25). These investigators suggested that the 3α-hydroxy and 17β- polar groups interact with the receptor, whereas the hydrophobic backbones are linked with fatty acyl chains of membrane phospholipids by hydrogen bonding.

More recently, Majewska and colleagues demonstrated that the anesthetically "inactive" steroid pregnenolone sulfate can antagonize pentobarbital anesthesia; this finding may offer one possible avenue for the design of chemically related agonist and antagonist steroid anesthetic agents (26).

PHARMACOLOGIC AND CLINICAL PROPERTIES

The early studies with Althesin in animals demonstrated the drug to have a high therapeutic index, rapid onset, and short duration (27, 28). When the agent was given intravenously to animals, the therapeutic index of Althesin was 30.4, compared with values of 6.9, 7.4, and 8.5 for apnea, methohexital, and ketamine, respectively (28). The therapeutic index of hydroxydione in the same study was 17.3. The high therapeutic index had important applications for the use of Althesin in human patients; the drug caused only minimal cardiovascular depression when given at doses up to twice the median effective dose (ED_{50}) for induction (100 μl/kg compared with 50 μl/kg Althesin) (29). At the higher dose, the steroid caused decreases in systolic and diastolic blood pressures and a significant increase in heart rate. Stroke volume decreased, but cardiac output was unchanged (30). In all patients, induction of anesthesia was followed by a period of hyperventilation followed by apnea and then tachypnea. Arterial PO_2 fell, and there was a small increase in $PaCO_2$. At high doses (200 μl/kg), patients maintained blood pressure but required ventilatory assistance (31).

Althesin also had important effects on cerebral hemodynamics, cerebral metabolism, and intracranial pressure. Turner and colleagues showed that Althesin, 50 μl/kg, administered to patients receiving general anesthesia and controlled ventilation, caused a fall in intracranial pressure proportional to the initial pressure (32). This fall was assumed to be due to reductions in both cerebral blood flow and cerebral blood volume. Althesin also caused decreases in cerebrospinal fluid pressure (33). With infusions of Althesin (300 μg/kg/h), there were decreases in both cerebral blood flow and cerebral metabolic rate compared with the awake state. In conclusion, Althesin caused marked decreases in cerebral blood flow, cerebral oxygen utilization, and intracranial pressure in a manner similar to that of the barbiturates. However, only minimal effects on blood pressure, respiration, and temperature homeostasis were noted, a finding suggesting that the central depressive effect of Althesin may differ from the effects of other intravenous agents. In human patients, Althesin reduced brain blood flow homogenously to all cortical areas, but the technologies available when the study was conducted were inadequate to provide data on the effect of flow on subcortical and brain stem activity. These effects have been shown to be obtunded with large doses of barbiturates (34). When regional performance is assessed using the technique of glucose utilization, halothane, barbiturates, and benzodiazepines all reduce subcortical as well as cortical function. However, Althesin has little effect on the former areas (35), a finding that may explain the agent's minimal hemodynamic and respiratory effects compared with other anesthetic agents.

Althesin had no significant effects on either renal or hepatic function when given by bolus dose or infusions to patients undergoing various surgical procedures

(36-39). The drug was considered not to be safe when it was administered to patients with acute porphyria (both acute intermittent [Swedish] and variegate [South African] types) (40), but it was an important agent for the management of patients susceptible to malignant hyperpyrexia (41). Other reported advantages of Althesin included a transient decrease in intraocular pressure following induction of anesthesia and a relaxant effect on laryngeal muscle when given in large doses (42, 43).

Recovery

Following either single-dose administration (50 to 75 μl/kg) or incremental dosing to supplement N_2O anesthesia for short surgical procedures, immediate recovery after Althesin is more rapid than after thiopental and is comparable with that after methohexital (44, 45). In the few comparative studies existing between Althesin and propofol (formulated as the emulsion), the cardiovascular effects of the two drugs when used for induction of anesthesia were similar, although recovery to opening eyes to command and to giving correct date of birth were faster after propofol (46). At doses higher than 100 μl/kg, Althesin caused significant cardiorespiratory depression.

The main side effects of Althesin induction were a dose-related incidence of hiccups, coughing, laryngospasm, and involuntary muscle movements. Of advantage was the low incidence of postoperative nausea and vomiting, and venous sequelae.

Adverse Reactions to Althesin

The first reports of immediate adverse reactions to Althesia were published in March, 1973 (47-49). From these and other reports, three factors appeared to be significant in the predisposition to Althesin reactions: 1) history of asthma or other atopic manifestations; 2) known sensitivity to other drugs; and 3) previous administration of Althesin. In a review of the first 100 complete reports of Althesin reactions, Clarke and associates described three main types of response:

1. Histaminoid: peripheral vasodilatation, skin flushes, edema and wheals.
2. Bronchospasm: usually accompanied by vasodilatation or hypotension.
3. Cardiovascular collapse: not usually accompanied by other features of histaminoid reactions (50).

Subsequent incidences of reactions varied among different series of cases reported from 1 in 1000 (51) to 1 in 18,000 (52). The immunology of adverse reactions to Althesin may have been multietiologic; reactions on first exposure were either by to a direct nonimmunologic effect on mast cells, causing histamine and other autocoids to be released, or by an alternative pathway complement activation. Reactions to repeat exposure to Althesin resulted from classic complement pathway activation, indicating an antigen-antibody interaction. This latter group of reactions generally had more severe symptoms (53). IgE antibodies were not detected in affected individuals, but Moneret-Vautrin and associates found anti-Cremophor EL IgG antibodies (54). In a further in vitro study, Tachon and associates showed that Althesin (formulated in Cremophor EL), but not the individual steroids, was allergenic (55).

Another laboratory observation seen in patients receiving Althesin was complement activation in the absence of clinical symptoms (56). In a prospective study of 137 patients receiving a first exposure to Althesin, 2 had positive clinical signs of an adverse reaction in the absence of complement changes (i.e., probably anaphylactoid); 6 showed complement activation (C_3 conversion) with no clinical signs (i.e., subclinical reaction), and a further 2 showed both clinical and immunologic signs of an adverse reaction. No relationship was noted between the dose of Althesin and the incidence of either clinical or subclinical changes. In contrast, no changes were seen in the control group of 46 patients receiving thiopental. Of the 10 patients reacting to Althesin, 8 were pregnant at the time of surgery; therefore, the altered immunologic status of pregnant patients may possibly render them more susceptible to Cremophor-associated reactions. This study suggested that the overall rate of reactions to Althesin after an initial exposure may be as high as 1 in 14. Whether the reactions to Cremophor-formulated drugs such as Althesin were due to the pharmacologically active components, with the Cremophor acting as an adjuvant, or to the Cremophor itself must now remain a matter of conjecture.

Pharmacokinetics of Althesin

Initial studies with bolus doses of Althesin in human subjects by Dubois and associates indicated an elimination half-life for alphaxalone of about 30 minutes (57); however, this study was limited by the poor sensitivity of the gas-liquid chromatography assay. The subsequent studies of Simpson and associates (58) and of Sear and Sanders (59) determined the disposition of bolus doses of Althesin and determined a systemic clearance for alphaxalone of around 20 ml/kg/min and an apparent volume of distribution at steady state of 0.79 L/kg. The latter study also provides the only available data on the kinetics of alphadolone acetate following single-dose administration of Althesin to human subjects (Table 8-1). The protein binding of alphaxalone and alphadolone was mainly to albumin,

TABLE 8-1. Disposition Kinetics of Three Steroid Anesthetics (Althesin-Alphaxalone/Alphadolone Acetate; Minaxolone Citrate; and Eltanolone; Mean ± SD)

	$t_{1/2}\ \beta$ (min)	V_b (L)	V_{dss} (L)	Cl_p (L/min)
Bolus dosing				
Alphaxalone (Simpson[58])	34.2(2)	—	53.8(7.6)	1.44(0.27)
Alphaxalone (Sear and Sanders[59])	32(10)	65.3(11)	48.3(16)	1.52(0.50)
Alphadolone (Sear and Sanders[59])	36.4(10)	53.7(6)	44.0(8)	1.09(0.32)
Minaxolone (Dunn et al[125])	47.2(26)	98.2(23)	—	1.55(0.46)
Eltanolone (Carl et al[84])	73.0(10)	361(51)	—	3.46(0.53)
Eltanolone (Gray et al[94])	88.8(66)	—	134(69)	1.85(0.37)
Infusion continuous				
Alphaxalone (Sear et al[119])	90.5(27)	—	107.3(68)	0.84(0.47)
Minaxolone (Sear et al[119])	87.3(23)	—	149.1(27)	1.15(0.13)
Eltanolone (Schuttler et al[102])	182(27)	—	—	1.80(0.4)

$t_{1/2}\ \beta$, elimination half-life; V_b and V_{dss}, apparent volumes of distribution during the elimination phase and at steady state; Cl_p, systemic (plasma) clearance.

but also to β-lipoproteins. There were no good quantitative estimates of the magnitude of protein binding.

Metabolism of Althesin Steroids

The uptake and distribution of the Althesin steroids are similar to those of other nonanesthetic steroid compounds. By the third minute after intravenous injection, ^{14}C label appears within the liver, with subsequent excretion into the bile duct and duodenum (60). The main metabolites are 2α-hydroxy, 16α-hydroxy, and 2α-,16α-di-hydroxy alphaxalone (61).

The metabolism of the Althesin steroid is different in human subjects, with a greater percentage of labeled drug (> 59%) appearing in the urine over the first 24 hours (62). Using a gas chromatography-mass spectrometry technique to detect the parent compounds and their metabolites in blood, bile, and urine, the kinetics of alphaxalone and alphadolone has been found to be similar in patients with normal liver function and in patients with primary biliary cirrhosis (Child's grades A and B) (59, 63). When the agent was given by continuous infusion, plasma concentrations of 20α-hydroxy alphaxalone remained low despite changes in the Althesin infusion rate and plasma alphaxalone concentration. Pooled urine collected over 24 hours after operation revealed most of the alphaxalone (90 to 95%) to be eliminated in the glucuronide fraction of the urine as the 20α-reduced alphaxalone glucuronide. The other urinary metabolite was alphadolone glucuronide; no alphadolone acetate, as free steroid or glucuronide or any 11-reduced compounds, or 20-reduced alphadolone was found in any urine sample. The metabolic clearance rate of these glucuronide conjugates approximated to the glomerular filtration rate. There were also no metabolites with additional hydroxyl groups (which increase hydrophilicity) in the plasma, bile, or urine (64). No evidence of the presence of either steroid or its metabolites in any of the bile samples was noted, in contrast to the findings of Strunin and associates, who detected radiolabeled compounds in bile within 10 minutes of a single dose of 10 to 20 μCi ^{14}C alphaxalone (62).

Further studies by Desmet and colleagues (65) studied the excretion of alphaxalone after a 90-minute infusion of a dose of 25.2 mg/kg. The total urinary alphaxalone excretion (free and glucuronide conjugated) was less than 1%, indicating the significant role of systemic metabolism in drug elimination. Evidence also indicates extrahepatic metabolism of Althesin steroids when examined in vitro using the isolated rat lung (66). In this study, the major metabolites were 11-hydroxy alphaxalone and the 5α-pregnane, 3α,11,20-triol. Other studies have suggested that the lung may have a storage role for lipophilic drugs. This role has been demonstrated for alphaxalone where, after a 10-minute infusion, the rate of efflux of the steroid does not follow that of a drug that remains solely in the vascular compartment. If such storage occurs in human patients, it may be one of the mechanisms for the occurrence of secondary peaks in the plasma drug concentration during the elimination phase.

Infusions of Althesin

Because of the relatively high clearance and short duration of action of the Althesin steroids, the drug is appropriate for use by continuous infusion. The first reports involving Althesin infusions for neuroradiologic and orthopedic procedures came from du Cailar and associates (43). Many other authors described further developments of the technique using the steroid to supplement either opioids or extradural blockade (67) or N_2O (68-70). Typical alphaxalone infusion rates ranged from 15 to 30 μg/kg/min. Side effects (e.g., muscle twitching, hiccups, salivation) were minimal, and cardiovascular stability was remarkable even at eight times the maintenance rate when given to patients receiving 67% N_2O and controlled ventilation.

One of the major drawbacks preventing a comparison of the dynamic properties of Althesin by infusion with those of the volatile agents was the absence of any indices of equipotency. As a result, the concept of the minimum infusion rate (MIR) for an intravenous hypnotic agent that would suppress movement in response to a defined surgical stimulus (the initial surgical incision) in 50% of patients was described (70). The MIR has an associated plasma drug concentration (EC_{50}). For the Althesin steroids, the reported ED_{50} rate in opioid premedicated patients receiving the drug with 67% N_2O was between 13.7 and 14.6 μg/kg/min (71, 72), and the associated alphaxalone concentration was about 1.9 μg/ml. In benzodiazepine-premedicated patients, the ED_{50} was higher (18.5 to 20.0 μg/kg/min). However, hindsight has shown possible fallacies and flaws in this approach, which failed to confirm the relationship between blood and brain (or effector site) concentration; hence the concentration-effect relationships is true only if equilibration between the input and effector sites is rapid.

In a review article describing the cardiovascular effects of Althesin and the three available inhalational agents, an Althesin infusion supplemented with 67% N_2O was compared with halothane. Hemodynamic depression was greater at equianesthetic doses in subjects receiving the volatile agent (73) (Fig. 8-2).

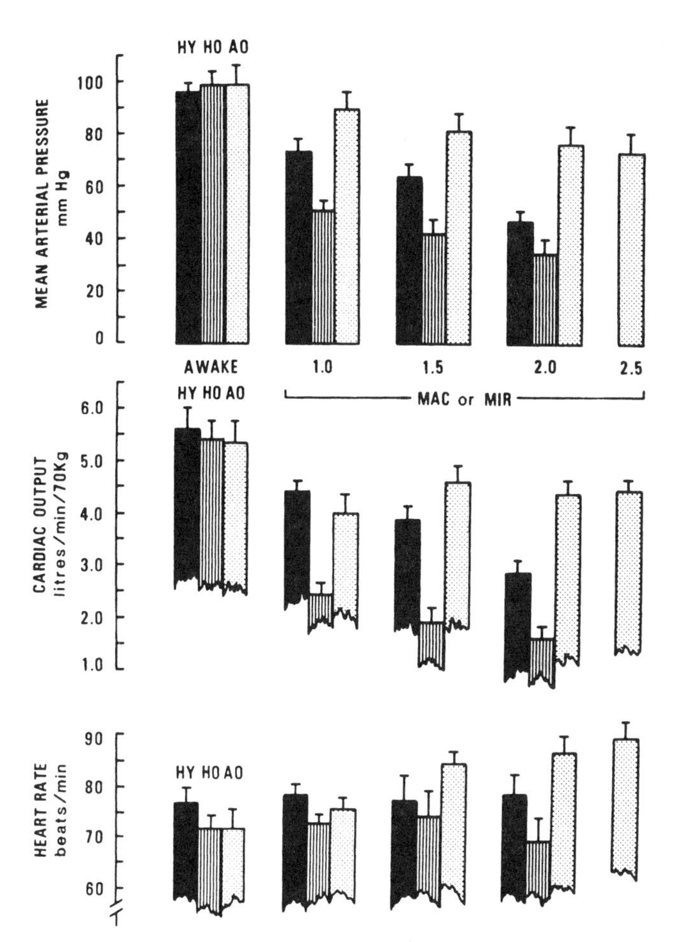

FIGURE 8-2. The influence of age on the dose-dependent cardiovascular effects of halothane-oxygen (HO) anesthesia and a comparison with the dose-dependent effects of Althesin-nitrous oxide (AO) anesthesia. The effects of halothane (HY) in young volunteers (mean age 23 [1] years) are contrasted with those (HO) in patients aged 53 (6) years. The data on Althesin infusions were obtained from a study of older patients (mean age 55 [7] years). MAC, Minimum alveolar concentration; MIR, minimum infusion rate. (From Prys-Roberts C. Cardiovascular effects of continuous intravenous anaesthesia compared with those of inhalational anaesthesia. Acta Anaesthesiol Scand 1982;26 (suppl 75):10–17.)

Veterinary Uses

Although the steroid anesthetics were principally developed for clinical practice in humans patients, Althesin has been widely used in various animal species. It can be used in most domesticated animals (except the dog), without any major problems (74, 75). In most animals, the cardiorespiratory effects are similar to those seen in human patients, apart from a lower incidence of respiratory upsets (e.g., coughing, hiccuping, laryngospasm) and increased cardiovascular sensitivity to Althesin in sheep. In the cat, Althesin produces muscle relaxation without respiratory depression.

SIDE EFFECTS AND SAFETY

Animals recovering from Althesin may show muscle tremors and paddling and, if stimulated, excited behavior and occasional convulsions. Another side effect is the development of edema or hyperemia of the ear pinnae and paws in cats, and these effects appear to be idiosyncratic responses to the solvent (Cremophor EL). Studies with a cyclodextrin-formulated preparation of Althesin have been described, together with preliminary data regarding its administration to dogs (76, 77). It does not appear to offer any significant advantages over the original formulation and has been associated with pain on injection in some animals. Despite these side effects, Althesin has been used safely in many species including budgerigars, birds of prey, rabbits, hamsters and guinea pigs, horses, goats, pigs, sheep, and nonhuman primates.

NEWER STEROID ANESTHETIC AGENTS

Investigators have known for many years that ovarian steroids affect CNS activity. Estrogens increase brain excitability, whereas large doses of progesterone can produce sedation (or deep sleep) in human subjects (78), although the onset is slow, as seen with hydroxydione. 3α-hydroxy, A ring reduced C_{19} and C_{21} steroids bind to the $GABA_A$ complex. Figdor and colleagues (79) demonstrated that progesterone (PG), 5α-pregnanedione (5α-P), and 3α-OH, 5α-pregnan-20-one (5α- or allo pregnanolone) are all potent hypnotic agents. However, the first two steroids convert to 3α-OH, 5α-pregnan-20-one in the brain, and this metabolite is responsible for PG and 5α-P anesthesia in animals (80-

82). Both 5α-pregnanolone and its β-enantiomer are anesthetically active in animals and humans (83, 84).

Compared with the stereochemical requirements generally associated with steroid endocrine effects, substantial differences in the spatial conformation of the A and B rings (*cis, trans*) cause little difference in anesthetic potency and toxicity. However *cis*-AB C_{21} esters are usually less toxic than allo-C_{21} esters or compounds solubilized at C_3. In general, the free alcohol aqueous suspensions are more potent than the derived water-soluble succinate esters. Additional nuclear substitutions in either A or B rings, or at C_{17} or C_{21}, have typically reduced or abolished the depressant activity of the steroids, often with the occurrence of central stimulant or excitatory properties. Because of their high hydrophobicity, 5α-pregnanolone and 5β-pregnanolone need to be formulated in lipid or similar solvents. McKeen and associates (85) and Grimes and Abel (86) have shown that Intralipid has a negative inotropic effect in animals. In an attempt to overcome this disadvantage, Wang and associates examined the anesthetic properties of 5α-pregnanolone solvented in albumin, and compared them with pregnanolone in Intralipid (87). These investigators determined the dose of each formulation needed to achieve 1 second or more of electroencephalographic (EEG) burst suppression. Regional concentrations of 5α-pregnanolone in various parts of the brain at burst suppression were greater after dosing with 5α-pregnanolone in albumin, at a common infusion rate. The greatest steroid levels were found in the striatum, and considerable interregional variations in drug levels were noted. These variations paralleled the known regional differences in neuroactive steroid modulation of $GABA_A$ receptor complexes.

When compared with thiopental, pregnanolone has a potency ratio for induction of hypnosis of between 3.2 and 5. Furthermore, the duration of this "anesthetic" parallels the uptake of the steroid into the brain, with a subsequent redistribution phase in which drug passes from the brain to the liver, intestines, and fatty tissues. The main metabolites appear to be steroid glucuronides and sulfates, with the possibility of enterohepatic recycling of unchanged pregnanolone excreted in the bile (88). Another important property of 5β-pregnanes is thermogenesis, with increases in body temperature to 102 to 105°F.

Animal Pharmacology of 5β-Pregnanolone

In 1987, Norberg and associates evaluated the anesthetic properties of 3α-hydroxy, 5α-pregnanolone and 5β-pregnanolone formulated as an emulsion in Intralipid (83). Both showed excitatory movements during infusions to EEG burst suppression. In a subsequent series of rat experiments, the 5β-isomer of pregnanolone was found to have an anesthetic dose in 50% of animals (AD_{50}) for loss consciousness of 3.64 mg/kg, compared with 21.8 mg/kg for apnea (89). Induction of anesthesia was rapid with both drugs, but recovery was faster after pregnanolone than after thiopental at doses of 1.25 and 5 times the AD_{50}.

5β-pregnanolone has also been evaluated in various animal species and has been shown to have a high therapeutic index (>40). It is isotonic in 10% Intralipid and has a pH of 7.5. There is rapid hepatic metabolism to inactive glucuronide and sulfate conjugates, with excretion by both the kidney and biliary tract. In rats, induction leads to minimal cardiovascular depression, but recovery is not as rapid as following propofol or Althesin (90, 91). In studies of pregnanolone emulsion in dogs receiving fentanyl (0.2 mg/kg/min), pregnanolone doses of 0.5 to 4 mg/kg produced anesthesia lasting 10 to 15 minutes. Cardiac output, systolic arterial pressure, and myocardial contractility only decreased after doses higher than 2 to 4 mg/kg. Systemic vascular resistance also decreased, but pulmonary vascular resistance appeared to increase (92).

Further evaluation of pregnanolone in instrumented dogs has demonstrated that pregnanolone has negative inotropic properties. At high doses (2.5 to 5 mg/kg), pregnanolone caused a dose-dependent decrease in hepatic arterial blood flow, while producing only minimal changes in portal venous flow or renal arterial flow (93). Although both propofol and pregnanolone are partitioned into the oil phase of a fat emulsion, the constituents differ in that the latter contains 7% diacetylated monoglycerides. Further investigation of the effects of pregnanolone on hepatic hemodynamics and on the possible alteration in clearance of concurrently administered flow-dependent drugs is clearly needed.

Studies in Volunteers

Pregnanolone emulsion caused anesthesia with doses of 0.4 to 0.6 mg/kg when it was given to six healthy male volunteers (84). Loss of verbal contact occurred before loss of the eyelash reflex (unlike with thiopental). Hemodynamic effects were minimal, and there was only mild ventilatory depression. Significant side effects included excitation of short duration during the induction of sleep and minor involuntary movements. Following venous blood sampling for up to 4 hours after anesthesia, pharmacokinetic analysis showed a high clearance (2.16 to 4.40 L/min) and a terminal half-life of 0.91 to 1.44 hours (see Table 8-1). The drug has a high degree of protein binding (>99%) to albumin. Balance studies recovered less than 1% unchanged pregnanolone and only 8 to 16% as conjugated pregnanolone in the urine over 24 hours after anesthesia. The main reduced pregnanolone metabolite in human subjects was 5β-pregnan-3α,20α-diol. Total urinary excretion accounts for about 57% of the steroid, with 28% appearing in the feces.

In a second volunteer study, Gray and colleagues gave 0.5 to 1.0 mg/kg to males (94) and observed dose-related depression of cardiorespiratory function, with involuntary movements during 13 of the 33 administrations. The duration of hypnosis was also dose-related. The kinetic profile was similar to that described by Carl (84), with a mean clearance between 1.23 and 1.54 L/kg/h, an elimination half-life 1.48 to 1.65 hours, and apparent volume of distribution of 2 L/kg. However, both this study and that of Carl and associates had poorly designed venous sampling regimens, such that the clearance was overestimated.

In more recent pharmacokinetic studies in adults, children, and the elderly, the mean values of the elimination half-life range from 3.1 to 4.3 hours, clearance ranges from 1.38 to 1.90 L/kg/h, and apparent volume of distribution is between 1.20 and 2.30 L/kg.

All these preliminary studies had a similar dynamic profile. Hemodynamic and respiratory effects were minimal, and the cardiovascular and respiratory depression was dose-related. Significant side effects included transient excitation during the induction of anesthesia and minor involuntary movements. Following a single dose of pregnanolone, 0.6 mg/kg, investigators also noted decreases in cerebral blood flow (−34%) and a comparable fall in oxygen consumption, thereby maintaining a coupling between metabolism and blood flow (95).

Clinical Studies of Eltanolone (5β-Pregnanolone)

Three studies have defined the ED_{50} induction dose in benzodiazepine and opioid premedicated patients to be between 0.33 and 0.44 mg/kg, respectively. Induction caused only minimal hemodynamic depression, with mean decreases in systolic and diastolic arterial pressure of 12% and an increase in heart rate of +9% (Fig. 8-3). A low incidence of pain on injection was observed, with primary effects being involuntary movements, mild apnea, and hypertonus (96-98). Compared with eltanolone, the relative potency of propofol in benzodiazepine-premedicated patients is 0.313; however, recovery appears slower after eltanolone than after propofol (99). In children, the ED_{50} for the loss of response to verbal commands was 0.68 mg/kg in unpremedicated children aged 6 to 10 years, and 0.53 mg/kg between 11 and 15 years (100). In an unpublished study, a significant effect of aging was found on the induction dose of eltanolone needed to produce loss of verbal contact within 120 seconds of the start of drug administration. In young patients (18 to 40 years), the ED_{50} dose was 0.27 mg/kg, compared with 0.13 mg/kg for patients over 65 years of age.

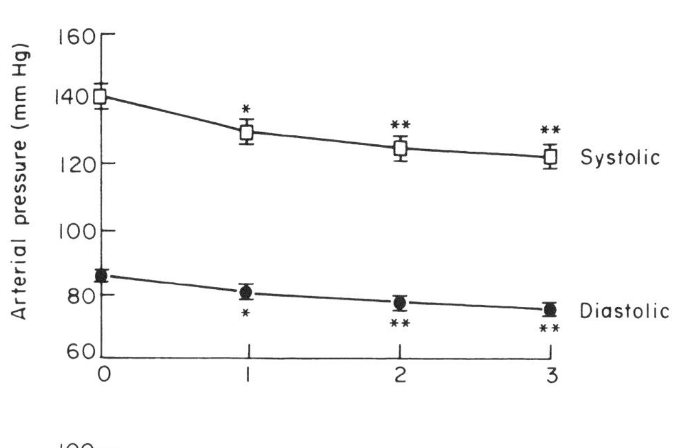

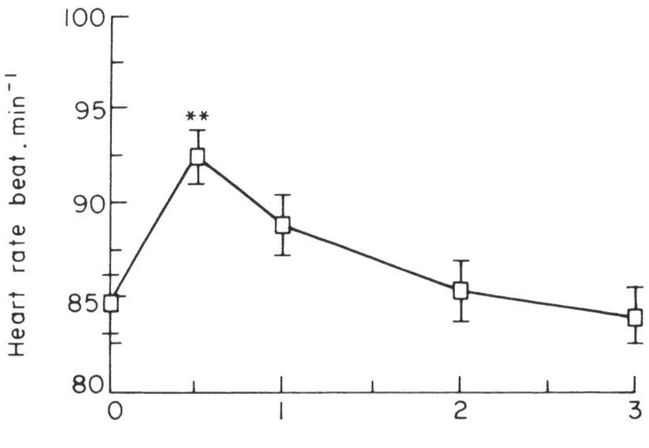

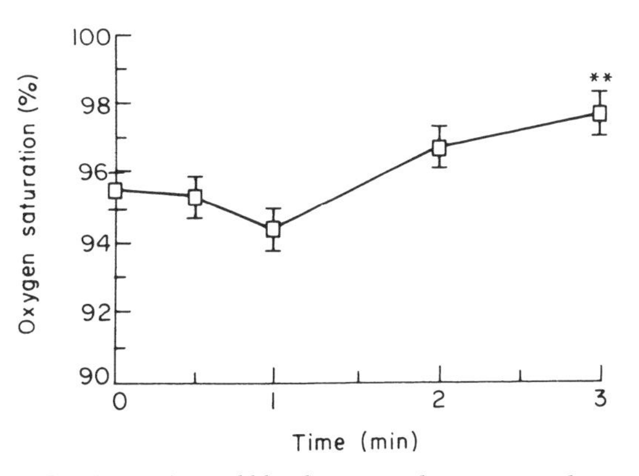

FIGURE 8-3. Arterial blood pressure, heart rate, and oxygen saturation during the 3 minutes following successful induction of anesthesia with eltanolone. Values are shown as mean (SEM). Statistically significant changes from preinduction values (time 0), *$p < 0.05$; **$p < 0.01$ (ANOVA). (From Powell H, Morgan M, Sear JW. Pregnanolone, a new steroid intravenous anesthetic: dose-finding study. Anaesthesia 1992;47:74–80.).

However, at the ED_{50} dose, some patients showed awakening within the 4-minute period following the start of injection.

Myint and associates compared the efficacy of induction of anesthesia using three different rates of administration of eltanolone to patients older than 60 years of age (101). When this agent was infused at 300, 600, or 1200 ml/h, the induction doses (for loss of consciousness) were 0.59, 0.70, and 0.89 mg/kg, respectively, and the induction times were 112, 73, and 50 seconds, respectively. Hence, with a 75% decrease in the eltanolone infusion rate, there was a 120% increase in the induction time and a 33% decrease in the dose required. If we compare these data for eltanolone with comparable data for propofol, etomidate, and thiopental, important differences are noted. For eltanolone, investigators saw a smaller reduction in the induction dose with an increase in the induction time, suggesting a slower response time of the kinetic-dynamic model for the steroid anesthetic. This slower response has been confirmed in a recent study by Schuttler and associates, who demonstrated a $t_{1/2}\,k_{e0}$ (the time required for the biophase concentration to reach 50% of the plasma concentration) of 6.9 minutes and an index of steepness of the concentration-response curve of about 6 (102). These values are similar to those described previously for fentanyl and sufentanil, but they are greater than the values for thiopental and propofol.

The cardiovascular effects of eltanolone associated with induction of anesthesia, laryngoscopy, and intubation have been studied in benzodiazepine-premedicated ASA (American Society of Anesthesiologists classification) I and II patients (103). Anesthesia was induced with either eltanolone or propofol in doses of 1.33 times the ED_{50}, while the patients breathed 67% N_2O in oxygen supplemented by enflurane. Patients were intubated after vecuronium, 0.1 mg/kg. Blood pressure values were recorded noninvasively, and cardiac output was measured using thoracic bioimpedance. At induction doses of 0.58 and 1.7 mg/kg, for the groups receiving eltanolone and propofol, respectively, responses to induction and intubation in both groups were similar, although there was a significantly greater increase in heart rate after laryngoscopy and intubation in those patients receiving eltanolone (103) (Fig. 8-4).

Further studies of the clinical cardiovascular effects of eltanolone have been conducted in patients undergoing coronary artery bypass surgery. These investigators compared the effects of three doses of eltanolone (0.5 to 1.0 mg/kg) and thiopental (3 mg/kg) when coadministered with fentanyl 3 mg/kg and pancuronium (0.1 mg/kg). The decrease in arterial pressure was greater after eltanolone than thiopental, although cardiac output was unaltered by the pregnanolone emulsion. These data suggest a greater effect of eltanolone on systemic vascular resistance than on myocardial contractility (104). In subsequent studies, patients received either eltanolone, 0.5 mg/kg, or thiopental, 3 mg/kg, followed by fentanyl-vecuronium. A comparison of these groups demonstrated a lower mean arterial pressure and systemic vascular resistance in the eltanolone-treated group, as well as a lower pulmonary capillary wedge pressure and left ventricular stroke work index. When administered in combination with fentanyl, eltanolone appeared to have a greater vasodilator effect than thiopental (105).

When eltanolone is administered alone, the hemodynamic effects of eltanolone (0.5 mg/kg) and incidence of thiopental is similar to thipoental (3 mg/kg) are comparable, although the former treatment group showed greater peripheral vasodilation and less depression of myocardial contractility (personal communication, P Tassani). The latter characteristic of eltanolone in preserving contractility has been confirmed in vitro by Riou and colleagues, who found that eltanolone perfusate concentrations of up to 10 μg/ml (therapeutic concentrations are of the order of 500 to 2500 ng/ml) did not significantly alter contraction-relaxation coupling under both low and high loading conditions in the rat myocardium (106). There was no significant negative inotropic effect, although higher concentrations caused a decrease in calcium release from the sarcoplasmic reticulum. Furthermore, in contrast to the in vivo effects seen in the studies by Wouters and colleagues (107) in chronically instrumented dogs, Riou and associates were unable to demonstrate any significant negative inotropic effect of the solvent. Studies by Mulier and coworkers examined peak systolic pressure-end systolic volume (PSP-ESV) relationships in human patients using transesophageal echocardiography (108). These investigators failed to show differences in the extent of negative inotropism between eltanolone, 0.5 and 1.0 mg/kg, and propofol, 1.25 and 2.5 mg/kg, with all patients showing a decrease in PSP-ESV of between 13 and 18%. Thus, the hemodynamic effects of eltanolone and propofol at equipotent doses appear comparable in healthy patients and in those undergoing coronary artery graft procedures when the ejection fraction is greater than 30%.

In a study involving 69 patients, the respiratory effects of eltanolone appeared favorable when compared with propofol. Ventilatory performance following eltanolone (0.75 mg/kg), thiopental (4.0 mg/kg), and propofol (2.5 mg/kg) was assessed using a pneumotachograph and differential pressure transducer in unpremedicated volunteers. After breathing 35% oxygen for 3 minutes, subjects received the hypnotic agent over 30 seconds (109). The main results in terms of changes in tidal volume (V_t) and minute ventilation are shown in Figure 8-5. The overall incidence of apnea was 57% for eltanolone, 74% for thiopental, and 100% for propofol. Apnea lasting longer than 30 seconds occurred in 30% of patients receiving eltanolone, 39% of those receiving thiopental, and 74% of those receiving propofol. The duration of apnea was least with eltanolone and greatest with propofol, with median and interquartile ranges of 6 seconds (0 to 41 seconds) and 88 seconds (30 to 113 seconds), respectively.

The pattern of breathing was assessed by measuring breath-to-breath inspiratory (T_i) and expiratory times. The decrease in T_i was greater with eltanolone and propofol than with thiopental. There was also a tendency for inspiratory drive (expressed as the gradient of the inspiratory line [V_t/T_i]) to be more greatly reduced following propofol than after the other two induction agents. Thus, eltanolone appears to cause less ventilatory depression than propofol and to be comparable with thiopental. No available data are currently available on whether eltanolone affects the central control of respiration.

Maintenance of Anesthesia with Eltanolone

In few studies eltanolone has been used by incremental dosing or infusion to supplement either N_2O or opioid anesthesia. In a preliminary study using incremental doses of eltanolone, Rajah and colleagues achieved satisfactory "surgical anesthesia" in 42 of 50 patients; however, the remaining 8 patients required isoflurane to supplement N_2O (110). Maintenance anesthetic requirements ranged between 0.015 and 0.025 mg/kg/min (similar to those described for the Althesin steroids and minaxolone). The complication rate in this study was low, but most patients showed a slow rate of recovery to orientation in time and space and the

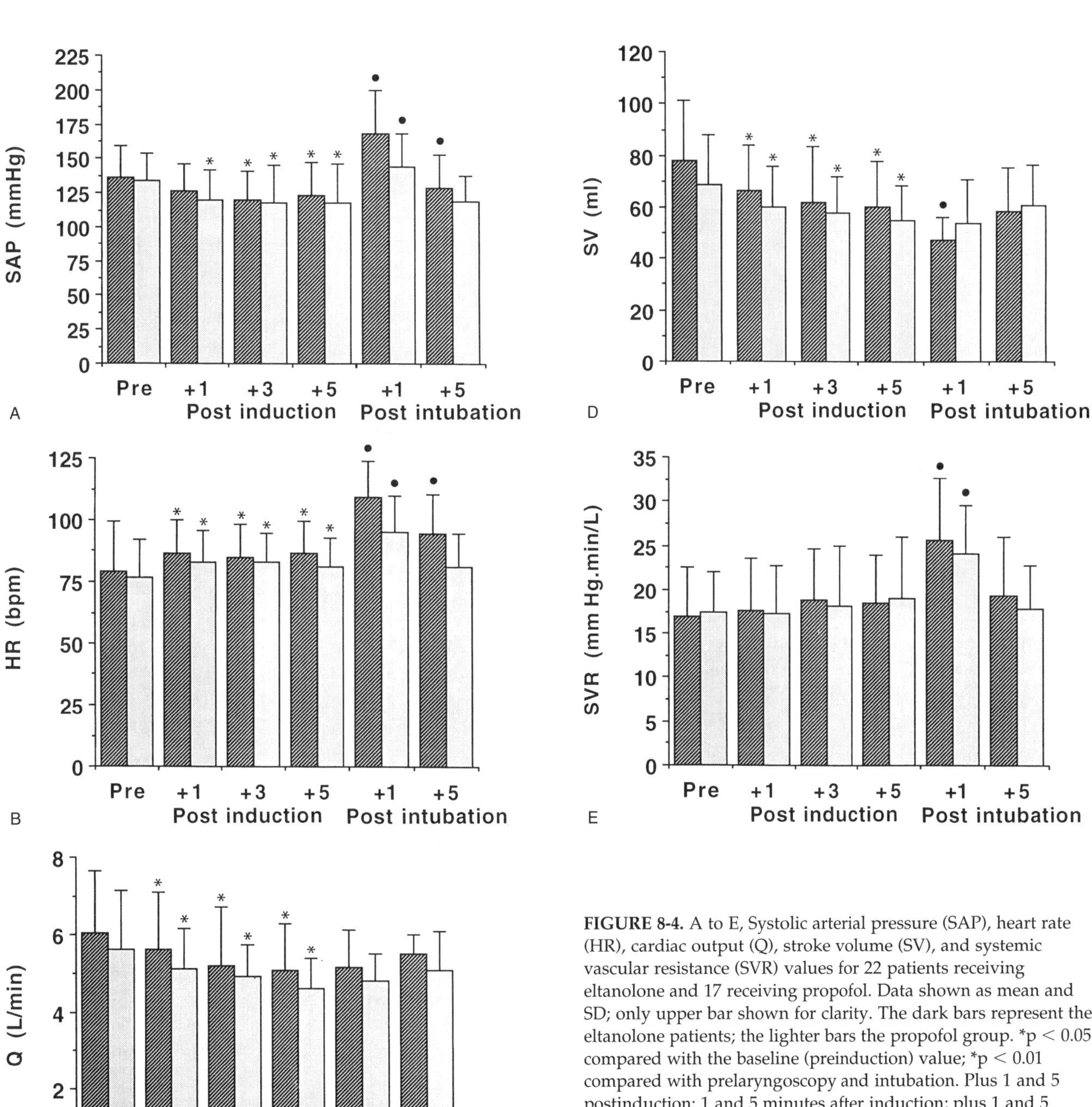

FIGURE 8-4. A to E, Systolic arterial pressure (SAP), heart rate (HR), cardiac output (Q), stroke volume (SV), and systemic vascular resistance (SVR) values for 22 patients receiving eltanolone and 17 receiving propofol. Data shown as mean and SD; only upper bar shown for clarity. The dark bars represent the eltanolone patients; the lighter bars the propofol group. *$p < 0.05$ compared with the baseline (preinduction) value; *$p < 0.01$ compared with prelaryngoscopy and intubation. Plus 1 and 5 postinduction: 1 and 5 minutes after induction; plus 1 and 5 postintubation: 1 and 5 minutes after intubation. (From Sear JW, Jewkes C, Wanigasekera V. Hemodynamic effects during induction, laryngoscopy and intubation with eltanolone (5β-pregnanolone) or propofol: a study in ASA I and II patients. J Clin Anesth 1995;7:126–131.)

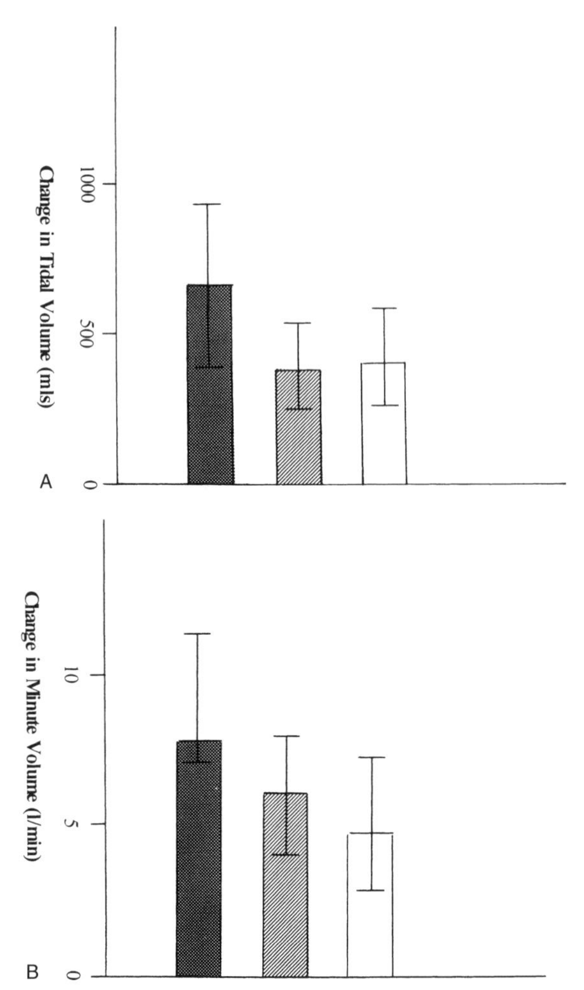

FIGURE 8-5. A and B, Ventilatory effects of eltanolone (0.75 mg/kg, propofol 92.5 mg/kg, or thiopentone (4.0 mg/kg) during induction of anaesthesia in healthy volunteers. Data shown as median and interquartile ranges for the maximum change in tidal and minute volumes from baseline (preinduction) values. (Data from Spens HJ, Drummond GB. Ventilatory effects of eltanolone on induction of anaesthesia: a comparison with propofol and thiopentone. Br J Anaesth 1995;74 (suppl 1):A164.)

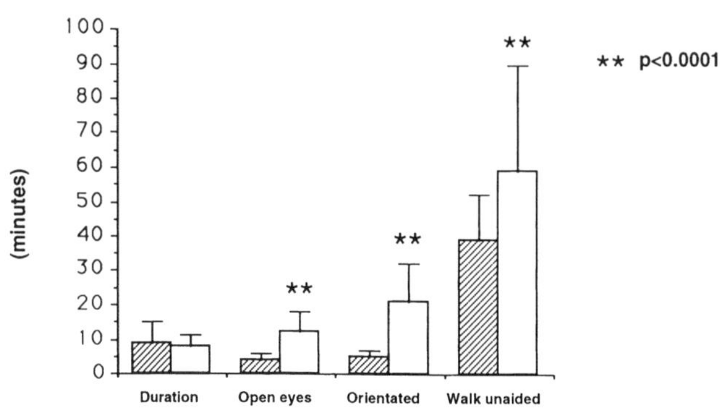

FIGURE 8-6. Comparison of recovery in patients receiving either eltanolone 0.8 mg/kg or propofol 2 mg/kg for induction of anaesthesia. All patients received alfentanil, 10 mg/kg, before induction. Anesthesia was maintained with 67% nitrous oxide and increments of eltanolone (0.2 mg/kg) or propofol (0.5 mg/kg). Data shown as mean and SD. **$p < 0.001$ compared with propofol. (Data from Kallela H, Haasio J, Korttila K. Comparison of eltanolone and propofol in anesthesia for termination of pregnancy. Anesth Analg 1994;79:512–516.)

ability to sit unaided. These data support the earlier findings of Kallela and Eriksson and their associates, who used either thiopental or propofol as the comparator drug (99, 111). When eltanolone was used to supplement N_2O, it was associated with a slower recovery than that after propofol and a recovery similar to that after thiopental (Fig. 8-6). However, in light of the slower dynamic response to eltanolone and steep concentration-effect relationship, overdosing may have occurred in the preliminary studies by Kallela.

Infusions of eltanolone appear to display unique dynamic properties compared with the other available hypnotic drugs in that there is a steep concentration-response curve and marked concentration-effect hysteresis. In more recent studies involving the use of eltanolone as a maintenance anesthetic agent, intermittent bolus administration techniques have been utilized (112). Compared with an induction (2.4 mg/kg) and maintenance (0.6 mg/kg) technique involving propofol and 67% N_2O, eltanolone (0.75 or 1 mg/kg), followed by intermittent bolus doses of 0.2 mg/kg in combination with N_2O, produced acceptable surgical conditions. Although cardiorespiratory stability was similar with both induction agents, propofol was associated with a more rapid emergence and improved cognitive abilities in the first 30 to 60 minutes after surgery than eltanolone. Late recovery times (e.g., ambulation and discharge and postoperative nausea and vomiting) were similar with eltanolone and propofol. Unfortunately, the occurrence of minor allergic-type reactions (e.g., skin rash, urticaria) resulted in the withdrawal of eltanolone (Careltan) from clinical development in early 1996 (112).

Water-Soluble Aminosteroid Anesthetics

Investigators have been interested in finding suitable solvents for water-insoluble steroids since the initial studies of Selye (2). Figdor and colleagues demonstrated that aminoesters of 21-hydroxypregnanedione were water soluble and had general anesthetic properties (79).

In 1964, Hewett and associates investigated the animal pharmacology of certain derivatives of androstane or pregnane with aminoradicals attached at C_2, C_6, or C_{16}. The most potent in causing the loss of righting reflex was a C_2 morpholinosteroid (3α-hydroxy, 2β-morpholino, 5α-pregnan-20-one: SAV 1710) (113). Although the therapeutic index of this aminosteroid was 4.69, it had some disadvantages, including a long time to onset of anesthesia and a long duration of effect. Introduction of an 11-keto group shortened the duration of the ED_{50} dose from 30 to 17 minutes without altering the potency. The steroid anesthetic SAV 1710 had other interesting effects, including the antagonism of the convulsant action of leptazol at low (sedative) doses.

Subsequent studies by Phillips and colleagues examined a range of steroids carrying a basic constituent at the 11 position (114). Compounds with 11α or 11β-dialkylaminoacyloxy- or dialkylamino-substituents formed water-soluble salts that displayed anesthetic activity in animals. Minaxolone citrate had the same pregnane ring structure as alphaxalone and alphadolone, but with introduction of 11α-dimethyl amino and 2β-ethoxy groups, and a 3α-hydroxy group in the A ring of the steroid molecule. The addition of the 2β-ethoxy group was associated with an increased potency compared with alphaxalone, whereas the dimethyl amino group at the 11 position in the C ring in place of the dione group conferred water solubility.

Minaxolone has a high therapeutic index (>5) and is two to three times as potent as Althesin and eight times more potent than thiopental (115). The properties of minaxolone and Althesin appear similar with less respiratory depression and more rapid recovery than after thiopental. Although excitatory movements occur during induction of anesthesia, minaxolone is similar to Althensin and thiopental with respect to its CNS depressant effects. Minaxolone prevents maximal electroshock seizures at subanesthetic doses, and, like Althesin, it can completely abolish cortical electrical activity without associated respiratory depression. In contrast, thiopental produces apnea while the EEG still shows spike and wave activity.

Unfortunately, clinical studies with minaxolone showed a slower onset of action and a more prolonged recovery when compared with Althesin (116-119). The ED_{50} induction dose of minaxolone was 0.52 mg/kg (117). When it was given by incremental dosing to supplement N_2O, the incidence of excitatory movements and hypertonus was greater in the patients receiving minaxolone than in the comparator group (120). The cardiovascular and ventilatory effects of an induction dose of minaxolone (0.5 mg/kg) were of similar magnitude to those seen following equipotent doses of Althesin (118, 121, 122). Both agents are associated with a low incidence of postoperative nausea and vomiting.

When given by continuous infusion, minaxolone infusion rates of 10 to 15 μg/kg/min were needed to supplement 67% N_2O in oxygen anesthesia (119). In comparisons of the cardiovascular and respiratory effects of infusions of minaxolone, Althesin, propofol, and methohexital displayed only minor differences among the four drugs (73). In a subgroup of patients receiving minaxolone to supplement N_2O for vascular surgery, nine patients had no significant effects on hepatic function. However, the other two patients developed signs of postoperative obstructive jaundice, with increases in alkaline phosphatase and serum bilirubin in the first month after surgery (39).

Disposition of Minaxolone

The pharmacokinetics of minaxolone was studied in volunteers by Mather and colleagues (123, 124), who showed a greater whole blood clearance and volume of distribution than seen with alphaxalone. Renal clearance was low (<0.5% of total systemic clearance), and the disposition kinetics following a bolus dose of minaxolone could best be described by a two-compartment kinetic model with an elimination half-life of 47 minutes and clearance of 25.9 ml/kg/min (125). Similar kinetics was determined when the drug was given by infusion to supplement 67% N_2O in oxygen (119) (see Table 8-1).

In contrast to Althesin, the greater water solubility of minaxolone resulted in a greater percentage of the drug's being excreted unchanged by the kidney. The main metabolites in human subjects were the unconjugated steroid (50%) and the N-desmethyl, O-desethyl, and N-desmethyl O-desethyl compounds. The urinary excretion of minaxolone appeared to be pH-dependent with increased elimination under acidic conditions. No data indicated whether minaxolone was excreted by the biliary route in human subjects. Analysis of the acidic fraction of bile suggested that the metabolism of minaxolone was similar to that of PG, with C_{21} oxidation to the corresponding carboxylic acid. Of those products excreted in the bile, about 30% underwent enterohepatic reabsorption and subsequent urinary excretion.

The main undesirable features of minaxolone were the high incidence of excitatory side effects during induction, increased muscle tone intraoperatively, and involuntary movements during recovery. Minaxolone was withdrawn from clinical studies in late 1979 because of these adverse features, as well as concern over toxicologic effects of large doses of the drug and an absence of any clear advantage over the other agents available in clinical practice.

Other Water-soluble Steroid Hypnotic Agents

Other water-soluble agents were evaluated by Organon. In 1993, Gemmell and associates described the anesthetic properties of a water-soluble 2-substituted aminosteroid (ORG 20599) (126, 127). This drug appeared to have an efficacy similar to that of Althesin, a high therapeutic index of 13, and a hypnotic effect of short duration. However, this drug was not evaluated in human subjects because of problems relating to the stability and solubility of the methanesulphonate salt.

More recently, another water-soluble 2-substituted aminosteroid was evaluated in animals (ORG 21465: base; ORG 21256: citrate salt) (128). This steroid also displayed a high therapeutic index in animals (13.8) when compared with propofol or thiopental (4-5). ORG 21465 was compared with propofol in doses of 4 and 3 mg/kg, respectively. Both anesthetics displayed a rapid onset of hypnosis, but the duration of sleep and recovery was slower with the aminosteroid. In the dog, the effective hypnotic induction dose of ORG 21465 was 3 mg/kg, and maintenance doses were 2.8 mmol/kg/min, giving a potency ratio of 1:8 with respect to propofol.

Preliminary data from human volunteers revealed that, with doses in excess of 1 mg/kg, loss of consciousness occurred within 1 minute in unpremedicated subjects, and the duration of effect was dose-dependent over the range 1.0 to 1.8 mg/kg. However, as with many of the other steroids investigated in human subjects (120, 122), the incidence (70%) of excitatory side effects was high. However, no accompanying EEG spike activity was evident, and cardiovascular and respiratory depression was absent.

In conclusion, at the time of this review, no steroid agents seem to have the advantages of Althesin or the low incidence of side effects seen after thiopental. With the prospects of generic propofol as the "leader" in the intravenous anesthesia market, it is difficult to envision eltanolone (or any other steroid anesthetic) taking over from propofol as the leader in our quest for the ideal intravenous anesthetic. Although eltanolone may produce less cardiorespiratory depression, an absence of pain following injection, and a comparable incidence of postoperative nausea and vomiting, the higher incidence of excitatory phenomena, airway irritability, and cutaneous reactions (e.g., flush, rash, and urticaria) will limit its acceptance as a cost-effective alernative to the currently available agents. Thus, the future of steroid anesthesia is questionable.

REFERENCES

1. Cashin MF, Moravek V. The physiological action of cholesterol. Am J Physiol 1927;82:294–298.
2. Selye H. The anesthetic effect of steroid hormones. Proc Soc Exp Biol Med 1941;46:116–121.
3. Laubach GD, P'An SY, Rudel HW. Steroid anesthetic agent. Science 1955;122:78.
4. Taylor N, Shearer WM. The anesthetic properties of 21-hydroxypregnanedione sodium hemisuccinate (hydroxydione), a pharmacological and clinical study of 130 cases. Br J Anaesth 1956;28:67–76.
5. Galley AH, Rooms M. An intravenous steroid anaesthetic: experiences with Viadril. Lancet 1956;1:990–994.
6. Montmorency FA, Chen A, Rudel H, et al. Evaluation of cardiovascular and general pharmacologic properties of hydroxydione. Anesthesiology 1958;19:450–456.
7. Phillips GH. Structure-activity relationships in steroidal anaesthetics. J Steroid Biochem 1975;6:607–613.
8. Atkinson RM, Davis B, Pratt MA, et al. Action of some steroids on the central nervous system. J Med Chem 1965;8:426–432.
9. P'An SY, Gardocki JF, Hutcheon DE, et al. General anesthetic and other pharmacological properties of a soluble steroid, 21-hydroxy-pregnanedione sodium succinate. J Pharmacol Exp Ther 1955;115:432–441.
10. Gyermek L, Iriarte J, Crabbe P. Structure-activity relationship of some steroid hypnotic agents. J Med Chem 1968;11:117–125.
11. Feldman S, Todt J, Porter R. Effect of adrenocortical hormones on evoked potentials in the brain stem. Neurology 1961;11:109–115.
12. Barraclough CA, Cross BA. Unit activity in the hypothalamus of the cyclic female rat: effect of genital stimuli and progesterone. J Endocrinol 1963;26:339–359.
13. Kawakami M, Sawyer CH. Induction of behavioral and electroencephalographic changes in the rabbit by hormone administration or brain stimulation. Endocrinology 1959;65:631–643.
14. Kawakami M, Sawyer CH. Neuroendocrine correlates changes in brain activity thresholds by sex hormones and pituitary hormones. Endocrinology 1959;65:652–668.
15. Gyermek L, Soyka LF. Steroid anesthetics. Anesthesiology 1975;42:331–344.
16. Makriyannis A, Fesik S. Mechanism of steroid anesthetic action: interaction of alphaxalone and Δ-16 alphaxalone with bilayer vesicles. J Med Chem 1983;26:463–465.
17. Harrison NL, Simmonds MA. Modulation of the GABA receptor complex by a steroid anaesthetic. Brain Res 1984;323:287–292.
18. Cottrell GA, Lambert GG, Peters JA. Modulation of $GABA_A$ receptor activity by alphaxalone. Br J Pharmacol 1987;90:491–500.
19. Majewska MD. Neurosteroids: endogenous bimodal modulators of the $GABA_A$ receptor. Mechanism of action and physiological significance. Prog Neurobiol 1992;38:379–395.
20. Barker JL, Harrison NL, Lange GD, Owen DG. Potentiation of γ-aminobutyric acid activated chloride conductance by a steroid anaesthetic in cultured rat spinal neurones. J Physiol (Lond) 1987;386:485–501.
21. Simmonds MA, Turner JP, Harrison NL. Interactions of steroids with the $GABA_A$ receptor complex. Neuropharmacology 1984;23:877–878.
22. Majewska MD, Harrison NL, Schwartz RD, et al. Steroid hormone metabolites are barbiturate-like modulators of the $GABA_A$ receptor. Science 1986;232:1004–1007.
23. Peters JA, Kirkness EF, Callachan H, et al. Modulation of the $GABA_A$ receptor by depressant barbiturates and pregnane steroids. Br J Pharmacol 1988;94:1257–1269.
24. Harrison NL, Majewska MD, Harrington JW, Barker JL. Structure activity relationships for steroid interaction with the gamma-aminobutyric acid-A receptor complex. J Pharmacol Exp Ther 1987;241:346–353.
25. Im WB, Blakeman DP, Davis JP, Ayer ED. Studies on the mechanism of interaction between anesthetic steroids and $GABA_A$ receptors. Mol Pharmacol 1990;37:429–434.
26. Majewska MD, Bluet-Pajot M-T, Robel P, Baulieu E-E. Pregnenolone sulfate antagonizes barbiturate-induced hypnosis. Pharmacol Biochem Behav 1989;33:701–703.
27. Child KJ, Davis B, Dodds MG, Twissel DJ. Anaesthetic, cardiovascular and respiratory effects of a new steroidal agent CT 1341: a comparison with other intravenous anaesthetic agent in the unrestrained cat. Br J Pharmacol 1972;46:189–200.
28. Child KJ, Currie JP, Davis B, et al. The pharmacological properties in animals of CT 1341: a new steroid anaesthetic agent. Br J Anaesth 1971;43:2–13.
29. Campbell D, Forrester AC, Miller DC, et al. A preliminary clin-

ical study of CT 1341, a steroid anaesthetic agent. Br J Anaesth 1971;43:14–24.
30. Savege TM, Foley EI, Ross L, Maxwell MP. A comparison of the cardiorespiratory effects during induction of anaesthesia of Althesin with thiopentone and methohexitone. Postgrad Med J 1972;48 (suppl 2):66–72.
31. Clarke RSJ, Montgomery SJ, Dundee JW, Bovill JG. Clinical studies of induction agents: XXXIX:CT 1341, a new steroid anaesthetic. Br J Anaesth 1971;43:947–952.
32. Turner JM, Coroneos NJ, Gibson RM, et al. The effect of Althesin on intracranial pressure in man. Br J Anaesth 1973; 45:168–172.
33. Takahashi T, Takasaki M, Namiki A, Dohi A. Effects of Althesin on cerebrospinal fluid pressure. Br J Anaesth 1973;45:179–184.
34. Wechsler RL, Dripps RD, Kety SS. Blood flow and oxygen consumption of the human brain during anesthesia produced by thiopental. Anesthesiology 1951;12:308–314.
35. Davis DW, Hawkins RA, Man AM, et al. Regional cerebral glucose utilization during Althesin anesthesia. Anesthesiology 1984;61:362–368.
36. Clarke RSJ, Dundee JW, Doggart JR, Lavery T. The effects of single and intermittent administrations of Althesin and other intravenous anesthetic agents on liver function. Anesth Analg 1974;53:461–468.
37. Park GR, Wilson J. Althesin infusion and regional blockade anaesthesia for major gynaecological surgery. Br J Anaesth 1978; 50:1219–1226.
38. Blunnie WP, Zacharias M, Dundee JW, et al. Liver enzyme studies with continuous intravenous anaesthesia. Anaesthesia 1981; 36:152–156.
39. Sear JW, Prys-Roberts C, Dye A. Hepatic function after anaesthesia for major vascular reconstructive surgery: a comparison of four anaesthetic techniques. Br J Anaesth 1983;55:603–609.
40. Harrison GG, Meissner PN, Hift RJ. Anaesthesia for the porphyric patient. Anaesthesia 1993;48:417–421.
41. Harrison GG. Althesin and malignant hyperpyrexia. Br J Anaesth 1973;45:1019–1021.
42. Fordham RMM, Awdry PN, Paterson GM. The suitability of Althesin for use as an induction agent in intra-ocular surgery. Postgrad Med J 1972;48 (suppl 2):129.
43. Du Cailar J. The effects in man of infusion of Althesin with particular regard to the cardiovascular system. Postgrad Med J 1972;48 (suppl 2):72–79.
44. Craig JG, Cooper GM, Sear JW. Recovery from day case anaesthesia: comparison between methohexitone, Althesin and etomidate. Br J Anaesth 1982;54:447–453.
45. Hannington-Kiff JG. Comparative recovery rates following induction of anaesthesia with Althesin and methohexitone in outpatients. Postgrad Med J 1972;48 (suppl 2):116–119.
46. Uppington J, Kay NH, Sear JW. Propofol (Diprivan) as a supplement to nitrous oxide-oxygen for the maintenance of anaesthesia. Postgrad Med J 1985;61 (suppl 3):80–83.
47. Horton JN. Adverse reaction to Althesin. Anaesthesia 1973; 28:182–183.
48. Avery AF, Evans A. Reactions to Althesin. Br J Anaesth 1973; 45:300–302.
49. Hester JB. Reaction to Althesin. Br J Anaesth 1973;45:303.
50. Clarke RSJ, Dundee JW, Garrett RT, et al. Adverse reactions to intravenous anaesthetics: a survey of 1000 reports. Br J Anaesth 1975;47:575–585.
51. Fisher MM. Severe histamine mediated reactions to Althesin. Anaesth Intensive Care 1976;4:33–35.
52. Sutton JA, Garrett RT, McArdle GK. A survey of adverse reactions to Althesin [ARS abstract]. Br J Anaesth 1974;46:806.
53. Radford SG, Lockyer JA, Simpson PJ. Immunological aspects of adverse reactions to Althesin. Br J Anaesth 1982;54:859–863.
54. Moneret-Vautrin DA, Laxenaire MC, Viry-Babel F. Anaphylaxis caused by anti-Cremophor EL IgG STS antibodies in a case of reaction to Althesin. Br J Anaesth 1983;55:469–471.
55. Tachon P, Descotes J, Laschi-Loquerie A, et al. Assessment of the allergenic potential of Althesin and its constituents. Br J Anaesth 1983;55:715–717.
56. Simpson PJ, Radford SG, Lockyer JA, Sear JW. Some predisposing factors to hypersensitivity reactions following first exposure to Althesin. Anaesthesia 1985;40:420–423.
57. Dubois M, Allison J, Geddes IC. The determination of alphaxalone in human blood by gas-liquid chromatography [ARS abstract]. Br J Anaesth 1975;47:902.
58. Simpson ME. Pharmacokinetics of Althesin:comparison with lignocaine. Br J Anaesth 1978;50:1231–1234.
59. Sear JW, Sanders RS. Intra-patient comparison of the kinetics of alphaxalone and alphadolone in man. Eur J Anaesthesiol 1984;1:113–121.
60. Card B, McCullough RJ, Pratt DAH. Tissue distribution of CT 1341 in the rat: an autoradiographic study. Postgrad Med J 1972; 48 (suppl 2):34–37.
61. Child KJ, Gibson W, Harnby G, Hart JW. Metabolism and excretion of Althesin (CT 1341) in the rat. Postgrad Med J 1972; 48 (suppl 2):37–42.
62. Strunin L, Strunin JM, Knights KM, Ward ME. Metabolism of ^{14}C-labelled alphaxalone in man. Br J Anaesth 1977;49:609–614.
63. Sear JW, Makin HLJ, Stafford MA, et al. Disposition and metabolism of Althesin in patients with cirrhotic liver disease [ARS abstract]. Br J Anaesth 1981;53:1093–1094.
64. Holly JMP, Trafford DJH, Sear JW, Makin HLJ. The in vivo metabolism of Althesin (alphaxalone + alphadolone acetate) in man. J Pharm Pharmacol 1981;33:427–433.
65. Desmet G, Nemitz B, Biotieux JL, et al. Dosage de l'alphaxalone dans le serum et les urines par chromatographie gaz-liquide. Ann Biol Clin (Paris) 1979;37:83–88.
66. Nicholas TE, Jones ME, Johnson DW, Phillippi G. Metabolism of the steroid anaesthetic alphaxalone by the isolated perfused rat lung. J Steroid Biochem 1981;14:45–51.
67. Savege TM, Ramsay MAE, Curran JPJ, et al. Intravenous anaesthesia by infusion. A technique using alphaxalone/alphadolone (Althesin). Anaesthesia 1975;30:757–764.
68. Dechene JP. Alfathesin by continuous infusion supplemented with intermittent pentazocine. Can Anaesth Soc J 1977;24:706–713.
69. Sear JW, Prys-Roberts C. Plasma alphaxalone concentrations during continuous infusion of Althesin. Br J Anaesth 1979; 51:861–865.
70. Sear JW, Prys-Roberts C. Dose-related haemodynamic effects of continuous infusions of Althesin in man. Br J Anaesth 1979; 51:867–873.
71. Sear JW, Phillips KC, Andrews CJH, Prys-Roberts C. Dose-response relationships for infusions of Althesin or methohexitone. Anaesthesia 1983;38:931–936.
72. Sear JW, Prys-Roberts C, Phillips KC. Age influences the minimum infusion rate (ED_{50}) for continuous infusions of Althesin and methohexitone. Europ J Anaesthesiol 1984;1:319–325.
73. Prys-Roberts C. Cardiovascular effects of continuous intravenous anaesthesia compared with those of inhalational anaesthesia. Acta Anaesthesiol Scand 1982;26 (suppl 75):10–17.
74. Hall LW. Althesin in the larger animal. Postgrad Med J 1972; 48 (suppl 2):55–58.
75. Eales FA, Small J. Alphaxalone/alphadolone anaesthesia in the lamb. Vet Rec 1982;110:273–275.
76. Brewster ME, Estes KS, Bodor N. Development of a non-surfactant formulation for alfaxalone through the use of chemically-modified cyclodextrins. J Parenter Sci Technol 1989; 43:262–265.
77. Clarke KW, White RN, England GCW, Bryant CE. Alphaxalone/cyclodextrin anaesthesia in the dog. In Abstracts of the

Fourth International Congress of Veterinary Anaesthesia, Utrecht, 1991:59.
78. Merryman W, Bioman R, Barnes L, Rothchild I. Progesterone "anaesthesia" in human subjects. J Clin Endocrinol 1954; 14:1567–1569.
79. Figdor SK, Kodet MJ, Bloom BM, et al. Central activity and structure in a series of water-soluble steroids. J Pharmacol Exp Ther 1957;119:299–309.
80. Mok WM, Herschkowitz S, Krieger NR. In vivo studies identify 5α-pregnan-3α-ol-20-one as an active anesthetic agent. J Neurochem 1991;57:1296–1301.
81. Mok WM, Herschkowitz S, Krieger NR. Evidence that 3α-hydroxy-5α-pregnan-20-one is the metabolite responsible for anesthesia induced by 5α-pregnanedione in the mouse. Neurosci Lett 1992;135:145–148.
82. Krieger NR, Mok WM. Steroid brain levels at specified behavioral endpoints for general anesthesia. Ann N Y Acad Sci 1991; 625:556–557.
83. Norberg L, Wahlstrom G, Backstrom T. The anaesthetic potency of 3α-hydroxy-5α-pregnan-20-one and 3α-hydroxy-5β-pregnan-20-one determined with an intravenous EEG-threshold method in male rats. Pharmacol Toxicol 1987;61:42–47.
84. Carl P, Hogsklide S, Nielsen JW, et al. Pregnanolone emulsion: a preliminary pharmacokinetic and pharmacodynamic study of a new intravenous anaesthetic agent. Anaesthesia 1990;45:189–197.
85. McKeen CR, Brigham KL, Bowers RE, Harris TR. Pulmonary vascular effects of fat emulsion infusion in unanaesthetized sheep. J Clin Invest 1978;501:1291–1297.
86. Grimes JB, Abel RM. Acute hemodynamic effects of intravenous fat emulsion in dogs. J Parenter Enteral Nutr 1979;3:40–44.
87. Wang MD, Wahlstrom G, Gee KW, Backstrom T. Potency of lipid and protein formulation of 5α-pregnanolone at induction of anaesthesia and the corresponding regional brain distribution. Br J Anaesth 1995;74:553–557.
88. Raisinghani KH, Dorfman RI, Forchielli E, et al. Uptake of intravenously administered progesterone, pregnanedione and pregnanolone by the rat brain. Acta Endocrinol 1968;57:395–404.
89. Larsson-Backstrom C, Lutteman Lustig L, Eklund A, Thorstensson M. Anaesthetic properties of pregnanolone in mice in an emulsion preparation for intravenous administration: a comparison with thiopentone. Pharmacol Toxicol 1988;63:143–149.
90. Hogskilde S, Nielsen JA, Carl P, Sorensen MB. Pregnanolone emulsion. A new steroid preparation for intravenous anaesthesia: an experimental study. Anaesthesia 1987;42:586–590.
91. Hogskilde S, Wagner J, Carl P, Sorensen MB. Anaesthetic properties of pregnanolone emulsion: a comparison with alphaxalone/alphadolone, propofol, thiopentone and midazolam in a rat model. Anaesthesia 1987;42:1045–1050.
92. Hogsklide S, Wagner J, Strom J, et al. Cardiovascular effects of pregnanolone emulsion: an experimental study in artificially ventilated dogs. Acta Anaesthesiol Scand 1991;35:669–675.
93. Wouters PF, Van de Velde MA, Marcus MAE, et al. Hemodynamic changes during induction of anesthesia with eltanolone and propofol in dogs. Anesth Analg 1995;81:125–131.
94. Gray H StJ, Holt BL, Whitaker DK, Eadsforth P. Preliminary study of a pregnanolone emulsion (KABI 2213) for i.v. induction of general anaesthesia. Br J Anaesth 1992;68:272–276.
95. Wolff J, Carl P, Bo Hansen P, et al. Effects of eltanolone on cerebral blood flow and metabolism in healthy volunteers. Anesthesiology 1994;81:623–627.
96. Powell H, Morgan M, Sear JW. Pregnanolone: a new steroid intravenous anaesthetic. Dose-finding study. Anaesthesia 1992; 47:287–290.
97. Hering W, Biburger G, Rugheimer E. Induction of anaesthesia with the new steroid intravenous anaesthetic eltanolone (pregnanolone): dose finding and pharmacodynamics. Anaesthetist 1993;42:74–80.
98. van Hemelrijck J, Muller P, Van Aken H, White PF. Relative potency of eltanolone, propofol, and thiopental for induction of anesthesia. Anesthesiology 1994;80:36–41.
99. Kallela H, Haasio J, Korttila K. Comparison of eltanolone and propofol in anesthesia for termination of pregnancy. Anesth Analg 1994;79:512–516.
100. Beskow A, Westrin P, Werner O. Induction of general anesthesia with eltanolone in children 6–15 years of age [ASA abstract]. Anesthesiology 1994;81:A 1336.
101. Myint Y, Peacock JE, Reilly CS. Induction of anaesthesia with eltanolone at different rates of infusion in elderly patients. Br J Anaesth 1994;73:771–774.
102. Schuttler J, Hering W, Ihmsen H, et al. Pharmacokinetic dynamic modeling of the new intravenous anesthetic eltanolone [ASA abstract]. Anesthesiology 1994;81:A 409.
103. Sear JW, Jewkes C, Wanigasekera V. Hemodynamic effects during induction, laryngoscopy and intubation with eltanolone (5β-pregnanolone) or propofol: a study in ASA I and II patients. J Clin Anesth 1995;7:126–131.
104. Tassani P, Groh J, Ott E, et al. Eltanolone, a new induction agent: hemodynamic effects in patients with coronary artery disease compared to thiopentone [ASA abstract]. Anesthesiology 1993;79:A328.
105. Tassani P, Janicke U, Ott E, et al. Hemodynamic effects of anesthetic induction with eltanolone-fentanyl versus thiopental-fentanyl in coronary artery bypass patients. Anesth Analg 1995; 81:469–473.
106. Riou B, Ruel P, Hanouz J-L, et al. In vitro effects of eltanolone on rat myocardium. Anesthesiology 1995;83:792–798.
107. Wouters PF, Van de Velde M, Marcus M, Van Aken H. Negative inotropic properties of pregnanolone in dogs due to the lipid emulsion [IARS abstract]. Anesth Analg 1995;80:S559.
108. Mulier JP, Van Aken H. Cardiodynamic effects of eltanolone as an induction agent in comparison with propofol: assessment with a transesophageal echocardiographic approach [ASA abstract]. Anesthesiology 1995;83:A70.
109. Spens HJ, Drummond GB. Ventilatory effects of eltanolone on induction of anaesthesia: a comparison with propofol and thiopentone. Br J Anaesth 1995;74 (suppl 1):A164.
110. Rajah A, Powell H, Morgan M. Eltanolone for induction of anaesthesia and to supplement nitrous oxide for minor gynaecological surgery. Anesthesia 1993;48:951–954.
111. Eriksson H, Haasio J, Korttila K. Comparison of eltanolone and thiopental in anaesthesia for termination of pregnancy. Acta Anaesthesiol Scand 1995;39:479–484.
112. QI J, Tang J, Wang B, White PF, et al. Clinical use of eltanolone, a new steroid anesthetic, as an alternative to propofol for ambulatory anesthesia. Anesth Analg (submitted for publication).
113. Hewett CL, Savage DS, Lewis JJ, Sugrue MF. Anticonvulsant and interneuronal blocking activity in some synthetic aminosteroids. J Pharm Pharmacol 1964;16:765–767.
114. Phillips GH, Ayres BE, Bailey EJ, et al. Water-soluble steroidal anaesthetics. J Steroid Biochem 1979;11:79–86.
115. Davis B, Dodds MG, Dolamore PG, et al. Minaxlone: a new water-soluble steroid anaesthetic [ARS abstract]. Br J Anaesth 1979;51:564.
116. Aveling W, Sear JW, Fitch W, et al. Clinical evaluation of minaxolone, a new intravenous steroid anaesthetic agent. Lancet 1979;2:71–73.
117. Punchihewa VG, Morgan M, Lumley J, Whitwam JG. Initial experience with minaxolone, a water-soluble steroid intravenous anaesthetic agent. Anaesthesia 1980;35:214–217.
118. Sear JW, Cooper GM, Williams NB, et al. Minaxolone or Althesin supplemented by nitrous oxide: a study in anaesthesia for short operative procedures. Anaesthesia 1980;35:169–173.

119. Sear JW, Prys-Roberts C, Gray AJG, et al. Infusions of minaxolone to supplement nitrous oxide-oxygen anaesthesia: a comparison with Althesin. Br J Anaesth 1981;53:339–350.
120. McNeill HG, Clarke RSJ, Dundee JW, Briggs LP. Minaxolone: an evaluation with and without premedication. Anaesthesia 1981;36:239–244.
121. Sear JW, Prys-Roberts C, Dye J. Cardiovascular studies during induction with minaxolone. Acta Anaesthesiol Belg 1979;30 (suppl):161–168.
122. Gray AJG, Cooper GM, Chapman J, et al. Studies on premedication and ventilatory responses of minaxolone. Acta Anaesthesiol Belg 1981;32;121–130.
123. Mather LE, Gourlay GK, Parkin KS, Roberts JG. Pharmacodynamics of minaxolone, a new steroidal anesthetic. J Pharmacol Exp Ther 1981;217:481–488.
124. Mather LE, Seow LT, Roberts JG, et al. Development of a model for integrated pharmacokinetic and pharmacodynamic studies of intravenous anaesthetic agents: application to minaxolone. Eur J Clin Pharmacol 1981;19:371–381.
125. Dunn GL, Morison DH, McChesney J, et al. The pharmacokinetics and pharmacodynamics of minaxolone. J Clin Pharmacol 1981;22:452–455.
126. Venning-Hill C, Callachan H, Peters JA, et al. Modulation of the $GABA_A$ receptor by ORG 20599: a water-soluble steroid [BPS abstract]. Br J Pharmacol 1994;111 (suppl):183.
127. Gemmell DK, Campbell AC, Anderson A, et al. ORG 20599: a new water soluble aminosteroid intravenous anaesthetic [BPS abstract]. Br J Pharmacol 1994:111 (suppl):189.
128. Gemmell DK, Byford A, Anderson A, et al. The anaesthetic and $GABA_A$ modulatory actions of ORG 21465, a novel water soluble steroidal intravenous anaesthetic agent [BPS abstract]. Br J Pharmacol 1995;116 (suppl):443.

9 Ketamine and Its Isomers

Jürgen Schüttler, Elemer K. Zsigmond, and Paul F. White

Ketamine is a phencyclidine derivative that was synthesized by Stephens in 1963 (1). The first pharmacologic studies in humans were performed by Corssen and Domino in 1965. To describe the unique anesthetic state produced by ketamine, these investigators introduced the term "dissociative anesthesia" (2), a unique state of unconsciousness in which the patient is in a cataleptic trance-like state (often with eyes open), disconnected from the surroundings, and apparently profoundly analgesic.

PHYSICOCHEMICAL PROPERTIES

Ketamine has a molecular weight of 238 and a pKa of 7.5. Its hydrochloride is a white crystalline salt that is water soluble. The pH values of pharmaceutical solutions of ketamine range between 3.5 and 5.5. The solution is stable at room temperature, clear, and colorless. Ketamine is an optically active compound that is commercially available as a racemic mixture of its two optically active isomers, S(+) ketamine and R(−) ketamine (Fig. 9-1) (3).

PHARMACOKINETICS

Ketamine has a low degree of plasma protein binding. Although Chang and Glazko (4) reported no significant protein binding, Wieber and associates (5) reported that 12% of ketamine was plasma protein bound, whereas Dayton and colleagues (6) described variable binding (22 to 47%) depending on the pH value. Because of its high lipid solubility and low degree of protein binding, ketamine is extensively distributed in the body, with apparent distribution volumes of 100 to 400 L. The initial (central) volume of distribution is large, with values of 20 to 100 L. The high elimination capacity of the human organism for ketamine, with a total body clearance of 1000 to 1600 ml/min, has only limited effect on its terminal half-life value (with $t_{1/2}\beta$ values of 2.5 to 3.1 hours) (Tables 9-1 and 9-2). In children, the pharmacokinetic data were not significantly different compared with adults when corrected for body weight, although most investigators have reported higher clearance rates, smaller volumes of distribution, and shorter elimination half-lives values in children (7).

The bioavailability of ketamine administered intramuscularly is high (93%); however, only 17% is available following oral administration because of first-pass metabolism (8). The maximum plasma concentration is reached immediately after intravenous injection and within 5 minutes after intramuscular application. A bolus dose of ketamine, 2 mg/kg intravenously, induces unconsciousness within 20 to 60 seconds, with emergence occurring 10 to 15 minutes after a single bolus dose. As with thiopental, redistribution of ketamine from the brain and other highly perfused vital organs to more poorly vascularized tissues is the main factor in terminating ketamine's action on the central nervous system (CNS).

The plasma ketamine concentration 10 to 15 minutes after a bolus dose of 2.2 mg/kg is approximately 1 μg/ml, with the minimal effective anesthetic concentration reported to be between 0.65 and 1.3 μg/ml (9). Norketamine (N-demethylated ketamine), the first important metabolite in the chain of ketamine metabolism, is mediated by hepatic microsomal enzymes. Norketamine appears in the plasma 2 to 3 minutes after ke-

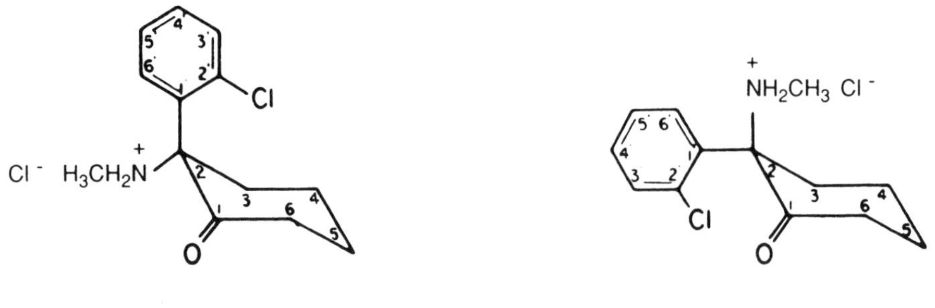

S (+) Ketamine hydrochloride

R (−) Ketamine hydrochloride

Figure 9-1. Structural configuration of the two optical isomers of ketamine. The commercial formulation consists of equal amounts of the two isomers. (From White PF, Ham J, Way WL, Trevor AJ. Pharmacology of ketamine isomers in surgical patients. Anesthesiology 1980; 52:231–239.)

TABLE 9-1. Pharmacokinetic Variables for Racemic Ketamine Mean Values ± S.D. (in Parentheses)

Study	Subjects	Model	Sampling	V_1 (l)	V_{dss} (l)	V_{darea} (l)	Cl_{tot} (ml/min)	$t_{1/2\beta}$ (min)
Wieber et al, 1975 (5)	Patients, bolus injection (n=5)	2-KM	720	60.3 (4.1)	204 (22)	214 (35)	1277 (285)	151 (27)
Clements et al, 1981 (8)	Volunteers, bolus injection (n=5)	2-KM	420	90.1 (11.3)	158 (23)	384 (20)	1429 (75)	186 (10)
Grant et al, 1983 (7)	Patients, bolus injection (n=8)	2-KM	540		206 (28)	228 (35)	869 (152)	182 (25)
	Children, 4–9 y, 20 kg (n=9)	2-KM	420		38 (12)	52 (9)	336 (66)	108 (15)
Schüttler et al, 1987 (12)	Volunteers, infusion, (n=5) racemic ketamine	3-KM	360	73.0 (28.3)	175 (20)	221 (40)	1209 (345)	132 (163)

V_{dss}, volume of distribution at steady state; V_{darea}, area volume of distribution; Cl_{tot}, total clearance; $t_{1/2\beta}$, elimination half-life.

TABLE 9-2. Pharmacokinetic Parameters of Racemic Ketamine and S(+) Ketamine in Volunteers When Both Drugs Were Administered Using a Crossover Design After a Minimum Period of 14 Days*

Parameter	Racemic Ketamine	S(+) Ketamine
$k_{12}[min^{-1}]$	0.096±0.010	0.096±0.0014
$k_{21}[min^{-1}]$	0.023±0.003	0.026±0.003
Cl[l/min]	1.29±0.09	2.18±0.09*
V_c[k/kg]	0.31±0.05	0.41±0.05*
σ^2_{Cl}	20%	16%
σ^2_{Vc}	45%	21%
σ^2_{ε}	21%	22%

Data refer to arterial blood sampling.

σ^2_{Cl}, σ^2_{Vc}, Interindividual variation of clearance (Cl) and central volume of distribution (Vc); σ^2_{ε}, all other random variation.

(From Schüttler J, Kloos S, Ihmsen H, Pelzer E. Pharmacokinetic-pharmacodynamic properties of S(+)-ketamine versus racemic ketamine: a randomized double-blind study in volunteers. Anesthesiology 1992;77:A330.)

tamine administration and reaches its peak level of approximately 0.3 μg/ml in 30 minutes. Norketamine is hydroxylated at two different positions on the cyclohexanone ring to hydroxynorketamine metabolites III and IV (Fig. 9-2) (10). Metabolites III and IV may be dehydrated by heat to metabolite II, or they may be conjugated with glucuronic acid and excreted as a water-soluble metabolite in the urine. Renal excretion of unchanged ketamine accounts for 4% of the eliminated drugs, with 16% eliminated as hydroxylated derivatives. Chang and associates (4) showed that, within a period of 5 days, 91% of the total dose appeared in urine, whereas fecal excretion accounted for only 3%. The primary metabolite, norketamine, is pharmacologically active with an anesthetic and analgesic potency one-third to one-tenth that of ketamine itself (11).

Coadministration of ketamine with benzodiazepines (or barbiturates) may prolong the terminal half-life of ketamine (10). Simultaneous administration of diazepam with ketamine results in increased plasma concentrations of ketamine because diazepam is a competitive inhibitor of N-demethylation of ketamine and thereby decreases its hepatic clearance rate.

EFFECTS ON THE CENTRAL NERVOUS SYSTEM

Electroencephalographic Effects

The morphologic changes in the electroencephalogram (EEG) produced by ketamine can be described by three sequential phases (12, 13) (Fig. 9-3). Phase I is associated with loss of α activity that is combined with a decrease in amplitude and an increase or decrease in frequency, and the median EEG frequency can range between 6 and 15 Hz. Phase II is characterized by per-

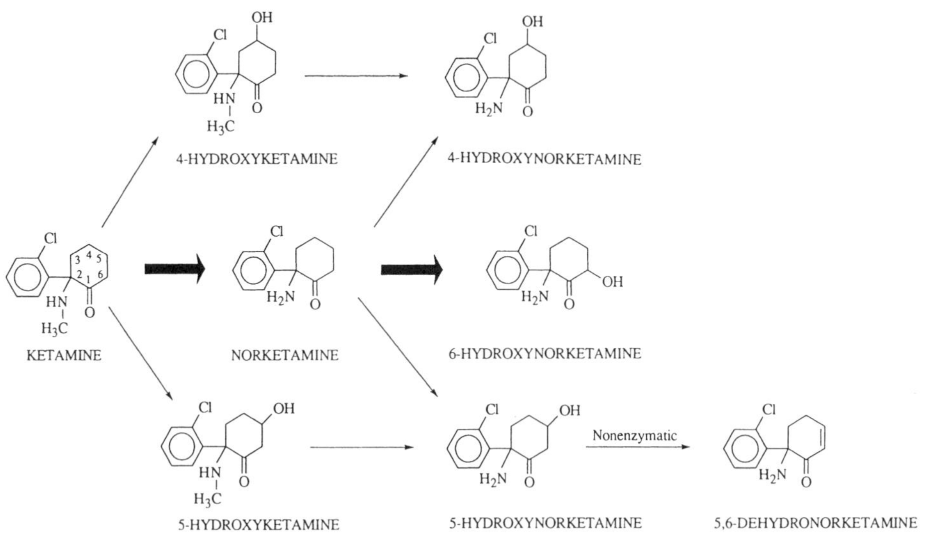

KETAMINE

NORKETAMINE

4-HYDROXYKETAMINE

4-HYDROXYNORKETAMINE

6-HYDROXYNORKETAMINE

5-HYDROXYKETAMINE

5-HYDROXYNORKETAMINE

Nonenzymatic

5,6-DEHYDRONORKETAMINE

Figure 9-2. Biotransformation pathway of ketamine in humans. (From Park GR, Manara AR, Mendel L, et al. Ketamine infusion: its use as a sedative, inotrope, and bronchodilator in a critically ill patient. Anaesthesia 1987;42:980.)

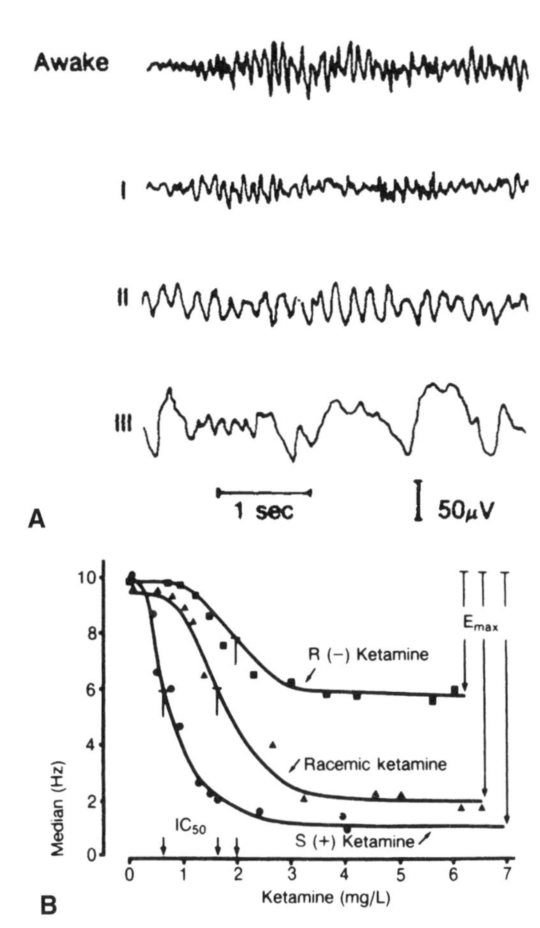

Figure 9-3. A, Progressive changes in the electroencephalogram (EEG) produced by ketamine; phases I to III were seen with racemic ketamine and its S (+) isomer. With R(−) ketamine, the maximal EEG effect was phase III. B, Relationship between the changes in the electroencephalographic median frequency and serum ketamine concentrations in a volunteer receiving racemic ketamine, S(+), and R(−) ketamine on separate occasions. (From Schüttler J, Stanski DR, White PF, et al. Pharmacodynamic modeling of the EEG effects of ketamine and its enantiomers in man. J Pharmacokinet Biopharm 1987;15:241–253.)

sistent rhythmic activity (4 to 6 Hz) with an increased amplitude. Phase III consists of intermittent high-amplitude polymorphic δ activity (0.5 to 2 Hz). Ketamine differs from other intravenous anesthetic agents that simultaneously depress all CNS areas. In contrast, ketamine depresses some regions of the neocortex and subcortical structures (e.g., thalamus) while activating other parts of the limbic system (e.g., hippocampus). Miyasaka and Domino (14) demonstrated that ketamine anesthesia was associated with hypersynchronous δ wave activity in neocortical and thalamic areas and, paradoxically, arousal waves in the hippocampus, which were interpreted as showing a functional dissociation between the limbic and the thalamoneocortical systems.

Domino and associates (15) demonstrated a flattening of visually evoked potentials after hypnotic doses of ketamine. Similarly, ketamine affects acoustic evoked responses in children. Somatosensory evoked potentials recorded from the postrolandic region during electrical stimulation of the contralateral median nerve demonstrated enhancement of all components and minimal effect on discharge after administration of a hypnotic dose of ketamine. In a more recent study, Schwender and his colleagues (16) investigated midlatency auditory evoked potentials (MLAEP), with peaks and valleys occurring between 10 and 100 seconds after the stimulus as a result of the primary cortical responses to the stimulus. However, these investigators did not find a change of MLAEP after ketamine, 2 mg/kg intravenously, compared with the awake (control) group.

Miscellaneous Actions

Transient increases of intracranial pressure (ICP) have been reported after administration of ketamine to patients with intracranial tumors. However, spontaneously breathing animals with normal ICP values showed no increase in ICP compared with a group with preexisting increased ICP (17). Shapiro and associates (18) observed increases in ICP of 1 to 60 mm Hg after ketamine, 2 mg/kg intravenously, or ketamine, 4 mg/kg intramuscularly, in patients with intracranial disease. In general, acute increases in ICP are not accompanied by corresponding increases in systemic arterial pressure. Gardener and colleagues (19) observed elevated ICP in healthy volunteers; however, the extent of ICP increase was less pronounced than in patients with intracranial disease. Investigators have also shown that ketamine increases cerebral blood flow from 47 to 76 ml/min/100 g secondary to a decrease in cerebral vascular resistance from 1.9 to 1.4 mm Hg/ml/min/100 g (20). Therefore, investigators have suggested that ketamine should be avoided in patients with intracranial disease or abnormal cerebral perfusion (17).

Following the introduction of ketamine into clinical practice, controversy has surrounded the complex profile of CNS effects produced by this agent, including conflicting reports regarding its epileptogenic properties. Bennett and colleagues (21) and Ferrer-Allado and associates (22) suggested that ketamine could precipitate seizures or accentuate EEG abnormalities in patients with preexisting convulsive disorders. Corssen and colleagues (23) and Celesia and associates (24) administered ketamine to healthy volunteers and to patients with a history of active epilepsy and found no evidence that ketamine aggravated or precipitated seizures. In fact, Celesia and colleagues found ketamine to be less effective than natural sleep as an activator of epileptic discharges in patients with a history of focal or generalized epilepsy (24). Given that ketamine is an N-methyl-D-aspartate (NMDA)-receptor antagonist, other anesthetic drugs may accentuate the anticonvulsant properties of ketamine (25). Velisek and Mares (26) found that ketamine possessed an anticonvulsant profile in animals. Hypnotic doses of ketamine suppressed generalized tonic-clonic seizures without influencing pure clonic seizures. These investigators concluded that ketamine exhibits a potent anticonvulsant action against generalized tonic-clonic seizures.

NON-CNS PHARMACODYNAMIC EFFECTS

In a double-blind, placebo-controlled trial comparing the circulatory effects and catecholamine levels in gynecologic patients receiving either ketamine, 2.2 mg/kg, or thiamylal, 5 mg/kg intravenously, significant increases in heart rate, mean arterial pressure, and plasma free norepinephrine and epinephrine levels were noted at 2, 5, 10, and 20 minutes after ketamine, in contrast to a marked reduction in mean arterial pressure and no compensatory changes in heart rate and norepinephrine levels in the thiamylal-treated group (27, 28). The circulatory effects of ketamine are likely caused by central sympathetic stimulation (29). In situations where central sympathetic stimulation is advantageous (e.g., hypovolemia, massive hemorrhage), ketamine may have an advantage over the thiobarbiturates. In addition to the well-known cardiac depressant effect of thiobarbiturates, peripheral vasodilatation and occasional histamine release have been described. In contrast to ketamine, cardiac arrest has been reported after rapid injection of thiobarbiturates in hypovolemic patients, patients in hemorrhagic shock, and burn patients who were highly dependent on an intact sympathetic autoregulatory system for the maintenance of adequate circulation (30-32).

A direct depressant effect of ketamine on the myocardium has been observed following large bolus doses (>1.5 mg/kg) or rapid injection (<30 seconds), but it is less than 15% even after a large dose of 2.2 mg/kg intravenously when given over 30 to 60 seconds. When large doses of ketamine were given over several minutes to cardiac patients premedicated with diazepam, no reduction in ejection fraction or stroke index was noted. However, other investigators reported a significant myocardial depressant effect following ketamine administration (32-36). Cabbabe and associates (37) suggested that ketamine was responsible for the dysrrhythmias that occurred in patients undergoing plastic surgery who were receiving large volumes of subcutaneous lidocaine containing epinephrine. However, other factors may have contributed to the occurrence of arrhythmias in this patient population (38). Clinical experience suggests a potentiation of epinephrine-induced arrhythmias by ketamine rather than the antiarrhythmic effect reported in early animal experiments.

Ketamine directly dilates vascular smooth muscle and produces sympathetically mediated vasoconstriction, the net effect being a minimal change in systemic vascular resistance. Although ketamine increases coronary blood flow, it may not be sufficient to meet the oxygen demands of the heart in the presence of ketamine-induced tachycardia and hypertension; therefore, circulatory stimulation should be minimized by premedication with a benzodiazepine. Sudden decreases in blood pressure may also occur following ketamine administration in critically ill patients (39). Pulmonary arterial pressure and right ventricular stroke are increased by ketamine because of an increase in pulmonary vascular resistance. Therefore, ketamine is contraindicated in patients with reduced right ventricular reserve. In patients without intrinsic heart disease, ketamine caused a 40% increase in pulmonary vascular resistance and a transient 20% increase in intrapulmonary shunts (40). However, hypoxic pulmonary vasoconstrictor response is well-maintained during ketamine anesthesia in patients undergoing one-lung anesthesia (41).

Increases in ICP occur after intravenous ketamine injection, but lesser changes are observed after intramuscular injection. The ketamine-induced increase in cerebral blood flow is likely responsible for the increase in cerebrospinal fluid (CSF) pressure. Prior administration of thiopental (or a benzodiazepine) blunts the increase in cerebral blood flow (42). Therefore, ketamine should be avoided in patients with abnormal CSF pressure or cerebral blood flow or with intracranial disease. Mayberg and associates (43) reported no increase in cerebral blood flow velocity or ICP after ketamine administration to a patient undergoing craniotomy with isoflurane-nitrous oxide (N_2O) anesthesia.

Commonly used doses of ketamine, 0.5 to 1.0 mg/kg intravenously, cause minimal respiratory depression. However, the rapid injection of large bolus doses of ketamine, more than 2 mg/kg intravenously, over 30 seconds produced significant reductions in PaO_2, increases in $PaCO_2$, and decreases in pH in healthy patients (44). Premedication with diazepam, 0.2 to 0.3 mg/kg intravenously, infused over 3 minutes markedly increased the respiratory depressant effect of ketamine in healthy volunteers (45). On the other hand, no significant change was observed in either PaO_2 or $PaCO_2$ with slower intravenous infusion of ketamine in adult patients premedicated with diazepam, 10 to 15 mg intramuscularly (46). During vaginal deliveries, ketamine, 1.0 mg/kg, produced no significant changes in the blood gas values of either the parturient or the neonate (47). In fact, Morel and associates (48) reported respiratory stimulation by small doses of ketamine (<1 mg/kg). Manikikian and colleagues (49) reported that administration of ketamine was associated with maintenance of normal functional residual capacity, minute ventilation, tidal volume, and increases in the intercostal muscle contribution to ventilatory function.

Corssen and colleagues (50) reported a beneficial effect of ketamine in patients with asthma secondary to its sympathetic stimulant effects. This bronchodilating effect was present after β blockade with propranolol or when the catecholamine release was blocked by diazepam premedication (51). Ketamine-induced bronchodilatation appears to be mediated by the direct smooth muscle relaxant effects of ketamine (52, 53). Because this effect was also present in endothelium-denuded tracheal strips (54), it is unlikely that the smooth muscle relaxation was mediated by endothelin or inhibition of the calcium channels.

Both salivary and tracheobronchial secretions are increased by ketamine. Therefore, administration of an antisialogogue (e.g., glycopyrrolate, 0.1 to 0.2 mg intravenously) should be considered before ketamine administration. Both laryngeal and pharyngeal airway reflexes are well maintained, and patients may be capable of maintaining an intact airway and swallowing during ketamine anesthesia. Therefore, pulmonary aspiration is less likely to occur with ketamine than with other general anesthetics. Nonetheless, normal safety precautions should be used when ketamine anesthesia is given to patients "at risk" of pulmonary aspiration. In one study conducted with the jet-injector (55), 20% of the children developed laryngospasm after ketamine, 2.5 to 3.5 mg/kg jet injected. Intravenous atropine promptly stopped the spasm in all children except two, who required muscle relaxants and tracheal intubation.

The nonpurposeful tonic, clonic, athetoid movements frequently seen during and after ketamine administration can be disturbing to surgeons and recovery room nurses. Nystagmus and phonation routinely occur, and the conventional ocular signs of adequate anesthesia are not present because the eyes remain open, pupils are dilated, and nystagmus is frequently present. Because the purposeless movements, unusual eye signs, and circulatory stimulation associated with ketamine make evaluation of the depth of anesthesia difficult, the practitioner must rely on empirically or pharmacokinetically-derived infusion rates for adjustments in the dosage of ketamine during the intraoperative period.

Ketamine has been safely used in patients with myopathies and a history of malignant hyperthermia (56). Use of a ketamine infusion for induction and maintenance of anesthesia was associated with higher muscle relaxant requirement than during a thiopental-N_2O-meperidine "balanced" anesthetic technique in healthy gynecologic patients undergoing abdominal laparoscopy (57). However, when ketamine was given during volatile anesthesia, muscle relaxant requirements were decreased. Ketamine has no effect on directly stimulated skeletal muscle, but it increases the indirectly evoked twitch response, suggesting a postsynaptic action (58).

Both pleasant and unpleasant dreams, visual disturbances and hallucinations, illusions, "weird trips," floating sensations, alterations in mood and body image, and delirium have been reported during the recovery phase following ketamine anesthesia. Although flashbacks several weeks following ketamine anesthesia have been reported, a multi-institutional study could not detect any long-lasting psychomimetic sequelae related to postoperative excitement and illusions induced by ketamine (17). When ketamine, 2.0 mg/kg intravenously, was administered over 30 seconds to unpremedicated patients, the incidences of visual disturbances, unpleasant dreams, and pleasant dreams were 80%, 90%, 40%, and 15%, respectively, after gynecologic surgery (59). Neither covering the eyes nor allowing the patients to emerge from anesthesia in a dark, quiet room reduced the incidence of CNS side effects. Factors associated with a higher incidence of emergence reactions included age older than 14 years, female gender, habitual dreaming, history of psychologic problems, and excessive doses of ketamine (17). Certainly, the incidence of psychotomimetic emergence reactions is higher with ketamine than with other general anesthetics (59, 60). In healthy volunteers, no adverse psychic behavioral changes were detected after ketamine-induced hallucinations, as compared with a thiopental-treated control group, despite the high incidence of psychotomimetic side effects associated with ketamine (60). Centrally-active vagolytic drugs (e.g., atropine) increase rather than decrease the incidence of psychotomimetic side effects. Droperidol proved to be inadequate in reducing the psychotomimetic effects of ketamine; however, it was effective in reducing the cardiostimulant effects of ketamine. Concomitant use of thiobarbiturates, N_2O, and volatile anesthetics led to a reduction in the incidence of the psychotomimetic reactions. With a reduction in the induction (1 to 1.5 mg/kg) and maintenance (25 to 100 μg/kg/min) dosages of ketamine and the concomitant use of a benzodiazepine (or other antipsychotic drug), a low incidence (<20%) of psychotomimetic reactions has been reported. Benzodiazepines provide the most complete protection against both the circulatory and psychotomimetic side effects of ketamine.

Ketamine increases uterine tone and the intensity of uterine contractions (61). Analgesic doses of ketamine, 0.2 to 0.4 mg/kg intravenously, produce no discernible effects, whereas larger doses (1 to 2 mg/kg intravenously) increased the intensity of uterine contractions without increasing basal uterine tone. Oats and associates (62) reported that, in the first-trimester pregnant uterus, ketamine was similar to ergometrine in enhancing uterine contractions. On the obstetric ward, ketamine can be used for induction of anesthesia for precipitous forceps delivery or emergency cesarean delivery to maintain blood pressure and uterine contractility in the presence of acute hemorrhage while allowing for the administration of 100% oxygen.

Ketamine's effects on intraocular pressure are similar to those of thiopental and etomidate (63). Ketamine was claimed to inhibit platelet aggregation irreversibly in animals (64); however, Heller and associates (65) could not confirm this antiplatelet effect in humans. Ketamine causes less elevation in blood glucose (12%) than either halothane (55%) or thiopental (72%). Thyroid function tests are not altered by ketamine. Similarly, liver enzymes (e.g., alkaline phosphates, SGOT, and SGPT) plasma cholinesterase, and creatine phosphokinase levels were not changed following ketamine, 2.2 mg/kg intravenously (66). Ketamine increases plasma renin and alanine (ALA) synthetase activity in animals, although the drug has been used safely in patients with acute intermittent porphyria.

Idvall and colleagues (67) and Clements and associates (68) studied the relationship between the plasma concentrations of ketamine and its effects on the CNS. The analgesic level of ketamine was found to be 0.2 μg/ml, and the minimum hypnotic level of ketamine alone was 1.5 to 2.5 μg/ml. However, concomitant administration of N_2O reduced the ketamine levels necessary for anesthesia by approximately 50% (9). The context-sensitive half-time of ketamine after a 40 μg/kg/min infusion was 79 minutes. White and associates (9), using a variable-rate ketamine infusion titrated to the patient's response to a painful stimulus during balanced anesthia, reported maintenance infusion rates between 2 and 6 mg/min, resulting in a mean plasma ketamine level of 1.1 μg/ml. Lower infusion rates of ketamine provide adequate analgesia and sedation for patients being ventilated in the intensive care unit (69).

Ketamine Isomers

The currently available pharmaceutical formulation of ketamine is a racemic mixture containing both S(+)-ketamine and R(−)-ketamine enantiomers mixed in a 1:1 ratio. Marietta and Ryder and Trevor and their associates (70, 71) were the first to study the individual isomers of ketamine in animals. The S(+) isomer of ketamine was shown to elicit periods of hypnosis lasting nearly twice as long as the R(−) isomer following administration of equimolar doses, with the racemate being of intermediate potency. This difference appeared to have a pharmacodynamic basis, because differences were not found in plasma or brain ketamine concentrations for either the individual isomers or the racemate. Furthermore, at equipotent doses, S(+) ketamine produced more profound analgesia and caused significant less postanesthetic stimulation of locomotor activity in animals. White and associates were the first to investigate the pharmacology of ketamine in volunteers and in surgical patients (3, 13). These investigators studied doses of 2 mg/kg of racemic ketamine, 1 mg/kg of S(+) ketamine, and 3 mg/kg of R(−) ketamine in a randomized double-blind fashion in 60 healthy patients undergoing elective outpatient surgery (3). In this study, S(+) ketamine was judged to produce more effective anesthesia than racemic or R(−) ketamine. Assessments of the verbal responses in the postanesthetic period suggested significantly more psychic emergence reactions after R(−) ketamine (37%) than after racemic (15%) or S(+) ketamine (5%). R(−) ketamine also produced more agitated behavior than did racemic or S(+) ketamine (26% versus 10% versus 0%). In addition, postoperative pain occurred more commonly in the R(−) and racemic groups than in the S(+) group. This favorable outcome for the S(+) ketamine led to more systematic clinical pharmacologic studies to characterize S(+) ketamine, with the ultimate goal of developing S(+) ketamine as a new anesthetic drug.

In preliminary studies, investigators showed that R(−) ketamine was not able to depress cortical EEG activity to the same degree as S(+) ketamine or the racemic mixture (12, 13) (see Fig. 9-3B). Racemic ketamine and S(+) ketamine were able to decrease median

EEG frequency to below 2 Hz, whereas R(−) ketamine was only able to decrease median EEG frequency to 4 to 6 Hz. In a more recent randomized double-blind study in volunteers, the pharmacokinetic and pharmacodynamic properties of S(+) ketamine and the racemic mixture were examined in volunteers (72). The double-blind crossover design was performed in volunteers who received S(+) ketamine and racemic ketamine on two different occasions (separated by at least 14 days) using a computer-controlled infusion device to achieve linearly increasing plasma levels with an anticipated slope of 0.1 mg/ml/min for S(+) ketamine and 0.2 mg/ml/min for the racemic ketamine (based on previously published pharmacodynamic potency calculations). During and after the ketamine infusions, the EEG was recorded, and the median frequency of the EEG power spectrum was calculated as a continuous pharmacodynamic measurement of the hypnotic effect. Ketamine administration was discontinued after 20.5 ± 5.2 minutes when a deep anesthetic effect was achieved as quantified by the EEG behavior (i.e., the occurrence of burst suppression and slow δ waves) (see Fig. 9-3) (72).

After a recovery period of 21 to 62 minutes (mean 36 ± 12 minutes), which was determined by a return to full orientation, a second infusion loop was administered. The time course of the arterial ketamine levels and the median frequencies of a representative case are shown in Figure 9-4. Both two- and three-compartment models were used for fitting the arterial and venous blood concentration decay curves. Denoting by i the individual number and by j the jth blood sample drawn, the error model specified was assumed to be:

$$Cl_i = Cl(1+\eta_i^{(Cl)}) \quad E(\eta_i^{(Cl)}) = 0 \quad Var(\eta_i^{(Cl)}) = \sigma_{Cl}^2$$
$$V_{ci} = V_c(1+\eta_i^{(Vc)}) \quad E(\eta_i^{(Vc)}) = 0 \quad Var(\eta_i^{(Vc)}) = \sigma_{Vc}^2$$
$$c_{ij} = c_{pij}(1+\varepsilon_{ij}) \quad E(\varepsilon_{ij}) = 0 Var(\varepsilon_{ij}) = \sigma_\varepsilon^2$$

As a pharmacodynamic model, the median EEG frequency was related inversely to the blood concentration of the S(+) ketamine by the generalized Hill equation:

$$E(t) = E_0^- E_i \frac{c_e^\gamma(t)}{c_{50}^\gamma + c_e^\gamma(t)}$$

E(t) denotes the actual median EEG frequency, E_0 baseline median EEG frequency, and E_1 the maximum dynamic range of the pharmacodynamic effect. C_{50} is the concentration at half-maximum effect, and γ an index for modeling the steepness of the concentration-response relationship. Biophase (or effect compartment) concentrations (C_e) were determined by convolution of the measured concentration with a distribution in the form k*exp(-kt).

$$c_e(t) = k_{e0} \cdot \int e^{-k_{eo} \cdot (t-t')} \cdot c(t')dt'$$

With respect to both the central volume of distribution and clearance, a significant difference exists between racemic ketamine and the S(+) isomer. The central volume of distribution proved to be proportional, dependent on body weight. If one compares the parameters that emerged from fitting a two- or three-compartment model to venous ketamine levels, two aspects deserve to be mentioned. First, fitting a three-compartment model to the data did not significantly improve the fit with respect to a two-compartment model, and second, the difference between racemic ketamine and S(+) isomer was no longer apparent.

Significant differences were found between both drugs with respect to their concentrations at half-maximum effects (C_{50}) and the steepness of the parameter. The clinical signs (i.e., loss and return of orientation, response, and reflexes) were correlated with the blood concentrations and median EEG frequency (Fig. 9-5). The arterial concentrations are virtually identical to the concentrations in the effect-compartment because of the high k_{e0} for ketamine and its S(+) isomer (Tables

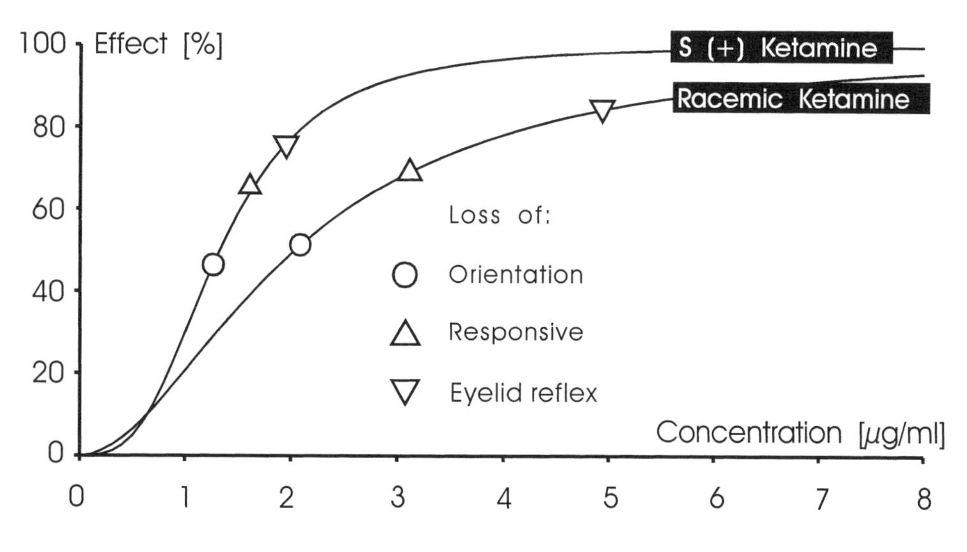

Figure 9-4. Concentration-response relationship for racemic ketamine and S(+)-ketamine in relation to specific clinical end points. The slowing of the median electroencephalographic (EEG) frequency was used as the effect (end point) and was related to the arterial blood concentrations of ketamine. (From Schüttler J, Kloos S, Ihmsen H, Pelzer E. Pharmacokinetic-pharmacodynamic properties of S(+)-ketamine versus racemic ketamine: a randomized double-blind study in volunteers. Anesthesiology 1992;77:A330.)

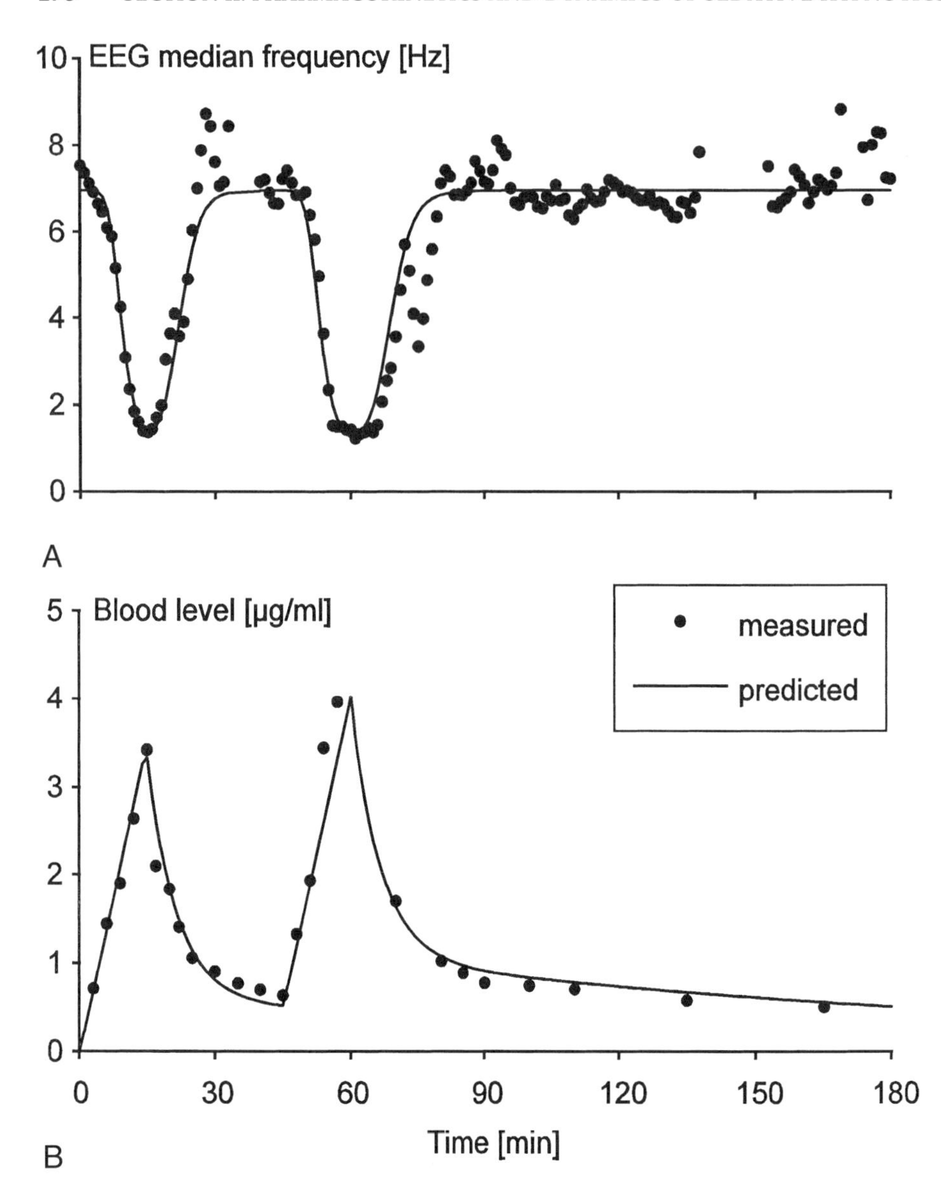

Figure 9-5. Time course of the two infusion loops in a representative case. Upper panel, Measured (filled dots) and predicted (solid lines) EEG median frequencies. Lower panel, Calculated (solid line) and measured (filled dots) concentrations of ketamine. (From Schüttler J, Kloos S, Ihmsen H, Pelzer E. Pharmacokinetic-pharmacodynamic properties of S(+)-ketamine versus racemic ketamine: a randomized double-blind study in volunteers. Anesthesiology 1992;77:A330.)

9-3 and 9-4). As expected, the required concentrations for loss of orientation and loss of the reflexes are lower for S(+) ketamine when compared with the racemic mixture, whereas the median frequencies are similar (see Fig. 9-5). The loss of orientation to person, place, and time occurred in close succession at effect levels of 40%, 50%, and 60%, respectively, followed by loss of response to verbal commands and loss of eyelid reflex (at 75%).

The pharmacokinetic-pharmacodynamic data comparing racemic ketamine and S(+) ketamine suggest that S(+) offers better controllability because S(+) ketamine has a higher clearance than the racemic mixture and a steeper concentration-effect curve. An interesting feature observed by Geisslinger and colleagues (73) and Kharasch and Labroo (74) is that the pharmacokinetics of the racemic mixture is less favorable than that of the S(+) isomer not only because of the presence

TABLE 9-3. Pharmacodynamic Parameters with the Rate Constant for the Distribution of the Biophase k_{e0} Following Administration of Either Racemic Ketamine or the S(+) Ketamine Isomers*

Parameter	Racemic Ketamine	S(+) Ketamine
$k_{e0}[min^{-1}]$	1.03±1.61	1.02±0.58
$C_{50}[\mu g/ml]$	2.76±0.49	1.42±0.29
γ	1.32±0.57	2.08±0.41
$E_0[Hz]$	8.3±1.6	7.8±0.3
$E_1[Hz]$	6.3±1.0	6.0±1.5
σ^2_{E0}	8%	11%
σ^2_{E1}	45%	42%
σ^2_{ε}	26%	21%

Data refer to arterial blood sampling and the median EEG frequency as a pharmacodynamic signal.

E_0, Baseline median EEG frequency; E_1, maximum dynamic range. σ^2_{E0}, σ^2_{E1}, interindividual of E_1 and E_0, respectively; σ^2_{ε}, all other random variation.

(From Schüttler J, Kloos S, Ihmsen H, Pelzer E. Pharmacokinetic-pharmacodynamic properties of S(+)-ketamine versus racemic ketamine: a randomized double-blind study in volunteers. Anesthesiology 1992;77:A330.)

TABLE 9-4. Comparison of the Arterial Blood Concentrations of Racemic Ketamine and S(+) Ketamine at Different Clinical End Points.

End Point	Phase	Racemic Ketamine (Blood Level [μg/ml])	S(+) Ketamine (Blood Level [μg/ml])
Orientation to time	Loss	1.61±0.57	0.87±0.26
	Return	0.88±0.22	0.45±0.15
Orientation to place	Loss	1.72±0.53	0.94±0.29
	Return	0.87±0.21	0.45±0.14
Orientation to person	Loss	1.84±0.73	0.98±0.34
	Return	1.10±0.35	0.52±0.16
Response to verbal command	Loss	2.41±0.90	1.11±0.30
	Return	1.48±0.46	0.75±0.21
Eyelid reflex	Loss	3.68±1.43	1.56±0.32
	Return	2.42±0.84	1.14±0.33

(From Schüttler J, Kloos S, Ihmsen H, Pelzer E. Pharmacokinetic-pharmacodynamic properties of S(+)-ketamine versus racemic ketamine: a randomized double-blind study in volunteers. Anesthesiology 1992;77:A330.)

of the R(−) isomer, but also because there seems to be an intrinsic S(+) and R(−) interaction. Using a stereoselective assay, Geisslinger and colleagues demonstrated that the clearance of S(+) ketamine was significantly greater (15%) than that of R(−) ketamine when the two were administered as a racemic mixture. When the isomers were administered individually, the plasma clearance of S(+) ketamine was 22% greater than that of R(−) ketamine.

Because anesthetic recovery from racemic ketamine appears to be significantly slower than recovery from the S(+) enantiomer, White and associates (13) suggested that the presence of R(−) ketamine in the racemate could exert an inhibitory influence on the recovery from the more potent S(+) enantiomer. Inhibition of S(+) ketamine metabolism by the R(−) enantiomer could account for the more prolonged recovery from the racemate. Kharasch and Labroo (74) tested the hypothesis that differences in hepatic ketamine enantiomer metabolism can account for observed differences the enantiomer pharmacokinetics of ketamine. At ketamine concentrations typically achieved during clinical anesthesia, the S(+) ketamine demethylation was 20% greater than that of R(−) ketamine and 10% greater than that of the racemate. At all ketamine concentrations, the rate of racemate demethylation was less than the sum of the individual enantiomers, suggesting that one ketamine enantiomer (R[ms]) inhibits the metabolism of the other enantiomer (S[+]).

CLINICAL USES

Since its introduction into clinical practice in the early 1970s, the clinical usefulness of ketamine has been limited because of its cardiovascular-stimulating properties and high incidence of psychomimetic emergence

TABLE 9-5. Clinical Uses of Ketamine in the Practice of Anesthesiology.

- Induction of anesthesia in high-risk patients
  - Shock or cardiovascular instability
  - Severe dehydration
  - Bronchospasm
  - Severe anemia
  - One-lung anesthesia
- Obstetric patients
  - Induction of general anesthesia
    - Severe hypovolemia
    - Acute hemorrhage
    - Acute bronchospasm
  - Low-dose for analgesia
    - To supplement regional anesthetic techniques
  - At the time of delivery or during the postpartum period
- Adjunct to local and regional anesthetic techniques
  - For sedation and analgesia during performance of nerve block procedures
  - To supplement an inadequate block
- Outpatient surgery
  - For brief diagnostic and therapeutic procedures
  - To supplement local and regional block techniques
- Use outside the operating room
  - In burn units (e.g., debridement, dressing changes)
  - In emergency rooms (e.g., closed reductions)
  - In intensive care units (e.g., sedation, painful procedures)
  - In recovery rooms (e.g., postoperative sedation and analgesia)

(From Gajraj N, White PF. Clinical pharmacology and applications of ketamine. In: Bowdle, et al, eds. The pharmacologic basis of anesthesiology. New York: Churchill Livingstone, 1994:375–392.)

reactions. However, supplementation with other sedative-hypnotic drugs (e.g., diazepam, midazolam, thiopental, and propofol) has reduced the incidence of these side effects. Therefore, ketamine has become a valuable drug in specific clinical situations (Table 9-5) (75).

Ketamine is an ideal anesthetic agent for anesthesia for catastrophic surgery (e.g., war, mass casualties, accidents, massive hemorrhage, inaccessibility to the victim's body). In the latter situations, ketamine can be given safely by a jet injector because of its high therapeutic index. In children, ketamine is well-suited for magnetic resonance imaging because an infusion of ketamine can be easily titrated from a remote area. Given its pulmonary and circulatory effects, ketamine may be the anesthetic of choice in areas where trained anesthesiologists are not readily available during the performance of brief, painful procedures (e.g., for burn dressing changes, bone marrow biopsies and spinal taps in children, for insertion of invasive monitors, intubation for of status asthmaticus, pericardiotomy).

Cardiothoracic Anesthesia

The cardiostimulatory properties of ketamine can produce serious sequelae in patients with cardiac disease. Although labetalol (1 mg/kg intravenously) is effective in attenuating the ketamine-induced rise in heart rate and blood pressure, benzodiazepines are also used for this purpose (76). When a ketamine infusion was administered in combination with high-dose diazepam and N_2O for cardiac anesthesia, adequate anesthetic conditions were produced with minimal effect on the cardiorespiratory system (77). Results showed excellent anterograde amnesia, satisfactory analgesia, and no postoperative emergence reactions. Diazepam (0.3 to 0.5 mg/kg intravenously) effectively prevents the increase in the rate-pressure product following administration of ketamine (78). As mentioned earlier, ketamine-induced cardiovascular stimulation and the concomitant rise in plasma norepinephrine levels can be significantly decreased by premedication with diazepam (79). Flunitrazepam and midazolam also effectively attenuate the cardostimulatory response produced by ketamine.

In a study comparing a morphine-diazepam-N_2O combination with ketamine-N_2O-induced anesthesia for coronary bypass surgery, Reves and associates (80) found that, although the overall number of changes in this rate-pressure product was similar, the mean maximal increases in systolic blood pressure and rate-pressure product would have been less if diazepam had also been incorporated as part of the ketamine regimen. Nevertheless, these investigators found no significant difference between the two treatment groups with respect to perioperative morbidity and mortality rates.

In a controlled study of the circulatory responses during induction and maintenance of anesthesia in patients undergoing heart valve replacement, Dhadphale and associates (81) found no significant differences between the diazepam-ketamine-N_2O and morphine-N_2O techniques. These investigators believed that high-dose diazepam (0.5 mg/kg intravenously) combined with ketamine (1 to 2 mg/kg for induction and 15 to 30 μg/kg/min for maintenance) was a satisfactory alternative to morphine-N_2O-induced anesthesia for patients with coronary artery disease and for those undergoing heart valve replacement. A potential advantage of the diazepam-ketamine technique is that the N_2O concentration is not critical, and therefore, 100% oxygen can be used. As with any "balanced" anesthetic technique, the patient may recall intraoperative events during cardiac surgery with a diazepam-ketamine anesthetic technique. Apart from its intrinsic anesthetic properties, ketamine produces minimal, if any, anterograde amnesia. The adjunctive use of either lorazepam or midazolam would be expected to decrease the possibility of intraoperative recall when ketamine is used without N_2O.

High-dose opioid techniques (e.g., fentanyl 50 to 150 μg/kg or sufentanil 5 to 15 μg/kg) have been popular for anesthetic induction of hemodynamically unstable patients undergoing cardiac surgery. In a comparison of ketamine and sufentanil for the induction of anesthesia in patients with severe cardiomyopathy who were undergoing cardiac transplantation, Gutzke and colleagues (82) reported that ketamine maintained a stable cardiac index and heart rate at the expense of increased wall tension. In patients undergoing elective coronary bypass surgery, fentanyl (50 μg/kg) effectively obtunded the sympathomimetic actions of ketamine (1.5 mg/kg) (83). In contrast to the commonly used sedative hypnotics (thiopental and etomidate), the use of ketamine to supplement fentanyl-induced anesthesia was not associated with significant hemodynamic changes. Furthermore, when ketamine or fentanyl was administered as an intravenous adjunct during thoracic surgery, ketamine was associated with more prolonged postoperative analgesia than fentanyl (84).

Many cardiac anesthesiologists have considered ketamine the drug of choice for inducing and maintaining anesthesia in patients with cardiac tamponade or constrictive pericarditis because ketamine maintains sympathetic nervous system activity, even though ketamine may further increase the pulmonary vascular resistance. In these patients, the hemodynamic response to ketamine varies considerably, especially if the pulmonary capillary wedge pressure exceeds 15 mm Hg. Further studies are needed in these surgical populations.

Extensive experience with the use of ketamine for pediatric cardiac catheterizations suggests that it provides adequate sedative-hypnotic conditions with fewer catheter-associated arrhythmias than the volatile anesthetics. Compared with propofol, the mean systolic blood pressure is better maintained, although the recovery time is longer (85). Yet, clinical evidence suggests that ketamine can sensitize the myocardium to circulating catecholamines. Nevertheless, a combination of midazolam and low-dose ketamine has been used successfully for sedation and analgesia during electrical cardioversions. When ketamine is used for cardiac catheterization in adults, it can produce significant decreases in blood pressure.

Critically Ill Patients

Ketamine has been used in critically ill patients, in whom a period of hypotension or apnea can be life-threatening. Park and associates (10) described the use of a ketamine infusion as a sedative, inotrope, and bronchodilator in a critically ill patient. Sharma (86) also reported on the use of intravenous ketamine in two patients with acute severe asthma who did not respond to conventional therapy. An infusion of ketamine at a rate of 0.15 mg/kg/min was used in each case to prevent a recurrence of bronchospasm. When ketamine was used in critically ill patients, it was reported to provide good surgical anesthesia with a greater margin of safety than "conventional" anesthesia.

The use of ketamine during major surgical procedures in elderly patients has been associated with hemodynamic stability and a rapid emergence, with a low incidence of unpleasant dreams. Stefansson and colleagues (87) reported that using ketamine as the sole anesthetic for hip fracture surgery in the geriatric patient resulted in a survival rate that did not differ significantly from that seen with other common anesthetic techniques, including epidural and volatile anesthetics. Furthermore, Pedersen and associates (88) reported that ketamine, in contrast to thiopental, did not decrease cardiac output when the drug was used for the induction of anesthesia in critically ill patients. The so-called "slow-dose" ketamine technique, which consists of a benzodiazepine (e.g., diazepam 2 to 5 mg intravenously) followed by an infusion of ketamine (2 to 4 mg/min) can also be extremely useful in aged patients and in those at high risk (89).

Ketamine is regarded by some clinicians as advantageous for patients in hemorrhagic shock; others dispute its usefulness in this situation. In contrast to the marked pressor response following ketamine administration in normovolemic subjects, induction with ketamine in patients who are hypovolemic secondary to acute hemorrhage causes no significant change or even a slight decrease in blood pressure. Rather than clarifying the cardiovascular and metabolic actions of ketamine, animal studies have produced conflicting results.

In experimental hemorrhagic and septic shock, ketamine significantly increases systolic and diastolic blood pressure. Compared with hypovolemic barbiturate anesthetized rats, hypovolemic rats anesthetized with ketamine had significantly greater perfusion to their vital organs. Using a dog model, ketamine was found more effective than either thiopental or diazepam in maintaining renal blood flow (90). Furthermore, a higher survival rate was reported in hypotensive rats anesthetized with ketamine compared with halothane. In contrast to the volatile anesthetics, Longnecker and associates (91) demonstrated that ketamine diminished the arteriolar response to hemorrhage, and therefore, tissue hypoxia did not occur. On the other hand, Weiskopf and colleagues (92) found that ketamine produced a greater base deficit and larger increases in arterial lactate concentration than did the volatile agents. These investigators reported that, in spite of its ability to increase catecholamine levels, the use of ketamine was associated with cardiovascular depression and metabolic acidosis (93).

Critically ill patients occasionally respond to ketamine with an unexpected drop in blood pressure, which may result from the inability of the sympathomimetic actions of ketamine to counterbalance its direct myocardial depressant and vasodilatory effects. A diminished catecholamine response to ketamine following prolonged stress can result in a maldistribution of systemic blood flow. Waxman and associates (39) observed occasional decreases in cardiac and pulmonary performance when ketamine was used to induce anesthesia in critically ill and acutely traumatized patients.

Patients with Pulmonary Disease

As a result of its salutary effects on airway resistance, ketamine may be the agent of choice for the rapid induction of anesthesia in patients with reactive airway disease. Furthermore, ketamine is an alternative to the volatile agents for maintenance of anesthesia in patients who are receiving parenteral bronchodilators. However, concurrent administration of ketamine and aminophylline may decrease the seizure threshold (94).

Ketamine is an excellent alternative to the volatile agents for one-lung anesthesia in patients with preexisting pulmonary disease and abnormal preoperative blood gas values. When one-lung anesthesia was used during thoracic surgery, patients with impaired pulmonary function had improved oxygenation and decreased pulmonary shunt fractions when a diazepam-ketamine infusion-muscle relaxant anesthetic technique was used as an alternative to conventional inhalation techniques (41). The difference appeared to be a result of ketamine's ability to preserve the hypoxic vasoconstrictor reflex. Ketamine would also be advantageous in clinical situations in which a high inspired oxygen concentration is required to maintain adequate tissue oxygenation (e.g., severe anemia and cerebrovascular insufficiency).

Obstetric Anesthesia and Analgesia

Early studies using ketamine anesthesia for routine vaginal deliveries reported an unacceptably high incidence of maternal complications and depressed infants with low Apgar scores. These problems were shown to be dose related. When lower doses of ketamine (0.2 to 0.5 mg/kg intravenously) were used, neonates were not depressed, and complications were minimal, with high patient acceptance. Nevertheless, even when subanesthetic doses of ketamine are used to produce obstetric analgesia, most of these patients experience a dream-like state.

Ketamine, given in combination with N_2O for obstetric anesthesia, produces virtually no recall of pain during delivery, and although dreaming occurs in many patients, a majority of the dreams are pleasant, with excellent patient acceptance. The use of larger doses of ketamine (more than 1.5 mg/kg intravenously) for inducing anesthesia in unpremedicated parturients produces good surgical anesthesia; however, recovery from anesthesia is often unpleasant. In a large obstetric series comparing low-dose ketamine

(0.5 mg/kg intravenously) with methoxyflurane (0.25 to 10%), ketamine produced a more rapid onset of action and was the superior analgesic; patient acceptance was similar for the two groups. The use of droperidol as an adjunct to ketamine prolonged the recovery period without decreasing the incidence of adverse emergence reactions.

Compared with thiopental for induction of anesthesia before cesarean section, ketamine provided rapid induction and greater analgesia and amnesia, with a similar incidence of unpleasant emergence reactions. However, the incidence of undesirable psychotomimetic reactions was low following both induction agents. Using ketamine as the sole anesthetic for cesarean section in developing countries has been reported to result in lower fetal mortality rates than with other general anesthetic techniques.

In comparison with thiopental, ketamine is advantageous for hypovolemic patients (e.g., abruptio placentae, placenta previa) and for patients with acute bronchospasm. Some investigators suggest that ketamine may be a useful analgesic for managing the hemodynamically unstable preeclamptic patient because of its anticonvulsant properties; however, this agent should be used with caution in this situation because its cardiostimulatory properties can precipitate a hypertensive crisis.

No clinical reports have been published regarding fetal acid-base changes following ketamine anesthesia; however, animal studies indicate that ketamine increases uterine blood flow without adversely affecting fetal cardiovascular or acid-base status. Using a chronic sheep preparation with induced fetal acidosis, Pickering and associates (95) found better preservation of blood pressure and cerebral blood flow following administration of ketamine compared with thiopental. Arterial blood gas evaluations in mothers and infants receiving ketamine-induced analgesia for vaginal delivery showed no significant differences compared with those in patients who received regional anesthesia. In a comparative study of ketamine and thiopental for rapid intravenous induction before cesarean section, ketamine-treated patients showed higher maternal umbilical artery and vein pH and base excess values (96).

Neonatal arterial blood pressure has been reported to be less depressed after maternal ketamine anesthesia compared with a similar group receiving thiopental (97). Neonatal neurobehavioral scores following vaginal delivery with ketamine, 0.7 mg/kg intravenously, and 50% N_2O or 2% chloroprocaine epidural anesthesia revealed the greatest percentage of high scores in the epidural group, intermediate values following ketamine-N_2O, and the lowest scores after thiopental-N_2O (98).

The reduced blood loss that has been reported when ketamine was used as an induction agent for first-trimester abortions may be related to its ability to increase both uterine tone and the intensity of uterine contractions. However, a study comparing ketamine-midazolam with methohexital found no difference in blood loss (99). In parturients, ketamine has been reported to have variable effects on uterine tone and contractility. Ketamine can induce contractions equal to those induced by ergonovine when ketamine is administered during the first trimester of pregnancy, and it produces dose-related changes in uterine activity in the full-term pregnant uterus. So called "analgesic" doses of ketamine (0.2 to 0.4 mg/kg intravenously) increase the intensity of uterine contractions. Similarly, ketamine increases both basal uterine tone and the intensity of contractions in the nonpregnant uterus.

Pediatric Anesthesia

Ketamine has been used by the oral route to premedicate pediatric patients. In one study, 6 mg/kg of ketamine mixed with 0.2 ml/kg of cola-flavored drink was well accepted (100). Predictable sedation occurred within 20 to 25 minutes without significant side effects. Intramuscular ketamine (4 to 8 mg/kg) was also extremely useful for induction of anesthesia before administering an inhalational agent and for diagnostic and minor surgical procedures not requiring intravenous cannulae or endotracheal intubation.

Ketamine has been used successfully for oral surgical procedures and diagnostic muscle biopsies lasting from 5 to 30 minutes (doses, 1 to 3 mg/kg intramuscularly or 0.5 to 1.0 mg/kg intravenously). However, the reported side effects include cardiovascular stimulation, partial airway obstruction, and minor postanesthetic complications, including unpleasant dreams. Diazepam (5 to 10 mg orally) combined with ketamine (3 mg/kg intramuscularly) can provide excellent sedation with few side effects for children requiring oral surgical procedures lasting 45 to 60 minutes (101).

In children undergoing minor otolaryngologic procedures, ketamine (2 mg/kg intravenously) compared favorably with thiopental (4 mg/kg) (102). Although the operating conditions were similar, thiopental produced more cardiorespiratory depression and a greater need for postoperative analgesics; ketamine was associated with a higher incidence of restlessness and a more prolonged recovery period. Ketamine (10 mg/kg intramuscularly) has also been used for bronchoscopy in children without significant complications. However, ketamine stimulated the production of copious amounts of upper airway secretions, necessitating concomitant use of an antisialagogue. Furthermore, anecdotal reports indicate that ketamine may produce "hyperreactive" airway reflexes, especially when the upper respiratory tract is inflamed (e.g., in burned patients).

Finally, rectal ketamine (7.5 to 15 mg/kg) has been used successfully as an induction agent in pediatric anesthesia. Compared with rectal methohexital (25 mg/kg), the use of ketamine (15 mg/kg per rectum) for induction was associated with a higher incidence of airway complications during the preoperative period (103). Although there is a high degree of acceptance of ketamine in children undergoing repeated anesthesia for radiotherapy anesthesia, tolerance to its CNS effects may develop.

Anesthesia for Burned Patients

Ketamine has also been used extensively in burn units for dressing changes and skin grafting procedures in children and adults. Intramuscular ketamine (2 to 6 mg/kg) produces excellent surgical conditions for eschar excision. The relatively rapid recovery from ketamine causes minimal delays in resuming nutritional intake. Rare emergence reactions (mild excitement or illusions) have been noted in unpremedicated burned patients. In premedicated patients, even lower doses of ketamine (1 to 2 mg/kg intramuscularly) can produce good operating conditions, amnesia, and satisfactory analgesia with a rapid recovery and resumption of normal activities. However, tolerance to ketamine has appeared to develop in all patients receiving more than two exposures, and the dose requirement increases progressively in patients receiving repeated doses of ketamine.

Sedation and Analgesia

During the performance of a painful nerve block, the ideal adjunctive drug would provide analgesia, sedation, and amnesia without cardiorespiratory depression. In comparing the clinical effectiveness and acceptability of diazepam, droperidol-fentanyl, and ketamine for sedation and analgesia before intercostal nerve blocks, ketamine was reported to produce more optimal conditions during the block procedure and higher patient acceptance (104). Furthermore, the use of a diazepam (0.15 mg/kg)-ketamine (0.5 mg/kg) combination was not associated with increased side effects or a greater need for postoperative care than an unpremedicated group undergoing similar nerve block procedures. More important, patient acceptance was significantly better in the diazepam-ketamine group. Low-dose ketamine combined with a benzodiazepine has become increasingly popular during the injection of local anesthetics for outpatient cosmetic procedures. Patients are reported to be more comfortable and cooperative with this drug combination (38).

In a randomized double-blind study, midazolam was compared with diazepam for sedation when administered as an adjuvant to ketamine during local anesthesia (105). Midazolam (0.05 to 0.15 mg/kg intravenously) was found to produce a spectrum of CNS activity similar to that of diazepam (0.1 to 0.3 mg/kg intravenously). However, the slope of midazolam's dose-response curve for sedation appeared to be steeper (i.e., a narrower therapeutic dosage range). In a comparative evaluation, midazolam (0.1 mg/kg intravenously) produced more profound sedation and amnesia than diazepam (0.2 mg/kg intravenously). Midazolam was associated with significantly less pain on injection and a lower incidence of postoperative venoirritation. Although recovery characteristics were similar for the two benzodiazepines when used as adjuvants to ketamine, overall patient acceptance was higher with midazolam than with diazepam.

Ketamine infusions (1 to 1.5 mg/min) have been used during the early postoperative period for sedation and analgesia. In achieving adequate postoperative analgesia with ketamine, profound sedation also is produced. When used to sedate patients requiring postoperative ventilatory support, ketamine was reported to decrease agitation and the analgesic requirements (69).

Outpatient Anesthesia

It appears that ketamine can be used for induction and maintenance of outpatient anesthesia if the minimal effective dose of ketamine (0.5 to 1.0 mg/kg for induction followed by continuous infusion of 15 to 30 μg/kg/min) is administered in combination with N_2O and thiopental (1 to 3 mg/kg) or midazolam (0.7 to 0.15 mg/kg). To provide for a more rapid recovery following brief outpatient procedures, a combination of propofol (1 to 3 mg/kg intravenously) for induction followed by a continuous infusion of ketamine (3 to 6 mg/min) and N_2O (70% in oxygen) is recommended. The use of a continuous infusion of ketamine significantly decreases the drug dosage requirement, improves intraoperative conditions, and decreases recovery time compared with the traditional intermittent bolus technique (106). Although ketamine and N_2O produced superior intraoperative conditions compared with a fentanyl-N_2O combination, recovery times were more prolonged, and side effects were more frequent with the ketamine-based technique (9).

Ketamine Infusions

The titration of intravenous anesthetics such as ketamine using small incremental bolus doses has been performed by anesthesiologists for many years. Continuous infusion is a logical extension of this method of titration because it minimizes the fluctuations in blood and hence brain ketamine concentrations following intermittent bolus injections (107). To achieve a therapeutic blood level more rapidly, it is necessary to

TABLE 9-6. Use of Ketamine Infusion as Part of a Balanced Anesthetic Technique for Major Abdominal Surgery, Cardiac Surgery, and Gynecologic Surgery

		Induction				
Investigator	Premedication	Adjunct	(mg/kg)	Ketamine (mg/kg)	Nitrous Oxide (%)	Maintenance Ketamine (μg/kg/min)
Major abdominal surgery						
Hatano et al (1979)	Diazepam	Diazepam	0.2–0.3	1.3–2.0	66	10–15
Houlton and Downing (1978)	Omnopon (papaveretum)	Flunitrazepam	0.3	—	—	33
Idvall et al (1979)	Atropine/meperidine, droperidol/fentanyl	—	—	2.0	50	41
Cardiac surgery						
Hatano et al (1976)	Diazepam		0.5–0.5	1.0	50	12
Jackson et al (1978)	Morphine		0.4	2.0	—	90
Dhadphale et al (1979)	Morphine		0.4	2.0	50	17
Gynecologic surgery						
El-Naggar et al (1977)	Diazepam	Diazepam	0.2	0.5–1.0	66	17–34
Liburn et al (1978)	Lorazepam		—	1.0	—	66–83
Barclay et al (1980)	Papaveretum, atropine	Flunitrazepam, atropine	0.3	—	40–60	16–81
Freuchen et al (1981)	Flunitrazepam	Flunitrazepam	0.3	1.0	60	18

(From Gajraj N, White PF. Clinical pharmacology and applications of ketamine. In: Bowdle, et al, eds. The pharmacologic basis of anesthesiology. New York: Churchill Livingstone, 1994:375–392.)

administer a loading dose (LD). To maintain a desired drug concentration, it is necessary to infuse the drug continuously. Although infusions are usually administered on an empiric basis, a knowledge of basic pharmacokinetic principles may allow the anesthesiologist to predict more accurately the dosage requirements (108). Pharmacokinetic data for ketamine can be used to calculate the LD and the initial maintenance infusion rate (MIR).

Two simple equations can be used to estimate the LD and MIR for ketamine, as follows:

$$\text{LD } (\mu g/kg) = \text{Cp } (\mu g/ml) \times \text{V } (ml/kg)$$

$$\text{MIR } (\mu g/kg/min) = \text{Cp } (\mu g/ml) \times \text{CL } (ml/kg/min)$$

where Cp = plasma drug concentration, V = volume of distribution, and CL = clearance of drug.

The ranges of ketamine population pharmacokinetic values are Cp = 0.2 to 2.5 μg/ml, V = 0.6 to 3.0 ml/kg, and CL = 15 to 20 ml/kg/min.

The loading dose can be administered as either a bolus or as a rapid "priming" infusion. Because side effects appear to be more severe with rapid fluctuations in plasma drug concentrations, a loading infusion may be preferred to a loading bolus. The required plasma drug concentration depends on the desired pharmacologic effect (e.g., sedation and hypnosis), the presence of other centrally active drugs, the type of operation, and the individual's sensitivity to the drug (e.g., age, level of anxiety, and drug history). The influence of premedication, adjunctive drugs, N_2O, and type of operation on the maintenance requirement for ketamine is shown in Table 9-6.

Which clinical signs are most useful in deciding whether to increase or decrease the MIR of ketamine? Although the most sensitive clinical signs of depth of anesthesia appear to be changes in muscle tone and ventilatory pattern, the physician must rely on evidence of autonomic hyperactivity (e.g., sweating, lacrimation, tachycardia, hypertension, and pupillary dilatation) if the patient has received a muscle relaxant. Although the blood pressure response to surgical stimulation may be a useful guide in judging the depth of anesthesia with volatile anesthetics, it is a less reliable index when intravenous anesthetics are used. Table 9-7 summarizes an approach to using a ketamine infusion as part of a "balanced" anesthetic technique as well as for sedation and analgesia during local and regional anesthesia.

Epidural Ketamine

Theoretically, the administration of ketamine by the epidural or intrathecal route should be able to produce analgesia without sympathetic blockade or respiratory depression (109). Epidural ketamine was reported to be effective in producing postoperative analgesia. In an uncontrolled study of 50 patients, Islas and colleagues (110) claimed potent analgesia from 4 mg epidural ketamine. Naquib and associates (111) reported using up to 30 mg epidural ketamine in patients who underwent cholecystectomy, with 54% of patients receiving 30 mg having adequate analgesia for up to 24 hours. In a more recent study, ketamine was compared with bupivacaine for caudal analgesia in 50 children undergoing inguinal herniotomy (112). Caudal administration of ketamine, 0.5 mg/kg, produced postoperative analgesia comparable to that associated with cau-

TABLE 9-7. Recommendations for Using Ketamine as a Sedative, Analgesic, or Anesthetic During the Perioperative Period

Premedication
- A benzodiazepine administered either orally (e.g., diazepam, 15–30 mg or lorazepam, 2–5 mg) 60–90 min before surgery or IV (e.g. midazolam 0.05–0.1 mg/kg) immediately before induction of anesthesia as an adjunctive agent
- If preoperative sedation is contraindicated, a benzodiazepine can be administered IV after induction of anesthesia but before termination of surgery; An antisialagogue (e.g., glycopyrrolate, 0.005 mg/kg IV) can effectively decrease secretions if administered 5–10 min before induction

Induction of anesthesia
- Ketamine, 0.5–1.5 mg/kg IV, or 4–6 mg/kg IM
- Lower doses of ketamine are used if thiopental (1–2 mg/kg IV) midazolam (0.075–0.15 mg/kg), or propofol (0.75–1.5 mg/kg IV) is used as a coinduction agent in place of the premedicant or if the patient is elderly or critically Ill.

Maintenance of anesthesia
- Ketamine 15–45 μg/kg/min (1–3 mg/min) by continuous IV infusion with supplemental nitrous oxide, 70%; following a barbiturate (or propofol) induction, a higher initial maintenance infusion rate is required (e.g., 30–90 μg/kg/min)

Sedation and analgesia
- Ketamine, 0.2–0.8 mg/kg IV (over 2–3 min) or 2–4 mg/kg IM, followed by a continuous ketamine infusion (5–20 μg/kg/min) with or without supplemental oxygen

(From Gajraj N, White PF. Clinical pharmacology and applications of ketamine. In: Bowdle T, et al, eds. The pharmacologic basis of anesthesiology. New York: Churchill Livingstone, 1994:375–392.)

dal injection of 0.25% bupivacaine, 1 ml/kg. Two studies comparing epidural ketamine with epidural morphine, however, found that morphine was the more potent and longer-acting analgesic (Fig. 9-6) (113, 114).

Patients With Uncommon Diseases

Although ketamine can increase skeletal muscle tone and can occasionally produce muscle spasms, it has been used safely in patients with various myopathies and in those with a history compatible with malignant hyperthermia (115). Even though ketamine increases ALA synthetase activity in animals, it was used successfully to anesthetize patients with acute intermittent porphyria and hereditary coproporphyria (116, 117). A diazepam and ketamine combination was used successfully to provide anesthesia for a patient with malignant carcinoid syndrome and associated tricuspid valvular disease (118). Ketamine was also used for a patient with Shy-Drager syndrome (119).

In summary, ketamine is a safe, rapid-acting, intravenous anesthetic and analgesic agent. Ketamine alone increases blood pressure and heart rate and produces profuse salivation, lacrimation, sweating, skeletal muscle hypertonus, involuntary purposeless movements, and agitation or even transient delirium during emergence. The use of a continuous infusion technique allows the anesthesiologist to titrate the drug more closely and, thereby, to reduce the total amount of drug required. Benzodiazepines are highly effective in preventing the marked cardiovascular responses and unpleasant emergence reactions associated with ketamine anesthesia. A combination of ketamine and midazolam was useful for rapid induction of anesthesia and can also be used for maintenance of anesthesia and sedation during total intravenous anesthesia.

Numerous clinical studies have appeared in the literature over the last 15 years using ketamine infusion techniques. The clinical pharmacology and therapeutic uses of ketamine were initially reviewed in 1982 (17) and were subsequently updated in 1989 (120) and 1994 (75). Clinical applications for ketamine in anesthesia include a role in total intravenous anesthesia for major surgery, in the management of acute trauma, and in ambulatory surgery. Ketamine is widely used for sedation and analgesia during procedures using local anesthesia. In addition, ketamine can be used in intensive care units and emergency rooms for providing acute pain relief during brief procedures or painful manipulations. Although ketamine apparently does not possess all the physicochemical and pharmacologic properties of an ideal intravenous anesthetic (17), its diverse pharmacologic properties provide important insights in the continuing search for an intravenous drug that will be closer to the ideal. The availability of S(+) ketamine for clinical use would be a step in the right direction. However, this isomer of ketamine still possesses many of the side effects associated with the currently available racemic mixture.

REFERENCES

1. Corssen G. Historical aspects of ketamine: first clinical experience. In: Domino EF, ed. Status of ketamine in anesthesiology. NPP Books, 1990:1–5.
2. Corssen G, Domino EF. Dissociative anesthesia: further pharmacologic studies and first clinical experience with the phencyclidine derivative CI-581. Anesth Analg 1966;42:29–40.
3. White PF, Ham J, Way WL, Trevor AJ. Pharmacology of ketamine isomers in surgical patients. Anesthesiology 1980;52:231–239.
4. Chang T, Glazko AJ. Biotransformation and disposition of ketamine. Int Anesthesiol Clin 1974;12:157–177.
5. Wieber J, Gugler R, Hengstmann JH, Dengler HJ. Pharmacokinetics of ketamine in man. Anaesthesist 1975;24:260–263.
6. Dayton PG, Stiller RL, Cook DR, Perel JM. The binding of ketamine to plasma proteins: emphasis on human plasma. Eur J Clin Pharmacol 1983;24:825–831.
7. Grant IS, Nimmo WS, McNicol LR, Clements JA. Ketamine disposition in children and adults. Br J Anaesth 1983;55:1107–1111.
8. Clements JA, Nimmo WS. The pharmacokinetics and analgesic effect of ketamine in man. Br J Anaesth 1981;53:27–30.
9. White PF, Dworsky WA, Horai Y, Trevor AJ. Comparison of continuous infusion fentanyl or ketamine versus thiopental: determining the mean effective serum concentrations for outpatient surgery. Anesthesiology 1983;59:564–569.

10. Park GR, Manara AR, Mendel L, et al. Ketamine infusion: its use as a sedative, inotrope, and bronchodilator in a critically ill patient. Anaesthesia 1987;42:980.
11. White PF, Johnston RR, Pudwill CR. Interaction of ketamine and halothane in rats. Anesthesiology 1975;42:179–207.
12. Schüttler J, Stanski DR, White PF, et al. Pharmacodynamic modeling of the EEG effects of ketamine and its enantiomers in man. J Pharmacokinet Biopharm 1987;15:241–253.
13. White PF, Schüttler J, Shafer A, et al. Comparative pharmacology of the ketamine isomers. Br J Anaesth 1985;57:197–203.
14. Miyasaka M, Domino EF. Neuronal mechanisms of ketamine-induced anesthesia. Int J Neuropharmacol 1968;7:557–573.
15. Domino EF, Chodoff P, Corssen G. Pharmacologic effects of CI-581, a new dissociative anesthetic in man. Clin Pharmacol Ther 1965;6:279.
16. Schwender D, Faber-Züllig E, Fett W, et al. Akustisch evozierte potentiale mittlerer Latenz. Anaesthesist 1993;42:280–287.
17. White PF, Way WL, Trevor AJ. Ketamine: its pharmacology and therapeutic uses. Anesthesiology 1982;56:119–136.
18. Shapiro HM, Wyte SR, Harris AB. Ketamine anesthesia in patients with intracranial pathology. Br J Anaesth 1972;44:1200–1204.
19. Gardener AE, Olson BE, Lichtiger M. Cerebrospinal fluid pressure during dissociative anesthesia with ketamine. Anesthesiology 1971;35:226–229.
20. Takeshita H, Okuda Y, Sari A. The effects of ketamine on cerebral circulation and metabolism in man. Anesthesiology 1972; 36:69–75.
21. Bennett DR, Madsen JA, Jordan WS, Wiser WC. Ketamine anesthesia in brain-damaged epileptics. Neurology 1973;23:449–460.
22. Ferrer-Allado T, Brechner VL, Dymond A, et al. Ketamine-induced electroconvulsive phenomena in the human limbic and thalamic region. Anesthesiology 1973;38:333–344.
23. Corssen G, Little EB, Tavakoli M. Ketamine and epilepsy. Anesth Analg 1974;53:319–335.
24. Celesia GG, Chen RC, Bamforth BJ. Effects of ketamine in epilepsy. Neurology 1975;25:169–172.
25. Church J. The anticonvulsant activity of ketamine and other phencyclidine receptor ligands, with particular reference to N-methyl-D-aspartate receptor mediated events. In: Domino EF, ed. Status of ketamine in anesthesiology. NPP Books, 1990:521–540.
26. Velisek L, Mares P. Anticonvulsant action of ketamine in laboratory animals. In: Domino EF, ed. Status of ketamine in anesthesiology. NPP Books, 1990:541–547.
27. Zsigmond EK, Kelsch RC, Kothary SP, Vadnay L. Plasma norepinephrine concentrations during anesthetic induction with ketamine. Rev Brasil Anest 1972;22:443–451.
28. Stanley TH. Blood pressure and pulse rate responses to ketamine during general anesthesia. Anesthesiology 1973;648–649.
29. Chodoff P. Evidence for central adrenergic action of ketamine. Anesth Analg 1972;51:247–250.
30. Slogoff S, Allen GW. The role of baroreceptors in the cardiovascular response to ketamine. Anesth Analg 1974;53:704–707.
31. McGrath JC, MacKenzie JE, Miller RAL. Effects of ketamine on central sympathetic discharge and the baroreceptor reflex during mechanical ventilation. Br J Anaesth 1975;47:1141–1147.
32. Traber DL, Wilson RD, Priano LL, et al. Blockade of the hypertensive response to ketamine. Anesth Analg 1970;49:420–426.
33. Traber DL, Wilson RD, Priano LL. Differentiation of the cardiovascular effects of CI581. Anesth Analg 1968;47:769–778.
34. Schwatz DA, Horwitz LD. Effects of ketamine on left ventricular performance. J Pharmacol Exp Ther 1975;194:410–414.
35. Goldberg AH, Keane PW, Phear WPC. Effects of ketamine on contractile performance and excitability of isolated heart muscle. J Pharmacol Exp Ther 1970;175:388–394.
36. Davies AE, McCane JL. Effects of barbiturate anesthetics and ketamine on the force-frequency relation of cardiac muscle. Eur J Pharmacol 1979;26:65–73.
37. Cabbabe EB, Behbahani PM. Cardiovascular reactions associated with the use of ketamine and epinephrine in plastic surgery. Ann Plast Surg 1985;15:50.
38. White PF. Use of ketamine for sedation and analgesia during injection of local anaesthetics. Ann Plast Surg 1985;15:53–56.
39. Waxman K, Shoemaker WC, Lippmann M. Cardiovascular effects of anesthetic induction with ketamine. Anesth Analg 1989; 59:355–358.
40. Gooding JM, Dimick AR, Tavakoli M. A physiologic analysis of cardiopulmonary responses to ketamine anesthesia in noncardiac patients. Anesth Analg 1977;56:813.
41. Lumb PD, Silvay G, Weinreich AI, et al. A comparison of the effects of continuous ketamine infusion and halothane on oxygenation during one-lung anesthesia. Can Anaesth Soc J 1979; 26:394.
42. Dawson B, Michenfelder D, Theye A. Effects of ketamine on canine cerebral blood flow and metabolism: modification by prior administration of thiopental. Anesth Analg 1971;50:443.
43. Mayberg TS, Lam AM, Matta BF, et al. Ketamine does not increase cerebral blood flow velocity or intracranial pressure during isoflurane/nitrous oxide anesthesia in patients undergoing craniotomy. Anesth Analg 1995;81:84–89.
44. Zsigmond EK, Matsuki A, Kothary SP, Jallad M. Arterial hypoxemia caused by intravenous ketamine. Anesth Analg 1976; 55:311–314.
45. Zsigmond EK, Kothary SP, Matsuki A, Flynn KB. Comparison of the effect of ketamine with three structurally unrelated analgesics on arterial blood gases. In: Langrehr E, ed. Ketamine and the cardiovascular system. Amsterdam: Excerpta Medica, 1980:41–47.
46. Rust M, Landauer B, Kolb E. Stellwert von ketamin in der notfallsituationen. Anaesthesist 1978;27:205.
47. Maduska AL, Hajghassemali M. Arterial blood gases in mothers and infants during ketamine anesthesia for surgical delivery. Anesth Analg 1978;57:121–123.
48. Morel DR, Foster A, Gemperle M. Noninvasive evaluation of breathing pattern and thoraco-abdominal motion following the infusion of ketamine or droperidol in humans. Anesthesiology 1986;65:392.
49. Manikikian B, Cantineau JP, Sartene R, et al. Ventilatory pattern and chest wall mechanics during ketamine anesthesia in humans. Anesthesiology 1986;65:492.
50. Corssen G, Gutierrez J, Reves JG, Huber FC. Ketamine in the anesthetic management of asthmatic patients. Anesth Analg 1972;51:588.
51. Hirshman CA, Downes H, Farbood A, et al. Ketamine block of bronchospasm in experimental canine asthma. Br J Anaesth 1979;51:713–718.
52. Zsigmond EK. Invited comment on Corssen G. Ketamine in the anesthetic management of asthmatic patients. Anesth Analg 1972;51:595–596.
53. Hirota K, Sato T, Rabito SF, et al. Relaxant effect of ketamine and its isomers on histamine-induced contraction of tracheal smooth muscle in guinea pigs. Br J Anaesth 1996;76:266–270.
54. Sato T, Hirota K, Matsuki A, et al. NMDA receptors are not involved in the relaxant effect of ketamine on airway smooth muscle. Anesthesiology 1995;83;A359.
55. Zsigmond EK, Kovacs V, Fekete G. A new route, jet-injection for anesthetic induction in children. II. Ketamine dose-range finding studies. Int J Clin Pharmacol Ther 1996:34:84–88.
56. Zsigmond EK. Malignant hyperthermia with subsequent uneventful general anesthesia. Anesth Analg 1971;50:1111–1112.
57. Johnston RR, Miller RD, Way WL. The interaction of ketamine wth *d*-tubocurarine, pancuronium, and succinylcholine. Anesth Analg 1974;53:496–501.
58. Marwaha J. Some mechanisms underlying actions of ketamine

on electromechanical coupling in skeletal muscle. J Neurosci Res 1980;5:43.
59. Albin MS. Evaluation in patients subjected to ketamine anesthesia and other anesthetic agents [Abstract]. Proceedings of the Meeting of the American Society of Anesthesiologists, New York, 1970.
60. Moretti RJ, Hassan SZ, Goodman LI, et al. Comparison of ketamine and thiopental in healthy volunteers: effects on mental status, mood and personality. Anesth Analg 1984;63:1087.
61. Marx GF, Hwang HS, Chandra P. Postpartum uterine pressure with different doses of ketamine. Anesthesiology 1979;50:163.
62. Oats JN, Vasey OP, Waldren BA. Effects of ketamine on the pregnant uterus. Br J Anaesth 1979;51:1163.
63. Badrinath Sk, Vazeery A, McCarthy RJ, Ivankovich AD. The effect of different methods of inducing anesthesia on intraocular pressure. Anesthesiology 1986;65:431.
64. Atkinson PM, Taylor DI, Chetty N. Inhibition of platelet aggregation by ketamine hydrochloride. Thromb Res 1985;40:227.
65. Heller W, Fuhrer G, Kuhner M, et al. Haemastaseologische Untersuchungen unter der Anwendung von Midazolam/Ketamin. Anaesthesist 1986;35:419.
66. Zsigmond EK, Domino EF, Goulet JR. Ketamine on the hepatic function in healthy prisoneer volunteers. Excerpta Med Int Cong Ser 1980;533:78.
67. Idvall J, Ahlgren I, Aronson KF, et al. Ketamine infusions: pharamacokinetics and clinical effects. Br J Anaesth 1979;51:1167–1172.
68. Clements A, Nimmo WS, Grant IS. Bioavailability, pharmacokinetics and analgesic activity of ketamine in humans. J Pharm Sci 1979;71:539–541.
69. Joachimsson PO, Headstrand U, Ekland A. Low dose ketamine infusion for analgesia during postoperative ventilator treatment. Acta Anaesthesiol Scand 1986;30:697–700.
70. Marietta MP, Way WL, Castagnoli N, Trevor AJ. On the pharmacology of the ketamine enantiomorphs in the rat. J Pharmacol Exp Ther 1977;202:157–165.
71. Ryder S, Way WL, Trevor AJ. Comparative pharmacology of the optical isomers of ketamine in mice. Eur J Pharmacol 1978; 49:15–23.
72. Schüttler J, Kloos S, Ihmsen H, Pelzer E. Pharmacokinetic-pharmacodynamic properties of S(+)-ketamine versus racemic ketamine: a randomized double-blind study in volunteers. Anesthesiology 1992;77:A330.
73. Geisslinger G, Menzel-Soglowek S, Kamp HD, Brune K. Stereoselective high-performance liquid chromatographic determination of the enantiomers of ketamine and norketamine in plasma. J Chromatogr 1991;568:165–176.
74. Kharasch ED, Labroo R. Metabolism of ketamine stereoisomers by human liver microsomes. Anesthesiology 1992;77:1201–1207.
75. Gajraj N, White PF. Clinical pharmacology and applications of ketamine. In: Bowdle T, et al, eds. The pharmacologic basis of anesthesiology. New York: Churchill Livingstone, 1994:375–392.
76. Spotoft H, Korshin JD, Sorensen MB, et al. The cardioavascular effects of ketamine used for induction of anaesthesia in patients with valvular heart disease. Can Anaesth Soc J 1979;26:463–467.
77. Hatano S, Keane DM, Boggs RE, et al. Diazepam-ketamine anaesthesia for open heart surgery: a micro-mini drip administration technique. Can Anaesth Soc J 1976;23:648–656.
78. Jackson APF, Dhadphale PR, Callaghan ML. Haemodynamic studies during induction of anaesthesia for open-heart surgery using diazepam and ketamine. Br J Anaesth 1978;50:375–377.
79. Kumar SM, Kothary SP, Martinez OA, et al. Plasma free norepinephrine and epinephrine concentrations following diazepam-ketamine induction in patients undergoing cardiac surgery. Acta Anaesthesiol Scand 1978;22:593–600.
80. Reves JG, Lell WA, McCraken LE, et al. Comparison of morphine and ketamine. Anesthetic techniques for coronary surgery: a randomized study. South Med J 1978;71:33.
81. Dhadphale PR, Jackson APF, Alseri S. Comparison of anesthesia with diazepam and ketamine vs morphine in patients undergoing heart-valve replacement. Anesthesiology 1979;51:200.
82. Gutzke GE, Shah K, Glisson SN, et al. Sufentanil or ketamine: induction in cardiomyopathy patients. Anesthesiology 1986; 67:84.
83. Newsome LR, Moldenhauer CC, Hug CC, et al. Hemodynamic interactions of moderate doses of fentanyl with etomidate and ketamine. Anesth Analg 1985;64:260.
84. Benumof JL, Canada ED, Scanlon TS. Intravenous anesthesia and postoperative analgesia. Anesth Analg 1981;60:240.
85. Lebovic S, Reich DL, Steinberg LG, et al. Comparison of propofol versus ketamine for anesthesia in pediatric undergoing cardiac catheterization. Anesth Analg 1992;74:490.
86. Sharma VJ. Use of ketamine in acute severe asthma. Acta Anaesthesiol Scand 1992;36:106.
87. Stefannsson T, Wickstom I, Haljamae H. Hemodynamic and metabolic effects of ketamine anesthesia in the geriatric patient. Acta Anaesthesiol Scand 1982;26:371.
88. Pedersen T, Engback J, Klausen NO, et al. Effects of low-dose ketamine and thiopentone on cardiac performance and myocardial oxygen balance in high risk patients. Acta Anaesthesiol Scand 1982;26:235.
89. Sher MH. Slow dose ketamine: a new technique. Anaesth Intensive Care 1980;8:359.
90. Priano LL. Alterations of renal hemodynamics by thipental: diazepam and ketamine in conscious dogs. Anesth Analg 1982; 61:853.
91. Longnecker DE, Ross DC, Silver IA. Anesthetic influence on arteriolar diameters and tissue oxygen tension in hemorrhaged rats. Anesthesiology 1982;57:177.
92. Weiskopf RB, Townsley MI, Riordan KK, et al. Comparison of cardiopulmonary responses to graded hemorrhage during enflurane: halothane, isoflurane and ketamine anesthesia. Anesth Analg 1981;60:481.
93. Bogetz MS, Weiskopf RB, Roizen MF. Ketamine increases catecholamines but causes cardiovascular depression and acidosis in hypovolemic swine. Anesthesiology 1982;57:29.
94. Hirshman CA, Krieger W, Littlejohn G, et al. Ketamine aminophylline induced decrease in seizure threshold. Anesthesiology 1982;56:464.
95. Pickering BG, Palahniuk RJ, Cote J, et al. Cerebral vascular responses to ketamine and thiopentone during foetal acidosis. Can J Anaesth 1982;29:463.
96. Dich-Nielsen J, Holasek J. Ketamine as induction agent for cesarean section. Acta Anaesthesiol Scand 1982;26:139.
97. Levinson G, Shnider SM, Gildea JE, et al. Maternal and foetal cardiovascular and acid-base changes during ketamine anaesthesia in pregnant ewes. Br J Anaesth 1973;45:1111–1115.
98. Hodgkinson K, Marx GF, Kim SS, et al. Noenatal neurobehavorial tests following vaginal delivery under ketamine, thiopental, and extradural anesthesia. Anesth Analg 1977;56:548–553.
99. Coad NR, Mills PJ, Verma R, Ramasubramanian R. Evaluation of blood loss during suction termination of pregnancy: ketamine compared with methohexitone. Acta Anaesthesiol Scand 1986;30:253.
100. Gutstein HB, Johnson KL, Heard MB, et al. Oral ketamine preanesthetic medication in children. Anesthesiology 1992;76:28.
101. Duperon DF, Jedrychowski JR. Preliminary report on the use of ketamine in pediatric dentistry. Pediatr Dentist 1983;5:75.
102. Saarnivaara L. Comparison of thiopentone, althesin and ketamine in anesthesia for otolaryngological surgery in children. Br J Anaesth 1977;49:363.
103. Jantzen JP, Tzanova I, Klein AM, et al. A clinical evaluation of

methohexitone and ketamine for anorectal induction of anesthesia in children. Anasthesiol Intensivmed Notfallmed Schmerzther 1987;28:56.
104. Thompson GE, Moore DC. Ketamine, diazepam, and Innovar: a computerized comparative study. Anesth Analg 1971;50:458–505.
105. White PF, Vasconez LE, Mathes S, et al. Comparison of midazolam and diazepam for sedation during plastic surgery. Plast Reconstr Surg 1988;81:703–710.
106. White PF. Use of continuous infusions versus intermittent bolus administration of fentanyl or ketamine during outpatient anesthesia. Anesthesiology 1983;59:294.
107. White PF. Clinical uses of intravenous anesthetic and analgesic infusions. Anesth Analg 1989;68:161–171.
108. Pace NA, Victory RA, White RF. Anesthetic infusion techniques: how to do it. J Clin Anesth 1992;4:45S–52S.
109. Tung S, Yaksh TL. Analgesic effect of intrathecal ketamine in the rat. Reg Anesth 1981;6:91.
110. Islas JA, Astorga J, Loredo M. Epidural ketamine for control of postoperative pain. Anesth Analg 1985;64:1161.
111. Naquib M, Adu-Gyamfi Y, Absood GM, et al. Epidural ketamine for postoperative analgesia. Can J Anaesth 1986;33:16.
112. Naquib M, Sharif AM, Seraj M, et al. Ketamine for caudal analgesia in children: comparison with caudal bupivacaine. Br J Anaesth 1991;67:559.
113. Ravat F, Dorne R, Baechle JP, et al. Epidural ketamine or morphine for postoperative analgesia. Anesthesiology 1987;66:819.
114. Kawana Y, Sato H, Shimada H. Epidural ketamine for postoperative pain relief after gynecologic operations. Anesth Analg 1987;66:735.
115. Lees DE, Kim YD, MacNamara TE. The safety of ketamine in pediatric neuromuscular disease. Anesth Rev 1982;9:17.
116. Bancroft GH, Lauria JI. Ketamine induction for cesarian section in a patient with acute intermittent porphyria and achondroplastic dwarfism. Anesthesiology 1983;53:143.
117. Capouet V, Dernovoi B, Azagra JS. Induction of anesthesia with ketamine during an acute crisis of hereditary coproporphyria. Can J Anaesth 1987;34:388.
118. Eisenkraft JB, Dimich I, Miller R. Ketamine-diazepam anesthesia in a patient with carcinoid syndrome. Anaesthesia 1981; 36:881.
119. Saarnivaara L, Kautto U-M, Teravainen H. Ketamine anesthesia for a patient with the Shy-Drager syndrome. Acta Anaesthesiol Scand 1983;27:123.
120. Reich DL, Silvay G. Ketamine: an update on the first twenty-five years of clinical experience. Can J Anaesth 1989;36:186.

III PHARMACOKINETICS AND DYNAMICS OF OPIOID AND NONOPIOID ANALGESICS

10 Morphine Compounds

Douglas V. Brown, Kenneth J. Tuman

HISTORY

Opium, derived from the oriental poppy (*Papaver somniferum*), was first described by Theophrastus in the third century B.C. Although the drug was initially utilized for treatment of dysentery, the analgesic properties of opium were well recognized (1). In 1680, Sydenham reported that "among the remedies which it has pleased Almighty God to give to man to relieve his sufferings, none is so universal and so efficacious as opium." Although more than 20 different alkaloids are contained in opium, morphine is the most abundant. Morphine was the first of the opium alkaloids isolated and was named after Morpheus, the Greek god of dreams. Other opium alkaloids were isolated soon after the discovery of morphine in 1803, including codeine in 1832, and papaverine in 1848 (2). The terminology applied to this group of alkaloids persists to this day, with the term *opioid* referring to all natural and synthetic drugs with morphine-like qualities and to drugs that bind with opiate receptors. The word *opiate* is currently interchangeable for opioid, but originally it referred only to true opium derivatives. The term *narcotic* is derived from the Greek word for stupor, and it nonspecifically describes any drug resulting in sedation and sleep, although the term often is used in reference to opioids.

In 1869, Bernard utilized morphine in the perioperative period as a premedicant, and he noted that the drug decreased the chloroform requirements. Schneiderlein subsequently administered large doses of morphine and scopolamine without inhaled agents to provide anesthesia. This early use of morphine with an anticholinergic agent as the sole anesthetic for various surgical procedures was apparently associated with little recall and reduced the induction and emergence "excitation" phenomenon reported with inhalation agents. Because neither muscle relaxant medication nor positive pressure ventilation was utilized at that time, however, this technique was limited by intraoperative patient movement (necessitating restraints), as well as the occurrence of deaths due to ventilatory depression (3). Morbidity and mortality related to morphine-induced ventilatory depression restricted the early application of high-dose opiate anesthesia, and opioids were used primarily as adjuvants to inhalational agents or to supplement regional anesthesia.

In 1938, meperidine, the first synthetic opioid, was produced (1). Nitrous oxide and meperidine were administered with curare and barbiturates as part of a "balanced" anesthetic technique as described by Neff and associates in 1947 (4). Nitrous oxide-opioid anesthesia became a popular alternative to inhaled anesthetics. In 1958, Bailey and colleagues utilized meperidine and oxygen for cardiac anesthesia (5). Subsequent reports of enhanced hemodynamic stability in patients with compromised cardiovascular function prompted the use of high-dose morphine, 0.5 to 1.0 mg/kg, for cardiac anesthesia (6). Further experience with this technique revealed problems related to intraoperative recall, failure to prevent intraoperative hypertension, histamine-related hypotension, and increased perioperative fluid requirements. In an effort to prevent recall and to provide a deeper level of anesthesia, even higher doses of morphine were administered (10 mg/kg); however, this produced greater hemodynamic instability (7). Use of high-dose meperidine did not eliminate the problems of high-dose morphine anesthesia for cardiac surgery, but it was associated with other problems such as tachycardia and cardiac depression (8). Attempts to find a more potent opioid with fewer cardiovascular side effects led to the development of fentanyl and its related congeners.

The side effects of opiates including the potential for addiction and respiratory depression prompted the search for alternative drugs with greater analgesic selectivity. Synthesized in 1942, nalorphine was found to antagonize the effects of morphine. When given alone postoperatively, however, nalorphine was noted to possess analgesic properties (9). Pentazocine, butorphanol, and buprenorphine were subsequently found to possess similar mixed agonist-antagonist activity. The advent of opiates with mixed agonist-antagonist activity suggested the existence of more than one type of opiate receptor (10).

In addition, clinicians and investigators now recognize three distinct types of endogenous opioid peptides: the endorphins; the enkephalins; and the dynorphins. The most potent of the endogenous opioids, β-endorphins, are derived from the precursor peptide pro-opiomelanocortin, found in highest concentrations in the pituitary gland. Pro-opiomelanocortin also contains adrenocorticotropic hormone (ACTH) and melanocyte stimulating hormone (MSH), whereas breakdown of the precursor proenkephalin yields both met- and leu-enkephalins. Unlike β-endorphins, enkephalins are widely distributed throughout the central nervous system (CNS), with their highest concentrations in areas of importance for nociception including the periaqueductal gray, rostroventral medulla, and spinal cord laminae I, II, V, and X. These peptides are also found outside the CNS (e.g. the adrenal medulla). Dynorphins, the least potent endogenous opioid peptides, are also widely distributed.

OPIATE RECEPTOR SUBTYPES

Opiates exert their activity by discrete transmembrane stereoselective opioid receptors, namely, μ, κ, and δ receptor subtypes. ε and σ receptors bind opiates, as well as other moieties (e.g., ketamine) and are not classified as "true" opiate receptors. Stimulation of each receptor type elicits a characteristic physiologic response (Table 10-1), and considerable effort has been directed toward synthesis of opioids that act more selectively, in an effort to separate the desirable analgesic effects from side effects such as ventilatory depression, ileus, pruritus, nausea, and vomiting.

The μ receptor mediates many of the clinical effects of morphine-like compounds. The μ receptors comprise two subpopulations, μ–1 and μ–2, which mediate analgesia and ventilatory depression, respectively (11, 12). μ–1 Receptors appear at a later developmental stage than μ–2 receptors, so ventilatory depression from μ agonists may occur in the neonate before analgesia is achieved (13). Although they have similar affinities at the μ–1 site (14), morphine and other exogenous opiates have a greater affinity for μ–2 receptors than do endogenous opiate peptides. Currently, no μ–1-selective opiate is available, although drugs such as meptazinol have been investigated in the hope of identifying an opioid with such specificity (15, 16). In addition to its opiate properties, meptazinol appears to have another distinct analgesic mechanism that is not mediated by opioid receptors (17). Meptazinol is associated with acetylcholine release in the CNS, and the analgesic effect of cholinergic drugs is well established in animals (18, 19). The anticholinergic agent scopolamine partially antagonizes meptazinol's analgesic effects (17).

Analgesia, the most important pharmacologic property of opiates, has been demonstrated to be supraspinally, spinally, and peripherally modulated. Supraspinal analgesia is the most prominent site of activity after intravenous administration and is mediated primarily by the μ receptor. High densities of μ–1 recep-

TABLE 10-1. Characteristics of Opioid Receptor Subtype

	μ Receptor				
Effect	μ1	μ2	κ Receptor	δ Receptor	σ Receptor
Analgesia	Primarily supraspinal	Primarily spinal	Yes	Primarily spinal	—
Ventilatory effects	—	Depression	—	Depression	Stimulation
Cardiovascular effects	—	Bradycardia	—	—	Vasomotor stimulation (tachycardia, hypertension)
Central nervous system effects	Sedation, prolactin release	Euphoria, pruritis	Sedation, dysphoria, psychotomimetic reactions (hallucinations, delirium), diuresis (inhibition of vasopressin release)	—	Psychotomimetic reactions (hallucinations, delirium)
Pupil	—	Miosis	—	—	Mydriasis
Gastrointestinal effects	—	Inhibition of peristalsis; nausea, vomiting	—	—	—
Genitourinary effects	—	Urinary retention	—	—	—
Pruritus	—	Yes	—	Yes	—
Physical dependence	No	Yes	—	—	—

tors are found in areas important for pain transmission, including the periaqueductal gray matter, corpus striatum, and hypothalamus (20). Intraspecies differences in μ–1-receptor density in these areas correlate well with morphine's analgesic activity (21). Although spinal analgesia had been attributed to the κ receptor, μ-receptor activation may also play a significant role because μ receptors make up the largest population of opiate receptors in the spinal cord (22). Peripheral analgesic effects of opiates are mediated by μ, κ, and δ receptors (23). In addition to analgesia and respiratory depression, μ-receptor activity is responsible for intestinal ileus and constipation, urinary hesitancy, euphoria, and physical dependence (24).

κ receptors were named after the drug ketocyclazocine, which was originally found to bind to this receptor (25). The endogenous opiates, dynorphins, are specific κ-receptor ligands (26). The κ receptor and dynorphin-containing nerves are concentrated in the substantia gelatinosa of the spinal cord and in the periaqueductal gray matter and thalamus in the brain, important CNS areas for modulating afferent nociceptive impulses (27). Whereas μ-receptor agonists are effective analgesics for all types of noxious stimuli, including chemical stimuli, pressure, or heat, opiates acting at the κ receptor have a limited ability to relieve pain elicited by thermal stimuli (28). κ Agonists at least partially mediate dysphoria and cause psychotomimetic effects that have classically been attributed to the σ receptor (29). These properties may confer to κ agonists a reduced abuse potential compared with μ agonists, which cause euphoria (30). κ-Receptor activity also produces sedation and inhibits antidiuretic hormone (ADH) release, resulting in diuresis (22). Pure κ agonists do not cause respiratory depression (31).

Partial opiate agonists, including nalorphine, pentazocine, butorphanol, nalbuphine, and dezocine, are also thought to provide analgesia by κ-receptor activity. These opiates are often referred to as mixed agonist-antagonists because the pharmacologic response to nalorphine-like agents can be explained by κ-receptor agonist activity and μ-receptor antagonist activity. More recent data, however, suggest that nalorphine-like opiates actually possess partial agonist activity at both κ and μ receptors (32-35). The affinity and activity currently available at the μ and κ receptors are summarized in Table 10-2. Respiratory depression can occur with nalorphine-like agents as a result of partial μ agonism (31). Prior administration of a selective μ-antagonist drug shifts the analgesia dose-response curve for nalorphine-like agents to the right, suggesting that some of the analgesic activity must occur at the μ receptor (33). Because only partial agonist activity occurs, a plateau (ceiling) is reached where increasing the drug levels does not produce additional opiate effects. Dezocine and buprenorphine are also partial μ agonists, and their binding with κ and δ opiate receptors is less than butorphanol or nalbuphine. Dezocine's μ-agonist activity is probably greater than that of the agonist-antagonist opioids. Buprenorphine exhibits high affinity for the μ receptor that is difficult to antagonize, and incomplete reversal with naloxone can result in increased μ activity with an enhancement of analgesia and ventilatory depression (36).

TABLE 10-2. Affinity and Activity of Morphine and Related Compounds at μ and κ Receptors

Agent	μ Receptor		κ Receptor	
	Affinity	Activity	Affinity	Activity
Morphine	High	High	Low	Low
Meperidine	Moderate	Moderate	Low	Low
Fentanyl	Very high	Very high	—	—
Pentazocine	Moderate	—	High	High
Nalbuphine	Moderate	—	High	High
Butorphanol	Moderate	—	High	Moderate
Buprenorphine	High	Low	Moderate	Very low
Dezocine	High	Low	Low	Very low
Tramadol	Moderate	Low	—	—

When an agonist-antagonist opioid is administered following a μ agonist, the effect of the mixed agonist-antagonist opioid depends on the μ-agonist dose. After a small dose of a μ agonist (with low μ-receptor occupancy) administration of a partial agonist increases opiate effects. Nalbuphine enhances ventilatory depression when the drug is given in adults after 15 mg of morphine (37). After a large dose of a morphine-like agent (with μ receptors more fully occupied), a partial agonist usually antagonizes μ effects, including respiratory depression and analgesia (37-39). The intrinsic analgesic activity of the nalorphine-like agents prevents complete antagonism of analgesia, and thus, nalorphine-like drugs are perhaps better alternatives to naloxone for reversal of perioperatively administered morphine-like opiates (37) and their side effects (e.g., pruritus, nausea, and vomiting). These agents may precipitate withdrawal and reverse the effects of previously administered agonists in opioid-dependent patients, however (40).

δ receptors are located spinally and supraspinally, but they are sparsely distributed in the areas typically associated with opiate analgesia (41, 42). Enkephalins have been shown to bind to δ receptors more avidly than exogenous opioids. Selective δ-receptor agonists are weak supraspinal analgesics but are important in mediating analgesia at the spinal level (43). Activation of δ receptors may produce analgesia synergistically with the μ receptor or may mediate μ-receptor activity (44). An interaction between μ and δ receptors may account for the bell-shaped analgesic response curve of buprenorphine (45), with increasing analgesia at doses up to 3.0 mg/kg and attenuated analgesic efficacy at larger doses (46-48).

Along with the μ and κ receptors, the σ receptor is one of Martin's originally proposed opiate receptors (10). The D isomer of phencyclidine is inactive at μ, δ, and κ receptors, but it preferentially binds to the σ receptor (Only L isomers of opioids are recognized at opiate receptors.) σ Receptors are not specifically considered opiate receptors, and naloxone does not antagonize opiate or phencyclidine effects at σ receptors (49). The physiologic significance of opiate binding to these receptors is unknown. Investigators have postulated that the σ receptors modulate presynaptic catecholamine release (50, 51), and their activation results in psychotomimetic effects as well as tachycardia and hypertension commonly observed with ketamine.

Tramadol is a drug that binds with weak affinity at σ and κ receptors while having modest activity at μ receptors (52). Unlike the traditional morphine-like analgesics, tramadol is an atypical centrally-acting binary analgesic with a dual mechanism of action, also blocking reuptake of the monoamines norepinephrine and serotonin (similar to the tricyclic antidepressants) (53). The effects of tramadol have been isolated to its different enantiomers, with (+) tramadol exhibiting a greater affinity at μ receptors, as well as inhibiting serotonin uptake and enhancing its release, whereas (−) tramadol inhibits norepinephrine reuptake (54). Because of this dual mechanism of action, the analgesic effects of tramadol are only partially antagonized by naloxone (55). α–2 antagonists (e.g., yohimbine) and serotonin antagonists also partially attenuate tramadol's analgesic effect (56).

The ϵ receptor is poorly understood, and whether the ϵ receptor represents a unique opiate receptor is debated (57). β-Endorphins appear to have agonist activity at the ϵ receptor under specific conditions. Morphine does not bind to this receptor, and κ agonists antagonize the binding of β-endorphin to ϵ receptors (58). Among the endogenous opiate peptides, the enkephalins are relatively δ specific, but they also exert μ activity. β-Endorphins exert similar activity at both μ and δ receptors, whereas dynorphins bind primarily to κ receptors.

OPIATE RECEPTORS: MECHANISM OF ACTION

Although activation of opioid receptors results in a spectrum of well-recognized pharmacologic effects, uniform inhibitory action is associated with this system (59). This inhibitory action can increase nerve transmission when inhibitory interneuron opiate receptors are activated. Opiate receptor effects are mediated by guanine nucleotide binding proteins (G proteins), and adenyl cyclase acts as a second messenger for some, but probably not all, opiate activity. Both μ and δ receptors are similar in that they mediate an influx of potassium ions resulting in cell hyperpolarization. Opiate receptors are located both postsynaptically, where hyperpolarization of postsynaptic membranes inhibits nerve transmission, and presynaptically, where decreases in calcium influx inhibit neurotransmitter release. κ Receptors differ from μ and δ receptors by causing closure of calcium channels (60).

STRUCTURE-ACTIVITY RELATIONSHIPS

The opiate structure produces its pharmacodynamic effects by determining the molecules' affinity and activity at specific receptor subtypes. Additionally, the physical characteristics of opiates (e.g., pKa, lipid solubility, and protein binding) depend on molecular structure and determine the pharmacokinetic profile by influencing their absorption, disposition, and metabolism.

Morphine and other naturally occurring analgesic alkaloids contain a five-ring partially hydrogenated phenanthrene structure (Fig. 10-1). Alteration of morphine's major functional groups while preserving the five-ring morphine skeleton (which is not essential for opiate activity) results in semisynthetic opiates. When

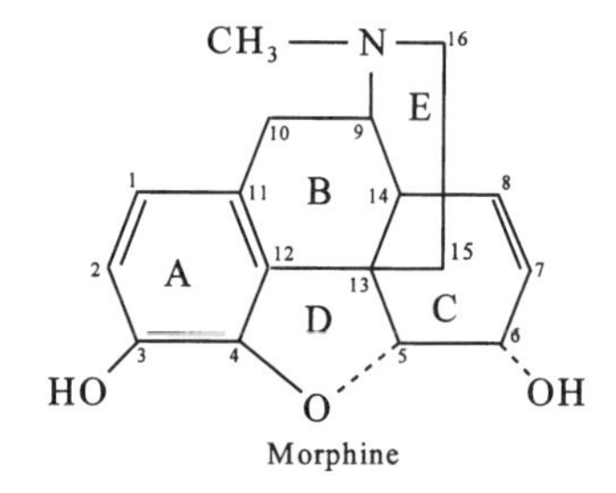

	Position of Substitution						
	3	4-5	6	14	-N	7	8
Agonists							
Morphine	-OH	O	-OH	--	$-CH_3$	--	--
Heroin	$-OCOCH_3$	O	$-OCOCH_3$	--	$-CH_3$	--	--
Hydromorphone	-OH	O	=O	--	$-CH_3$	-H	-H
Levorphanol	-OH	--	-H	--	$-CH_3$	-H	-H
Codeine	$-OCH_3$	O	-OH	--	$-CH_3$	--	--
Hydrocodone	$-OCH_3$	O	=O	--	$-CH_3$	-H	-H
Oxycodone	$-OCH_3$	O	=O	-OH	$-CH_3$	-H	-H
Mixed Agonists/Antagonists							
Nalorphine	-OH	O	-OH	--	$-CH_2CH{=}CH_2$	--	--
Buprenorphine*	-OH	O	$-OCH_3$		$-CH_2$ —◁	-H	-H
Butorphanol	-OH	--	-H	-OH	$-CH_2$ —◇	--	--
Nalbuphine	-OH	O	-OH	-OH	$-CH_2$ —◇	-H	-H
Antagonists							
Naloxone	-OH	O	=O	-OH	$-CH_2CH{=}CH_2$	-H	-H

* contains endoetheno bridge between C-6 and C-14 and 1-hydroxy-1,2,2-trimethylpropyl substitution on C-7

FIGURE 10-1. Structural modifications of the parent morphine molecule and the resulting related compounds.

TABLE 10-3. Pharmacokinetic Variables for Morphine-Related Opioids

	Elimination Half-Life (h)	Volume of Distribution at Steady State (L/Kg)	Clearance (ml/kg/ min)	Protein Bound (%)	Bioavailability (%)	Equivalent Analgesic Dosing		Metabolism
AGONISTS:								
NATURALLY OCCURRING								
Morphine	1.7–2.2	3–5	15–20	23–26	20	10	60	phase I
Codeine	2–4	2.5–3.5	10–15	7–25	40–80	130	200	phase II
SEMISYNTHETIC DERIVATIVES OF MORPHINE: ALTERED FUNCTIONAL GROUPS								
Hydromorphone	2.4–3	1.2–2.4	14–23	7–14	50–60	1.5	7.5	phase I
Hydrocodone	3.3–4.5	nd	nd	nd	nd	nd	nd	phase II
Oxycodone	3.7	2.6	13	nd	60	15	30	phase II
SYNTHETIC DERIVATIVES								
MORPHINANS								
Levorphanol	11	12	15	60	nd	2	4	phase I
PHENYLPIPERIDINES								
Meperidine	3–5	3–5	5–17	70	60	75	300	phase II
Meptazinol†	1.6–2	3–5	20–30	30	9	75–150	nd	phase I
Tramadol†	5.1–7	3–5	7–10	20	68	75	150	phase II
DIPHENYLPROPYLAMINES								
Methadone	15	5	2	90	75–95	10	20	phase II
Propoxyphene	8–12	2.5	7–20	80	30–70	240	500	phase II
MIXED AGONISTS-ANTAGONISTS: ALTERED FUNCTIONAL GROUPS								
SEMISYNTHETIC DERIVATIVES								
Buprenorphine	3	2.8	19	96	15–30	0.4	nd	phase I & II
Nalbuphine	2.3–5	2.2–4.3	16–21	25–40	12–25	10	nd	phase I
SYNTHETIC DERIVATIVES								
MORPHINANS								
Butorphanol	2–4	5	40–67	80	17	2	nd	phase II
BENZOMORPHANS								
Pentazocine	2–4	5	18	60–70	18	60	180	phase I
Dezocine†	2.5	10	50	nd	nd	10	nd	phase I
ANTAGONISTS								
Naloxone	0.9–1.0	2.6–3	20–30	40	nd			phase I & II
Naltrexone	3–9	16	20	20	5–60			phase I & II
Nalmefene	8–9	2.3	14	nd	nd			phase I & II

†*Contains some but not all structural characteristics of group*
nd, No data available.

the five-ring structure is altered, the resultant opioid compounds are classified as synthetic. The four synthetic opiate classes are morphinans, benzomorphans, piperidines, and diphenylpropylamines (Table 10-3). In the morphinan class, which includes levorphanol, the D-ring is eliminated. Benzomorphans, including pentazocine, are missing the C and D rings. Meperidine and the fentanyl analogs are piperidines in which, in addition to missing the C and D ring of morphine, the B ring is opened. Only the A ring of morphine remains intact in the diphenylpropylamines such as methadone and propoxyphene.

Viewed in a single dimension, the structures of these agents appear unrelated; however, the three-dimensional structure of most opiates contains a common feature. The piperidine ring is typically perpendicular to the aromatic ring, forming a T shape (61). In this configuration (Fig. 10-2), the spacing between the aromatic group and the nitrogen atom remains at a

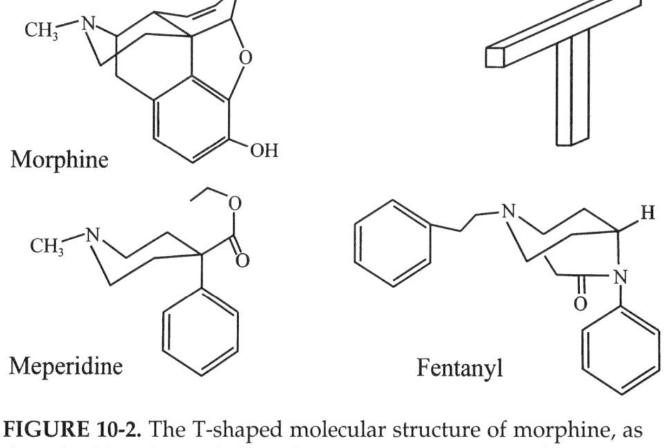

FIGURE 10-2. The T-shaped molecular structure of morphine, as described by Thorpe (61), and analogous projections of representative phenylpiperidine molecules.

two-carbon distance. Comparison of spatial models of the exogenous opioid alkaloids and the endogenous opiate peptides also reveals the presence of a positively charged tertiary nitrogen separated by two carbon atoms from a phenolic hydroxyl moiety. The opiate receptor is stereospecific and recognizes only the L isomer; therefore, the D isomer of clinically available compounds is devoid of analgesic activity (62, 63).

The various side chain substituents of the opiate molecule are more important in determining opiate activity than the molecular skeleton (see Fig. 10-1). Maximal opiate potency is achieved with a free phenolic group at position 3. Masking the phenolic function at position 3 decreases opioid potency. For example, morphine becomes 10-fold less potent by adding a methyl to the hydroxyl group of the phenolic ring to form codeine. In contrast, when a larger side chain is appended to the 6-hydroxyl group, opioid potency is generally increased (most likely a result of enhanced lipophilicity, facilitating transfer across the blood-brain barrier). The highly lipophilic opioid heroin has acetyl groups at both positions 3 and 6. The increased potency afforded by the larger acetyl group at position 6 is reduced by altering the free phenolic group at the 3 position, resulting in a compound only moderately more potent than morphine.

Altering the basic amino group at position 17 results in profound changes in opiate activity. Replacing morphine's nitrogen methyl group with an allyl side chain ($CH_2CH{=}CH_2$) results in the partial agonist nalorphine, whereas opiates with κ-agonist properties have other similar nitrogen substituents. Nalbuphine and butorphanol both have N-cyclobutylmethyl side chains, and pentazocine has a structurally similar amino side chain. Substitution of larger N-alkyl side chains (e.g., fentanyl) results in an increase in potency (see Fig. 10-2). The addition of a 14-hydroxyl substituent to an oxymorphone derivative of nalorphine rigidifies its molecular structure and results in the formation of naloxone, a pure opioid antagonist. Naloxone's allyl nitrogen substituent sterically inhibits interaction with the opiate receptor, and the addition of the hydroxyl group at C–14 sufficiently alters binding such that opiate receptor activation is not possible (64). The long-acting opioid antagonist, naltrexone, shares the same hydroxyl side chain. Nalmefene, a long-acting opioid antagonist recently made available for intravenous administration, contains a methylene group rather than a hydroxyl group at position 14.

PHARMACOKINETIC FACTORS

The pharmacokinetics of morphine has been extensively described in the anesthesia literature. Morphine is used as a prototype to discuss opiate absorption, distribution, metabolism, and elimination. The other opiates are only discussed if they demonstrate significant differences from the prototypic compound. Opiate pharmacokinetics depends primarily on physical characteristics including protein binding, lipid solubility, and pKa, which depend on structural differences among the morphine-like agents (see Table 10-3).

Absorption

Absorption is the process of a drug leaving the site of administration and entering the systemic circulation. Following oral administration, peak plasma levels of morphine occur an average of 50 minutes after ingestion of morphine in liquid form and 140 minutes after ingestion of tablets (65, 66). Peak serum drug levels occur 1 to 1.3 hours after oral codeine (67-69) and 2.5 to 4 hours following oral methadone (70) administration. The prolonged absorption time of some opiates has been implicated in a longer "biologic" half-life compared with intravenously administered opiates.

Although intestinal absorption of morphine and most other opiates is near complete, over 80% of enteral morphine is metabolized before reaching the systemic circulation ("first-pass" effect); the result is that only 20% of the administered dose remains available for systemic activity (71). First-pass metabolism occurs both in the intestinal mucosa and the liver, with over 50% occurring in the intestine (72, 73). Codeine has a much greater bioavailability (60%) and consequently is more easily dosed orally than morphine (see Table 10-3). Methylation at the 3 position is thought to protect codeine from rapid first-pass metabolism (74). Tramadol also has a high bioavailability (68%) after oral administration (75).

When administered intramuscularly, morphine-like opioids are 100% bioavailable. Peak plasma concentrations are attained between 7 and 20 minutes after morphine injection (76) and at approximately 30 minutes following intramuscular meperidine injection in volunteers (77). Postoperatively, repeated intramuscular injections of meperidine result in peak plasma concentrations approximately 45 minutes after injection, although peak plasma concentrations can vary fivefold among patients. The large variability in meperidine plasma concentrations is probably accounted for by differences in intramuscular absorption, whereas intravenous administration results in a much narrower range of blood concentrations (78).

Distribution and Redistribution

The decline in serum morphine concentration following intravenous injection is typically described by a bi- or triexponential plasma decay function. The redistribution half-life is rapid (approximately 1 minute) and by 10 minutes, 96 to 98% of intravenously administered morphine is cleared from the plasma (76, 79, 80). During the initial redistribution phase, morphine-like opioids are distributed to visceral organs and muscle tissue, with first-pass uptake by the lung further reducing the peak arterial blood concentration. Although less than 3% of morphine undergoes pulmonary extraction, uptake by the lung affects a much greater fraction of the more lipophilic opioids. Meperidine and fentanyl are 65 and 75% extracted, respectively (81). Previous administration of other basic lipophilic amines such as propranolol and lidocaine may saturate lung binding sites and may result in decreased uptake of opiates (82). The lung-bound opiate is later released, with 60% of absorbed fentanyl reentering the circulation over the next 10 minutes (83). Similarly, a second peak in plasma opiate concentration occurs after oral ingestion of morphine and probably represents enterohepatic circulation. After morphine is hepatically conjugated with glucuronide, it is excreted in bile. Intestinal bacteria subsequently break down the conjugated metabolite yielding the parent compound, which is then available for reabsorption (84).

Distribution and redistribution of morphine and related opioids depend on certain physicochemical characteristics (see Table 10-3). As with other drugs, the protein-bound fraction of morphine is devoid of pharmacologic activity, and the rate of diffusion of morphine from blood to its sites of action is proportional to the concentration of free drug, not the total drug concentration. Morphine's limited degree of protein binding (23 to 26%) makes the free fraction relatively insensitive to alteration of serum protein levels (85, 86). This is also true of tramadol, which is approximately 20% protein bound (87). With more highly protein-bound opiates (e.g., fentanyl and its analogs), a change in plasma protein concentration expectedly alters the free opioid level to a greater extent. Whereas morphine is primarily bound to albumin, methadone and meperidine bind preferentially to α acid-glycoprotein, an acute-phase reactant that is produced in increasing amounts in association with stress, malignancy, pregnancy, and inflammation. In cancer patients receiving methadone, the bound-to-free methadone ratio correlates linearly with the plasma α acid-glycoprotein concentration (88).

Lipid solubility is a major determinant of the rate and extent to which an opiate traverses the blood-brain barrier to reach its primary effect sites in the CNS. Highly lipophilic opioids (e.g., fentanyl and its analogs) accumulate in fat and generally are associated with a high volume of distribution. Morphine, with an octanol-water solubility ratio of 0.7 to 1.0, is one of the most hydrophilic opiates (89, 90) and therefore has a relatively small volume of distribution (3.2 to 3.4 L/kg) (76, 79, 80). Morphine crosses lipid membranes poorly and tends to bind to less lipophilic tissues. Lipophilic opioids tend to equilibrate between the central compartment and the effect site (brain) more rapidly than hydrophilic opioids.

The nonionized form of a drug is able to cross most biologic membranes readily, and the degree of ionization of a drug is determined by its pKa, as well as blood and tissue pH. Less than 10% of morphine is nonionized in blood at physiologic pH (90, 91). Because opioids are bases, the nonionized fraction increases with increased pH, as well as decreased pKa. A concentration gradient for the opioid develops when a transmembrane pH difference exists, with a higher concentration equilibrating on the relatively acidic side of the membrane. This phenomenon is known as ion trapping and under certain circumstances can result in significant opiate accumulation in the stomach, the CNS, and the in utero fetus. Brain accumulation is exaggerated during respiratory alkalosis, and fetal opioid accumulation is accentuated during fetal distress (92-94).

Concentrations of morphine in the CNS do not parallel serum concentrations. After intravenous administration of morphine, cerebrospinal fluid (CSF) morphine concentration remains significantly less than serum levels and less than the morphine concentration in other vessel-rich organ groups. Peak CSF concentration does not occur until 15 to 30 minutes after intravenous administration, reflecting the slow and limited ability of the poorly lipid soluble morphine to cross the blood-brain barrier (Fig. 10-3) (95). When administered intracerebrally or intraventricularly, morphine is a much more potent opiate than when administered systemically because the blood-brain barrier no longer inhibits entry into the CNS (96). In newborn rats, intravenous morphine becomes progressively less potent with age, and this is thought to be partly the result of a maturing blood-brain barrier (97). In addition to concentration gradients across the CNS, the distribution of morphine within the CNS is not uniform. The cellular (gray) portions of the brain initially have a greater concentration than the acellular (white) regions, and over time, the situation is reversed, with more opiate partitioned into the white than the gray areas (98).

The decay of CSF morphine levels is slow, with an elimination half-life value in the CSF twice that in blood (95). An increased ionized fraction of morphine in the relatively acidic CSF contributes to its slow elimination. As a result, CNS morphine concentrations exceed plasma morphine concentrations beginning approximately 1 hour after intravenous injection, and this phenomenon explains why the biologic actions of morphine are longer than predicted from its serum half-life value (1.7 to 2.2 hours). Clinical effects of morphine correlate well with CSF morphine concentrations, although actual brain opiate concentration lags behind the CSF concentration.

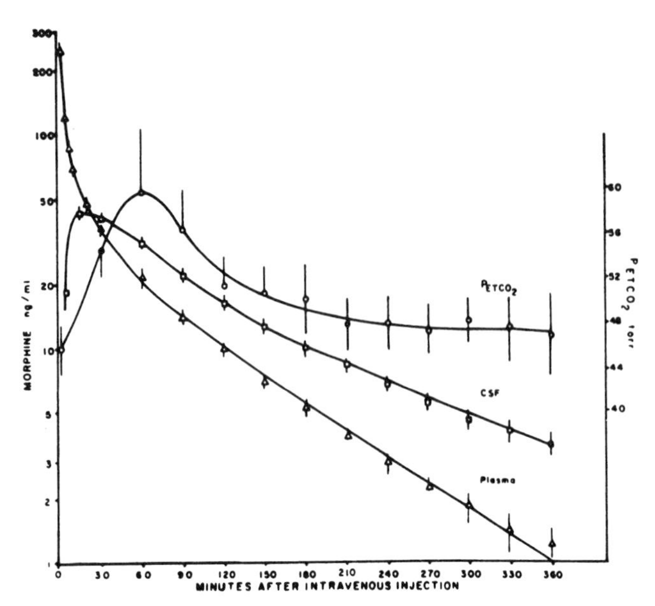

FIGURE 10-3. Cerebrospinal fluid (CSF) and plasma levels of morphine and end-tidal carbon dioxide levels during spontaneous ventilation after intravenous morphine, 0.3 mg/kg. Neither peak plasma levels nor peak CSF levels of morphine correlated with maximum ventilatory depression. (Adapted from Hug CC, Murphy MR, Rigel EP, Olson WA. Pharmacokinetics of morphine injected intravenously into the anesthetized dog. Anesthesiology 1981;54:38–47.)

Although serum levels of morphine do not closely correlate with its analgesic effects (76, 95), therapeutic serum opioid levels have been defined for other more lipophilic opiates. For example, the relationship between blood meperidine concentrations and analgesic effect has been described, with a mean minimal effective analgesic concentration of 0.46 μg/ml (0.24 to 0.76 μg/ml) in postsurgical patients (99). The individual blood concentration-effect curves for meperidine are steep, with a difference of as little as 0.05 μg/ml separating severe pain from effective analgesia. A blood concentration of 0.7 μg/ml has been predicted to provide effective analgesia in 95% of postsurgical patients (99).

Most lipophilic opiates do not demonstrate as great a disparity as morphine between serum levels and clinically important biologic effects. The clinical effects of the lipophilic partial μ and κ receptor agonist buprenorphine also bear little relationship to its serum concentration, (100, 101). Buprenorphine is associated with a slow onset and termination of its CNS effects, with ventilatory depression peaking 3 hours after intravenous administration. Buprenorphine's prolonged duration of action has been attributed to its slow dissociation from the μ receptors. Buprenorphine's high affinity for the μ receptor makes reversal of its opiate effects difficult. Even large doses of naloxone (2.4 to 16 mg) only partially reverse buprenorphine-induced ventilatory depression (102, 103).

Metabolism and Elimination

For most opioids, multiple or continuous dosing methods influence the time required for serum drug concentration to decrease by a fixed fraction, and they prolong the duration of the opioid's effect. The concentration of drug in a peripheral compartment depends on the dose of drug previously administered, as well as the capacity of the compartment to continue absorbing drug from the central compartment. The concentration gradient between peripheral and central compartments determines the direction and extent of drug movement. The terminal elimination half-life of opiates has traditionally been determined following single bolus dose administration. Although longer half-lives have been reported (76), the elimination half-life of morphine is generally considered to be 1.7 to 2.2 hours (79, 80). Interstudy differences of reported terminal half-lives have been accounted for by differences in assays and by the finding that most radioimmunoassay techniques are not specific for morphine but also detect morphine metabolites. When the concentration of morphine metabolites greatly exceeds the concentration of the parent compound, "actual" serum morphine concentrations may be overestimated (104, 105).

The concept of context-sensitive half-life describes the terminal half-life of an opioid after termination of a continuous infusion (106, 107). Context-sensitive half-life values of most opioids typically increase with a prolonged duration of infusion. Computer simulation has been used to characterize the decay in the serum concentration of the potent opiates in the fentanyl family (108).

Clearance of morphine is primarily a result of hepatic metabolism. In healthy volunteers and in surgical patients, clearance is 15 to 23 ml/kg/min and approaches hepatic blood flow (76, 79). Clearance has been reported to exceed hepatic blood flow in at least one study, suggesting extrahepatic metabolism (109). Morphine is metabolized predominately by a phase II conjugation reaction, with morphine–3-glucuronide and, to a lesser extent, morphine–6-glucuronide being the primary metabolites. Morphine metabolism is efficient, and morphine–3-glucuronide is detectable in the plasma 1 minute after intravenous morphine injection, with plasma levels exceeding the parent compound within 10 minutes (110). In animals, evidence indicates modest opiate antagonist activity of morphine–3-glucuronide, resulting in hypesthesia and ventilatory stimulation (111). Conversely, morphine–6-glucuronide has been found to be 13 times more potent as a μ agonist than the parent compound when administered intrathecally (112). Despite greater hydrophilicity than morphine, morphine–6-glucuronide crosses the blood-brain barrier (113), and intravenous morphine–6-glucuronide produces clinical analgesia (114). The ability of the brain to transform morphine to morphine–6-glucuronide is limited (115); however, glucuronyl transferase (the enzyme responsible for morphine metabolism to morphine–6-glucuronide) is located close to opioid receptors (116). The plasma concentration of morphine–6-glucuronide exceeds morphine concentrations by nearly an order of magnitude within 30 minutes after intravenous administration of morphine (110). Although the elimination half-life of morphine–6-glucuronide is only slightly longer than the parent compound, its elimination from the CSF is significantly slower than morphine (117). At 1 hour after administration of intravenous morphine, morphine–6-glucuronide probably contributes more to ventilatory depression than morphine itself (118). Peak respiratory depression does not occur for almost 1 hour after intravenous morphine injection, temporally much later than when the peak CSF morphine concentration is achieved (see Fig. 10-3) (95). Similarly, the return to normocarbia lags behind the decline in CSF morphine levels. The plasma metabolite-to-morphine ratio is greater after oral administration than after intravenous administration, probably because of extensive first-pass metabolism (114).

Most other opioid analgesics are metabolized by hepatic phase I reactions and often have active metabolites (see Table 10-3). Although not definitively established, codeine's opiate activity may be primarily mediated by its metabolism to morphine (69, 80, 119-121). One of the primary metabolites of tramadol produced by O-demethylation is pharmacologically active and contributes to its analgesic efficacy (122). Normeperidine is a metabolite of meperidine that possesses weak opiate agonist properties but also causes CNS excitability, which can result in restlessness, agitation, and seizure activity (123). Propoxyphene's main metabolite, norpropoxyphene, has weak opiate properties but also causes central excitatory effects and cardiac conduction disturbances (124). Naltrexone's metabolite, 6-β-hydroxynaltrexone, is an active opioid antagonist with an elimination half-life slightly longer than that of its parent compound.

Renal excretion of morphine accounts for less than 15% of the total morphine elimination. Following a single oral or parenteral dose of morphine, renal excretion accounts for approximately 2 and 8% of the initial morphine dose, respectively (125). Renal excretion, however, is the primary elimination route of morphine glucuronides. Urinary excretion is also important in the elimination of other opiates, contributing 20% to meperidine clearance (126) and 34% to methadone clearance (127). In both instances, renal elimination depends on urinary pH, and it increases as urine becomes acidified. Administration of an opiate itself may theoretically increase its own renal excretion because opioid-induced ventilatory depression produces respiratory acidosis, resulting in compensatory metabolic alkalosis mediated by renal hydrogen ion elimination, thereby acidifing the urine and increasing opiate excretion (127).

PATIENT FACTORS INFLUENCING PHARMACOKINETICS

Age

Neonates are more susceptible to respiratory depression from morphine (128) because the permeability of the blood-brain barrier is increased, resulting in higher brain concentrations. Decreased α acid-glycoprotein levels in the neonate result in a greater free drug fraction of several opiates (129). In addition, neonatal morphine clearance is decreased primarily because morphine glucuronidation in the liver proceeds at a much slower rate, and immature renal function limits the rate of opiate and opiate metabolite elimination (130). In preterm infants, the clearance rate of morphine increases almost fivefold from 26 to 40 weeks' gestation (131). Although morphine clearance is decreased in neonates, it quickly approaches adult morphine clearance (as early as 1 month of age) (132). The pharmacokinetics of morphine is similar in adults and in children older than 1 year (80). As previously noted, differential μ-receptor development may predispose the neonate to ventilatory depression before effective analgesia is achieved (11). The paucity of μ–1 receptors and the decrease in formation of the active metabolite morphine–6-glucuronide appear to be responsible for the greater morphine serum concentration requirements for adequate analgesia in neonates (133, 134). Limited hepatic metabolic capacity in the neonate also leads to prolonged serum meperidine and normeperidine half-lives values (13 and 63 hours, respectively) after maternal drug administration (135). Meperidine-induced neurobehavioral deficits have been observed up to 3 days after birth (136), probably related to decreased clearance of neonatal normeperidine (137).

Similarly, opiate pharmacokinetics is altered in the elderly. Both the hepatic clearance rate and the volume of distribution are decreased (138, 139). Decreased serum albumin concentration, increased fraction of body fat, and decreased hepatic blood flow contribute to these alterations and result in significant prolongation of plasma opiate concentrations in elderly patients (140). In addition to altered pharmacokinetics, the elderly also appear to have a steeper dose-response curve for these drugs (141).

Acid-Base Disturbances

Alterations in blood pH affect the pharmacokinetics of opioids, and both respiratory acidosis and respiratory alkalosis have been demonstrated to increase the brain concentrations of morphine (93, 94). Alkalosis increases the un-ionized opiate fraction, facilitating transfer across lipophilic membranes and decreasing morphine clearance. Brain levels of morphine increased by 30 to 70% when the $PaCO_2$ was reduced from 40 to 20 mm Hg (94). Acidosis decreases protein binding and increases cerebral blood flow, so increases of $PaCO_2$ from 40 to 70 mm Hg are accompanied by a 20% elevation in cerebral cortex morphine concentration (93) and a significant prolongation of the morphine half-life in the CNS.

Renal Dysfunction

Although morphine's elimination half-life is not altered by renal failure (142-144), prolonged ventilatory depression and miosis have been reported in patients with chronic renal failure (145, 146). Furthermore, the morphine analgesic requirement appears to be decreased in patients with renal dysfunction (147). This disparity between pharmacokinetic and clinical effects is largely accounted for by the accumulation of active morphine metabolites in renal failure, especially morphine–6-glucuronide (144, 148). Renal excretion is the primary route of elimination for morphine glucuronides, with their elimination rate approaching glomerular filtration rate. A nearly linear relationship exists between creatinine clearance and renal clearance of morphine-glucuronides, and their elimination half-life values increase from 4 hours to 14 to 119 hours in the presence of renal failure (149).

Meperidine and propoxyphene also have active metabolites that are renally excreted. Normeperidine, a meperidine metabolite with weak analgesic activity, has a half-life value that is markedly prolonged in renal failure (>1.5 days) (150). The resultant elevated plasma concentrations of normeperidine have been associated with irritability, agitation, and seizures in patients with renal failure (123). These CNS effects are probably not opiate receptor mediated, and naloxone administration is unable to reverse these effects (151). The propoxyphene metabolite norpropoxyphene also depends on renal elimination and, in addition to analgesic effects, may cause cardiac conduction abnormalities when elevated levels occur in the presence of renal dysfunction (124). Although 20% of methadone is eliminated unchanged in the urine (152), limited data suggest that renal failure does not significantly alter its elimination half-life value (153).

Hepatic Dysfunction

Morphine clearance occurs primarily by hepatic metabolism. Severe liver disease decreases total body morphine clearance by approximately 50%, resulting in a doubling of its elimination half-life (154-156). Altered portal blood flow and decreased hepatic function also increase the bioavailability of orally administered morphine (157, 158). Morphine's volume of distribution and plasma protein binding are not significantly altered even in the presence of significant liver disease. Phase II metabolic reactions, including glucuronidation, are well preserved until end-stage liver failure (155). Therefore, mild liver disease does not profoundly affect morphine clearance. Approximately 10% of morphine glucuronidation normally occurs in extrahepatic tissues (probably the intestine and kidney) (159), and with liver failure this proportion increases to 30% (155).

Unlike phase II reactions, phase I reactions are confined to the liver and are more significantly affected by milder degrees of hepatic dysfunction (160-162). Therefore, unlike with morphine, mild hepatic disease alters the pharmacokinetics of other opioids that depend on hepatic phase I reactions for their metabolism. Acute viral hepatitis not resulting in prothrombin time elevation has been associated with prolonged meperidine elimination (163). Predictably, severe hepatic cirrhosis doubles the elimination half-life of meperidine and methadone.

PHARMACODYNAMIC CONSIDERATIONS

Cardiac Effects

Opiate-based anesthesia is often selected for patients with compromised cardiac status. Morphine and morphine-like drugs, however, can have significant effects on the cardiovascular system, including alteration of heart rate, contractility, and peripheral vascular resistance. Most opioids decrease heart rate by a central vagally mediated mechanism (164). Opiate binding in the medulla causes vagal stimulation (165), and opiate heart rate effects are abolished following bilateral vagotomy (166). The negative chronotropic effects of opiates are influenced by both the dose and the rate of drug administration (166) and may be attenuated with slow drug administration, as well as by anticholinergic premedication (167). The vagotonic effects of morphine may also increase the ventricular fibrillation threshold (168). Morphine has a direct negative chronotropic effect on the sinoatrial node, but this effect is not significant at clinically relevant doses (169). Morphine-mediated histamine release may partially offset the opioid's central and direct heart rate effects, because histamine causes an increase in heart rate as well as stimulating catecholamine release.

Meperidine differs from other μ agonists in that it produces a direct positive chronotropic effect. This probably results from the structural similarity meperidine shares with atropine, but also it may result from the central stimulatory effects of meperidine and normeperidine (170). Meperidine also has nonopiate mediated effects on cardiac conduction and can prolong the action potential duration. Cardiac conduction disturbances have not been reported with morphine, but toxic doses of propoxyphene may result in conduction abnormalities, which are probably related to the local anesthetic properties of propoxyphene and its primary metabolite, norpropoxyphene (171).

In extremely high doses, morphine can cause a negative inotropic effect (172), although myocardial function is not depressed at clinically relevant serum concentrations (173). In fact, with morphine doses of 1 to 2 mg/kg, a positive inotropic effect has been demonstrated and is probably related to increased circulating catecholamine and histamine levels (174, 175). Meperidine is unique among opiates in directly depressing myocardial contractility. Even at low doses of 2.0 to 2.5 mg/kg, meperidine decreases cardiac output (176, 177). The time course of the negative inotropy following meperidine administration parallels myocardial meperidine concentrations (178).

The primary cardiovascular effects of morphine depend on the peripheral vasculature. Morphine-induced histamine release, altered sympathetic tone, and direct vasodilation can result in profound hypotension. Morphine's release of histamine may be the most important of these effects (179), because the cardiovascular response to morphine is significantly attenuated by premedication with H_1 and H_2 blocking drugs (180). The extent of the histamine release is determined in part by the speed of morphine's administration. Meperidine and codeine also may cause clinically significant histamine release. Histamine itself causes hypotension by arterial and venous dilation, and it also causes receptor-mediated increases of both cardiac chronotropy and inotropy (181).

Baseline vascular resistance influences morphine's effect on arterial resistance. If baseline vascular resistance is greater than normal, morphine can cause a decrease in vascular resistance. If baseline resistance is less than normal, the resistance may actually increase with morphine (182). Therefore, a larger fall in resistance and blood pressure would be expected when morphine is administered in conditions associated with increased sympathetic activity (e.g., congestive heart failure or hypovolemia), in contrast to conditions of normal basal sympathetic activity. Direct morphine-mediated vasodilation has also been demonstrated on denervated vessels and may contribute to decreases in blood pressure at clinically relevant doses (182).

Whereas transient arteriolar vasodilation can be produced by morphine, persistent venous dilation is more common (Fig. 10-4) (183). Standard doses of morphine effectively block neurally and hormonally mediated venoconstriction (184). Fluid requirements following an "anesthetic" dose of morphine, 9.3 mg/kg, are twice those after a 2.7-mg/kg dose (185). During cardiopulmonary bypass, morphine, 1 mg/kg, decreases systemic vascular resistance by about 50% within 2 minutes and returns to baseline values with 15 minutes. An equally rapid but sustained 600-ml increase in vascular capacitance occurs after the same dose of morphine (186).

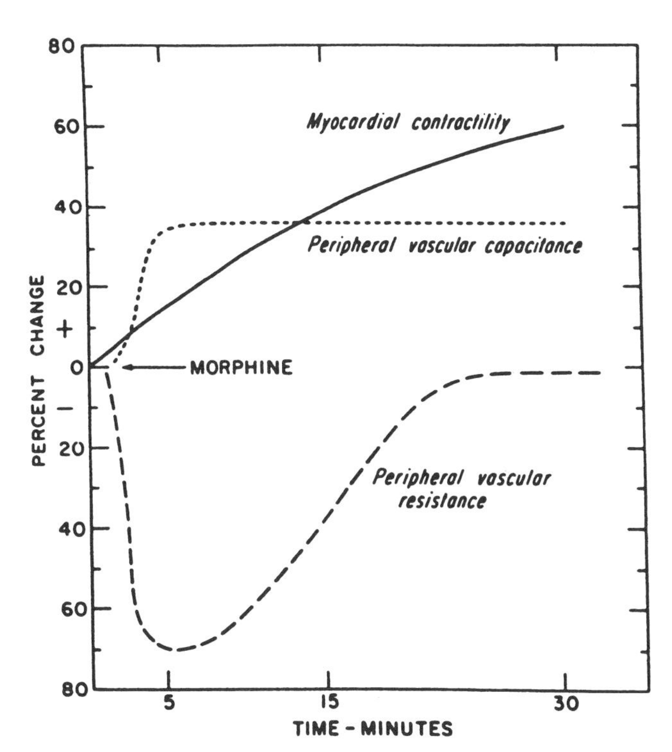

FIGURE 10-4. Time course of effects of intravenous morphine on myocardial contractility, peripheral vascular resistance, and venous capacitance. (From Vasko J, Henney R, Oldham N, et al. Am J Cardiol 1966;18:876-883.)

The cardiovascular effects of opioid agonist-antagonists are more diverse. Nalorphine and pentazocine alter hemodynamic parameters, resulting in increased arterial blood pressure, heart rate, systemic vascular resistance, pulmonary artery pressure, and left ventricular work index (187, 188). Increased serum catecholamine levels have been reported to occur with these agents, independent of the effects of opioid-induced hypercarbia. Although butorphanol has been reported to induce similar changes in patients with preexisting cardiac disease (189), other data demonstrate lack of hemodynamic response to high-dose butorphanol (190) or nalbuphine (191, 192). In large doses, dezocine causes cardiac depression (193, 194); however, excellent hemodynamic stability has been reported at analgesic doses (195).

In small doses, opioid antagonists have no acute cardiovascular effects in normal, opioid-naive patients (196). High doses of naloxone can increase blood pressure and heart rate, however (197). Pressor effects have been reported when large doses of naloxone were administered to patients in septic shock (198). When administered after opioids, naloxone has been reported to increase blood pressure, heart rate, contractility, and oxygen consumption (199). The short-term cardiovascular effects of naloxone are compounded by the presence of opioid-induced hypercarbia (200). Although investigators have speculated that these cardiovascular effects result from an increased perception of pain, physiologic alterations after naloxone have occurred without coexisting painful stimuli (200) and have been reported in patients deeply anesthetized with inhaled agents. Increased serum catecholamine levels following naloxone administration can result in markedly elevated systemic (201) and pulmonary artery pressures, pulmonary edema (202), ventricular arrhythmias (203), myocardial ischemia, and even cardiac arrest (204). These acute cardiovascular effects do not appear to be dose related and can occur even in young, healthy individuals (205). Cardiovascular instability and pulmonary edema have also been reported when the mixed agonist-antagonist drugs were administered after opiate agonists (206, 207).

Ventilatory Effects

Ventilatory depression secondary to μ-receptor binding in the medulla is the opiate side effect of greatest concern to clinicians. The μ–2 receptor mediates opiate ventilatory effects (12) and has a higher affinity for opiates than μ–1 receptors (208, 209). Additionally, tolerance to the analgesic effect of opiates occurs before tolerance develops to the respiratory depressant effects of opiates (210). Opiates cause a decrease in minute ventilation, and the resultant hypoventilation may be associated with hypercarbia and ventilatory acidosis, as well as hypoxemia. Opiate-induced decreases in the ventilatory response to carbon dioxide (CO_2) is quantified by comparing changes in minute ventilation with changes in arterial CO_2 tension. At low doses, morphine causes a rightward shift of this relationship (i.e., the set point is changed, but not the relative change in ventilatory response to an increased CO_2 concentration). At higher doses of morphine, the right shift is accompanied by a decreased slope of the ventilatory response curve for CO_2 (211). In addition, the hypoxic ventilatory drive is also decreased by opiate administration (212, 213), Following long-term opioid administration, tolerance to hypercarbic ventilatory depression occurs earlier than to hypoxic pulmonary drive, suggesting different opiate receptor mechanisms (214). After morphine administration, sleep results in a change in the slope of the CO_2 response curve (215).

Although ventilatory depression without a decrease in ventilatory rate has been described (216), morphine-induced ventilatory depression is typically associated with a reduced ventilatory rate. The resting tidal volume decreases significantly after large doses of opiates, as a result of a decrease in rib cage motion (217). Morphine does not change pulmonary dead space, but it does decrease bronchociliary motion. Although opioid analgesics decrease flow rate (217), inspiratory time as a fraction of the ventilatory cycle is not altered. As arterial CO_2 tension initially rises, a compensatory increase in minute ventilation occurs (with increased tidal volumes) (217). Periodic and irregular ventilatory patterns may occur with opiate administration, especially in older patients (218). Opiate administration can depress the drive to breathe such that apnea ensues in the conscious patient, but the ability to breathe on command persists. Opiates also blunt the typical increase in ventilatory effort associated with an imposed increase in the work of breathing (211).

Although agonist-antagonist drugs also produce ventilatory depression, the extent of ventilatory depression is limited by their ceiling effect at the μ receptor. The ceiling for ventilatory depression for butorphanol, nalorphine, nalbuphine, and dezocine is equivalent to that resulting from 30 mg of morphine in the average adult (219-222). Larger doses of butorphanol do not alter the CO_2 response curve but do prolong the duration of ventilatory depression (223). Pentazocine exhibits a less steep dose-response for ventilatory depression compared with morphine; however, a true ceiling phenomenon has not been demonstrated in patients because dysphoria limits the dosing of this drug (224). A ceiling effect with respect to the ventilatory response to buprenorphine is also likely, but it has not been proven (225). Meptazinol (226) and tramadol (227) appear to exert less ventilatory depression than morphine or the agonist-antagonist compounds.

Opioids are cough suppressants, and their antitussive effects are believed to be primarily mediated at the medulla. The receptor mediating this activity appears to be less stereospecific than other opiate receptors (1). Evidence suggests that opiate-induced antitussive activity may also be mediated peripherally (228), and opiate receptors are known to exist on the vagus nerves, which partially mediate the cough reflex. Synthetic opioids that do not cross the blood-brain barrier demonstrate antitussive activity.

Central Nervous System Effects

Anesthetic and Analgesic Properties

Unlike the generalized CNS depression resulting from potent inhaled anesthetics, opiates depress the CNS activity by a specific receptor mechanism. Consequently, even profoundly increased doses of opioids do not produce electroencephalographic (EEG) silence (229). EEG slowing does occur with morphine and some of its congeners, but to a lesser extent than with the more potent phenylpiperidines (230). In view of these effects, opiates are not considered to be complete anesthetics. Opioid analgesics decrease the minimum alveolar concentration (MAC) of the potent inhaled agents in a dose-related fashion (231, 232). However, even large doses of opioid analgesics produce a maximal 60 to 70% decrease in the anesthetic requirement. Therefore, supplementation inhaled agent (or other anesthetic drugs) may be required to prevent movement in response to surgical stimulation (231, 232). Not surprisingly, intraoperative awareness and recall after opiate-oxygen anesthesia have been reported to occur with greater frequency with "high-dose" opioid techniques than when other anesthetic techniques were used. Limited data are available regarding the risk of awareness compared with other anesthetic regimens employing either benzodiazepines or inhaled agents.

Despite the limitations of μ agonists to decrease the anesthetic requirement for inhaled agents, to prevent awareness, and to produce muscle relaxation, high doses of opioid analgesics are more effective than other drugs in preventing the neurohumoral stress response to surgery and trauma. Surgical stimulation commonly produces a generalized neurohumoral response consisting of an increase in serum levels of cortisol, glucose, catecholamines, growth hormone, aldosterone, and ADH (vasopressin). This response may be detrimental to patients with preexisting cardiovascular disease because it can increase cardiac demands, accelerate protein catabolism, and decrease immune function. Whereas potent inhaled agents are unable to suppress the neurohumoral response effectively, high doses of opiates more effectively suppress this response to noxious stimuli (233).

In contrast, opiate agonist-antagonists have less anesthetic-sparing effects than large doses of μ agonists. Butorphanol, nalbuphine, and pentazocine produce only a 10 to 20% decrease in the anesthetic requirement (231, 234), similar to that achieved with low doses of the pure μ agonists (190, 235). Patients receiving a benzodiazepine and nalbuphine have higher serum catecholamine levels and require greater use of vasodilators to control blood pressure than patients receiving a benzodiazepine and fentanyl for cardiac surgery (236). Nalbuphine is also less effective than a pure μ agonist in attenuating responses to noxious stimuli such as laryngoscopy (237). Large doses of dezocine (6 to 20 mg/kg) have been reported to decrease the anesthetic requirement by 50%, however (193, 238). After arthroscopic surgery under general anesthesia, dezocine has been shown to be similar in efficacy to morphine and superior to nalbuphine in alleviating pain (239). In general, postoperative analgesia can usually be effectively managed with either pure or partial opiate agonists (240).

The profound sedative effects of agonist-antagonist drugs with significant κ receptor activity limit their use as analgesics. When nalbuphine or fentanyl was administered as analgesics after surgery, the primary side effect of fentanyl was ventilatory depression, whereas nalbuphine produced increased sedation (237). Butorphanol produces sedation that is qualitatively similar to that induced by midazolam and occurs even at subanalgesic doses (241). The agonist-antagonist agents also cause variable degrees of psychotomimetic and dysphoric effects, mediated by κ-receptor activity. The dysphoric effects of nalorphine and pentazocine are troublesome and limit their use in clinical practice (22, 242, 243). Opioid-induced euphoria is less likely to occur with the agonist-antagonist agents than with pure μ agonists. Therefore, the abuse potential for agonist-antagonist opioids appears to be reduced (244, 245). Nonetheless, physical dependence can result after prolonged administration of agonist-antagonist drugs, and withdrawal can be precipitated if the drug is abruptly discontinued (223, 246).

Other CNS Properties

The effects of opiates on cerebral blood flow and metabolism in the anesthetized patient have not been thoroughly investigated. It is known, however, that morphine-like analgesics cause a modest reduction in cerebral blood flow and cerebral metabolic rate, related in large part to a decrease in the level of CNS arousal (247). Autoregulation (248) and cerebrovascular reactivity to CO_2 are well maintained in the presence of opioid analgesics. The effect of opiates on cerebrovascular tone is not completely understood. μ- or δ- receptor agonists applied directly to cerebral vessels result in vasodilation (249), and reports have implicated sufentanil and fentanyl in directly vasodilating cerebral vessels resulting in increasing intracranial pressure (250, 251). In contrast, other studies have found neither increased cerebral blood flow nor increased intracranial pressure following opioid administration (252).

Seizure-like movements have also been reported following opiate administration, but EEG seizure activity associated with opioids has not been firmly established, and these movements may represent opiate-related rigidity (253). Normeperidine, the primary metabolite of meperidine, is a CNS stimulant and in high concentration can cause seizure activity when it accumulates after repeated dosing in patients with impaired renal function (254). Increased muscular tone and neuromuscular rigidity may occur with opioid administration. Rigidity predominantly involves the thoracic and abdominal muscles and can make ventilation extremely difficult. Whereas all opiates can elicit this side effect, rigidity occurs less frequently with morphine and related compounds compared with the more potent fentanyl derivatives. The speed of injection of potent opiates is thought to be a contributing factor (255), and opiate-induced unconsciousness almost always precedes rigidity. Rigidity typically occurs immediately following anesthetic induction when large doses of opiates are utilized, although intraoperative or even postoperative muscle tightness can develop as a result of a secondary peak in the opiate concentration (256). Although full neuromuscular blockade prevents (or reverses) this phenomenon, pretreatment with a defasiculating dose of a nondepolarizing muscle relaxant is also effective in decreasing the incidence and severity of opioid-induced rigidity (255, 257). Benzodiazepine premedication has also been found to decrease the incidence of rigidity (255). The mechanism of opiate-induced rigidity is not certain, but it probably involves interactions with γ-aminobutyric acid and dopaminergic neurons in the brain (258).

Other opiate side effects that are centrally mediated include pupillary miosis, pruritus, and decreased shivering. Miosis is due to an excitatory action of opiates at the Edinger-Westphal nucleus. Although the degree of miosis has been found to correlate with plasma codeine concentration (259), pupil size is not uniformly useful in assessing the extent of opiate activity (260). Pruritus may result after opiate administration and is observed in the absence of histamine release. Pruritus is opiate receptor mediated, can be reversed with small doses of opiate antagonists, and is particularly marked around the nares, although the reason is unclear. Administered intravenously, meperidine is uniquely effective among the opiates in its ability to diminish or terminate shivering from hypothermia, from blood transfusion reactions, or related to epidural anesthesia (261, 262), and intraoperative administration of this drug (as well as morphine or alfentanil) may also decrease the incidence of postoperative shivering (263).

Gastrointestinal and Renal Effects

Morphine and related compounds decrease gastrointestinal motility by both central and peripheral mechanisms mediated by opiate receptors that can be reversed with naloxone (264). Intraventricular morphine administration decreases bowel motility (265), and morphine also decreases acetylcholine release from gastrointestinal nerve endings (266), although vagotomy does not prevent opiate-induced gastrointestinal effects(267). Opiate-induced slowing of gastric emptying as well as reduction of lower esophageal sphincter activity (268) may theoretically increase the risk of regurgitation and aspiration during anesthetic induction in certain patients. Opiates not only decrease intestinal propulsive action but also increase intestinal tone and spasm (269). The severity of spasm is higher in patients with ulcerative colitis than in other patients, and toxic megacolon may be related to use of opioids in this population (270).

Opiates cause sphincter of Oddi contraction and result in dose-related increases in biliary duct pressures (Fig. 10-5) (271-273). Opioid-induced biliary spasm may present diagnostic problems during performance of cholangiograms (272) and may cause pain that has even been confused with angina (274). Morphine-induced biliary spasm is reversible with naloxone, glucagon, or nitroglycerin and less reliably with atropine (275). Meperidine is often the opioid selected in patients with biliary tract disease because its anticholinergic activity decreases sphincter of Oddi contraction frequency (while morphine increases the frequency of contraction) (276), although elevated biliary pressures still can result from meperidine (272). The mixed agonist-antagonist opiates butorphanol and pentazocine cause significantly less biliary pressure elevation than pure μ-agonist agents and may be advantageous in patients with biliary tract disease (277).

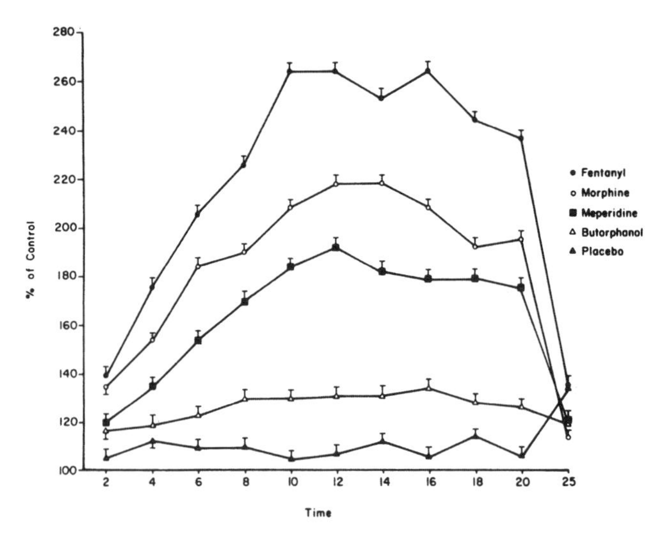

FIGURE 10-5. The effect of morphine and related compounds on common bile duct pressure and the response to naloxone administered after 20 minutes. (From Radnay PA, Duncalf D, Novakovic M, Lesser ML. Common bile duct pressure changes after fentanyl, morphine, meperidine, butorphanol, and naloxone. Anesth Analg 1984;63:441–444.)

Nausea and vomiting are common postoperative problems, and many factors, including opiate administration, contribute to their occurrence. Opioids promote emesis by stimulating the chemoreceptor trigger zone. They probably increase vestibular sensitivity as well, and nausea following morphine is typically more common in ambulatory than in resting patients (278). The emetogenic effects of opioids are unfortunately not susceptible to naloxone reversal (279, 280).

Morphine administration has been associated with a decrease in urine output. An increase in ADH has been implicated, and although μ-receptor agonists do result in increased serum ADH levels in animals, morphine-like opiates do not elicit this effect in humans (Fig. 10-6) (281). Surgical stimulation itself produces a marked increase in serum ADH, and opiates may actually diminish the extent of intraoperative ADH elevation by decreasing the neurohumoral response to surgery. Although μ agonists have little direct effect on serum ADH levels, κ-receptor agonists may cause

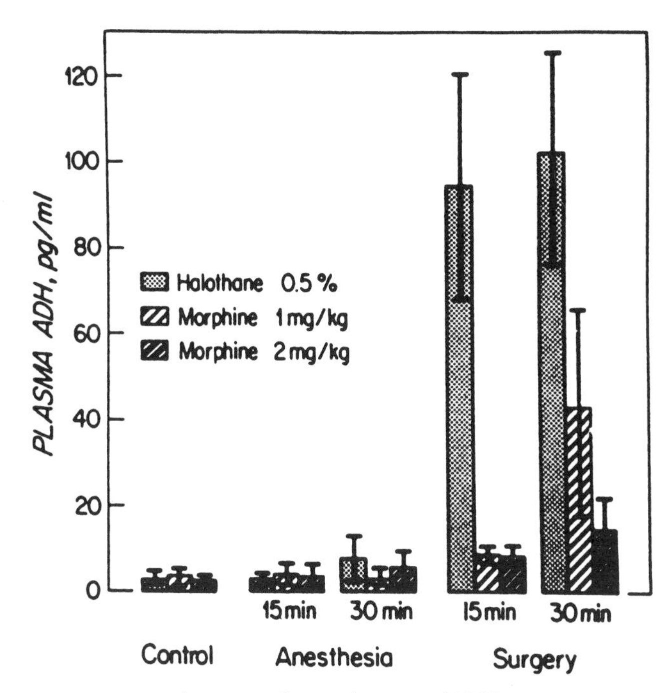

FIGURE 10-6. Plasma antidiuretic hormone (ADH) responses to surgery with an inhaled anesthetic (halothane) in comparison with morphine. (From Philbin DM, Coggins CH. Plasma antidiuretic hormone levels in cardiac surgical patients during morphine and halothane anesthesia. Anesthesiology 1978;49:95–98.)

a decrease in plasma ADH levels resulting in diuresis (282). Decreased urine output following μ-agonist administration may be related to changes in cardiac output or renal blood flow (283). Morphine may also contribute to a decrease in urine output because of enhanced proximal renal tubular sodium reabsorption modulated by an opiate receptor mechanism (284). Morphine-like opiates effect the genitourinary smooth muscle, producing increased urethral tone and peristaltic activity. Simultaneously, detrusor muscle tone is augmented, and vesicular sphincter tone is increased, resulting in urinary urgency as well as urinary retention (227).

DRUG INTERACTIONS

The effects of morphine-like drugs can be altered by concomitant administration of other drugs. In addition to variable degrees of MAC reduction when combined with potent inhaled anesthetics, morphine and related compounds can produce decreases in blood pressure and cardiac output when coadministered with nitrous oxide (285-288). These hemodynamic effects are significantly greater than those observed with either agent alone and are more pronounced in patients with poor cardiac function (289). Opiates reduce the dose of barbituates and propofol required for induction of anesthesia (290, 291), and these induction agents potentiate opiate-induced ventilatory depression (292).

Small doses of benzodiazepines are often added to an opioid-based anesthetic to provide perioperative amnesia. Subanalgesic doses of opioids increase the hypnotic effect of benzodiazepines, and synergistic hypnotic effects have been demonstrated between opiates and benzodiazepines (293). Combining benzodiazepines and opioids also markedly increases ventilatory depression (294). Although hemodynamic instability is unusual with administration of either class of drugs alone, hypotension and a decrease in systemic vascular resistance can result from their coadministration (295-297).

Selection of a nondepolarizing muscle relaxant is often determined by cardiovascular side effect profiles. For example, the vagolytic property of pancuronium offsets the vagotonic effect of large doses of morphine. When administered alone, vecuronium is considered to have no effect on heart rate, although it may potentiate the bradycardia associated with opiates (298). Subsequently greater sympathomimetic use may be required with vecuronium than with pancuronium during opioid anesthesia (299, 300).

Combining meperidine with monoamine oxidase inhibitors can produce life-threatening reactions ranging from hypotension and ventilatory depression to hypertension and hyperpyrexia. Decreased metabolism of meperidine secondary to monoamine oxidase inhibition may explain the exaggerated responses to meperidine (301). The hyperdynamic responses are probably due to potentiation of the central serotonin uptake inhibition of monoamine oxidase inhibitors by meperidine. Other opioids are probably safe to administer with monoamine oxidase inhibitors (302, 303). Monoamine oxidase inhibitor treatment, however, may result in potentiation and prolongation of opiate effects and has been described with morphine, meperidine, and pentazocine (301, 304, 305).

SUMMARY

In summary, morphine and its related compounds have been utilized widely in the practice of anesthesia for many years. Although not currently administered as a major component of intravenous anesthesia techniques, these compounds remain useful adjuncts in the perioperative period and in aggregate have provided much insight into the clinical relevance of the opiate receptor subtypes. Adequate knowledge of the pharmacokinetic and pharmacodynamic characteristics of these agents as described in this chapter is necessary for optimal application in clinical anesthesia, especially when these drugs are combined with other anesthetic or analgesic agents.

REFERENCES

1. Jaffe JH, Martin WR. Opioid analgesics and antagonists. In: Goodman AG, Gilman LS, eds. Goodman and Gilman's The pharmacological basis of therapeutics. 8th ed. New York: Pergamon Press, 1990:485–521.
2. Brownstein MJ. A brief history of opiates, opioid peptides, and opioid receptors. Proc Natl Acad Sci U S A 1993;90:5391–5393.
3. Foldes FF, Swerdlow M, Siker ES, eds. Narcotics and narcotic antagonists: chemistry, pharmacology, and applications in anesthesiology and obstetrics. Springfield, IL:Charles C Thomas, 1964.
4. Neff W, Mayer EC, de la Luz Perales M. Nitrous oxide and oxygen anesthesia with curare relaxation. Calif Med 1947; 66:67–73.
5. Bailey P, Gerbode F, Garlington L. An anesthetic technique for cardiac surgery which utilizes 100% oxygen as the only inhalant. Arch Surg 1958;76:437–443.
6. Lowenstein E, Hallowell P, Levine FH, et al. Cardiovascular response to large doses of intravenous morphine in man. N Engl J Med 1969;281:1389–1393.
7. Stanley TH, Gray NG, Stanford W, Armstrong R. The effects of high-dose morphine on fluid and blood requirements in open-heart operations. Anesthesiology 1973;38:536–541.
8. Stanley TH, Liu WS. Cardiovascular effects of nitrous oxide-meperidine anesthesia before and after pancuronium. Anesth Analg 1977;56:669–673.
9. Lasagna L, Beecher HK. The analgesic effectiveness of nalorphine and nalorphine-morphine combinations in man. J Pharmacol Exp Ther 1965;112:356–363.
10. Martin WR. Opioid antagonists. Pharmacol Rev 1967;19:463–521.
11. Pasternak GW, Zhang A, Tecott L. Developmental differences between high and low affinity opiate binding sites: their relationship to analgesia and respiratory depression. Life Sci 1980; 27:1185–1190.
12. Ling GSF, Spiegel K, Lockhart SH, Pasternak GW. Separation of opioid analgesia from respiratory depression: evidence for different receptor mechanisms. J Pharmacol Exp Ther 1985;232; 149–155.
13. Zhang A, Pasternak GW. Ontogeny of opioid pharmacology and receptors: high and low affinity site differences. Eur J Pharmacol 1981;73:29–40.
14. Wolozin BL, Pasternak GW. Classification of multiple morphine and enkephalin blinding sites in the central nervous system. Proc Natl Acad Sci U S A 1981;78:6181–6185.
15. Spiegel K, Pasternak GW. Meptazinol: a novel mu–1 selective opioid analgesic. J Pharmacol Exp Ther 1984;228:414–419.
16. Jordan C, Lehane JR, Robson PJ, Jones JG. Comparison of the respiratory effects of meptazinol, pentazocine and morphine. Anaesthesia 1979;51:497–501.
17. Bill DJ, Hartley JE, Stephens RJ, Thompson AM. The antinociceptive activity of meptazinol depends on both opiate and cholinergic mechanisms. Br J Pharmacol 1983;79:191–199.
18. Ireson JD. A comparison of the antinociceptive actions of cholinomimetic and morphine-like drugs. Br J Pharmacol 1970; 40:90–101.
19. Leslie GB. The effect of anti-parkinsonian drugs on oxotremorine-induced analgesia in mice. J Pharm Pharmacol 1969; 21:248–250.
20. Goodman RR, Pasternak GW. Visualization of μ_1 opiate receptors in rat brain by using a computerized autoradiographic subtraction technique. Proc Natl Acad Sci U S A 1985; 82:6667–6671.
21. Moskowitz AS, Goodman RR. Autoradiographic analysis of mu_1 mu_2 and delta opioid binding in the central nervous system of C57BL/6BY and CXBK (opioid receptor-deficient) mice. Brain Res 1985;360:108–116.
22. Millan MJ. μ-opioid receptors and analgesia. Trends Pharmacol Sci 1990;11:70–76.
23. Stein C. Peripheral mechanisms of opioid analgesia. Anesth Analg 1993;76:182–191.
24. Goldstein DJ, Meador-Woodruff JH. Opiate receptors: opioid agonist-antagonist effects. Pharmacotherapy 1991;11:164–167.
25. Itzhak Y. Multiple opioid binding sites. In: Pasternak GW, ed. The opiate receptors. Clifton, NJ: Humana Press, 1988:95–142.
26. Chavkin C, James IF, Goldstein A. Dynorphin is a specific endogenous ligand of the opioid receptor. Science 1982;215:413–415.
27. Mansour A, Khachaturian H, Lewis ME, et al. Anatomy of CNS opioid receptors. Trends Neurosci 1988;11:309–314.
28. Millan MJ. Kappa-opioid receptor-mediated antinociception in the rat. I. Comparative actions of mu- and kappa-opioids against noxious thermal, pressure and electrical stimuli. J Pharmacol Exp Ther 1989;251:334–341.
29. Pfeiffer A, Branti V, Herz A, Emrich HM. Psychotomimesis mediated by opiate receptors. Science 1986;233:774–776.
30. Unterwald E, Sasson S, Kornetsky C. Evaluation of the supraspinal analgesic activity and abuse liability of ethylketocyclazocine. Eur J Pharmacol 1987;133:275–281.
31. Freye E, Hartung E, Schenk GK. Bremazocine: an opiate that induces sedation and analgesia without respiratory depression. Anesth Analg 1983;62:483–438.
32. Dykstra LA. Butorphanol, levallorphan, nalbuphine and nalorphine as antagonists in the squirrel monkey. J Pharmacol Exp Ther 1990;254:245–252.
33. Zimmerman DM, Leander JD, Reel JK, Hynes MD. Use of β-funaltrexamine to determine mu opioid receptor involvement in the analgesic activity of various opioid ligands. J Pharmacol Exp Ther 1987;241:374–378.
34. Horan PJ, Ho IK. Comparative pharmacological and biochemical studies between butorphanol and morphine. Pharmacol Biochem Behav 1989;34:847–854.
35. Picker MJ, Negus SS, Craft RM. Butorphanol's efficacy at mu and kappa opioid receptors: inferences based on the schedule-controlled behavior of nontolerant and morphine-tolerant rats and on the responding of rats under a drug discrimination procedure. Pharmacol Biochem Behav 1990;36:563–568.
36. Pedersen JE, Chraemmer-Jørgensen B, Schmidt JF, Risbo A. Naloxone: a strong analgesic in combination with high-dose buprenorphine? Br J Anaesth 1985;57:1045–1046.
37. Bailey PL, Clark NJ, Pace NL, et al. Failure of nalbuphine to antagonize morphine: a double-blind comparison with naloxone. Anesth Analg 1986;65:605–611.
38. Bailey PL, Clark NJ, Pace NL, et al. Antagonism of postoperative opioid-induced respiratory depression: nalbuphine versus naloxone. Anesth Analg 1987;66:1109–1114.
39. Jaffe RS, Moldenhauer CC, Hug CC, et al. Nalbuphine antagonism of fentanyl-induced ventilatory depression: a randomized trial. Anesthesiology 1988;68:254–260.
40. Preston KL, Jasinski DR. Abuse liability studies of opioid agonist-antagonists in humans. Drug Alcohol Depend 1991;28:49–82.
41. Goodman RR, Snyder SH, Kuhar MJ, Young WS III. Differentiation of delta and mu opiate receptor localizations by light microscopic autoradiography. Proc Natl Acad Sci U S A 1980; 77:6239–6243.
42. Quirion R, Zajac JM, Morgat JL, Roques BP. Autoradiographic distribution of mu and delta opiate receptors in rat brain using highly selective ligands. Life Sci 1983;33:227–230.
43. Moulin DE, Max MB, Kaiko RF, et al. The analgesic efficacy of intrathecal d-ala^2-d-leu^5-enkephalin in cancer patients with chronic pain. Pain 1985;23:213–221.
44. Millan MJ. Multiple opioid systems and pain. Pain 1986;27:303–347.

45. Sadée W, Richards ML, Grevel J, Rosenbaum JS. In vivo characterization of four types of opioid binding sites in rat brain. Life Sci 1983;33:187–189.
46. Dum JE, Herz A. In vivo receptor binding of the opiate partial agonist, buprenorphine, correlated with its agonistic and antagonistic actions. Br J Pharmac 1981;74:627–633.
47. Cowan A, Lewis JW, MacFarlane IR. Agonist and antagonist properties of buprenorphine, a new antinociceptive agent. Br J Pharmacol 1977;60:537–545.
48. Pedersen JE, Chraemmer-Jørgensen B, Schmidt JF, Risbo A. Peroperative buprenorphine: do high dosages shorten analgesia postoperatively? Acta Anaesthesiol Scand 1986;30:660–663.
49. Walker JM, Bowen WD, Walker FO, et al. Sigma receptors: biology and function. Pharmacol Rev 1990;42:355–402.
50. Sonders MS, Keana JFW, Weber E. Phencyclidine and psychotomimetic sigma opiates: recent insights into their biochemical and physiological sites of actions. Trends Neurosci 1988; 11:37–40.
51. Deutsch SI, Weizman A, Goldman ME, Morihisa JM. The sigma receptor: a novel site implicated in psychosis and antipsychotic drug efficacy. Clin Neuropharmacol 1988;11:105–119.
52. Raffa RB, Friderichs E, Reimman W, et al. Opioid and nonopioid components independently contribute to the mechanism of action of tramadol, an "atypical" opioid analgesic. J Pharmacol Exp Ther 1992;260:275–285.
53. Hennies HH, Friderichs E, Wilsmann K, Flohé L. Effect of the opioid analgesic tramadol on inactivation of norepinephrine and serotonin. Biochem Pharmacol 1982;31:1654–1655.
54. Friderichs E, Reimann W, Selve N. Contribution of both enantiomers to antinociception of the centrally acting analgesic tramadol [Abstract]. Arch Pharm 1992;346:R36.
55. Collart L, Luthy C, Dayer P. Multimodal analgesic effect of tramadol [Abstract]. Clin Pharmacol Ther 1993;53:223.
56. Kayser V, Besson JM, Guilbaud G. Evidence for a noradrenergic component in the antinociceptive effect of the analgesic agent tramadol in an animal model of clinical pain, the arthritic rat. Eur J Pharmacol 1992;224:83–88.
57. Pleuvry BJ. Opioid receptors and their relevance to anaesthesia. Br J Anaesth 1993;71:119–126.
58. Wüster M, Schulz R, Herz A. Specificity of opioids towards the μ-, δ- and ϵ-opiate receptors. Neurosci Lett 1978;15:193–198.
59. North RA. Drug receptors and the inhibition of nerve cells. Br J Pharmacol 1989;98:13–28.
60. McFadzean I. The ionic mechanisms underlying opioid actions. Neuropeptides 1988;11:173–180.
61. Thorpe DH. Opiate structure and activity: a guide to understanding the receptor. Anesth Analg 1984;63:143–151.
62. Janssen PAJ. A review of the chemical features associated with strong morphine-like activity. Br J Anaesth 1962;34:260–268.
63. Janssen PAJ, Vander Eycken CAM. The chemical anatomy of potent morphine-like analgesics. In: Burger A, ed. Drugs affecting the central nervous system. vol. 2. New York: Marcel Dekker, 1968:25–60.
64. Kolb VM. New opiate-receptor model. J Pharm Sci 1978;67:999–1002.
65. Säwe J, Svensson JO, Rane A. Morphine metabolism in cancer patients on increasing oral doses-no evidence for autoinduction or dose-dependence. Br J Clin Pharmacol 1983;16:85–93.
66. Brunk SF, Delle M. Morphine metabolism in man. Clin Pharmacol Ther 1974;16:51–57.
67. Findlay JWA, Butz RF, Welch RM. Codeine kinetics as determined by radioimmunoassay. Clin Pharmacol Ther 1977; 22:439–446.
68. Shah JC, Mason WD. Plasma codeine and morphine concentrations after a single oral dose of codeine phosphate. J Clin Pharmacol 1990;30:764–766.
69. Persson K, Hammarlund-Udenaes M, Mortimer O, Rane A. The postoperative pharmacokinetics of codeine. Eur J Clin Pharmacol 1992;42:663–666.
70. Inturrisi CE, Verebely K. Disposition of methadone in man after a single oral dose. Clin Pharmacol Ther 1972;13:923–930.
71. Iwamoto K, Klaassen CD. First-pass effect of morphine in rats. J Pharmacol Exp Ther 1977;200:236–244.
72. Rance MJ, Shillingford JS. The role of the gut in the metabolism of strong analgesics. Biochem Pharmacol 1976;25:735–741.
73. Dahlström BE, Paalzow LK. Pharmacokinetic interpretation of the enterohepatic recirculation and first-pass elimination of morphine in the rat. J Pharmacokinet Biopharm 1978;6:505–519.
74. Beaver WT, Wallenstein SL, Rogers A, Houde RW. Analgesic studies of codeine and oxycodone in patients with cancer. II. Comparisons of intramuscular oxycodone with intramuscular morphine and codeine. J Pharmacol Exp Ther 1978;207:101–108.
75. Dayer P, Collart L, Desmeules J. The pharmacology of tramadol. Drugs 1994;47:3–7.
76. Stanski DR, Greenblatt DJ, Lowenstein E. Kinetics of intravenous and intramuscular morphine. Clin Pharmacol Ther 1978; 24:52–59.
77. Stambaugh JE, Wainer IW, Sanstead JK, Hemphill DM. The clinical pharmacology of meperidine-comparison of routes of administration. J Clin Pharmacol 1976;16:245–256.
78. Austin KL, Stapleton JV, Mather LE. Multiple intramuscular injections: a major source of variability in analgesic response to meperidine. Pain 1980;8:47–62.
79. Murphy MR, Hug CC. Pharmacokinetics of intravenous morphine in patients anesthetized with enflurane-nitrous oxide. Anesthesiology 1981;54:187–192.
80. Dahlström B, Bolme P, Feychting H, et al. Morphine kinetics in children. Clin Pharmacol Ther 1979;26:354–365.
81. Roerig DL, Kotrly KJ, Vucins ED, et al. First pass uptake of fentanyl, meperidine, and morphine in the human lung. Anesthesiology 1987;67:466–472.
82. Geddes DM, Nesbitt K, Trial T, Blackburn JP. First pass uptake of ^{14}C propranolol by the lung. Thorax 1979;34:810–813.
83. Taeger K, Weninger E, Franke N, et al. Uptake of fentanyl by human lung [Abstract]. Anesthesiology 1984;61:A246.
84. Hanks GW, Hoskin PJ, Aherne GW, et al. Enterohepatic circulation of morphine. Lancet 1988;1:469.
85. Olsen GD. Morphine binding to human plasma proteins. Clin Pharmacol Ther 1974;17:31–35.
86. Hollt V, Teschemacher H-J. Hydrophobic interactions responsible for unspecific binding of morphine-like drugs. Naunyn Schmiedebergs Arch Pharmacol 1975;288:163–177.
87. Lee CR, McTavish D, Sorkin EM. Tramadol: a preliminary review of its pharmacodynamic and pharmacokinetic properties, and therapeutic potential in acute and chronic pain states. Drugs 1993;46:313–340.
88. Abramson FP. Methadone plasma protein binding: alterations in cancer and displacement from $_1$-acid glycoprotein. Clin Pharmacol Ther 1982;32:652–658.
89. Hertz A, Teschemacher H-J. Activities and sites of antinociceptive action of morphine-like analgesics. In: Harper NJ, Simmonds AB, eds. Advances in drug research. New York: Academic Press, 1971:79–86.
90. Roy SD, Flynn GL. Solubility and related physicochemical properties of narcotic analgesics. Pharm Res 1988;5:580–586.
91. Kaufman JJ, Semo NM, Koski WS. Microelectrometric titration measurement of the pK_as and partition and drug distribution coefficients of narcotics and narcotic antagonists and their pH and temperature dependence. J Med Chem 1975;18:647–655.
92. Benson DW, Kaufman JJ, Koski WS. Theoretic significance of pH dependence of narcotics and narcotic antagonists in clinical anesthesia. Anesth Analg 1976;55:253–256.
93. Finck AD, Berkowitz BA, Hempstead J, Ngai SH. Pharmacokinetics of morphine: effects of hypercarbia on serum and brain morphine concentrations in the dog. Anesthesiology 1977; 47:407–410.
94. Nishitateno K, Ngai SH, Finck AD, Berkowitz BA. Pharmacokinetics of morphine: concentrations in the serum and brain of

the dog during hyperventilation. Anesthesiology 1979;50:520–523.
95. Hug CC, Murphy MR, Rigel EP, Olson WA. Pharmacokinetics of morphine injected intravenously into the anesthetized dog. Anesthesiology 1981;54:38–47.
96. Von Cube B, Teschemacher H, Herz A, et al. Permeation morphinartic wirksamer substanzen an den Ort der antinociceptiven Wirkung im Gehirn in Abhängigkeit von ihrer Lipoidlöslichkeit nach intravenöser und nach intraventriculärer Applikation. Naunyn Schmiedebergs Arch Pharmacol 1970; 265:455–473.
97. Kupfberberg HJ, Way EL. Pharmacologic basis for the sensitivity of the newborn rat to morphine. J Pharmacol Exp Ther 1963; 141:105–112.
98. Mule SJ, Woods LA. Distribution of N-C^{14}-methyl labeled morphine. I. In central nervous system of nontolerant and tolerant dogs. J Pharmacol Exp Ther 1962;136:232–241.
99. Austin KL, Stapleton JV, Mather LE. Relationship between blood meperidine concentrations and analgesic response: a preliminary report. Anesthesiology 1980;53:460–466.
100. Boas RA, Villiger JW. Clinical actions of fentanyl and buprenorphine: the significance of receptor binding. Br J Anaesth 1985; 57:192–196.
101. Villiger JW. Binding of buprenorphine to opiate receptors: regulation by guanyl nucleotides and metal ions. Neuropharmacology 1984;23:373–375.
102. Orwin JM. Buprenorphine pharmacological aspects in man. In: Harcus AW, et al, eds. Pain: new perspectives in measurement and management. Edinburgh: Churchill Livingstone, 1977.
103. Orwin JM, Robson PJ, Orwin J, Price M. Antagonist action of naloxone on the acute effects of buprenorphine. In: Proceedings of the 6th World Congress of Anesthesiology, Mexico City, April 1976;sect 5:189.
104. Stanski DR, Paalzow L, Edlund PO. Morphine pharmacokinetics: GLC assay versus radioimmunoassay. J Pharm Sci 1982; 71:314–316.
105. Catlin DH. Pharmacokinetics of morphine by radio-immunoassay: the influence of immunochemical factors. J Pharmacol Exp Ther 1977;200:224–235.
106. Hughes MA, Glass PSA, Jacobs JR. Context-sensitive half-time in multicompartment pharmacokinetic models for intravenous anesthetic drugs. Anesthesiology 1992;76:334–341.
107. Shafer SL, Varvel JR. Pharmacokinetics, pharmacodynamics, and rational opioid selection. Anesthesiology 1991;74:53–63.
108. Youngs EJ, Shafer SL. Pharmacokinetic parameters relevant to recovery from opioids. Anesthesiology 1994;81:833–842.
109. Mazoit JX, Sandouk P, Scherrmann JM, Roche A. Extrahepatic metabolism of morphine occurs in humans. Clin Pharmacol Ther 1990;48:613–618.
110. Osborne R, Joel S, Trew D, Slevin M. Morphine and metabolite behavior after different routes of morphine administration: demonstration of the importance of the active metabolite morphine–6-glucuronide. Clin Pharmacol Ther 1990;47:12–19.
111. Smith MT, Watt JA, Cramond T. Morphine–3-glucuronide: a potent antagonist of morphine analgesia. Life Sci 1990;47:579–585.
112. Sullivan AF, McQuay HJ, Bailey D, Dickenson AH. The spinal antinociceptive actions of morphine metabolites morphine–6-glucuronide and normorphine in the rat. Brain Res 1989; 482:219–224.
113. Hand CW, Blunnie WP, Claffey LP, et al. Potential analgesic contribution from morphine–6-glucuronide in CSF. Lancet 1987:2;1207–1208.
114. Osborne R, Thompson P, Joel S, et al. The analgesic activity of morphine–6-glucuronide. Br J Clin Pharmacol 1992;34:130–138.
115. Bigler D, Christensen CB, Eriksen J, Jensen NH. Morphine, morphine–6-glucuronide and morphine–3-glucuronide concentrations in plasma and cerebrospinal fluid during long-term high-dose intrathecal morphine administration. Pain 1990;41:15–18.
116. Wahlström A, Winblad B, Bixo M, Rane A. Human brain metabolism of morphine and naloxone. Pain 1988;35:121–127.
117. Hanna MH, Peat SJ, Woodham M, et al. Analgesic efficacy and CSF pharmacokinetics of intrathecal morphine–6-glucuronide: comparison with morphine. Br J Anaesth 1990;64:547–550.
118. Pelligrino DA, Riegler FX, Albrecht RF. Ventilatory effects of fourth cerebroventricular infusions of morphine–6- or morphine–3-glucuronide in the awake dog. Anesthesiology 1989; 71:936–940.
119. Findlay JWA, Jones EC, Butz RF, Welch RM. Plasma codeine and morphine concentrations after therapeutic oral doses of codeine-containing analgesics. Clin Pharmacol Ther 1978;24:60–68.
120. Guay DR, Awni WM, Findlay JW, et al. Pharmacokinetics and pharmacodynamics of codeine in end-stage renal disease. Clin Pharmacol Ther 1988;43:63–71.
121. Shah J, Mason WD. Pharmacokinetics of codeine after parenteral and oral dosing in the rat. Drug Metab Dispos 1990;18:670–673.
122. Hennies HH, Friderichs E, Schneider J. Receptor binding, analgesic and antitussive potency of tramadol and other selected opioids. Arzneimittelforschung 1988;38:877–880.
123. Kaiko RF, Foley KM, Grabinski PY, et al. Central nervous system excitatory effects of meperidine in cancer patients. Ann Neurol 1983;13:180–185.
124. Nickander R, Smits SE, Steinberg MI. Propoxyphene and norpropoxyphene: pharmacologic and toxic effects in animals. J Pharmacol Exp Ther 1977;200:245–253.
125. Säwe J. High-dose morphine and methadone in cancer patients: clinical pharmacokinetic considerations of oral treatment. Clin Pharmacokinet 1986;11:87–106.
126. Verbeeck RK, Branch RA, Wilkinson GR. Meperidine disposition in man: influence of urinary pH and route of administration. Clin Pharmacol Ther 1981;30:619–628.
127. Nilsson MI, Widerlöv E, Meresaar U, Änggård E. Effect of urinary pH on the disposition of methadone in man. Eur J Clin Pharmacol 1982;22:337–342.
128. Way WL, Costley EC, Way EL. Respiratory sensitivity of the newborn infant to meperidine and morphine. Clin Pharmacol Ther 1965;6:454–461.
129. Notarianni LJ. Plasma protein binding of drugs in pregnancy and in neonates. Clin Pharmacokinet 1990;18:20–36.
130. Choonara IA, McKay P, Hain R, Rane A. Morphine metabolism in children. Br J Clin Pharmacol 1989;28:599–604.
131. Bhat R, Chari G, Gulati A, et al. Pharmacokinetics of a single dose of morphine in preterm infants during the first week of life. J Pediatr 1990;117:477–481.
132. Lynn AM, Slattery JT. Morphine pharmacokinetics in early infancy. Anesthesiology 1987;66:136–139.
133. Chay PCW, Duffy BJ, Walker JS. Pharmacokinetic-pharmacodynamic relationships of morphine in neonates. Clin Pharmacol Ther 1992;51:334–342.
134. Olkkola KT, Maunuksela EL, Korpela R, Rosenberg PH. Kinetics and dynamics of postoperative intravenous morphine in children. Clin Pharmacol Ther 1988;44:128–136.
135. Kuhnert BR, Kuhnert PM, Philipson EH, Syracuse CD. Disposition of meperidine and normeperidine following multiple doses during labor. Am J Obstet Gynecol 1985;151:410–415.
136. Hodgkinson R, HU S, Ain FJ. The duration of effect of maternally administered meperidine on neonatal neurobehavior. Anesthesiology 1982;56:51–52.
137. Wittels B, Scott DT, Sinatra RS. Exogenous opioids in human breast milk and acute neonatal neurobehavior: a preliminary study. Anesthesiology 1990;73:864–869.
138. Baillie SP, Bateman DN, Coates PE, Woodhouse KW. Age and the pharmacokinetics of morphine. Age Aging 1989;18:258–262.
139. Chan K, Kendall MJ, Mitchard M, Will WDE. The effect of aging on plasma pethidine concentration. Br J Clin Pharmacol 1975; 2:297–303.

140. Greenblatt DJ, Sellers EM, Shader RI. Drug disposition in old age. N Engl J Med 1982;306:1081–1086.
141. Singleton MA, Rosen JI, Fisher DM. Pharmacokinetics of fentanyl in the elderly. Br J Anaesth 1988;60:619–622.
142. Aitkenhead AR, Vater M, Achola K, et al. Pharmacokinetics of single-dose I.V. morphine in normal volunteers and patients with end-stage renal failure. Br J Anaesth 1984;56:813–818.
143. Woolner DF, Winter D, Frendin TJ, et al. Renal failure does not impair the metabolism of morphine. Br J Clin Pharmacol 1986; 22:55–59.
144. Chauvin M, Sandouk P, Scherrmann JM, et al. Morphine pharmacokinetics in renal failure. Anesthesiology 1987;66:327–331.
145. Don HF, Dieppa RA, Taylor P. Narcotic analgesics in anuric patients. Anesthesiology 1975;42:745–747.
146. Mostert JW, Evers JL, Hobika GH, et al. Cardiorespiratory effects of anaesthesia with morphine or fentanyl in chronic renal failure and cerebral toxicity after morphine. Br J Anaesth 1971; 43:1053–1060.
147. Regnard CFB, Twycross RG. Metabolism of narcotics [Letter]. Br Med J 1984;288:860.
148. D'Honneur G, Gilton A, Sandouk P, et al. Plasma and cerebrospinal fluid concentrations of morphine and morphine glucuronides after oral morphine. Anesthesiology 1994;81:87–93.
149. Säwe J, Odar-Cederlöf I. Kinetics of morphine in patients with renal failure. Eur J Clin Pharmacol 1987;32:377–382.
150. Szeto HH, Inturrisi CE, Houde R, et al. Accumulation of normeperidine, an active metabolite of meperidine, in patients with renal failure or cancer. Ann Intern Med 1977;86:738–741.
151. Gilbert PE, Martin WR. Antagonism of the convulsant effects of heroin, d-propoxyphene, meperidine, normeperidine and thebaine by naloxone in mice. J Pharmacol Exp Ther 1975; 192:538–541.
152. Inturrisi CE, Verebely K. Disposition of methadone in man after a single oral dose. Clin Pharmacol Ther 1972;13:923–930.
153. Kreek MJ, Schecter AJ, Gutjahr CL, Hecht M. Methadone use in patients with chronic renal disease. Drug Alcohol Depend 1980;5:197–205.
154. Hasselström J, Eriksson S, Persson A, et al. The metabolism and bioavailability of morphine in patients with severe liver cirrhosis. Br J Clin Pharmacol 1990;29:289–297.
155. Crotty B, Watson KJR, Desmond PV, et al. Hepatic extraction of morphine is impaired in cirrhosis. Eur J Clin Pharmacol 1989; 36:501–506.
156. Mazoit JX, Sandouk P, Zetlaoui P, Scherrmann JM. Pharmacokinetics of unchanged morphine in normal and cirrhotic subjects. Anesth Analg 1987;66:293–298.
157. Neal EA, Meffin PJ, Gregory PB, Blaschke TF. Enhanced bioavailability and decreased clearance of analgesics in patients with cirrhosis. Gastroenterology 1979;77:96–102.
158. Pond SM, Tong T, Benowitz NL, Jacob P. Enhanced bioavailability of pethidine and pentazocine in patients with cirrhosis of the liver. Aust N Z J Med 1980;10:515–519.
159. Yue Q, Odar-Cederlöf I, Säwe J. Glucuronidation of morphine in human kidney. Pharmacol Toxicol 1988;63:337–341.
160. Pond SM, Tong T, Benowitz NL, et al. Presystemic metabolism of meperidine to normeperidine in normal and cirrhotic subjects. Clin Pharmacol Ther 1981;30:183–188.
161. Klotz U, McHorse TS, Wilkinson GR, Schenker S. The effect of cirrhosis on the disposition and elimination of meperidine in man. Clin Pharmacol Ther 1974;16:667–675.
162. Novick DM, Kreek MJ, Fanizza AM, et al. Methadone disposition in patients with chronic liver disease. Clin Pharmacol Ther 1981;30:353–362.
163. McHorse TS, Wilkinson GR, Johnson RF, Schenker S. Effect of acute viral hepatitis in man on the disposition and elimination of meperidine. Gastroenterology 1975;68:775–780.
164. Urthaler F, Isobe JH, James TN. Direct and vagally mediated chronotropic effects of morphine studied by selective perfusion of the sinus node of awake dogs. Chest 1975;68:222–228.
165. Laubie M, Schmitt H, Vincent M. Vagal bradycardia produced by microinjections of morphine-like drugs into the nucleus ambiguus in anaesthetized dogs. Eur J Pharmacol 1979;59:287–291.
166. Reitan JA, Stengert KB, Wymore ML, Martucci RW. Central vagal control of fentanyl-induced bradycardia during halothane anesthesia. Anesth Analg 1978;57:31–36.
167. Liu WS, Bidwai AV, Stanley TH, Isern-Amaral J. Cardiovascular dynamics after large doses of fentanyl and fentanyl plus N_2O in the dog. Anesth Analg 1976;55:168–172.
168. DeSilva RA, Verrier RL, Lown B. Protective effect of the vagotonic action of morphine sulphate on ventricular vulnerability. Cardiovasc Res 1978;12:167–172.
169. Urthaler F, Isobe JH, Gilmour KE, James TN. Morphine and autonomic control of the sinus node. Chest 1973;64:203–211.
170. Huang YF, Upton RN, Rutten AJ, Mather LE. The hemodynamic effects of intravenous bolus doses of meperidine in conscious sheep. Anesth Analg 1994;78:442–449.
171. Holland DR, Steinberg MI. Electrophysiologic properties of propoxyphene and norpropoxyphene in canine cardiac conducting tissues in vitro and in vivo. Toxicol Appl Pharmacol 1979;47:123–133.
172. Strauer BE. Contractile responses to morphine, piritramide, meperidine, and fentanyl: a comparative study of effects on the isolated ventricular myocardium. Anesthesiology 1972;37:304–310.
173. Goldberg AH. Myocardial depression by fentanyl and morphine. Anesthesiology 1973;38:600–602.
174. Vatner SF, Marsh JD, Swain JA. Effects of morphine on coronary and left ventricular dynamics in conscious dogs. J Clin Invest 1975;55:207–217.
175. Vasko JS, Henney RP, Brawley RK, et al. Effects of morphine on ventricular function and myocardial contractile force. Am J Physiol 1966;210:329–334.
176. Freye E. Cardiovascular effects of high dosages of fentanyl, meperidine, and naloxone in dogs. Anesth Analg 1974;53:40–47.
177. Stanley TH, Bidwai AV, Lunn JK, Hodges MR. Cardiovascular effects of nitrous oxide during meperidine infusion in the dog. Anesth Analg 1977;56:836–841.
178. Huang YF, Upton RN, Mather LE. The pharmacokinetics of meperidine in the myocardium of conscious sheep. Anesth Analg 1994;79:987–992.
179. Rosow CE, Moss J, Philbin DM, Savarese JJ. Histamine release during morphine and fentanyl anesthesia. Anesthesiology 1982;56:93–96.
180. Philbin DM, Moss J, Akins CW, et al. The use of H_1 and H_2 histamine antagonists with morphine anesthesia: a double-blind study. Anesthesiology 1981;55:292–296.
181. Moss J, Rosow CE. Histamine release by narcotics and muscle relaxants in humans. Anesthesiology 1983;59:330–339.
182. Lowenstein E, Whiting RB, Bittar DA, et al. Local and neurally mediated effects of morphine on skeletal muscle vascular resistance. J Pharmacol Exp Ther 1972;180:359–366.
183. Henney RP, Vasko JS, Brawley RK, et al. The effects of morphine on the resistance and capacitance vessels of the peripheral circulation. Am Heart J 1966;72:242–250.
184. Ward JM, McGrath RL, Weil JV. Effects of morphine on the peripheral vascular response to sympathetic stimulation. Am J Cardiol 1972;29:659–665.
185. Stanley TH, Gray NH, Stanford W, Armstrong R. The effects of high-dose morphine on fluid and blood requirements in open-heart operations. Anesthesiology 1973;38:536–541.
186. Hsu HO, Hickey RF, Forbes AR. Morphine decreases peripheral vascular resistance and increases capacitance in man. Anesthesiology 1979;50:98–102.
187. Alderman EL, Barry WH, Graham AF, Harrison DC. Hemodynamic effects of morphine and pentazocine differ in cardiac patients. N Engl J Med 1972;287:623–627.

188. Jewitt DE, Maurer BJ, Hubner PJB. Increased pulmonary arterial pressures after pentazocine in myocardial infarction. Br Med J 1970;1:795–796.
189. Popio KA, Jackson DH, Ross AM, et al. Hemodynamic and respiratory effects of morphine and butorphanol. Clin Pharmacol Ther 1978;23:281–287.
190. Aldrete JA, de Campo T, Usubiaga LE, et al. Comparison of butorphanol and morphine as analgesics for coronary bypass surgery: a double-blind, randomized study. Anesth Analg 1983; 62:78–83.
191. Lake CL, Duckworth EN, DiFazio CA, Magruder MR. Cardiorespiratory effects of nalbuphine and morphine premedication in adult cardiac surgical patients. Acta Anaesthesiol Scand 1984:28:305–309.
192. Lee G, Low RI, Amsterdam EA, et al. Hemodynamic effects of morphine and nalbuphine in acute myocardial infarction. Clin Pharmacol Ther 1981;29:576–581.
193. Hall RI, Murphy MR, Szlam F, Hug CC Jr. Dezocine: MAC reduction and evidence for myocardial depression in the presence of enflurane. Anesth Analg 1987;66:1169–1174.
194. Lewis AJ, Kirchner T. A comparison of the cardiorespiratory effects of cinamadol, dezocine, morphine and pentazocine in the anaesthetised dog. Arch Int Pharmacodyn Ther 1981; 250:73–83.
195. Rothbard RL, Schreiner BF, Yu PN. Hemodynamic and respiratory effects of dezocine, ciramadol, and morphine. Clin Pharmacol Ther 1985;38:84–88.
196. Estilo AE, Cottrell JE. Hemodynamic and catecholamine changes after administration of naloxone. Anesth Analg 1982; 61:349–353.
197. Cohen MR, Cohen RM, Pickar D, et al. Physiological effects of high dose naloxone administration to normal adults. Life Sci 1982;30:2025–2031.
198. Bonnet F, Bilaine J, Lhoste F, et al. Naloxone therapy of human septic shock. Crit Care Med 1985;13:972–975.
199. Patschke D, Eberlein HJ, Hess W, et al. Antagonism of morphine with naloxone in dogs: cardiovascular effects with special reference to the coronary circulation. Br J Anaesth 1977;49:525–531.
200. Mills CA, Flacke JW, Miller JD, et al. Cardiovascular effects of fentanyl reversal by naloxone at varying arterial carbon dioxide tensions in dogs. Anesth Analg 1988;67:730–736.
201. Estilo AE, Cottrell JE. Naloxone, hypertension, and ruptured cerebral aneurysm [Letter]. Anesthesiology 1981;54:352.
202. Prough DS, Roy R, Bumgarner J, Shannon G. Acute pulmonary edema in healthy teenagers following conservative doses of intravenous naloxone. Anesthesiology 1984;60:485–486.
203. Michaelis LL, Hickey PR, Clark TA, Dixon WM. Ventricular irritability associated with the use of naloxone hydrochloride. Ann Thorac Surg 1974;18:608–614.
204. Andree RA. Sudden death following naloxone administration. Anesth Analg 1980;59:782–784.
205. Partridge BL, Ward CF. Pulmonary edema following low-dose naloxone administration. Anesthesiology 1986;65:709–710.
206. Blaise GA, Nugent M, McMichan JC, Durant PAC. Side effects of nalbuphine while reversing opioid-induced respiratory depression: report of four cases. Can J Anaesth 1990;37:794–797.
207. DesMarteau JK, Cassot AL. Acute pulmonary edema resulting from nalbuphine reversal of fentanyl-induced respiratory depression [Letter]. Anesthesiology 1986;66:237.
208. Johnson N, Pasternak GW. Binding of [^{3}H] naloxonazine to rat brain membranes. Mol Pharmacol 1984;26:477–483.
209. McGilliard KL, Takemori AE. Antagonism by naloxone of narcotic-induced respiratory depression and analgesia. J Pharmacol Exp Ther 1978;207:494–503.
210. Martin WR, Jasinski DR, Sapira JD, et al. The respiratory effects of morphine during a cycle of dependence. J Pharmacol Exp Ther 1968;162:182–189.
211. Gal TJ, DiFazio CA, Moscicki J. Analgesic and respiratory depressant activity of nalbuphine: a comparison with morphine. Anesthesiology 1982;57:367–374.
212. Amin HM, Sopchak AM, Foss JF, et al. Efficacy of methylnaltrexone versus naloxone for reversal of morphine-induced depression of hypoxic ventilatory response. Anesth Analg 1994; 78:701–705.
213. Weil JV, McCullough RE, Kline JS, Sodal IE. Diminished ventilatory response to hypoxia and hypercapnia after morphine in normal man. N Engl J Med 1975;292:1103–1106.
214. Santiago TV, Pugliese AC, Edelman NH. Control of breathing during methadone addiction. Am J Med 1977;62:347–354.
215. Forrest WH Jr, Bellville JW. The effect of sleep plus morphine on the respiratory response to carbon dioxide. Anesthesiology 1984;25:137–141.
216. Camporesi EM, Nielsen CH, Bromage PR, Durant PAC. Ventilatory CO_2 sensitivity after intravenous and epidural morphine in volunteers. Anesth Analg 1983;62:633–640.
217. Rigg JRA, Rondi P. Changes in rib cage and diaphragm contribution to ventilation after morphine. Anesthesiology 1981; 55:507–514.
218. Arunasalam K, Davenport HT, Painter S, Jones JG. Ventilatory response to morphine in young and old subjects. Anaesthesia 1983;38:529–533.
219. Keats AS, Telford T. Studies of analgesic drugs. X. Respiratory effects of narcotic antagonists. J Pharmacol Exp Ther 1966; 112:126–132.
220. Gal TJ, DiFazio CA. Ventilatory and analgesic effects of dezocine in humans. Anesthesiology 1984;61:716–722.
221. Romagnoli A, Keats AS. Ceiling effect for respiratory depression by nalbuphine. Clin Pharmacol Ther 1980;27:478–485.
222. Romagnoli A, Keats AS. Ceiling respiratory depression by dezocine. Clin Pharmacol Ther 1984;35:367–373.
223. Heel RC, Brogden RN, Speight TM, Avery GS. Butorphanol: a review of its pharmacological properties and therapeutic efficacy. Drugs 1978;16:473–505.
224. Nagashima H, Karamanian A, Malovany R, et al. Respiratory and circulatory effects of intravenous butorphanol and morphine. Clin Pharmacol Ther 1976;19:738–745.
225. De Klerk G, Mattie H, Spierdijk J. Comparative study on the circulatory and respiratory effects of buprenorphine and methadone. Acta Anaesthesiol Belg 1981;32:131–139.
226. Jones JG. The respiratory effects of meptazinol. Postgrad Med J 1983;59:72–77.
227. Vickers MD, O'Flaherty D, Szekely SM, et al. Tramadol: pain relief by an opioid without depression of respiration. Anaesthesia 1992;47:291–296.
228. Adcock JJ. Peripheral opioid receptors and the cough reflex. Respir Med 1991;85:43–46.
229. Chi OZ, Sommer W, Jasaitis D. Power spectral analysis of EEG during sufentanil infusions in humans. Can J Anaesth 1991; 38:275–280.
230. Smith NT, Dec-Silver H, Sanford TJ, et al. EEGs during high-dose fentanyl-, sufentanil-, or morphine-oxygen anesthesia. Anesth Analg 1984;63:386–393.
231. Murphy MR, Hug CC Jr. The enflurane sparing effect of morphine, butorphanol and nalbuphine. Anesthesiology 1982; 57:489–492.
232. Lake CL, DiFazio CA, Moscicki JC, Engle JS. Reduction in halothane MAC: comparison of morphine and alfentanil. Anesth Analg 1985;64:807–810.
233. Weissman C. The metabolic response to stress: an overview and update. Anesthesiology 1990;73:308–327.
234. Hoffman JC, DiFazio CA. The anaesthesia sparing effect of pentazocine, meperidine and morphine. Arch Int Pharmacodyn Ther 1970;186:261–268.
235. Zsigmond EK, Winnie AP, Raza SMA, et al. Nalbuphine as an

analgesic component in balanced anesthesia for cardiac surgery. Anesth Analg 1987;66:1155–1164.
236. Weiss BM, Schmid ER, Gattiker RI. Comparison of nalbuphine and fentanyl anesthesia for coronary artery bypass surgery: hemodynamics, hormonal response, and postoperative respiratory depression. Anesth Analg 1991;73:521–529.
237. Rawal N, Wennhager M. Influence of perioperative nalbuphine and fentanyl on postoperative respiration and analgesia. Acta Anaesthesiol Scand 1990;34:197–202.
238. Rowlingson JC, Moscicki JC, DiFazio CA. Anesthetic potency of dezocine and its interaction with morphine in rats. Anesth Analg 1983;62:899–902.
239. Cohen RI, Edwards WT, Kezer EA, et al. Serial intravenous doses of dezocine, morphine, and nalbuphine in the management of postoperative pain for outpatients. Anesth Analg 1993;77:533–539.
240. Hoskin PJ, Hanks GW. Opioid agonist-antagonist drugs in acute and chronic pain states. Drugs 1991;41:326–344.
241. Dershwitz M, Rosow CE, DiBiase PM, Zaslavsky A. Comparison of the sedative effects of butorphanol and midazolam. Anesthesiology 1991;74:717–724.
242. Rosow C. Agonist-antagonist opioids: theory and clinical practice. Can J Anaesth 1989;36:S5-S8.
243. Musacchio JM. The psychotomimetic effects of opiates and the sigma receptor. Neuropsychopharmacology 1990;3:191–200.
244. Vandam L. Drug therapy: butorphanol. N Engl J Med 1980;302:381–384.
245. Jasinski DR, Mansky PA. Evaluation of nalbuphine for abuse potential. Clin Pharmacol Ther 1971;13:78–90.
246. Jaskinski DR, Marin WR, Hoeldtke RD. Effects of short- and long-term administration of pentazocine in man. Clin Pharmacol Ther 1969;11:385–403.
247. Moyer JH, Pontius R, Morris G, Hirshberger R. Effect of morphine and *N*-allylnormorphine on cerebral hemodynamics and oxygen metabolism. Circulation 1957;15:379–387.
248. Jobes DR, Kennell E, Bitner R, et al. Effects of morphine-nitrous oxide anesthesia on cerebral autoregulation. Anesthesiology 1975;42:30–34.
249. Wahl M. Effects of enkephalins, morphine, and naloxone on pial arteries during perivascular microapplication. J Cereb Blood Flow Metab 1985;5:451–457.
250. Milde LN, Milde JH, Gallagher WJ. Effects of sufentanil on cerebral circulation and metabolism in dogs. Anesth Analg 1990;70:138–146.
251. Sperry RJ, Bailey PL, Reichman MV, et al. Fentanyl and sufentanil increase intracranial pressure in head trauma patients. Anesthesiology 1992;77:416–420.
252. Weinstabl C, Mayer N, Richling B, et al. Effect of sufentanil on intracranial pressure in neurosurgical patients. Anaesthesia 1991;46:837–840.
253. Smith NT, Benthuysen JL, Bickford RG, et al. Seizures during opioid anesthetic induction: are they opioid-induced rigidity? Anesthesiology 1989;71:852–862.
254. Mather LE, Meffin PJ. Clinical pharmacokinetics of pethidine. Clin Pharmacokinet 1978;3:352–368.
255. Bailey PL, Wilbrink J, Zwanikken P, et al. Anesthetic induction with fentanyl. Anesth Analg 1985;64:48–53.
256. Goldberg M, Ishak S, Garcia C, McKenna J. Postoperative rigidity following sufentanil administration. Anesthesiology 1985;63:199–201.
257. Jaffe TB, Ramsey FM. Attenuation of fentanyl-induced truncal rigidity. Anesthesiology 1983;58:562–564.
258. Blasco TA, Lee D, Amalric M, et al. The role of the nucleus raphe pontis and the caudate nucleus in alfentanil rigidity in the rat. Brain Res 1986;386:280–286.
259. Peacock JE, Henderson PD, Nimmo WS. Changes in pupil diameter after oral administration of codeine. Br J Anaesth 1988;61:598–600.
260. Bailey PL, Rhondeau S, Schafer PG, et al. Dose-response pharmacology of intrathecal morphine in human volunteers. Anesthesiology 1993;79:49–59.
261. Casey WF, Smith CE, Katz JM, et al. Intravenous meperidine for control of shivering during caesarean section under epidural anaesthesia. Can J Anaesth 1988;35:128–133.
262. Friedlander M, Noble WH. Meperidine to control shivering associated with platelet transfusion reaction. Can J Anaesth 1989;36:460–462.
263. Crossley AW. Six months of shivering in a district general hospital. Anaesthesia 1992;47:845–848.
264. Thoren T, Sundberg A, Wettwil M, et al. Effects of epidural bupivacaine and epidural morphine on bowel function and pain after hysterectomy. Acta Anaesthesiol Scand 1989;33:181–185.
265. Parolaro D, Sala M, Gori E. Effect of intracerebroventricular administration of morphine upon intestinal motility in rat and its antagonism with naloxone. Eur J Pharmacol 1977;46:329–338.
266. Lamki L, Sullivan S. A study of gastrointestinal opiate receptors: the role of the mu receptor on gastric emptying: concise communication. J Nucl Med 1983;24:689–692.
267. Stewart JJ, Weisbrodt NW, Burks TF. Central and peripheral actions of morphine on intestinal transit. J Pharmacol Exp Ther 1978;205:547–555.
268. Hill SA, Quinn K, Shelly MP, Park GR. Reversible renal failure following opioid administration. Anaesthesia 1991;46:938–939.
269. Chapman WP, Rowlands EN, Jones CM. Multiple-balloon kymographic recording of the comparative action of Demerol, morphine and placebos in the motility of the upper small intestine in man. N Engl J Med 1950;243;171–177.
270. Garrett JM, Sauer WG, Moertel CG. Colonic motility in ulcerative colitis after opiate administration. Gastroenterology 1967;53:93–100.
271. Radnay PA, Duncalf D, Novakovic M, Lesser ML. Common bile duct pressure changes after fentanyl, morphine, meperidine, butorphanol, and naloxone. Anesth Analg 1984;63:441–444.
272. Cushieri A, Hughes JH, Cohen M. Biliary-pressure studies during cholecystectomy. Br J Surg 1972;59:267–273.
273. Borody TJ, Quigley EMM, Phillips SF, et al. Effects of morphine and atropine on motility and transit in the human ileum. Gastroenterology 1985;89:562–570.
274. Maltby JR, Williams RT. Morphine-induced cardiac pain? Anesthesiology 1986;64:527–528.
275. Salik JO, Siegel CI, Mendeloff AI. Biliary duodenal dynamics in man. Radiology 1973;106:1–11.
276. Thune A, Baker RA, Saccone GTP, et al. Differing effects of pethidine and morphine on human sphincter of Oddi motility. Br J Surg 1990;77:992–995.
277. Radnay PA, Brodman E, Mankikar D, Duncalf D. The effect of equi-analgesic doses of fentanyl, morphine, meperidine and pentazocine on common bile duct pressure. Anaesthetist 1980;29:26–29.
278. Watcha MF, White PF. Postoperative nausea and vomiting: its etiology, treatment and prevention. Anesthesiology 1992;77:162–184.
279. Costello DJ, Borison HL. Naloxone antagonizes narcotic self-blockade of emesis in the cat. J Pharmacol Exp Ther 1977;203:222–230.
280. Longnecker D, Grazis P, Eggers G. Naloxone antagonism of morphine induced respiratory depression. Anesth Analg 1973;52:447–453.
281. Philbin DM, Coggins CH. Plasma antidiuretic hormone levels in cardiac surgical patients during morphine and halothane anesthesia. Anesthesiology 1978;49:95–98.

282. Leander JD, Hart JC, Zerbe RL. Kappa agonist-induced diuresis: evidence for stereoselectivity, strain differences, independence of hydration variables and a result of decreased plasma vasopressin levels. J Pharmacol Exp Ther 1987;242:33–39.
283. Stanley TH, Gray NH, Bidwai AV, Lordon R. The effects of high dose morphine and morphine plus nitrous oxide on urinary output in man. Can J Anaesth 1974;21:379–384.
284. El-Awady E, Walker LA. Effects of morphine on the renal handling of sodium and lithium in conscious rats. J Pharmacol Exp Ther 1990;254:957–961.
285. McDermott RW, Stanley TH. The cardiovascular effects of low concentrations of nitrous oxide during morphine anesthesia. Anesthesiology 1974;41:89–91.
286. Wong KC, Martin WE, Hornbein TF, et al. The cardiovascular effects of morphine sulfate with oxygen and with nitrous oxide in man. Anesthesiology 1973;38:542–548.
287. Stowe DF, Monroe SM, Marijic J, et al. Effects of nitrous oxide on contractile function and metabolism of the isolated heart. Anesthesiology 1990;73:1220–1226.
288. Lawson D, Frazer MJ, Lynch C III. Nitrous oxide effects on isolated myocardium: a reexamination in vitro. Anesthesiology 1990;73:930–945.
289. Stoelting RK, Gibbs PS. Hemodynamic effects of morphine and morphine-nitrous oxide in valvular heart disease and coronary-artery disease. Anesthesiology 1973;38:45–52.
290. Epstein B, Levy ML, Thein M, Coakley C. Evaluation of fentanyl as an adjunct to thiopental-nitrous oxide-oxygen anesthesia for short procedures. Anesthesiol Rev 1985;2:24–29.
291. Short TG, Plummer JL, Chui PT. Hypnotic and anaesthetic interactions between midazolam, propofol and alfentanil. Br J Anaesth 1992;69:162–167.
292. Taylor MB, Grounds RM, Mulrooney PD, Morgan M. Ventilatory effects of propofol during induction of anaesthesia. Anaesthesia 1986;41:816–820.
293. Kissin I, Vinik HR, Castillo R, Bradley EL Jr. Alfentanil potentiates midazolam-induced unconsciousness in subanalgesic doses. Anesth Analg 1990;71:65–69.
294. Bailey PL, Pace NL, Ashburn MA, et al. Frequent hypoxemia and apnea after sedation with midazolam and fentanyl. Anaesthetist 1990;73:826–830.
295. Hoar PF, Nelson NT, Mangano DT, et al. Adrenergic response to morphine-diazepam anesthesia for myocardial revascularization. Anesth Analg 1981;60:406–411.
296. Lowenstein E, Hallowell P, Levine FH, et al. Cardiovascular response to large doses of intravenous morphine in man. N Engl J Med 1969;281:1389–1393.
297. Hasbrouck JD. Morphine anesthesia for open-heart surgery. Ann Thorac Surg 1970;10:364–369.
298. Inoue K, El-Banayosy A, Stolarski L, Reichelt W. Vecuronium induced bradycardia following induction of anaesthesia with etomidate or thiopentone, with or without fentanyl. Br J Anaesth 1988;60:10–17.
299. Oikkonen M. Alfentanil combined with vecuronium or pancuronium: haemodynamic implications. Acta Anaesthesiol Scand 1992;36:406–409.
300. Gravlee GP, Ramsey FM, Roy RC, et al. Pancuronium is hemodynamically superior to veuronium for narcotic/relaxant induction [Abstract]. Anesthesiology 1986;65:A46.
301. Wells DG, Bjorksten AR. Monoamine oxidase inhibitors revisited. Can J Anaesth 1989;36:64–74.
302. El-Ganzouri AR, Ivankovich AD, Braverman B, McCarthy RJ. Monoamine oxidase inhibitors: should they be discontinued preoperatively? Anesth Analg 1985;64:592–596.
303. Michaels I, Serrings M, Shier N, Barash PG. Anesthesia for cardiac surgery in patients receiving monoamine oxidase inhibitors. Anesth Analg 1984;63:1041–1044.
304. Rogers KJ, Thorton JA. The interaction between monoamine oxidase inhibitors and narcotic analgesics in mice. Br J Pharmacol 1969;36:470–480.
305. Clark B, Thompson JW. Analysis of the inhibition of pethidine N-demethylation by monoamine oxidase inhibitors and some other drugs with special reference to drug interactions in man. Br J Pharmacol 1972;44:89–99.

11 Fentanyl and Congeners

Peter Bailey and Talmage Egan

Opioids are a key component of intravenous anesthesia. They are unique in their ability to control pain and a host of physiologic responses to noxious stimuli. In modern anesthetic practice, fentanyl or one of its congeners (i.e., the phenylpiperidines, Fig. 11-1) dominates as the opioid of choice for intravenous anesthesia, as well as most other types of "balanced" anesthetic techniques. The pharmacology of these compounds, with regard to both pharmacokinetic and pharmacodynamic properties, renders them most suitable of all the available opioids for the practice of intravenous anesthesia.

The phenylpiperidine class of opioid compounds includes meperidine, which was synthesized in 1939. This drug serendipitously resulted from research for a synthetic substitute for atropine (1). Combining meperidine with other new intravenous agents (barbiturates), and the popularization of the concept of balanced anesthesia (2), resulted in a resurgent interest in the intraoperative use of opioid compounds. Other investigators (3) also reported an anesthetic technique that supplemented nitrous oxide-oxygen with meperidine for analgesia and curare for muscle relaxation. Although the greater lipid solubility of meperidine produced a faster onset of opioid action compared with morphine, meperidine was less potent, and it still produced significant adverse effects.

In 1953, Paul Janssen became interested in developing more potent opioids (4). He believed that increased potency would enhance the specificity and efficacy of opioid action, improve safety, and decrease adverse effects. His research led to a better understanding of opioid structure-activity relationships and resulted in the synthesis of fentanyl in 1960. Depending on the species studied, fentanyl was found to be 100 to 300 times as potent as morphine, possessed a higher therapeutic index than morphine or meperidine, and produced fewer adverse side effects. The use of fentanyl was additionally popularized by DeCastro and Mundeleer, who developed the concept of neuroleptanalgesia and neuroleptanesthesia. Neuroleptanalgesia is produced by combining a major tranquilizer such as droperidol with an opioid such as fentanyl. Adding nitrous oxide as an inhaled agent results in neuroleptanesthesia. These techniques can be considered the conceptual forerunners of total intravenous anesthesia (TIVA). They were intended to produce analgesia, amnesia, absence of overt motor activity, suppression of autonomic reflexes, and the maintenance of cardiovascular stability.

In the early 1970s, fentanyl also became widely employed in cardiac anesthesia. High doses of morphine, initially reported to produce anesthesia successfully in cardiac surgical candidates (5), ultimately proved inadequate as a sole anesthetic agent. Fentanyl, however, in high doses (75 to 125 μg/kg), showed greater promise. This was because of a combination of factors, including greater potency and reduced side effects, especially those related to histamine release. To date, fentanyl remains popular as an opioid that has withstood the test of time and is inexpensive. It also has drawbacks, however, including incomplete efficacy as a primary anesthetic and, perhaps most notably, a prolonged duration of effect when used in high doses or by continuous infusion. Newer fentanyl congeners have been developed (Fig. 11-2), and they continue to be developed in attempts to produce the optimal opioid for anesthesia.

Sufentanil, synthesized in the mid–1970s (6), is a fentanyl congener that is approximately 7 to 10 times as potent as its parent compound. It has been demonstrated in numerous studies to be more effective than fentanyl when sufentanil is employed either as a sole anesthetic or as a supplement in a balanced technique. Although the latency to peak effect after intravenous injection is similar for fentanyl and sufentanil, sufentanil has a shorter duration of action compared to fentanyl, especially after multiple doses or continuous infusions (7). In the late 1970s alfentanil was synthesized. While less potent than fentanyl by a factor of approximately five, it was demonstrated to be much shorter acting. The short latency to peak effect (1 minute) of alfentanil after intravenous injection also affords anesthesiologists greater control.

Other fentanyl congeners, including carfentanil and lofentanil, do not possess enough new advantages to find their way into the clinician's armamentarium. Remifentanil, formally known as GI87084B, is a novel, short-acting fentanyl congener now approved for clinical use. A member of the 4-anilidopiperidine class, this drug is unique among currently marketed agents because of its ester structure. Remifentanil undergoes widespread extrahepatic metabolism by blood and tissue nonspecific esterases, resulting in an extremely rapid clearance and a ultrashort duration of action (8, 9) (Fig. 11-3). Remifentanil is somewhat less potent than fentanyl and demonstrates a rapid onset of action, similar to that of alfentanil (10). Like remifentanil, trefentanil is a fentanyl congener under development that may offer clinical advantages because of its unusual pharmacokinetic profile. Although its potency and onset time are similar to those of alfentanil, trefentanil is pharmacokinetically unique in that the time required for a 50% decrease in plasma concentration after cessation of a variable-length infusion is relatively short, although not as short as the newer fentanyl derivatives (11).

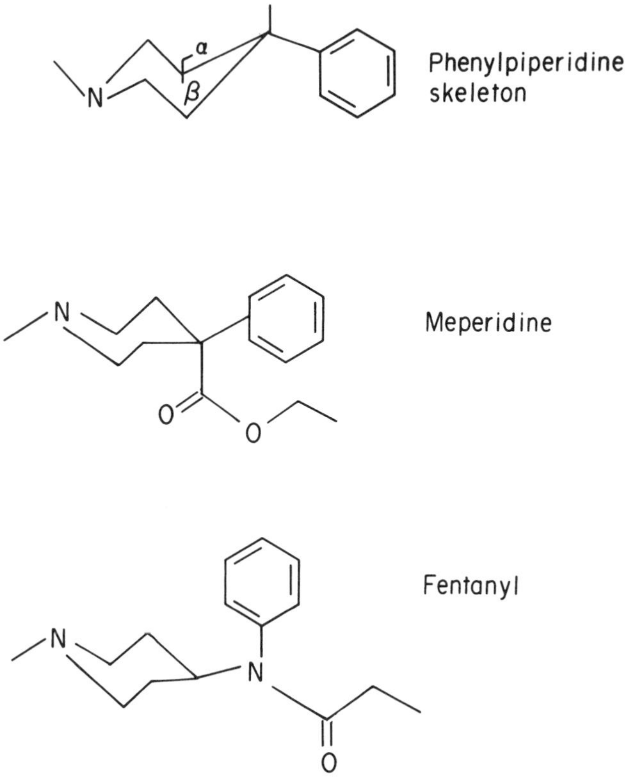

Phenylpiperidine skeleton

Meperidine

Fentanyl

FIGURE 11-1. The phenylpiperidine skeleton structure and the synthetic phenylpiperidine opioids meperidine and fentanyl.

With the advent of remifentanil, drugs with a full range of pharmacokinetic characteristics, from long-acting to ultrashort-acting, are now available. The cost of developing a new drug, estimated at $200 to $300 million, becomes increasingly prohibitive as each new drug possesses fewer advantages and is less likely to be successfully marketed. It remains to be seen, especially under current economic conditions, whether further refinements in chemical structure will result in new fentanyl congeners with enough advantages and potential benefits to merit full research, development, and marketing. The fentanyl congener series of opioids has been progressively tailored to produce nearly optimal drug pharmacokinetics. The potential remains enormous, however, if manipulation of the chemical structure of opioids could change their pharmacodynamic profile. The adverse effects of opioids, most importantly respiratory depression, as well as postoperative nausea and vomiting, remain a significant limitation to their clinical use. The synthesis of an opioid that could produce potent analgesia with little to no respiratory depression would represent a great advance. To date, however, the possibility of such pharmacologic action has only been suggested (12).

This chapter reviews the general pharmacology of

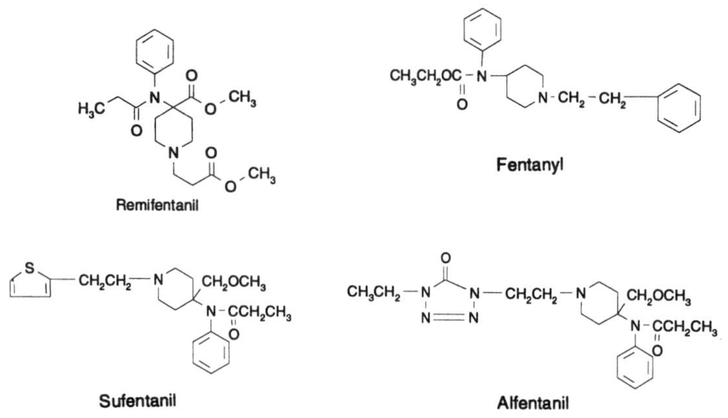

Remifentanil

Fentanyl

Sufentanil

Alfentanil

FIGURE 11-2. Modern-day opioids of clinical importance in the phenylpiperidine series.

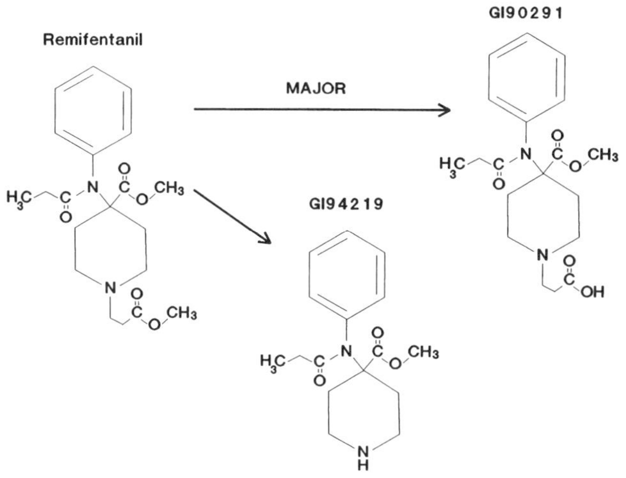

FIGURE 11-3. The chemical structure and proposed metabolic pathways of remifentanil.

the fentanyl congeners. In addition, their pharmacokinetic and pharmacodynamic properties as well as common side effects are discussed. Finally, important drug interactions involving these opioid compounds in clinical practice are reviewed.

GENERAL PHARMACOLOGY

Potency

The relative affinities of sufentanil, fentanyl, and alfentanil for μ opioid receptors coincide with their potency ratios and predict sufentanil to be the most potent of the three (13–15). Traditionally, relative potency has been a simple concept. It has been based on drug dose, especially for intravenous agents, and often one drug effect, frequently in animal models. This approach permits clinicians to have a concrete idea of the relative doses and safety of various drugs that can be easily remembered. For the fentanyl series of opioids most commonly employed, fentanyl is approximately 5 times as potent as alfentanil, and sufentanil is about 10 times more potent than fentanyl. Remifentanil is 20 to 30 times as potent as alfentanil. This type of comparison is now recognized not only as inadequate, but also at times as misleading, however. For example, comparing opioids by dose alone is inadequate because of the tremendous variability (4- to 6-fold) in the plasma drug level achieved in different individuals after a given dose. In addition, drug concentrations change at differing rates depending on the drug's pharmacokinetic profile. Comparisons based on dose alone are not likely to represent plasma concentration ratios accurately for a similar level of effect. Moreover, determining the relative potency among various opioids for one drug effect (e.g., analgesia) does not necessarily predict that the same potency ratios will exist for other drug actions (e.g., anesthesia). Experienced clinicians rapidly move beyond simplistic potency ratios when using opioids and other drugs in anesthetic practice.

Significant advances have been made in the description of relative drug potencies by exploring other relationships besides clinical dose-response pharmacology, thereby eliminating much of the intrinsic variability. For example, comparisons of the plasma drug levels necessary to produce equal (half-maximal) slowing of the electroencephalogram (EEG) (10, 16, 17) have demonstrated that, in humans, sufentanil is 12 times as potent as fentanyl, and fentanyl and remifentanil are 75 and 16 times as potent as alfentanil, respectively. When determining the plasma (or whole blood) drug levels of each opioid necessary to reduce the minimum alveolar concentration (MAC) of isoflurane by 50%, the calculated potency ratio for sufentanil:fentanyl:remifentanil:alfentanil is 1:10:10:80 (18–23). Based on EEG studies and experimental pain studies performed in humans, trefentanil has a potency similar to that of alfentanil (11, 24).

Most clinicians believe all the potent μ agonist opioids have similar if not identical pharmacodynamic profiles; however, evidence can be found to support the notion that some opioids are better "anesthetics." For example, Bowdle and Ward (25) found sufentanil, compared with fentanyl in doses reflecting a potency

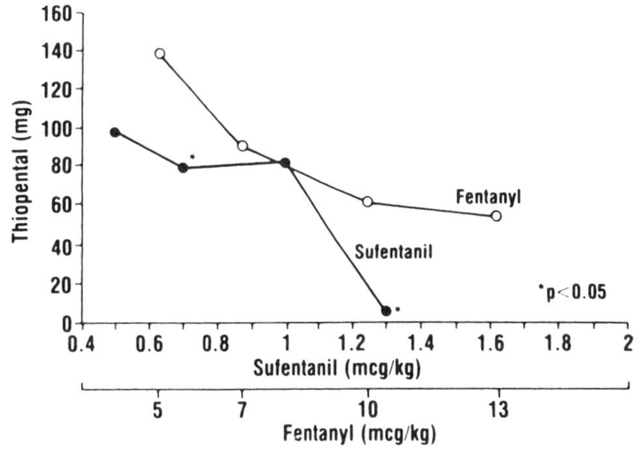

FIGURE 11-4. Thiopental requirement for induction of sleep versus opioid dose in surgical patients. Thiopental was administered intravenously in 25-mg increments every 30 seconds until the subject was unconscious. Sufentanil and fentanyl doses were plotted on the same scale, using a potency ratio of 1:8. Thiopental requirements were significantly less ($p < 0.0001$) for sufentanil (0.7 and 1.3 μg/kg) than for equipotent doses of fentanyl (5 and 10 μg.kg). Only 1 in 10 patients receiving sufentanil, 1.3 μg/kg, required any thiopental compared with 10 of 10 in the fentanyl 10 μg/kg group and 8 of 10 in the fentanyl 13 μg/kg group ($p < 0.0001$). (From Bowdle TA, Ward RJ. Induction of anesthesia with small doses of sufentanil or fentanyl: dose versus EEG response, speed of onset and thiopental requirement. Anesthesiology 1989;70:26–30.)

ratio of 80:1, to require much less sodium thiopental supplementation to produce sleep (Fig. 11-4). Other investigators have found sufentanil, compared with other fentanyl congeners, to be a more effective component of balanced analgesia. The use of sufentanil can provide greater hemodynamic stability, reduce the need for supplementation, and permit a more rapid emergence characterized by better analgesia and less respiratory depression than other opioids (26–29). Although some investigators report sufentanil to be a more "complete" anesthetic in high doses for cardiac anesthesia and surgery (30–33), others disagree (34–36).

Pharmacokinetic Considerations

Anesthesiologists are now inundated with a host of pharmacokinetic parameters and models. Classic pharmacokinetic information is still routinely published, including terminal elimination half-lives ($t_{1/2}\,\beta$), although many of these parameters are of little clinical utility to the practitioner of anesthesia (37, 38). $t_{1/2}\,\beta$, for example, does not accurately predict the duration of drug effect in anesthesia. New insights and descriptions of drug behavior have led to improved understanding and clinical pharmacologic practice (7, 37, 39, 40). Unfortunately, no simple description or single pharmacokinetic parameter permits the clinical prediction of the important aspects of pharmacology that concern anesthesiologists, such as the duration of drug effect. What has emerged with these new approaches is a different and, one hopes, better, albeit complex, way of describing what happens to intravenously administered drugs. The ongoing process of drug distribution, as well as the factors affecting equilibrium between plasma and effect site, play significant roles in the termination of clinical drug action (37, 38). Various pharmacologic terms ("relevant effect-site decrement time") (7, 37, 39) derived from mathematical models are utilized to better predict recovery from drug effect. Although they are useful, these new concepts are not yet widely appreciated and have not yet been fully validated (41).

Although recent advances are noteworthy, the inability to measure or to quantify plasma or effect site drug concentrations inexpensively in real time in vivo is considered by some experts to be a major limitation to the advancement of the practice of intravenous anesthesia. The large variability that exists from patient to patient with regard to the plasma drug concentration that a given opioid dose produces, as well as the effect that a given plasma opioid concentration elicits, continues to present significant challenges to practitioners. The following section describes conventional and newer pharmacokinetic information with the recognition that it constitutes the scientific basis of a medical practice that must still rely on clinical skills.

MEPERIDINE

The plasma concentration versus time decay curve of meperidine is best characterized by a biexponential equation with a distribution half-life ($t_{1/2}\,\alpha$) that varies from 5 to 15 minutes (42–47). After intravenous injection, first-pass uptake of meperidine by the lungs is approximately 65%, and although most meperidine is re-released into the blood within 1 minute, such uptake buffers the plasma from higher drug levels (48). Meperidine is 70% bound to plasma proteins, primarily α_1-acid glycoprotein. Meperidine binds only to a minor extent to plasma albumin. Meperidine is less than 10% un-ionized at physiologic pH and is less lipid soluble than fentanyl (Table 11-1). The volume of distribution of meperidine is similar to that of morphine (4 ± 1 L/kg) (42–46), as is its clearance (8 to 18 mg•kg^{-1}•min^{-1}) (42, 43). A high hepatic extraction ratio results in meperidine biotransformation that depends on hepatic blood flow.

The principal metabolic pathways of meperidine are N-demethylation and hydrolysis, which produce normeperidine, meperidinic acid, and normeperidinic

TABLE 11-1. Physiochemical and Pharmacokinetic Data of Commonly Used Opioid Agonists

Parameter	Meperidine	Fentanyl	Sufentanil	Alfentanil	Remifentanil
pKa	8.5	8.4	8.0	6.5	7.1
Percentage un-ionized at pH 7.4 (%)	<10	<10	20	90	67
Octanol:H_2O partition/coefficient	39	813	1,778	129	18
Percentage bound to plasma protein (%)	70	84	93	92	70
$t_{1/2}\,\beta$ (h)	3–5	2–4	2–3	1–2	0.1–0.6
V_{dcc} L/kg	1–2	0.5–1.0	0.2	0.1–0.3	0.1–0.2
V_{dss} L/kg	3–5	3–5	2.5–3.0	0.4–1.0	0.3–0.4
Clearance ml•min^{-1}•kg^{-1}	8–18	10–20	10–15	4–9	40–60
Hepatic extraction ratio	0.7–0.9	0.8–1.0	0.7–0.9	0.3–0.5	—
$t_{1/2}\,k_{e0}$ (min)	—	4–5	4–5	0.6–1.2	1.0–1.5

$T_{1/2}\,\beta$, Terminal elimination half-life; $T_{1/2}\,k_{e0}$ (min), half-time for equilibration between plasma and effect site; V_{dcc}, volume of distribution, central compartment; V_{dss}, volume of distribution at steady state.

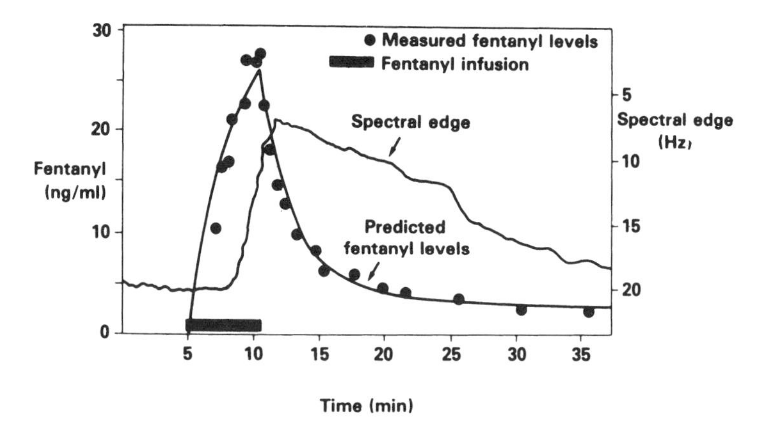

FIGURE 11-5. Time course of spectral edge and serum fentanyl concentrations. Note the inverted spectral edge axis. The spectral edge changes lag behind the serum concentrations changes. Fentanyl infusion rate is 150 $\mu g \cdot min^{-1}$ (solid bar). (From Scott JC, Ponganis KV, Stanski DR. EEG quantitation of narcotic effect: the comparative pharmacodynamics of fentanyl and alfentanil. Anesthesiology 1985;62:234–241.)

acid as the major metabolites. Little meperidine (<5%) is excreted unchanged in the urine. Normeperidine has some opioid action and is roughly twice as potent as its parent compound in producing seizures in animals (49). The greater epileptogenic properties of normeperidine are not reversible by naloxone. The $t_{1/2}\ \beta$ for meperidine is approximately 4 ± 1 hours (42–46), and excretion of its metabolites occurs predominantly by the kidney. The $t_{1/2}\ \beta$ of normeperidine is considerably longer than that of meperidine. Repeated doses of meperidine can easily produce normeperidine accumulation and toxicity in patients with renal disease (50).

FENTANYL

The pharmacokinetics of fentanyl has been studied by numerous investigators (51–58). A three-compartment model is often used to describe plasma fentanyl concentration decay (51, 52, 54, 55). The lungs exert a significant first-pass effect and take up approximately 75% of an injected dose of fentanyl. Fentanyl is rapidly released from the lung in a bimodal fashion (48, 59). After intravenous administration in human patients, fentanyl rapidly disappears from the plasma. More than 98% of an injected dose is eliminated from the plasma after 1 hour. Rapid distribution ($t_{1/2}\ \pi$) of fentanyl takes 1 to 2 minutes, and a second distribution phase ($t_{1/2}\ \alpha$) takes 10 to 30 minutes. Brain fentanyl levels parallel plasma levels with a lag time (hysteresis) of approximately 5 minutes. The hysteresis may result from the lipophilicity of fentanyl and the drug's uptake by nonreceptor fatty tissue in the central nervous system (CNS). Spectral edge analysis of the EEG in patients receiving fentanyl, 8.8 $\mu g/kg$ administered over 6 minutes (Fig. 11-5), suggests that the drug is best administered approximately 5 minutes before a painful stimulus (16). (Another alternative is to administer a larger dose to saturate brain opioid receptors rapidly as well as nonreceptor storage sites.) In rats, muscle tissue is found to hold the most fentanyl after redistribution (56%), whereas maximum fat tissue content

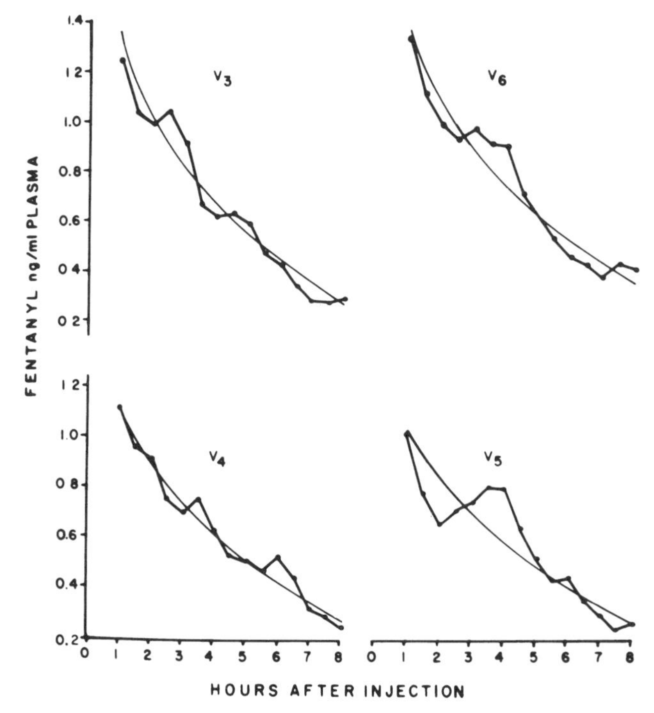

FIGURE 11-6. Arithmetic plot of fentanyl level/time after a single bolus intravenous injection (3.2 or 6.4 $\mu g/kg$) in each of four subjects. The thin line represents the curve determined by nonlinear least-squares analysis of the data for each subject. Note the occurrence of second peaks. (From McClain DA, Hug CC Jr. Intravenous fentanyl kinetics. Clin Pharmacol Ther 1980;28:106–114.)

is only 17% (60). At steady state, fentanyl's volume of distribution (3 to 6 L/kg) and clearance (10 to 20 $ml \cdot kg^{-1} \cdot min^{-1}$) are both high.

Fentanyl's lipid solubility is high (see Table 11-1) and results in its large volume of distribution. Björkman and associates (61) found the tissue-blood partition coefficients of fentanyl to range from 2- to 30-fold higher than those of alfentanil. The large volume of distribution for fentanyl causes rapid and continued peripheral tissue uptake of the drug from the blood and limits hepatic access and metabolism. Fentanyl must ultimately be returned to the blood to be metabolized and eliminated from the body. Hudson and Stanski (62) suggest that fentanyl's large volume of distribution results in more variability in plasma levels during the elimination phase. Such variability in plasma concentrations may be due in part to surges in muscle blood flow. Resultant fluctuations in the amount of fentanyl returned to the blood may contribute to second peaks in plasma fentanyl levels (Fig. 11-6) (52).

The high hepatic clearance of fentanyl (approaching hepatic blood flow) and high hepatic extraction ratio (approaching 1.0) minimize the contribution of enterohepatic circulation to secondary peaks in drug plasma levels (63). Decreases in hepatic blood flow can decrease fentanyl elimination. Fentanyl is primarily metabolized in the liver by N-dealkylation and hydroxylation (57). Metabolites begin to appear in the plasma as early as 1.5 minutes after injection (60). Norfentanyl is detectable in the urine for up to 48 hours after intravenous fentanyl administration in human patients (64).

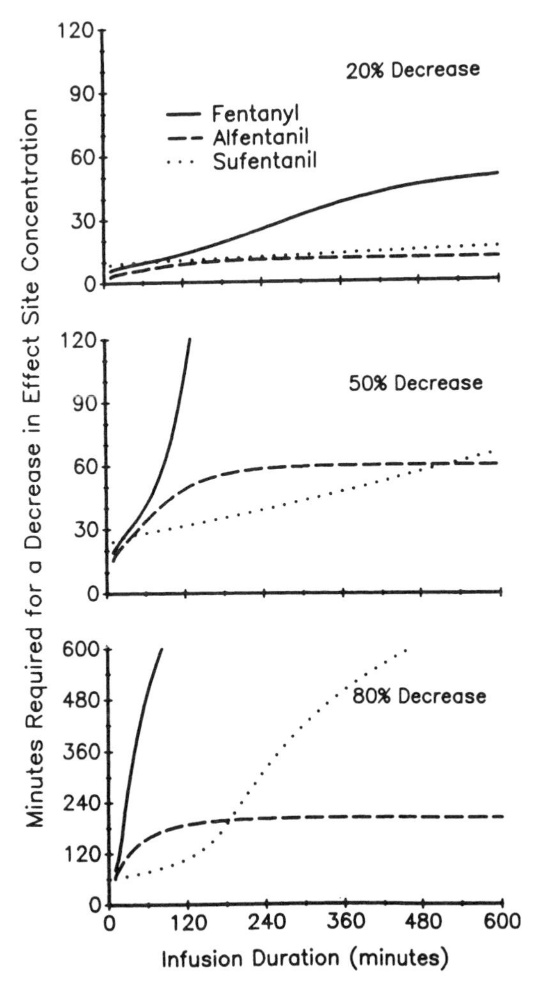

FIGURE 11-7. Computer simulation recovery curves for fentanyl, alfentanil and sufentanil describing the time required (y axis) for 20%, 50%, and 80% decreases in effect site concentrations after intravenous infusions of variable duration (x axis). (Adapted from Shafer SL, Varvel JR. Pharmacokinetics, pharmacodynamics, and rational opioid selection. Anesthesiology 1991;74:53–63.)

The receptor binding of fentanyl metabolites does not demonstrate different selectivity (14). The activity of fentanyl's metabolites is unclear, but it is thought to be minimal. Little fentanyl is excreted in the urine unchanged (52).

Approximately 80% of fentanyl is bound to plasma proteins, and significant amounts (40%) are taken up by red blood cells (65). Approximately half of fentanyl binds to α_1-acid glycoprotein. Because the negative log of dissociation constant (pKa) of fentanyl is high (8.4) at physiologic pH, it exists mostly in the ionized form (>90%). As noted previously, fentanyl's high lipid solubility and volume of distribution contribute to variability in reported pharmacokinetic profiles (62). Indeed, Reilly and colleagues (66) noted a 13-fold range in peak plasma levels (8.4 to 113.6 ng/ml) after a 500-μg intravenous injection in adults. These investigators also reported significant variability in other pharmacokinetic parameters. Other reasons for the large differences in reported fentanyl pharmacokinetics include small study sample size, differences in the duration of fentanyl infusion, inadequate duration of plasma drug sampling, different fentanyl assay methods, and studies using patients on cardiopulmonary bypass. The time it takes for blood fentanyl levels to decrease 50% is affected by the method and length of time of drug delivery (Fig 11-7) (7).

SUFENTANIL

Like fentanyl, sufentanil is supplied as an aqueous solution of the citrate salt in a preservative-free solution containing 50 μg/ml. Sufentanil is approximately 10 times as potent as fentanyl and, like fentanyl, is a basic amine. Its pKa is 8.0 at physiologic pH. Therefore, after administration of the drug, only a small amount (20%) exists in the un-ionized form. After intravenous injection, first-pass pulmonary extraction and retention are similar to those of fentanyl. This phenomenon is of little clinical import (67). Sufentanil is approximately twice as lipid soluble as fentanyl and is highly bound (93%) to plasma proteins, mostly to α_1-acid glycoprotein. Bovill and associates (68) have reported the pharmacokinetic profile for sufentanil. In 9 of 10 patients studied, the plasma decay curves conformed to a three-compartment model. The $t_{1/2}\ \pi$ was 1.4 ± 0.3 minutes, and $t_{1/2}\ \alpha$ was 17.7 ± 2.6 minutes. After intravenous injection, 98% of sufentanil had left the plasma within 30 minutes. The $t_{1/2}\ \beta$ was 164 ± 22 minutes, and the apparent volume of the central compartment 0.16 ± 0.02 L/kg. The apparent volume of distribution at steady state was 2.86 ± 0.25 L/kg, and hepatic clearance was high (12.7 ± 0.8 ml•kg^{-1}•min^{-1}).

Other investigators have reported pharmacokinetic data for sufentanil (69). Gepts and colleagues (70) have tried to resolve conflicts in reported sufentanil pharmacokinetics and have recognized the impact of length of sampling and assay sensitivity. Pharmacokinetics were determined over a range of sufentanil doses (250 to 1500 μg) administered over 10 to 20 minutes in surgical patients. Plasma samples were obtained for 48 hours after drug administration. A linear three-compartmental model adequately described sufentanil pharmacokinetics. The central volume of distribution was 14.3 L, the rapidly equilibrating volume was 261.6 L, and the steady-state distribution volume was 339 L. Metabolic clearance was 0.92 L/min, rapid distribution clearance was 1.55 L/min, slow distribution clearance was 0.33 L/min, and $t_{1/2}$ β was 769 minutes.

Sufentanil's hepatic extraction ratio is high (0.8), and thus changes in liver blood flow can significantly alter its elimination. The major metabolic pathways of sufentanil include N-dealkylation, oxidative N-dealthylation, oxidative O-demethylation, and aromatic hydroxylation (71). Major resultant metabolites include N-phenylpropanamide. Metabolic pathways of sufentanil also appear to be similar in humans, rats, and dogs. Extensive renal tubular reabsorption leads to little unchanged sufentanil in the urine.

Sufentanil is more tightly bound to receptors (mostly μ) than fentanyl and has only minimal nonspecific brain tissue binding (15). These properties, along with its high degree of plasma protein binding and lower volume of distribution, are the probable explanation for sufentanil's shorter $t_{1/2}$ β and duration of effect compared with fentanyl even though it is highly lipophilic (octanol:water partition coefficient of 1788). In fact, after intraoperative infusions of sufentanil of less than 6 to 8 hours in duration, opioid effects may dissipate at least as rapidly as those produced by similar infusions of alfentanil (see Fig. 11-7) (7).

ALFENTANIL

The pharmacokinetics of alfentanil has been extensively evaluated (63, 72–84). Following intravenous injection, alfentanil plasma concentrations fit either two-compartment (63, 72, 74, 75, 78) or three-compartment models (73, 76, 77). As with fentanyl and sufentanil, transient pulmonary retention occurs after intravenous alfentanil administration. Distribution (range of mean $t_{1/2}$ α reported is 4 to 17 minutes; see Table 11-1) and elimination of alfentanil (range of mean $t_{1/2}$ β reported is 70 to 112 minutes; see Table 11-1) are rapid. Clearance (4 to 9 ml•min^{-1}•kg^{-1}) is less than that of fentanyl. A small volume of distribution at steady state (0.4 to 1.0 L/kg) limits distribution and tissue accumulation of alfentanil and is largely responsible for the short $t_{1/2}$ β of alfentanil despite its lower clearance than fentanyl.

Alfentanil is lipid soluble enough to permit rapid brain penetration (heptane-water partition coefficient 2.5), but it is significantly less lipid soluble than fentanyl (heptane-water partition coefficient 9.0) (81, 82). Thus, little alfentanil is taken up by and stored in nonreceptor brain tissue. This helps to explain alfentanil's rapid onset of action as well as its decline in activity after cessation of drug administration (16, 40, 82). At physiologic pH, alfentanil is mostly (90%) un-ionized because of its relatively low pKa (6.5) (85). This, too, aids tissue (brain) penetration. Alfentanil is highly bound to plasma proteins (90%), predominantly to α_1-acid glycoproteins (63, 75, 77). Binding and dissociation from plasma proteins are usually not rate-limiting reactions, however (82). Little alfentanil (<1%) appears in the urine unchanged because of its protein binding, renal tubular reabsorption, and hepatic metabolism. Reported hepatic extraction ratios vary from 0.3 to 0.5 (63, 77, 86). The main metabolic pathways of alfentanil are similar to those of sufentanil and include oxidative N-dealkylation and O-demethylation, aromatic hydroxylation, and ether glucuronide formation (87). Oxidative-N-dealkylation of alfentanil produces its major metabolite, noralfentanil. Other metabolites include desmethylalfentanil, desmethylnoralfentanil, and several other products (88–90). The degradation products of alfentanil have little-known opioid activity. Patients deficient in the cytochrome P450 form involved in debrisoquin metabolism do not have an altered disposition of alfentanil (89, 90). This is consistent with the finding that human alfentanil metabolism may be predominantly, if not exclusively, by cytochrome P450 3A3/4 (91).

REMIFENTANIL

Compared with the currently marketed fentanyl congeners, the pharmacokinetic profile of remifentanil is unique. After injection, remifentanil is subject to widespread extrahepatic hydrolysis by nonspecific blood and tissue esterases. Incubation of remifentanil in fresh, human whole blood demonstrates that the drug can undergo ester cleavage in vitro, suggesting that such metabolism is also operative in vivo. The primary metabolic pathway of remifentanil is de-esterification to form a weakly active carboxylic acid metabolite, GI90291. The red blood cell appears to be the main location of remifentanil's metabolic pathway (92). Almost 90% of the drug is recovered in the urine in the form of this metabolite (93). A summary of remifentanil's metabolic pathway is depicted in Figure 11-3.

Representative, model-independent, pharmacokinetic parameters for remifentanil, determined by an area under the curve analysis of data from healthy adult male volunteers who received a brief infusion of the drug, provide compelling evidence of widespread extrahepatic metabolism. Egan and colleagues reported a mean clearance of 2.9 ± 0.4 L/min, a value that is well above typical adult hepatic blood flow rates. Other parameters reported included a mean residence time (MRT) of 10.9 ± 2.3 minutes and a volume of distribution at steady state of 31.8 ± 7.4 L (8).

Remifentanil's concentration decay in whole blood can be described by a three-compartment model (8, 94). Like the model-independent parameters, analysis of the compartmental parameters for remifentanil reveals a strikingly high clearance. Egan and colleagues reported a central clearance of 2.8 L/min as estimated by a population analysis of data from adult male volunteers (8). Westmoreland and associates (94) reported similar findings in adult male and female patients undergoing elective surgery, with clearances ranging from 4.1 to 5.0 L/min. Remifentanil's rapid clearance implies that, unlike the other fentanyl congeners, termination of drug effect is primarily a result of clearance rather than redistribution.

The rapid clearance of remifentanil has been confirmed in prospective comparison studies with alfentanil. Glass and colleagues (93) reported a mean central clearance of 41.2 ml•kg^{-1}•min^{-1} for remifentanil versus 9.0 ml•kg^{-1}•min^{-1} for alfentanil in a randomized, parallel group comparison study in adult male volunteers. Similarly, in a randomized, crossover comparison study in adult male volunteers, Egan and colleagues reported a remifentanil central clearance of 34.7 ml•kg^{-1}•min^{-1} versus 4.2 ml•kg^{-1}•min^{-1} for alfentanil (10).

Remifentanil undergoes extensive extravascular distribution. The mean volume of distribution at steady-state, determined by an area under the curve analysis, is 31.8 ± 7.4 L (8). Compartmental analysis of the same data from volunteers and other data collected from patients is consistent with extensive tissue distribution. In these studies, the volume of distribution at steady state was 32.8 L and 25 to 40 L, respectively (8, 94).

The relative similarity of remifentanil and alfentanil with respect to distribution has been confirmed in prospective comparison studies with alfentanil. Glass and colleagues (93) reported a mean central volume of 0.153 ± 0.099 L/kg for remifentanil versus 0.152 ± 0.098 L/kg for alfentanil in a randomized, parallel group comparison study in adult male volunteers (93). Similarly, in a randomized, crossover comparison study in adult male volunteers, Egan and associates reported a remifentanil volume of distribution at steady state of 22.4 L versus 38.2 L for alfentanil (8, 94). Unlike with the other fentanyl congeners, the lung is not a site of significant clearance or sequestration of remifentanil (95).

Because remifentanil's major metabolite, GI90291, is not subject to extrahepatic hydrolysis, its clearance is not nearly so high. Based on area under the curve ratios of GI90291 to remifentanil, Westmoreland and colleagues (94) concluded that steady-state concentrations of the metabolite would be, on average, 12 times greater than remifentanil concentrations. Under normal circumstances, however, because the metabolite is thought to be at least several orders of magnitude less potent than remifentanil, the pharmacodynamic significance of the metabolite is likely negligible. Nevertheless, because the metabolite is eliminated principally unchanged in the urine, its accumulation in patients in renal failure is an issue of some importance that is currently under investigation.

TREFENTANIL

Comparatively little has been published regarding trefentanil's pharmacokinetics. Like the other fentanyl congeners (except remifentanil), its metabolism depends on the liver. Trefentanil's concentration decay in the plasma can be adequately described by a three-compartment model. Trefentanil's elimination clearance is approximately 0.4 L/min (11). Its steady-state distribution volume is similar to that of alfentanil and has been reported to be 37 L (11).

FACTORS INFLUENCING PHARMACOKINETICS

Dose

Changes in dose generally do not alter classic opioid pharmacokinetic profiles (79, 80). This finding suggests that biotransformation and excretion mechanisms are not easily saturated by clinical doses of opioids, and kinetics usually remain first order (drug concentration independent). For example, Gepts and associates (70) reported no impact of sufentanil dose (250 to 1500 μg) on its pharmacokinetics. In other words, the pharmacokinetics of opioids is linear in that the shape of the concentration versus time curve dose not change with increasing doses. Altered alfentanil pharmacokinetics has, however, been reported with increasing doses (96).

Drug infusion duration also influences the subsequent rate of decline in plasma opioid concentrations once opioid administration is discontinued, hence the concept of "context-sensitive half times" (37). After a single bolus dose, computer simulations predict equivalent plasma declines for fentanyl, sufentanil, and alfentanil (7). Increases in the size of a single bolus dose of fentanyl, as well as repeated sequential doses, are more likely to delay recovery from drug action. The decline of plasma fentanyl concentrations is significantly affected as drug infusion time is increased. After a 2-hour infusion, the time required for a 50% decrease in plasma fentanyl levels quadruples (to 2 hours) compared with the time required for a similar decrease after a 1-hour infusion (7). Sufentanil and alfentanil are, on the other hand, much less affected by dose and infusion duration (37).

Like the other fentanyl congeners, remifentanil's

pharmacokinetic profile appears to be unaltered by dose. Westmoreland and associates (94) demonstrated that the total clearance and steady-state distribution volume of remifentanil were independent of bolus doses ranging from 5 to 30 $\mu g/kg$ administered to adults undergoing elective surgery. Egan and colleagues (8) published similar findings involving larger total doses given by infusion to adult male volunteers. These investigators observed no change in the overall shape of the dose-normalized concentration versus time curves in subjects who received from 1 to 8 $\mu g{\bullet}kg^{-1}{\bullet}min^{-1}$ for 20 minutes. Thus, over a large dose range for both boluses and infusions, the pharmacokinetics of remifentanil appears to be independent of dose.

Acid-base Changes

The overall clinical impact of acid-base changes on opioid pharmacokinetics is complex. For example, respiratory acidosis during fentanyl administration has multiple effects including increases in ionization and cerebral blood flow (CBF) and decreases in plasma protein binding (97–100). When mechanical ventilation is abruptly terminated, respiratory acidosis rapidly decreases the pH of the extracellular (blood and interstitial) space. More fentanyl in the interstitial compartment becomes ionized as determined by the Henderson-Hasselbach equation for weak bases:

$$pH = pKa + log \frac{proton\ acceptor\ (B)}{proton\ donor\ (BH^+)}$$

More opioid receptors, on cell membranes that interact with ionized fentanyl, are stimulated, producing an enhanced opioid effect. Additional respiratory acidosis because of opioid-induced depression of respiratory centers could produce a vicious cycle of ventilatory depression-acidosis-increased ionized fentanyl and increased ventilatory depression. Alfentanil, with a pKa of 6.5, is not as strongly influenced by either pH changes or tissue accumulation (100).

Intraoperative hyperventilation can also increase the duration of opioid-induced respiratory depression (101). Brain fentanyl levels are higher with respiratory alkalosis (102). Alkalosis also increases the lipophilicity (increased octanol:water partition coefficient) of several opioids. Schwartz and colleagues (103) reported an increased volume of distribution for sufentanil after hyperventilation. Thus, both intraoperative respiratory alkalosis and respiratory acidosis in the immediate postoperative period can prolong and exacerbate opioid-induced respiratory depression.

Plasma Protein Binding

Opioids are basic drugs and bind to certain plasma proteins including α_1-acid glycoprotein, lipoproteins, and albumin. Protein binding of opioids limits tissue penetration and drug availability at receptor sites. Fentanyl, sufentanil, and alfentanil are 84.4%, 92.5%, and 92.1% protein bound after injection in humans (65). Approximately 50% of circulating fentanyl and sufentanil are bound to albumin, whereas only 33% of alfentanil is bound to albumin. Fentanyl and sufentanil, and to a lesser extent alfentanil, are also bound to α and β globulins. All three opioids are bound to α_1-acid glycoprotein, but changes in α_1-acid glycoprotein concentration seem to affect unbound alfentanil the most. Increases in α_1-acid glycoprotein occur with inflammatory diseases, myocardial infarct, renal failure, surgery, rheumatoid arthritis, cancer, and pneumonia and can lead to an increase in opioid binding. Belpaire and Bogaert (104) found myocardial infarction but not renal failure, rheumatoid arthritic, or intensive care problems to increase alfentanil binding in patients, however. Pregnancy and oral contraceptives decrease α_1-acid glycoprotein. Dilution of plasma proteins by one-third increases plasma free fentanyl, sufentanil, and alfentanil by 50%, 35%, and 25%, respectively (65). α_1-Acid glycoprotein binds other drugs including propranolol, imipramine, and lidocaine. Increases in α_1-acid glycoprotein cause increased binding of alfentanil, limit distribution, and decrease the volume of distribution (24%) and clearance in patients with cancer (105). The $t_{1/2}\ \beta$ is minimally altered because these changes in distribution volume and clearance have opposite effects on elimination. Acidosis also impairs plasma protein binding of opioids, with fentanyl more strongly affected than sufentanil (105).

Although protein binding may seem only remotely important to anesthetic considerations in healthy individuals, Lemmens and associates (106) have reported that up to 45% of the variability found in Cp_{50} (the plasma concentration for which 50% of patients had no response to surgical stimulation) for alfentanil can be explained by variability in protein binding of the opioid. Moreover, free drug fractions represent unbound drug and are responsible for drug effect.

Remifentanil is estimated to be 70% bound to plasma proteins, but the exact nature or extent of remifentanil's propensity for plasma protein binding has not yet been fully determined (9).

Hepatic Disease

The primary site of opioid metabolism is the liver. It follows that decreases in drug delivery (e.g., hepatic blood flow) or hepatic function could prolong opioid effects. Liver changes associated with cirrhosis can result in altered or decreased hepatic blood flow and impaired drug handling. The metabolism of drugs with high hepatic extraction ratios (e.g., most opioids) is more likely to be decreased if hepatic blood flow is impaired. Acute viral hepatitis and alcoholic liver injury predominantly affect the pericentral regions of the liner and are more likely to affect drugs metabolized by oxidative processes. In contrast, chronic active hepatitis and primary biliary cirrhosis affect mainly the periportal regions and have little effect on drug metabolism (107). Preservation of glucuronidation in patients with chronic liver disease is due to the large reserve of this transferase enzyme and its location throughout the liver parenchyma, especially in the more protected locale of the periportal region. Extrahepatic glucuronidation may also take place; however, in the absence of liver function, as during the anhepatic phase of liver transplantation, fentanyl $t_{1/2}\ \beta$ is markedly prolonged (108).

Meperidine clearance is reduced and $t_{1/2}\ \beta$ increased in patients with cirrhosis compared with age-matched healthy volunteers (109, 110), although volumes of distribution and plasma protein binding are unchanged. Abnormalities in biochemical liver function tests do not correlate with alterations in $t_{1/2}\ \beta$ or clearance. The kinetics of meperidine are also altered in patients with acute viral hepatitis or a history of heavy alcohol consumption (42, 111). Investigators have suggested that an increased volume of distribution and lower initial plasma concentrations contribute to an apparent decrease in affect of meperidine in alcoholics.

The disposition of fentanyl is not altered in patients with cirrhosis during general anesthesia (56). Only with severe hepatic dysfunction and perhaps high doses of fentanyl is altered pharmacokinetics observed. Decreases in hepatic blood flow may account for the prolonged $t_{1/2}\ \beta$ (8.7 hours) of fentanyl (100 μg/kg) and sufentanil in patients undergoing abdominal aortic surgery (112, 113). A positive correlation exists between alcohol consumption and the need for fentanyl supplementation during nitrous oxide-oxygen-relaxant anesthesia (114). Up to 70% more fentanyl (6.4 versus 3.8 $\mu g{\bullet}kg^{-1}{\bullet}h^{-1}$) was needed in individuals with a mean annual consumption of 31 L pure alcohol.

Alfentanil clearance is also reduced, and its $t_{1/2}\ \beta$ is prolonged in cirrhotic patients undergoing general anesthesia (115). In addition, in one study, although α_1-acid glycoprotein concentrations were not decreased, the plasma free fraction of alfentanil was increased (18.6 versus 11.5%). Chemical alteration of α_1-acid glycoprotein alfentanil binding sites may occur. Thus, an augmented and prolonged alfentanil effect can be anticipated in patients with cirrhosis. Children with cholestatic liver disease who were scheduled to undergo orthotopic liver transplantation showed no changes in alfentanil $t_{1/2}\ \beta$, clearance, and volume of distribution at steady state; after liver transplantation, alfentanil clearance was impaired and elimination prolonged (116). Patients with high alcohol consumption rates require higher plasma alfentanil levels than nondrinking patients. Ventilation is also adequate at higher alfentanil plasma concentrations in patients with a history of high alcohol consumption. Decreased CNS sensitivity to opioid effects is likely in alcoholic patients (117).

Because alfentanil has an intermediate hepatic extraction ratio (0.3 to 0.5), decreases in hepatic blood flow can still result in a decrease in its elimination (86). Thus, indocyanine green clearance (a measure of hepatic blood flow) has been found to correlate with alfentanil clearance (86). Major intra-abdominal surgery has been shown to prolong alfentanil effects by reducing clearance from 6.8 to 2.6 $ml{\bullet}min^{-1}{\bullet}kg^{-1}$ (118). A greater $t_{1/2}\ \beta$ (3.7 ± 2.6 hours) has also been observed for alfentanil in patients undergoing abdominal aortic surgery (119). Hudson and associates (119) believe, however, that alfentanil is eliminated faster than fentanyl or sufentanil in such patients. Although this may be true, alfentanil appears to be more susceptible to alterations in its pharmacokinetic profile in cirrhotic individuals than fentanyl and sufentanil (107).

Sufentanil (3 μg/kg) pharmacokinetics appears to be minimally changed in cirrhotic patients (120). Major intra-abdominal surgery can increase the volume of distribution at steady state and the $t_{1/2}\ \beta$ of sufentanil (112).

In contrast to the other fentanyl congeners, preliminary evidence indicates that, as may be theoretically expected based on the its unique metabolic pathway, hepatic disease and changes in liver blood flow do not alter remifentanil's pharmacokinetic profile. Dershwitz and colleagues (121) prospectively compared the pharmacokinetics of remifentanil in patients awaiting liver transplantation for end-stage hepatic failure with healthy control subjects. These investigators concluded that remifentanil's pharmacokinetics is unaltered by severe hepatic disease at doses up to 0.025 $\mu g{\bullet}kg^{-1}{\bullet}min^{-1}$. Dershwitz and colleagues (121) reported a clearance of 39.8 ± 5.7 $ml{\bullet}kg^{-1}{\bullet}min^{-1}$ and a distribution volume of 0.29 ± 0.07 L/kg in patients in liver failure and similar values of 32.9 ± 8.2 $ml{\bullet}kg^{-1}{\bullet}min^{-1}$ and 0.23 ± 0.13 L/kg in healthy subjects. In fact, remifentanil's clearance is not appreciably altered during the anhepatic phase of human liver transplatation (122).

In summary, initial doses of opioids need not necessarily be decreased or increased unless patients have CNS symptoms (encephalopathy) or a history of heavy alcohol consumption. Prolonged duration of opioid action may occur, however, especially in patients with severe liver disease, and maintenance doses should be decreased accordingly.

Renal Insufficiency

The accumulation of opioid metabolites excreted by the kidney occurs in proportion to the degree of renal impairment. Normeperidine, a major meperidine metabolite, is normally eliminated more slowly than meperidine. It possesses twice the convulsant activity of meperidine but half the analgesic potency (50). In renal failure, or in the presence of chlorpromazine (123) (which may enhance N-demethylation), normeperidine and normeperidinic acid levels may rise and produce toxic (CNS, cardiac) effects. No data are available to evaluate the pharmacokinetics of meperidine in patients with impaired renal function.

Renal failure should not alter fentanyl pharmacokinetics. Fentanyl metabolites may accumulate, but they are largely inactive and nontoxic. Patients with hyperlipoproteinemia bind more fentanyl to plasma proteins, but without significantly changing drug kinetics (124).

Sufentanil pharmacokinetics is not altered in any consistent fashion by kidney disease, although greater variability in its clearance and $t_{1/2}\ \beta$ may result (125). No sufentanil dose modification appears necessary in patients with renal insufficiency (69, 126).

Two studies have reported alfentanil's pharmacokinetics in patients with renal failure (127, 128). Both studies suggested that an increase in clinical effect was likely with alfentanil because of a decreased initial volume of distribution and an increased alfentanil free fraction (127, 128). Discrepancies exist in the results of the two studies, but clearance was unchanged in both. Variations in plasma protein abnormalities (hypoproteinemia, abnormal structure, hyperlipoproteinemia, and various accumulated endogenous and exogenous substances) could possibly explain the differing results. Both reports concluded no delay in recovery after alfentanil should be expected. The clearance of alfentanil may be increased in patients with diabetic renal failure (129). Children with end-stage renal disease do not have significant alterations in alfentanil pharmacokinetics (116).

Remifentanil's pharmacokinetics is not substantially altered by renal insufficiency. Hoke and associates compared the pharmacokinetics of remifentanil administered by infusion for 4 hours in patients undergoing renal dialysis versus healthy volunteers (130). These investigators reported a clearance of 34.2 $ml \cdot kg^{-1} \cdot min^{-1}$ in healthy volunteers and 36.0 $ml \cdot kg^{-1} \cdot min^{-1}$ in patients in renal failure, a statistically insignificant difference. Remifentanil's volume of distribution was also unaltered by renal failure, as reported by Hoke and associates (130). As expected, $t_{1/2}\ \beta$ of the metabolite GI90291 was markedly prolonged in patients in renal failure. Although the metabolite is thought to be essentially inactive, whether some as yet unknown pharmacodynamic activity or toxicity will be observed in patients in renal failure who receive large doses or prolonged administration of remifentanil is unknown.

Obesity

Overweight, and especially morbidly obese, individuals have many significant abnormalities in organ system function that can alter the disposition of drugs. Lipophilic drugs should accumulate in obese individuals (because the peripheral compartment has a high percentage of adipose tissue), resulting in a prolongation of $t_{1/2}\ \beta$. Unfortunately, limited data are available to document this assumption. Bentley and colleagues (131) studied the pharmacokinetics of fentanyl (10 μg/kg) in obese and nonobese individuals. No difference was found, yet the authors suggested administering fentanyl on a lean weight basis.

The pharmacokinetics of sufentanil is altered in the obese. Compared with control patients, obese neurosurgical candidates (94 ± 14 versus 70 ± 13 kg) had increased volumes of distribution (9098 ± 2793 versus 5073 ± 1673 ml/kg ideal body weight) and prolonged $t_{1/2}\ \beta$ (208 ± 82 versus 135 ± 42 minutes). The magnitude of the changes in the these values correlated with the severity of obesity. Clearance was similar between the groups (132). The effects of obesity on alfentanil pharmacokinetics have been evaluated (131). Alfentanil clearance was reduced by 45% (321 to 179 ml/min), and $t_{1/2}\ \beta$ was nearly doubled (92 to 172 minutes). Alfentanil apparently should be administered on the basis of lean body mass, and maintenance doses should be decreased in anticipation of impaired clearance. Simlarly, remifentanil pharmacokinetics is also influenced by weight. Egan and colleagues reported that weight-normalized central clearance and steady-state distribution volume are significantly smaller in obese patents (132a). This finding suggests that remifentanil dosage should be based on ideal body weight.

PHARMACODYNAMICS

Opioids are routinely administered during anesthesia to relieve pain, to blunt or eliminate various responses to noxious stimuli, to maintain cardiovascular stability, and to reduce requirements for other anesthetics. The spectrum of opioid-induced effects is wide and usually dose dependent. Opioid actions can be beneficial or deleterious, depending on the patient and the circumstances. For the purposes of discussion, opioid actions are divided into those that are therapeutic and those that are not.

Therapeutic Actions

Central Nervous System

Neurologic therapeutic opioid actions that accompany analgesia include sedation, anxiolysis (especially elicited by pain or fear of pain), cough suppression, and the relief of dyspnea. High doses of opioid agonists produce unconsciousness and possibly anesthesia. Whereas inhaled anesthetics produce a dose-dependent continuum of EEG changes eventually resulting in burst suppression and a silent EEG, opioids produce minimal changes at low doses and high-voltage slow (δ) waves with high doses. These EEG effects have been documented to be consistent with anesthesia (133, 134).

Whether opioids alone are anesthetics, capable of producing anesthesia, including amnesia, continues to be debated. Although it is an academic point of pharmacologic interest on one hand, the responsibility of anesthesiologists to ensure amnesia for their patients makes this issue real on the other. Opioids do not possess significant amnestic properties, and amnesia can and should be achieved with other agents. Data that demonstrate that sufentanil can be substituted for halothane support the notion that opioids such as sufentanil may be anesthetic (Fig. 11-8) (135). Unconsciousness and amnesia have also been produced by fentanyl (15 μg/kg, intravenously) alone in volunteers, who became both rigid and apneic (136). Unconsciousness accompanied by apnea and rigidity have also been observed with remifentanil.

The impact of opioids on cerebral hemodynamics and metabolic rate is most often small. Many animal experiments but few adequate human studies have evaluated this action. Fentanyl- and sufentanil-based anesthetic techniques result in little or modest decreases in cerebral metabolic rate (CMR) and CBF. At certain doses, opioids activate subcortical structures and increase regional CMR and CBF in animal models. Whether these findings are clinically relevant is unknown. The impact of the potent synthetic opioids on intracranial pressure (ICP), especially in patients at risk (e.g., patients with brain tumors or head trauma), is controversial. Evidence suggests that opioids may possess direct cerebrovasodilatory properties. This action may underlie the increases in ICP observed by some investigators in victims of head trauma who received either fentanyl (3 μg/kg) or sufentanil (0.6 μg/kg) (137). Other investigators have not found sufentanil to exert an effect on ICP in neurosurgical candidates (138). Remifentanil produces a decrease in CBF and ICP in dogs, with EEG changes characteristic for potent opioids (139).

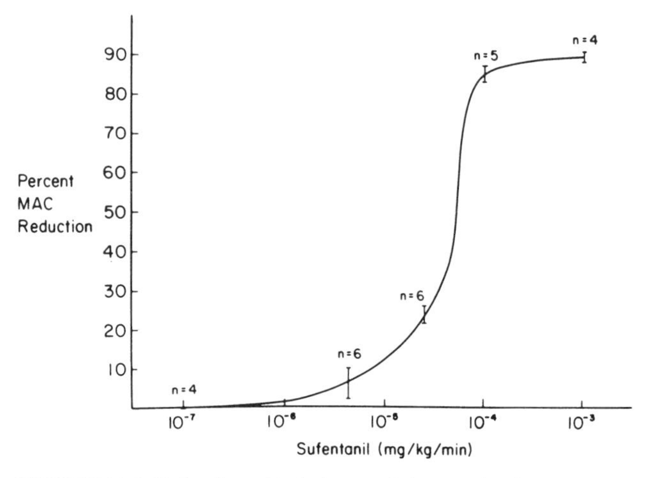

FIGURE 11-8. Reduction of halothane minimum alveolar concentration in the rat observed with progressively increased sufentanil dosage. (From Hecker BR, Lake CL, DiFazio CA, et al. The decrease of the minimum alveolar anesthetic concentration produced by sufentanil in rats. Anesth Analg 1983;62:987–990.)

Cardiovascular System

The rationale behind the application of opioids in anesthesia is not only to provide analgesia, but also to produce stable hemodynamics in the presence and in the absence of noxious stimuli. Opioids are arguably superior to most other agents in achieving this goal. Central cardiovascular regulatory centers, the spinal cord, the sympathetic nervous system, vagal nuclei, and the adrenal medulla are among the key sites that possess opioid receptors and contribute to the ability of opioids to blunt or eliminate significant hemodynamic responses to noxious stimuli (140). The potent opioids applied in anesthesia produce minimal cardiac depression, with modest to no decreases in preload and afterload (141–143), little depression of great vessel and atrial baroreceptors (144), and no effect on coronary vasomotion. Although opioids (excluding meperidine) exert a significant slowing effect on heart rate, hemodynamic stability is usually not threatened during periods of little or no surgical stimulation.

Respiratory System

Some significant therapeutic respiratory benefits can be obtained by the use of opioids in anesthesia as well as in certain pathophysiologic states. Pain or anxiety and stress can induce excessive spontaneous ventilation and respiratory alkalosis. At an extreme, such hyperventilation can reduce CBF to the point of unconsciousness. Opioids, by decreasing both pain and central ventilatory drive, are effective agents in such conditions. Lack of adequate postoperative pain relief can also cause significant respiratory dysfunction (145).

Opioids are also excellent agents for depressing upper airway and tracheal reflexes. This action is beneficial not only during anesthesia, but also in the intensive care (ICU) setting. Opioids allow patients to tolerate endotracheal tubes without coughing or "bucking," which when pronounced can lead to hypoxemia, hypercarbia, hemodynamic instability, increased ICP, and other deleterious effects. Impaired gas exchange results from marked disturbances in ventilation as well as loss of lung volume that bucking produces. Thus, on emergence from general anesthesia, patients anesthetized with a potent inhalation agent and no opioid often cough and buck before they regain consciousness and responsiveness, whereas patients adequately treated with opioids can awaken without such disturbances, even while they are still tracheally intubated.

Opioids can also help to quiet the lower respiratory

tract and to avoid increases in bronchomotor tone. Fentanyl may relax airway smooth muscle (146), and opioids have long been used in the treatment of acute asthma. Opioids also do not alter pulmonary gas exchange (147). The minimal impact of opioids on hypoxic pulmonary vasoconstriction (148) (in contrast to the effects of the potent inhalation agents) coupled with associated hemodynamic stability and the stability of bronchomotor tone all contribute to minimal interference with pulmonary gas exchange.

Endocrine System

The endocrine response to surgery results in augmented metabolism and increased mobilization of energy stores. This "stress response," although at times appropriate and beneficial, can contribute to perioperative hemodynamic and metabolic instability (149). Under the assumption that prevention, reduction, or elimination of the stress response benefits patients, numerous studies have evaluated the impact of opioids on various indices of this phenomenon. Opioids may possibly control stress responses because opioid receptors exist at multiple sites and levels in the neuraxis and in some endocrine organs (e.g., the adrenal gland). Moreover, some endogenous opioids (β-endorphin) are cosynthesized with adrenocorticotropic hormone, and endogenous opioids may modulate the secretion of other hormones.

Opioids, especially in high doses, can blunt perioperative, stress-induced increases in blood levels of cortisol, catecholamines, vasopressin, and growth hormone (150–152). Metabolic catabolism may also be reduced. Only a few recent clinical studies suggest the possible outcome benefits of applying high doses of opioids in anesthesia. Significant associations between the maintenance of intense analgesia or anesthesia with sufentanil into the postoperative period and reductions in morbidity and mortality have been found (153, 154). Future studies may confirm these findings and determine which patient populations and procedures are most susceptible to this intervention.

Nontherapeutic Pharmacodynamic Actions

Central Nervous System

Lethargy, dysphoria, euphoria, pruritus, and meiosis are some of the most frequent nontherapeutic opioid neurophysiologic actions. Nausea and vomiting and respiratory depression are often of greatest concern and are discussed later under the specific organ systems. Two additional neurophysiologic adverse effects merit discussion.

Muscle Rigidity

Opioids can cause increases in skeletal muscle tone that may be severe. At least one central neurologic site including the nucleus raphe pontis is responsible for this opioid effect (155). The occurrence of opioid-induced rigidity is dose dependent, as well as related to the patient's age. In healthy, young adult volunteers, 15 μg/kg of fentanyl intravenously produces rigidity 50% of the time, is not predicted to occur at a certain plasma level, and abates spontaneously in 10 to 20 minutes with decreasing blood drug levels (136). Older patients experience a higher incidence of rigidity after intravenous opioids (156). The potent or rapid-acting opioids sufentanil, fentanyl, and alfentanil are likely to trigger some rigidity in patients as single bolus doses approach 0.3, 3.0, and 30 μg/kg, respectively. The concomitant use of nitrous oxide also exacerbates opioid-induced rigidity.

Opioid-induced rigidity is characterized by upper extremity flexion, especially at the fingers, wrist, and elbow, significant decreases in abdominothoracic compliance, vocal cord closure, and, when associated with apnea, unconsciousness. Rarely, patients may verbally relate some mild musculoskeletal symptoms (tight chest) consistent with mild rigidity following intravenous administration of an opioid. When rigidity is moderate to severe, ventilation by bag and mask, and even manually or mechanically by an endotracheal tube, may be difficult or impossible. Although various agents may possibly attenuate or prevent rigidity, only the administration of neuromuscular blockers is consistently effective in anesthetic practice. Naloxone, too, can antagonize opioid-induced rigidity. Rigidity rarely occurs postoperatively, probably in association with second peaks in plasma opioid levels and respiratory acidosis. If this effect is unrecognized or inadequately treated, respiratory arrest rapidly follows the onset of significant rigidity.

In addition to markedly impairing ventilation, opioid-induced rigidity can increase pulmonary artery and central venous pressures, as well as ICP (157, 158). These adverse effects are reversed with adequate treatment of rigidity. Avoidance or minimizing of rigidity and its effects during anesthesia is best approached by administering nondepolarizing muscle relaxants as defasciculating or "priming" doses before opioid administration and being prepared to complete the induction of anesthesia along with muscle relaxation rapidly once significant rigidity occurs.

Neuroexcitatory Effects

Neuroexcitatory phenomena occasionally occur after opioid administration. These effects range from nystagmus and nonspecific eye movements to single extremity myoclonus or tonus to grand mal seizure-like activity. Although these effects are clinically perturbing to witness, detailed studies have failed to document any superficial electrode-based EEG evidence of seizure activity in humans after high doses of fentanyl, alfentanil, or sufentanil (133, 134, 158). In addition, no permanent neurologic deficit has ever been reported to be associated with opioid-induced neuroexcitation. Nevertheless, some concerns remain. In particular, focal increases in CBF (159) and metabolism (160) can occur with opioids in animal models. Moreover, recent deep electrode (e.g., hippocampal) EEG studies in humans suggest some epileptogenic effect of opioids (161). The significance of these observations for patients at risk for CNS injury is incompletely understood.

Cardiovascular Actions

Although certain opioid actions (e.g., negative chronotropy) are desirable in some patients, they may not be in others. Thus, whereas opioids are chosen to promote hemodynamic stability, sometimes their effects may be exaggerated or unwanted, resulting in untoward hemodynamic sequelae.

Hypotension can occur after opioid administration as a result of direct vascular smooth muscle effects (162) or reductions in sympathetic tone. Vasoconstricted hypovolemic patients may be at greater risk for opioid-induced hypotension. Opioids may also exert a direct local anesthetic-like effect on the myocardium that is not reversible by naloxone and that results in some depression of contractility (163). Direct myocardial depression may occur after meperidine administration. Augmented parasympathetic and vagal tone may exacerbate cardiovascular instability. Moreover, meperidine can release histamine, resulting in vasodilatation and hypotension. Fentanyl, alfentanil, sufentanil, and remifentanil do not stimulate histamine release (164–167), but they too can cause hypotension. The rate of drug administration, as well as the administration of other anesthetics (see the discussion of drug interactions later in this chapter), can contribute to hypotension. Although sufentanil alone may be a more complete anesthetic compared with fentanyl (30), this effect may also account for reports documenting lower blood pressures and decreases in myocardial contractility associated with it (168). High-dose alfentanil anesthesia may produce greater hypotension than either fentanyl or sufentanil (168).

Hypertension may occur during high-dose opioid anesthesia or other anesthetic techniques. This can be due to an inadequate dose of opioid, improper timing of drug administration, or failure to recognize the need for other anesthetic supplements. Patients with good left ventricular function become hypertensive more frequently during opioid-based anesthesia (169). Occasionally, sympathetic activation occurs even after administration of nonhistamine-releasing opioids (170). This effect may be related to sufentanil's ability to cause adrenal gland catecholamine release (171). Specific cardiogenic reflexes elicited during aortic root manipulation may also underlie hypertensive episodes during opioid anesthesia (172). The reported incidences of hypertension associated with fentanyl and sufentanil vary, but they are likely to be less with the latter drug (31). Alfentanil is less reliable in controlling hypertensive episodes when it is used for cardiac anesthesia (168).

All opioids except meperidine decrease heart rate by means of vagal stimulation. Opioids can induce sinus bradycardias, with heart rates as low as 30 to 40 beats per minute. This condition alone usually results in little hemodynamic deterioration. Slow junctional rhythms occasionally occur and can result in hypotension. Sinus arrest or asystole has been reported after opioid administration, especially in conjunction with other vagal stimuli such as laryngoscopy and nasal stimulation (173) or with other medications such as succinylcholine (174). Alfentanil and sufentanil seem to carry higher greater risks for this complication. Alfentanil may also carry a greater risk for bradycardia compared with sufentanil and fentanyl when it is used to induce anesthesia in patients with known coronary artery disease (168).

Respiratory Actions

All μ-receptor opioid agonists produce dose-dependent depression of ventilation, primarily through a direct action on the medullary respiratory center (175, 176). The responsiveness of the respiratory center to CO_2 is significantly reduced by opioids. The slope (or "gain") of the ventilatory response to CO_2 is decreased, and minute ventilatory responses to increases in $PaCO_2$ are shifted to the right (Fig. 11-9). The apneic

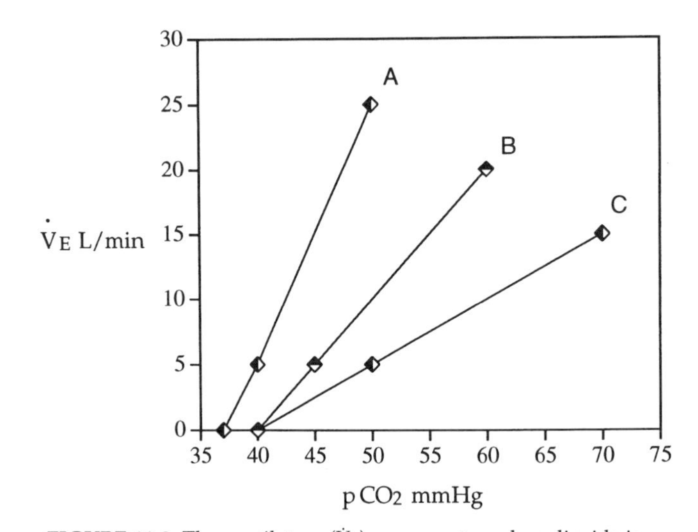

FIGURE 11-9. The ventilatory ($\dot{V}_E$) response to carbon dioxide is typically assessed by a "modified Read" rebreathing method. A graphic representation of the ventilatory response to progressive hypercapnia can be constructed by a regression of ($\dot{V}_E$) versus PCO_2. The slope of line A is approximately 2 $L{\cdot}min^{-1}{\cdot}mm\ Hg^{-1}$, though a wide range of responses in humans exists. The slope of the ventilatory response to CO_2 is reduced to 1 and 0.5 in lines B and C, respectively. Lines B and C are also "shifted" to the right of line A. Lines C and B have the same intercept along the x axis, indicating no displacement or shift of line C compared with line B.

threshold and resting arterial PCO_2 are also increased by opioids. Thus, the mechanism whereby the body protects itself from significant increases in CO_2 and respiratory acidosis is markedly impaired. Opioids also decrease hypoxic ventilatory drive (177, 178) and blunt the increase in respiratory drive normally associated with increased loads such as increased airway resistance (178). Opioid-induced effects on the control of respiratory rhythm and pattern include increased respiratory pauses, delays in expiration, and irregular or periodic breathing. Tidal volume can increase after small increments of opioids, or it can decrease or remain unchanged. Opioids cause a marked slowing of the respiratory rate and can produce apnea without producing unconsciousness. Patients may still respond to verbal commands or tactile prompts to breathe when so affected.

Many factors can change both the magnitude and the duration of respiratory depression after opioid administration (Table 11-2). Even small doses of opioids markedly potentiate the normal right shift of the $PaCO_2$-alveolar ventilation curve that occurs during natural sleep (179, 180). In addition, sleep also impairs tonic and phasic upper airway muscle activity that accompanies breathing (181). This combination of factors can be worrisome when patients have an opioid-based anesthetic and an operation that results in little or no postoperative pain or receive another analgesic regimen or regional anesthetic that leaves opioid actions unopposed by pain. In these patients, apparently adequate breathing may become insufficient when they fall asleep.

Delayed or recurrent respiratory depression can occasionally occur with most opioids including fentanyl (182, 183), meperidine (184), alfentanil (185), and sufentanil (186). Explanations for this phenomenon include the lack of stimulation or pain, administration of supplemental analgesics and other medications, activity causing release of opioids from muscles, hypothermia, hypovolemia, and hypotension. Investigators

TABLE 11-2. Factors Increasing the Magnitude and/or Duration of Opioid-Induced Respiratory Depression

Factor
↑ Dose
Intermittent bolus (versus continuous infusion)
↑ Brain penetration/drug delivery
↓ Distribution (↓ cardiac output)
↑ Unionized fraction (respiratory alkalosis)
↓ Reuptake from the brain (intraoperative respiratory alkalosis)
↓ Clearance (↓ hepatic blood flow, e.g., intraabdominal surgery)
Secondary peaks in plasma opioid levels (reuptake of opioid from muscle, lung, fat, intestine)
↑ Ionized opioid at receptor site (postoperative respiratory acidosis)
Sleep
↑ Age
Metabolic alkalosis

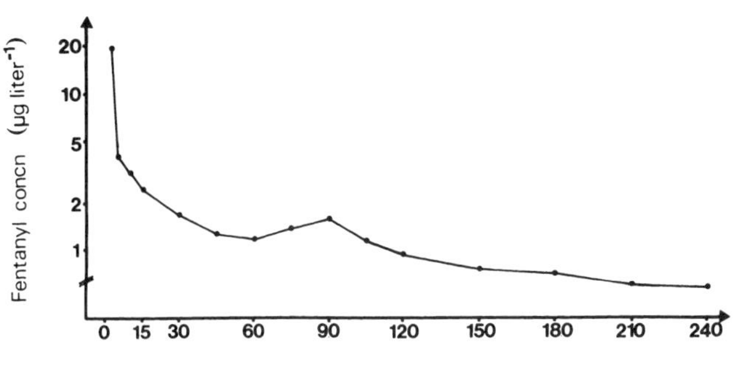

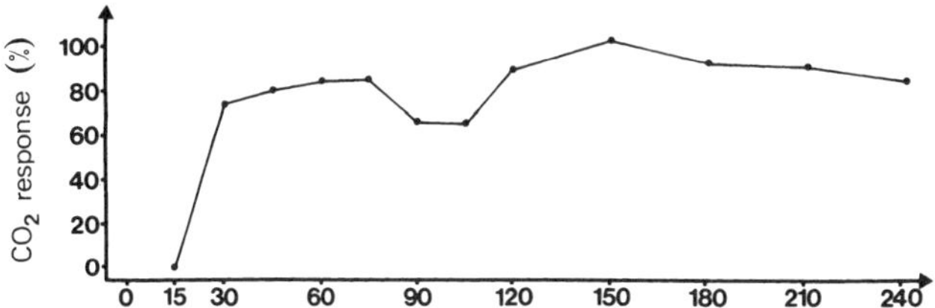

FIGURE 11-10. Fentanyl plasma concentrations (upper panel) after a single bolus injection of fentanyl, 0.5 mg, and the CO_2 ventilatory response slopes as percentages of the control slope (lower panel) in a volunteer with a second, delayed decrease in the response to CO_2. (From Stoeckel H, Schuttler J, Magnussen H, Hengstmann JH. Plasma fentanyl concentrations and occurrence of respiration depression in volunteers. Br J Anaesth 1982;54:1087–1095.)

have noted second peaks in plasma fentanyl levels during the drug's elimination phase (see Fig. 11-6) (52). Investigations have also shown secondary peaks in fentanyl plasma levels to coincide with decreases in brain stem sensitivity to CO_2 (Fig. 11-10) (187).

Some authors suggest and the perception exists that the intraoperative use of opioids leads to an increased incidence of postoperative respiratory problems such as hypoxemia (188). Most studies to date, however, have failed to isolate the use of opioids in anesthesia as especially hazardous compared with other anesthetic agents (189).

Gastrointestinal Effects

Opioids have many gastrointestinal actions that most often represent undesirable side effects in anesthesia. Chief among these effects are nausea and vomiting. Postoperative nausea and vomiting are frequently of great concern to many patients (190). The use of opioids in a balanced anesthetic technique contributes to the significant incidence (15 to 60%) of nausea and vomiting after surgery. Many other factors, however, predispose patients to this problem (190). No one particular opioid agonist has proved more or less emetogenic than others. In fact, the specific opioid receptor type in the chemoreceptor trigger zone of the area postrema of the medulla that is responsible for the potent effect of opioids at this site is unclear. Because it is necessary to treat pain, which can also cause nausea, the adequate application of opioids or other analgesics is appropriate. The use of a continuous opioid infusion may further increase the incidence of vomiting (191). Reducing opioid requirements by administering nonsteroidal anti-inflammatory drugs, when they are appropriate, can help reduce nausea and vomiting (192).

Other opioid-induced gastrointestinal effects that may contribute to nausea and vomiting include the ability of these drugs to increase gastrointestinal secretions, decrease gastrointestinal activity and lower esophageal sphincter tone, and delay gastric emptying. The last effect may increase the risk of a "full stomach" in patients receiving opioids before surgery. Naloxone, and to a lesser degree metoclopramide, can reverse the effect of opioids on gastric emptying. The clinical significance, if any, of the constipating effect of opioids (resulting from decreased propulsion and augmented resting tone) administered in the perioperative period is uncertain, but postoperative ileus is probably increased by opioid use in certain circumstances. Opioid-induced increases in biliary duct pressure and sphincter of Oddi tone can produce biliary spasm and colic and can also contribute to nausea and vomiting.

Other Pharmacodynamic Nontherapeutic Opioid Actions

The renal effects of fentanyl congeners used in modern anesthetic practice are benign. The lower urinary tract, however, can be significantly affected by opioids. Disturbances in micturition include increased detrusor muscle tone, sometimes resulting in urgency, and increased vesical sphincter and ureteral tone, sometimes making urination difficult. Such disturbances are often responsive to naloxone or mixed agonist-antagonist opioids.

Opioids, like most anesthetics, may exacerbate hepatic injury associated with hypoxia (193). Small degrees of hepatic dysfunction may be associated with most anesthetics including fentanyl (194). Nevertheless, little evidence implicates opioids in any significant adverse hepatic effect in humans. As mentioned previously, opioid agonists, in a dose-dependent fashion, can increase biliary tree pressure by an opiate receptor-mediated mechanism. Rarely, such actions can result in a failed intraoperative cholangiogram or epigastric pain that mimics angina (195). Naloxone fully antagonizes this adverse action, except when it is induced by meperidine, which has direct, nonopioid receptor-mediated effects on the biliary tract (196, 197).

SIDE EFFECTS AND THEIR MANAGEMENT

A broad definition of side effects includes nontherapeutic drug actions discussed previously. Most notable among these effects are excessive respiratory depression and muscle rigidity. Bradyarrhythmias can also be considered a side effect. Nausea and vomiting, and not infrequently pruritus, are also annoying adverse opioid-induced side effects. Pruritus is not indicative of an allergic response to opioids, although medical records commonly indicate this as so. Opioid-induced pruritus is centrally mediated. Urinary retention and biliary spasm are occasionally problematic after intravenous opioid administration. Serious allergic responses to opioids are rare, although anaphylaxis after fentanyl and meperidine has been reported (198, 199). Wheal and flare responses to opioids vary, are independent of analgesic potency, and depend on both mast cell-related histamine release and direct vascular effects (200). The most troublesome side effects associated with the use of opioids in intravenous anesthesia are respiratory depression and nausea and vomiting.

Excessive opioid-induced respiratory depression can occur when preoperative medication includes an opioid. The intravenous administration of fentanyl, and especially sufentanil or alfentanil, can be particularly hazardous in settings outside the operating room. Significant respiratory depression frequently accompanies the use of fentanyl derivatives during the induction of anesthesia and is usually anticipated. Normally, in such circumstances, the induction of anesthesia is completed, the airway secured, and ventilation controlled. In patients in whom a difficult airway is anticipated or suspected, caution should be taken to avoid excessive opioid-induced respiratory depression and muscle rigidity before securing the airway. Toward the latter part of an anesthetic administration, excessive opioid-induced respiratory depression may interfere with emergence from anesthesia. Postoperatively, opioid-induced respiratory depression or the recurrence of excessive respiratory depression can produce troubling, if not dangerous, situations.

Regardless of the circumstance, excessive opioid-induced respiratory depression must be recognized and treated appropriately and expeditiously. Under all circumstances, the patient's oxygenation must be ensured immediately. Pulse oximetry remains the best method for assessing oxygenation in most circumstances. Some patients may only require verbal or tactile prompts to breathe. Anesthetized patients may require moderately high but usually benign $PaCO_2$ levels (50 to 60 mm Hg) to breathe spontaneously, even during emergence from anesthesia. Nonintubated patients who experience opioid-induced apnea and rigidity rapidly become cyanotic and hypoxic. They require immediate establishment of an airway and artificial ventilation. In some circumstances, the administration of an opioid antagonist can be helpful.

Naloxone remains the opioid antagonist of choice in most circumstances. Naloxone was introduced into clinical practice in the 1960s. Reports of side effects (e.g., increases in heart rate and blood pressure) and more serious complications (e.g., pulmonary edema)

TABLE 11-3. Reported Severe Complications Following Naloxone Administration

Author (Reference)	Naloxone Dose (IV, mg)	Complication
Azar & Turndorf (201)	0.4	Hypertension (270/140)
Estilo & Cottrell (202)	0.4	Hypertension (260/140); cerebrovascular accident
Flacke et al. (203)	0.4	Pulmonary edema
Tanaka (204)	0.4	Hypertension (340/150)
Andree (205)	0.4	Cardiac arrest, death
	0.4	Cardiac arrest, death
Prough et al. (206)	0.1	Pulmonary edema
	0.2 (+0.3 IM)	Pulmonary edema
Michaelis et al. (207)	0.1	Ventricular tachycardia ventricular fibrillation
	0.4	Ventricular fibrillation
Partridge & Ward (208)	0.08	Pulmonary edema
Taff (209)	0.3	Pulmonary edema

soon followed (Table 11-3) (201–209). Initial naloxone dose recommendations ranged from 0.4 to 0.8 mg. These doses are now recognized as necessary only in emergencies (210).

The mechanisms producing increases in arterial blood pressure, heart rate, and other significant hemodynamic alterations after naloxone reversal of opioids are not well defined. Possibilities include pain, rapid awakening, and sympathetic activation, not only from pain, but also from other causes such as hypercarbia. Because of the potential for undesired hemodynamic changes, opioid reversal is perhaps best avoided in patients with significant cardiovascular risks. Although naloxone has been used safely in neuroanesthesia (211), significant increases in CBF and CMR of oxygen ($CMRO_2$) can occur (212), and careful titration is required. Opioid reversal may be particularly hazardous in patients with pheochromocytoma or chromaffin tissue tumors (213).

Onset of action after the intravenous administration of naloxone is rapid (1 to 2 minutes). The $t_{1/2}\ \beta$ and duration of effect of naloxone are short (30 to 60 minutes) (214, 215). Naloxone is primarily metabolized in the liver by glucuronidation. Attempts to compensate for naloxone's short duration of action by increasing the dose are associated with an increased incidence and severity of unwanted side effects. Most often, 1.0 to 2.0 μg/kg titrated in 0.5- to 1.0-μg/kg boluses every 2 to 3 minutes restores adequate spontaneous ventilation (210, 211, 216). Careful titration of naloxone may not be possible if patients are hypoxic. Recurrence of respiratory depression after naloxone administration is due to the agent's short $t_{1/2}\ \beta$, reuptake of opioid from peripheral compartment tissues (e.g., muscle), and other factors, as discussed previously. Remifentanil is not as likely to be associated with renarcotization because, although its respiratory depressant effects are known to be reversible by naloxone (217), they are also known to be shorter lived. Kapila and associates (218) reported that, after a 3-hour infusion, 50% recovery of spontaneous minute ventilatory volume took just 5 ± 2 minutes with remifentanil but much longer (54 ± 48 minutes) after alfentanil.

"Renarcotization" occurs more frequently when naloxone is used to reverse longer-acting opioids such as fentanyl. In these circumstances, an additional intramuscular dose or continuous infusion of naloxone may be helpful. In the immediate postoperative setting, these modes of administering naloxone should not supplant good nursing care and attentive observations of respiratory function. Shorter-lasting opioids pose a danger of renarcotization less frequently, because of their rapid plasma decay curve. Second peaks in plasma alfentanil or remifentanil levels are also less likely because of their small volume of distribution and metabolism, respectively. Alfentanil opiate receptor binding is also weaker than that of fentanyl and sufentanil (13).

A rational use of opioid antagonists includes the following:

1. Use opioids during anesthesia such that antagonists are rarely necessary.
2. Avoid inducing unnecessary intraoperative hypocapnia such that body CO_2 stores are not depleted and adequate ventilatory drive remains after anesthesia and surgery.
3. Carefully titrate opioid antagonists to specific endpoints.
4. Avoid antagonists in patients with cardiovascular risk factors such as hypertension and cardiac or cerebrovascular disease.

Although naloxene is active at μ, δ, κ, and σ receptors, it has greatest affinity for μ receptors. Thus, it is unlikely, with the current agents available, that analgesia can be reliably spared following reversal of respiratory depression with naloxone. Careful titration of naloxone can, however, usually restore adequate spontaneous ventilation without completely reversing analgesia. Nalbuphine can also be employed to reverse excessive opioid-induced respiratory depression (210, 219, 220). However, significant pain, hypertension, and tachycardia can occur following opioid reversal with nalbuphine (210, 221–224). As with naloxone, patients at risk for cardiac events are not good candidates for opioid reversal. Restoration of spontaneous ventilation using small titrated doses of nalbuphine (2.5 mg every 2 to 3 minutes) may result in less pain and renarcotization compared with naloxone (0.08 mg titrated similarly) after fentanyl (mean dose 25 μg/kg), isoflurane, and nitrous oxide anesthesia (210).

Opioids can increase the incidence of nausea and

vomiting when these agents are used as premedicants, intraoperative agents, or postoperative analgesics (190). Many other factors contribute to postoperative nausea and vomiting, including age (emesis is greater in pediatric patients), female gender, surgery during the first 8 days of the menstrual cycle (225), obesity, history of motion sickness, anxiety, gastroparesis, certain operative procedures (e.g., laparoscopy), duration of surgery, oral intake, hydration status, pain, and ambulation. Anesthesia-associated factors that increase nausea and vomiting include opioid premedication, gastric distention, balanced anesthesia, and drugs like etomidate and nitrous oxide, although the effect of nitrous oxide is still debated (190, 226, 227). The use of propofol in balanced or TIVA reduces the incidence of nausea and vomiting (228). Many studies report a low incidence (5 to 20%) of nausea and vomiting after TIVA with propofol-alfentanil.

Some of the more efficacious antiemetics commonly used in anesthesia are as follows:

1. Drugs with anticholinergic activity, in particular scopolamine and to a lesser degree atropine. Glycopyrrolate is not effective because it penetrates the blood-brain barrier poorly.
2. Butyrophenones (e.g., droperidol), which are most likely effective because of antidopaminergic properties.
3. Dopamine antagonists (e.g., metoclopramide), which act both centrally at the chemoreceptor trigger zone and peripherally, by increasing gastrointestinal motility.
4. Serotonin antagonists (e.g., ondansetron), which may be among the most efficacious drugs available (229).

DRUG INTERACTIONS

Although the introduction of drugs with greater specificity of action purportedly improves safety, it has also led to the administration of many different drugs during a single anesthetic. The potential for and existence of significant drug interactions frequently determine the impact of an anesthetic technique more than the effect of any one particular agent.

The clinical effects of opioids can be greatly altered by the concomitant administration of many other drugs. Most notably, hemodynamic stability can be compromised and respiratory depression exacerbated. Some drug interactions can be advantageous; the administration of modest doses of opioids, for example, usually reduces the requirements for other agents used to induce loss of consciousness. Thus, alfentanil, 50 μg/kg, reduces the required induction dose of propofol from 2 to 3 mg/kg (230) to less than 1 mg/kg (231). In a similar vein, fentanyl and, to an even greater degree sufentanil, decrease the sleep-inducing dose of thiopental in a dose-dependent fashion (see Fig. 11-4) (25). Whether similar-type drug interactions are additive (232) or synergistic (233) is not entirely clear. Although other drug interactions may also be employed toward favorable ends (e.g., adding a benzodiazepine to increase amnesia or to reduce hypertensive episodes during opioid anesthesia), the purpose of this section is to illustrate potentially unfavorable or undesirable drug interactions.

Monoamine oxidase inhibitors (MAOIs) can lead to a serious and potentially fatal adverse drug interaction with meperidine. The safety of other opioids, such as morphine and fentanyl, has been documented in many patients receiving MAOIs and needs to be highlighted (234, 235). Two forms of the MAOI-meperidine interaction exist. One is an "excitatory" form characterized by agitation, rigidity, hyperpyrexia, convulsions, hemodynamic instability, and coma. It is thought to be related to the blockade of neuronal uptake of serotonin by meperidine. The second type of interaction is "depressive" and manifests as respiratory depression, hypotension, and coma, perhaps because of hepatic microsomal enzyme inhibition by MAOI and resultant meperidine accumulation. Successful therapies for these conditions are unsubstantiated but include common supportive measures.

The respiratory depression produced by opioids can be markedly exacerbated by other drugs, especially CNS depressants. Benzodiazepines, as well as other sedative-hypnotic anesthetic induction agents such as propofol (236), even in small doses, can result in significant respiratory depression when combined with opioids. For example, in human volunteers, either fentanyl (2.0 μg/kg intravenously) or midazolam (0.05 mg/kg intravenously) administered alone results in no apnea, but these agents in combination produce apnea 50% of the time (237). The administration of even small doses of benzodiazepines in the immediate preinduction phase of anesthesia can increase the incidence of inadequate postoperative ventilation (238). The preservation of ventilatory function associated with ketamine anesthesia is also reduced by the concomitant administration of opioids. Other CNS-acting drugs such as droperidol, tricyclic antidepressants, and α_2 agonists (such as clonidine) do not significantly potentiate opioid-induced ventilatory depression (239).

Although considered to have mild respiratory depressant properties, nitrous oxide can worsen opioid-induced respiratory effects (240). In the presence of a potent inhalation agent such as isoflurane, sufentanil has been shown to reduce ventilation significantly while minimally affecting hemodynamics in dogs (241). In humans, even small doses of fentanyl (0.3 μg/kg intravenously) administered during inhalation anesthesia (enflurane plus nitrous oxide) significantly depress ventilation by increasing expiratory time and thus decreasing minute ventilatory volume (242). Apnea can occur in patients who are spontaneously ventilating during general anesthesia with a potent inhalation agent if more than 25, 2.5, and 250 μg of fentanyl, sufentanil, or alfentanil respectively, is administered intravenously as a bolus.

Although the loss of adequate respiratory drive can usually be easily managed intraoperatively, drug-induced hemodynamic effects are not always so readily addressed. In addition, drug actions that result in myocardial dysfunction or ischemia may require significant interventions to treat or prevent irreversible and significant morbidity. Thus, whereas the effects of drug combinations are usually sought for patient benefit (e.g., improved amnesia), they can be undesirable (e.g., hypotension). The physical condition of a patient also affects the severity of drug interactions. The exact result of drugs simultaneously administered can be difficult to predict.

Many intravenous sedative-hypnotic agents are concomitantly administered with opioids. The list primarily includes barbiturates, droperidol, benzodiazepines, ketamine, etomidate, and propofol. Hypotension frequently results after barbiturate administration. This is due to venodilatation and decreased cardiac filling. Other mechanisms include myocardial depression and decreased sympathetic nervous system activity. Attempts to ensure amnesia by combining barbiturates with opioids can significantly compromise hemodynamic stability and can result in hypotension and reduced cardiac output (243, 244). Reducing induction doses of barbiturate administered concomitantly with opioids, to 0.5 to 1.0 mg/kg of sodium thiopental, for example, is recommended.

Much information exists on benzodiazepine-opioid combinations and hemodynamic effects. This drug combination is useful, not only because the benzodiazepines are potent amnestics, but also because their interaction with opioids is synergistic when these agents are administered to achieve anesthesia (245, 246). Thus, unconsciousness and prevention of responses to noxious stimuli may be better achieved by such a drug combination. Nevertheless, hemodynamic stability can be compromised by combining opioids and benzodiazepines, especially in patients with little to no cardiovascular reserve. Hypotension can result from combinations of diazepam, midazolam, or lorazepam with virtually all opioids, including fentanyl (141, 156) and sufentanil (247). Hemodynamic consequences include decreases in heart rate, mean arterial and central venous pressure, and cardiac output. Mechanisms include decreases in sympathetic tone (248), decreases in circulating catecholamines (249, 250), additive negative inotropic effects (251), baroreflex function depression (252), and higher opioid plasma levels secondary to the pharmacokinetic consequences of decreased cardiac output (253). In addition, the order of drug administration has been suggested to be important. Lorazepam-sufentanil combinations result in hypotension when lorazepam precedes sufentanil (247, 254, 255) but not when it follows both anesthetic induction with sufentanil and endotracheal intubation (256, 257).

The administration of propofol-opioid combinations follows the same logic as benzodiazepine-opioid combinations: together they can provide unconsciousness and block responses to noxious stimuli, whereas alone neither drug reliably does both. Propofol does, however, produce significant cardiovascular depression that may not resolve immediately with decreasing blood drug levels (258). Although propofol-fentanyl (259) and propofol-sufentanil (260) anesthesia for coronary artery bypass surgery may provide acceptable conditions, mean arterial pressure can decrease, especially during induction of anesthesia, to levels that may jeopardize coronary perfusion (259). Other anesthetic induction agents such as etomidate and ketamine can be combined with opioids and can result in little cardiovascular instability. Alone, these agents inadequately block responses to noxious stimuli, but in low doses (e.g., 4 to 8 mg of etomidate), they can enhance amnesia and preserve the hemodynamic stability sought with opioid-based anesthetic techniques.

Frequently, nitrous oxide or one of the potent inhaled anesthetic gases is administered in conjunction with low- or high-dose opioid anesthesia. Nitrous oxide often, but not always, preserves cardiovascular function (261). When nitrous oxide is combined with fentanyl in human patients, concentration-dependent decreases in cardiac output and arterial blood pressure can result (262). Deterioration of cardiac function with nitrous oxide-opioid combinations may be due to increases in afterload (systemic and pulmonary vascular resistance increases) (263, 264), increases in coronary vascular resistance resulting in impaired coronary blood flow (265), lower inspired oxygen concentration associated with the use of nitrous oxide (266), or direct myocardial depression (267, 268). The use of nitrous oxide in conjunction with fentanyl for anesthesia in cardiac surgery has been found not to be associated with increases in myocardial ischemia (269, 270), however.

Potent inhalation anesthetics are frequently administered in low to moderate concentrations along with opioids (271–273). Ideally, the cardiovascular depressant properties of the inhalation agents improves the myocardial oxygen supply-demand ratio. Thus, low doses of isoflurane can control hypertensive episodes during high-dose sufentanil anesthesia for cardiac surgery (274). Excessive hemodynamic depression can occur with the use of potent inhaled anesthetics and result in significant decreases in cardiac output and blood pressure (275), however. Patients with poor left ventricular function and minimal cardiovascular reserve may be at greater risk for these problems. Good hemodynamic control also does not guarantee the absence of ischemia (275).

Muscle relaxants are frequently administered to patients anesthetized with opioids to eliminate rigidity, to facilitate tracheal intubation, and to provide surgical relaxation. Some muscle relaxants, but in particular older agents, can produce undesirable effects. Pancuronium causes vagal blockade and some sympathetic stimulation and can increase heart rate and blood pressure. Pancuronium-high-dose opioid anesthetic techniques can result in increases in heart rate and myocardial ischemia (255, 276–278). Some clinicians recommend that pancuronium not be given to patients who are candidates for coronary artery surgery (276), but at times it may be employed to advantage if increases in heart rate and blood pressure are desirable (279).

Vecuronium, although devoid of autonomic and cardiac effects alone, can cause hemodynamic depression when it is combined with fentanyl (280). A vecuronium-opioid combination can result in a greater need for vasopressor support than pancuronium-opioid anesthetic techniques (279, 281).

Metocurine alone can result in hypotension (278, 282), but metocurine-pancuronium mixtures may reduce side effects associated with either muscle relaxant alone (283). Newer muscle relaxants have been developed and marketed with the aim of eliminating any relaxant-induced cardiovascular changes. These newer agents include doxacurium, pipecuronium, mivacurium, and rocuronium. These agents, in doses less than or equal to twice the ED_{95}, usually produce minimal to no hemodynamic alterations (284–287). Atracurium, too, at doses lower than 0.5 mg/kg, is usually free of cardiovascular effects (288).

Erythromycin can inhibit the metabolism of several compounds including theophylline and the H_2 blockers. It supposedly reduces the oxidizing activity of cytochrome P450. Alfentanil, but not sufentanil, may have its action prolonged by impaired metabolism in patients receiving erythromycin (289, 290).

Cimetidine can prolong opioid effects by decreasing hepatic blood flow or by diminishing hepatic metabolism. Ranitidine can also reduce hepatic blood flow, but it binds less to the P450 system and has less impact on opioid metabolism than cimetidine (291).

CLINICAL APPLICATIONS

Sedation and Analgesia

Whether for the relief of perioperative pain, for use during monitored anesthesia care, for sedation or supplementation during regional anesthesia, or for general anesthesia, opioids are frequently administered. For short but painful procedures not requiring general anesthesia (e.g., awake nasotracheal intubation) (292), a single bolus injection of an opioid can provide significant or even complete analgesia. Intravenous meperidine, 50 to 100 mg, produces variable degrees of pain relief and is not always effective in patients with severe pain (50, 293). Meperidine plasma levels of 0.5 to 0.8 μg/ml are usually necessary for relief of severe pain (50, 293). Minimally effective meperidine plasma concentrations are 0.1 to 0.2 μg/ml. Intravenous boluses of fentanyl (1 to 3 μg/kg), alfentanil (10 to 30 μg/kg), or sufentanil (0.1 to 0.3 μg/kg) can produce potent, short-lasting analgesia. Plasma concentrations of these opioids that produce analgesia are detailed in Table 11-6. For certain procedures (e.g., awake craniotomy for epilepsy) requiring monitored anesthesia care, small doses of opioids followed by an infusion titrated to effect can produce satisfactory conditions (294). When these drugs are supplemented with an agent such as droperidol, infusion rates range from 0.01 to 0.05 $\mu g \cdot kg^{-1} \cdot min^{-1}$ for fentanyl, 0.0015 to 0.01 $\mu g \cdot kg^{-1} \cdot min^{-1}$ for sufentanil, and 0.25 to 0.75 $\mu g \cdot kg^{-1} \cdot min^{-1}$ for alfentanil (294).

Balanced Anesthesia

Induction of Anesthesia

Opioids are frequently administered just before the induction of balanced anesthesia. This approach may be particularly desirable in patients who require laryngoscopy and tracheal intubation, because of the stimulatory nature of these procedures and the well-documented ability of intravenous opioids to help control resultant cardiovascular responses (295–297). Fentanyl remains popular as the opioid chosen for this purpose. For example, fentanyl is superior to esmolol for heart rate control during laryngoscopy after induction of anesthesia (298). Preinduction intravenous bolus doses of fentanyl shown to be effective when combined with reduced doses of a sedative-hypnotics range from 2 to 8 μg/kg.

The median effective dose (ED_{50}) for the loss of verbal response to command for alfentanil alone in unpremedicated adult volunteers is 111 μg/kg (299). Significant synergism between alfentanil and propofol and midazolam as well as most other induction agents frequently permits much lower doses of any of these agents to be used when they are combined (300, 301). Smith and colleagues (302) found that alfentanil (16 μg/kg) more effectively blunted the hemodynamic response to intubation than esmolol (2 mg/kg) after induction of anesthesia with propofol. Peak opioid action occurs within 1 to 2 minutes after intravenous administration of alfentanil, but it takes several more minutes after fentanyl or sufentanil. Figure 11-11 illustrates the plasma alfentanil concentrations over time from four different studies (74, 75, 77, 78). Bolus injections of alfentanil (80 to 200 μg/kg) produce initial

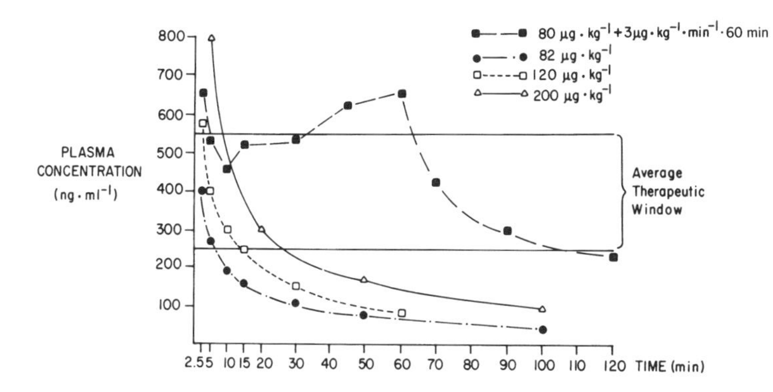

FIGURE 11-11. Plasma alfentanil levels after three different bolus injections and one bolus plus continuous infusion for 1 hour.

plasma levels proportional to the dose. Because alfentanil penetrates the brain so rapidly, equilibration of alfentanil between the plasma and the CNS can be achieved while plasma alfentanil levels are relatively high compared with sufentanil and fentanyl (Fig. 11-12). If alfentanil maintenance infusions are not instituted, plasma levels rapidly decline and may be subtherapeutic (e.g., less than 400 ng•ml^{-1}) for endotracheal intubation. After 50 μg/kg, plasma levels of alfentanil are less than 300 ng•ml^{-1} within 3 to 5 minutes (76).

Sufentanil, 0.25 to 2.0 μg/kg, administered several minutes before induction of anesthesia, can also effectively prevent significant hemodynamic responses to laryngoscopy and intubation. Marty and associates (303) studied 14 patients who were premedicated with lorazepam (2.5 mg) and then anesthetized with sufentanil (2-μg/kg bolus plus 0.66 μg•kg^{-1}•h infusion). These patients were ventilated with 66% nitrous oxide in oxygen and received vecuronium or succinylcholine for muscle relaxation. The mean plasma sufentanil concentration reported to be the Cp_{50} for prevention of hemodynamic responses to laryngoscopy and tracheal intubation was 1.08 ng/ml, with a range of 0.73 to 2.55 ng/ml.

Although detailed reports are not yet available, preliminary evidence indicates that remifentanil, like the other fentanyl congeners, will serve as an effective adjunctive agent for induction of general anesthesia. Remifentanil has been used, for example, in bolus doses of 1 μg/kg in combination with propofol for induction of anesthesia with favorable results (304). Remifentanil's short duration of action after bolus dosing (1 to 5 μg/kg) mandates that an infusion (0.1 to 1.0 μg/kg/min) be started before or soon after the bolus dose to ensure sustained opioid effect.

For procedures of short duration, additional opioid administration may not be necessary, depending on the intensity of surgical stimulation and the degree of immediate postoperative pain. Residual analgesia produced by the foregoing doses of fentanyl and sufentanil may be adequate, whereas patients who receive alfentanil are more likely to require further opioid or analgesic supplementation if postoperative pain will be significant. Remifentanil is so short acting that residual analgesia is minimal unless a continuous infusion is employed.

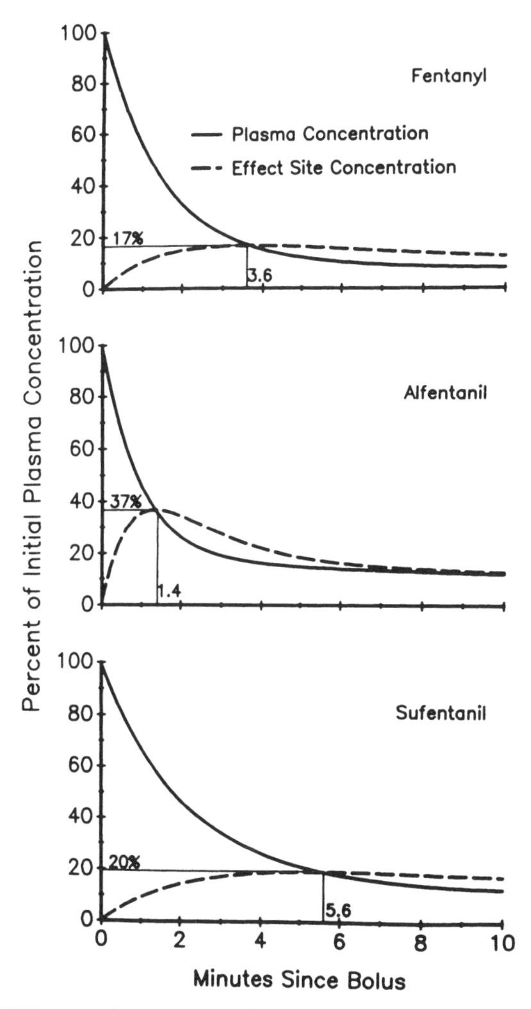

FIGURE 11-12. Computer-simulated plasma and effect site concentrations for fentanyl, alfentanil, and sufentanil, for the first 10 minutes after a bolus injection, as a percentage of initial plasma concentrations. (Adapted from Shafer SL, Varvel JR. Pharmacokinetics, pharmacodynamics, and rational opioid selection. Anesthesiology 1991;74:53–63.)

Maintenance of Anesthesia

In many circumstances, additional opioid doses are given intraoperatively to prevent or blunt responses to surgical stimulation, to contribute to the maintenance of anesthesia, and to provide postoperative analgesia. Fentanyl, for example, can attenuate heart rate responses to isoflurane and desflurane (305). Intermittent boluses of fentanyl (25 to 100 μg) are commonly employed. Preemptive administration of such doses before stimulation of the patient are likely to be more effective than similar doses given after responses to noxious stimuli are manifested. Fentanyl plasma concentrations of 1.0 to 2.0 ng/ml are associated with basal analgesia (306), and 50 and 63% reductions in the MAC of isoflurane are produced by fentanyl plasma concentrations of 1.67 and 3.0 ng/ml, respectively (21). Other investigators have reported the fentanyl plasma concentration that reduces the MAC of isoflurane 50% to be lower (0.5 ng/ml), but they have also noted a wide range of effective concentrations (18). In unpremedicated patients who were anesthetized with a fentanyl infusion and 70% nitrous oxide in oxygen, the Cp_{50} and the Cp_{50} BAR (which are the steady-state plasma drug concentrations that prevent somatic and adrenergic responses to skin incision, respectively, in 50% of patients), for fentanyl at skin incision were 3.26 and 4.17 ng/ml, respectively (307). Although certain reports suggest a good dose-response relationship between fentanyl dose and potent inhalation MAC reduction (308), others suggest that with greater doses or plasma fentanyl concentrations, further MAC reductions become proportionately less. For example, McEwan and colleagues (21) found that increasing plasma fentanyl concentrations from 3.0 to 10 ng/ml only further reduced the MAC of isoflurane from 63 to 82%.

Except for the shortest procedures, anesthesiologists should administer alfentanil by continuous infusion to maintain its clinical effects. Infusion rates typically range from 0.5 to 3.0 $\mu g \cdot kg^{-1} \cdot min^{-1}$, with 1.0 to 2.0 $\mu g \cdot kg^{-1} \cdot min^{-1}$ most frequently necessary for maintenance. Alfentanil requirements vary greatly, depending on many factors including the type and doses of other anesthetic agents employed, the surgical procedure, and patient-related characteristics. Superimposed small boluses of alfentanil (5 to 10 μg/kg) rapidly produce increases in plasma drug levels of approximately 50 to 150 ng/ml in anticipation of stronger stimuli or if anesthesia is inadequate. Ausems and associates (309) have determined the plasma alfentanil concentrations required to supplement nitrous-oxide anesthesia for several types of strong noxious stimuli (Table 11-4). Premedication with a benzodiazepine or the use of propofol can reduce alfentanil requirements by 50 to 75% (310). Anesthetic induction with alfentanil (50 μg/kg) and propofol (1.0 mg/kg) followed by infusions of 1.0 to 1.5 $\mu g \cdot kg^{-1} \cdot min^{-1}$ of alfentanil and 80 to 120 $\mu g \cdot kg^{-1} \cdot min^{-1}$ of propofol will produce complete anesthesia in patients ventilated with nitrous oxide and oxygen for a variety of procedures. Although many alternatives to propofol exist, the similarity between propofol's pharmacokinetic profile and that of alfentanil and the ability of propofol to reduce any nausea and vomiting associated with the use of alfentanil make it a particularly desirable agent.

TABLE 11-4. Stimuli and Corresponding Alfentanil Plasma Concentration at 50% Response (CP_{50})

Stimulus	CP_{50} ng/ml (mean ± SE)
Intubation	475 ± 28
Skin incision	279 ± 20
Skin closure	150 ± 23
Breast surgery	270 ± 63
Lower abdominal surgery	309 ± 44
Upper abdominal surgery	412 ± 135

(From Ausems M, Hug CC, Stanski D, Burm A. Plasma concentrations of alfentanil required to supplement nitrous oxide anesthesia for general surgery. Anesthesiology 1986;65:362–373.)

Vuyk and colleagues have evaluated propofol-alfentanil pharmacodynamic interactions in women undergoing lower abdominal surgery (301). These investigators documented significant synergism between the two agents and explored numerous combinations of blood drug concentrations. They proposed that alfentanil concentrations as low as 85 ng/ml, when combined with blood propofol concentration of 3.5 μg/ml, can produce both optimal anesthetic conditions and speed of recovery. In an accompanying editorial, Stanski and Shafer (311) suggested that bolus doses and initial infusion rates for alfentanil and propofol would be 30 μg/kg and 0.35 $\mu g \cdot kg^{-1} \cdot min^{-1}$ and 0.7 mg/kg and 180 $\mu g \cdot kg^{-1} \cdot min^{-1}$, respectively. Recognizing that these calculations were based on EC_{50} data in patients undergoing only moderately painful procedures, clinicians should adjust these doses accordingly. Further, studies of these type should help define optimal alfentanil doses and blood levels for a variety of noxious stimuli and surgical conditions.

In balanced anesthetic techniques in which potent inhalation agents are also employed, relatively low plasma alfentanil concentrations (e.g., 29 ng/ml) can reduce the MAC of isoflurane approximately 50% (18). As illustrated in Figure 11-11, excessive plasma levels can occur if high alfentanil infusion rates are empirically employed.

Sufentanil, administered either by intermittent bolus (2.5 to 10 μg) or by continuous infusion (0.3 to 1.0 $\mu g \cdot kg^{-1} \cdot h^{-1}$), can be employed to provide the opioid component in balanced anesthesia. The Cp_{50} for prevention of motor responses to skin incision in patients anesthetized only with sufentanil and nitrous oxide has been reported to be 2.08 ng/ml (19). Plasma sufentanil concentrations of less than 0.5 ng/ml can lead to an increase in the need for other supplements (312). Maintaining the cumulative amount of sufentanil infused to less than 1.0 $\mu g \cdot kg^{-1} \cdot h^{-1}$ is recommended for

TABLE 11-5. Approximate Opioid Loading (Bolus) Doses, Maintenance Infusion Rates, and Additional Maintenance Doses for Balanced Anesthesia or Total Intravenous Anesthesia

Agent	Loading Dose (μg/kg)	Maintenance Infusion Rate	Additional Boluses
Alfentanil	25–100	1–3 μg/kg/min	5–10 μg/kg
Sufentanil	0.25–2	0.25–1.5 μg/kg/h	2.5–10 μg
Fentanyl	4–20	2–10 μg/kg/h	25–100 μg
Remifentanil	0.5–1.0	0.25–2 μg/kg/min	0.25–1.0 μg/kg

TABLE 11-6. Approximate Plasma (or Whole Blood for Remifentanil) Opioid Concentrations (ng/ml) Required for Total Intravenous Anesthesia

Use	Fentanyl	Sufentanil	Alfentanil	Remifentanil
Predominant agent	15–30	5–10	400–800	13–25
Major surgery	4–10	1–3	300–500	5–1
Minor surgery	3–6	0.25–1	150–300	1–7
Spontaneous ventilation	1–3	<.4	<200	0.5–5.0
Analgesia	1–2	0.2–0.4	50–150	0.5–5.0

patients and procedures requiring immediate postoperative tracheal extubation (313). Tables 11-5 and 11-6 depict the range of loading and maintenance doses and plasma levels required for fentanyl, alfentanil, sufentanil, and remifentanil in balanced anesthesia.

Emergence from Balanced Anesthesia

Troublesome opioid-induced respiratory depression needs to be avoided if fentanyl and its congeners are to be optimally employed in most patients. In balanced anesthesia, this means that, at the appropriate time, adequate spontaneous ventilation has returned without the frequent use of opioid antagonists. Among the fentanyl congeners, repeated doses or continuous infusions of fentanyl are most likely to result in significant depression of spontaneous ventilation (7, 28, 29, 314). This is especially likely if fentanyl dosage is empiric, without titration to some clinical end point. Administering fentanyl boluses toward the latter part of an operation also increases the likelihood of troublesome respiratory actions. Other investigators have reported that fentanyl, 1 to 2 μg/kg, administered at the time of peritoneal closure in women undergoing gynecologic surgery, can significantly attenuate hemodynamic responses to tracheal extubation (315). Another useful clinical approach is to wait for spontaneous ventilation to resume, then to administer additional titrated doses (10 to 25 μg) of fentanyl to produce a respiratory rate of 8 to 12 breaths per minute before tracheal extubation. Adequate analgesia and cardiovascular stability are often achieved with this approach. Plasma fentanyl levels associated with adequate analgesia after abdominal surgery have been reported to range fivefold from 0.23 to at least 1.18 ng/ml (306).

Similarly, repeated doses or high infusion rates of alfentanil administered near the end of an operation are likely to depress spontaneous ventilation significantly. On the other hand, if no alfentanil is administered toward the latter part of an anesthetic administration, inadequate analgesia will exist in many patients shortly after they regain consciousness, unless steps have been taken to ensure analgesia. Although alfentanil infusions should be reduced as permitted during balanced anesthesia, they should not be terminated until the operation is nearly finished. Alfentanil plasma concentrations that permit the return of spontaneous ventilation have been reported to be 223 ± 13 ng/ml (309). Alfentanil infusion rates of 0.5 ± 0.25 $\mu g \cdot kg^{1} \cdot min^{-1}$, administered until surgery is nearly complete, do not frequently interfere with the return of adequate spontaneous ventilation and emergence from anesthesia.

The same precautions with regard to the timing and amount of opioid dosage hold true for sufentanil. Infusion rates of less than 1.0 $\mu g \cdot kg^{-1} \cdot h^{-1}$ are associated with fewer problems during emergence and in the immediate postoperative period (313, 316, 317). Administering any sufentanil bolus near the end of surgery is likely to interfere with adequate spontaneous ventilation unless the drug is titrated in the smallest of doses (e.g., 2.5 μg). Such dosing is best done once spontaneous ventilation has already been established. Plasma levels of sufentanil of less than 0.25 ng/ml often permit spontaneous ventilation (303).

Remifentanil administration should permit a rapid and trouble-free emergence in light of its extremely short duration of action. Infusion rates of 0.05 ± 0.025 μg/kg/min should permit the return of spontaneous ventilation and emergence with maintenance of analgesia. A unique problem associated with emergence from remifentanil anesthesia is the possibility of an excessively rapid dissipation of opioid effect with undesirable consequences (e.g., excessive pain). The need for alternative analgesic therapies should be anticipated and administered in a timely fashion.

Choosing an Opioid for Balanced Anesthesia

The ideal opioid would permit rapid titration to effect, successfully prevent unwanted responses to noxious stimuli, require little supplementation, not depress cardiovascular function, permit the return of adequate spontaneous ventilation in a timely manner, and produce residual postoperative analgesia. Numerous studies have evaluated one or more of these facets for the fentanyl congeners. Alfentanil and remifentanil provide the greatest ability to titrate drugs rapidly because of their extremely rapid onset of effect. The administration of these two agents can be timed much like other anesthetic induction agents. In addition, increases in the depth of anesthesia can be most rapidly achieved with alfentanil or remifentanil, compared with sufentanil or fentanyl. Sufentanil, on the other hand, frequently provides better hemodynamic stability and conditions that least often require additional or repeated supplementation (26, 27, 318, 319). Computer simulations (7) and studies in volunteers (29) as well as in patients (28, 314) indicate that sufentanil and alfentanil are better than fentanyl with regard to producing conditions that permit trouble-free emergence with adequate spontaneous ventilation and analgesia.

If the goal when employing opioids as part of an anesthetic regimen is to provide only basal analgesia and to minimize drug costs, then fentanyl may be the best choice. The latter issue can no longer be ignored in light of the significant drug cost differences between fentanyl and sufentanil or alfentanil. On the other hand, anesthesia-related costs should not be calculated in oversimplified ways (e.g., summation of drug costs), but they should also reflect associated costs (e.g., prolonged emergence). If opioids are to be employed as an "anesthetic" agent, sufentanil, alfentanil, and remifentanil offer significant advantages over fentanyl. Whether these benefits outweigh the disadvantage of increased drug cost depends on their optimal application in appropriately selected patients. Proof of such differences remains difficult.

Total Intravenous Anesthesia (TIVA)

Although TIVA does not necessarily require an opioid component, especially in minimally stimulating procedures, the fentanyl congeners most often are an important part of TIVA. In procedures in which marked stimulation is produced, the inclusion of an opioid as a component of TIVA not only provides analgesia, but also permits reductions in the required doses of other agents and contributes significantly to hemodynamic stability. For example, fentanyl plasma concentrations ranging from 0.63 to 3.0 ng/ml have reduced propofol requirements to prevent motor responses to skin incision from 50 to 89% (320). Profound synergism also exists when several agents such as propofol, alfentanil, and midazolam are combined (300, 301). Indeed, although several different sedative-hypnotic agents can be employed in TIVA to provide hypnosis and amnesia (e.g., midazolam, propofol), the fentanyl congeners are arguably essential components of TIVA.

Continuous infusions of intravenous opioids should be employed but for the shortest of procedures (321). Although the delivery of intravenous anesthetics by intermittent bolus injection will always retain a role and is appealing because of its simplicity, only by employing continuous infusions can the use of opioids in anesthesia be optimized (Table 11-7) (322–325). Although high-dose opioid anesthesia can conveniently be administered by intermittent injections, several factors have diminished the popularity of this technique even in cardiac anesthesia, in which it has been most commonly employed. These include the lack of evidence substantiating any significant outcome benefit associated with the use of large doses of opioids (326, 327), the added drug costs (especially with large doses of sufentanil), and the trend toward "fast track" approaches to the cardiac patient. "Fast track" care includes early (within 2 to 8 hours postoperatively) tracheal extubation, which can be impeded by large doses of fentanyl (328). The use of continuous infusions of opioids, even at doses required in cardiac anesthesia, can permit significant and stable opioid actions to be produced without prolonged postoperative respiratory depression.

Many factors must be considered when choosing an opioid for infusion during TIVA including the drug's pharmacodynamics and pharmacokinetics, target plasma concentrations, patient factors and the type and duration of the surgical procedure. Additive or synergistic effects resulting from various drug combinations must also be considered, as discussed previously. In addition, approaches to producing, and maintaining, appropriate drug levels must be considered. The gap with regard to the tools (e.g., computer technology, drug assays) employed in research versus those available to clinicians is still large. Some investigators validate the accuracy of pharmacokinetic model-driven opioid infusions and suggest that simple pocket calculators can be employed to predict drug concentrations from pharmacokinetic data (329, 330). Others have failed to verify the ability of population pharmacokinetic data to predict plasma opioid concentrations adequately (331). Undoubtedly, variability from patient to patient with regard to opioid pharmacokinetics as well as pharmacodynamics remains a large part of the problem (332).

TABLE 11-7. Potential Advantages of Continuous Infusions Over Intermittent Boluses of Opioids in Anesthesia (325)

Decreased total dose
Greater hemodynamic stability
Decreased side effects (e.g., rigidity)
Decreased need for supplementation
More rapid recovery of consciousness
Respiratory depression and need for antagonists
Pain in the immediate postoperative period
Decreased discharge time

Induction and Maintenance of Tiva

Many clinicians administer TIVA with the use of an infusion pump with which drug delivery rate is manually set. Initially, clinicians can administer one or several titrated drug boluses during the induction of anesthesia to achieve effective plasma opioid concentrations (see Tables 11-5 and 11-6). The dose of opioid required to establish a specific plasma concentration has traditionally been determined by the central volume of distribution. This "loading" dose equals the desired concentration times that volume of distribution. In a 70-kg individual with a central volume of distribution for sufentanil of 3 L/kg, 84 μg would be estimated as a loading dose to produce a plasma concentration of 0.4 μg/L or 0.4 ng/ml. Because plasma opioid levels can decrease rapidly (see Fig. 11-12), appropriate steps should be taken. Often, it is best to initiate a continuous drug infusion before inducing anesthesia. In this manner, anesthesia can be maintained, and clinicians can direct their full attention to airway management or other tasks. Infusion rates can be estimated by multiplying the target plasma concentration times the clearance rate. In an individual with an estimated sufentanil clearance rate of 0.8 $L{\cdot}kg^{-1}{\cdot}h^{-1}$, a sufentanil concentration of 0.4 μg/L (or 0.4 ng/ml) would be achieved with an infusion of 22.4 μg/h. The foregoing loading dose and infusion rate calculations are oversimplifications at best. They do not take into consideration important factors such as the disequilibrium between blood and effect site concentrations or other tissue compartments. More modern approaches to understanding and determining drug infusion schemes are being developed.

Required opioid doses and plasma concentrations during TIVA may equal those suggested for balanced anesthesia with nitrous oxide, they may be less depending on concomitant sedative-hypnotic administration (333), or they may be greater when the predominant or sole anesthetic is the opioid. Fragen and colleagues (78) suggest 176 μg/kg of alfentanil as an induction dose followed by an infusion of 1.3 $\mu g{\cdot}kg^{-1}{\cdot}min^{-1}$ as a reasonable guideline to achieve a plasma level of approximately 400 ng/ml. Terminating the alfentanil infusion 10 to 30 minutes before the end of surgery allows enough time for plasma levels to decrease 50%. As mentioned earlier, Vuyk and associates (301) reported in detail on the synergism between different plasma levels of propofol and alfentanil.

TIVA for cardiac or other large operations is also popular. Frequently, in such cases, immediate postoperative tracheal extubation is not necessary, and opioid dosing is not constrained by the need for spontaneous ventilation at the end of surgery. Many opioid regimens have been reported. Hall and associates (334), employing a modified Wagner method (335), suggest that a 20-minute loading infusion of fentanyl (2.4 $\mu g{\cdot}kg^{-1}{\cdot}min^{-1}$), started simultaneously with a fentanyl maintenance infusion of 0.3 $\mu g{\cdot}kg^{-1}{\cdot}min^{-1}$, produces plasma fentanyl concentrations between 20 and 27 ng/ml and minimizes the need for other supplements. Other clinicians argue that no plasma opioid concentration can eliminate the need for supplements entirely (34).

Clinicians administering TIVA may frequently initiate anesthesia with doses derived in part by the foregoing or other formulas. Similarly, initial maintenance doses may be calculated. No matter what tools clinicians do or do not have at their disposal (EEG monitoring, computer software), the titration of anesthetic agents, drug infusion rate determinations, and administration of additional bolus injections all require anticipation of noxious stimuli and their intensity, as well as close scrutiny of patient responses. No clinically available and reliable monitor of depth or adequacy of anesthesia exists. The clinical signs of inadequate anesthesia are either autonomic or motor. Opioid actions can blunt or eliminate most hemodynamic and autonomic signs of inadequate anesthesia. Because a motor response may be the earliest sign of inadequate anesthesia, neuromuscular blockade should be employed only to produce necessary surgical relaxation or to protect the patient. Fear of patient movement in and of itself does not justify the administration of neuromuscular blockers.

In anticipation of noxious stimuli, additional small doses of an opioid (e.g., alfentanil, 5 to 10 μg/kg) can be administered preemptively. This may be particularly appropriate early on in surgical procedures when stimuli tend to be great, and time for the dissipation of profound opioid action exists. As the operation and anesthetic administration proceed, a lack of any sign of inadequate anesthesia provides the opportunity for the clinician to decrease infusion rates gradually by decrements of 10 to 25% to reduce the possibility of drug overdose. This approach of searching for the lowest opioid (or other drug) infusion rate necessary may actually result in too light a level of anesthesia. It has been recommended as perhaps the only clinically available method to determine appropriate infusion rates, however (309). When clinical titration forms the basis of TIVA administration, the advantages of alfentanil and remifentanil lie in their more rapid onset of action.

Emergence From TIVA

Once surgery is nearly complete, continuous opioid infusions should be terminated. The actual time required for patients to regain adequate spontaneous ventilatory drive and consciousness depends on a host of factors. These include the length of the procedure, the intensity of residual pain, patient-specific characteristics that may have affected drug pharmacokinetics, anesthetic requirements of the patient, and the skill and experience of the clinician. With most procedures of 1 to 2 hours' duration, ensuring that appropriate opiate doses have been employed, 10 to 30 minutes are usually required for sufentanil or alfentanil plasma concentrations to decrease to levels that permit adequate spontaneous ventilation and emergence from anesthesia (37). For example, spontaneous ventilation usually resumes below a plasma alfentanil concentration of 150 ng/ml. However, significant respiratory depression can still occur with plasma alfentanil levels of 100 to 200 ng/ml (336).

TIVA techniques employing infusions of fentanyl are likely to require longer periods of time for adequate decreases in plasma drug levels following termination of the infusion (7, 37). Sufentanil may possess an advantage over alfentanil in that its plasma level may decrease more rapidly after infusions of less than 6 to 8 hours' duration (37). In addition, compared with fentanyl, sufentanil may produce better analgesia with less respiratory depression (29). The potential advantages and disadvantages of remifentanil have already been mentioned. When TIVA techniques employing an opioid combined with a sedative-hypnotic are properly administered, emergence from anesthesia can be nearly ideal. Patients awaken tolerant of endotracheal tubes with good analgesia. Almost immediately after regaining consciousness and tracheal extubation, patients are appropriately responsive. Nausea and vomiting are frequently minimal, and patients have few (if any) unpleasant side effects.

REFERENCES

1. Brownstein MJ. A brief history of opiates, opioid peptides, and opioid receptors. Proc Natl Acad Sci U S A 1993;90:5391–5393.
2. Lundy JS. Balanced anesthesia. Minn Med 1926;9:399.
3. Neff W, Mayer EC, de la Luz Perales M. Nitrous oxide and oxygen anesthesia with curare relaxation. Calif Med 1947;66:67.
4. Stanley TH. The history and development of the fentanyl series. J Pain Symptom Management 1992;7:S3-S7.
5. Lowenstein E, Hallowell P, Levine FH, et al. Cardiovascular response to large doses of intravenous morphine in man. N Engl J Med 1969;281:1389–1393.
6. Janssen PAJ. Potent, new analgesics, tailor-made for different purposes. Acta Anaesthesiol Scand 1982;26:262–268.
7. Shafer SL, Varvel JR. Pharmacokinetics, pharmacodynamics, and rational opioid selection. Anesthesiology 1991;74:53–63.
8. Egan TD, Lemmens HJM, Fiset P, et al. The pharmacokinetics of the new short-acting opioid remifentanil (GI87084B) in healthy adult male volunteers. Anesthesiology 1993;79:881–892.
9. Glass PS. Remifentanil: a new opioid. J Clin Anesth 1995;7:558–563.
10. Egan TD, Minto C, Hermann DJ, et al. Remifentanil versus alfentanil: comparative pharmacokinetics and pharmacodynamics in healthy adult male volunteers. Anesthesiology 1996; 84:821-833.
11. Lemmens HJM, Dyck JB, Shafer SL, Stanski DR. Pharmacokinetic-pharmacodynamic modeling in drug development: application to the investigational opioid trefentanil. Clin Pharmacol Ther 1994;56:261–271.
12. Pasternak GW, Zhang AZ, Tecott L. Developmental differences between high and low affinity opiate binding sites: their relationship to analgesia and respiratory depression. Life Sci 1980; 27:1185.
13. Brown JH, Pleuvry BJ. Antagonism of the respiratory effects of alfentanil and fentanyl by naloxone in the conscious rabbit. Br J Anaesth 1981;53:1033–1037.
14. Yeadon M, Kitchen I. Comparative binding of m and d selective ligands in whole brain and pons/medulla homogenates from rat: affinity profiles of fentanyl derivatives. Neuropharmacology 1988;27:345–348.
15. Leysen JE, Gommeren W, Niemegeers CJE. [3H]sufentanil, a superior ligand for μ-opiate receptors: binding properties and regional distribution in rat brain and spinal cord. Eur J Pharmacol 1983;87:209–225.
16. Scott JC, Ponganis KV, Stanski DR. EEG quantitation of narcotic effect: the comparative pharmacodynamics of fentanyl and alfentanil. Anesthesiology 1985;62:234–241.
17. Scott JC, Cooke JE, Stanski DR. Electroencephalographic quantitation of opioid effect: comparative pharmacodynamics of fentanyl and sufentanil. Anesthesiology 1991;74:34–42.
18. Westmoreland CL, Sebel PS, Gropper A. Fentanyl or alfentanil decreases the minimum alveolar anesthetic concentration of isoflurane in surgical patients. Anesth Analg 1994;78:23–28.
19. Glass PSA, Doherty MA, Jacobs JR, et al. CP_{50} for sufentanil. Anesthesiology 1990;73:A378.
20. Westmoreland CW, Sebel PS, Gropper A, Hug CC Jr. Reduction of isoflurane MAC by fentanyl or alfentanil. Anesthesiology 1992;77:A394.
21. McEwan AI, Smith C, Dyar O, et al. Isoflurane minimum alveolar concentration reduction by fentanyl. Anesthesiology 1993;78:864–869.
22. Kapila A, Lang E, Glass P, et al. MAC reduction of isoflurane by remifentanil. Anesthesiology 1994;81:A378.
23. Brunner MD, Braithwaite P, Jhaveri R. MAC reduction of isoflurane by sufentanil. Br J Anaesth 1994;72:42–46.
24. Cambareri JJ, Afifi MS, Glass PSA, et al. A–3665, a new short-acting opioid: a comparison with alfentanil. Anesth Analg 1993; 76:812–816.
25. Bowdlc TΛ, Ward RJ. Induction of anesthesia with small doses of sufentanil or fentanyl: dose versus EEG response, speed of onset and thiopental requirement. Anesthesiology 1989;70:26–30.
26. Ghoneim MM, Dhanaraj J, Choi WW. Comparison of four opioid analgesics as supplements to nitrous oxide anesthesia. Anesth Analg 1984;63:405–412.
27. Flacke JW, Bloor BC, Flacke WE, et al. Comparison of morphine, meperidine, fentanyl, and sufentanil in balanced anesthesia: a double-blind study. Anesth Analg 1985;64:897–910.
28. Clark NJ, Meuleman T, Liu W, et al. Comparison of sufentanil-N_2O and fentanyl-N_2O in patients without cardiac disease undergoing general surgery. Anesthesiology 1987;66:130–135.
29. Bailey PL, Streisand JB, East KA, et al. Differences in magnitude and duration of opioid-induced respiratory depression and analgesia with fentanyl and sufentanil. Anesth Analg 1990;70:8–15.
30. Lake CL, DiFazio CA. Sufentanil versus fentanyl: hemodynamic effects in valvular heart disease. Anesth Analg 1987; 66:S99.
31. de Lange S, Stanley TH, Boscoe MJ, Pace NL. Comparison of sufentanil-O_2 and fentanyl-O_2 for coronary artery surgery. Anesthesiology 1982;56:112–118.
32. Benthuysen JL, Foltz BD, Smith NT, et al. Prebypass hemodynamic stability of sufentanil–O_2, fentanyl-O_2 and morphine-O_2 anesthesia during cardiac surgery: a comparison of cardiovascular profiles. J Cardiothorac Anesth 1988;12:749–757.

33. Howie MB, Smith DF, Reiley TE, et al. Postoperative course after sufentanil or fentanyl anesthesia for coronary artery surgery. J Cardiothorac Vasc Anesth 1991;5:485–489.
34. Philbin DM, Rosow CE, Schneider RC, et al. Fentanyl and sufentanil anesthesia revisited: how much is enough? Anesthesiology 1990;73:5–11.
35. Sonntag H, Stephan H, Lange H, et al. Sufentanil does not block sympathetic responses to surgical stimuli in patients having coronary artery revascularization surgery. Anesth Analg 1989; 68:584–592.
36. Moore RA, Yang SS, McNicholas KW, et al. Hemodynamic and anesthetic effects of sufentanil as the sole anesthetic for pediatric cardiovascular surgery. Anesthesiology 1985;62:725–731.
37. Hughes MA, Glass PSA, Jacobs JR. Context-sensitive half-time in multicompartment pharmacokinetic models for intravenous anesthetic drugs. Anesthesiology 1992;76:334–341.
38. Shafer SL, Stanski DR. Improving the clinical utility of anesthetic drug pharmacokinetics [Editorial]. Anesthesiology 1992; 76:327–330.
39. Bailey J. Technique for quantifying the duration of intravenous anesthetic effect. Anesthesiology 1995;83:1095–1103.
40. Ebling WF, Lee EN, Stanski DR. Understanding pharmacokinetics and pharmacodynamics through computer simulation: I. The comparative clinical profiles of fentanyl and alfentanil. Anesthesiology 1990;72:650–658.
41. Schnider TW, Shafer SL. Evolving clinically useful predictors of recovery from intravenous anesthetics. Anesthesiology 1995; 83:902–905.
42. Mather LE, Tucke GT, Pflug AE, et al. Meperidine kinetics in man: intravenous injection in surgical patients and volunteers. Clin Pharmacol Ther 1975;17:21–30.
43. Klotz U, McHorse TS, Wilkinson GR, Schenker S. The effect of cirrhosis on the disposition and elimination of meperidine in man. Clin Pharmacol Ther 1974;16:667–675.
44. Verbeeck RK, Branch RA, Wilkinson GR. Meperidine disposition in man: influence of urinary pH and route of administration. Clin Pharmacol Ther 1981;30:619–628.
45. Stambaugh JE, Wainer IW, Sanstead J, Hemphill DM. The clinical pharmacology of meperidine: comparison of routes of administration. J Clin Pharmacol 1976;16:245–256.
46. Austin KL, Stapleton JV, Mather LE. Multiple intramuscular injections: a major source of variability in analgesic response to meperidine. Pain 1980;8:47.
47. Fung DL, Asling JH, Eisele JH, et al. A comparison of alphaprodine and meperidine pharmacokinetics. J Clin Pharmacol 1980;20:37.
48. Roerig DL, Kotrly KJ, Vucins EJ, et al. First pass uptake of fentanyl, meperidine, and morphine in the human lung. Anesthesiology 1987;67:466–472.
49. Miller JW, Anderson HH. The effect of N-demethylation on certain pharmacologic actions of morphine, codeine and meperidine in the mouse. J Pharmacol Exp Ther 1954;112:191–196.
50. Szeto HH, Inturrisi CE, Houde R, et al. Accumulation of normeperidine, an active metabolite of meperidine, in patients with renal failure or cancer. Ann Intern Med 1977;86:738–741.
51. Bentley JB, Borel JD, Nenad REJ, Gillespie TJ. Age and fentanyl pharmacokinetics. Anesth Analg 1982; 61:968–971.
52. McClain DA, Hug CC Jr. Intravenous fentanyl kinetics. Clin Pharmacol Ther 1980;28:106–114.
53. Hengstmann JH, Stockel H, Schüttler J. Infusion model for fentanyl based on pharmacokinetic analysis. Br J Anaesth 1980; 52:1021–1025.
54. Fung DL, Eisele JH. Fentanyl pharmacokinetics in awake volunteers. J Clin Pharmacol 1980;20:652–658.
55. Schleimer R, Benjamin E, Eisele J, Henderson G. Pharmacokinetics of fentanyl as determined by radioimmunoassay. Clin Pharmacol Ther 1978;23:188–194.
56. Haberer JP, Schoeffler P, Couderc E, Duvaldestin P. Fentanyl pharmacokinetics in anaesthetized patients with cirrhosis. Br J Anaesth 1982;54:1267–1270.
57. Mather LE. Clinical pharmacokinetics of fentanyl and its newer derivatives. Clin Pharmacokinet 1983;8:422–446.
58. Shafer SL, Varvel JR, Aziz N, Scott JC. Pharmacokinetics of fentanyl administered by computer-controlled infusion pump. Anesthesiology 1990;73:1091–1102.
59. Taeger K, Weninger E, Schmelzer F, et al. Pulmonary kinetics of fentanyl and alfentanil in surgical patients. Br J Anaesth 1988; 61:425–434.
60. Hug CC, Murphy MR. Tissue redistribution of fentanyl and termination of its effects in rats. Anesthesiology 1981;55:369–375.
61. Björkman S, Stanski DR, Verotta D, Harashima H. Comparative tissue concentration profiles of fentanyl and alfentanil in humans predicted from tissue/blood partition data obtained in rats. Anesthesiology 1990;72:865–873.
62. Hudson RJ, Stanski DR. Metabolism versus redistribution of fentanyl and alfentanil. Anesthesiology 1983;59:A243.
63. Bower S, Hull CJ. Comparative pharmacokinetics of fentanyl and alfentanil. Br J Anaesth 1982;54:871–877.
64. Silverstein JH, Reiders MF, McMullin M, et al. Norfentanyl is detectable in urine for>48 hours; an advance for urine drug testing in anesthesia. Anesthesiology 1991;75:A895.
65. Meuldermans WEG, Hurkmans RMA, Heykants JJP. Plasma protein binding and distribution of fentanyl, sufentanil, alfentanil and lofentanil in blood. Arch Int Pharmacodyn Ther 1982; 257:4–19.
66. Reilly CS, Wood AJJ, Wood M. Variability of fentanyl pharmacokinetics in man: computer predicted plasma concentrations for three intravenous dosage regimens. Anaesthesia 1984; 40:837–843.
67. Boer F, Bovill JG, Burm AGL, Mooren RAG. Uptake of sufentanil, alfentanil and morphine in the lungs of patients about to undergo coronary artery surgery. Br J Anaesth 1992;68:370–375.
68. Bovill JG, Sebel PS, Blackburn CL, et al. The pharmacokinetics of sufentanil in surgical patients. Anesthesiology 1984;61:502–506.
69. Sear JW. Sufentanil disposition in patients undergoing renal transplantation: influence of choice of kinetic model. Br J Anaesth 1989;63:60–67.
70. Gepts E, Shafer SL, Camu F, et al. Linearity of pharmacokinetics and model estimation of sufentanil. Anesthesiology 1995; 83:1194–1204.
71. Lavrijsen K, Van Houdt J, Van Dyck D, et al. Biotransformation of sufentanil in liver microsomes of rats, dogs, and humans. Drug Metab Dispos 1990;18:704–710.
72. Shafer A, Sun M-L, White PF. Pharmacokinetics and pharmacodynamics of alfentanil infusions during general anesthesia. Anesth Analg 1986;65:1021–1028.
73. Bovill JG, Sebel PS, Blackburn CL, Heykants J. Kinetics of alfentanil and sufentanil: a comparison. Anesthesiology 1981; 55:A174.
74. McDonnell TE, Bartkowski RR, Bonilla FA, et al. Evidence for polymorphic oxidation of alfentanil in man. Anesthesiology 1984;61:A284.
75. Schüttler J, Stoeckel H. Alfentanil (R 39209) ein neues kurwirkendes opioid. Anaesthetist 1982;31:10–14.
76. Bovill JG, Sebel PS, Blackburn CL, Heykants J. The pharmacokinetics of alfentanil (R39209): a new opioid analgesic. Anesthesiology 1982;57:439–443.
77. Camu F, Gepts E, Rucquoi M, Keykants J. Pharmacokinetics of alfentanil in man. Anesth Analg 1982;61:657–661.
78. Fragen RJ, Booij LHD, Braak GJJ, et al. Pharmacokinetics of the infusion of alfentanil in man. Br J Anaesth 1983;55:1077–1081.
79. Persson MP, Nilsson A, Hartvig P. Pharmacokinetics of alfentanil in total IV anaesthesia. Br J Anaesth 1988;60:755–761.

80. Stanski DR, Hug CC Jr. Alfentanil: a kinetically predictable narcotic analgesic. Anesthesiology 1982;57:435–438.
81. Waud BE, Waud DR. Dose-response curves and pharmacokinetics. Anesthesiology 1986;65:355–358.
82. Hug CC Jr. Lipid solubility, pharmacokinetics, and the EEG: are you better off today than you were four years ago? Anesthesiology 1985;62:221–226.
83. Grevel J, Whiting B. The relevance of pharmacokinetics to optimal intravenous anesthesia. Anesthesiology 1987;66:1–2.
84. Brater DC. Bayesian dosing of anesthetic agents: esoteric or practical? Anesthesiology 1988;69:641–642.
85. Hull CJ. The pharmacokinetics of alfentanil in man. Br J Anaesth 1983;55:157S–164S.
86. Chauvin M, Bonnet F, Montembault C, et al. The influence of hepatic plasma flow on alfentanil plasma concentration plateaus achieved with an infusion model. Anesth Analg 1986; 65:999–1003.
87. Meuldermans W, Hendrickx J, Lauwers W, et al. Excretion and biotransformation of alfentanil and sufentanil in rats and dogs. Drug Metab Dispos 1987;15:905–913.
88. Bovill J, Odoom J, Heykants J. Biotransformation of alfentanil in man. Anesthesiology 1988;69:A467.
89. Lavrijsen KLM, Van Houdt JMG, Van Dyck DMJ, et al. Is the metabolism of alfentanil subject to debrisoquine polymorphism? Anesthesiology 1988;69:535–540.
90. Meuldermans W, van Peer A, Hendricks J, et al. Alfentanil pharmacokinetics and metabolism in humans. Anesthesiology 1988;69:527–534.
91. Kharasch ED, Thummel KE. Human alfentanil metabolism by cytochrome P450 3A3/4: an explanation for the interindividual variability in alfentanil clearance? Anesth Analg 1993;76:1033–1039.
92. Stiller RL, Davis PJ, McGowan FX, et al. In vitro metabolism of remifentanil the effects of pseudocholinesterase deficiency. Anesthesioloy 1995;83:A381.
93. Glass PSA, Hardman D, Kamiyama Y. Preliminary pharmacokinetics and pharmacodynamics of an ultra-short acting opioid: remifentanil (G187084B). Anesthesiology 1993;77:1031–1040.
94. Westmoreland CL, Hoke JF, Sebel PS, et al. Pharmacokinetis of remifentanil (G187084B) and its major metabolite (G19029) in patients undergoing elective impatient surgery. Anesthesiology 1993;79:893.
95. Duthie DJR, Muir KT, Baddoo H, et al. Remifentanil is not metabolised by the lung. Anesthesiology 1995;83:A324.
96. Robbins R, Whalley DG, Donati F, et al. Altered pharmacokinetics of alfentanil. Can Anaesth Soc J 1986;33:S103-S104.
97. Nishitateno K, Ngai SH, Finck AD, Berkowitz BA. Pharmacokinetics of morphine: concentrations in the serum and brain of the dog during hyperventilation. Anesthesiology 1979;50:520–523.
98. Benson DW, Kaufman JJ, Koski WS. Theoretic significance of pH dependence of narcotics and narcotic antagonists in clinical anesthesia. Anesth Analg 1976;55:253.
99. Finck AD, Berkowitz BA, Hempstead J, et al. Pharmacokinetics of morphine: effects of hypercarbia on serum and brain morphine concentrations in the dog. Anesthesiology 1977;47:407–410.
100. Lüllmann H, Martins B-S, Peters T. pH-dependent accumulation of fentanyl, lofentanil, and alfentanil by beating guinea pig atria. Br J Anaesth 1985;57:1012–1017.
101. Cartwright P, Prys-Roberts C, Gill K, et al. Ventilatory depression related to plasma fentanyl concentrations during and after anesthesia in humans. Anesth Analg 1983;62:966–974.
102. Ainslie SG, Eisele JH, Corkill G. Fentanyl concentrations in brain and serum during respiratory acid-base changes in the dog. Anesthesiology 1979;51:293–297.
103. Schwartz AE, Matteo RS, Ornstein E, et al. Pharmacokinetics of sufentanil in neurosurgical patients undergoing hyperventilation. Br J Anaesth 1989;63:385–388.
104. Belpaire FM, Bogaert MG. Binding of alfentanil to human a_1-acid glycoprotein, albumin and serum. Int J Clin Pharmacol Ther Toxicol 1991;29:96–102.
105. Meistelman C, Levron JC, Barre J, et al. Effects of increased alpha–1-acid glycoprotein in cancer patients on pharmacokinetics of alfentanil. Anesthesiology 1988;69:A602.
106. Lemmens HJ, Burm AGL, Bovill JG, et al. Pharmacodynamics of alfentanil. Anesthesiology 1992;76:65–70.
107. Bower S, Sear JW, Roy RC, Carter RF. Effects of different hepatic pathologies on disposition of alfentanil in anaesthetized patients. Br J Anaesth 1992;68:462–465.
108. Hug CC Jr, Murphy MR, Sampson JF, et al. Biotransformation of morphine and fentanyl in anhepatic dogs. Anesthesiology 1981;55:A261.
109. Klatz U, McHorse TS, Wilkinson GR, Schenker S. The effect of cirrhosis on the disposition and elimination of meperidine in man. Clin Pharmacol Therapeutics 1974;16:669.
110. Neal EA, Meffin PJ, Gregory PB, et al. Enhanced bioavailability and decreased clearance of analgesics in patients with cirrhosis. Gastroenterology 1979;77:96–102.
111. Pond SM, Tong T, Benowitz NL, et al. Presystemic metabolism of meperidine to normeperidine in normal and cirrhotic subjects. Clin Pharmacol Ther 1981;30:183–188.
112. Hudson RJ, Bergstrom RG, Thomson IR, et al. Pharmacokinetics of sufentanil in patients undergoing abdominal aortic surgery. Anesthesiology 1989;70:426–431.
113. Hudson RJ, Thomson IR, Cannon JE, et al. Pharmacokinetics of fentanyl in patients undergoing abdominal aortic surgery. Anesthesiology 1986;64:334–338.
114. Tammisto T, Tigerstedt I. The need for fentanyl supplementation of N_2O-O_2 relaxant anaesthesia in chronic alcoholics. Acta Anaesthesiol Scand 1977;21:216–221.
115. Ferrier C, Marty J, Bouffard Y, et al. Alfentanil pharmacokinetics in patients with cirrhosis. Anesthesiology 1985;62:480–484.
116. Davis PJ, Stiller RL, Cook DR, et al. Effects of cholestatic hepatic disease and chronic renal failure on alfentanil pharmacokinetics in children. Anesth Analg 1989;68:579–583.
117. Lemmens HJM, Bovill JG, Hennis PJ, et al. Alcohol consumption alters the pharmacodynamics of alfentanil. Anesthesiology 1989;71:669–674.
118. Reitz J, MacKichan JJ, Hoffer L, et al. Reduced plasma clearance of alfentanil associated with prolonged major intra-abdominal surgery. Anesth Analg 1984;63:265.
119. Hudson RJ, Thomson IR, Burgess PM, Rosenbloom M. Alfentanil pharmacokinetics in patients undergoing abdominal aortic surgery. Can J Anaesth 1991;38:61–67.
120. Chauvin M, Ferrier C, Haberer JP, et al. Sufentanil pharmacokinetics in patients with cirrhosis. Anesth Analg 1989;68:1–4.
121. Dershwitz M, Rosow CE, Michalowski P, et al. Pharmacokinetis and pharmacodynamics of remifentanil in volunteer subjects with severe liver disease compared with normal subjects [Abstract]. Anesthesiology 1994;81:A377.
122. Navapurkar VU, Archer S, Frazer NM, et al. Pharmacokinetics of remifentanil during hepatic transplantation. Anesthesiology 1995;83:A382.
123. Stambaugh JE Jr, Wainer IW. Drug interaction: meperidine and chlorpromazine, a toxic combination. J Clin Pharmacol 1981; 21:140–146.
124. Bower S. Plasma protein binding of fentanyl: the effect of hyperlipoproteinaemia and chronic renal failure. J Pharm Pharmacol 1981;34:102–106.
125. Davis PJ, Stiller RL, Cook DR, et al. Pharmacokinetics of sufentanil in adolescent patients with chronic renal failure. Anesth Analg 1988;67:268–271.
126. Fyman PN, Reynolds JR, Moser F, et al. Pharmacokinetics of

sufentanil in patients undergoing renal transplantation. Can J Anaesth 1988;35:312–315.
127. van Peer A, Vercauteren M, Noorduin H, et al. Alfentanil kinetics in renal insufficiency. Eur J Clin Pharmacol 1986;30:245–247.
128. Chauvin M, Lebrault C, Levron JC, Duvaldestin P. Pharmacokinetics of alfentanil in chronic renal failure. Anesth Analg 1987;66:53–56.
129. Koehntop DE, Noormohamed SE, Fletcher CV. Pharmacokinetics of alfentanil during renal transplantation in diabetic and non-diabetic patients. Anesth Analg 1990;70:S212.
130. Hoke J, Muir K, Glass P, et al. Pharmacokinetics of remifentanil and its metabolite (G190291) in subjects with renal disease [Abstract]. Clin Pharmacol Ther 1995;57:148.
131. Bentley JB, Borel JD, Gillespie TJ, et al. Fentanyl pharmacokinetics in obese and nonobese patients. Anesthesiology 1981; 55:A177.
132. Schwartz AE, Matteo RS, Ornstein E, et al. Pharmacokinetics of sufentanil in obese patients. Anesth Analg 1991;73:790–793.
132a. Egan TD, Gupta SK, Sperry RJ, et al. The pharmacokinetics of remifentanil in obese versus lean elective surgery patients [Abstract]. Anesth Analg 1996;82:S99.
133. Smith NT, Dec-Silver H, Sanford TJ, et al. EEGs during high-dose fentanyl-, sufentanil-, or morphine-oxygen anesthesia. Anesth Analg 1984;63:386–393.
134. Sebel PS, Bovill JG, Wauquier A, Rog P. Effects of high dose fentanyl anesthesia on the electroencephalogram. Anesthesiology 1981;55:203–211.
135. Hecker BR, Lake CL, DiFazio CA, et al. The decrease of the minimum alveolar anesthetic concentration produced by sufentanil in rats. Anesth Analg 1983;62:987–990.
136. Streisand JB, Bailey PL, LeMaire L, et al. Fentanyl-induced rigidity and unconsciousness in human volunteers. Anesthesiology 1993;78:629–634.
137. Sperry RJ, Bailey PL, Reichman MV, et al. Fentanyl and sufentanil increase intracranial pressure in head trauma patients. Anesthesiology 1992;77:416–420.
138. Weinstabl C, Mayer N, Richling B, et al. Effect of sufentanil on intracranial pressure in neurosurgical patients. Anaesthesia 1991;46:837–840.
139. Hoffman WE, Cunningham F, James MK, et al. Effects of remifentanil a new short-acting opoioid, on cerebral blood flow brain electrical activity and intracranial pressure in dogs anesthetized with isoflurane and nitrous oxide. Anesthesiology 1993;79:107–113.
140. Parratt JR. Opioid receptors in the cardiovascular system. In: van Zwielen P, Schönbaum E, eds. Progress in pharmacology. Stuttgart: Gustav Fischer, 1986.
141. Stanley TH, Webster LR. Anesthetic requirements and cardiovascular effects of fentanyl-oxygen and fentanyl-diazepam-oxygen anaesthesia in man. Anesth Analg 1978;57:411.
142. Sebel PS, Bovill JG. Cardiovascular effects of sufentanil anesthesia: a study in patients undergoing cardiac surgery. Anesth Analg 1982;61:115.
143. Nauta J, Stanley TH, de Lange S, et al. Anaesthetic induction with alfentanil: comparison with thiopental, midazolam, and etomidate. Can Anaesth Soc J 1983;30:53–60.
144. Ebert TJ, Kotrly KJ, Madsen KE, et al. Fentanyl-diazepam anesthesia with or without N_2O does not attenuate cardiopulmonary baroreflex-mediated vasoconstrictor responses to controlled hypovolemia in humans. Anesth Analg 1988;67:548–554.
145. Tyler DC. Respiratory effects of pain in a child after thoracotomy. Anesthesiology 1989;70:873.
146. Toda N, Hatano Y. Contractile responses of canine tracheal muscle during exposure to fentanyl and morphine. Anesthesiology 1980;53:93–100.
147. Anjou-Lindskog E, Broman L, Broman M, et al. Effects of intravenous anesthesia on Va/Q distribution: a study performed during ventilation with air and with 50% oxygen, supine and in the lateral position. Anesthesiology 1985;62:485–492.
148. Bjertraes LJ. Hypoxia-induced vasoconstriction in isolated perfused lungs exposed to injectable or inhalation anesthetics. Acta Anaesthesiol Scand 1977;21:133–147.
149. Oyama T, Wakayama S. The endocrine responses to general anesthesia. Int Anesthesiol Clin 1988;26:176–181.
150. Reier CE, George JM, Kilman JW. Cortisol and growth hormone response to surgical stress during morphine anesthesia. Anesth Analg 1973;52:1003–1009.
151. Haxholdt O, Kehlet H. Effect of fentanyl on the cortisol and hyperglycaemic response to abdominal surgery. Acta Anaesthesiol Scand 1981;25:434–436.
152. Anand K. The stress response to surgery and trauma: from physiological basis to therapeutic implications. Prog Food Nutr Sci 1986;10:67–132.
153. Mangano DT, Siliciano D, Hollenberg M, et al. Postoperative myocardial ischemia: therapeutic trials using intensive analgesia following surgery. Anesthesiology 1992;76:342–353.
154. Anand KJS, Philbin D, Hickey PR. Halothane-morphine compared with high-dose sufentanil for anesthesia and postoperative analgesia in neonatal cardiac surgery. N Engl J Med 1992; 326:1–9.
155. Blasco TA, Lee D, Amalric M, et al. The role of the nucleus raphe pontis and the caudate nucleus in alfentanil rigidity in the rat. Brain Res 1986;386:280–286.
156. Bailey PL, Wilbrink J, Zwanikken P, et al. Anesthetic induction with fentanyl. Anesth Analg 1985;64:48.
157. Benthuysen JL, Kien ND, Quam DD. Intracranial pressure increases during alfentanil-induced rigidity. Anesthesiology 1988;68:438–440.
158. Benthuysen JL, Smith NT, Sanford TJ, et al. Physiology of alfentanil-induced rigidity. Anesthesiology 1986;64:440–446.
159. Safo Y, Greenberg J, Young M, et al. Effects of high dose fentanyl on regional cerebral blood flow. Anesthesiology 1983; 59:A306.
160. Tommasino C, Mackawa T, Shapiro HM. Fentanyl-induced seizures activate subcortical brain metabolism. Anesthesiology 1984;60:283–290.
161. Tempelhoff R, Modica PA, Bernardo KL, Edwards I. Fentanyl-induced electrocorticographic seizures in patients with complex partial epilepsy. J Neurosurg 1992;77:201–208.
162. Lowenstein E, Whiting RB, Bittar DA, et al. Local and neurally mediated effects of morphine on skeletal muscle vascular resistance. J Pharmacol Exp Ther 1972;180:359–367.
163. Rendig SV, Amsterdam EA, Henderson GL, Mason DT. Comparative cardiac contractile actions of six narcotic analgesics: Morphine meperidine, pentazocine, fentanyl, methadone and I-a-acetylmethadol (LAAM). J Pharmacol Exp Ther 1980; 215:259–265.
164. Flacke JW, Van Etten AP, Bloor BC, et al. Histamine release by four narcotics: a double blind study in humans. Anesth Analg 1987;66:723–730.
165. Rosow CE, Moss J, Philbin DM, Savarese JJ. Histamine release during morphine and fentanyl anesthesia. Anesthesiology 1982;56:93–96.
166. Moss J, Rosow CE. Histamine release by narcotics and muscle relaxants in humans. Anesthesiology 1983;59:330–339.
167. Sebel PS, Hoke JF, Westmoreland C, et al. Histamine concentrations and hemodynamic responses after remifentamil. Anesth Analg 1995;80:990–993.
168. Miller DR, Wellwood M, Teasdale SJ, et al. Effects of anaesthetic induction on myocardial function and metabolism: a comparison of fentanyl, sufentanil and alfentanil. Can J Anaesth 1988; 35:219–233.
169. Wynands JE, Wong P, Whalley DG, et al. Oxygen-fentanyl an-

esthesia in patients with poor left ventricular function, hemodynamics and plasma fentanyl concentrations. Anesth Analg 1983;62:476–482.
170. Thomson IR, Putnins CL, Friesen RM. Hyperdynamic cardiovascular response to anesthetic induction with high dose fentanyl. Anesth Analg 1986;65:91–95.
171. Gaumann DM, Yaksh TL, Tyce GM, Lucas DL. Opioids preserve the adrenal medullary response evoked by severe hemorrhage: studies on adrenal catecholamines and met-enkephalin secretion in halothane anesthetized cats. Anesthesiology 1988;68:743–753.
172. James TN, Isobe JH, Urthaler F. Analysis of components in a cardiogenic hypertensive chemoreflex. Circulation 1975;52:179–192.
173. Bailey PL. Sinus arrest induced by trivial nasal stimulation during alfentanil-nitrous oxide anesthesia. Br J Anaesth 1990; 65:718–720.
174. Sherman EP, Lebowitz PW, Street WC. Bradycardia following sufentanil-succinylcholine. Anesthesiology 1987;66:106.
175. Ngai SH. Effects of morphine and meperidine on the central respiratory mechanisms in the cat, the action of levallorphan in antagonizing these effects. J Pharmacol Exp Ther 1961;131:91–99.
176. Hickey RF, Severinghaus JW. Regulation of breathing: drug effects. In: Hornbein T, ed. Lung biology in health and disease. New York: Marcel Dekker, 1981:1251–1298.
177. Weil JV, McCullough RE, Kline JS, Sodal IE. Diminished ventilatory response to hypoxia and hypercapnia after morphine in normal man. N Engl J Med 1975;292:1103–1106.
178. Kryger MH, Yacoub O, Dosman J, et al. Effect of meperidine on occlusion pressure responses to hypercapnia and hypoxia with and without external inspiratory resistance. Am Rev Respir Dis 1976;114:333–340.
179. Reed DJ, Kellog RH. Changes in respiratory response to CO_2 during natural sleep at sea level and at altitude. J Appl Physiol 1958;13:325–330.
180. Forrest WH, Bellville JW. The effect of sleep plus morphine on the respiratory response to carbon dioxide. Anesthesiology 1964;25:137–141.
181. Longobardo GE, Gothe B, Goldman MD, Cherniak NS. Sleep apnea considered as a control system instability. Respir Physiol 1982;50:311–333.
182. Becker LD, Paulson BA, Miller RD, et al. Biphasic respiratory depression after fentanyl-droperidol or fentanyl alone used to supplement nitrous oxide anesthesia. Anesthesiology 1976; 44:291–296.
183. Adams AP, Pybus DA. Delayed respiratory depression after use of fentanyl during anaesthesia. Br Med J 1978;1:278–279.
184. Chan K, Kendall MJ, Mitchard M, Will WDE. The effect of aging on plasma pethidine concentration. Br J Clin Pharmacol 1975; 2:297–302.
185. Mahla ME, Maj MC, Maj SEW, Moneta MD. Delayed respiratory depression after alfentanil. Anesthesiology 1988;69:593–595.
186. Chang J, Fish KJ. Acute respiratory arrest and rigidity after anesthesia with sufentanil: a case report. Anesthesiology 1985; 63:710–711.
187. Stoeckel H, Schuttler J, Magnussen H, Hengstmann JH. Plasma fentanyl concentrations and occurrence of respiration depression in volunteers. Br J Anaesth 1982;54:1087–1095.
188. Severinghaus JW, Kelleher JF. Recent developments in pulse oximetry. Anesthesiology 1992;76:1018–1038.
189. Bailey PL. The use of opioids in anesthesia is not especially associated with nor predictive of postoperative hypoxemia [Letter]. Anesthesiology 1992;77:1235.
190. Watcha MF, White PF. Postoperative nausea and vomiting: its etiology, treatment, and prevention. Anesthesiology 1992; 77:162–184.
191. Okum GS, Colonna-Romano P, Horrow JC. Vomiting after alfentanil anesthesia: effect of dosing method. Anesth Analg 1992;75:558–569.
192. Watcha MF, Jones MB, Lagueruela RG, et al. Comparison of ketorolac and morphine as adjuvants during pediatric surgery. Anesthesiology 1992;76:368–372.
193. Shingu K, Eger EI, Brynte H, et al. Effect of oxygen concentration, hyperthermia, and choice of vendor on anesthetic-induced hepatic injury in rats. Anesthesia Analg 1983;62:146–150.
194. Baden JM, Kundomal YR, Luttropp ME Jr, et al. Effects of volatile anesthetics or fentanyl on hepatic function in cirrhotic rats. Anesth Analg 1985;64:1183–1188.
195. Maltby JR, Williams RT. Morphine-induced cardiac pain? [Letter]. Anesthesiology 1986;64:527–528.
196. Radnay PA, Duncalf D, Novakovic M, Lesser ML. Common bile duct pressure changes after fentanyl, morphine, meperidine, butorphanol, and naloxone. Anesth Analg 1984;63:441–444.
197. Goldberg M, Vatashsky E, Haskel Y, et al. The effect of meperidine on the guinea pig extrahepatic biliary tract. Anesth Analg 1987;66:1282–1286.
198. Levy JH, Rockoff MA. Anaphylaxis to meperidine. Anesth Analg 1982;61:301–303.
199. Bennett MJ, Anderson LK, McMillar JC, et al. Anaphylactic reaction during anaesthesia associated with positive intradermal skin test to fentanyl. Can Anaesth Soc J 1986;33:75–78.
200. Levy JH, Brister NW, Shearin A, et al. Wheal and flare responses to opioids in humans. Anesthesiology 1989;70:756–760.
201. Azar I, Turndorf H. Severe hypertension and multiple atrial premature contractions following naloxone administration. Anesth Analg 1979;58:524.
202. Estilo AE, Cottrell JE. Naloxone, hypertension, and ruptured cerebral aneurysm. Anesthesiology 1981;54:352.
203. Flacke JW, Flacke WE, Williams GD. Acute pulmonary edema following naloxone reversal of high-dose morphine anesthesia. Anesthesiology 1977;47:376–378.
204. Tanaka GY. Hypertensive reaction to naloxone. JAMA 1974; 228:25–26.
205. Andree RA. Sudden death following naloxone administration. Anesth Analg 1980;59:782–784.
206. Prough DS, Roy R, Bumgarner J, Shannon G. Acute pulmonary edema in healthy teenagers following conservative doses of intravenous naloxone. Anesthesiology 1984;60:485–486.
207. Michaelis LL, Hickey PR, Clark TA, Dixon WM. Ventricular irritability associated with the use of naloxone hydrochloride. Ann Thorac Surg 1974;18:608–614.
208. Partridge BL, Ward CF. Pulmonary edema following low-dose naloxone administration. Anesthesiology 1986;65:709–710.
209. Taff RH. Pulmonary edema following naloxone administration in a patient without heart disease. Anesthesiology 1983;59:576–577.
210. Bailey PL, Clark NJ, Pace NL, et al. Antagonism of postoperative opioid induced respiratory depression: nalbuphine vs. naloxone. Anesth Analg 1987;66:1109–1114.
211. Shupak RC, Harp JR, Stevenson-Smith W, et al. High-dose fentanyl for neuroanesthesia. Anesthesiology 1983;58:579–582.
212. Keykhah MM, Smith DS, Englebach I, Harp JR. Effects of naloxone on cerebral blood flow and metabolism. Anesthesiology 1983;59:A309.
213. Mannelli M, Maggi M, De Feo ML, et al. Naloxone administration releases catecholamines. N Engl J Med 1982;308:654–655.
214. Ngai SH, Berkowitz BA, Yang JC, et al. Pharmacokinetics of naloxone in rats and man. Anesthesiology 1976;44:398–401.
215. Kaufman R. Relative potencies and durations of action with respect to respiratory depression of intravenous meperidine, fentanyl and alphaprodine in man. J Pharmacol Exp Ther 1979; 208:73–79.
216. Andersen R, Dobloug I, Refstad S. Postanaesthetic use of nal-

oxone hydrochloride after moderate doses of fentanyl. Acta Anaesthesiol Scand 1976;20:255–258.
217. Amin HM, Sopchak AM, Esposito BF, et al. Naloxone reversal of depressed ventilatory response to hypoxia during continuous infusion of remifentanil [Abstract]. Anesthesiology 1993; 79:A1203.
218. Kapila A, Peter SA, Glass MB, et al. Measured context-sensitive half-times of remifentanil an alfentanil. Anesthesiology 1995; 83:968–975.
219. Tabatabai M, Kitahata LM, Collins JG. Disruption of the rhythmic activity of the medullary inspiratory neurons and phrenic nerve by fentanyl and reversal with nalbuphine. Anesthesiology 1989;70:489–495.
220. Latasch L, Probst S, Duziak R. Reversal by nalbuphine of respiratory depression caused by fentanyl. Anesth Analg 1984; 63:814–816.
221. Blaise GA, McMichan JC, Nugent M, Hollier LH. Nalbuphine produces side-effects while reversing narcotic-induced respiratory depression. Anesth Analg 1986;65:S19.
222. Ramsay JG, Wynands JE, Robbins R, Townsend GE. Early extubation after high-dose fentanyl anaesthesia for aortocoronary bypass surgery: reversal of respiratory depression with low-dose nalbuphine. Can Anaesth Soc J 1985;32:597–606.
223. Tabatabai M, Javadi P, Tadjziechy M, Mazloomdorst M. Effect of nalbuphine hydrochloride on fentanyl-induced respiratory depression and analgesia. Anesthesiology 1984;61:A475.
224. Jaffe RS, Moldenhauer CC, Hug CC Jr, et al. Nalbuphine antagonism of fentanyl-induced ventilatory depression: a randomized trial. Anesthesiology 1988;68:254–260.
225. Beattie WS, Lindblad T, Buckley DN, Forrest JB. Menstruation increases the risk of nausea and vomiting after laparoscopy. Anesthesiology 1993;78:272–276.
226. Hartung J. Nitrous oxide: it's enough to make you vomit [Letter]. Anesthesiology 1993;78:403–404.
227. Watcha MF, White PF. Correspondence. Anesthesiology 1993; 78:405–406.
228. Raftery S, Sherry E. Total intravenous anaesthesia with propofol and alfentanil protects against postoperative nausea and vomiting. Can J Anaesth 1992;39:37–40.
229. Alon E, Himmelseher S. Ondansetron in the treatment of postoperative vomiting: a randomized, double-blind comparison with droperidol and metoclopramide. Anesth Analg 1992; 75:561–565.
230. Leslie K, Crankshaw DP. Potency of propofol for loss of consciousness after a single dose. Br J Anaesth 1990;64:734–736.
231. Richards MJ, Skues MA, Jarvis AP, Prys-Roberts C. Total I.V. anaesthesia with propofol and alfentanil: dose requirements for propofol and the effect of premedication with clonidine. Br J Anaesth 1990;65:157–163.
232. Tverskoy M, Fleyshman G, Ezry J, et al. Midazolam-morphine sedative interaction in patients. Anesth Analg 1989;68:282–285.
233. Kissin I, Brown P, Bradley E, et al. Diazepam-morphine hypnotic synergism in rats. Anesthesiology 1989;70:689–694.
234. Stack CG, Rogers P, Linter SPK. Monoamine oxidase inhibitors and anaesthesia. Br J Anaesth 1988;60:222–227.
235. Wells DG, Bjorksten AR. Monoamine oxidase inhibitors revisited [Review article]. Can J Anaesth 1989;36:64–74.
236. Taylor MB, Grounds RM, Mulrooney PD, Morgan M. Ventilatory effects of propofol during induction of anaesthesia. Anaesthesia 1986;41:816–820.
237. Bailey PL, Pace NL, Ashburn MA, et al. Frequent hypoxemia and apnea after sedation with midazolam and fentanyl. Anesthesiology 1990;73:826–830.
238. Silbert B, Rosow CE, Keegan CR, et al. The effect of diazepam on induction of anesthesia with alfentanil. Anesth Analg 1986; 65:71–77.
239. Bailey PL, Sperry RJ, Johnson GK, et al. Respiratory effects of clonidine and morphine, alone and in combination. Anesthesiology 1991;73:43–48.
240. Andrews CJH, Sinclair M, Dye A, et al. The additive effect of nitrous oxide on respiratory depression in patients having fentanyl or alfentanil infusion. Br J Anaesth 1982;54:1129.
241. Abdul-Rasool IH, Ward DS. Ventilatory and cardiovascular responses to sufentanil infusion in dogs anesthetized with isoflurane. Anesth Analg 1989;69:300–306.
242. Drummond GB. Comparison of decreases in ventilation caused by enflurane and fentanyl during anesthesia. Br J Anaesth 1983; 55:825–835.
243. Takkunen O, Meretoja OA. Thiopentone reduces the haemodynamic response to induction of high-dose fentanyl-pancuronium anaesthesia in coronary artery surgical patients. Acta Anaesthesiol Scand 1988;32:222–227.
244. Pomane C, Paulin M, Lena P, et al. Comparison of the haemodynamic effects of a midazolam-fentanyl and thiopental-fentanyl combination for induction of general anesthesia. Anesthesiology 1983;2:75–79.
245. Vinik HR, Bradley EL, Kissin I. Midazolam-alfentanil synergism for anesthetic induction in patients. Anesth Analg 1989; 69:213–217.
246. Ben-Shlomo I, Abd-El-Khalim H, Ezry J, et al. Midazolam acts synergistically with fentanyl for induction of anaesthesia. Br J Anaesth 1990;64:45–47.
247. Spiess BD, Sathoff RH, El-Ganzouri ARS, Ivankovich AD. High-dose sufentanil: four cases of sudden hypotension on induction. Anesth Analg 1986;65:703–705.
248. Flacke JW, David LJ, Flacke WE, et al. Effects of fentanyl and diazepam in dogs deprived of autonomic tone. Anesth Analg 1985;64:1053–1059.
249. Hoar PF, Nelson NT, Mangano DT, et al. Adrenergic response to morphine-diazepam anesthesia for myocardial revascularization. Anesth Analg 1981;60:406–411.
250. Tomichek RC, Rosow CE, Philbin DM, et al. Diazepam-fentanyl interaction: hemodynamic and hormonal effects in coronary artery surgery. Anesth Analg 1983;62:881–884.
251. Reves JG, Kissin I, Fournier SE, Smith LR. Additive negative inotropic effect of a combination of diazepam and fentanyl. Anesth Analg 1984;63:97–100.
252. Marty J, Gauzit R, Lefevre P, et al. Effects of diazepam and midazolam on baroreflex control of heart rate and on sympathetic activity in humans. Anesth Analg 1986;65:113–119.
253. Thomson IR, Bergstrom RG, Rosenbloom M, Meatherall RC. Premedication and high-dose fentanyl anesthesia for myocardial revascularization: a comparison of lorazepam versus morphine-scopolamine. Anesthesiology 1988;68:194–200.
254. Butterworth JF, Bean VE, Royster RL. Premedication profoundly influences hemodynamics during rapid sequence induction with sufentanil-succinylcholine for aortocoronary bypass grafting. Anesthesiology 1988;69:A65.
255. Thomson IR, MacAdams CL, Hudson RJ, Rosenbloom M. Drug interactions with sufentanil: hemodynamic effects of premedication and muscle relaxants. Anesthesiology 1992;76:922–929.
256. Heikkilä H, Jalonen J, Laaksonen V, et al. Lorazepam and high-dose fentanyl anaesthesia: effects on haemodynamics and oxygen transportation in patients undergoing coronary revascularization. Acta Anaesthesiol Scand 1984;28:357–361.
257. Benson KT, Tomlinson DL, Goto H, Arakawa K. Cardiovascular effects of lorazepam during sufentanil anesthesia. Anesth Analg 1988;67:996–998.
258. Coetzee A, Fourie P, Coetzee J, et al. Effect of various propofol plasma concentrations on regional myocardial contractility and left ventricular afterload. Anesth Analg 1989;69:473–483.
259. Lepage J-Y, Pinaud M, Helias J, et al. Left ventricular function during propofol and fentanyl anesthesia in patients with coronary artery disease: assessment with a radionuclide approach. Anesth Analg 1988;67:949–955.

260. Hall RI, Murphy JT, Moffitt EA, et al. A comparison of the myocardial metabolic and haemodynamic changes produced by propofol-sufentanil and enflurane-sufentanil anaesthesia for patients having coronary artery bypass graft surgery. Can J Anaesth 1991;38:996–1104.
261. Eisele JH, Smith NT. Cardiovascular effects of 40 percent nitrous oxide in man. Anesth Analg 1972;51:956–962.
262. Stoelting RK, Gibbs PS, Creasser CW, Peterson C. Hemodynamic and ventilatory response to fentanyl, fentanyl-droperidol, and nitrous oxide in patients with acquired valvular heart disease. Anesthesiology 1975;42:319.
263. Lunn JK, Stanley TH, Webster LR, et al. High dose fentanyl anesthesia for coronary artery surgery: plasma fentanyl concentration and influence of nitrous oxide on cardiovascular responses. Anesth Analg 1979;58:390.
264. Wong KC, Martin WE, Hornbein TF, et al. The cardiovascular effects of morphine sulfate with oxygen and with nitrous oxide in man. Anesthesiology 1973;38:542–549.
265. Moffitt EA, Scovil JE, Barker RA, et al. Myocardial metabolism and hemodynamics of nitrous oxide in fentanyl or enflurane anesthesia in coronary patients. Anesthesiology 1983;59:A31.
266. Michaels I, Barash PG. Does nitrous oxide or a reduced FiO_2 alter hemodynamic function during high-dose sufentanil anesthesia? Anesth Analg 1983;62:275.
267. Stowe DF, Monroe SM, Marijic J, et al. Effects of nitrous oxide on contractile function and metabolism of the isolated heart. Anesthesiology 1990;73:1220–1226.
268. Lawson D, Frazer MJ, Lynch C. Nitrous oxide effects on isolated myocardium: a reexamination in vitro. Anesthesiology 1990; 73:930–943.
269. Cahalan MK, Lurz FW, Eger EI, et al. Narcotics decrease heart rate during inhalational anesthesia. Anesth Analg 1987;66:166–170.
270. Mitchell MM, Prakash O, Rulf EN, et al. Nitrous oxide does not induce myocardial ischemia in patients with ischemic heart disease and poor ventricular function. Anesthesiology 1989; 71:526–534.
271. Moffitt EA, McIntyre AJ, Glenn JJ, et al. Myocardial metabolism and haemodynamic responses with fentanyl-halothane anaesthesia for coronary patients. Can Anaesth Soc J 1985;32:S86-S87.
272. Hillel Z, Thys D, Goldman ME, et al. Halothane produces dose-dependent myocardial depression in man during fentanyl anesthesia. Anesth Analg 1986;65:S71.
273. Heikkilä H, Jalonen J, Arola M, et al. Low-dose enflurane as adjunct to high-dose fentanyl in patients undergoing coronary artery surgery: stable hemodynamics and maintained myocardial oxygen balance. Anesth Analg 1987;66:111–116.
274. O'Young J, Mastrocostopoulas G, Hilgenberg A, et al. Myocardial circulatory and metabolic effects of isoflurane and sufentanil during coronary artery surgery. Anesthesiology 1987; 66:653–658.
275. O'Brien DJ, Moffitt EA, McIntyre AJ, et al. Myocardial metabolism and hemodynamic responses with fentanyl-halothane anaesthesia in hypertensive patients undergoing coronary arterial surgery. Can Anaesth Soc J 1986;33:S101-S102.
276. Thomson IR, Putnins CI. Adverse effects of pancuronium during high-dose fentanyl anesthesia for coronary artery bypass grafting. Anesthesiology 1985;62:708–713.
277. Sethna DH, Starr NJ, Estafanous FG. Cardiovascular effects of non-depolarizing neuromuscular blockers in patients with coronary artery disease. Can Anaesth Soc J 1986;33:280–286.
278. Atlee JL, Laravuso RB. Muscle relaxants and high-dose fentanyl: hemodynamics during coronary bypass surgery. Anesth Analg 1984;63:181.
279. Oikkonen M. Alfentanil combined with vecuronium or pancuronium: haemodynamic implications. Acta Anaesthesiol Scand 1992;36:406–409.
280. Salmenperä M, Peltola K, Takkunen O, Heinonen J. Cardiovascular effects of pancuronium and vecuronium during high-dose fentanyl anesthesia. Anesth Analg 1983;62:1059–1064.
281. Gravlee GP, Ramsey FM, Roy RC, et al. Pancuronium is hemodynamically superior to vecuronium for narcotic/relaxant induction. Anesthesiology 1986;65:A46.
282. Hill AEG, Muller BJ. Optimum relaxant for sufentanil anesthesia. Anesthesiology 1984;61:A393.
283. Lebowitz PW, Ramsey FM, Savarese JJ, et al. Combination of pancuronium and metocurine: neuromuscular and hemodynamic advantages over pancuronium alone. Anesth Analg 1981;60:12–17.
284. Emmott RS, Bracey BJ, Goldhill DR, et al. Cardiovascular effects of doxacurium, pancuronium and vecuronium in anaesthetized patients presenting for coronary artery bypass surgery. Br J Anaesth 1990;65:480–486.
285. Murray DJ, Mehta MP, Choi WW, et al. The neuromuscular blocking and cardiovascular effects of doxacurium chloride in patients receiving nitrous oxide narcotic anesthesia. Anesthesiology 1988;69:472–477.
286. Savarese JJ, Ali HH, Basta SJ, et al. The cardiovascular effects of mivacurium chloride (BW B1090U) in patients receiving nitrous oxide-opiate-barbiturate anesthesia. Anesthesiology 1989; 70:386–394.
287. Wierda JMKH, Richardson FJ, Agoston S. Dose-response relation and time course of action of pipecuronium bromide in humans anesthetized with nitrous oxide and isoflurane, halothane, or droperidol and fentanyl. Anesth Analg 1989;68:208–213.
288. Rupp SM, Fahey MR, Miller RD. Neuromuscular and cardiovascular effects of atracurium during nitrous oxide-fentanyl and nitrous oxide-isoflurane anaesthesia. Br J Anaesth 1983; 55:67S–70S.
289. Bartowski RR, McDonnell TE. Prolonged alfentanil effect following erythromycin administration. Anesthesiology 1990; 73:566–568.
290. Bartkowski RR, Goldberg ME, Huffnagle S, Epstein RH. Sufentanil disposition: is it affected by erythromycin administration? Anesthesiology 1993;78:260–265.
291. Sedman AJ. Cimetidine: drug interactions. Am J Med 1984; 76:109–114.
292. Randell T, Valli H, Lindgren L. Effects of alfentanil on the responses to awake fiberoptic nasotracheal intubation. Acta Anaesthesiol Scand 1990;34:59–62.
293. Austin KL, Stapleton JV, Mather LE. Relationship between blood meperidine concentrations and analgesic response: a preliminary report. Anesthesiology 1980;53:460.
294. Gignac E, Manninen PH, Gelb AW. Comparison of fentanyl, sufentanil and alfentanil during awake craniotomy for epilepsy. Can J Anaesth 1993;40:421–424.
295. Martin DE, Rosenberg H, Aukberg SJ, et al. Low-dose fentanyl blunts circulatory responses to tracheal intubation. Anesth Analg 1982;61:680–684.
296. Lawes EG, Downing JW, Duncan PW, et al. Fentanyl-droperidol supplementation of rapid sequence induction in the presence of severe pregnancy-induced and pregnancy-aggravated hypertension. Br J Anaesth 1987;59:1381–1391.
297. Van Aken H, Meinshausen E, Prien T, et al. The influence of fentanyl and tracheal intubation on the hemodynamic effects of anesthesia induction with propofol/N_2O in humans. Anesthesiology 1988;68:157–163.
298. Ebert JP, Pearson JD, Gelman S, et al. Circulatory responses to laryngoscopy: the comparative effects of placebo, fentanyl and esmolol. Can J Anaesth 1989;36:301–306.
299. McDonnell TE, Bartkowski RR, Williams JJ. ED_{50} of alfentanil for induction of anesthesia in unpremedicated young adults. Anesthesiology 1984;60:136–140.

300. Vinik HR, Bradley EL Jr, Kissin I. Triple anesthetic combination: propofol-midazolam-alfentanil. Anesth Analg 1994;78:354–358.
301. Vuyk J, Lim T, Engbers F, et al. The pharmacodynamic interaction of propofol and alfentanil during lower abdominal surgery in women. Anesthesiology 1995;83:8–22.
302. Smith I, Jan Hemelrijck J, White PF. Efficacy of esmolol versus alfentanil as a supplement to propofol-nitrous oxide anesthesia. Anesth Analg 1991;73:540–546.
303. Marty J, Couderc E, Servin F, et al. Plasma concentrations of sufentanil required to suppress hemodynamic responses to noxious stimuli during nitrous oxide anesthesia. Anesthesiology 1988;69:A631.
304. Randel GI, Fragen RJ, Librojo ES. Remifentanil blood concentration effect relationship at intubation and skin incision in surgical patients compared to alfentanil [Abstract]. Anesthesiology 1994;81:A375.
305. Pacentine GC, Muzi M, Ebert TJ. Effects of fentanyl on sympathetic activation associated with the adminstration of desflurane. Anesthesiology 1995;82:823–831.
306. Gourlay GK, Kowalski SR, Plummer JL, et al. Fentanyl blood concentration-analgesic response relationship in the treatment of postoperative pain. Anesth Analg 1988;67:329–337.
307. Glass PSA, Doherty M, Jacobs JR, et al. Plasma concentration of fentanyl, with 70% nitrous oxide, to prevent movement at skin incision. Anesthesiology 1993;78:842–847.
308. Ghouri AF, White PF. Effect of fentanyl and nitrous oxide on the desflurane anesthetic requirement. Anesth Analg 1991; 72:377–381.
309. Ausems ME, Hug CC Jr, Stanski DR, Burm AG. Plasma concentrations of alfentanil required to supplement nitrous oxide anesthesia for general surgery. Anesthesiology 1986;65:362–373.
310. Vuyk J, Lim T, Engbers FHM, et al. The pharmacodynamics of alfentanil as a supplement to propofol or nitrous oxide for lower abdominal surgery. Anesthesiology 1992;77:A402.
311. Stanski DR, Shafer SL. Quantifying anesthetic drug ineraction. Anesthesiology 1995;83:1–5.
312. O'Connor M, Sear JW. Sufentanil to supplement nitrous oxide in oxygen during balanced anaesthesia. Anaesthesia 1988; 43:749–752.
313. Murkin JM. Multicentre trial: sufentanil anaesthesia for major surgery: the multicentre Canadian clinical trial. Can J Anaesth 1989;36:343–349.
314. Kalenda Z, Scheijground HW. Anaesthesia with sufentanil-analgesia in carotid and vertebral arteriography: a comparison with fentanyl. Anaesthetist 1976;25:380–383.
315. Nishina K, Mikawa K, Markawa N, Obara H. Fentanyl attenuates cardiovascular responses to tracheal extubation. Acta Anesthesiologica Scandinavica 1995;39:85–89.
316. Cheng DCH, Chung F, Chapman KR, Romanelli J. Low-dose sufentanil and lidocaine supplementation of general anaesthesia. Can J Anaesth 1990;37:521–527.
317. Glenski JA, Friesen RH, Lane GA, et al. Low-dose sufentanil as a supplement to halothane/N_2O anesthesia in infants and children. Can J Anaesth 1988;35:379–384.
318. Kuperwasser B, Dahl M, McSweeney TD, Howie MB. Comparison of alfentanil and sufentanil in the ambulatory surgery procedure when used in balanced anesthesia technique. Anesth Analg 1988;67:S122.
319. van de Walle J, Lauwers P, Adriaensen H. Double blind comparison of fentanyl and sufentanil in anesthesia. Acta Anaesthesiol Belg 1976;27:129.
320. Smith C, McEwan AI, Jhaveri R, et al. The interaction of fentanyl on the Cp_{50} of propofol for loss of consciousness and skin incision. Anesthesiology 1994;81:820–828.
321. Ausems ME, Vuyk J, Hug CC Jr, Stanski DR. Comparison of a computer-assisted infusion versus intermittent bolus administration of alfentanil as a supplement to nitrous oxide for lower abdominal surgery. Anesthesiology 1988;68:851–861.
322. Cork RC, Gallo JA, Weiss LB. Sufentanil infusion: pharmacodynamics compared to bolus. Anesth Analg 1988;67:S40.
323. Alvis JM, Reves JG, Govier AV, et al. Computer assisted continuous infusions of fentanyl during cardiac anesthesia: comparison with a manual method. Anesthesiology 1985;63:41–49.
324. Pathak KS, Brown RH, Nash CL Jr, Cascorbi HF. Continuous opioid infusion for scoliosis fusion surgery. Anesth Analg 1983; 62:841–845.
325. White PF. Use of continuous infusion versus intermittent bolus administration of fentanyl or ketamine during outpatient anesthesia. Anesthesiology 1983;59:294–300.
326. Tuman KJ, McCarthy RJ, Spiess BD, et al. Does choice of anesthetic agent significantly affect outcome after coronary artery surgery? Anesthesiology 1989;70:189–198.
327. Slogoff S, Keats AS. Randomized trial of primary anesthetic agents on outcome of coronary artery bypass operations. Anesthesiology 1989;70:179–188.
328. Bell J, Sartain J, Wilkinson GAL, Sherry KM. Propofol and fentanyl anaesthesia for patients with low cardiac output state undergoing cardiac surgery: comparison with high-dose fentanyl anaesthesia. Br J Anaesth 1994;73:162–166.
329. Glass PSA, Jacobs JR, Smith LR, et al. Pharmacokinetic model-driven infusion of fentanyl: assessment of accuracy. Anesthesiology 1990;73:1082–1090.
330. Maitre PO, Shafer SL. A simple pocket calculator approach to predict anesthetic drug concentrations from pharmacokinetic data. Anesthesiology 1990;73:332–336.
331. Jenstrup M, Fruegard K, Nielsen J, et al. Alfentanil infusion in total intravenous anaesthesia (TIVA): population pharmacokinetics fails to predict plasma concentration of alfentanil. Acta Anaesthesiol Scand 1992;36:846–847.
332. Wood M. Variability of human drug response [Editorial]. Anesthesiology 1989;71:631–634.
333. Desiderio DP, Thorne AC, Shah NK, et al. Alfentanil-midazolam by continuous infusion: a total intravenous anaesthetic technique for general surgery. Anesthesiology 1988;69:A557.
334. Hall RI, Molderhauer CC, Hug CC Jr. Fentanyl plasma concentrations maintained by a simple infusion scheme in patients undergoing cardiac surgery. Anesth Analg 1993;76:957–963.
335. Wagner JG. A safe method for rapidly achieving plasma concentration plateaus. Clin Pharmacol Ther 1974;16:691–700.
336. Lu J, Schafer PG, Zhang J, et al. Respiratory depression with low levels of alfentanil is significant and dose related [Abstract]. Anesthesiology 1993;79:A374.

12 Nonsteroidal Anti-inflammatory Drugs

Andrew J. Souter

Nonsteroidal anti-inflammatory drugs (NSAIDs) are among the oldest in Western medicine. Salicin was identified as the active ingredient of willow bark in 1829, a finding that led to the commercial production of synthetic acetylsalicylic acid (aspirin) by Bayer in 1899. However, only the recent availability of injectable preparations of this class of drugs has produced a surge of interest in their perioperative use (1). NSAIDs are devoid of the unwanted side effects characteristic of the other major group of systemic perioperative analgesics (e.g., respiratory depression, nausea, vomiting, urinary retention, tolerance, addiction, and abuse by health care professionals). Furthermore, both NSAIDs and opioid analgesics may have a role in balanced analgesia, a multimodality approach to improving pain relief while reducing side effects from any single analgesic compound (2-4).

MECHANISM OF ACTION

Traditionally NSAIDs have been thought to produce analgesia by acting in the periphery to inhibit prostaglandin synthesis (Fig. 12-1) (5). In response to trauma, a cascade of tissue responses results in nociception, inflammation, and hyperalgesia (6-8). Peripheral nerves play an important role by releasing prostaglandins, substance P, and other nociceptive peptides. The resultant inflammatory process is characterized by vasodilatation, increased vascular permeability, and hyperalgesia, an altered functional state of the nervous system in which sensitization of nociceptors decreases the pain threshold (6). These sensitization processes are associated with changes in the spinal dorsal horn neurons thought to be mediated by activation of N-methyl-D-aspartate (NMDA) receptors and are characterized by expansion of their receptive field, a reduction in firing threshold, and a disruption of the normal pattern of processing (9, 10). Consequently, a windup phenomenon has been described in which a positive feed forward circuit is established modulating responses to pain and resulting in a hyperalgesic state that may outlast the initial injury (8). Primary and secondary hyperalgesia occurs; primary hyperalgesia refers to sensitization within the boundaries of injury, whereas secondary hyperalgesia describes the sensitization of adjacent uninjured tissue as a result of altered central processing of peripheral impulses.

Although a reduction in peripheral synthesis of prostaglandins decreases the inflammatory tissue response to trauma and hence nociception and pain perception, in vivo animal studies have suggested a centrally mediated role for NSAIDs in pain modulation. NSAIDs produce a dose-dependent depression in rat thalamic responses to peripheral nociceptor input (11). They also appear to prevent the rise in prostaglandins found in the cerebrospinal fluid (CSF) following activation of NMDA receptors (12). Furthermore, ketorolac given intrathecally to rats inhibits the first and second phase of the rat formalin test (the first phase relating to immediate pain and the second to hyperalgesia) (13, 14).

However, although NSAIDs may show centrally mediated activity in animal models, this may be irrelevant following parenteral administration of NSAIDs in humans. The central analgesic activity of these agents may in part depend on the sensitivity of prostaglandin synthetase in the central nervous system (CNS), because the ratio of plasma to CSF ketorolac concentrations is approximately 1000:1 following parenteral administration (15). Because clinical studies on intrathecal or other central routes of administration have not been performed, the clinical efficacy of NSAIDs in the CNS is yet to be proven.

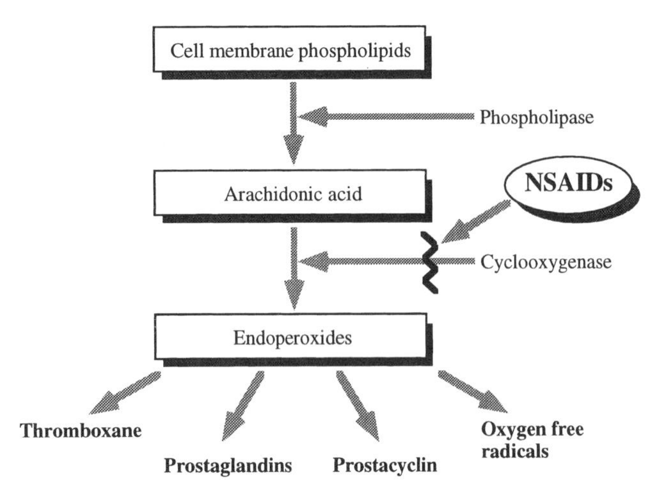

FIGURE 12-1. The peripheral mechanism of action of the nonsteroidal anti-inflammatory drugs (NSAIDs).

Ketorolac Tromethamine

Diclofenac Sodium

Ketoprofen

Tenoxicam

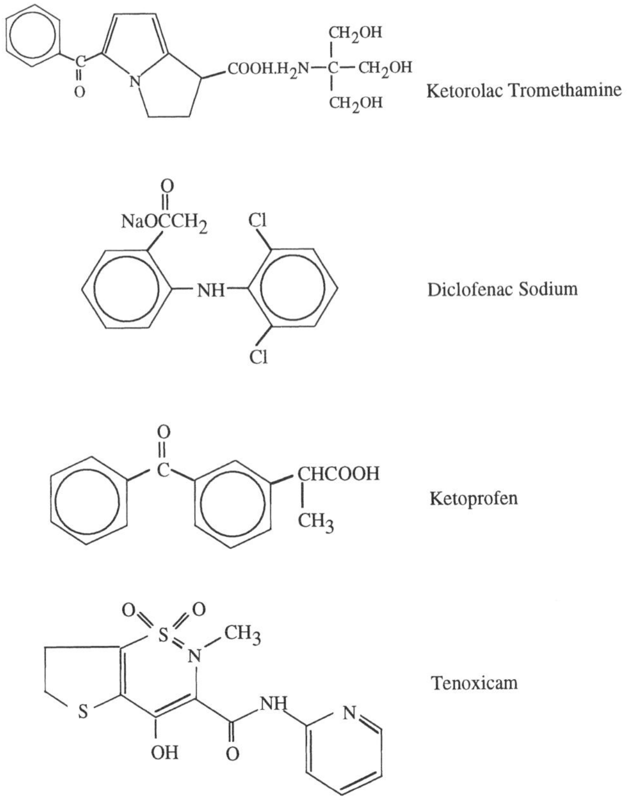

FIGURE 12-2. Chemical structures of the nonsteroidal anti-inflammatory drugs (NSAIDs) available in parenteral formulations.

PHARMACOKINETICS OF PARENTERAL AGENTS

Ketorolac

Ketorolac tromethamine (Toradol) was released onto the market in the United States in March 1990, as the first NSAID licensed for postoperative analgesia. Ketorolac is a member of the carboxylic acid group of NSAIDs, structurally related to tolmetin and zomepirac (Fig. 12-2). This agent is the most potent analgesic in the NSAID group available for use in humans; it is 800 times more potent than aspirin in standard animal models (16). Initially approved for intramuscular use, ketorolac is now licensed for intravenous and oral administration in most of the Western world. That it was the first to gain widespread use as an intravenous analgesic seems to account for the greater level of interest it has attracted compared with other injectable NSAIDs.

Ketorolac is rapidly absorbed and undergoes negligible levels of presystemic metabolism when administered orally or intramuscularly; it takes 30 to 45 minutes to achieve maximum plasma concentrations (Table 12-1). When given intravenously, ketorolac has a time to onset of approximately 20 minutes, demonstrating a delay between reaching adequate plasma levels and its pharmacodynamic effect (17). The majority of the drug is excreted by the kidney, 60% unchanged and 40% in conjugated and hydroxylated forms. This metabolism is thought to occur in the kidney rather than the liver (18). Plasma half-life at 5.4 hours is intermediate within the NSAID group and ranges from 0.8 hours for tolmetin to 72 hours for phenylbutazone. Volume of distribution for ketorolac is low and protein binding is high (99%), in common with other NSAIDs (16, 18). Displacement of drugs such as anticoagulants, digoxin, and methotrexate from plasma proteins accounts for most of the potentially dangerous drug interactions. Plasma clearance ranges from 0.021 to 0.037 L/kg/h in young, healthy volunteers (19, 20). However, these pharmacokinetic values are altered in the elderly and in the presence of renal dysfunction, with plasma half-life and decreased clearance rates in these patient populations (20, 21).

Ketorolac, in common with other NSAIDs, is transferred from the maternal to the fetal circulation, but the ratio of 0.12 (fetal-maternal) is low compared with the opioid analgesics (22). Small amounts of ketorolac are excreted in breast milk, in which it has been calculated that the newborn receives between 0.1 and 0.4% of the daily maternal dose (23).

Diclofenac

The parenteral form of diclofenac sodium (Voltarol, Voltaren) predates ketorolac. However, diclofenac has only recently been licensed for intravenous use in the United Kingdom, Finland, and Sweden. Diclofenac is a phenylacetic acid, a relatively new class of NSAIDs (see Fig. 12-2). Although less potent than ketorolac, diclofenac has analgesic, anti-inflammatory, and anti-

TABLE 12-1. Pharmacokinetics of Parenteral Nonsteroidal Anti-inflammatory Drugs

Drug	Daily Dose (mg)	Dosing Interval (h)	Elimination Half-Life (h)	Volume of Distribution (L/kg)	Clearance (L/kg/h)	Metabolism (%)
Ketorolac tromethamine	150 mg (first day) 120 mg (subsequently)	4–8	5.4	0.11–0.25	0.02–0.03	40
Diclofenac sodium	150	8–12	1–2	0.12	0.04–0.08	99
Ketoprofen	200	4–12	1.5–2	0.11	0.07	99
Tenoxicam	20	24	72	0.14	0.0017	99

pyretic effects approximately 100 times greater than those of aspirin (24). Diclofenac is supplied in 3-ml ampules containing 25 mg/ml and, being poorly water soluble, it is dissolved in propylene glycol. Intravenous injection of diclofenac in its undiluted form is associated with an unacceptably high incidence of venous sequelae within 72 hours after intravenous injection (with a 60 to 80% incidence of venous thrombosis). Vein irritation can be reduced by a fivefold dilution in saline or dextrose or slow injection (25), or it can be avoided entirely by addition to at least 100 ml of intravenous fluid and infusion over 30 minutes (26). The drug does not precipitate on addition to aqueous solutions, but it is unstable, requiring infusion within a short time of preparation.

When diclofenac is administered intravenously, it adheres to a three-compartment or triphasic pharmacokinetic model with a short elimination half-life of 1 to 2 hours (see Table 12-1). Diclofenac is well absorbed but undergoes significant presystemic metabolism (approximately 40%) when given orally. Once in the circulation, the agent undergoes extensive metabolism to phenolic compounds conjugated with glucuronide or sulfate groups and excreted by the kidney. Less than 1% of the parent compound is excreted as unchanged diclofenac. Analogous to ketorolac, diclofenac is extensively bound to plasma proteins (99.5%), reflected in a low volume of distribution of 0.12 L/kg and similar to ketorolac with respect to its potential drug interactions. Only insignificant amounts of diclofenac are excreted into breast milk (27).

Ketoprofen

Analogous to diclofenac, ketoprofen (Orudis, Oruvail) has been available in injectable form for more than a decade in many parts of the world. In common with other NSAIDs, ketoprofen is analgesic, antipyretic, and anti-inflammatory. It belongs to the propionic acid group of NSAIDs along with ibuprofen, fenoprofen, and flurbiprofen (see Fig. 12-2), and it is slightly less potent than diclofenac. Although this agent is not widely licensed for intravenous use, intravenous administration has been extensively reported in the literature without noted adverse effects.

Overall, the pharmacokinetics of ketoprofen is similar to that of ketorolac and diclofenac (see Table 12-1). The drug is well absorbed by the gastric mucosa and undergoes minimal presystemic metabolism, resulting in high bioavailability after oral administration. Ketoprofen has a short elimination half-life of 1.5 to 2 hours, because extensive metabolism takes place in the liver, where the agent is conjugated, and it is mainly excreted in the urine, with less than 1% appearing as free ketoprofen. Unlike with ketorolac and diclofenac, a significant amount of ketoprofen (10 to 20%) is excreted in bile (28). Because ketoprofen is highly protein bound with a low volume of distribution, it has the potential to produce many drug interactions.

Tenoxicam

Tenoxicam (Mobiflex) is a much more recent addition to the class of injectable NSAIDs and is widely licensed for intravenous use. Along with piroxicam, tenoxicam belongs to the thienothiazine or oxicam group of NSAIDs (see Fig. 12-2). Because of its instability in solution, this drug is supplied as a powder that must be reconstituted with a small volume (2 ml) of water. Like other NSAIDs, it has profound antipyretic, analgesic, and anti-inflammatory properties.

Following intravenous administration, the tenoxicam plasma concentration decay curve fits a biexponential or two-compartment pharmacokinetic model, with a rapid first phase of redistribution and a slow elimination phase (see Table 12-1). An elimination half-life of 72 hours distinguishes it from the other parenterally active NSAIDs. Tenoxicam can be administered using a once-daily dosing regimen. Metabolism is extensive, and only negligible amounts are excreted unchanged in the urine (<1%) (29). Plasma clearance is low, with values ranging from 1.3 to 4.2 ml/min, and plasma protein binding is high (99%), contributing to a small volume of distribution (0.2 to 0.4 L/kg). No data are available on transfer from maternal to fetal circulations or excretion into breast milk.

PHARMACODYNAMICS

Intraoperative Use

Adjuvants to General Anesthesia

Potent short-acting opioid analgesics are an important part of a balanced anesthetic technique. They attenuate pressor responses to laryngoscopy and intubation and produce a dose-dependent reduction in the minimum alveolar concentration (MAC) of volatile anesthetics (30). However, the use of ketorolac is not associated with a significant reduction in MAC (31). Therefore, one could predict that NSAIDs would not provide the intraoperative benefits of opioid analgesics.

Several end points have been studied in which NSAIDs have been used as adjuvants during the intraoperative period. The use of these agents as sole intraoperative analgesics has been associated with an unacceptably high incidence of purposeful movement in response to surgical stimulus (32). Conversely, these drugs appear to have a more favorable profile with respect to cardiorespiratory effects, causing less reduction in blood pressure, heart rate, respiratory rate, tidal volume, and minute ventilation than potent short-acting opioids during volatile anesthesia (33, 34) or intravenous sedation (35). Furthermore, intraoperative use of NSAIDs confers benefits extending into the immediate postoperative period. When compared with short-acting opioids alone, ketorolac is associated with greater residual analgesia following more painful ambulatory surgery such as laparoscopic tubal ligation (36, 37). Finally, the intraoperative use of NSAIDs may be associated with other benefits following ambulatory surgery, including a more rapid recovery profile (38) and a reduction in postoperative nausea and vomiting when compared with opioid compounds (36, 39).

Another possible advantage of perioperative NSAID administration relates to the effects of these drugs on the surgical stress response. Perioperative NSAID administration has improved nitrogen balance (40), resulted in significantly lower plasma cortisol levels (39), and when used in combination with an epidural block, it has reduced postsurgical elevations in body temperature and granulocyte production (41). However, research has failed to show any reduction in the postoperative elevations of the acute-phase reactants C-reactive protein, α_1-acid glycoprotein, haptoglobin, α_1-chymotrypsin, and ceruloplasmin (42). Although it is not clear whether changes in these acute-phase reactants are associated with alterations in postoperative morbidity (43), any observed NSAID-induced changes in the metabolic or endocrine response to surgery seem to be beneficial.

Thus, although NSAIDs may be inadequate as sole intraoperative analgesics, when used in combination with opioids and local anesthetics, they can reduce unwanted cardiorespiratory effects, significantly improve analgesia and reduce morbidity in the immediate postoperative period, and attenuate the stress response to surgery.

Adjuvants to Local Anesthesia During Monitored Anesthesia Care

Patients undergoing ambulatory procedures under local anesthesia with a monitored anesthesia care (MoAC) technique have traditionally received opioid analgesics for intraoperative pain and discomfort refractory to local anesthetic drugs. Because NSAIDs appear to be devoid of opioid-related side effects, their use as intraoperative adjuvants may be advantageous in this day-case setting.

Similar to their effect on the anesthetic requirement during volatile anesthesia, intravenous opioids significantly reduce propofol dosage requirements during sedation techniques, whereas NSAIDs do not (44). However, intravenous NSAID are efficacious for the management of intraoperative pain refractory to local anesthesia, and when compared with opioid analgesics, NSAIDs are associated with decreased postoperative pain and analgesic requirements, significantly less pruritus and nausea, and the potential for earlier discharge (44, 45).

During extracorporeal shock wave lithotripsy with an MoAC technique, the administration of diclofenac was associated with only a marginal reduction in opioid requirement (46). However, the combination of ketorolac with patient-controlled fentanyl administration resulted in improved analgesia and lower opioid requirements after these procedures compared with fentanyl alone (47).

Postoperative Use

Early clinical studies suggested that parenteral NSAID alone could provide analgesia comparable to morphine- or meperidine-induced analgesia in the postoperative period (48, 49). Unfortunately, these early studies suffered from methodologic problems (e.g., differing patient populations undergoing many procedures with different associated pain levels and using excessively large doses of the NSAID. Furthermore, subsequent studies have cast doubt on the ability of NSAIDs alone to provide effective pain relief following major surgery (50-52). More recent work has focused on the ability of these agents to augment analgesia provided by opioids or local anesthetic techniques, and the studies suggest a useful role in this area (53).

Use of NSAIDs Alone

Theoretically, NSAIDs should be most efficacious when pain is a result of minor-to-moderate tissue damage. It is therefore not surprising that the use of parenteral NSAIDs alone provides adequate analgesia in the postoperative period following minor procedures (e.g., dental, arthroscopic, nasal, and various other outpatient operations) (54-57).

However, following major painful surgery such as laparotomy or thoracotomy, the use of parenteral NSAIDs is clearly inadequate in the immediate postoperative period when pain is most severe (50-52). Furthermore, ketorolac when used in an intravenous patient-controlled analgesia (PCA) system for the management of postoperative abdominal pain provides inadequate analgesia with a correspondingly high withdrawal rate compared with a standard morphine PCA technique (58). This finding is not surprising because intravenous ketorolac has a slow onset time (20 to 40 minutes) compared with morphine, a property that renders ketorolac less suitable for PCA, which requires a rapid onset time for the feedback loop to be efficient (17). Furthermore, unless extremely small PCA ketorolac doses are used, potential overdosage can produce serious toxicity.

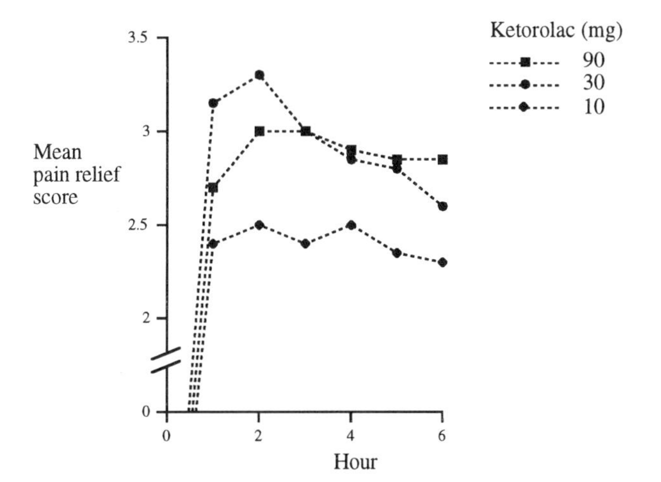

FIGURE 12-3. The ceiling effect of nonsteroidal anti-inflammatory drugs (NSAIDs). (From O'Hara DA, Fragen RJ, Kinzer M, Pemberton D. Ketorolac tromethamine as compared with morphine sulfate for treatment of postoperative pain. Clin Pharmacol Ther 1987;41:556-561.)

The failure to control severe postoperative pain when NSAIDs are used alone may in part be explained by the ceiling effect with respect to analgesia that is exhibited by most NSAIDs (Fig. 12-3) (49). Opioid analgesics, in contrast, do not exhibit this phenomenon. Later in the postoperative period, when pain is less severe, parenteral NSAIDs alone may provide analgesia superior to small intravenous doses of the opioid (morphine 2 to 4 mg) and equivalent to a larger intramuscular dose (morphine 12 mg) (59, 60). Although possessing similar mechanisms of action, some NSAIDs may be more effective than others in alleviating pain in specific situations. For example, investigators have suggested that ketorolac is more effective than diclofenac following arthroscopy, whereas diclofenac is associated with less supplemental opioid analgesia following maxillofacial surgery than ketoprofen (61, 62).

Combination of NSAIDs with Opioids

Many studies have compared the use of postoperative NSAIDs with placebo when opioids are used for supplemental analgesia by a PCA delivery system. These studies have examined the combination of an NSAID and an opioid analgesic versus the opioid analgesic alone. Results are expressed in terms of pain and pain relief scores, as well as effects on the PCA opioid requirements. In this area, results consistently demonstrate that NSAIDs plus opioids improve postoperative analgesia while decreasing the opioid requirement (Table 12-2).

Various NSAID-opioid combinations have been used following major surgery including spinal, thoracic, and abdominal surgery, in which these regimens have been shown to reduce pain and opioid require-

TABLE 12-2. Use of Combinations of Nonsteroidal Anti-inflammatory Drugs (NSAIDs) and Opioids Following Major Surgery and the Effect on Pain Scores and Opioid Use

Reference	Type of Surgery	Postoperative NSAID	Route	Postoperative Opioid	Route	Pain Scores	Opioid Use
Hodsman et al, 1987[69]	Abdominal	Diclofenac	IM	Morphine	PCA/IV	↓	↓
Sevarino et al, 1992[71]	Abdominal	Ketorolac	IM	Morphine	PCA/IV	↓	↓
Sevarino et al, 1994[72]	Abdominal	Ketorolac	IV	Morphine	PCA/IV	↓	↓
Kinsella et al, 1992[73]	Orthopedic	Ketorolac	IM	Morphine	PCA/IV	↓	↓
Gillies et al, 1987[74]	Abdominal	Ketorolac	IM	Morphine	PCA/IV	↓	↓
Burns et al, 1991[75]	Abdominal	Ketorolac	IM	Morphine	PCA/IV	↓	↓
Blackburn et al, 1995[77]	Abdominal	Ketorolac	IV	Morphine	PCA/IV	↓	↓
Liu et al, 1993[78]	Laparoscopic cholecystectomy	Ketorolac	IM/IV	Fentanyl	IV	↓	↓
McLoughlin et al, 1990[81]	Arthroscopy	Diclofenac	IM	Codeine	Oral	↓	↓
Parker et al, 1994[88]	Abdominal hysterectomy	Ketorolac	IV	Morphine/meperidine	IV	↓	↓
Ready et al, 1994[89]	Various major	Ketorolac	IV	Morphine	PCA/IV	↓	↓

IM, Intramuscular; IV, intravenous; PCA, patient-controlled analgesia.

ments (39, 63-78). When ketorolac was given by intravenous infusion, pain scores and PCA opioid requirements were reduced early in the postoperative period (39, 77), whereas these effects were limited to a later time in the recovery period when ketorolac (or diclofenac) was administered by the intramuscular route (74-76). Many studies have suggested a beneficial effect for NSAIDs in reducing pain and opioid requirements, as well as emetic symptoms (79-81), after ambulatory surgery. NSAIDs have also been used as adjuvants to epidural and intrathecal opioid-induced analgesia. Administration of parenteral ketorolac (or diclofenac) to patients undergoing abdominal surgery or cesarean delivery in combination with epidural fentanyl or morphine has also reduced pain scores and opioid requirements (82-84). Similar effects have been seen when combining parenteral ketorolac with intrathecal opioids (85, 86).

Reduction in postoperative opioid use should in theory have beneficial effects with respect to a decrease in opioid-related side effects. In healthy volunteers, morphine significantly delayed gastric emptying and prolonged small bowel transit time. Ketorolac, on the other hand, had no adverse effects on bowel function (87). Not surprisingly, therefore, intravenous ketorolac given as an adjuvant to PCA-administered morphine resulted in a more rapid return of bowel function in patients who had undergone laparotomy (88), and it provoked less vomiting following surgery (89). Similarly, because opioids can exacerbate spasm of the sphincter of Oddi in patients undergoing biliary tract surgery, NSAIDs are useful adjuncts when increased biliary tract pressure is undesirable (90).

Combination of NSAIDs with Local Anesthetics

NSAIDs have been combined with local anesthetic techniques in an attempt to enhance postoperative analgesia. When parenteral ketorolac was combined with intra-articular bupivacaine, pain and opioid requirements were decreased following knee arthroscopy compared with the local anesthetic technique alone (91). In contrast, piroxicam failed to enhance analgesia when combined with continuous epidural bupivacaine and morphine following laparotomy or thoracotomy (92, 93). The explanation for this effect may be, in part, that pain scores were already low in the control group receiving continuous epidural morphine and bupivacaine.

Novel uses of parenteral ketorolac have been reported in combination with local anesthetics. Following intra-articular administration of the NSAID with bupivacaine, patients undergoing knee arthroscopy benefited from improved quality and length of analgesia and decreased supplementary analgesic requirements (94). These authors also described an intravenous regional anesthetic technique combining ketorolac and lidocaine with similarly improved intra- and postoperative pain control and decreased postoperative analgesic requirements (95).

When analgesia resulting from a local or regional anesthetic technique is already profound, little benefit may be gained from the addition of NSAIDs. However, when local analgesia is incomplete, NSAIDs may be extremely beneficial. Finally, the combination of local anesthetics and NSAIDs may prolong the period of analgesia.

Perioperative Use in Children

Inadequate postoperative pain relief in the pediatric population not only is distressing to the child, but also is unacceptable to parents and medical staff. Although opioids provide effective analgesia, postoperative care unit discharge can be delayed as a result of the associated somnolence, urinary retention, and nausea and vomiting. Therefore, administration of analgesic drugs such as the NSAIDs, which are devoid of these unwanted side effects, may be advantageous in this patient population.

Intraoperative parenteral administration of NSAIDs has been compared with local and opioid analgesia in children. In one study, caudal local analgesia exhibited a greater volatile anesthetic-sparing effect than intravenous ketorolac, whereas in the postoperative period, pain scores were similar, and the NSAID-treated group experienced less nausea (96). Conversely, following inguinal herniorrhaphy, rectal diclofenac produced less analgesia in the immediate postoperative period than did caudal bupivacaine. However, the analgesic effect of the NSAID was more prolonged, and it was more effective than the one-shot local anesthetic technique in the later postoperative period (97). When compared with opioids, intraoperative use of parenteral NSAIDs has consistently produced favorable results. Ketorolac has demonstrated analgesic properties similar to those of morphine in children undergoing ambulatory surgery, whereas it causes less nausea and emesis in the early postoperative period (98, 99). Following tonsillectomy, NSAID administration has resulted in similar levels of analgesia when compared with shorter-acting opioids (100). However, concerns have been raised regarding the risks of postoperative hemorrhage resulting from the antiplatelet effects of the NSAIDs (101).

In the postoperative period, intramuscular injections are painful and frightening to children; therefore, the intravenous route would seem to offer advantages. One large retrospective study of the use of intravenous ketorolac in children for postoperative pain has found it to be safe (2 minor allergic reactions following 3420 doses) and effective (102). As with intraoperative use, the postoperative use of NSAIDs has been compared with standard opioid analgesia with favorable results.

NSAIDs administered by a variety of routes (namely, parenteral, rectal, and oral) have provided analgesia similar to that achieved with opioid analgesics (103-105). Furthermore, when used in conjunction with opioids, NSAIDs have improved objective pain assessments, while allowing a reduction in the amount of opioid administered to children (106).

NSAIDs seem to have a firm place in the management of perioperative pain in children. These compounds are well tolerated, safe, and effective, especially when given intravenously. As with adults, when these agents are used as part of a balanced analgesic technique in conjunction with opioids or local anesthetics, superior postoperative analgesia with reduction in opioid use (and potentially opioid-related side effects) can be achieved.

ADVERSE EFFECTS

Serious concerns have been raised regarding the effects of NSAIDs on the renal, gastrointestinal, and coagulation systems following the perioperative use of these agents. Anecdotal case reports of adverse effects including deaths ascribed to acute renal toxicity and bleeding diatheses have begun to appear in the medical literature. These concerns have led to analysis of risks versus benefits with subsequent suspension of licenses for perioperative use of ketorolac in some European countries (107-109). Furthermore, because prostaglandins are ubiquitous local hormones, they have the potential for adverse effects throughout the body.

Effects on Renal Function

By virtue of their ability to inhibit prostaglandin synthetase, all NSAIDs can adversely affect renal function (110, 111). In an authoritative review in 1984, clinicians were advised to withhold NSAIDs before surgery because of the risk of acute renal failure (112). Despite this warning, the widespread use of these drugs in the perioperative period has led to few case reports of renal toxicity. Furthermore, clinically significant renal impairment associated with the use of NSAIDs has only been reported in patients with risk factors for developing acute renal failure (e.g., hypovolemia, sepsis, cardiac failure, cirrhosis, and preexisting renal dysfunction) or following the concurrent use of NSAIDs with other nephrotoxic drugs (e.g., antibiotics) (113-115).

Although renal function can be altered secondary to a reduction in the synthesis of renal prostaglandins, NSAIDs appear to have a low potential for clinically significant renal toxicity in the presence of adequate hydration because renal function does not depend on synthesis of prostaglandins in this situation. However, because prostaglandins control renal blood flow during hypovolemic conditions, as well as in the presence of cardiac failure and cirrhosis, cyclooxygenase inhibition can result in renal vasoconstriction and subsequent alterations in renal function (116).

When studied over a 72-hour period after abdominal hysterectomy procedures, intravenous ketorolac caused no significant changes in serum creatinine levels (88). However, during prolonged postoperative administration (5 days) of ketorolac to elderly patients with impaired renal function, transient increases in serum creatinine were demonstrated (117). Following upper abdominal surgery in patients with normal renal function, administration of intramuscular ketorolac resulted in a small but significant reduction in potassium excretion (118). However, the clinical relevance of the latter finding is unknown. Perioperatively, NSAIDs should be used with caution in the elderly and avoided in those patients with known renal risk factors and to whom nephrotoxic drugs are administered. When no such contraindications exist, these drugs appear to be safe and effective analgesic adjuvants during the postoperative period.

Effect on Hemostasis

Because of their reversible inhibition of cyclooxygenase activity, NSAIDs can also inhibit platelet aggregation. Although the administration of indomethacin resulted in increased perioperative blood loss following abdominal hysterectomy (119), diclofenac had no significant effect on blood loss following transurethral prostatectomy or knee replacement (120, 121). The intramuscular administration of ketorolac was associated with a clinically insignificant increase in bleeding time and resulted in local ecchymosis. However, ketorolac had no effect on thromboelastographic parameters (122). Furthermore, no synergism was demonstrated when ketorolac was administered in combination with low-dose heparin to healthy volunteers (123).

One area where bleeding would be of particular concern is microvascular reconstructive surgery. An anecdotal report has noted an increase in the incidence of significant postoperative hematomas in association with ketorolac in patients undergoing plastic surgery (124). It should therefore be reassuring that, in an animal model of a skin flap, high doses of ketorolac had no effect on flap ischemia or necrosis (125). Alternatively, NSAID-induced inhibition of platelet aggregation has been used therapeutically to improve perfusion following microvascular surgery (126), although when studied in a rat model, ketorolac only produced a short-lived increase in microartery patency, a finding that questions the efficacy of this therapeutic maneuver (127).

Effects on the Gastrointestinal Mucosa

Although gastrointestinal bleeding in the postoperative period has been reported following the perioperative use of ketorolac (115, 128, 129), the multifactorial nature of the bleeding in these cases makes it difficult to ascribe this complication to ketorolac alone (130, 131). Perioperative use of NSAIDs is also implicated in the pathogenesis of peptic ulceration (132). In light of these case reports, one should limit the dose and duration of use of perioperative NSAIDs and avoid them altogether in patients with a history of peptic ulcer disease or gastrointestinal bleeding.

Effect on the Cardiovascular System

Prostaglandins are potent local regulators of vascular tone and, therefore, of local blood flow. In particular, prostacyclin is a potent vasodilator, whereas PGE_2 and $PGF_2\alpha$ are potent vasoconstrictors and can induce coronary vasoconstriction. Despite their abilities to affect vascular tone profoundly, these compounds appear to have little effect on cardiovascular parameters including arterial blood pressure, systemic vascular resistance, and cardiac output (133). A possible explanation for the lack of NSAID-induced cardiovascular toxicity relates to the balanced reduction in prostaglandins with opposing actions. Despite limited effects, NSAIDs should be used with caution in patients with coronary ischemia or hypertension (134).

In conclusion, the use of NSAID compounds has been extensively studied during the perioperative period. Although these agents are clearly less efficacious than opioids in the intraoperative and early postoperative period, NSAIDs have proven useful for ambulatory surgery and as adjuvants to opioids following major surgery, by improving pain relief and reducing opioid use. Benefits arising from reduced opioid use have been less readily demonstrated. For example, despite NSAIDs' opioid-sparing effects, reports of a significant reduction in emetic sequelae have only appeared in a few studies. However, trends toward fewer adverse effects associated with the opioid-sparing effect of NSAIDs suggest that a meta-analysis of the available literature may find a statistically significant effect.

Concerns regarding adverse events associated with perioperative NSAID administration have led to more cautious utilization in recent years. Licensing authorities have reduced approved dosages and have limited their length of use. These agents should be used with care in the elderly and should be avoided in patients who are at risk of developing renal, cardiac, or bleeding disorders in the postoperative period.

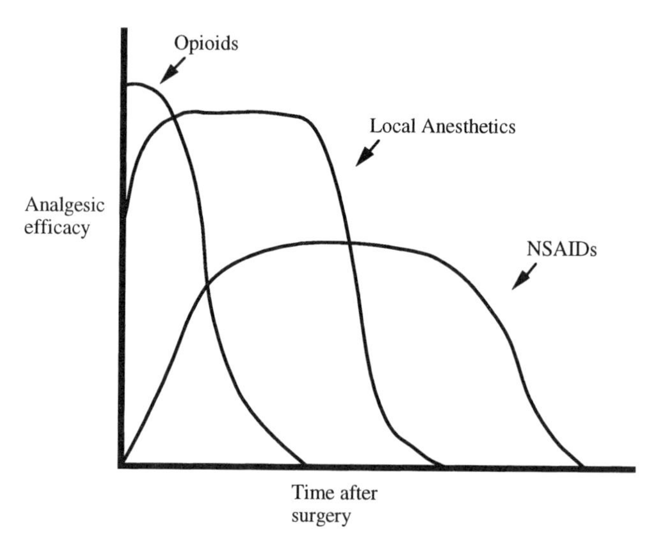

FIGURE 12-4. Proposed time course and efficacy of drugs used in the postoperative period. (From Souter A, Fredman B, White PF)

After an initial period of enthusiasm associated with the introduction of NSAIDs as intravenous perioperative analgesics, more rational indications for the use of these drugs now apply. The NSAIDs are especially appropriate for ambulatory surgery, in which they can eliminate or reduce the need for opioid analgesia and can facilitate earlier discharge. Elsewhere, NSAID administration has demonstrated an important role in multimodal analgesia, by improving pain relief and potentially decreasing opioid-related side effects. At present, the optimal regimen for the management of perioperative pain appears to include the selective use of NSAIDs in combination with opioid analgesics and local anesthetics (Fig. 12-4).

REFERENCES

1. Souter A, Fredman B, White PF. Controversies in the perioperative use of non-steroidal antiinflammatory drugs. Anesth Analg 1994;79:1178–1190.
2. Code W. NSAIDs and balanced analgesia. Can J Anaesth 1993; 40:401–405.
3. Dahl JB, Rosenberg J, Dirkes WE, et al. Prevention of postoperative pain by balanced analgesia. Br J Anaesth 1990;64:518–520.
4. Kehlet H, Dahl JB. The value of multimodal or balanced analgesia in postoperative pain treatment. Anesth Analg 1993; 77:1048–1056.
5. McCormack K, Brune K. Dissociation between the antinociceptive and anti-inflammatory effects of the non-steroidal anti-inflammatory drugs. Drugs 1991;41:533–547.
6. Dahl JB, Kehlet H. Non-steroidal anti-inflammatory drugs: rationale for use in severe postoperative pain. Br J Anaesth 1991; 66:703–712.
7. Dahl JB, Kehlet H. The value of pre-emptive analgesia in the treatment of postoperative pain. Br J Anaesth 1993;70:434–439.
8. Woolf CJ. Recent advances in the pathophysiology of acute pain. Br J Anaesth 1989;63:139–146.
9. Davies SN, Lodge D. Evidence for involvement of N-methyl-

aspartate receptors in wind-up of class 2 neurones in the dorsal horn of the rat. Brain Res 1987;424:402–406.
10. Coderre TJ, Melzack R. The contribution of excitatory amino acids to central sensitization and persistent nociception after formalin-induced tissue injury. J Neurosci 1992;12:3665–3670.
11. Jurna I, Brune K. Central effect of the nonsteroidal anti-inflammatory agents indomethacin, ibuprofen and diclofenac, determined in C fibre-evoked activity in single neurones of the rat thalamus. Pain 1990;41:71–80.
12. Sorkin LS. IT Ketorolac blocks NMDA-evoked spinal release of prostaglandin E2 (PGE2) and thromboxane B2 (TXB2) [Abstract]. Anesthesiology 1993;79:A909.
13. Malmberg AB, Yaksh TL. Pharmacology of the spinal action of ketorolac, morphine, U50488H, and L-PIA on the formalin test and an isobolographic analysis of the NSAID interaction. Anesthesiology 1993;79:270–281.
14. Malmberg AB, Yaksh TL. Antinociceptor actions of spinal nonsteroidal anti-inflammatory agents on the formalin test in the rat. J Pharmacol Exp Ther 1992;263:136–146.
15. Rice ASC, Lloyd J, Bullingham RES, O'Sullivan G. Ketorolac penetration into the cerebrospinal fluid of humans. J Clin Anesth 1993;5:459–462.
16. Buckley MM, Brogden RN. Ketorolac: a review of its pharmacodynamic and pharmacokinetic properties, and therapeutic potential. Drugs 1990;39:86–109.
17. Rice AS, Whitehead EM, O Sullivan G, et al. Speed of onset of analgesic effect of intravenous ketorolac compared to morphine and placebo. Eur J Anaesthesiol 1995;12:313–317.
18. Mroszczak EJ, Lee FW, Combs D, et al. Ketorolac tromethamine absorption, distribution, metabolism, excretion, and pharmacokinetics in animals and humans. Drug Metab Dispos 1987; 15:618–626.
19. Jung D, Mroszczak E, Bynum L. Pharmacokinetics of ketorolac tromethamine in humans after intravenous, intramuscular and oral administration. Eur J Clin Pharmacol 1988;35:423–425.
20. Martinez JJ, Garg DC, Pages LJ, et al. Single dose pharmacokinetics of ketorolac in healthy young and renal impaired subjects [Abstract]. J Clin Pharmacol 1987;27:722.
21. Montoya-Iraheta C, Garg DC, Jallad SN, et al. Pharmacokinetics of single dose oral and intramuscular ketorolac tromethamine in elderly vs young healthy subjects [Abstract]. J Clin Pharmacol 1986;26:545.
22. Walker JJ, Johnstone J, Lloyd J, Rocha CL. The transfer of ketorolac tromethamine from maternal to foetal blood. Eur J Clin Pharmacol 1988;34:509–511.
23. Wischnik A, Manth SM, Lloyd J, Bullingham R. The excretion of ketorolac tromethamine into breast milk after multiple oral dosing. Eur J Clin Pharmacol 1989;36:512–514.
24. Menasse R, Hedwell PR, Kraetz I. Pharmacological properties of diclofenac sodium and its metabolites. Scand J Rheumatol Suppl 1978;22:5–16.
25. Campbell WI, Watters CH. Venous sequelae following i.v. administration of diclofenac. Br J Anaesth 1989;62:545–547.
26. Gopinath R. Venous sequelae after i.v. diclofenac. Br J Anaesth 1991;67:803.
27. Todd PA, Sorkin EM. Diclofenac sodium: a reappraisal of its pharmacodynamic and pharmacokinetic properties and therapeutic efficacy. Drugs 1988;35:244–285.
28. Debruyne D, Hurault DLB, Ryckelynck JP, et al. Clinical pharmacokinetics of ketoprofen after single intravenous administration as a bolus or infusion. Clin Pharmacokinet 1987;12:214–221.
29. Heintz RC, Guentert TW, Enrico JF, et al. Pharmacokinetics of tenoxicam in healthy human volunteers. Eur J Rheumatol Inflamm 1984;7:33–44.
30. Hoffman JC, DiFazio CA. The anesthesia sparing effect of pentazocine, meperidine and morphine. Arch Int Pharmacodyn Ther 1970;186:261–268.
31. Rich GF, Schacterle R, Moscicki JC, DiFazio CA. Ketorolac does not decrease the MAC of halothane or depress ventilation in rats. Anesth Analg 1992;75:99–102.
32. Ding Y, Fredman B, White PF. Use of ketorolac and fentanyl during outpatient gynecologic surgery. Anesth Analg 1993; 77:205–210.
33. Murray AW, Brockway MS, Kenny GN. Comparison of the cardiorespiratory effects of ketorolac and alfentanil during propofol anaesthesia. Br J Anaesth 1989;63:601–603.
34. Reinhart DJ, Klein K, Griffin JD, et al. Comparison of effects of intravenous ketorolac vs fentanyl on spontaneous ventilation during isoflurane anesthesia: a double-blind, randomized study [Abstract]. Anesthesiology 1992;77:A32.
35. Ramirez-Ruiz M, Smith I, White PF. Use of analgesics during propofol sedation: a comparison of ketorolac, dezocine and fentanyl. J Clin Anesth 1995;7:481–485.
36. Ding Y, White PF. Comparative effects of ketorolac, dezocine, and fentanyl as adjuvants during outpatient anesthesia [see comments]. Anesth Analg 1992;75:566–571.
37. Badrinath SK, Braverman B, Ivankovich AD, et al. Comparison of dezocine, ketorolac and alfentanil analgesia in outpatients receiving propofol anesthesia [Abstract]. Anesthesiology 1992; 77:A25.
38. Bosek V, Smith DB, Endicott J, et al. Comparison of intravenous ketorolac and alfentanil as supplements to propofol anesthesia for diagnostic panendoscopy. J Clin Anesth 1995;7:40–43.
39. Varrassi G, Panella L, Piroli A, et al. The effects of perioperative ketorolac infusion on postoperative pain and endocrine-metabolic response. Anesth Analg 1994;78:514–519.
40. Asoh T, Shirasaka C, Uchida I, Tsuji H. Effects of indomethacin on endocrine responses and nitrogen loss after surgery. Ann Surg 1987;206:770–776.
41. Schulze S, Schierbeck J, Sparso BH, et al. Influence of neural blockade and indomethacin on leukocyte, temperature and acute-phase protein response to surgery. Acta Chir Scand 1987; 153:255–259.
42. Claeys MA, Camu F, Maes V. Prophylactic diclofenac infusions in major orthopedic surgery: effects on analgesia and acute phase proteins. Acta Anaesthesiol Scand 1992;36:270–275.
43. Kehlet H. Surgical stress: the role of pain and analgesia. Br J Anaesth 1989;63:189–195.
44. Ramirez-Ruiz M, Newson CD, White PF. Monitored anesthesia care: use of ketorolac, dezocine and fentanyl. Anesthesiology 1992;77 (suppl 3A):A27.
45. Bosek V, Smith DB, Cox C. Ketorolac or fentanyl to supplement local anesthesia? J Clin Anesth 1992;4:480–483.
46. Fredman B, Jedeikin R, Olsfanger D, Aronheim M. The opioid-sparing of diclofenac sodium in outpatient extracorporeal shock wave lithotripsy (ESWL). J Clin Anesth 1993;5:141–144.
47. McCallion CF, McCallion J, Shulman MS. The effect of ketorolac on fentanyl PCA requirements in patients undergoing lithotripsy [Abstract]. Anesth Analg 1993;76 (suppl 2S):S253.
48. Yee JP, Koshiver JE, Allbon C, Brown CR. Comparison of intramuscular ketorolac tromethamine and morphine sulfate for analgesia of pain after major surgery. Pharmacotherapy 1986; 6:253–261.
49. O'Hara DA, Fragen RJ, Kinzer M, Pemberton D. Ketorolac tromethamine as compared with morphine sulfate for treatment of postoperative pain. Clin Pharmacol Ther 1987;41:556–561.
50. Folsland B, Skulberg A, Halvorsen P, Helgesen KG. Placebo-controlled comparison of single intramuscular doses of ketorolac tromethamine and pethidine for post-operative analgesia. J Int Med Res 1990;18:305–314.
51. Peirce RJ, Fragen RJ, Pemberton DM. Intravenous ketorolac tromethamine versus morphine sulfate in the treatment of immediate postoperative pain. Pharmacotherapy 1990;10:111–115.
52. Power I, Noble DW, Douglas E, Spence AA. Comparison of IM

ketorolac trometamol and morphine sulphate for pain relief after cholecystectomy. Br J Anaesth 1990;65:448–455.
53. Singh H, Bossard RF, White PF, Yeatts RW. Effects of ketorolac versus bupivacaine supplementation of hydromorphone epidural analgesia following thoracotomy. Anesthesiology (submitted for publication).
54. Vallane J, Kortila K, Ylikorkala O. Intravenous diclofenac sodium decreases prostaglandin synthesis and postoperative symptoms after general anaesthesia in outpatients undergoing dental surgery. Acta Anaesth Scand 1987;31:722–727.
55. Honig WJ, Van OJ. A multiple-dose comparison of ketorolac tromethamine with diflunisal and placebo in postmeniscectomy pain. J Clin Pharmacol 1986;26:700–705.
56. El Hakim M. A comparison of intravenous ketoprofen with pethidine for postoperative pain relief following nasal surgery. Acta Anaesthesiol Scand 1991;35:279–282.
57. Wong HY, Carpenter RL, Kopacz DJ, et al. A randomized, double-blind evaluation of ketorolac tromethamine for postoperative analgesia in ambulatory surgery patients [see comments]. Anesthesiology 1993;78:6–14.
58. Cepeda MS, Vargas L, Ortegon G, et al. Comparative analgesic efficacy of patient-controlled analgesia with ketorolac versus morphine after elective intraabdominal operations. Anesth Analg 1995;80:1150–1153.
59. Brown CR, Mazzulla JP, Mok MS, et al. Comparison of repeat doses of intramuscular ketorolac tromethamine and morphine sulfate for analgesia after major surgery. Pharmacotherapy 1990;10:45–50.
60. Brown CR, Moodie JE, Wild VM, Bynum LJ. Comparison of intravenous ketorolac tromethamine and morphine sulfate in the treatment of postoperative pain. Pharmacotherapy 1990; 10:116–121.
61. Morrow BC, Bunting H, Milligan KR. A comparison of diclofenac and ketorolac for postoperative analgesia following day-case arthroscopy of the knee joint [see comments]. Anaesthesia 1993;48:585–587.
62. Niemi L, Tuominen M, Pitkanen M, Rosenberg PH. Comparison of parenteral diclofenac and ketoprofen for postoperative pain relief after maxillofacial surgery. Acta Anaesthesiol Scand 1995;39:96–99.
63. Segstro R, Morley-Foster PK, Lu G. Indomethacin as a postoperative analgesic for total hip arthroplasty. Can J Anaesth 1991;38:578–581.
64. Rhodes M, Conacher I, Morritt G, Hilton C. Nonsteroidal antiinflammatory drugs for postthoracotomy pain: a prospective trial after lateral thoracotomy. J Thorac Cardiovasc Surg 1992; 103:17–20.
65. Pavy T, Medley C, Murphy DF. Effect of indomethacin on pain relief after thoracotomy. Br J Anaesth 1990;65:624–627.
66. McGlew IC, Angliss DB, Gee GJ, et al. A comparison of rectal indomethacin with placebo for pain relief following spinal surgery. Anaesth Intensive Care 1991;19:40–45.
67. Nissen I, Jensen KA, Öhrström JK. Indomethacin in the management of postoperative pain. Br J Anaesth 1992;69:304–306.
68. Reasbeck PG, Rice ML, Reasbeck JC. Double blind controlled trial of indomethacin as an adjunct to narcotic analgesia after major abdominal surgery. Lancet 1982;2:115–118.
69. Hodsman NBA, Burns J, Blyth A, et al. The morphine sparing effects of diclofenac following abdominal surgery. Anaesthesia 1987;42:1005–1008.
70. Bush DJ, Lyons G, MacDonald R. Diclofenac for analgesia after caesarean section. Anaesthesia 1992;47:1075–1077.
71. Sevarino FB, Sinatra RS, Paige D, et al. The efficacy of intramuscular ketorolac in combination with intravenous PCA morphine for postoperative pain relief. J Clin Anesth 1992;4:285–288.
72. Sevarino FB, Sinatra RS, Paige D, Silverman DG. Intravenous ketorolac as an adjunct to patient-controlled analgesia (PCA) for management of postgynecologic surgical pain. J Clin Anesth 1994;6:23–27.
73. Kinsella J, Moffat AC, Patrick JA, et al. Ketorolac trometamol for postoperative analgesia after orthopaedic surgery. Br J Anaesth 1992;69:19–22.
74. Gillies GW, Kenny GN, Bullingham RE, McArdle CS. The morphine sparing effect of ketorolac tromethamine:a study of a new, parenteral non-steroidal anti-inflammatory agent after abdominal surgery. Anaesthesia 1987;42:727–731.
75. Burns JW, Aitken HA, Bullingham RE, et al. Double-blind comparison of the morphine sparing effect of continuous and intermittent i.m. administration of ketorolac. Br J Anaesth 1991; 67:235–238.
76. Perttunen K, Kalso E, Heinonen J, Salo J. IV diclofenac in post-thoracotomy pain. Br J Anaesth 1992;68:474–480.
77. Blackburn A, Stevens JD, Wheatley RG, et al. Balanced analgesia with intravenous ketorolac and patient-controlled morphine following lower abdominal surgery. J Clin Anesth 1995; 7:103–108.
78. Liu J, Ding Y, White PF, et al. Effects of ketorolac on postoperative analgesia and ventilatory function after laparoscopic cholecystectomy. Anesth Analg 1993;76:1061–1066.
79. Fricke JJ, Angelocci D, Fox K, et al. Comparison of the efficacy and safety of ketorolac and meperidine in the relief of dental pain. J Clin Pharmacol 1992;32:376–384.
80. Dueholm S, Forrest M, Hjorts E, Lemvigh E. Pain relief following herniotomy: a double blind randomized comparison between naproxen and placebo. Acta Anaesth Scand 1989;33:391–394.
81. McLoughlin C, McKinney MS, Fee JPH, Boules Z. Diclofenac for day-care arthroscopy surgery: comparison with standard opioid therapy. Br J Anaesth 1990;65:620–623.
82. Grass JA, Sakima NT, Valley M, et al. Assessment of ketorolac as an adjuvant to fentanyl patient-controlled epidural analgesia after radical retropubic prostatectomy [see comments]. Anesthesiology 1993;78:642–648.
83. Mok MS, Tzeng JI. Intramuscular ketorolac enhances the analgesic effect of low dose epidural morphine [Abstract]. Anesth Analg 1993;76 (suppl 2S):S269.
84. Sun H-L, Wu C-C, Lin M-S, et al. Combination of low-dose epidural morphine and intramuscular diclofenac sodium in postcesarean analgesia. Anesth Analg 1992;75:64–68.
85. Gwirtz KH, Helvie JE, Young JV, Li W. Ketorolac enhances intrathecal analgesia after major surgery. Anesth Rev 1993; 20:222–228.
86. Gershon RY, Manning-Williams D, Zikowski DM, Westbrook HD. Prophylactic intravenous ketorolac tromethamine and intrathecal fentanyl for post-partum tubal ligation pain [Abstract]. Anesth Analg 1993;76 (suppl 2S):A1014.
87. Yee MK, Evans WD, Facey PE, et al. Gastric emptying and small bowel transit in male volunteers after IM ketorolac and morphine. Br J Anaesth 1991;67:426–431.
88. Parker RK, Holtmann B, Smith I, White PF. Use of ketorolac after lower abdominal surgery: effect on analgesic requirement and surgical outcome. Anesthesiology 1994;80:6–12.
89. Ready LB, Brown CR, Stahlgren LH, et al. Evaluation of intravenous ketorolac administered by bolus or infusion for treatment of postoperative pain: a double-blind, placebo-controlled, multicenter study. Anesthesiology 1994;80:1277–1286.
90. Krimmer H, Bullingham RES, Lloyd J, Bruch HP. Effects on biliary tract pressure in humans of intravenous ketorolac tromethamine compared with morphine and placebo. Anesth Analg 1992;75:204–207.
91. Smith I, Shively RA, White PF. Effects of ketorolac and bupivacaine on recovery after outpatient arthroscopy. Anesth Analg 1992;75:208–212.

92. Mogensen T, Vegger P, Jonsson T, et al. Systemic piroxicam as an adjunct to combined epidural bupivicaine and morphine for postoperative pain relief: a double blind study. Anesth Analg 1992;74:366–370.
93. Bigler D, M ller J, Kamp-Jensen M, et al. Effect of piroxicam in addition to continuous thoracic epidural bupivicaine and morphine on postoperative pain and lung function after thoracotomy. Acta Anaesth Scand 1992;36:647–650.
94. Reuben SS, Connelly NR. Postoperative analgesia for outpatient arthroscopic knee surgery with intraarticular bupivacaine and ketorolac. Anesth Analg 1995;80:1154–1157.
95. Reuben SS, Steinberg RB, Kreitzer JM, Duprat KM. Intravenous regional anesthesia using lidocaine and ketorolac. Anesth Analg 1995;81:110–113.
96. Cohen IT, Latta K, Weiner ES, Davis PJ. A study of ketorolac for intraoperative and postoperative analgesia for herniorrhaphy in children [Abstract]. Anesth Analg 1993;76 (suppl 2S):S50.
97. Moores MA, Wandless JG, Fell D. Paediatric postoperative analgesia: a comparison of rectal diclofenac with caudal bupivicaine after inguinal herniotomy. Anaesthesia 1990;45:156–158.
98. Watcha MF, Jones MB, Lagueruela RG, et al. Comparison of ketorolac and morphine as adjuvants during pediatric surgery [see comments]. Anesthesiology 1992;76:368–372.
99. Munro HM, Riegger LQ, Reynolds PI, et al. Comparison of the analgesic and emetic properties of ketorolac and morphine for paediatric outpatient strabismus surgery. Br J Anaesth 1994; 72:624–628.
100. Desparmet JF, MacArthur C, MacArthur A, Grillas B. Pain and vomiting after tonsillectomy in children: a comparison of intraoperative ketorolac and fentanyl. Anesthesiology 1993; 79:A1194.
101. Gunter JB, Barughese AM, Harrington JF, et al. Recovery and complications after tonsillectomy in children: a comparison of ketorolac and morphine. Anesth Analg 1995;81:1136–1141.
102. Houck CS, Wilder RT, McDermott J, Berde CB. Intravenous ketorolac in children following surgery: safety and cost savings using a unit dosing system [Abstract]. Anesthesiology 1993; 79:A1137.
103. Bean JD, Hunt R. Effects of ketorolac on postoperative analgesia and bleeding time in children [Abstract]. Anesthesiology 1993; 79:A1190.
104. Bone ME, Fell D. A comparison of rectal diclofenac with intramuscular papaveretum or placebo for pain relief following tonsillectomy. Anaesthesia 1988;43:277–280.
105. Watters CH, Patterson CC, Mathews HML, Campbell W. Diclofenac for post-tonsillectomy pain in chidren. Anaesthesia 1988;43:641–643.
106. Maunuksela E-L, Ryhänen P, Janhunen L. Efficacy of rectal ibuprofen in controlling postoperative pain in children. Can J Anaesth 1992;39:226–230.
107. Committee on Safety of Medicine. Current problems in pharmacovigilance. Med Control Agency 1993;19:5–6.
108. Choo V, Lewis S. Ketorolac doses reduced [News]. Lancet 1993; 342:8836.
109. Lewis S. Ketorolac in Europe. Lancet 1994;343:784.
110. Whelton A, Stout RL, Spilman PS, Klassen DK. Renal effects of ibuprofen, piroxicam and sulindac in patients with asymptomatic renal failure. Ann Intern Med 1990;112:568–576.
111. Passmore AP, Copeland S, Johnston GD. The effects of ibuprofen and indomethacin on renal function in the presence and absence of furosemide in healthy volunteers on a restricted sodium diet. Br J Clin Pharmacol 1990;29:311–319.
112. Clive DM, Stoff JS. Renal syndromes associated with nonsteroidal antiinflammatory drugs. N Engl J Med 1984;310:563–572.
113. Schoch PH, Ranno A, North DS. Acute renal failure in an elderly woman following intramuscular ketorolac administration. Ann Pharmacother 1992;26:1233–1236.
114. Pearce CJ, Gonzalez FM, Wallin JD. Renal failure and hyperkalemia associated with ketorolac tromethamine. Arch Intern Med 1993;153:1000–1002.
115. Murray RP, Watson RC. Acute renal failure and gastrointestinal bleed associated with postoperative toradol and vancomycin. Orthopedics 1993;16:1361–1363.
116. Orme ML. Nonsteroidal anti-inflammatory drugs and the kidneys. Br Med J 1986;292:1621–1622.
117. Kenny GNC. Ketorolac trometamol: a new non-opioid analgesic. Br J Anaesth 1990;65:445–447.
118. Aitken HA, Burns JW, McArdle CS, Kenny GN. Effects of ketorolac trometamol on renal function. Br J Anaesth 1992;68:481–485.
119. Engel C, Lund B, Kristensen SS, et al. Indomethacin as an analgesic after hysterectomy. Acta Anaesthesiol Scand 1989; 33:498–501.
120. Bricker SRW, Savage ME, Kenny GNC. Perioperative blood loss and nonsteroidal anti-inflammatory drugs. Eur J Anaesthesiol 1987;4:429–434.
121. Fragen RJ, Stulberg SD, Wixson R, et al. Effect of ketorolac tromethamine on bleeding and on requirements for analgesia after total knee arthroplasty. J Bone Joint Surg Am 1995;77:998–1002.
122. Koenig HM, Cunningham FE, Andrews C, et al. The effect of ketorolac vs placebo on thrombolelastogram in patients undergoing surgery [Abstract]. Anesth Analg 1994;78:S210.
123. Spowart K, Greer TA, McLaren M, et al. Haemostatic effects of ketorolac with and without concomitant heparin in normal volunteers. Thromb Haemost 1988;60:382–386.
124. Garcha IS, Bostwick J. Postoperative hematomas associated with Toradol (Letter). Plast Reconstr Surg 1991;88:19–20.
125. Davis RE, Cohen JI, Robinson JE, et al. Ketorolac (Toradol) and acute random-pattern skin flap survival in rat. Arch Otolaryngol Head Neck Surg 1995;121:673–677.
126. Concannon MJ, Meng L, Welsh CF, Puckett CL. Inhibition of perioperative platelet aggregation using Toradol (ketorolac). Ann Plast Surg 1993;30:264–266.
127. Buckley RC, Davidson SF, Das SK. Effects of ketorolac tromethamine (Toradol) on a functional model of microvascular thrombosis [see comments]. Br J Plast Surg 1993;46:296–299.
128. Fleming BM, Coombs DW. Bleeding diathesis after perioperative ketorolac [Letter] [see comments]. Anesth Analg 1991; 73:235.
129. McCann KJ, Irish J. Postoperative gastrointestinal bleeding: a case report involving a non-steroidal anti-inflammatory drug. J Can Dent Assoc 1994;60:124–128.
130. O'Hara DA. Bleeding diathesis after perioperative ketorolac (Letter). Anesth Analg 1992;74:167–168.
131. Horswell JL. Bleeding diathesis after perioperative ketorolac (Letter). Anesth Analg 1992;74:168–169.
132. Wolfe PA, Polhamus CD, Kubik C, et al. Giant duodenal ulcers associated with the postoperative use of ketorolac: report of three cases. Am J Gastroenterol 1994;89:1110–1111.
133. Camu F, Van OL, Bullingham R, Lloyd J. Hemodynamic effects of two intravenous doses of ketorolac tromethamine compared with morphine. Pharmacotherapy 1990;10:122–126.
134. Camu F, Van LC, Lauwers MH. Cardiovascular risks and benefits of perioperative nonsteroidal anti-inflammatory drug treatment. Drugs 1992;5:42–51.

13 Local Anesthetics

Robert J. McCarthy and Kenneth J. Tuman

HISTORY

Local anesthetics are drugs that temporarily block neural conduction along an axon in a predictable and reversible manner. The first local anesthetic discovered was cocaine, an alkaloid that occurs naturally in the shrub *Erythroxylon coca*; the leaves of the coca plant are chewed by inhabitants of the Peruvian highlands to relieve fatigue and to obtain a feeling of well-being. The native Peruvians have also found that this effect is intensified if the leaves of the plant are mixed with a dash of lime, which aids in the extraction of the alkaloid; this approach continues to have clinical application (1).

After the isolation of cocaine by Niemann in 1860, much interest was generated in the clinical application of this agent (2). Initially used as a stimulant, cocaine was reported to be beneficial for the treatment of consumption, asthma, and psychosis, as well as opium and alcohol withdrawal. Carl Koller obtained crystalline cocaine from Sigmund Freud, who had extensively investigated its properties, and studied its use as a local ophthalmologic anesthetic agent (3, 4). Shortly after the clinical introduction of cocaine as a local anesthetic for ophthalmologic procedures in 1884, physicians began to recognize the ability of this agent to produce local antinociception in other tissues. Aided by the advent of the hypodermic syringe, cocaine-induced local infiltration nerve blockade for minor surgical procedures was reported by Halsted 1 year after Koller's discovery (5, 6). In the same year, cocaine-induced epidural anesthesia was described by Corning, and the ability of this drug to produce subarachnoid block was reported by Bier in 1899 (7, 8). Following introduction into clinical practice, use of cocaine in various tonic and elixir forms was widespread until its physical and social hazards were recognized, when the search began for a less toxic substitute (1). After elucidation of the chemical structure of cocaine, other synthetic benzoic acid esters including benzocaine (1890), procaine (1905), tetracaine (1930) and 2-chloroprocaine (1955) were introduced into clinical practice (9).

Dibucaine, the first aminoamide local anesthetic, was introduced in 1929, and in 1943 Lofgren discovered lidocaine, the first synthetic aminoacyl amide-linked local anesthetic from a series of aniline derivatives (10). This represented a major step leading to the development and introduction of other local anesthetics with amide linkages including mepivacaine (1957), prilocaine (1960), bupivacaine (1963), etidocaine (1972), and most recently, ropivacaine (9). Although the differences in chemical structure between the amide- and ester-linked local anesthetics determines their pharmacokinetic and pharmacodynamic properties, the molecular basis of local anesthetic action has only recently been elucidated.

MECHANISM OF ACTION

In the resting state, neural membranes are 25 to 30 times more permeable to potassium (K^+) than sodium (Na^+) and are maintained at ionic disequilibrium by the active pumping of Na^+ ions out of the cell and K^+ into the cell by the energy-dependent activity of the membrane-bound enzyme Na^+-K^+ adenosine triphosphatase (ATPase). The ionic gradient created by concentrating K^+ inside the cell is counterbalanced by membrane impermeable anions that impart a net negative charge to membrane interior. The electrical potential of the cell, created by this K^+ gradient, is maintained at −40 to −80 mV (near the K^+ equilibrium potential) by the active exchange of three Na^+ ions for two K^+ ions and the voltage independent leak of K^+ or chloride (Cl^-) ions.

During depolarization, the voltage change across the membrane occurs rapidly, up to 500 volts per second. To achieve such a high ionic flux, ions must move at rates approximating 100,000,000 ions per second, which exceeds by severalfold the maximum turnover rates of the fastest enzyme systems. The surface of plasma membranes including neural cells is formed by a bilayer phospholipid matrix that is relatively impermeable to ion passage, and conformational changes occurring in the structure of the cell membrane during the process of depolarization facilitate the movement of these ions. Transmembrane ionophores, frequently referred to as ion channels, are formed by one or more glycoprotein subunits, probably in an α-helical conformation, and are oriented in the membrane by attachment to long-chain fatty acids (11-13) (Fig. 13-1). The transmembrane ionophores are selective for specific ions, with Na^+ channels 20 times more permeable to Na^+ than K^+, whereas K^+ ionophores are 100 times more selective for K^+ than Na^+ (14, 15). During depolarization, the channels that faciliate passage of Na^+ are briefly opened and then closed, allowing for rapid changes in transmembrane potential and propagation of an impulse along the nerve axon (16).

The permeability of the channel is controlled by a gating mechanism, and these channels may exist in resting (closed), open (permeable), or inactive (closed) conformation (17, 18). Activation of resting channels can occur as a result of ion current flow (voltage gating), receptor ligand binding (chemical gating), phosphorylation of gating proteins, or mechanical forces resulting from channel cytoskeleton interactions (Fig. 13-2). In addition to neural impulse propagation, this process also results in the opening of outward-flowing K^+ channels that serve to restore electrical neutrality (19). The Na^+ channels remain in the open conformation for only a brief period. After closing, they may again reopen briefly or may change conformation and

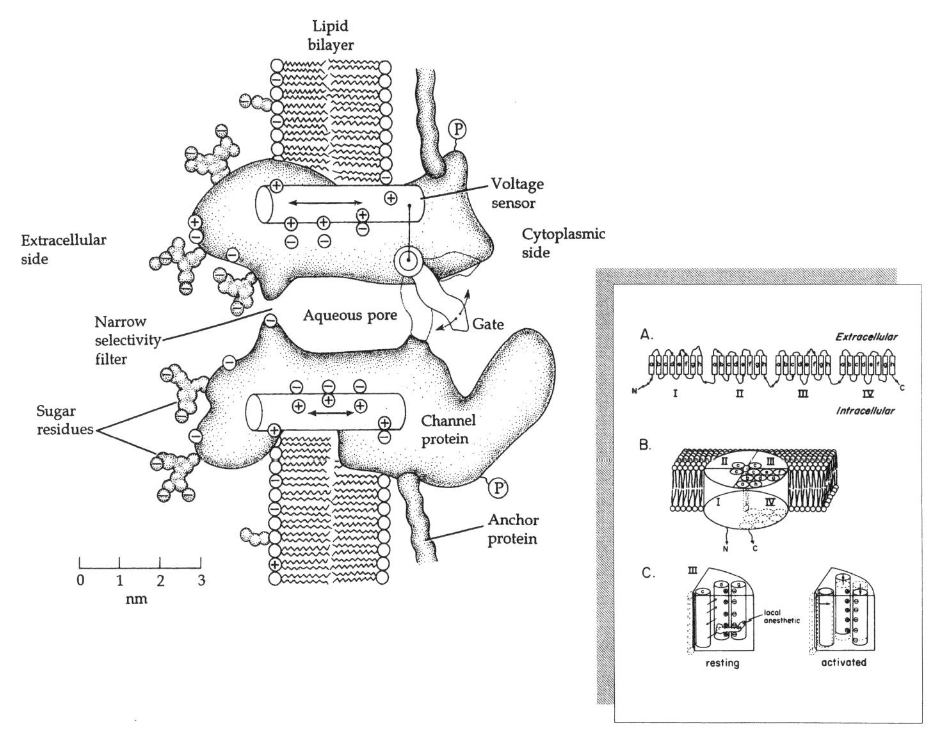

FIGURE 13-1. Hypothesized model of an ion channel. The transmembrane ionophore is attached to the bilayer lipid matrix of the cell membrane as well as to other membrane proteins. Functional regions of the channel include the selectivity filter, which limits ion entry based on size and hydration status, the gate that opens the channel to allow ion flow, and the sensor that responds to energy change and controls the opening of the gate. (From Hille B. Ionic channels of excitable membranes. 2nd ed. Sunderland, MA: Sinauer, 1992.) The inset details a model of the mechanism by which local anesthetics interact with the channel. A, The amino acid sequences in an α-helical structure span the membrane and are repeated in each of four domains I to IV. B, Six to eight of these units are arranged such that the polar edges of the "c" subunits come together to form the pore lining. C, A view of the third quadrant depicts the conformational changes that may accompany depolarization. In the resting conformation, helices d and g are held in ionic balance by arranging their outer surfaces with oppositely charged moieties. During depolarization, helix g is pulled in, pushing helix d out, which causes the c helices in the four quadrants to separate and open the channel. Local anesthetics likely interact with these gating helices near the inner surface of the cell, thereby preventing or slowing the conformational changes that occur during depolarization. (Inset from Butterworth JF, Strichartz GR. Molecular mechanisms of local anesthesia: a review. Anesthesiology 1990;72:711–734.)

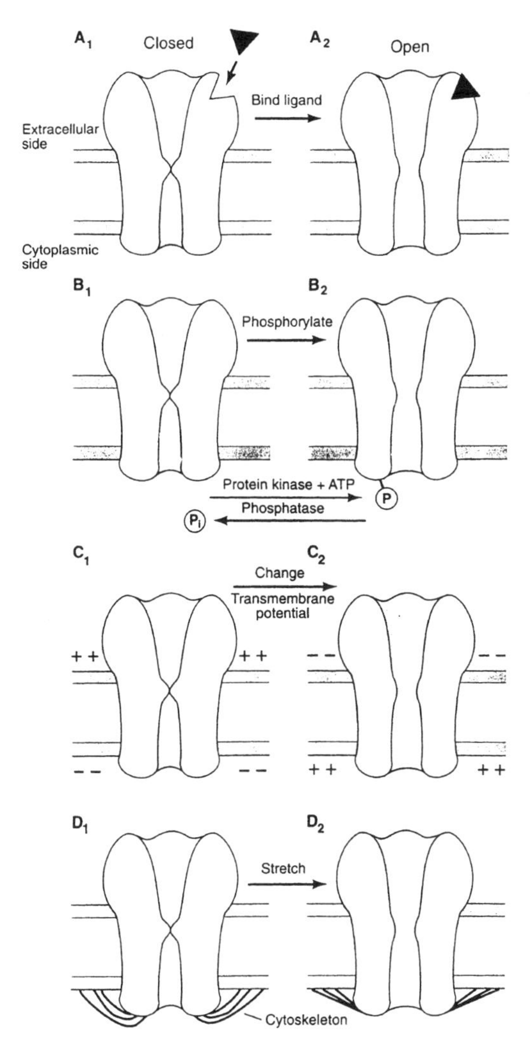

FIGURE 13-2. Permeability of ion channels is mediated by gating mechanisms controlled by several types of stimuli. A, Receptor ligand binding can result in activation of resting channels, with the energy from ligand binding driving the gating to an open state. B, Protein phosphorylation and dephosphorylation with the subsequent transfer of high-energy phosphate (P) result in the opening and closing of some channels. C, Changes in electrical potential difference across membranes can modulate channel opening and closing for channels such as the Na^+ channel where local anesthetics are active. D, Pressure or stretch can activate some channels utilizing energy derived from mechanical perturbations of the membrane. (From Siegelbaum SA, Koester J. Ion channels. In: Kandel ER, Schwartz JH, Jessell TM, eds. Principles of neural science. 3rd ed. New York: Elsevier, 1991:66–94.)

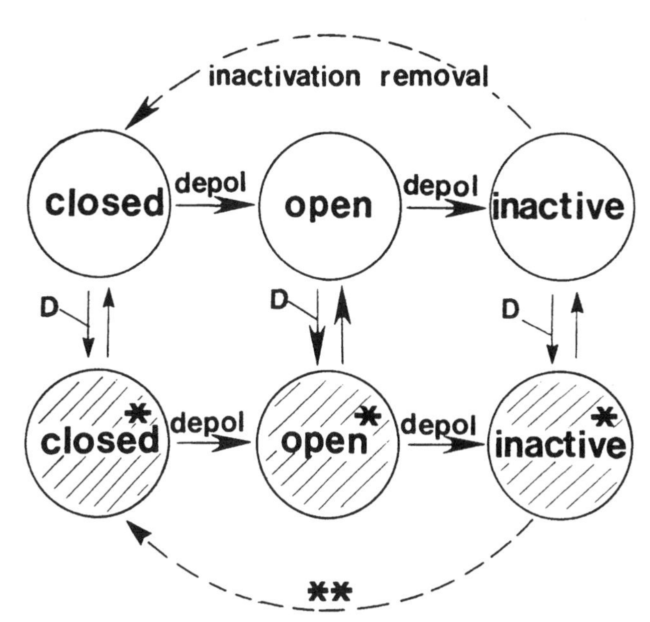

FIGURE 13-3. Diagram of modulated receptor mechanism of local anesthetic action. Following depolarization (depol), the sodium channel cycles from a closed to open state, then into an inactive conformation (upper circles). Drug can bind to each state of the channel, but affinity is the lowest for the resting closed conformation. When bound by drug (asterisk, shaded circles), channel voltage-dependent kinetics are altered as a result of drug effect on channel gating mechanisms. Recovery of channel from state of inactivation is rapid (tenths of milliseconds) in the absence of bound drug; however, with drug block, recovery may be delayed and may require additional gating or unblocking steps before returning to resting conformation. (From Courtney KR. Local anesthetics. Int Anesthesiol Clin 1988;26:239–247.)

become inactive before returning to the resting (closed) state (20, 21) (Fig. 13-3). In the inactive conformational state, they can only be reopened by a supramaximal stimulus.

Local anesthetics block the conduction of neural impulses by inhibiting the conformational change necessary for Na^+ channel activation and the movement of Na^+ through the cell membrane (22). This effect, which occurs even at low impulse conduction rates (tonic block), is intensified as the depolarization rate of the nerve is increased (phasic block), either as a result of recruitment of additional channels for drug binding or because channel conformations during depolarization result in greater drug affinity (23-25) or better drug receptor access (26, 27). Although the exact mechanism of channel inhibition has yet to be elucidated, data suggest that local anesthetics inhibit multiple conformational states of the ion channel (22, 25). In addition to altering the usual sequence of conformational changes in Na^+ channels that occur during membrane depolarization, local anesthetics also modify channel kinetics, resulting in an increased state of channel inactivation (28, 29). These effects are likely a result of local anesthetic interference with the gating mechanism that controls the conformational kinetics of the Na^+ channel (18, 30). Once activation occurs, however, local anesthetics have little influence on the Na^+ flux through open channels (22).

Although no single site of local anesthetic action has been identified, evidence points to a single binding region for tertiary amine local anesthetics (22, 31), with a second lower affinity site for neutral compounds such as benzocaine (32, 33). The local anesthetic binding region can accommodate many amphipathic bases and is not rigidly structurally specific, although it has some molecular size and stereospecificity requirements. Hydrophobic interactions appear to be involved in local anesthetic binding to Na^+ channels in their closed state (34). Although the exact location of this binding site is undefined, the site appears to be located near the inner portion of the membrane (35) and contains two hydrophobic binding domains (36, 37), which can accommodate up to a 12-hydrocarbon chain. Dissociation of large molecules from the binding site is known to be hindered in certain conformational states of the ion channel, so molecular size in conjunction with other factors such as the degree of lipophilicity and ionization influence the neurophysiologic actions of local anesthetics (38). A proposed model of the molecular mechanisms of local anesthetic action is depicted in Figure 13-1.

Local anesthetics affect other membrane proteins and enzymes including adenylyl cyclase (39, 40), guanylate cyclase (41), calmodulin-sensitive proteins (42, 43), Na^+-K^+ ATPase (44), and calcium-magnesium (Ca^{2+}-Mg^{2+}) ATPase (45), in addition to their effects on voltage-dependent Na^+ channels. Cytoplasmic enzymes such as phospholipase A_2, phospholipase C, and secondary messenger systems are also directly or indirectly inhibited by local anesthetics (46, 47). Local anesthetics inhibit the actions of the nicotinic acetylcholine receptor (nAChR), a prototypical postsynaptic receptor involved in chemical transmission at the neuromuscular junction (48, 49), and they also inhibit presynaptic nerve transmission at the spinal cord level. Local anesthetics are likely to produce similar inhibition at other chemically gated ion channels. Local anesthetic inhibition of Ca^{2+} and K^+ currents in myocardial tissues has been demonstrated (50, 51), and an external site for local anesthetic binding in myocardial tissue has been identified (52). The nonspecific nature of local anesthetic actions confers clinically useful properties as well as contributes to their toxicity.

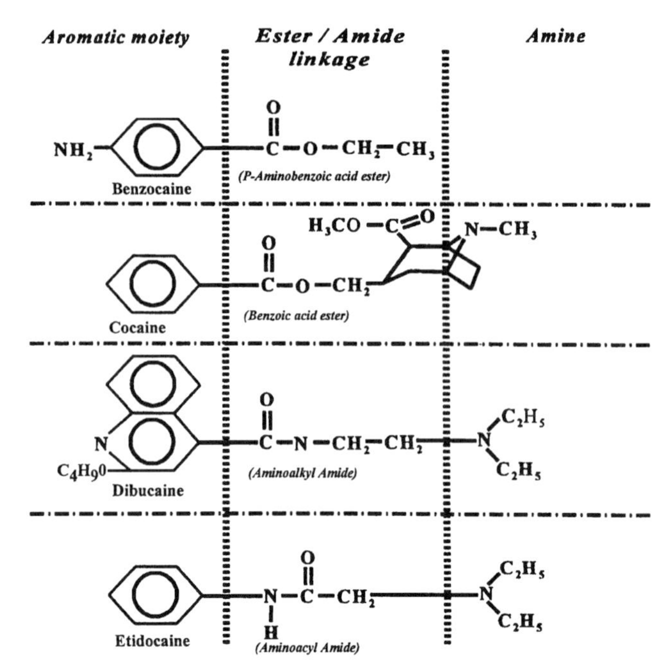

FIGURE 13-4. Representative structures of aminoester and aminoamide local anesthetics illustating the three fundamental structural molecular components. Most local anesthetics consist of an amine moiety connected to an aromatic ring of varying complexity by either ester or amide intermediate linkage. Benzocaine lacks an amino terminus, resulting in essentially no ionization at physiologic pH. Structures of other local anesthetics are displayed in Figure 13-6.

PHYSICOCHEMICAL PROPERTIES

Local anesthetics are a relatively homogeneous group of compounds in terms of both physical behavior and chemical structure. Most local anesthetics are weakly basic tertiary amines containing three fundamental structural molecular components. Clinically useful agents typically consist of an amine moiety connected to an aromatic ring of varying complexity by either an ester or an amide intermediate linkage (Fig. 13-4). The classification of local anesthetics into those containing ester versus amide linkages is important primarily in differentiating their mode of metabolism. Aminoesters (e.g., cocaine, procaine, tetracaine, and chloroprocaine) possess an ester linkage between the benzene ring and the intermediate chain that can be metabolized by ester hydrolysis, primarily in the plasma by the enzyme pseudocholinesterase, whereas aminoamides (e.g., lidocaine, mepivacaine, prilocaine, bupivacaine, etidocaine, and ropivacaine) have an amide link between the benzene ring and the intermediate chain and are degraded mainly in the liver by microsomal enzymes.

Alteration of any segment of the molecular structure of either aminoamides or aminoesters results in modification of protein-binding characteristics, potency, duration of action, rapidity of onset, negative logarithm of the acid ionization constant (pKa), and lipid and water distribution (Table 13-1). Increasing the molecular weight of local anesthetics tends to enhance potency and duration of action, but activity is diminished as molecular size further increases. Although a receptor specific for local anesthetics has not been identified, the location of their interaction within the ion channel places some structural limitations on drugs that can act as local anesthetics. Size constraints therefore result in a cluster of molecular weights for the clinically available local anesthetics between 200 and 300 daltons. The typical local anesthetic molecule is amphipathic, with the polar amine end of these molecules being hydrophilic and conferring water solubility as well as protein-binding affinity. Greater protein-binding capacity occurs with the substitution of large polar radicals to the amine end or with the addition of larger chemical radicals to the aromatic end of the local anesthetic molecule, resulting in prolongation of the duration of action. In the ester series, the addition of a butyl group

TABLE 13-1. Physiochemical Properties of Local Anesthetic Agents

Agent	Molecular Weight (daltons)	pKa (25° C)	Percentage of Drug in Base Form at pH = 7.0 (%)	pH = 7.4 (%)	pH = 7.8 (%)	Partition Coefficient*	Protein Binding (%)	Relative Potency†	Relative Latency†	Relative Duration†
Esters										
Procaine	236	8.9	1.2	3.1	7.4	0.02	5.8‡	1	1	1
2-Chloroprocaine	271	8.7	2.0	4.8	11.2	0.14	—	4	2	0.75
Tetracaine	264	8.4	3.8	9.1	20.1	4.1	70–76‡	16	0.8	8
Amides										
Lidocaine	234	7.9	11.2	24.0	44.3	2.9	58–75§	4	0.8	1.5
Prilocaine	220	7.6	20.1	38.7	61.3	0.9	~55§	3	1	1.5
Mepivacaine	246	7.6	20.1	38.7	61.3	0.8	68–84§	2	1	1.5
Ropivacaine	274	8.1	7.4	16.6	33.4	6.1	~92‖	N/A	N/A	N/A
Bupivacaine	288	8.1	7.4	16.6	33.4	28	88–96§	16	0.6	8
Etidocaine	276	7.7	16.6	33.4	55.7	141	94§	16	0.4	8

*N-heptane/water pH = 7.4.
†Relative properties determined in rat sciatic nerve.
‡Nerve homogenate binding.
§Human plasma.
‖Sheep plasma.
N/A, Comparable data not available.

to the aromatic ring of procaine results in 10-fold greater protein binding and a 3- to 4-fold greater duration of action for the homologue tetracaine. In the amide series, the replacement of an ethyl group by a propyl group at the amine end of lidocaine increases protein binding from 65% to greater than 90% for etidocaine, in conjunction with near doubling of anesthetic duration. The amide local anesthetics of the pipecolyl xylidide (PPX) class such as mepivacaine, ropivacaine, and bupivacaine all contain a heterocyclic amine differing in their n-substitution by a methyl, propyl, or butyl group, respectively. Bupivacaine has greater protein binding and twice the duration of action as its homologue mepivacaine, solely related to replacement of a methyl group with a butyl group on the amine moiety (9). The protein binding of the PPX class of local anesthetics is also influenced by the presence of a chiral carbon atom that confers stereospecificity to these molecules. R(+) bupivacaine has greater plasma protein binding than its S(−) enantiomer (53), whereas the R(+) form of mepivacaine has more rapid clearance and a smaller volume of distribution than its S(−) stereoisomer (54), perhaps because of similar stereospecific differences in protein binding. In addition, stereochemistry is an important determinant of the toxicity of the PPX agents, as discussed later in this chapter.

Alteration of the aromatic moiety, the amine group, and, to a lesser extent, the intermediate chain can influence lipophilicity and the ability to traverse lipid membranes encountered in neural tissues, which, in turn, affect intrinsic anesthetic potency (see Table 13-1). For example, among the amide compounds, the addition of a butyl group to the terminal amine of mepivacaine results in the formation of bupivacaine, which is more than 30 times more lipid soluble and 4 times more potent than mepivacaine (55). The intermediate length of ropivacaine's side chain (propyl) results in lipid solubility and potency somewhat less than those of bupivacaine. Similarly, etidocaine differs from lidocaine by the addition of an ethyl group at the α carbon in the intermediate chain as well as the substitution of a propyl group for an ethyl group at the amine end. These relatively minor structural alterations result in etidocaine's possessing a 50-fold greater lipophilicity and a 4-fold greater anesthetic potency than lidocaine (56). In the ester series, the addition of a butyl group to the aromatic ring of procaine results in tetracaine, which has a lipid:water partition coefficient more than 125 times that of procaine and a 4-fold greater potency (56).

Tertiary amine bases are poorly soluble in water and are chemically unstable, and most local anesthetics are produced commercially as their salts with strong acids, which are generally highly soluble and stable. In aqueous solution, the salt ionizes:

$$R - N + HCL \leftrightharpoons RNA^{+} + CL^{-}$$

The protonated or charged form is capable of donating its proton, and local anesthetics exist in reversible equilibrium with a weak base form:

$$R - NH^{+} \leftrightharpoons H^{+} + R - N$$

(or more simply $BH^{+} \leftrightharpoons B + H^{+}$)

The equilibrium constant (Ka) for this reaction is

$$Ka = [B][H^{+}]/[BH^{+}]$$

so

$$pKa = pH + Log_{10}\,[BH^{+}]/[B]$$

The pKa is thus the pH at which the charged and uncharged forms of the local anesthetic occur in equal concentrations. The ratio of the concentration of the charged, protonated cationic form of a local anesthetic $[BH^+]$ to the concentration of the local anesthetic in free base or uncharged form [B] in a solution can be calculated if the pH and pKa are known because

$$[BH^+]/[B] = 10^{(pKa - pH)}$$

The fraction of a local anesthetic that is in the protonated form can therefore be readily determined because

$$[BH^+]/\{[B]+[BH^+]\} = 10^{(pKa - pH)}/\{1 + 10^{(pKa - pH)}\}$$

The base form of the local anesthetic molecule is believed to traverse lipid neural tissues most readily and thereby allow the local anesthetic molecule to reach the site of action at the ion channel, so lower pKa and higher pH in solution and greater lipid solubility are associated with a more rapid onset of action. Agents such as mepivacaine and lidocaine with lower pKa values (7.6 to 7.9) and greater fractions of free base at physiologic pH (~30%) tend to have more rapid onset of action than agents such as bupivacaine or tetracaine with higher pKa values (8.1 to 8.4) and less available free base (~15%) (see Table 13-1). Consistent with the requirement for aqueous solubility and sufficient lipophilicity to traverse the hydrophobic neural tissues, most clinically useful local anesthetics have a dissociation constant (pKa) in the 7.5 to 9.0 range, permitting both molecular forms to coexist at physiologic pH.

Although desheathed nerves are more readily blocked by acidic anesthetic solutions that contain relatively greater proportions of the cationic form (BH^+), alkaline anesthetic solutions containing relatively greater fractions of the free base (B) tend to be more active in producing neural blockade in preparations with an intact epineurium (57, 58). This finding has long provided a scientific rationale for the clinical practice of alkalinizing local anesthetic solutions to speed onset of action by increasing the proportion of free base available to penetrate lipophilic neural structures. Commonly used preparations of local anesthetics such as lidocaine are often commercially supplied at a pH as low as 6.5, resulting in 95% ionization and only 5% free base (59). When a small amount of sodium bicarbonate ($NaHCO_3$) is added to increase the pH of the solution, however, the fraction of uncharged form significantly increases (at a pH of 8.0, a lidocaine solution contains 60% available free base). Alkalization of local anesthetics in clinical practice is limited by the relative insolubility of the free base form of some local anesthetic agents. For example, although clinicians commonly add 1 mEq (~1 ml) of $NaHCO_3$ to 10 ml lidocaine to improve speed of onset, similar practice results in precipitation of the less soluble bupivacaine free base.

The differential effects of acidic and alkaline solutions of local anesthetics on sheathed versus desheathed nerves have similarly suggested a basis for the traditional view that the protonated form of the molecule is the "active" form necessary for activity at the ion channel, whereas the more lipophilic uncharged free base form is important for diffusing to the site of action. The pharmacologic characteristics of benzocaine, however, suggest that both charged and uncharged forms of the local anesthetic molecule may be the "active" moieties that can block Na^+ channels and interrupt neural conduction. Benzocaine lacks the amino-terminus of procaine, its parent compound, and is highly lipid soluble and not ionizable. Nonetheless, it is highly effective as a local anesthetic despite the absence of a charged moiety, consistent with the concept that the aliphatic portion of the molecule is important for local anesthetic effect.

NEUROANATOMIC FACTORS INFLUENCING LOCAL ANESTHETIC BLOCKADE

Although local anesthetics act similarly to inhibit neural conduction and have remarkably homogeneous chemical structures, many factors influence the onset, extent, and duration of neural blockade. The dynamics of neural blockade are influenced by the interaction of the physical characteristics of the neural structures and the previously discussed pharmacologic properties of the specific agents that determine the absorption, diffusion, and extent of tissue binding of local anesthetics. The minimum blocking concentration of a local anesthetic (C_m) sufficient to suppress impulse conduction after a specified period is similar for all nerve fibers, independent of fiber diameter. The traditional concept that fiber diameter was a primary determinant of the effectiveness of local anesthetics at a specified concentration had its basis in a series of studies demonstrating that conduction block was slower to develop and required greater concentrations of local anesthetic in thicker fibers (60-63).

Anesthesiologists now appreciate that nerve length is the critical factor, and blockade of neural impulses depends on the ability of local anesthetics to block at least three nodes of Ranvier (64). Thicker nerve fibers have broader internodal distances, and the reduced number of nodes per exposure length makes large nerves harder to block. Therefore, when local anesthetic is applied in close proximity to *isolated* fibers of larger diameter, such as those responsible for motor activity, touch, and pressure, concentrations much greater than the C_m are required to achieve a similar reduction in impulse conduction than in isolated small nerve fibers, which typically conduct impulses for pain, temperature, and autonomic activity and which are blocked faster and at lower concentrations. These differences have clinical relevance to the concept of differential block of autonomic, sensory, and motor fibers.

The clinical situation most closely approximating the application of local anesthetics to isolated nerves is central neuraxial blockade, especially spinal anesthesia. In this setting, the differential functional blockade of neural fibers occurs in a fashion predicted from studies in isolated nerves, with sympathetic blockade occurring first, followed by sensory and then motor blockade after induction of spinal anesthesia. Regression of local anesthetic spinal conduction blockade is accompanied by functional recovery of these fibers in the reverse order. In addition, for a specified local anesthetic concentration, a transition phase typically occurs in which antinociceptive (small-diameter) fibers are blocked while touch and motor functions modulated by thick fibers are essentially intact. Although this pattern of onset and regression of differential sensory and motor nerve block is observed with most clinically available local anesthetics, etidocaine results in far less separation of motor and sensory effects, even when this agent is used for central neuraxial blockade (65).

In contrast to the differential blockade elicited by the diffusion of local anesthetics toward isolated nerve fibers, the structure of large peripheral nerves dramatically alters the characteristics of local anesthetic differential blockade. After injection around a peripheral nerve, local anesthetic molecules not only diffuse into surrounding tissues, but also move down a concentration gradient, diffusing inward toward the nerve core from the extraneuronal site of injection (Fig. 13-5). The net result of this diffusion is gradual dilution of the local anesthetic concentration as the drug molecules penetrate the nerve radially toward the central core. Onset of neural blockade is thus influenced not only by perineural tissue uptake, but also by the time required for the drug to diffuse to different sites within the nerve bundle. Because axons in the outer portions of peripheral nerve bundles supplying the body's limbs typically innervate the proximal portion of the extremity and those in the nerve's core innervate the distal extremity, onset of neural blockade does not follow dermatomal patterns as with central neuraxial block. In addition to this spatial discrepancy, the sequence of onset of sensory and motor block is the reverse of that predicted from fiber size. Hence, during brachial plexus block, motor paresis precedes sensory block because the motor innervation of the proximal arm courses through the mantle layers of the axillary portion of the brachial plexus, whereas the sensory innervation to the arm resides in the core portion of this nerve trunk. This example illustrates that anatomic factors can be exceedingly important in determining the clinical effects observed after extraneural injections of local anesthetics.

Intravenous injection of local anesthetics can effectively produce regional anesthesia when these agents are injected into a vascularly isolated limb after emptying the venous system with a compression bandage, and neural diffusion gradients are also important in this application of local anesthetics. Initial onset of cutaneous block after intravenous regional anesthesia is rapid and is probably related to the initial delivery of local anesthetic to cutaneous nerve endings and small nerve branches (66, 67). Simultaneously, local anesthetic molecules traverse the blood vessels supplying the larger nerve trunks that tend to be concentrated at the central core of the peripheral nerve bundles (67). Therefore, the local anesthetic diffusion gradient proceeds from the central core to the external mantle, so the gradient of analgesia proceeds from distal to proximal limb structures and occurs in a similar time frame to that required for extraneurally injected local anesthetics.

PHARMACOKINETIC PROPERTIES OF LOCAL ANESTHETIC AGENTS

The pharmacokinetics of the local anesthetics depends primarily on physical characteristics including protein

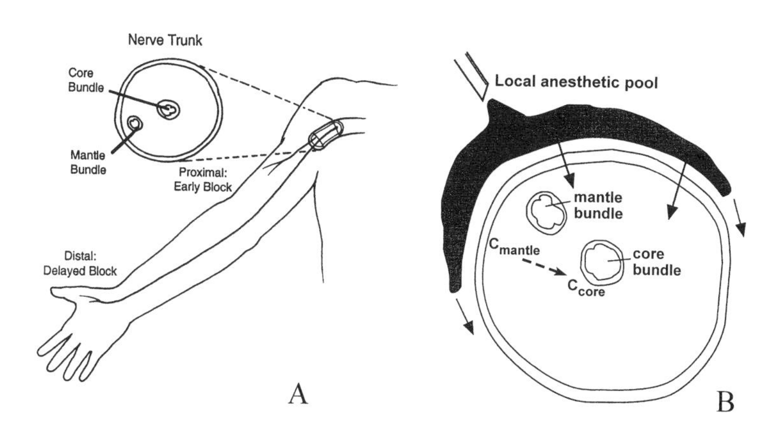

FIGURE 13-5. The actions of local anesthetics in producing peripheral nerve blockade are highly dependent on neuroanatomic factors. Axons in the outer mantle portions of peripheral nerve bundles typically innervate the proximal portion of a limb, and those in the nerve's core innervate the distal extremity (A). After injection around a peripheral nerve bundle, local anesthetic diffuses along a concentration gradient, so the concentration of local anesthetic around the mantle fibers (C_{mantle}) is initially greater than that in the core (C_{core}), resulting in onset of proximal limb motor blockade (mantle fibers) before distal limb (core fibers) sensory blockade (B). After the extraneural drug pool has been depleted by diffusion, dilution, absorption, and binding, the diffusion gradient reverses. (Adapted from de Jong RH. Local anesthetics. St. Louis: Mosby-Year Book, 1994.)

TABLE 13-2. Pharmacokinetic Properties of Some Local Anesthetic Agents after Intravenous Injection

Agent	$t_{1/2}$ (h)	V_{dss} (L/kg)	Cl (L/kg/h) Clearance	Hepatic Extraction Ratio	Free Fraction in Blood	Umbilical: Maternal Venous Ratio
Esters						
Procaine	0.1	0.93	5.62	—	—	—
2-Chloroprocaine	0.1	0.50	2.96	—	—	—
Amides						
Lidocaine	1.6	1.30	0.85	0.65	0.36	0.5–0.7
Prilocaine	1.6	2.73	2.03	N/A	N/A	1–1.1
Mepivacaine	1.9	1.20	0.67	0.52	0.22	0.7
Ropivacaine	2.0	0.91	0.63	N/A	0.07	N/A
Bupivacaine	2.7	1.02	0.41	0.38	0.07	0.2–0.3
Etidocaine	2.6	1.90	1.05	0.74	0.09	0.2–0.3

$T_{1/2}$, Half-Life; V_{dss}, volume of distribution at steady state.
N/A, comparable data not available.

binding, lipid solubility, and pKa, which, as noted previously, are influenced by structural differences among these agents (Table 13-2).

Absorption

Absorption is the process whereby a drug leaves the site of administration and enters the systemic circulation. Absorption of local anesthetics varies as a function of physiochemical properties of the agent, the site of injection, the dosage (both in terms of concentration and volume), and the presence of vasoconstrictor in the solution. Typically, measurements of the rate of change of serum concentrations of local anesthetics are utilized to assess the systemic uptake of these drugs after their parenteral administration.

Although the peak concentrations associated with the injection of these agents increase in direct proportion to the dose, the blood concentrations per 100 mg depend on the individual agent. For example, blood concentrations of approximately 1 μg/ml occur following peridural injection of lidocaine and mepivacaine without epinephrine, whereas concentrations of 0.4 to 0.7 μg/ml are achieved with similar amounts of bupivacaine or etidocaine (68) (Table 13-3). Although the time to peak concentration is similar, rates and extent of absorption vary among the local anesthetics. Systemic absorption of the more hydrophilic local anesthetics (lidocaine ≈ mepivacaine > prilocaine) is faster than that of the more lipophilic agents (bupivacaine > etidocaine) (69) and may reflect greater uptake of the latter agents by peripheral fat. Direct vasodilation by lidocaine and mepivacaine may enhance local blood flow and increase absorption compared with prilocaine. In addition, the use of carbonated local anesthetics may increase drug absorption compared with the injection of noncarbonated solutions, in part because of the vasodilating effect of carbon dioxide CO_2 (70).

Intrinsic vascularity of the site of injection is the primary determinant of systemic absorption of local anesthetics. Absorption increases in parallel with the vascularity of the following sites: subcutaneous < femoral-sciatic region < brachial plexus area < lumbar epidural space < caudal space < intercostal space. Absorption is rapid after deposition of local anesthetic at other highly vascularized regions such as intratracheal, paracervical, pudendal, and subcutaneous vaginal sites of injection. In addition, the presence of fat and connective tissue at the site of injection influences the absorption rate. Although many areas of the epidural space are more vascularized than the intercostal space, the much greater amount of fat in the epidural space acts to sequester local anesthetics, thereby reducing the rate of vascular uptake.

Addition of vasoconstrictors to solutions of local anesthetics reduces systemic absorption by direct vasomotor activity, which reduces local blood flow, as well as by attenuation of the direct vasodilator actions of some local anesthetics and blunting of increases in local blood flow resulting from local anesthetic-mediated sympathetic blockade. The influence of vasoconstrictor on prolongation of neural blockade as well as reduction in peak blood levels is the result of the interaction of intrinsic vascularity and other tissue characteristics with the physicochemical properties of the individual local anesthetic agents. Epinephrine 1:200,000 significantly reduces maximal blood levels of lidocaine and mepivacaine after both peripheral and epidural injection (71-73). For lidocaine and mepivacaine, a 75 to 90% increase in duration of brachial plexus blockade or epidural blockade is observed after the addition of epinephrine. In contrast, although peak blood levels of bupivacaine and etidocaine are reduced in the presence of epinephrine following peripheral nerve blocks, this effect is not observed after epidural administration (71, 72, 74, 75). Duration of brachial plexus blockade with bupivacaine is prolonged by about 50% with the addition of epinephrine, but duration of epidural blockade is prolonged only approximately 10 to 15%.

TABLE 13-3. Effect of Injection Site on Local Anesthetic Absorption

Agent	Site of Injection	Dose (mg)	Concentration (%)	Vasconstrictor	Peak Concentration (μg/ml/100 mg of drug)	Time to Peak Concentration (min)
Lidocaine*	Subcutaneous	400	2	No	0.49	~30
		400	2	Yes	0.26	~15
	Subcutaneous Vaginal	400	2	No	1.23	~15
		400	2	Yes	0.62	~15
	Intercostal	400	1	No	1.70	~15
		400	1	Yes	1.32	~20
	Peridural	400	2	No	1.07	~20
		400	2	Yes	0.74	~15
Mepivacaine†	Brachial Plexus	500	1	No	0.74	24(15–30)
		500	1	Yes	0.59	47(15–120)
	Sciatic Femoral	500	1	No	0.72	31(25–45)
		500	1	Yes	0.61	55(15–120)
	Intercostal	500	2	No	1.61	9(5–15)
		500	2	Yes	0.79	19(5–45)
		500	1	No	1.18	11(5–15)
		500	1	Yes	0.74	37(10–60)
	Peridural	500	2	No	0.99	16(10–20)
		500	2	Yes	0.64	26(1545)
	Caudal	500	2	No	1.10	13(10–15)
		500	2	Yes	0.92	40(25–60)
		500	1	No	0.91	25(10–60)
		500	1	Yes	0.48	72(30–120)
Bupivacaine‡	Brachial Plexus	150§	0.75	No	0.67	25
		150§	0.75	Yes	0.33	30
		150‖	0.75	No	0.47	30
		150‖	0.75	Yes	0.33	30
	Peridural	112.5§	0.75	No	0.89	25
		112.5§	0.75	Yes	0.71	25
		112.5‖	0.75	No	0.89	25
		112.5‖	0.75	Yes	0.44	25
Bupivacaine¶	Peridural	100	0.5	No	0.79	5
		100	0.5	Yes	0.74	15
Etidocaine¶	Peridural	200	1	No	0.43	20
		200	1	Yes	0.34	20

**Data from Scott DB, Jebsen PJR, Braid DP, et al. Factors affecting plasma levels of lignocaine and prilocaine. Br J Anaesth 1975;44:1040–1048.*

†Data from Tucker GT, Moore DC, Bridendaugh PO, et al. Systemic absorption of mepivacaine in commonly used regional block procedures. Anesthesiology 1972;37:277–287.

‡Data from Raj PP, Rosenblatt R, Miller J, et al. Dynamics of local anesthetic compounds in regional anesthesia. Anesth Analg 1977;56:110–117.

§With chloroprocaine.

‖With lidocaine.

¶Data from Abdel-Salam AR, Vonwiller JB, Scott DB. Evaluation of etidocaine in extradural block. Br J Anaesth 1975;47:1081–1086.

Similar reduction in local anesthetic absorption can be achieved with the use of phenylephrine or norepinephrine (76).

Alterations in regional blood flow are commonly associated with altered physiologic states that occur in pregnancy and disease states. Although peridural local anesthetic dosage requirements are reduced during pregnancy primarily because of peridural venous engorgement, this phenomenon is not associated with a significant difference in peak plasma drug levels or in the time required to reach peak levels (77). Alterations in systemic absorption of local anesthetics may not be reflected by plasma drug concentrations because other factors influencing drug disposition are often concomitantly altered. Changes in systemic absorption of local anesthetics have been observed in the presence of acute hypovolemia (slower rate of absorption of lidocaine) (78), as well as in patients in renal failure who have a hyperdynamic circulation (increased absorption and decreased duration of brachial plexus anesthesia) (79).

Distribution, Metabolism, and Elimination

Local anesthetics distribute throughout total body water, and the relationship of their blood concentration with time can be readily described using two- or three-compartmental pharmacokinetic models. After systemic absorption, the initial rapid decline in blood levels of local anesthetics is generally related to uptake by highly vascularized tissues such as skeletal muscle, lung, kidney, liver, and myocardium. As with other drugs, a subsequent slower decline in blood levels is often seen and reflects redistribution to slowly equilibrating tissues (e.g., peripheral fat), followed by a final phase reflecting metabolism and elimination. The ratio of plasma to whole blood drug concentration varies among the local anesthetic drugs because of differences in plasma protein binding, primarily to α_1-acid glycoprotein (80). Long-acting local anesthetics that are also more highly protein bound (e.g., etidocaine and bupivacaine) tend to have lower blood-to-plasma concentration ratios than less highly protein bound drugs (e.g., lidocaine and mepivacaine) (81). The greater free fraction of local anesthetics measured in neonatal compared with maternal plasma is probably related to lower neonatal α_1-acid glycoprotein levels (82). The reduced binding of local anesthetics in the fetal circulation also is largely responsible for the transplacental distribution gradient for local anesthetics, with umbilical cord-to-maternal concentration ratios in the range of 0.4 to 0.5 for bupivacaine and lidocaine, respectively (83-85) (see Table 13-2). In addition to influencing plasma protein binding, acid-base balance is also an important determinant of the circulating concentrations of local anesthetics, and fetal acidosis leads to ion trapping across the placenta (86, 87).

Total body clearance of local anesthetics is essentially equivalent to metabolic clearance because renal excretion of the parent compounds accounts for less than 5% of the total administered dose at physiologic urine pH (88, 89). Metabolic clearance of the amide-type local anesthetics is principally hepatic, whereas the ester-type agents are cleared both in plasma and, to a lesser extent, in the liver (Fig. 13-6). The ester-type local anesthetics are rapidly hydrolyzed by a plasma enzyme originally designated as procainesterase (90), subsequently found to be indistinguishable from serum pseudocholinesterase (91). Most ester-type local anesthetics have in vitro plasma half-lives of approximately 1 minute (92, 93), except in the presence of atypical pseudocholinesterase (homozygous), which can prolong the duration of toxic effects secondary to high plasma concentrations (92). Spinal fluid lacks esterases, so metabolism of aminoester local anesthetics depends on systemic uptake of the drug, a phenomenon that partially explains the discrepancy between the observed duration of spinal anesthesia and the rates of hydrolysis of aminoester local anesthetics.

The primary metabolites generated by the hydrolysis of the ester-type agents include diethylaminoethanol (DEAE) and paraaminobenzoic acid (PABA) (94), with allergic phenomena commonly attributed to PABA and its substituted analogues (95). PABA is ex-

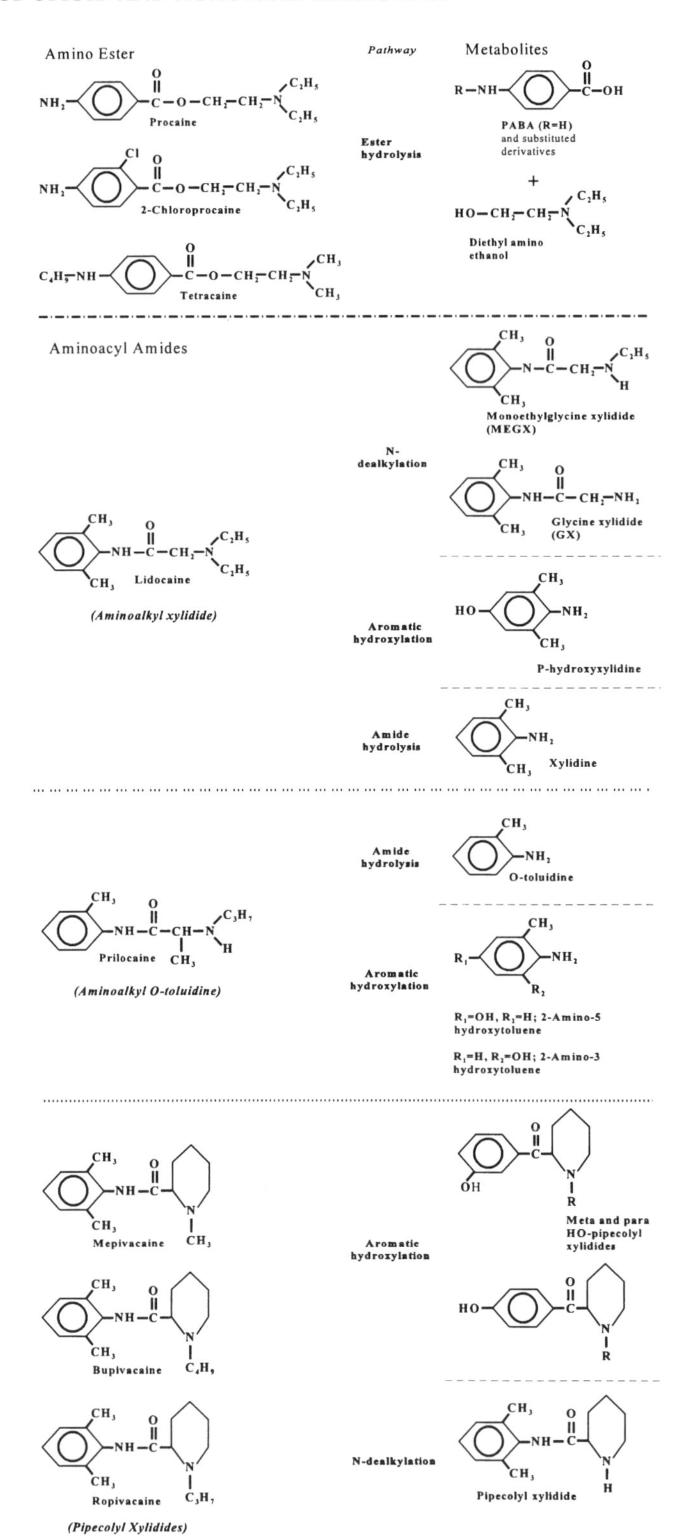

FIGURE 13-6. Representative metabolic pathways and the resulting metabolites for different structural classes of the local anesthetics.

creted unchanged or after conjugation, whereas DEAE undergoes further biodegradation. Unlike PABA, which has negligible anesthetic potency, DEAE has a blocking potency similar to that of procaine and about one-tenth that of tetracaine (96). Structural alterations of the aminoester local anesthetic molecule can result in significant changes in biotransformation rates. For example, orthochlorination of the aminobenzoic ring of procaine results in a four-fold greater hydrolysis rate for 2-chloroprocaine (92). Replacing the para-amino moiety of procaine with a larger parabutylamino group results in the formation of tetracaine and reduces the hydrolysis rate by a factor of 4 (92, 97).

Biotransformation of amide-type local anesthetics involves three major mechanisms: N-dealkylation; aromatic hydroxylation; and amide hydrolysis (68). Metabolism of aminoamide local anesthetics depends on whether the amide is linked to an aromatic acid (producing an aminolkyl amide) or an aromatic amine (yielding an aminoacyl amide). In general, aminoacyl amides such as lidocaine and mepivacaine are metabolized faster and more completely than aminoalkyl amides such as dibucaine, perhaps because conversion of the tertiary amines to secondary and primary amines occurs more readily in the former group. Although the conformation of the single-ringed aminoalkyl xylidides (e.g., lidocaine and etidocaine) partially resists amide hydrolysis, the aminoacyl PPX local anesthetics (e.g., bupivacaine, mepivacaine, and ropivacaine) contain a large piperidine ring that reduces the rate of conversion to secondary amines and inhibits hydrolytic enzymatic cleavage of the amide linkage (98).

Lidocaine metabolism has been extensively studied and serves as the model for metabolism of other amide-type local anesthetics. Lidocaine metabolism is limited by hepatic blood flow, and its high hepatic extraction ratio is reduced in the presence of advanced liver disease or hepatic congestion or after significant hepatic resection (99, 100). Lidocaine undergoes microsomal oxidative de-ethylation to the secondary amine monoethylglycinexylidide (MEGX) and subsequent amide hydrolysis to 2,6-xylidine, which is oxidized to 4-hydroxyxylidine, the predominant renally excreted lidocaine metabolite (65%) (101, 102). The oxidative pathways of lidocaine utilize the microsomal mixed-function oxidases and involve cytochrome P450, which is present in adequate amounts even in the neonatal liver but can be affected by certain commonly administered drugs (e.g., phenytoin, cimetidine, and barbiturates). Other biotransformation pathways include oxidative di-de-ethylation to glycinexylidide (GX), a primary amine, and aromatic hydroxylation of lidocaine and MEGX to 3-hydroxylidocaine and 3-hydroxy-MEGX (see Fig. 13-6).

Given that the pKa of lidocaine (7.9) is close to physiologic pH, renal elimination is increased by urinary acidification because of the resultant increased proportion of the protonated hydrophilic cationic species. MEGX and other conjugated products formed at aromatic ring sites are only minimally influenced by variations in urinary pH, however, and even decreased renal function does not result in significant accumulation of the primary metabolite or of the parent compound. Clearance of GX depends on renal secretion, and its long plasma half-life is further prolonged even with minor reductions in renal function (100), potentially resulting in significant accumulation of this metabolite after continuous lidocaine infusion (103).

Two-thirds of lidocaine delivered by the hepatic artery fails to return to the systemic circulation, although the rate of hepatic metabolism of the individual amide compounds (prilocaine $\gg$ etidocaine $>$ lidocaine $>$ mepivacaine $>$ bupivacaine) varies considerably (81, 104, 105). The unusually large clearance of prilocaine reflects extrahepatic elimination of this drug. In addition, the secondary amine prilocaine is unique in that it undergoes hydrolysis without prior N-dealklyation, and hydroxylation of the aromatic ring may take place at any time during the metabolic sequence. Conversion of prilocaine to n-propylalanine and orthotoluidine and its aminophenol metabolites (2-amino–5-hydroxytoluene and 2-amino–3-hydroxytoluene) can result in methemoglobinemia either after large doses of the parent drug are administered or in the presence of relative deficiency of the enzyme methemoglobin reductase, which occurs more commonly in neonates than in adults (106). Because of this potential toxicity, clinical use of prilocaine is primarily limited to topical application as a eutectic mixture with lidocaine, as discussed later. Although benzocaine, lidocaine, and mepivacaine are also metabolized to undesirable aminophenols, the dimethylated aniline ring of the xylidine series appears to suppress the tendency of the toluidine ring to oxidize hemoglobin, so clinically significant degrees of methemoglobinemia are uncommon with these agents (107, 108). Oxidative N-dealkylation in the liver serves as the major metabolic pathway for metabolism of bupivacaine and ropivacaine and a minor route of transformation for mepivacaine, resulting in the parent moiety PPX (109). As with the aminoalkyl xylidides, aromatic ring hydroxylation at the para and meta positions and subsequent conjugation with glucuronic acid comprise the major metabolic pathway for mepivacaine, with subsequent renal excretion (110).

PHARMACODYNAMIC PROPERTIES OF LOCAL ANESTHETICS

While local anesthetics primarily have nerve impulse conduction-blocking properties and are most commonly utilized to produce local or regional analgesia, the relatively nonspecific activity of these agents in inhibiting ion channel conduction in part results in other central nervous systems (CNS) actions that may be categorized as either therapeutic or toxic.

Systemic Therapeutic Effects of Local Anesthetics

In addition to providing local antinociception, local anesthetics can elevate pain thresholds and may produce analgesia when given intravenously (111). Lidocaine infusion has been shown to be effective in relieving central neuropathic pain (112, 113), acute ischemia-induced tourniquet pain (114), and the pain of diabetic neuropathy (115). The systemic analgesic properties of intravenous lidocaine, as well as those of procaine, are comparable to the effects of nitrous oxide, and these local anesthetics have also been utilized to supplement general anesthesia (116).

Antiarrhythmic activity is a more commonly utilized systemic therapeutic effect of some local anesthetics. Effects of local anesthetics on cardiac rhythm are predictable because of their actions on voltage-dependent ion channels and on the propagation of electrical impulses. With the discovery that local anesthetics applied directly to the heart could control arrhythmias, drugs such as procaine were also utilized as intravenous antiarrhythmic agents (117). The search for agents with longer duration of action lead to the development of procainamide (118), although its major side effect of hypotension after intravenous loading resulted in significant interest in alternatives such as lidocaine, which became popular as an antiarrhythmic in the 1960s (119). The widespread clinical acceptance of lidocaine to treat or to prevent serious ventricular arrhythmias prompted it to be studied more thoroughly in this regard than any other local anesthetic. At therapeutic concentrations, lidocaine has little effect on myocardial contractile function and does not alter sinus node or atrioventicular nodal function, except on rare occasions in the presence of preexisting significant disease of the conduction system (120). Therapeutic concentrations of lidocaine (1 to 5 μg/ml) decrease the slope of phase 4 depolarization primarily in the His-Purkinje system, and increase the threshold for ventricular fibrillation (121) without altering resting membrane potential or the voltage threshold (122).

Although all local anesthetics act at ion channels in the heart, differences in their effects depend on differences in their kinetic interactions with myocardial Na^+ channels. Although the effects of local anesthetics on neural conduction are primarily related to their ability to produce tonic (low-frequency) inhibition, their therapeutic as well as toxic effects on the heart are determined by the production of use-dependent (phasic) inhibition of Na^+ channels. The rate of association and of dissociation of local anesthetics from their binding sites during the transitions between various conformational states of the Na^+ channel is the predominant factor determining their cardiac pharmacology (123) (see Fig. 13-3). In contrast, the pharmacologic characteristics of neural block are more heavily determined by physical characteristics such as potency and lipophilicity.

As previously discussed, Na^+ channels can exist in three conformational states: resting (closed); open (permeable); and inactive (closed) (124). The resting state is most prevalent during the diastolic phase of the cardiac action potential, the open state is most common during systole, and the inactive state prevails during the plateau phase when the cell is depolarized (123). The affinity of Na^+ channel blocking drugs to interact with the various conformational states of the ion channel depends on drug concentration. At high concentrations, local anesthetics as well as other Na^+ channel blockers can bind to the channel receptor in any of its conformational states, although lower concentrations confer a relative conformational specificity. At therapeutic concentrations, all Na^+ channel blockers have a relatively low affinity for channels in the resting conformation, and blockade of activated (open) versus inactivated (closed) channels depends on the specific agent. Among the antiarrhythmic agents, lidocaine blocks Na^+ channnels in both the open and inactivated conformations, in contrast to drugs such as quinidine (open channel blockade) or amiodarone (inactivated channel blockade). In contrast to lidocaine, bupivacaine binds preferentially to the Na^+ channel in the inactive conformation (125).

Phasic inhibition occurs when drug binds to the Na^+ channel during open or inactive states and requires that drug dissociation is rapid so channels can recover during the diastolic resting phase. The dissociation time of lidocaine from cardiac Na^+ channels is on the order of 200 milliseconds, allowing recovery from channel blockade to occur with heart rates as high as 300 beats per minute (126). Conversely, ropivacaine and bupivacaine have dissociation times of approximately 1400 to 2000 milliseconds, which is insufficient time for dissociation from the channel even at normal resting heart rates (126). This marked difference in the dissociation time between lidocaine and other more potent local anesthetics such as bupivacaine and its congeners is responsible for the differences in their actions on cardiac conduction. Although lidocaine produces a phasic block, slows cardiac conduction, and acts as an antiarrhythmic, the longer dissociation times of bupivacaine-like drugs can result in tonic inhibition of conduction, facilitating the generation of arrhythmias by alternate pathways (127). Lidocaine primarily controls ventricular arrhythmias because it preferentially blocks inactivated channels in tissues with longer action potential durations, such as Purkinje fibers, in contrast to atrial tissues, which have shorter action potential duration. The antiarrhythmic action of lidocaine can be enhanced in ischemic myocardium primarily because of local tissue acidosis, which promotes a greater fraction of the cationic drug form that dissociates more slowly from the ion channel (128).

Prolonged intravenous infusions of lidocaine can exhibit decreased antiarrhythmic efficacy over time and this phenomena illustrates the importance of metabolites interacting with a parent compound. The lidocaine metabolite GX has both synergistic and antagonistic interactions with lidocaine at the ion channel (129). The competitive displacement of lidocaine by GX is related to the faster kinetics of onset and offset of blockade by GX compared with lidocaine (129). Because molecules with faster receptor kinetics tend to produce competitive antagonism, whereas those with slower kinetics may result in synergy, drugs such as bupivacaine can be displaced from cardiac ion channels by agents such as lidocaine (130), which may have clinical relevance when managing bupivacaine-induced arrhythmias.

Systemic Side Effects of Local Anesthetics

Although local anesthetics in high concentrations can be directly neurotoxic, the majority of side effects are related to CNS and cardiovascular effects. Other drug-induced adverse reactions occur as a result of systemic absorption from the site of injection. The factors influencing systemic absorption of local anesthetic are discussed previously and include anatomic characteristics of the site of injection, the mass of drug injected, the pH of the local anesthetic solution, and the physiochemical characteristics of the specific agents.

Central Nervous System Toxicity (CNS)

Blood concentrations of lidocaine similar to those in the therapeutic antiarrhythmic range (1 to 5 μg/ml) have been associated with anticonvulsant activity (131), whereas blood levels of lidocaine between 4.5 and 7 μg/ml increase cortical irritability, and levels higher than 7.5 μg/ml are associated with short ictal discharges (132). Anticonvulsant activity has been demonstrated for lidocaine, mepivacaine, procaine, and tetracaine (131), although this property is not utilized clinically because of the narrow therapeutic margin between neuroprotective and neurotoxic effects. The convulsant dose and associated threshold blood levels of local anesthetics are inversely related to their therapeutic potency (9, 133, 134) (Table 13-4), although mixtures of local anesthetics exhibit essentially additive toxicity (135).

As blood levels of local anesthetics increase, certain signs and symptoms of neurotoxicity are exhibited. Patients may be agitated and may describe lightheadedness, dizziness, circumoral paresthesias and numbness, and visual or auditory disturbances such as diplopia, blurred vision, or tinnitus (136). Dysarthria, confusion, nystagmus, and muscle tremors and twitches may be observed (136). These CNS effects correlate with local anesthetic blood levels, and mild symptoms such as lightheadedness can occur at levels above 4 to 4.5 μg/ml (97, 137, 138), which are commonly produced after rapid intravenous administration of at least 1 mg/kg lidocaine. As blood levels of local anesthetics increase, a generalized depressed response becomes manifest, and when blood concentrations exceed a drug-specific threshold, generalized tonic-clonic seizures occur. The initial stimulation associated with lower blood concentrations of local anesthetic occurs as a result of blockade of inhibitory cortical neurons and subsequent disinhibition of excitatory neurons (139). Local anesthetic can be distributed to body storage depots when drug slowly enters the systemic circulation, limiting the rate of rise of blood concentration to the neurotoxic threshold. The absolute blood concentration of local anesthetic at which seizures occur may be higher if the blood concentration rises slowly as during continuous intravenous infusion or after epidural administration, in contrast to rapidly rising levels observed with intravenous bolus administration (140). In addition, the blood concentration thresholds for systemic (including CNS) toxicity of local anesthetics can be modulated by the availability of free versus protein-bound drug. Gestational increases in the availability of the free fraction of bupivacaine are associated with enhanced toxicity, although serum protein binding of mepivacaine and hence its systemic toxicity are not altered in pregnancy (141).

TABLE 13-4. Comparative Central Nervous System (CNS) and Cardiovascular (CV) to Central Nervous System Ratio of Local Anesthetics

Agent	Convulsant Dose (mg/kg) CD_{100} in humans*	CV/CNS Toxicity Ratio in Sheep‡
Esters		
2-Chloroprocaine	22.8	N/A
Procaine	19	N/A
Amides		
Lidocaine	5–7	7.1
Mepivacaine	9.8	7.6
Ropivacaine	3.5† (sheep)	N/A
Bupivacaine	1.6	4.4
Etidocaine	3.4	3.7

**Data from Morishima HO, Pedersen H, Finster M, et al. Bupivacaine toxicity in pregnant and nonpregnant ewes. Anesthesiology 1985;63:134–139; and Morishima HO, Finster M, Arthur R, Covino BG. Pregnancy does not alter lidocaine toxicity. Am J Obstet Gynecol 1990;162:1320–1324.*

†Data from Garfield JM, Gugino L. Central effects of local anesthetic agents. Handb Exp Pharmacol 1987;81:253–284.

‡Nancarrow C, Rutten AJ, Runciman WB, Mather LE, Carapetis RJ, cLean c. Hipkins SF. Myocardial and cerebral drug concentrations and the mechanisms of death after fatal intravenous doses of lidocaine, bupivacaine, and ropivacaine in the sheep. Anesthesia & Analgesia. 1989;69:276–83.

N/A, Comparable data not available.

Threshold blood concentrations of local anesthetics for central nervous system toxicity can be influenced by tissue oxygenation, acid-base status as well as other factors such as the presence of other drugs that modify seizure threshold. Tissue hypoxia exacerbates local anesthetic CNS toxicity as well as cardiovascular side effects, decreasing the lethal dose (142). Reduction of $PaCO_2$ increases the cortical seizure threshold to local anesthetics (136, 143), whereas elevated blood CO_2 tension is associated with increased CNS toxicity (134). Hyperventilation therefore is a key initial step in management of CNS toxicity caused by local anesthetics, not only by increasing cerebral oxygenation, reducing cerebral excitability from CO_2, and reducing delivery of local anesthetic to the brain by decreasing cerebral blood flow, but also by reducing the intracerebral fraction of the active cationic species and therefore reducing ion trapping in the CNS.

The seizure-inducing dose of local anesthetics can be modified by coadministered drugs. In large doses, meperidine has been reported to enhance the CNS toxicity of lidocaine (144). Most other sedatives, tranquilizers, and general anesthetics increase the convulsant dose of local anesthetics (145). Effective reduction of seizure threshold by benzodiazepines makes this class of agents useful for prophylaxis of local anesthetic-induced seizures (146-148). The antagonism by flumazenil of the seizure prophylaxis produced by benzodiazepines is consistent with a relatively specific action of the latter class of drugs (149). Nondepressant doses of barbiturates and even conventional anticonvulsants such as phenytoin provide much less effective prophylaxis for local anesthetic-induced seizures (144, 150). Most local anesthetic-induced seizures are of brief duration because blood concentrations generally fall quickly as a result of rapid dilution and redistribution. In contrast to the disparity of benzodiazepines and other drugs in preventing local anesthetic-induced seizures, barbiturates, propofol, and benzodiazepines are all effective therapies for this complication (151, 152).

Cardiovascular Toxicity

In general, the adverse cardiovascular effects of local anesthetics occur at blood concentrations greater than those associated with CNS toxicity. Therefore, except when large amounts of extremely potent local anesthetics (e.g., bupivacaine) are injected directly intravascularly or when symptoms of CNS toxicity are masked (e.g., during general anesthesia), cardiovascular compromise typically is observed after adverse CNS sequelae. Cardiovascular toxicity of local anesthetics can be classified as direct cardiac effects or direct peripheral vascular effects, as well as indirect modulation of cardiovascular function by actions on the CNS. These effects are manifested clinically as ventricular arrhythmias, bradycardia, hypotension, hemodynamic instability, and cardiovascular collapse.

Like adverse CNS effects, cardiovascular toxicity of local anesthetics is inversely related to potency, and the enhanced protein binding of more potent agents facilitates high circulating blood levels as well as increased myocardial tissue binding. Unlike the ubiquitous ability of all clinically useful local anesthetics to induce CNS toxicity (seizures), the nature of serious cardiovascular complications varies profoundly among individual agents. For example, the ratio of the dose of local anesthetic associated with irreversible cardiovascular collapse (CV) to that resulting in CNS toxicity (seizures) is much lower for potent agents such as bupivacaine and etidocaine (CV:CNS dose ratios approximately 4) than for lidocaine (CV:CNS dose ratio approximately 7) (153).

In contrast to lidocaine and mepivacaine, bupivacaine and, to a lesser extent, etidocaine can produce severe ventricular arrhythmias and fatal ventricular fibrillation after rapid intravascular administration (154-156). As described earlier, the arrhythmogenicity of bupivacaine is likely related to its longer dissociation time from cardiac Na^+ channels and production of tonic conduction block (123). Elevated blood concentrations are associated with prolonged conduction through various cardiac impulse pathways (prolonged PR interval, QRS width, and QT interval), as well as an increase in diastolic threshold and an decrease in automaticity that may result in bradycardia (157). Coupled with blockade of slow Ca^+ channels, these electrophysiologic effects of bupivacaine may lead to reentry-type arrhythmias including torsades de pointes (158-161). In addition to bupivacaine's direct cardiac arrhythmogenic effects, the proarrhythmic effects of local anesthetics are neurogenically mediated (162). The CNS modulates cardiac conduction by autonomic pathways, consistent with the finding that microapplication of bupivacaine (and even lidocaine) at the nucleus of the tractus solitarius results in bradycardia and ventricular arrhythmias (163, 164). Centrally generated arrhythmias can therefore be attenuated with centrally acting drugs such as benzodiazepines (165). The blockade of sympathetic outflow at the first through fourth thoracic levels by epidurally administered local anesthetic is commonly associated with bradycardia related to inhibition of cardioaccelerator fibers.

Myocardial contractility is minimally affected by lidocaine when it is administered in therapeutic antiarrhythmic doses, although larger intravenous bolus doses of all local anesthetics including lidocaine can depress both atrial and ventricular contractility (166, 167). Analogous to its electrophysiologic effects, the potent negative inotropic effect of bupivacaine compared with that of lidocaine or ropivacaine is likely related to its slow release from Na^+ channel binding sites (168), as well as Ca^+ channel binding (126, 169,

170). Therefore, depression of cardiac contractility is predictably proportional to the conduction blocking potency of these agents (170), and the greater lipophilicity and protein binding of bupivacaine (as well as etidocaine) favors enhanced binding in myocardial tissue and makes cardiac resuscitation more difficult following bupivacaine-induced cardiovascular collapse (171-173). High lipophilicity facilitates direct transmembrane access to the ion channel binding sites, potentially overwhelming the effects of gating function or channel conformational state changes (168). Hypercarbia, acidosis, and hypoxemia all potentiate the negative inotropic action of bupivacaine or lidocaine (174), potentially exacerbating the cardiovascular depression that may occur in association with high blood concentrations of these agents (175).

Although local anesthetics bind with Na^+ channels in many different tissues, evidence indicates the stereospecificity of the cardiac Na^+ channel (176). The cardiotoxicity, especially the proarrhythmogenicity of bupivacaine, is severalfold greater for the R(+) enantiomer of bupivacaine than for S(−) bupivacaine (177). This finding is consistent with the fourfold faster diastolic dissociation of S(−) bupivacaine compared with that of R(+) bupivacaine (32). The reduced arrhythmogenicity and decreased cardiotoxicity of ropivacaine compared with bupivacaine have been postulated to be related at least partially to the drug's availability as a pure S(−) enantiomer rather than as a racemic mixture (178-180).

Other mechanisms mediating cardiovascular toxicity include CNS activation of sympathetic outflow contributing to the genesis of ventricular arrhythmias as well as CNS-mediated inotropic and chronotropic depression of the myocardium (163). Local anesthetic drugs also affect cardiovascular function by direct actions on peripheral vascular smooth muscle. With the exception of cocaine, local anesthetics at low concentrations can produce vasoconstriction and can reduce peripheral arterial flow, whereas at high concentrations, they cause vasodilation and augmented blood flow (181, 182). The vasoconstrictor effects of cocaine result from excess norepinephrine as a result of decreased reuptake by storage granules, whereas a CNS-stimulating effect (183) and impairment of endothelial formation of nitric oxide appear to be involved in the vasoconstrictive effects of other ester- as well as amide-type local anesthetics (184, 185).

Allergic Responses to Local Anesthetics

Allergic responses to local anesthetics are infrequent and have been best documented for the aminoester type local anesthetics (186). Cross sensitivity exists among the commonly used aminoesters (e.g., procaine, tetracaine, and benzocaine) (187). True allergic responses to aminoamide local anesthetics are exceedingly rare but have been documented (188-190). Local anesthetics are small molecules and are therefore unlikely to be primarily antigenic. These compounds are believed to initiate allergic responses by binding as haptens to larger proteins. Mediator release may be triggered when local anesthetics of the aminoester class form polyvalent crosslinks bridging two or more IgE antibody molecules (95). As noted previously, PABA and PABA-like compounds utilized as preservatives (e.g., methylparaben) are likely haptens for these reactions. Preservative-free local anesthetic solutions should therefore probably be utilized for known atopic patients, and aminoester drugs should probably be avoided in patients with known sensitivity to PABA-containing substances such as sunscreen.

NEW DEVELOPMENTS IN LOCAL ANESTHETIC PHARMACOLOGY

Long duration of action is a desirable characteristic of local anesthetics for postoperative analgesia, as well as for other areas of pain management, and the pharmacokinetic characteristics of currently available agents often necessitate the use of continuous infusions or repeated injections, which may increase the risk of systemic absorption and subsequent toxicity. Future developments for the use of local anesthetics to produce analgesia of long duration with minimal or low toxicity include introduction of new agents and new methods of local anesthetic drug delivery. The ongoing elucidation of the molecular structure of the Na^+ channel and of the structure-activity relationship of local anesthetic molecules has prompted study of a quaternary ammonium derivative of lidocaine (N-β-phenylethyl lidocaine quaternary ammonium bromide: tonicaine). Because of its permanent charge, tonicaine acts more slowly than lidocaine in blocking Na^+ currents but results in a prolonged tonic and phasic block (191). Tonicaine produces sensory block (7.7-fold longer thermal and 9.3-fold longer pinch analgesia than lidocaine) outlasting motor block (3.6-fold longer motor block than lidocaine) by a factor of 1.8 (191).

The development and introduction of the eutectic mixture of local anesthetics (EMLA) was one of the first alterations of drug delivery systems for local anesthetics that has become commercially available (192, 193). A cream containing equal portions of prilocaine and lidocaine crystalline bases (pH = 9.0) results in a mixture with a lower melting point than either compound, allowing this formulation to be liquid at room temperature (193). The liquid portion of the cream emulsion contains 80% local anesthetic base, facilitating penetration across membranes and permitting effective topical anesthesia as deep as 3 mm through the dermis (194). EMLA is limited primarily by the low-capacity dermal transport system and the requirement for prolonged application to achieve efficacy (193, 195, 196), as well as the potential for methemoglobinemia, especially in infants (193, 197, 198). Enhanced transdermal delivery may be achieved with a combination of transdermal local anesthetic base diffusion and cation electrophoretic transport to provide rapid onset and long-duration dermal analgesia (199, 200).

Liposomal delivery of local anesthetics, although not yet clinically available, offers the potential for slow release resulting in prolonged duration of action and reduction in systemic toxicity because of reduced peak blood concentrations (201, 202). Encapsulation has been widely employed for controlled delivery of biologically active agents. Although this route of delivery appears to offer significant advantages for local anesthetics, concerns about vehicle microembolization and antigenicity need to be resolved. Other approaches to providing substrates for prolonged local anesthetic delivery include the use of suspensions. The poorly water-soluble benzocaine congener, butyl paraamino benzoate (BAB) is slowly released from a suspended flocculate, resulting in ultra long-lasting analgesia (203, 204).

In addition to improving delivery systems for local anesthetics to reduce the need for multiple or repeated dosing, other efforts have been undertaken to widen the margin betweeen therapeutic efficacy and toxicity. Availability of stereoselective isomers of local anesthetics may provide clinical advantages over previously available racemic mixtures (e.g., bupivacaine and mepivacaine). As outlined earlier, S(−) ropivacaine has pharmacokinetic and pharmacodynamic properties similar to those of bupivacaine, although the potential for reduced CNS and cardiovascular toxicity conferred by the marketing of a pure preparation of the S(−) stereoisomer is likely to enhance its clinical application compared with bupivacaine.

SUMMARY

In summary, all clinically useful local anesthetics effectively produce neural blockade by a common mechanism involving ion movement through transmembrane channels. The nonspecific nature of this mechanism results in physiologically important actions at sites other than peripheral nerves, including cardiovascular and CNS effects. The latter actions are associated with clinically relevant side effects that occur in proportion to the blood concentrations of these agents. A thorough understanding of the pharmacokinetic and pharmacodynamic characteristics of these drugs is therefore necessary for optimal application of these compounds to maximize efficacy while limiting toxicity. Currently, the primary clinical application of local anesthetics by the intravenous route is the treatment of ventricular arrhythmias (lidocaine) and the establishment of regional anesthesia (Bier block) for isolated extremity nerve block. Nonetheless, topical, infiltrative, and regional applications of local anesthetics play a major role in modern anesthesia practice, permitting both minor and major operative procedures to be conducted with regional anesthesia and analgesia, often in combination with intravenous sedation or general anesthesia. Although still utilized in parts of Asia and South America, intravenous anesthesia with local anesthetics has been replaced by safer and more effective sedative-hypontic drugs.

REFERENCES

1. Musto DF. Opium, cocaine and marijuana in American history. Sci Am 1991;265:40–47.
2. Koller C. History of cocaine as a local anesthetic. JAMA 1941; 117:1284.
3. Becker HK. Carl Koller and cocaine. Psychoanal Q 1963;32:309–373.
4. Koller C. On the use of cocaine for producing anaesthesia on the eye. Lancet 1884;2:990–992.
5. Halsted WS. Practical comments on the use and abuse of cocaine: suggested by its invariably successful employment in more than a thousand minor surgical operations. NY Med J 1885;42:294.
6. Fink BR. Leaves and needles: the introduction of surgical local anesthesia. Anesthesiology 1985;63:77–83.
7. Corning JL. Spinal anaesthesia and local medication of the cord. NY Med J 1885;42:483–485.
8. Bier A. Versuche über Cocainisirung des Rueckenmarkes. Dtsch Z Chir 1899;51:361–369.
9. Covino BG, Vassallo HG. Local anesthetics: mechanisms of action and clinical use. New York: Grune & Stratton, 1976.
10. Lofgren N. Studies on local anesthetics. Xylocaine: a new synthetic drug. Stockholm: Hoeggstroms, 1948 [Thesis].
11. Smythies JR, Benington F, Bradley RJ, et al. The molecular structure of the sodium channel. J Theor Biol 1974;43:29–42.
12. Barchi RL. Biochemical studies of the excitable membrane sodium channel. Int Rev Neurobiol 1982;23:69–101.
13. Greenblatt RE, Blatt Y, Montal M. The structure of voltage sensitive sodium channels: inferences derived from computer-aided analysis of the *Electrophorus electricus* channel primary structure. FEBS Lett 1985;193:125–134.
14. Kaneda M, Oomura Y, Ishibashi O, Akaike N. Permeability to various cations of the voltage-dependent sodium channel of isolated rat hippocampal neurons. Neurosci Lett 1988;88:253–256.
15. Siegelbaum SA, Koester J. Ion channels. In: Kandel ER, Schwartz JH, Jessell TM, eds. Principles of neural science. 3rd ed. New York: Elsevier Science Publishing, 1991:66–79.
16. Hodgkin AL, Huxley AF, Katz B. Measurement of current-voltage relations in membrane of the giant axon of *Loligo*. J Physiol (Lond) 1952;116:424–448.
17. Armstrong CM, Bezanilla F. Charge movement associated with the opening and closing of the activation gates of Na channels. J Gen Physiol 1974;63:533–552.
18. Courtney KR. Local anesthetics. Int Anesthesiol Clin 1988; 26:239–247.
19. Hodgkin AL, Huxley AF. Currents carried by sodium and potassium ions through the membrane of the giant axon of *Loligo*. J Physiol (Lond) 1952;116:449–472.
20. Aldrich RW, Corey DP, Stevens CF. A reinterpretation of mammalian sodium gating based on single channel recording. Nature 1983;306:436–441.

21. Vanderberg CA, Horn R. Inactivation viewed through a single sodium channel. J Gen Physiol 1984;84:535–564.
22. Butterworth JF, Strichartz GR. Molecular mechanisms of local anesthesia: a review. Anesthesiology 1990;72:711–734.
23. Hille B. Local anesthetics: hydrophilic and hydrophobic pathways for the drug-receptor reaction. J Gen Physiol 1977;69:497–515.
24. Hondeghem LM, Katzung BG. Time- and voltage-dependent interactions of antiarrhythmic drugs with cardiac sodium channels. Biochim Biophys Acta 1977;472:373–398.
25. Chernoff DM. Kinetic analysis of phasic inhibition of neuronal sodium currents by lidocaine and bupivacaine. Biophys J 1990; 58:53–68.
26. Starmer CF, Grant AO, Strauss HC. Mechanisms of use-dependent block of sodium channels in excitable membranes by local anesthetics. Biophys J 1984;46:15–27.
27. Starmer CF, Grant AO. Phasic ion channel blockade: a kinetic model and parameter estimation procedure. Mol Pharmacol 1985;28:348–356.
28. Strichartz GR. The inhibition of sodium currents in myelinated nerve by quaternary derivatives of lidocaine. J Gen Physiol 1973;62:37–57.
29. Courtney KR. Mechanism of frequency-dependent inhibition of sodium currents in frog myelinated nerve by the lidocaine derivative GEA. J Pharmacol Exp Ther 1975;195:225–236.
30. Bekkers JM, Greeff NG, Keynes RD, Neumcke B. The effect of local anesthetics on the components of the asymmetry current in the squid giant axon. J Physiol 1984;352:653–668.
31. Schmidtmayer J, Ulbricht W. Interaction of lidocaine and benzocaine in blocking sodium channels. Pflügers Arch 1980; 387:47–54.
32. Lee-Son S, Wang GK, Concus A, et al. Stereoselective inhibition of neuronal sodium channels by local anesthetics: evidence for two sites of action? Anesthesiology 1992;77:324–35.
33. Wang GK, Mok WM, Wang SY. Charged tetracaine as an inactivation enhancer in batrachotoxin-modified Na^+ channels. Biophys J 1994;67:1851–1860.
34. Wang HH, Earnest J, Limbacher HP. Local anesthetic-membrane interaction: a multiequilibrium model. Proc Natl Acad Sci U S A 1983;80:5297–5301.
35. Watts A, Poile TW. Direct determination by ^{2}H-NMR of the ionization state of phospholipids and of a local anaesthetic at the membrane surface. Biochim Biophys Acta 1986;861:368–372.
36. Wang GK. Binding affinity and steroselectivity of local anesthetics in single batrachotoxin-activated Na^+ channels. J Gen Physiol 1990;96:1105–1127.
37. Wang GK, Simon R, Bell D, et al. Structural determinants of quaternary ammonium blockers in batrachotoxin-modified Na^+ channels. Mol Pharmacol 1993;44:667–676.
38. Courtney KR. Structure-activity relations for frequency-dependent sodium channel block in nerve by local anesthetics. J Pharamacol Exp Ther 1980;213:114–119.
39. Voeikov VL, Lefkowitz FJ. Effects of local anesthetics of guanyl nucleotide modulation of the catecholamine-sensitive adenylate cyclase system and beta-adrenergic receptors. Biochim Biophys Acta 1980;629:266–281.
40. Gordon LM, Dipple ID, Sauerheber RD, et al. The selective effects of charged local anaesthetics on the glucagon- and fluoride-stimulated adenylate cyclase activity of rat-liver plasma membranes. J Supramol Struct 1980;14:21–32.
41. Richelson E, Prendergast FG, Divinetz-Romero S. Muscarinic receptor-mediated cyclic GMP formation by cultured nerve cells: ionic dependence and effects of local anesthetics. Biochem Pharmacol 1978;27:2039–2048.
42. Volpi M, Sha'afi RI, Epstein PM, et al. Local anesthetics, mepacrine, and propranolol are antagonists of calmodulin. Proc Natl Acad Sci U S A 1981;78:795–799.
43. Tanaka T, Hidaka H. Interaction of local anesthetics with calmodulin. Biochem Biophys Res Commun 1981;101:447–453.
44. Anderson NB. The effect of local anesthetic and pH on sodium and potassium flux in human red cells. J Pharmacol Exp Ther 1968;163:393–406.
45. Henao F, de Foresta B, Orlowski S, et al. Kinetic characterization of the normal and porcaine-perturbed reaction cycles of the sarcoplasmic reticulum calcium pump. Eur J Biochem 1991; 202:559–567.
46. Scherphof G, Westenberg H. Stimulation and inhibition of pancreatic phospholipase A_2 by local anesthetics as a result of their interaction with the substrate. Biochim Biophys Acta 1975; 398:442–451.
47. Irvine RF, Hemington N, Dawson RM. The hydrolysis of phosphatidylinositol by lysosomal enzymes in the rat liver and brain. Biochem J 1978;176:475–484.
48. Ruff RL. The kinetics of local anesthetic blockade of end-plate channels. Biophys J 1982; 37:625–631.
49. Forman SA, Miller KW. Molecular sites of anesthetic action in postsynaptic nicotinic membranes. Trends Pharmacol Sci 1989; 10:447–452.
50. Karon BS, Geddis LM, Kutchai H, Thomas DD. Anesthetics alter the physical and functional properties of the Ca-ATPase in cardiac sarcoplasmic reticulum. Biophys J 1995;68:936–945.
51. Josephson IR. Lidocaine blocks Na, Ca, and K currents of chick ventricular myocytes. J Mol Cell Cardiol 1988;20:593–604.
52. Baumgarten CM, Makielski JC, Fozzard HA. External site for local anesthetic block of cardiac Na^+ channels. J Mol Cell Cardiol. 1991;23:85–93.
53. Rutten AJ, Mather LE, McLean CF, Nancarrow C. Tissue distribution of bupivacaine enantiomers in sheep. Chirality 1993; 5:485–91.
54. Vree TB, Beumer EM, Lagerwerf AJ, et al. Clinical pharmacokinetics of R(+)- and S(−)-mepivacaine after high doses of racemic mepivacaine with epinephrine in the combined psoas compartment/sciatic nerve block. Anesth Analg 1992;75:75–80.
55. Tucker GT, Boyes RN, Bridenbaugh PO, Moore DC. Binding of anilide-type local anesthetics in human plasma. I. Relationships between binding, physicochemical properties, and anesthetic activity. Anesthesiology 1970;33:287–303.
56. Boyes RN. Absorption, diffusion, fixation, metabolism and excretion of local anesthetic agents in animal and man. In: Anesthésiques locaux en anesthésie et réanimation. Paris: Librairie Arnette, 1974:127–135.
57. Ritchie JM, Ritchie B, Greengard P. The effect of the nerve sheath on the action of local anesthetics. J Pharmacol Exp Ther 1965;150:160–164.
58. Ritchie JM, Ritchie B, Greengard P. The active structure of local anesthetics. J Pharmacol Exp Ther 1965;150:152–159.
59. Moore DC. The pH of local anesthetic solutions. Anesth Analg 1981;60:833–834.
60. Gasser HS, Erlanger J. Role of fiber size in the establishment of a nerve block by pressure or cocaine. Am J Physiol 1929;88:581–591.
61. Nathan PW, Sears TA. Some factors concerned in differential nerve block by local anaesthetics. J Physiol (Lond) 1961; 157:565–580.
62. Franz DN, Perry RS. Mechanisms for differential block among single myelinated and non-myelinated axons by procaine. J Physiol 1974;236:193–210.
63. Ford DJ, Raj PP, Singh P, et al. Differential peripheral nerve block by local anesthetics in the cat. Anesthesiology 1984;60:28–33.
64. de Jong RH. Differential nerve block. In: de Jong RH, ed. Local anesthetics. St. Louis: CV Mosby, 1994.
65. Datta S, Corke BC, Alper MH, et al. Epidural anesthesia for cesarean section: a comparison of bupivacaine, chloroprocaine and etidocaine. Anesthesiology 1980;52:48–51.
66. Heavner JE, Leinonen L, Haasio J, et al. Interaction of lidocaine

and hypothermia in Bier blocks in volunteers. Anesth Analg 1989;69:53–59.
67. Raj PP, Garcia CE, Burleson JW, Jenkins MT. The site of action of intravenous regional anesthesia. Anesth Analg 1972;51:776–786.
68. Tucker GT, Mather LE. Clinical pharmacokinetics of local anaesthetics. Clin Pharmacokinet 1979;4:241–278.
69. Reynolds F. A comparison of the potential toxicity of bupivacaine, lignocaine and mepivacaine during epidural blockade for surgery. Br J Anaesth 1971;43:567–572.
70. Appleyard TN, Witt A, Atkinson RE, Nicholas AD. Bupivacaine carbonate and bupivacaine hydrochloride: a comparison of blood concentrations during epidural blockade for vaginal surgery. Br J Anaesth 1974;46:530–533.
71. Raj PP, Rosenblatt R, Miller J, et al. Dynamics of local anesthetic compounds in regional anesthesia. Anesth Analg 1977;56:110–117.
72. Mather LE, Tucker GT, Murphy TM, et al. The effects of adding adrenaline to etidocaine and lignocaine in extradural anaesthesia. II. Pharmacokinetics. Br J Anaesth 1976;48:989–994.
73. Tucker GT, Moore DC, Bridenbaugh PO, et al. Systemic absorption of mepivacaine in commonly used regional block procedures. Anesthesiology 1972;37:277–287.
74. Wilkinson GR, Lund PC. Bupivacaine levels in plasma and cerebrospinal fluid following peridural administration. Anesthesiology 1970;33:482–486.
75. Abdel-Salam AR, Vonwiller JB, Scott DB. Evaluation of etidocaine in extradural block. Br J Anaesth 1975;47:1081–1086.
76. Stanton-Hicks M, Berges PU, Bonica JJ. Circulatory effects of peridural block. IV. Comparison of the effects of epinephrine and phenylephrine. Anesthesiology 1973;39:308–314.
77. Morgan DJ, Cousins MJ, McQuillan D, Thomas J. Disposition and placental transfer of etidocaine in pregnancy. Eur J Clin Pharmacol 1977;12:359–365.
78. Morikawa KI, Bonica JJ, Tucker GT, Murphy TM. Effect of acute hypovolemia on lignocaine absorption and cardiovascular response following epidural block in dogs. Br J Anaesth 1974; 46:631–635.
79. Bromage PR, Gertel M. Brachial plexus anesthesia in chronic renal failure. Anesthesiology 1972;36:488–493.
80. Mather LE, Thomas J. Bupivacaine binding to plasma protein fractions. J Pharm Pharmacol 1978;30:653–654.
81. Tucker GT, Mather LE. Pharmacology of local anesthetic agents: pharmacokinetics of local anesthetic agents. Br J Anaesth 1975;47:213–224.
82. Mazoit JX, Denson DD, Samii K. Pharmacokinetics of bupivacaine following caudal anesthesia in infants. Anesthesiology 1988;68:387–391.
83. Mather LE, Long GJ, Thomas J. The binding of bupivacaine to maternal and foetal plasma proteins. J Pharm Pharmacol 1971; 23:359–365.
84. Thomas J, Long G, Moore G, Morgan D. Plasma protein binding and placental transfer of bupivacaine. Clin Pharmacol Ther 1976;19:426–434.
85. Tucker GT, Boyes RN, Bridenbaugh PO, Moore DC. Binding of anilide-type local anesthetics in human plasma. II. Implications in vitro with special reference to transplacental disposition. Anesthesiology 1970;33:304–314.
86. Biehl D, Shnider SM, Levinson G, et al. Placental transfer of lidocaine: effects of acidosis. Anesthesiology 1978;48:409–412.
87. Brown WU Jr, Bell GC, Alper MH. Acidosis, local anesthetics, and the newborn. Obstet Gynecol 1976;48:27–30.
88. Reynolds F. Metabolism and excretion of bupivacaine in man: a comparison with mepivacaine. Br J Anaesth 1971;43:33–37.
89. Adjepon-Yamoah KK, Prescott LF. Lignocaine metabolism in man. Br J Pharmacol 1973;47:672P–673P.
90. Kisch B, Koster H, Strauss E. Procaine esterase. Exp Med Surg 1943;1:51–65.
91. Kalow W. Hydrolysis of local anesthetics by human serum cholinesterase. J Pharmacol Exp Ther 1952;104:122–134.
92. Reidenberg MM, James M, Dring LG. The rate of procaine hydrolysis in serum of normal subjects and diseased patients. Clin Pharmacol Ther 1972;13:279–284.
93. Foldes FF, Davidson GM, Duncalf D, Kuwabarra S. The intravenous toxicity of local anesthetic agents in man. Clin Pharmacol Ther 1965;6:328–335.
94. Brodie BB, Lief PA, Poet R. The fate of procaine in man following its intravenous administration and methods for the estimation of procaine and diethylaminoethanol. J Pharmacol Exp Ther 1948;94:359–366.
95. Patterson R, Anderson J. Allergic reactions to drugs and biologic agents. JAMA 1982;248:2637–2645.
96. Butterworth JF, Cole LR. Low concentrations of procaine and diethylaminoethanol reduce the excitability but not the action potential amplitude of hippocampal pyramidal cells. Anesth Analg 1990;71:404–410.
97. Denson DD, Mazoit JX. Physiology, pharmacology and toxicity of local anesthetics: adult and pediatric considerations. In: Raj PP, ed. Clinical practice of regional anesthesia. New York: Churchill Livingstone, 1991.
98. Rosenberg PH, Heavner JE. Acute cardiovascular and central nervous system toxicity of bupivacaine and desbutylbupivacaine in the rat. Acta Anaesthesiol Scand 1992;36:138–141.
99. Aldrete JA, Homatas J, Boyes RN, Starzl TE. Effects of hepatectomy on the disappearance rate of lidocaine from blood in man and dog. Anesth Analg 1970;49:687–690.
100. Arthur GR. Pharmacokinetics of local anesthetics. Handb Exp Pharmacol 1987;81:165–186.
101. Mihaly GW, Moore RG, Thomas J, et al. The pharmacokinetics and metabolism of the anilide local anaesthetics in neonates. I. Lignocaine. Eur J Clin Pharmacol 1978;13:143–152.
102. Keenaghan JB, Boyes RN. The tissue distribution, metabolism and excretion of lidocaine in rats, pigs, dogs and man. J Pharmacol Exp Ther 1972;180:454–463.
103. Strong JM, Parker M, Atkinson AJ. Identification of glycinexylidide in patients treated with intravenous lidocaine. Clin Pharmacol Ther 1973;14:67–72.
104. Rowland M, Thomson PD, Guichard A, Melmon KL. Disposition kinetics of lidocaine in normal subjects. Ann NY Acad Sci 1971;179:383–398.
105. Moore RG, Thomas J, Triggs EJ, et al. The pharmacokinetics and metabolism of the anilide local anaesthetics in neonates. III. Mepivacaine. Eur J Clin Pharm 1978;14:203–212.
106. Ralston DH, Shnider SM. The fetal and neonatal effects of regional anesthesia in obstetrics. Anesthesiology 1978;48:34–64.
107. Hjelm M, Holmdahl MH. Methaemoglobinaemia following lignocaine. Lancet 1965;1:53–54.
108. McLean S, Starmer GA, Thomas J. Methaemoglobin formation by aromatic amines. J Pharm Pharmacol 1969;21:441–450.
109. Hansson E, Hoffman P, Kristerson L. Fate of mepivacaine in the body: II. Excretion and biotransformation. Acta Pharmacol (Kobenhavn) 1965;22:213–223.
110. Boyes RN. A review of the metabolism of amide local anaesthetic agents. Br J Anaesth 1975;47:225–230.
111. de Jong RH. Therapeutic properties of local anesthetics. In: de Jong RH, ed. Local anesthetics. St. Louis: CV Mosby, 1994.
112. Glazer S, Portenoy RK. Systemic local anesthetics in pain control. J Pain Symptom Manage 1991;6:30–39.
113. Backonja MM. Local anesthetics as adjuvant analgesics. J Pain Symptom Manage 1994;9:491–499.
114. Boas RA, Covino BG, Shahnarian A. Analgesic responses to i.v. lignocaine. Br J Anaesth 1982;54:501–505.
115. Kastrup J, Angelo H, Petersen P, et al. Treatment of chronic painful diabetic neuropathy with intravenous lidocaine infusion. Br Med J (Clin Res) 1986;292:173.
116. Garfield JM, Gugino L. Central effects of local anesthetic agents. Handb Exp Pharmacol 1987;81:253–287.

117. Mautz FR. Reduction of cardiac irritability by the epicardial and systemic administration of drugs as a protection in cardiac surgery. J Thorac Surg 1936;5:612–628.
118. Mark LC, Kayden HJ, Steele JM. The physiological disposition and cardiac effects of procaine amide. J Pharmacol Exp Ther 1951;102:5–15.
119. Harrison DC, Sprouse JH, Morrow AG. The antiarrythmic properties of lidocaine and procaine amide: clinical and physiologic studies of their cardiovascular effects in man. Circulation 1963;28:486–491.
120. Cheng TO, Wadhwa K. Sinus standstill following intravenous lidocaine administration. JAMA 1973;223,790–792.
121. Gerstenblith G. Spear JF, Moore EN. Quantitative study of the effect of lidocaine on the threshold for ventricular fibrillation in the dog. Am J Cardiol 1972;30:242–247.
122. Arnsdorf MF, Bigger JT. The effect of lidocaine on components of excitability in long mammalian cardiac Purkinje fibers. J Pharmacol Exp Ther 1975;195:206–215.
123. Hondeghem LM. Antiarrhythmic agents: modulated receptor applications. Circulation 1987;75:514–520.
124. Hondeghem LM, Katzung BG. Antiarrhythmic agents: the modulated receptor mechanism of action of sodium and calcium channel-blocking drugs. Annu Rev Pharmacol Toxicol 1984;24:387–423.
125. Clarkson CW, Hondeghem LM. Mechanism for bupivacaine depression of cardiac conduction: fast block of sodium channels during the action potential with slow recovery from block during diastole. Anesthesiology 1985;62:396–405.
126. Arlock P. Actions of three local anesthetics: lidocaine, bupivacaine and ropivacaine on guinea pig papillary muscle sodium channels (V_{max}). Pharmacol Toxiciol 1988:63:96–104.
127. Courtney KR. Sodium channel blockers: the size/solubility hypothesis revisited. Mol Pharmacol 1990;37:855–859.
128. Grant AO, Strauss LJ, Wallace AG, Strauss HC. The influence of pH on the electrophysiologic effects of lidocaine in guinea pig ventricular myocardium. Circ Res 1980;47:542–550.
129. Bennett PB, Woosley RL, Hondeghem LM. Competition between lidocaine and one of its metabolites, glycylxylidide, for cardiac sodium channels. Circulation 1988;78:692–700.
130. Clarkson CW, Hondeghem LM. Evidence for a specific receptor site for lidocaine, quinidine, and bupivacaine associated with cardiac sodium channels in guinea pig ventricular myocardium. Circ Res 1985;56:496–506.
131. Bernhard CG, Bohm E. Local anaesthetics as anticonvulsants. A study on experimental and clinical epilepsy. Stockholm: Almqvist & Wiksell, 1965.
132. Julien RM. Lidocaine in experimental epilepsy: correlation of anticonvulsant effect with blood concentrations. Electroencephalogr Clin Neurophysiol 1973;34:639–645.
133. Liu PL, Feldman HS, Giasi R, et al. Comparative CNS toxicity of lidocaine, etidocaine, bupivacaine and tetracaine in awake dogs following rapid intravenous administration. Anesth Analg 1983;62:375–379.
134. Englesson S. The influence of acid-base changes on central nervous system toxicity of local anaesthetic agents. I. An experimental study in cats. Acta Anaesth Scand 1974;18:79–87.
135. de Jong RH, Bonin JD. Mixtures of local anesthetics are no more toxic than the parent drugs. Anesthesiology 1981;54:177–181.
136. Scott DB. Toxic effects of local anaesthetic agents on the central nervous system. Br J Anaesth 1986;58:732–735.
137. Lie KI, Wellens HJ, van Capelle FJ, Durrer D. Lidocaine in the prevention of primary ventricular fibrillation: a double-blind, randomized study of 212 consecutive patients. N Engl J Med 1974;291:1324–1326.
138. Klein SW, Sutherland RI, Morch JE. Hemodynamic effects of intravenous lidocaine in man. Can Med Assoc J 1968;99:472–475.
139. Gilman AG, Rall TW, Nies AS, Taylor P. Local anesthetics. In: Goodman AG, Goodman LS, Gilman A, eds. The pharmacological basis of therapeutics. 8th ed. New York: Pergamon Press, 1990:311–329.
140. Malagodi MH, Munson ES, Embro WJ. Relation of etidocaine and bupivacaine toxicity to rate of infusion in rhesus monkeys. Br J Anaesth 1977;49:121–125.
141. Santos AC, Pedersen H, Harmon TW, et al. Does pregnancy alter the systemic toxicity of local anesthetics? Anesthesiology 1989;70:991–995.
142. Heavner JE, Dryden CF, Sanghani V, et al. Severe hypoxia enhances central nervous system and cardiovascular toxicity of bupivacaine in lightly anesthetized pigs. Anesthesiology 1992; 77:142–147.
143. de Jong RH, Wagman IH, Price DA. Effect of carbon dioxide on the cortical seizure threshold to lidocaine. Exp Neurol 1967; 17:221–232.
144. de Jong RH. Local anesthetics. 2nd ed. Springfield, IL: Charles C Thomas, 1977.
145. Modica PA, Tempelhoff R, White PF. Pro- and anticonvulsant effects of anesthetics. Anesth Analg 1990;70:433–444.
146. de Jong RH, Heavner JE. Diazepam prevents and aborts lidocaine convulsions in monkeys. Anesthesiology 1974;41:226–230.
147. de Jong RH, Bonin JD. Benzodiazepines protect mice from local anesthetic convulsions and death. Anesth Analg 1981;60:385–389.
148. Bernards CM, Carpenter RL, Rupp SM, et al. Effect of midazolam and diazepam premedication on central nervous system and cardiovascular toxicity of bupivacaine in pigs. Anesthesiology 1989;70:318–323.
149. Yokoyama M, Benson KT, Arakawa K, Goto H. Effects of flumazenil on intravenous lidocaine-induced convulsions and anticonvulsant property of diazepam in rats. Anesth Analg 1992; 75:87–90.
150. Wesseling H, Bovenhorst GH, Wiers JW. Effects of diazepam and pentobarbitone on convulsions induced by local anesthetics in mice. Eur J Pharmacol 1971;13:150–154.
151. Heavner JE, Arthur J, Zou J, et al. Comparison of propofol with thiopentone for treatment of bupivacaine-induced seizures in rats. Br J Anaesth 1993;71:715–719.
152. Hartung J, Ying H, Weinberger J, Cottrell JE. Propofol prevents or elevates the threshold for lidocaine-induced seizures in rats. J Neurosurg Anesthesiol 1994;6:254–259.
153. de Jong RH, Ronfeld R, DeRosa R. Cardiovascular effects of convulsant and supraconvulsant doses of amide local anesthetics. Anesth Analg 1982;61:3–9.
154. Tanz RD, Heskett T, Loehning W, Fairfax CA. Comparative cardiotoxicity of bupivacaine and lidocaine in the isolated perfused mammalian heart. Anesth Analg 1984;63:549–556.
155. Reiz S, Nath S. Cardiotoxicity of local anaesthetic agents. Br J Anaesth 1986;58:736–746.
156. Nath S, Haggmark S, Johansson G, Reiz S. Differential depressant and electrophysiologic cardiotoxicity of local anesthetics: an experimental study with special reference to lidocaine and bupivacaine. Anesth Analg 1986;65:1263–1270.
157. Collinsworth KA, Kalman SM, Harrison DC. The clinical pharmacology of lidocaine as an antiarrhythmic drug. Circulation 1974;50:1217–1230.
158. Coyle DE, Sperelakis N. Bupivacaine and lidocaine blockade of calcium-mediated slow action potentials in guinea pig ventricular muscle. J Pharmacol Exp Ther 1987;242:1001–1005.
159. Kotelko DM, Shnider SM, Dailey PA, et al. Bupivacaine induced cardiac arrhythmias in sheep. Anesthesiology 1984; 60:10–18.
160. Kasten GW, Martin ST. Bupivacaine cardiovascular toxicity: comparison of treatment with bretylium and lidocaine. Anesth Analg 1985; 64:911–916.
161. Kasten GW. Amide local anesthetic alterations of effective re-

fractory period temporal dispersion: relationship to ventricular arrhythmias. Anesthesiology 1986;65:61–66.
162. Heavner JE. Cardiac dysrhythmias induced by infusion of local anesthetics into the lateral cerebral ventricles of cats. Anesth Analg 1986;65:133–138.
163. Thomas RD, Behbehani MM, Coyle DE, Denson DD. Cardiovascular toxicity of local anesthetics: an alternative hypothesis. Anesth Analg 1986;65:444–450.
164. Denson DD, Behbehani MM, Gregg RV. Enantiomer-specific effects of an intravenously administered arrhythmogenic dose of bupivacaine on neurons of the nucleus tractus solitarius and the cardiovascular system in the anesthetized rat. Reg Anesth 1992;17:311–316.
165. Bernards CM, Artru AA. Hexamethonium and midazolam terminate dysrhythmias and hypertension caused by intracerebroventricular bupivacaine in rabbits. Anesthesiology 1991; 74:89–96.
166. Lynch C. Depression of myocardial contractility in vitro by bupivacaine, etidocaine, and lidocaine. Anesth Analg 1986; 65:551–559.
167. Itoh H, Minakuchi C, Hase K. The effect of local anesthetics on the isolated human right atrial appendages. 1. A comparison of inhibition of contractility with bupivacaine and lidocaine. Masui 1991;40:1198–203.
168. Courtney KR, Strichartz GR. Structural elements which determine local anesthetic activity. Handb Exp Pharmacol 1987; 81:53–94.
169. Eledjam JJ, de La Coussaye JE, Brugada J, et al. In vitro study on mechanisms of bupivacaine-induced depression of myocardial contractility. Anesth Analg 1989; 69:732–735.
170. Minakuchi C, Itoh H. The effect of local anesthetics on the isolated human right appendages. Part 2. Bupivacaine is different from lidocaine concerning the mechanism of inhibition of contractility. Masui 1991;40:1204–1209.
171. Albright GA. Cardiac arrest following regional anesthesia with etidocaine or bupivacaine. Anesthesiology 1979;51:285–287.
172. Prentiss JE. Cardiac arrest following caudal anesthesia. Anesthesiology 1979;50:51–53.
173. Rosen MA, Thigpen JW, Shnider S, et al. Bupivacaine-induced cardiotoxicity in hypoxic and acidotic sheep. Anesth Analg 1985;64:1089–1096.
174. Sage DJ, Feldman HS, Arthur GR, et al. Influence of lidocaine and bupivacaine on isolated guinea pig atria in the presence of acidosis and hypoxia. Anesth Analg 1984;63:1–7.
175. Moore DC, Crawford RD, Scurlock JE. Severe hypoxia and acidosis following local anesthetic-induced convulsions. Anesthesiology 1980;53:259–260.
176. Tucker GT, Lennard MS. Enantiomer specific pharmacokinetics. Pharmacol Ther 1990;45:309–329.
177. Denson DD, Behbehani MM, Gregg RV. Enantiomer-specific effects of an intravenously administered arrhythmogenic dose of bupivacaine on neurons of the nucleus tractus solitarius and the cardiovacsular system in the anesthetized rat. Reg Anesth 1992;17:311–316.
178. Rutten AJ, Nancarrow C, Mather LE, et al. Hemodynamic and central nervous system effects of intravenous bolus doses of lidocaine, bupivacaine, and ropivacaine in sheep. Anesth Analg 1989;69:291–299.
179. Feldman HS, Arthur GR, Covino BG. Comparative systemic toxicity of convulsant and supraconvulsant doses of intravenous ropivacaine, bupivacaine and lidocaine in the conscious dog. Anesth Analg 1989;69:794–801.
180. Scott DB, Lee A, Fagan D, et al. Acute toxicity of ropivacaine compared with that of bupivacaine. Anesth Analg 1989;69:563–569.
181. Johns RA, Seyde WC, DiFazio CA, Longnecker DE. Dose-dependent effects of bupivacaine on rat muscle arterioles. Anesthesiology 1986;65;186–191.
182. Johns RA, DiFazio CA, Longnecker DE. Lidocaine constricts or dilates rat arterioles in a dose-dependent manner. Anesthesiology 1985;62;141–144.
183. Lofstrom JB. 1991 Labat Lecture. The effect of local anesthetics on the peripheral vasculature [Review]. Reg Anesth 1992;17:1–11.
184. Johns RA. Local anesthetics inhibit endothelium-dependent vasodilation. Anesthesiology 1989;70:805–811.
185. Meyer P, Flammer J, Luscher TF. Local anesthetic drugs reduce endothelium-dependent relaxations of porcine ciliary arteries. Invest Ophthalmol 1993;34:2730–2736.
186. Adriani J. Etiology and management of adverse reactions to local anesthetics. Int Anesthesiol Clin 1972;10:127–151.
187. Aldrete JA, Johnson DA. Evaluation of intracutaneous testing for investigation of allergy to local anesthetic agents. Anesth Analg 1970;49:173–183.
188. Holty G, Hood FJC. An anaphylactoid reaction to lidocaine. Den Pract Den Res 1965;15:294–296.
189. Waldman HB, Binkley G. Lidocaine hypersensitivity: report of case. J Am Dent Assoc 1967;74:747–749.
190. Kennedy KS, Cave RH. Anaphylactic reaction to lidocaine. Arch Otolaryngol Head Neck Surg 1986;112:671–673.
191. Wang GK, Quan C, Vladimirov M, et al. Quaternary ammonium derivative of lidocaine as a long-acting local anesthetic. Anesthesiology 1995;83:1293–1301.
192. Lee JJ, Rubin AP. EMLA cream and its current uses Br J Hosp Med 1994;51:614–615.
193. Gajraj NM, Pennant JH, Watcha MF. Eutectic mixture of local anesthetics (EMLA) cream. Anesth Analg 1994;78:574–583.
194. Bjerring P, Arendt-Nielsen L. Depth and duration of skin analgesia to needle insertion after topical application of EMLA cream. Br J Anaesth 1990;64:173–177.
195. Maddi R, Horrow JC, Mark JB, et al. Evaluation of a new cutaneous topical anesthesia preparation. Reg Anesth 1990; 15:109–112.
196. Arendt-Neilsen L, Bjerring P, Nielsen J. Regional variations in analgesic efficacy of EMLA cream. Quantitatively evaluated by argon laser stimulation. Acta Dermatol Venereol 1990;70:314–318.
197. Nilsson A, Engerg G, Henneberg S, et al. Inverse relationship between age-dependent erythrocyte activity of methaemoglobin reductase and prilocaine-induced methaemoglobinaemia during infancy. Br J Anaesth 1990;64:72–76.
198. Nioloux C, Floch-Tudal C, Jaby-Sergent MP, Lejeune C. Local anesthesia with "EMLA" cream and risk of methemoglobinemia in a premature infant. Arch Pediatr 1995;2:291–292.
199. Gangarosa LP. Iontophoresis: a modality for expanding dental practice. Gen Dentistry 1988;36:402–404.
200. Greenbaum SS, Bernstein EF. Comparison of iontophoresis of lidocaine with a eutectic mixture of lidocaine and prilocaine (EMLA) for topically administered local anesthesia. J Dermatol Surg Oncol 1994;20:579–583.
201. Boogaerts J, Declercq A, Lafont N, et al. Toxicity of bupivacaine encapsulated into liposomes and injected intravenously: comparison with plain solutions. Anesth Analg 1993;76:553–555.
202. Grant GJ, Vermeulen K, Langerman L, et al. Prolonged analgesia with liposomal bupivacaine in a mouse model. Reg Anesth 1994;19:264–269.
203. Shulman M, Joseph NJ, Haller CA. Effect of epidural and subarachnoid injections of a 10% butamben suspension. Reg Anesth 1990;15:142–146.
204. Korsten HH, Ackerman EW, Grouls RJ, et al. Long-lasting epidural sensory blockade by n-butyl-p-aminobenzoate in terminally ill intractable cancer pain patient. Anesthesiology 1991; 75:950–960.

IV PHARMACOKINETICS AND DYNAMICS OF MUSCLE RELAXANTS

14 d-Tubocurarine and Succinylcholine

Burdett R. Porter and Martin D. Sokoll

d-TUBOCURARINE

Native Americans living in the Amazon region were the first to use curare for its neuromuscular effects. This benzylisoquinoline is found in the vine *Chondrodendron tomentosum* and is the key ingredient in poison arrows. Its application in hunting and fighting dates to at least the sixteenth century (1). In 1850, Pelouze and Bernard determined that curare blocked neuromuscular transmission, but it did not affect nerve or muscle excitability (2). T. Spencer Wells described the employment of curare to treat three cases of tetanus in 1859 (3). Other investigators used curare extracts to modify the convulsions associated with electroconvulsive therapy (ECT) (4). Lawen related his use of curarine as an anesthetic adjunct in a 1912 German publication (5). Unfortunately, the majority of the English-speaking anesthesia community did not read this article. In 1942, Griffith and Johnson of Montreal published their success with curare in *Anesthesiology* (6). The following year, Stuart C. Cullen reported curare-induced abdominal wall relaxation in his study of 131 patients (7).

In humans, each muscle cell receives innervation from one neuromuscular junction, with the exception of extraocular and facial muscles, which receive innervation from multiple junctions (8). The terminal end of the axon forms a synapse with the muscle cell. Nerve impulses produce an influx of ionized calcium at the nerve terminus that causes acetylcholine containing vesicles to adhere to the internal wall of the cell membrane and then release acetylcholine into the synaptic cleft (9). The action of ionized calcium at the presynaptic membrane is antagonized by magnesium. Acetylcholine migrates across the cleft to interact with nicotinic (cholinergic) receptors on the postsynaptic membrane (Fig. 14-1). Each nicotinic receptor is composed of two α subunits, one β subunit, one δ subunit, and one ϵ subunit. The acetylcholine molecules bind to each of the α subunits and cause the receptor to transform to allow passage of sodium ions through a central channel (10) (Fig. 14-2). The sodium influx results in depolarization of the muscle cell (11). Acetylcholinesterase within the cleft hydrolyzes the acetylcholine into choline and acetate. At low concentrations, d-tubocurarine (d-TC) competes with acetylcholine for α subunit binding sites. Acetylcholine must occupy both α subunits to open the channel. At high concentrations, d-TC produces a noncompetitive blockade by physically blocking the entrance of the open channel. This block cannot be reversed by increasing the concentration of acetylcholine.

The usual intubation dose of d-TC is 0.3 mg/kg; however, the bolus administration of doses as small as 0.25 mg/kg can cause significant histamine release (12). At high doses, d-TC produced hypotension as a result of sympathetic ganglionic block (13, 14). In 1954, Beecher and Todd (15) reported an increased mortality in patients who received muscle relaxants. However, their study design did not control for sicker patients accepted for surgery under "light" anesthetic. Gray and colleagues in Liverpool popularized the combination of oxygen, nitrous oxide, and large doses of muscle relaxant to provide an adequate surgical field (16). Unfortunately, widespread use of the so-called "Liverpool technique" led to the administration of muscle relaxants without adequate anesthesia or analgesia, leading to patient recall of intraoperative events (17, 18).

Anticholinesterases reverse neuromuscular block with d-TC by allowing acetylcholine to accumulate in the junctional cleft and to compete for the α subunits of the receptors. Edrophonium (0.5 to 1.0 mg/kg), neostigmine (0.035 to 0.070 mg/kg), or pyridostigmine (0.15 to 0.30 mg/kg) can be used to reverse residual paralysis. Larger doses of these reversal agents can block the ion channel (19, 20). Acetylcholinesterase hydrolyzes both neostigmine and pyridostigmine, and these agents bind by a covalent bond to the inhibitor. In contrast, edrophonium relies on electrostatic attraction for binding. Although each molecule occupies an enzyme site for only milliseconds, the molecule is quickly replaced by another edrophonium molecule. Duration of reversal depends on the renal clearance of edrophonium from the body, not on the duration of binding at the enzyme (21). Usually an anticholingergic (e.g., glycopyrrolate, 15 μg/kg or atropine, 20 μg/kg), is paired with the anticholinesterase to counter the muscarinic side effects.

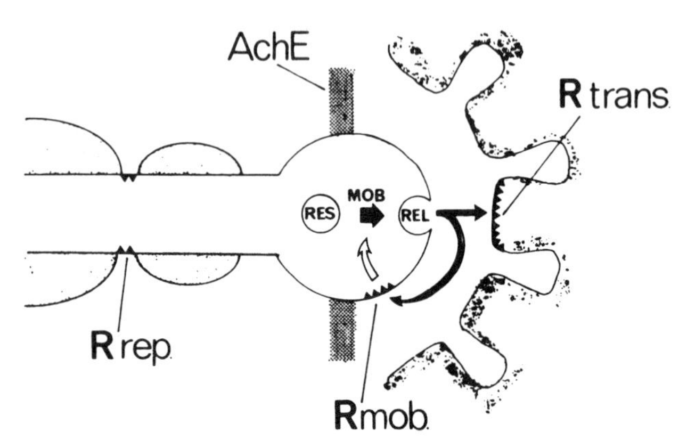

FIGURE 14-1. Nerve ending and the postjunctional membrane of the motor end plate. Transmission is mediated by acetylcholine stimulating the postjunctional receptors (R trans). The released acetylcholine also stimulates prejunctional receptors (R mob), which facilitate mobilization (MOB) of vesicles from the reserve (RES) to the readily releasable (REL) store, so output of acetylcholine can keep up with the demands of high-frequency stimulation. A second population of prejunctional receptors (R rep) located at the first node of Ranvier are represented. These mediate depolarization of the axonal membrane, which may give rise to repetitive firing of the nerve fibers. (Adapted from Bowman WC. Prejunctional and postjunctional cholinoceptors at the neuromuscular junction. Anesth Analg 1980;59:940.)

The effect of cholinesterase inhibitors can be evaluated by monitoring train-of-four stimulation and tetanic stimulation at 50 Hz sustained for 5 seconds at the adductor pollicis longus. Ideally, the train-of-four ratio should be greater than 0.70 (22, 23). Although this degree of reversal assures return of respiratory function, it may not result in patient comfort (24). A train-of-four ratio of 0.90 or greater before extubation is a more conservative approach.

After intravenous administration, d-TC distributes first into the extracellular fluid (i.e., from plasma to interstitial fluid). In the plasma, d-TC binds to both albumin (16%) and γ globulin (24%) (25). Aladjiemoff and associates (26) found a significant interpatient variation in plasma protein binding. Patients with the greatest binding were resistant to the effects of d-TC. The initial distribution from plasma to interstitial fluid requires 10 to 20 minutes and accounts for the initial rapid decrease in plasma levels (27). d-TC begins to act at the receptors before equilibration with the interstitial fluid because of the close proximity of capillaries to the neuromuscular junctions (27). Gibaldi and associates (28) asserted that the site of action lies within the central (pharmacokinetic) compartment and developed a three-compartment model to describe its pharmacokinetics. However, Ramzan and associates (29) and Ham and colleagues (30) preferred a two-compartment model. Sheiner and associates (31) presented a two-compartment pharmacodynamic model using the Hill equation (32) (Fig. 14-3). Although infants and children have a larger volume of distribution for d-TC than adults (i.e., pharmacokinetic differences), they also exhibit increased sensitivity to the drug (i.e., pharmacodynamic difference), such that the recommended dose on a per kilogram basis is unchanged (33). In pa-

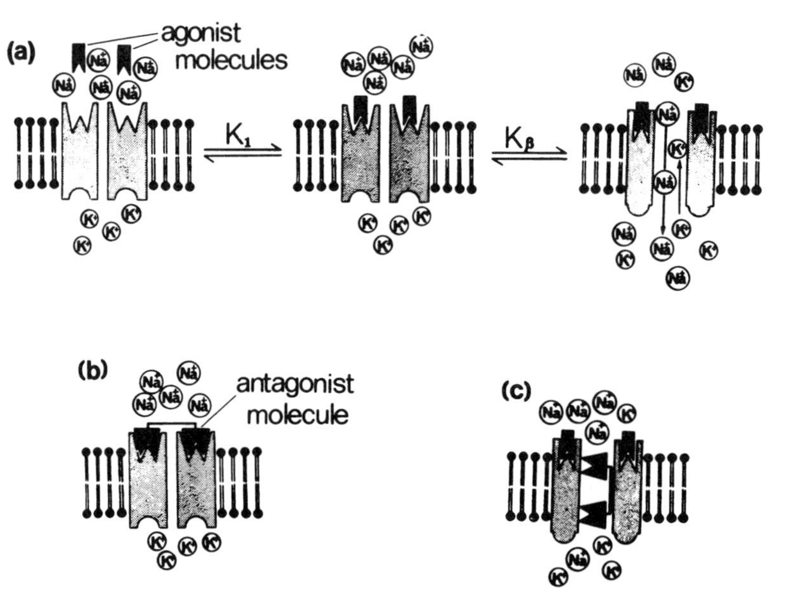

FIGURE 14-2. Diagrammatic representation of the interaction of an agonist (e.g., acetylcholine) and an antagonist (e.g., tubocurarine) with the end plate cholinoceptors. A, Agonist molecules combine with the recognition sites of the receptor and induce a conformational change in the ion conductance modulator protein. Ion channels open, allowing the diffusion of Na+ and K+ ions down their concentration gradients. B, An antagonist molecule has combined with the recognition sites of the closed-channel form of the receptor; no conformational change is induced. C, An antagonist molecule has combined with and blocked the open-channel form of the receptor, the ion channel having been opened by agonist molecules. (Adapted from Bowman WC. Peripheral cholinoceptors. In: Scurr C, Feldman S, eds. Scientific foundations of anaesthesia. London: William Heinemann Medical Books, 1982.)

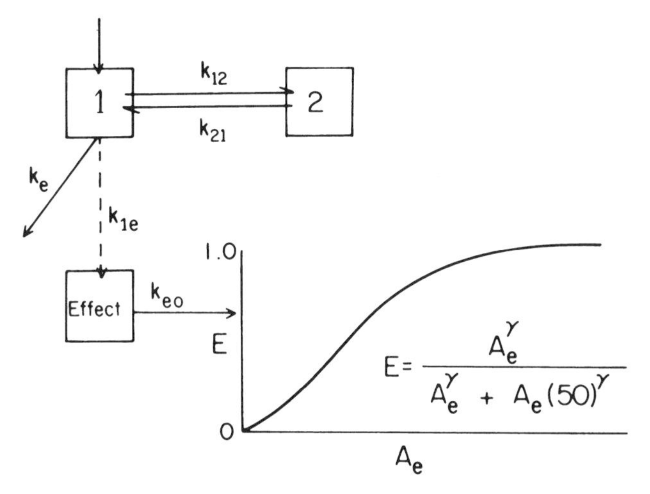

FIGURE 14-3. The pharmacokinetic and pharmacodynamic model as applied to d-tubocurarine (d-Tc). Plasma concentration data are treated as a two-compartment mamillary model, with k_{21} and k_{12} being rate constants of drug transfer between compartments 1 and 2. K_e is the rate constant for drug elimination from the body. The Hill equation shown is used to relate A_e, the amount of drug in the hypothetical effect compartment, to the effect, E, and generate a sigmoid concentration-effect curve. Model parameters that are determined in the nonlinear regression are k_{e0}, the first-order rate constant that characterizes the plasma concentration-effect dysequilibrium, g, a parameter of the Hill equation that allows sigmoidicity of response, and $A_e(50)$, a constant term in the Hill equation. (Adapted from Stanski DR, Ham J, Miller RD, et al. Pharmacokinetics and pharmacodynamics of d-TC during nitrous oxide-narcotic and halothane anesthesia in man. Anesthesiology 1979;51:237.)

tients over 70 years of age, Matteo and associates (34) found a decreased volume of distribution, decreased plasma clearance, and prolonged elimination half-life. Plasma concentration-response relationships remained unchanged. The prolonged effect of d-TC in patients over 70 years of age appears to be related to altered pharmacokinetic factors.

Miller and associates (35) determined that the kidneys eliminated 38% of d-TC unchanged in 24 hours. The ionized nature of the molecule impedes tubular resorption after filtration at the glomerulus. Meijer and associates (36) found that urinary excretion accounted for 45% of the drug's clearance in 24 hours and 63% in 48 hours. For both 24- and 48-hour measurements, biliary excretion cleared approximately 11% of curare unchanged. The fate of the remaining drug is unknown. The steady-state volume of distribution is approximately 300 ml/kg, with a clearance of 3 ml/kg/min, resulting in an elimination half-life of 120 minutes (37).

SUCCINYLCHOLINE

Hunt and de Taveau (38) reported on the first laboratory use of succinylcholine in 1906. They examined the cardiovascular effects of the drug on curarized felines and therefore did not appreciate the agent's profound neuromuscular blocking potential. In 1949, work by Bovet and associates (5) and by Phillips (5) documented the neuromuscular effect. Bruke and colleagues (5) introduced the clinical use of succinylcholine in Europe in 1951. Foldes and associates (39) described their experience in the United States in 1952. Foldes and his colleagues recognized that rapid changes in the degree of muscle relaxation was possible with succinylcholine as a result of its rapid and extensive clearance from the plasma. This property has led to widespread clinical use of succinylcholine in spite of its well-known side effects.

The molecular structure of succinylcholine consists of two acetylcholine molecules linked together by the acetyl moieties (i.e., diacetylcholine). Succinylcholine attaches to the α subunits of the cholinergic receptor and opens the ion channel. Because the cellular membranes depolarizes, this drug has been classified as a depolarizing muscle relaxant. Succinylcholine acts as an agonist at both nicotinic and muscarinic receptors. Succinylcholine's action on the presynaptic nicotinic receptor produces fasciculations, whereas its action on the postsynaptic receptor results in muscle relaxation. The most prominent muscarinic side effect is bradycardia (40-44) in children, or if the dose is repeated within 5 minutes. Succinylcholine owes its short duration of activity to rapid metabolism by butyrylcholinesterase (i.e., plasma cholinesterase). The succinylcholine molecule undergoes hydrolysis to form succinylmonocholine, a neuromuscular blocker with a low potency. Further metabolism of succinylmonocholine produces succinic acid and choline. Once succinylcholine reaches the neuromuscular junction, it cannot undergo metabolism by acetylcholinesterase within the synaptic cleft. The molecule must diffuse from the receptor and enter the plasma for further degradation (45).

The usual intubating dose of succinylcholine is 1 mg/kg, or 1.5 mg/kg if a defasciculating dose of nondepolarizing muscle relaxant has been administered. The onset is usually within 45 to 90 seconds, with a duration of action of 10 to 15 minutes.

Abnormalities in plasma cholinesterase activity can lead to prolonged block with succinylcholine. In 1957, Kalow and Genest (46) described the use of dibucaine, an amide local anesthetic, to detect abnormal plasma cholinesterase. Normally, dibucaine inhibits plasma cholinesterase activity by 80%. However, with atypical plasma cholinesterase, activity is only inhibited by 20%. Patients with 60% inhibition of plasma cholinesterase activity are considered to be genetic heterozygotes. Two other allelic expressions were reported by Harris and Whittaker (47) in 1961, namely, silent and fluoride-sensitive. These variants are rare. Homozygous normal occurs in approximately 96% of the population (48). These patients have qualitatively normal enzyme, but they may still have some prolongation of block if the quantitative amount of enzyme is less than normal (49).

In patients with normal quality and quantity of the enzyme, a single dose of succinylcholine larger than 2 to 5 mg/kg, or prolonged infusions of the drug, may lead to a transition phase and ultimately what appears to be a nondepolarizing neuromuscular block (50-53). This so-called phase II block is characterized by fading of both train-of-four stimulation and tetanus, post-tetanic potentiation, and tendency toward prolonged recovery (53, 54). Similar to nondepolarizing muscle relaxants, this block can be reversed with anticholinesterase drugs after succinylcholine is metabolized from the arterial blood by plasma cholinesterase (55). Ramsey and associates (54) recommend waiting at least 10 to 15 minutes after the bolus or infusion of succinylcholine is discontinued and then documenting spontaneous recovery of neuromuscular junction activity before reversing with anticholinesterase. Sokoll and Bastron (56) waited 30 minutes after terminating the infusion, documented improved myoneural conduction, and then administered edrophonium for further improvement.

In addition to bradycardia related to direct muscarinic receptor activation, succinylcholine can produce dysrhythmias related to hyperkalemia. The opening of acetylcholine receptor channels leads to an efflux of potassium concurrent with the influx of sodium. Following succinylcholine administration, Carter and associates (57) reported a serum potassium increase of 0.5 mEq/L in a control laboratory preparation. A much greater efflux occurs in pathologic conditions associated with nicotinic receptor proliferation or abnormal muscle membranes (e.g., burns, (58-61) trauma (62-64), neurologic injuries or neuromuscular diseases (65-67), and as well as intra-abdominal sepsis (68). In 1975 Gronert and Theye provided an extensive review of succinylcholine-induced hyperkalemia (69).

A side effect of succinylcholine that is possibly related to muscle fasiculations is muscle pain (myalgias) (70). The incidence of this complication ranges from 0.2 to 89% (71). Waters and Mapleson (72) hypothesized that unsynchronized muscle contractions in adjacent fibers damaged muscle tissue. Myoglobinuria following a single dose of succinylcholine is documented (73). Pretreatment with a nondepolarizing muscle relaxant before succinylcholine administration can prevent fasciculations (74), but its efficacy in preventing postoperative muscle pain remains less clear (71, 72, 74, 75).

Succinylcholine-related fasciculations also can increase intragastric and intraocular pressure. Miller and Way (76) reported that 5 of 30 patients studied had intragastric pressure increases greater than 30 cm H_2O. When fasciculations were prevented with nondepolarizing muscle relaxant pretreatment, no increase in intragastric pressure occurred. Smith and associates (77) questioned the clinical significance of this increase, arguing that fasciculation-related increases in intragastric pressure were matched by fasciculation-related increases in the high-pressure zone of the lower esophageal physiologic sphincter. Because the gradient between the two zones remained unchanged, there was no need for a defasciculating dose of nondepolarizing muscle relaxant.

The role played by extraocular muscle fasciculations with relation to increased intraocular pressure remains unclear. Miller and Way (78), as well as Libonati and associates (79), reported that a defasciculation dose before succinylcholine administration prevented the increase in intraocular pressure. In contrast, Meyers and colleagues (80) and Cook (81) were unable to stop the succinylcholine-associated increase in intraocular pressure. As an alternative, nondepolarizing muscle relaxants can be administered at two to three times their usual dose to provide rapid intubating conditions in patients with "open globe" injuries (82-85).

Succinylcholine-induced fasciculations also produce increases in intracranial pressure in patients with decreased intracranial elastance (86). Lanier and associates (87) demonstrated increased cerebral blood flow and intracranial pressure after succinylcholine administration. Increased muscle spindle activity produces increased cerebral afferent input, with resulting increased cerebral metabolism. Consequently, cerebral blood flow is increased. Stirt and colleagues (88) found that administration of metocurine before succinylcholine prevented the increase in intracranial pressure.

Succinylcholine is a trigger of malignant hyperthermia (MH) and is contraindicated in any patient with a family history positive for MH. Ombrédanne (89) first described anesthesia-induced postoperative hyperthermia with significant mortality in 1929. Denborough and Lovell (90) published their classic case study of anesthetic-related deaths in a family in 1960. In 1966, Hall and associates (91) reported the susceptibility of swine to succinylcholine and halothane. In 1975, Harrison (92) described the control of MH with dantrolene. The introduction of dantrolene reduced the mortality of MH from 70% in the early years to less than 10% (93).

With regard to pharmacokinetics, the majority of the injected dose of succinylcholine (80%) is hydrolyzed by plasma cholinesterase or is redistributed to the extracellular fluid in the first 5 minutes (94). Plasma protein binding and urinary elimination are negligible (94). Using high-performance liquid chromatography, Hoshi and associates (95) found the half-life to be 12 to 17 seconds and described the pharmacokinetics using a one-compartment model (Fig. 14-4 and Table 14-1). Nordgren and colleagues (96) demonstrated that re-

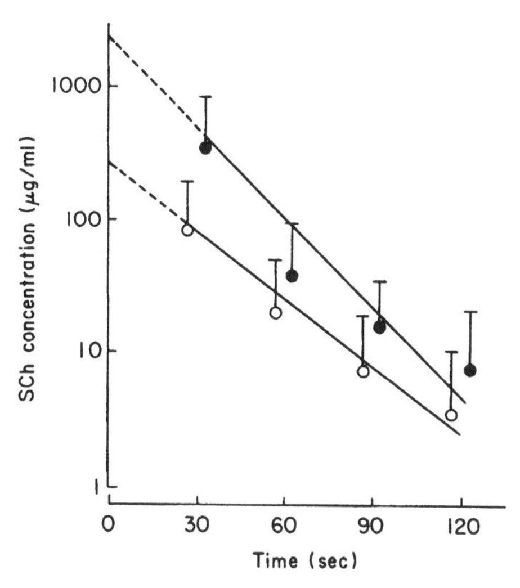

FIGURE 14-4. Semilogarithmic plot of mean arterial blood concentration versus time lines for succinylcholine. Open circles represent a 1-mg/kg dose, and solid circles represent a 2-mg/kg dose. The lines represent the best fit of an one-compartment model to each set of data. (Adapted from Hoshi K, Hashimoto Y, Matsukawa S. Pharmacokinetics of succinylcholine in man. Tohoku J Exp Med 1993;170:249.)

TABLE 14-1. Pharmacokinetic Parameters Derived by One-Compartment Model Analysis of Arterial Blood Succinylcholine Concentration Versus Time Data

	Succinylcholine	
	1 mg/kg (n = 8)	2 mg/kg (n = 6)
V_d (ml/kg)	16.4 ± 14.7	5.6 ± 6.8
Cl (L/min)	40.5 ± 38.3	15.0 ± 14.8
AUC (min μg/ml)	124.3 ± 163.2	695.3 ± 1008.9*
$t1k_2$ (sec)	16.6 ± 4.8	11.7 ± 4.5

*$p < 0.01$

V_d, Volume of distribution; Cl, clearance; AUC, area under the curve; $t1k_2$, rate constant.

(Adapted from Hoshi K, Hashimoto Y, Matsukawa S. Pharmacokinetics of succinylcholine in man. Tohoku J Exp Med 1993;170:248.)

distribution of succinylcholine also plays a significant role in decreasing its plasma concentration. Whether by metabolism or redistribution, the short plasma half-life of succinylcholine correlates with a brief duration of action in most patients. Succinylcholine remains the standard for muscle relaxants with a rapid onset and short duration of effect.

REFERENCES

1. Dittrick H. From the jungle to the operating room. Anesth Analg 1944;23:132.
2. Pelouze M, Bernard C. Recherches sur le curare. C R Acad Sci 1850;1850:533.
3. Wells TS. Three cases of tetanus in which "woorara" was used. Proc R Med Chir Soc Lond 1859;3:142–157.
4. Bennett AE. Preventing traumatic complications in convulsive shock therapy by curare. JAMA 1940;114:322–324.
5. Lee C. Succinylcholine: its past, present, and future. In: Katz RL, ed. Muscle relaxants. Orlando, FL: Grune & Stratton, 1984:69–85.
6. Griffith HR, Johnson GE. The use of curare in general anesthesia. Anesthesiology 1942;3:418.
7. Cullen SC. The use of curare for improvement of abdominal relaxation during halothane anesthesia: report on 131 cases. Surgery 1943;14:261.
8. Bowman WC. Pharmacology of neuromuscular function. Bristol, England: Wright, 1980.
9. Katz B. Nerve, muscle and synapse. New York: McGraw-Hill, 1966.
10. Dwyer T, Adams DJ, Hille B. The permeability of the endplate channel to organic cations in frog muscle. J Gen Physiol 1980; 75:469.
11. McArdle JJ. The neuromuscular junction. Mount Kisco, NY: Futura, 1984.
12. Moss J, Rosow CE, Savarese JJ, et al. Role of histamine in the hypotensive action of d-tubocurarine in humans. Anesthesiology 1981;55:19.
13. Bermingham AT, Hussein SZ. A comparison of skeletal neuromuscular and autonomic ganglion blocking potencies of five nondepolarizing relaxants. Br J Pharmacol 1980;70:501.
14. Healy TEJ, Palmer JP. In vitro comparison between the neuromuscular and ganglion blocking potency ratios of atracurium and tubocurarine. Br J Anaesth 1982;54:1307.
15. Beecher HK, Todd DP. A study of deaths with anesthesia and surgery. Ann Surg 1954;140:2.
16. Miller RD, Savarese JJ. Pharmacology of muscle relaxants and their antagonists. In: Miller RD, ed. Anesthesia. New York: Churchill Livingstone, 1990:390.
17. Bogetz MS, Katz JA. Recall of surgery for major trauma. Anesthesiology 1984;61:6.
18. Editorial. On being aware. Br J Anaesth 1979;51:711.
19. Payne JP, Hughes R, Azawi SA. Neuromuscular blockade by neostigmine in anaesthetized man. Br J Anaesth 1980;52:69.
20. Aracava Y, Deshpande S, Rickett D. The molecular basis of anticholinesterase actions on nicotinic and glutamatergic synapses. Ann N Y Acad Sci 1987;505:225.
21. Standaert FG. Neuromuscular physiology. In: Miller RD, ed. Anesthesia. New York: Churchill Livingstone, 1990:681.
22. Ali HH, et al. Stimulus frequency in the detection of NM block in man. Br J Anaesth 1970;42:967.
23. Brand JB, et al. Spontaneous recovery from non-depolarizing neuromuscular blockade: correlation between clinical and evoked responses. Anesth Analg 1977;56:55.
24. Howardy-Hansen P, et al. Pretreatment with non-depolarizing muscle relaxants: the influence on neuromuscular transmission and pulmonary function. Acta Anaesth Scand 1980; 24:419.
25. Ghoneim MM, Pandya H. Binding of d-tubocurarine to specific serum protein fractions. Br J Anaesth 1975;47:853.
26. Aladjiemoff L, Dikstein S, Shafrir E. Binding of d-tubocurarine chloride to plasma proteins. J Pharmacol 1958;123:43.
27. Kalow W. The distribution, destruction an elimination of muscle relaxants. Anesthesiology 1959;20:505–518.
28. Gibaldi M, Gerhard L, Hayton W. Kinetics of the elimination and neuromuscular blocking effect of d-tubocurarine in man. Anesthesiology 1972;36:213–218.
29. Ramzan IM, Shanks CA, Triggs EJ. Studies of d-tubocurarine pharmacokinetics in humans and dogs. Anaesth Intensive Care 1978;6:30–35.
30. Ham J, Miller RD, Sheiner LB, Matteo RS. Dosage schedule independence of d-tubocurarine pharmacokinetics and pharmacodynamics and recovery of neuromuscular function. Anesthesiology 1979;50:528–533.

31. Sheiner LB, Stanski DR, Vozeh S, et al. Simultaneous modeling of pharmacokinetics and pharmacodynamics: application to d-tubocurarine. Clin Pharmacol Ther 1979;25:358–371.
32. Stankski DR, Ham J, Miller RD, Sheiner LB. Pharmacokinetics and pharmacodynamics of d-tubocurarine during nitrous oxide-narcotic and halothane anesthesia in man. Anesthesiology 1979;51:235–241.
33. Fisher DM, O'Keeffe C, Stanski DR, et al. Pharmacokinetics and pharmacodynamics of d-tubocurarine in infants, children and adults. Anesthesiology 1982;57:203–208.
34. Matteo RS, Backus WW, McDaniel DD, Brotherton WP. Pharmacokinetics and pharmacodynamics of d-tubocurarine and metocurine in the elderly. Anesth Analg 1985;64:23–29.
35. Miller RD, Matteo RS, Benet LZ, Sohn YJ. The pharmacokinetics of d-tubocurarine in man with and without renal failure. J Pharmacol Exp Ther 1977;202:1–7.
36. Meijer DK, Weitering JG, Vermeer GA, Scaf AH. Comparative pharmacokinetics of d-tubocurarine and metocurine in man. Anesthesiology 1979;51:402–407.
37. Shanks CA. Pharmacokinetics of the nondepolarizing neuromuscular relaxants applied to the calculation of bolus and infusion dosage regimens. Anesthesiology 1986;64:72.
38. Hunt R, de Taveau R, et al. On the physiological action of certain cholin derivatives and new methods for detecting cholin. Br Med J 1906;2:1788–1791.
39. Foldes FF, Rendell-Baker L, Birch JH. Causes and prevention of prolonged apnea with succinylcholine. Anesth Analg 1956; 35:609.
40. Craythorne NWB, Turndorf H, Dripps RD. Changes in pulse rate and rhythm associated with the use of succinylcholine in anesthetized patients. Anesthesiology 1970;21:465.
41. Leigh MD, McCoy DD, Belton KM, et al. Bradycardia following intravenous administration of succinylcholine chloride to infants and children. Anesthesiology 1957,18:698.
42. Stoeltintg RK, Peterson C. Heart-rate slowing and junctional rhythm following intravenous succinylcholine with and without intramuscular atropine preanesthetic medication. Anesth Analg 1975;54:705.
43. Schoenstadt DA, Whitcher CE. Observations on the mechanism of succinylcholine-induced cardiac arrhythmias. Anesthesiology 1963;24:358.
44. Mathias JA, Evans-Prosser CDG, Churchill-Davidson HC. The role of nondepolarizing drugs in the prevention of suxamethonium bradycardia. Br J Anaesth 1970;42:609.
45. Basta SJ. Pharmacology of neuromuscular blocking agents. In: Rogers MC, Tinker JH, Covino BG, Longnecker DE. Principles and practice of anesthesiology. St. Louis: Mosby-Year Book, 1993:1521.
46. Kalow W, Genest K. A method for the detection of atypical forms of human serum cholinesterase: determination of dibucaine numbers. Can J Biochem 1957;35:339.
47. Harris H, Whittaker M. Differential inhibition of serum cholinesterase with fluoride: recognition of two new phenotypes. Nature 1961;191:496.
48. Whittaker M. Plasma cholinesterase variants and the anaesthetist. Anaesthesia 1971;26:127.
49. Viby-Mogensen J. Correlation of succinylcholine duration of action with plasma cholinesterase activity in subjects with normal enzyme. Anesthesiology 1980;53:517.
50. Donati F, Bevan DR. Long-term succinylcholine infusion during isoflurane anesthesia. Anesthesiology 1983;58:6.
51. Donati F, Bevan DR. Effect of enflurane and fentanyl on the clinical characteristics of long-term succinylcholine infusion. Can Anesth Soc J 1982;29:59.
52. Futter ME, Donati F, Bevan DR. Prolonged suxamethonium infusion during nitrous-oxide anaesthesia supplemented with halothane of fentanyl. Br J Anaesth 1983;55:947.
53. Lee C, Katz RL. Neuromuscular pharmacology. Br J Anaesth 1980;52:73.
54. Ramsey FM, Libowitz PW, Savarese JJ, et al. Clinical characteristics of long term succinylcholine neuromuscular blockade during balanced anesthesia. Anesth Analg 1980;59:110.
55. Gissen AJ, Katz RL, Karis JH, et al. Neuromuscular block in man during prolonged arterial infusion with succinylcholine. Anesthesiology 1966;27:242–249.
56. Sokoll MD, Bastron RD. Duration of desensitization (phase 2) block after succinylcholine infusion. Anesth Analg 1967;46: 682.
57. Carter JG, Sokoll MD, Gergis SD. Effect of spinal cord transection on neuromuscular function in the rat. Anesthesiology 1981; 55:542–546.
58. Schaner PJ, Brown RL, Kirksey TD, et al. Succinylcholine-induced hyperkalemia in burned patients. Anesth Analg 1969; 48:764.
59. Lowenstein E. Succinylcholine administration in the burned patient. Anesthesiology 1966;27:494.
60. Belin KP, Carleen CI. Cardiac arrest in the burned patient following succinylcholine administration. Anesthesiology 1966; 27:516.
61. Tolmie JD, Toyce TH, Mitchell GD. Succinylcholine danger in the burned patient. Anesthesiology 1967;28:467.
62. Birch AA, Mitchell GD, Playford GA, et al. Changes in serum potassium response to succinylcholine following trauma. JAMA 1969;210:490.
63. Kopriva C, Ratliff J, Fletcher JR, et al. Serum potassium changes after succinylcholine in patients with acute massive muscle trauma. Anesthesiology 1971;34:246.
64. Mazze RI, Escue HM, Houston JB. Hyperkalemia and cardiovascular collapse following administration of succinylcholine to the traumatized patient. Anesthesiology 1969;31:540.
65. Cooperman LH. Succinylcholine-induced hyperkalemia in neuromuscular disease. JAMA 1970;213:1867.
66. Cooperman LH, Strobel GE Jr. Kennell EM. Massive hyperkalemia after administration of succinylcholine. Anesthesiology 1970;32:161.
67. Stevenson PH, Birch AA. Succinylcholine induced hyperkalemia in a patient with a closed head injury. Anesthesiology 1979; 51:89.
68. Kohlshütter B, Baur H, Roth F. Suxamethonium-induced hyperkalemia in patients with severe intra-abdominal infections. Br J Anaesth 1976;48:557.
69. Gronert GA, Theye RA. Pathophysiology of hyperkalemia induced by succinylcholine. Anesthesiology 43:89;1975.
70. Dottori O, Loff BA, Ygge H. Muscle pains after suxamethonium. Acta Anaesth Scand 1965;9:247–256.
71. Brodsky JB, Brock-Unte JG, Samuels SI. Pancuronium pretreatment and post-succinylcholine myalgias. Anesthesiology 1979; 51:259.
72. Waters DJ, Mapleson WW. Suxamethonium pains: hypothesis and observation. Anaesthesia 1971;26:127.
73. Ryan JF, Kagen LJ, Hyman AI. Myoglobinemia after a single dose of succinylcholine. N Engl J Med 1971;285:824.
74. Jansen EC, Hansen PH. Objective measurement of succinylcholine-induced fasciculations and the effect of pretreatment with pancuronium or gallamine. Anesthesiology 1979;51:159.
75. Smith I, Ding Y, White PF. Comparison of induction, maintenance and recovery characteristics of sevoflurane-N_2O and propofol-sevoflurane-N_2O with propofol-isoflurane-N_2O anesthesia. Anesth Analg 1992;74:253–259.
76. Miller RD, Way WL. Inhibitor of succinylcholine-induced intragastric pressure by nondepolarizing muscle relaxants and lidocaine. Anesthesiology 1971;34:185.
77. Smith G, Dalling R, Williams TIR. Gastro-oesophageal pressure gradiant changes produced by induction of anesthesia and suxamethoniuim. Br J Anaesth 1978;50:1137.
78. Miller RD, Way WL. Inhibition of succinylcholine induced increased intraocular pressure by non-depolarizing muscle relaxant. Anesthesiology 1968;29:123–126.
79. Libonati MM, Leahy JJ, Ellison N. The use of succinylcholine in open eye surgery. Anesthesiology 1985;62:637.

80. Meyers EF, Krupin T, Johnson M, et al. Failure of non-depolarizing neuromuscular blockers to inhibit succinylcholine induced increased intracular pressure: a controlled study. Anesthesiology 1978;48:149–151.
81. Cook JH. The effect of suxamethonium on intraocular pressure. Anaesthesia 1981;36:359–365.
82. Badrinath SK, Vazecry A, McCarthy RJ, et al. The effect of different methods of inducing anesthesia on intraocular pressure. Anesthesiology 1986;65:431.
83. Lavery GG, McGalliard JN, Mirakhur RK, et al. The effects of atracurium on intraocular pressure during steady state anaesthesia and rapid sequence induction: a comparison with succinylcholine. Can Anaesth Soc J 1986;7:39.
84. Schneider MJ, Stirt JA, Finholt DA. Atracurium, vecuronium, and intraocular pressure in humans. Anesth Analg 1986;65:877.
85. Schwartz S, Ilias W, Lackner F, et al. Rapid tracheal intubation with vecuronium: the priming principle. Anesthesiology 1985; 62:388.
86. Minton MD, Grosslight K, Stirt JA, Bedford RF. Increases in intracranial pressure from succinylcholine: prevention by prior nondepolarizing blockade. Anesthesiology 1986;65:165.
87. Lanier WL, Milde JH, Michenfelder JD. Cerebral stimulation following succinylcholine in dogs. Anesthesiology 1986;64:551.
88. Stirt A, Grosslight KR, Bedford RF, et al. "Defasciculation" with metocurine prevents succinylcholine-induced increases in intracranial pressure. Anesthesiology 1987;67:50.
89. Ombrédanne L. De l'influence de l'anesthésique-employé dans la genèse des accidents post-opératoires de paleur-hyperthermie observés chez les nourrissons. Rev Med Fr 1929;10:617.
90. Denborough MA, Lovell RRH. Anaesthetic deaths in a family. Lancet 1960;2:45.
91. Hall LW, Woolf N, Bradley JWP, et al. Unusual reaction to suxamethonium chloride. Br Med J 1966;2:1305.
92. Harrison GG. Control of the malignant hyperpyrexic syndrome in MHS swine by dantrolene sodium. Br J Anaesth 1975;47:62.
93. Ranklev E, Fletcher R. Investigation of malignant hyperthermia in Sweden. Acta Anaesth Scand 1986;30:693.
94. Dal Santo G. Kinetics of distribution of radioactive labeled muscle relaxants. III. Investigatons with 14C-succinyldicholine and 14C-succinylmonocholine during controlled conditions. Anesthesiology 1969;29:435–443.
95. Hoshi K, Hashimoto V, Matsukawa S. Pharmacokinetics of succinylcholine in man. Tohoku J Exp Med 1993;170:245–250.
96. Nordgren I, Baldwin K, Forney R. Succinylcholine: tissue distribution and elimination from plasma in the dog. Biochem Pharmacol 1984;33:2519–2521.

15 Steroidal Compounds

Girish P. Joshi

HISTORY AND BACKGROUND

Following the introduction of curare (1), the use of neuromuscular blocking drugs increased significantly. Muscle relaxation was considered an essential part of balanced anesthesia by Gray and Holton (2). Neuromuscular blocking drugs have since become an important part of modern anesthetic practice. In one of the early clinical studies, Mushin and Mapleson tested a steroid bisquaternary ammonium salt (dipyrandium chloride) as a muscle relaxant, but found that the recovery from this drug was variable (3). Consequently, the search for new steroid-based muscle relaxants continued. Pancuronium bromide (Org NA 97) was the first synthetic aminosteroid muscle relaxant used in clinical practice (4). It was synthesized in 1964 by Hewett and Savage (4). Pancuronium provided an improved side effects profile because it did not release histamine or exhibit ganglionic blocking properties; however, it had prominent vagolytic activity. Although pancuronium remains in widespread use, the need still exists for a muscle relaxant with a rapid onset and short duration of action without cardiovascular side effects (5).

In the late 1970s and 1980s, the introduction of vecuronium (Org NC 45), an intermediate-acting steroidal relaxant, had a dramatic impact on clinical practice (6, 7). In addition to having a faster onset of relaxation and a more rapid and predictable recovery, this agent was devoid of cardiovascular effects over a wide dose range (8). Vecuronium was first synthesized more than 20 years ago by Savage and coworkers at the Organon Research Laboratories, in the same series of androstane compounds that yielded pancuronium (6).

Pipecuronium bromide, a long-acting muscle relaxant without cardiovascular side effects, was developed in Hungary in the late 1970s; however, it was not introduced in the United States until the early 1990s (9). More recently, rocuronium (Org 9426), an intermediate-acting relaxant with a more rapid onset of action, has been added to the anesthesiologist's armamentarium (10). Another steroidal muscle relaxant, Org 9487, an analog of vecuronium, is currently in early stages of clinical development. It is reported to have a rapid onset and a short duration of action (11). However, the search for a nondepolarizing neuromuscular blocking drug with a pharmacologic profile similar to that of succinylcholine continues.

Advances in our understanding of the pharmacokinetics and pharmacodynamics of neuromuscular blocking drugs, particularly the availability of more reliable analytic methods and improved understanding of the relationship between pharmacokinetics and structural properties important for muscle relaxant activity, have led to development of new and improved drugs (12-14). This chapter reviews the general pharmacology of the steroidal group of muscle relaxants, with emphasis on the new drugs. In addition, their pharmacokinetic and pharmacodynamic properties as well as the side effects are reviewed. Finally, the use of these drugs in special patient populations and important drug interactions involving these drugs in clinical practice are described.

STRUCTURE-ACTIVITY RELATIONSHIPS

Neuromuscular blocking drugs are quaternary ammonium compounds structurally related to acetylcholine because of the quaternary groups. Most muscle relaxants have two positive charges or at least two potential positive charges, separated by a bridging structure that is lipophilic and varies in size. The bridging structure is different for various neuromuscular blocking drugs and is a major determinant of potency. The structural characteristics of various neuromuscular blocking drugs, including the charge distribution, nature of substituents at the onium centers, and the interonium structure (between two quaternary nitrogen atoms) of the molecule, determine their interaction

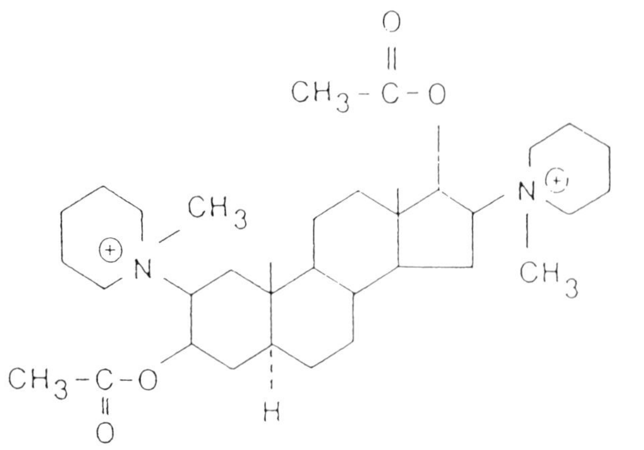

FIGURE 15-1. Chemical structure of pancuronium.

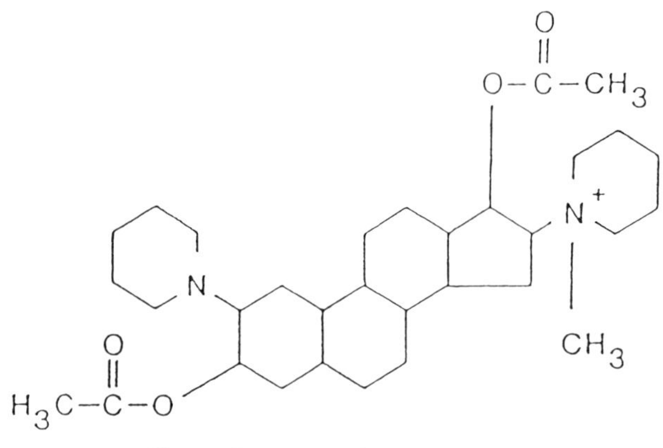

FIGURE 15-2. Chemical structure of vecuronium.

with acetylcholine receptors. The physicochemical features affect the transfer rate through biologic membranes, affinity for nonspecific binding sites and receptors, biotransformation, and excretion. Investigators originally thought that the distance between two quaternary nitrogen atoms (interonium distance) should be 1.2 to 1.4 nm for optimum neuromuscular blocking activity (15); however, this concept has been questioned.

Modification of steroidal nucleus with incorporation of acetylcholine-like structures into the molecule led to the development of potent nondepolarizing muscle relaxants (16). All currently available steroidal compounds are androstane derivatives with varying amino substitutes in positions 2 and 16. In an effort to develop an ideal muscle relaxant, Savage and coworkers incorporated into the steroid molecule chemical features that could theoretically contribute to the expected time-course of action and a more selective pharmacologic profile (6). Pancuronium bromide is a bisquaternary ammonium steroid compound with two quaternary ammonium groups separated by the 17-carbon atom ring structure common to all members of the steroid group of drugs (Fig. 15-1).

The muscarinic side effects of pancuronium were found to be due to the acetylcholine-like fragment A ring (2- to 3-position). The removal of the quaternizing methyl group in the 2-position eliminated the positive charge and reduced the acetylcholine-like character, which reduced the antimuscarinic property (6, 7, 17, 18). The newer steroidal muscle relaxants have been synthesized with a quaternary nitrogen in the D ring position. The lack of the second quaternary group did not affect potency, but a second nitrogen atom was essential for high activity. Thus, vecuronium, a monoquaternary analog of pancuronium without the N-methyl ammonium group at 2-position, was developed (Fig. 15-2). The tertiary amine in the A ring increases the lipophilicity of vecuronium, makes it susceptible to liver uptake, and reduces the duration of neuromuscular blockade (19).

Pipecuronium (Fig. 15-3) is a pancuronium derivative developed by changes in the quaternary groups, in which nitrogen atoms were moved to the distal (4-position) aspect of the 2,16-β-piperidino substitutions of pancuronium to 2,16-β-piperazino substitutions (20). The structural modifications of pipecuronium included a greater distance between the quaternary nitrogen moieties and were designed to improve its specificity thus, reducing the nicotinic side effects on the cardiac vagus nerve. This structural change increased the ratio of the vagolytic median effective dose (ED_{50}) to the neuromuscular ED_{50} from 2.5 for pancuronium to 25 for pipecuronium.

Improved understanding of the influence of structural modifications on the pharmacology of the neuromuscular blocking drugs resulted in the development of new muscle relaxants. However, until recently, investigators focused on potency rather than on the onset or duration of action of these drugs. Bowman and colleagues (21) observed that rapid onset with a nondepolarizing muscle relaxant was more likely with compounds that had low potency and rapid clearance. Similar observations were made by Kopman (22) in a clinical study comparing the onset of equipotent doses of gallamine, tubocurarine, and pancu-

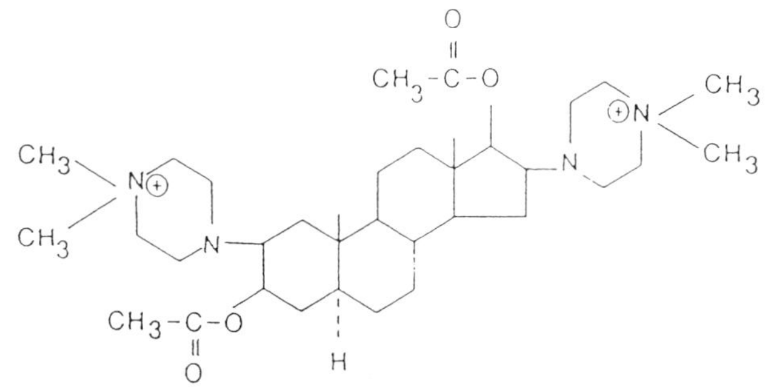

FIGURE 15-3. Chemical structure of pipercuronium.

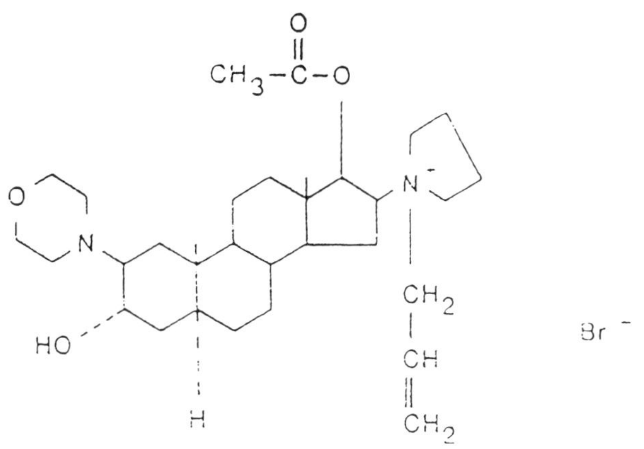

FIGURE 15-4. Chemical structure of rocuronium (Org 9426).

ronium. These findings led to modifications in the cycloamino structure of the androstne skeleton of aminosteroidal neuromuscular blocking drugs and resulted in the development of rocuronium (Org 9426) (23-25).

Rocuronium (Fig. 15-4) is a derivative of vecuronium with modification of the acetoxy substitution at position 3 to hydroxyl, substitution of piperidino group at position 2 by morphilino, and change of the position 16 substitution from piperidino with methyl quaternization to pyrrolidino with allyl quaternization. These structural changes result in a lower potency and faster onset of action than vecuronium; however, this does not change the duration of action or the rate of elimination. The lower potency of rocuronium also reduces the ratio of the vagolytic ED_{50} to neuromuscular ED_{50} from 50 for vecuronium to 5 for rocuronium (23). Thus, the possibility of vagolytic effects exists when high doses of rocuronium are administered.

Two new monoquaternary steroidal compounds, Org 7617 (16N-allyl, 17β-butyryl analog of vecuronium) and 9616 (differs from vecuronium only in possessing a 17α-butyryl group) with moderate potency and minor autonomic and cardiovascular side effects, are being investigated (26). In humans, Org 7617 has an rapid onset and a brief duration of action, but its low potency and the adverse effects suggestive of histamine release may prevent further clinical development of this drug (27). In animals, Org 9991, a 16-N-homopiperidinium substituted vecuronium analog, had an onset time of 1.2 to 1.9 minutes and a duration of 4.5 to 8.9 minutes (28). Effects on blood pressure or heart rate at 90% twitch blocking doses were either minor or absent (28). Org 9616 and Org 9991 have shorter duration of action than Org 9426 (rocuronium), but they decrease arterial blood pressure and increase heart rate with larger doses (29). Org 9273, a 2-morpholino, 3-desacetyl analog of vecuronium, has approximately 15 to 20% of the potency of vecuronium and a time course of action similar to that of vecuronium and rocuronium (30). However, three to four times ED_{90} of Org 9273 demonstrates a 20 to 25% increase in heart rate comparable to changes in heart rate after an intubation dose of pancuronium (30). Modifications in the 17-ester group of these compounds resulted in the development of Org 9453, Org 9489, and Org 9487. These compounds were rapid acting and had a short duration of action (31). Org 9487 (Fig. 15-5), the 16-N-allyl-17-β-propionate analog of vecuronium, has a fast onset and a short duration of action and is currently undergoing clinical trials.

PHARMACOKINETICS, METABOLISM, AND ELIMINATION

The pharmacokinetics of steroidal neuromuscular blocking drugs has been extensively reviewed (12-14, 32). Studies evaluating the pharmacokinetics of older muscle relaxants vary significantly in design, analytic technique, duration of sampling, and methodology of data analysis. The older analytic techniques such as the colorimetric and fluorometric assay lacked sensitivity and specificity because they did not discriminate between the unchanged drug and hydrolyzed, relatively inactive, metabolites (33). On the other hand, the mass spectrometry measures only the parent compound and not its metabolites (34). Other analytic techniques including gas chromatography and radioimmunoassay also have problems discriminating between the parent drug and its primary metabolites. However, sophisticated techniques including high-performance liquid chromatography methods are sensitive and specific for measuring levels of neuromuscular blocking drugs (35).

Neuromuscular blocking drugs have quaternary ammonium groups and have large molecules that are

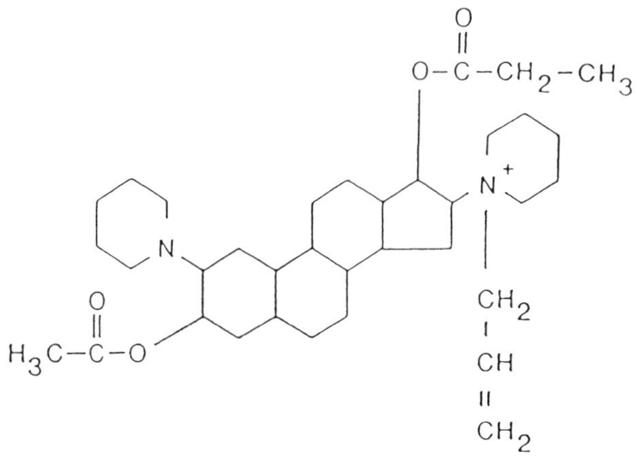

FIGURE 15-5. Chemical structure of Org 9487.

highly ionized regardless of pH, limiting their distribution to extracellular compartment (i.e., small volume of distribution). These drugs are highly water soluble, a property that prevents their passage across lipid membrane barriers, such as the blood-brain and placental barriers, renal tubular cells, hepatocytes, and nerve and muscle cells. Furthermore, neuromuscular blocking drugs are not significantly bound to plasma proteins (36, 37).

The disposition kinetics of pancuronium have been represented by multicompartment models (38-40). The volume of distribution at steady state for pancuronium is 230 ml/kg (180 to 300 ml/kg), whereas the plasma clearance is 1.3 ml/kg/min (0.8 to 3.0 ml/kg/min), and the elimination half-life is 145 minutes (90 to 250 minutes). Pharmacokinetic profile of pipecuronium is similar to that of pancuronium (Table 15-1) (9, 41-45). Khuenl-Brady and associates (43) studied the pharmacokinetics of pipecuronium in dogs using a two-compartment model and reported distribution and elimination half-life values of 3.9 and 44.8 minutes, respectively, with plasma clearance and mean residence time values of 0.9 ml/kg/min and 51.1 minutes, respectively. In humans, clearance of pipecuronium is 2.4 ml/kg/min (46). Plasma clearance rate is an important factor in determining the duration of action of a muscle relaxant (i.e., drugs that leave the plasma more rapidly have shorter duration of action).

Vecuronium fits the usual two- or three-compartment kinetic models with elimination occurring only from the central compartment. The initial volume of distribution is 51 ml/kg, steady-state volume of distribution is 260 ml/kg (191 to 510 ml/kg), and clearance is 4.6 ml/kg/min (3.6 to 6.7 ml/kg/min) (47-49). A shorter elimination half-life and more rapid clearance of vecuronium may be responsible for its shorter duration compared to pancuronium (49, 50). The elimination half-life of vecuronium in young adults is 70 to 90 minutes; liver uptake and biliary extraction contribute to a rapid clearance of vecuronium (19, 51). Fisher and Rosen (52), using a computer simulation, demonstrated that when a moderate dose of vecuronium (40 μg/kg) is administered, recovery occurs during the distribution phase. However, as the drug dose is increased, the recovery occurs further into the elimination phase.

The pharmacokinetic profile for rocuronium is similar to that of vecuronium and follows a three-compartment model (see Table 15-1). The distribution half-life is approximately 3 minutes, and the elimination half-life is 33 minutes (53). The volume of distribution at steady state is approximately 290 ml/kg, and the clearance is 3.0 ml/kg/min. The volume of the central compartment and the volume of distribution at steady state are smaller than those for vecuronium. However, the pharmacokinetic parameters vary.

Preliminary pharmacokinetic study of Org 9487 administered as a bolus (1.5 mg/kg) or infusion produced a plasma concentration decay described by a triexponential equation (31, 54), suggesting a relatively high plasma clearance (11.1 ml/kg/min) with a terminal half-life of 88 minutes (31). However, the terminal half-life values of Org 9487 were only slightly shorter than those of vecuronium (108 and 116 minutes) (49, 55) and rocuronium (94 and 97 minutes) (56, 57). The shorter duration of action of Org 9487 may be related to its higher rate of initial clearance.

Metabolism and Elimination

In contrast to the benzylisoquinolium group of muscle relaxants, the metabolism of the steroidal neuromuscular blocking drugs is generally independent of modifications in their structure. Steroidal muscle relaxants are less extensively metabolized and are excreted unchanged in the urine and bile. This group of drugs undergo deacetylation at 3 and 17 positions into three alcohol metabolites, 3-hydroxy, 17-hydroxy, or 3,17-dihydroxy compounds (Fig. 15-6).

Pancuronium does not undergo significant metabolism (58) and is predominantly excreted unchanged by the kidney, with 30 to 70% of the dose eliminated in the urine over 24 hours (38, 59-61). In animals, less than 25% of the injected pancuronium was detected unchanged in the liver (58, 62). Approximately 15 to 20% of pancuronium undergoes 3-deacetylation to 3-hydroxy pancuronium (33), and 10 to 20% of 3-hydroxy pancuronium is detected in the urine and 5% in

TABLE 15-1. Pharmacokinetics of Steroidal Neuromuscular Blocking Drugs

Muscle Relaxant	Volume of Distribution at Steady State (ml/kg)	Plasma Clearance (ml/kg/min)	Elimination Half-life (min)	Elimination (%)		References
				Urine	Bile	
Pancuronium	180–300	0.8–3	90–250	45–65	10	40, 49, 59, 61, 141, 183
Pipecuronium	250–350	2.4–3.5	90–160	20–25	40	44, 45, 46, 66
Vecuronium	190–510	3.6–6.7	35–100	15–40	30–50	55, 67, 141, 163, 183
Rocuronium	0.15–0.5	3.0–6.0	60–180	35	60	57, 73, 148, 203

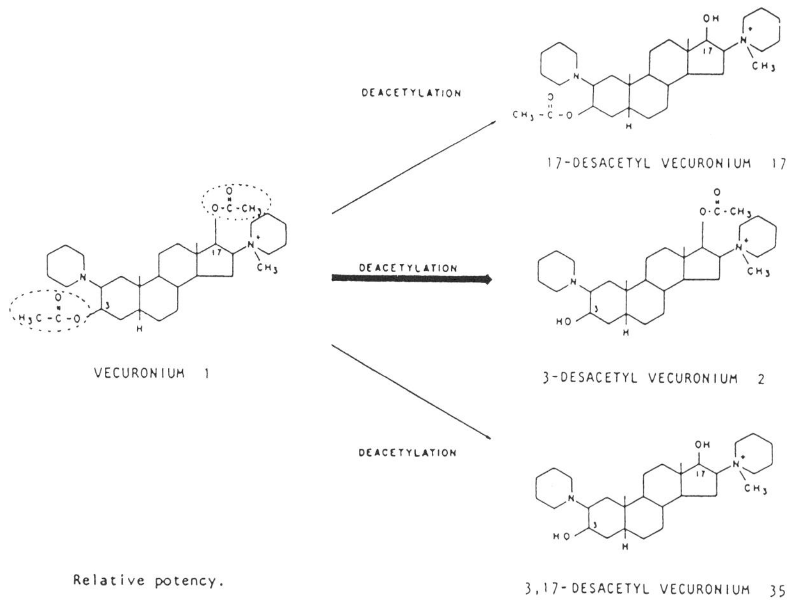

DEACETYLATION

17-DESACETYL VECURONIUM 17

VECURONIUM 1

DEACETYLATION

3-DESACETYL VECURONIUM 2

DEACETYLATION

Relative potency.

3,17-DESACETYL VECURONIUM 35

FIGURE 15-6. Metabolism of vecuronium as it occurs in the liver. Approximately 30 to 40% is deacetylated at the 3- and 17-positions. The major metabolite is 3-hydroxy vecuronium (heavy arrow). The metabolites are excreted in the urine and bile. The 3-hydroxy metabolite is nearly as potent as the parent drug and is probably cleared from blood at a rate slightly slower than that of vecuronium (From Agoston S, Seyr M, Khuenl-Brady K, et al. Use of neuromuscular blocking agents in the intensive care unit. Anesthesiol Clin North Am 1993;11:345–360.)

the bile (38, 59, 60). Only 5% of 17-hydroxy and 3,17-dihydroxy metabolites are recovered in the urine and bile (38). Pancuronium is three times more potent than its 3-hydroxy metabolite, 20 times more potent than the 17-hydroxy metabolite, and 45 times more potent than the 3,17-hydroxy metabolite (63). In humans, the corresponding values are 2, 50, and 54 times (33).

Pipecuronium, like pancuronium, is primarily excreted through the kidney. In animals, 45 to 80% of injected pipecuronium was detected unchanged in the urine (42, 43, 64), whereas only 8% is taken up by the liver and 5 to 10% is excreted in the bile (42). In humans, approximately 40% of the injected pipecuronium was detected in the urine within 24 hours (65). Although no metabolites were detected in the plasma or the bile, 4% of the injected pipecuronium is detected in the urine as the 3-hydroxy metabolite (66). The hepatic elimination of pipecuronium is minimal (41), with only 2% of the bolus dose of pipecuronium excreted in the bile (66).

Vecuronium is also minimally metabolized, with 30 to 50% of vecuronium excreted unchanged in the bile, and 20 to 30% is excreted unchanged in the urine (19, 67, 68). Vecuronium is rapidly taken up by the isolated rat liver and is excreted in the bile (58). After 2 hours, the rat liver contained 22% of the dose, whereas 70% was collected in the bile, of which 40% was the parent drug and 30% was the 3-hydroxy metabolite (58). Vecuronium undergoes a limited amount (30 to 40%) of deacetylation in the liver to 3-hydroxy vecuronium, 17-hydroxy vecuronium, and 3,17-dihydroxy vecuronium (6). The 3-hydroxy metabolite of vecuronium is approximately 50 to 80% as potent as the parent drug, whereas 17-hydroxy and 3,17 dihydroxy metabolites are far less potent (7, 63, 69). The major metabolite (3,17-dihydroxy analog) is only 2% as potent as the parent drug. The time course of neuromuscular blockade (i.e., onset, duration of action, and recovery rate) for both vecuronium and 3-hydroxy vecuronium is similar (63, 70). Only 5 to 10% of the metabolites of vecuronium are detected in the plasma, with less than 5% excreted as 3-hydroxy vecuronium (51, 55). The low plasma concentrations of 3-hydroxy vecuronium may be related to its storage in the liver or excretion through the bile (71).

Similar to vecuronium, rocuronium has an intermediate duration of action and undergoes little or no biotransformation (53). In animals, the major metabolite of rocuronium, 17-hydroxy rocuronium, is only 5% as potent as the parent drug (26). Rocuronium is primarily eliminated by the hepatobiliary route. Approximately 75% of injected rocuronium is eliminated in the bile within 360 minutes, and 9% is eliminated in the urine (53). Culture of human hepatocytes takes up rocuronium rapidly (72), thus suggesting that hepatic excretion may be important in humans. The elimination pathways of rocuronium remain uncertain in humans because only one-third of the dose is recovered nonmetabolized in urine (57). No detectable metabolites were demonstrated in bile, urine, or serum at the minimal level of sensitivity (5 ng/ml) following rocuronium, 1 mg/kg (53, 57). In humans, rocuronium does not depend on the kidney for its elimination (73).

Metabolism of Org 9487 is restricted to deacetylation on the 3 position, because only small amounts of the 3,17-didesacetyl metabolite are recovered from the urine (31). The renal excretion of Org 9487 appears to be of minor importance, with a urinary excreted fraction of the bolus dose of approximately 17% (parent compound and putative metabolites). This is similar to

TABLE 15-2. Pharmacodynamics of Steroidal Neuromuscular Blocking Drugs

Muscle Relaxant	Intubating Dose (mg/kg)	Onset (min)	Maintenance Dose (mg/kg)	Clinical Duration of Intubating Dose (min)	Clinical Duration of Maintenance Dose (min)	Infusion Rate (μg/kg/min)
Pancuronium	0.08–0.12	3.0–3.5	0.02	75–120	30–40	—
Pipecuronium	0.08–0.1	3.0–4.0	0.01	80–120	30–45	—
Vecuronium	0.1	2.5–3.0	0.02	35–45	15–30	0.8–2.0
Rocuronium	0.6	1.0–2.5	0.1	30–55	15–25	9–12
Org 9487	1.5	1.2–1.5	—	8–12	—	40–60

that of vecuronium (55) and rocuronium (57). The 3-hydroxy metabolite of Org 9487 was present in plasma, with concentrations varying from 10:1 (ratio of parent compound to metabolite) at the start of the measurement period to 1:10 at the end (31).

PHARMACODYNAMICS

The principal action of nondepolarizing neuromuscular blocking drugs is competitive antagonism of acetylcholine at nicotinic receptors on the postjunctional membrane of the neuromuscular junction. Neuromuscular blockade is assessed by measuring the muscular response (e.g., the adductor pollicis of the thumb) to supramaximal stimulation of a motor nerve (e.g., the ulnar nerve). The ED_{95} dose of a muscle relaxant is the dose required to achieve 95% depression of the twitch response of the adductor pollicis of the thumb following stimulation of the ulnar nerve. The paralysis exceeding 95% is associated with good conditions for tracheal intubation (74). The comparative pharmacodynamics of muscle relaxants is determined by measuring the onset and duration of neuromuscular blockade (Table 15-2). The dose-response relationship of muscle relaxants is constructed by performing linear regression over the linear portion of a semilogarithmic plot between 25 and 75% effect. More complex models relating the concentration of a muscle relaxant at the neuromuscular junction to its pharmacologic effect have also been developed (75). A relationship exists between the plasma concentration of pancuronium and the degree of neuromuscular blockade following administration of a bolus injection or infusion (76). Estimates of the ED_{50} values determined by dose-response analysis have been used to determine the relative potencies of rocuronium, pancuronium, pipecuronium, and vecuronium (1:4.5:5.4:6, respectively) (Table 15-3) (77). Dose-response relationship can be used to indicate drug efficacy or potency (78), enhancement of drug action, or antagonism (79, 80). The concentration-response curves are also used to study the effect of disease, drug interaction, or altered physiology on the pharmacodynamics of the muscle relaxant drugs (Fig. 15-7).

In contrast to the benzylisoquinolinium compounds, the steroidal group of drugs does not increase plasma histamine concentrations (81). The hemodynamic effects (i.e., increased heart rate and blood pressure) observed during the use of steroidal neuromuscular blocking drugs may be the result of their interactions with cardiac M2 muscarinic receptors (82). Appadu and Lambert evaluated the interaction of the steroidal neuromuscular blocking drugs with cardiac muscarinic receptors and found a rank order of potency of pancuronium > vecuronium > pipecuronium > rocuronium (82).

Kinetics and Dynamics of Neuromuscular Blockade in Various Muscles

The onset of neuromuscular blockade is not similar in all muscles groups (83). The onset and the recovery of neuromuscular blockade occurs earlier at the diaphragm compared with the peripheral muscles (84). However, the dose required for 90% blockade has been reported to be greater for the diaphragm than for the adductor pollicis muscle (85-87). These differences may be because the blood supply to the central muscle group (i.e., muscle of the larynx, the jaw, and the diaphragm) is significantly higher per unit weight compared with the peripheral muscle group (i.e., adductor pollicis of the thumb). These findings suggest that the dynamics of relaxant delivery and removal from the central muscle group occurs more rapidly than in the peripheral muscles. Therefore, the time course and potency of muscle relaxants differ at the laryngeal muscles and the diaphragm as compared with the adductor pollicis (88, 89).

TABLE 15-3. Potency of Steroidal Neuromuscular Blocking Drugs

Muscle Relaxant	95% Effective Dose (ED_{95}), (mg/kg)
Pancuronium	0.06–0.07
Pipecuronium	0.04–0.05
Vecuronium	0.05
Rocuronium	0.3
Org 9487	1.2

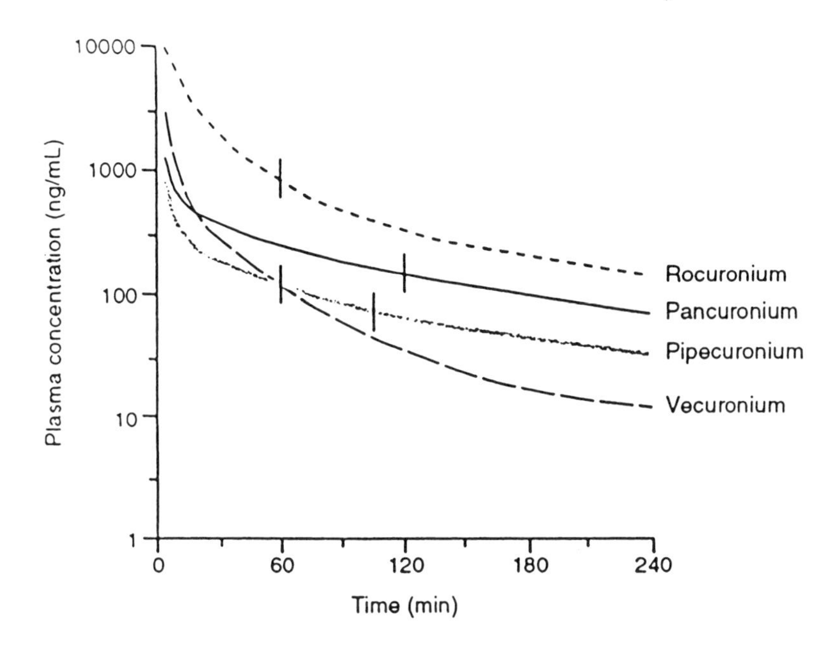

FIGURE 15-7. Mean venous plasma concentrations versus time, following intravenous administration of rocuronium 1 mg/kg, pancuronium 0.1 mg/kg, pipecuronium 0.07 mg/kg, and vecuronium 0.1 mg/kg. Vertical bars indicate 25% recovery of control twitch height. (From Ducharme J, Donati F. Pharmacokinetics and pharmacodynamics of steroidal muscle relaxants. Anesthesiol Clin North Am 1993; 11:283–307.)

Donati and his colleagues (88) showed that the orbicularis oculi response to facial stimulation reflects the extent of neuromuscular blockade of the diaphragm better than does the response of the adductor pollicis to ulnar nerve stimulation. These investigators also evaluated the differences between the neuromuscular blockade of the adductor muscles of the vocal cords and adductor pollicis (89). The onset of neuromuscular blockade at the larynx with vecuronium, 0.07 mg/kg, was 2.4 minutes earlier than that at the adductor pollicis (89). Similarly, the 90% recovery of the block following vecuronium, 0.07 mg/kg, was an average of 17 minutes earlier at the vocal cords (Fig. 15-8). These investigators concluded that the maximal effect at the vocal cords is reached more rapidly than at the adductor pollicis; however, total relaxation of the vocal cords required larger doses of vecuronium (89). Because of increased "resistance" of the vocal cords and diaphragm, a larger dose (2 × ED_{95}) of muscle relaxant is required for tracheal intubation.

Meistelman and associates (90) reported that the onset time, intensity of blockade, and duration of action of rocuronium were less at the larynx than at the adductor pollicis. After rocuronium, 0.25 mg/kg, the onset time was 1.4 minutes faster and the time to 90% recovery was 13 minutes earlier at the larynx as compared with the adductor pollicis (90). Similarly, with rocuronium, 0.5 mg/kg, the onset time was 1 minute faster and the duration of blockade was 15 minutes shorter at the larynx. The onset of maximum blockade was significantly shorter for rocuronium than for vecuronium both at the larynx and adductor pollicis (90). Wright and colleagues (91) observed a relative resistance to the effect of rocuronium at the larynx compared with the adductor pollicis. The onset of action was significantly faster at the laryngeal adductor muscles than at adductor pollicis with rocuronium, 0.4 mg/kg, but not with rocuronium, 0.8 and 1.2 mg/kg (91).

Pharmacodynamics of neuromuscular blocking drugs has traditionally been evaluated by stimulation of the ulnar nerve and monitoring of the response of the adductor pollicis of the thumb. However, monitoring the adductor pollicis response to determine the onset of blockade and optimal time for tracheal intubation can be misleading, but tracheal intubation may be accomplished after obtaining "weakening" of the adductor pollicis response. Ideally, orbicularis oculi monitoring is used for monitoring the onset of action of neuromuscular blockade, and the adductor pollicis is used for evaluating recovery. Once the adductor pol-

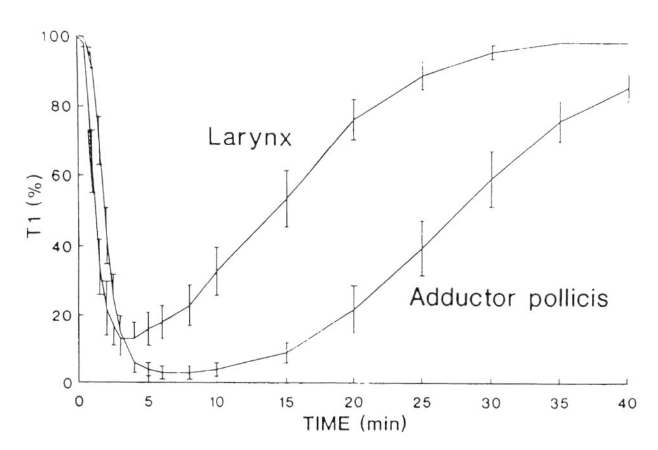

FIGURE 15-8. Twitch height (T_1) as a percentage of baseline versus time in minutes for larynx and adductor pollicis after administration of vecuronium, 0.07 mg/kg. (From Donati F, Meistelman C, Pland B. Vecuronium neuromuscular blockade at the adductor muscles of the larynx and adductor pollicis. Anesthesiology 1991;74:833–877.)

licis response has returned to normal values, the risk of residual depression of the twitch height of the geniohyoid muscle (one of the principal muscles contributing to airway patency) appears unlikely (92). Thus, if adductor pollicis function is recovered, the patient should have the neuromuscular power to protect the airway.

Onset of Neuromuscular Blockade

Investigators have long recognized the need for a nondepolarizing muscle relaxant to replace succinylcholine (5). This drug should have a rapid onset to complete paralysis and a short duration of action. Multiple factors may influence the onset of neuromuscular bockade. These factors include patient characteristics, such as cardiac output, circulation time, and muscle flow, volume of distribution, degree of protein binding, and rate of elimination. Donati (83) suggested that the speed of onset of muscle relaxants may be inversely related to potency. He hypothesized that a large proportion of receptors must be occupied before neuromuscular blockade is complete (93). Injection of a low potency drug entails the presence of more relaxant molecules in the circulation, leading to a faster occupancy of the number of receptors necessary to produce neuromuscular blockade (83). However, one study using a frog model suggested that the reverse relationship between onset (and offset) times of muscle relaxants and potency was due to events that occur at the motor end plate (94).

The relationship between potency and onset time has been observed in cats (21) and in humans (22). Bowman and associates (21) reported that, for steroid compounds administered to cats, onset time increased as ED_{95} decreased (Fig. 15-9). These authors suggested

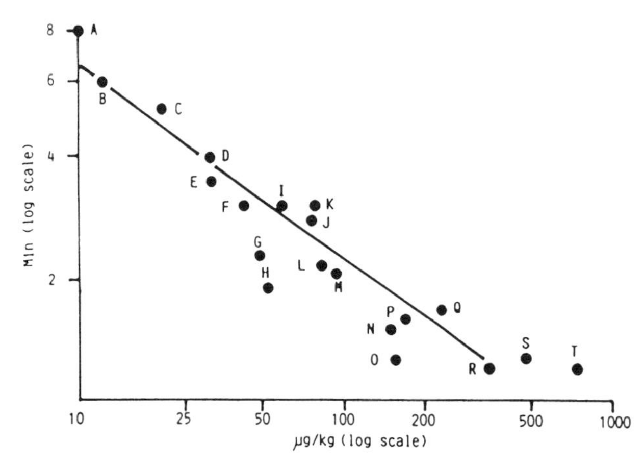

FIGURE 15-9. Time to onset of neuromuscular block (min) versus log dose for 50% neuromuscular block (ED_{50}) of steroidal neuromuscular blocking drugs. As the potency decreases (ED_{50} increase), (A to T) onset of action becomes shorter. (From Bowman WC, Rodger IW, Houston J, et al. Structure: action relationships among some desacetoxy analogues of pancuronium and vecuronium in the anesthetized cat. Anesthesiology 1988;69:57–62.)

that, because a larger number of molecules are administered when drug potency is low, according to the law of mass action, a higher concentration of molecules is expected to be necessary to achieve rapid receptor block and, therefore, rapid paralysis. In humans, Kopman (22) observed that the onset of action after administration of equipotent doses of gallamine, d-tubocurarine, and pancuronium was fastest with the least potent drug (gallamine) and slowest with the most potent drug (pancuronium). In animals, rocuronium is 20% as potent as vecuronium, and its onset of action is twice as fast as vecuronium (23). In humans, rocuronium is 7 to 8 times less potent than vecuronium (10, 24), and rocuronium has a significantly faster onset of action (95).

Onset of neuromuscular blockade may also be related to the pharmacokinetic behavior of the drug. A more rapid initial decay of the plasma concentration coincides with a more rapid equilibrium between the plasma and biophase, with a resultant decrease in the onset time (96). In addition, the rate of equilibrium between plasma and biophase may be enhanced by short-lasting blockade of calcium channels, which, in turn, increases the muscle blood flow (97). The high lipophilicity of Org 9487 may promote diffusion through membranes, resulting in a more rapid equilibrium between the plasma and biophase (96). Another possible mechanism contributing to a rapid onset is a pronounced inhibition of presynaptic nicotinic cholinoceptors, leading to a more pronounced decline in acetylcholine release (10, 98).

The onset time is dose dependent, with a minimum limit determined by the circulation time (because large dose reaches effective concentrations in the biophase on delivery by the circulation) (99). Increasing the size of the dose of muscle relaxants speeds the onset of action; however, the duration of action is also prolonged (100, 101). The onset times of nondepolarizing neuromuscular blocking drugs can also be shortened by using the "priming principle," which consists of administration of a small dose of the relaxant before a larger intubating dose (102-106). The size of the priming dose and the intubating dose, as well as the priming interval (time between the priming dose and the intubating dose) are all crucial in determining the efficacy of the priming technique (107). The "optimal" priming dose and priming interval should be adequate to hasten the onset of action without producing untoward side effects. A priming dose of 10% of a standard intubating dose ($2 \times ED_{95}$) and a priming interval of 3 to 4 minutes have been recommended as safe and effective. Some investigators have proposed a "timing" technique as an alternative to priming technique to achieve more rapid onset times (108). The timing technique uses a single bolus dose of nondepolarizing muscle relaxant, followed by administration of an induction agent timed to the onset of clinical weakness. The priming technique may be associated with side effects such as diplopia, difficulty in swallowing (109), and generalized discomfort secondary to difficulty in breathing leading to increased anxiety (110, 111). Respiratory compromise and dyspnea, although rare, may occur (112).

SPECIAL POPULATIONS

Pediatric Patients

Nondepolarizing muscle relaxants have been increasingly used in pediatric patients because of the possibility of malignant hyperthermia and cardiac arrhythmias associated with succinylcholine. Although the maturation of the neuromuscular junction occurs after the first 2 months of age (113), muscle relaxants can be safely used in infants. However, because of the greater sensitivity to muscle relaxants in neonates and infants, lower concentrations of the muscle relaxant are necessary to achieve the desired neuromuscular blockade compared with adults (114). The larger volume of distribution and slower clearance contribute to a longer elimination half-life of muscle relaxants in infants (115, 116). However, in children (2 to 10 years), the dosage requirements on the basis of milligrams per kilogram of body weight are higher than in adults, and the duration of effect is often shorter (117, 118).

The dose-response curves of pancuronium and vecuronium in infants and children are similar to those in the adults (115, 116, 119). However, the absence of observed differences in the results may be due to the small number of patients studied in these investigations. Some investigators have reported greater sensitivity to vecuronium in infants than in children (120). The ED_{95} values varied between 22 and 103 μg/kg, with lower values in neonates, infants, and adolescents compared with children between 3 and 10 years of age. The investigators concluded that the dose of vecuronium necessary for tracheal intubation was age dependent (120). The ED_{95} of vecuronium (0.64 mg/kg) in children is greater than in adults (117).

Compared with adults, the onset of neuromuscular blockade following pancuronium and vecuronium was found to be faster in infants and children (115, 120-122). The increased cardiac output and decreased circulation time in children may be responsible for the shorter onset times. The duration of action of vecuronium is prolonged in neonates and infants because of increase in the volume of distribution without a change in its clearance rate (115, 116, 123). On the other hand, the duration of action of pancuronium and vecuronium is shorter in children when compared with adults (115, 118, 120, 121). Vecuronium infusion requirements (μg/kg/min) in children aged 2 to 10 years were at least double those of adults during inhalation anesthesia, as well as during nitrous oxide-narcotic anesthesia (118). Compared with narcotic-nitrous oxide anesthesia, the vecuronium infusion requirements during inhalation anesthesia were significantly decreased after the first 30 minutes of infusion (118). These authors suggest that after a bolus of vecuronium to achieve 95% neuromuscular blockade, 2.0 to 2.5 μg/kg/min of vecuronium is a useful initial infusion rate that is likely to decrease to 1.5-1.8 μg/kg/min after 30 minutes in children anesthetized with a volatile agent and nitrous oxide (118). Vecuronium has been commonly used in children because of its faster onset, intermediate duration of action, and minimal residual postoperative paralysis (124).

In children, there is an 33% increase in ED_{95} of pipecuronium (79 versus 59 μg/kg) compared with adults during nitrous oxide-narcotic anesthesia (125). However, the neuromuscular potency of pipecuronium determined by electromyography is increased (48 versus 70 μg/kg) in infants younger than 1 year compared with children aged 2 to 9 years (126). In addition, the clinical duration of action of pipecuronium is shorter in infants and children, analogous to an intermediate-acting muscle relaxant (126). During halothane anesthesia there was no difference in the potency of pipecuronium between infants up to 3 months old, older infants (3 to 12 months), and children aged 2 to 9 years (127). The clinical duration of action and recovery index are similar for older children and adults (126).

Rocuronium has a rapid onset and an intermediate duration of action in infants (128) and children aged 1 to 5 years (129). The ED_{50} for rocuronium in children 1 to 5 years of age is 0.17 mg/kg, and the ED_{95} is 0.3 mg/kg (129). The clinical duration of rocuronium-induced neuromuscular blockade in children is similar to that reported in adults (129). A transient increase in heart rate (18%) has been observed with an intubating dose of 0.6 mg/kg in children (129). The potency of rocuronium is the same in children 1 to 4 years old as in those 5 to 10 years old (130). The clinical duration of action and recovery of rocuronium are significantly longer in the younger group (1 to 4 years) as compared with the older group (5 to 10 years). In children aged 4 to 11 years who are anesthetized with nitrous oxide and halothane, rocuronium's weight-normalized plasma clearance decreases with weight, and there are no maturational changes in weight-normalized distributional clearance or volumes of distribution (131).

Geriatric Patients

The physiologic changes that occur with aging, including a reduction in muscle mass (132) and total body water and an increase in fat, are responsible for many of the pharmacokinetic changes observed in the elderly (133). In addition, decreases in cardiac output, renal and hepatic blood flow, and plasma proteins may alter the kinetic responses of the elderly to neuromuscular blocking drugs. Anatomic and physiologic changes in the neuromuscular junction also occur with aging (134). However, the sensitivity of the acetylcholine receptors to muscle relaxants does not appear to be significantly altered with aging (135, 136). The steroidal muscle relaxants depend on the kidney or liver for metabolism and elimination. Therefore, the decreased splanchnic blood flow and the decrease in liver size and hepatic mass (137, 138) with age may significantly affect this group of drugs. Furthermore, hemodynamic changes associated with aging may delay the onset of neuromuscular blockade (83).

Pharmacokinetic and pharmacodynamic studies of pancuronium in the elderly have found decreased plasma clearance that prolongs the duration of action and slows recovery from pancuronium-induced neuromuscular block (61, 139). However, dose-response studies have reported no difference in the potencies of pancuronium and vecuronium in the young and the elderly (61, 136, 140). Although Rupp and colleagues (141) did not observe age-related changes in the elimination half-life of pancuronium, the plasma clearance and volume of distribution decreased in the elderly. Age-related differences in the kinetics and dynamics of pancuronium and vecuronium may be related to the finding that pancuronium is primarily eliminated by the kidney, whereas vecuronium is primarily eliminated by the liver (19). The drugs dependent on biliary excretion are influenced more by aging than are the relaxants dependent on the kidneys for their elimination (142).

A dose-response study demonstrated that the ED_{95} of pipecuronium in elderly patients (66 to 79 years) undergoing balanced anesthesia is smaller than in young adults (35 versus 45 μg/kg) (143). Ornstein and associates (144) examined the pharmacokinetics and dynamics of pipecuronium, 70 μg/kg, administered during balanced anesthesia and reported that the volume of distribution, clearance, elimination half-life, and recovery from pipecuronium were similar in young and elderly patients (144). The kinetics and dynamics of pipecuronium are not significantly altered in the elderly because the drug is exclusively dependent on the kidney for its elimination.

The onset of vecuronium-induced block is slower (122) and the duration of action and the rate of recovery of vecuronium prolonged in the elderly (145). These investigators used an infusion of vecuronium for studying its dosage requirements during steady state relaxation (145). Although they did not study the kinetics of vecuronium, their results suggested decreased elimination of the drug in the elderly. Rupp and associates (141) examined the pharmacokinetic and pharmacodynamic behavior of vecuronium administered as an infusion that was discontinued after achieving a twitch tension of 20 to 30% of the control. These authors reported that, although plasma clearance of vecuronium was reduced in the elderly, this was matched by a decrease in their volume of distribution. The elimination half-life and recovery index (time for twitch recovery from 25 to 75% of control tension) were unaffected by aging (141). Following bolus injections, the plasma clearance of vecuronium is reduced, and its elimination half-life is prolonged in the elderly (146). However, the duration of action of vecuronium is similar in elderly and young patients (147), and no age-related differences are observed in vecuronium's single dose-response relationships (136, 140). Because of reports of prolonged block with vecuronium in the elderly, the initial dose of vecuronium should be decreased, and subsequent doses should be administered according to monitoring of the neuromuscular function.

Rocuronium is structurally related to vecuronium and is eliminated primarily through the liver (57). Matteo and colleagues (148) evaluated the effects of age on the pharmacokinetic and dynamic responses to rocuronium, 0.6 mg/kg, during nitrous oxide-narcotic anesthesia. Although the onset times did not differ, the clinical duration of action of rocuronium was significantly prolonged in the elderly (43 versus 26 minutes). In addition, compared with younger patients, there was a significant decrease in plasma clearance (3.67 versus 5.03 ml/kg/min) and volume of distribution (399 versus 553 ml/kg) in the elderly (148). However, no significant difference was observed in the log plasma concentration versus twitch tension response relationship between 20 and 80% paralysis in young and elderly. In a similar study, Bevan and associates (149) reported slower onset and recovery of rocuronium-induced neuromuscular block in the elderly, but the potency of the drug did not differ from that in younger patients.

Obese Patients

Obesity is associated with changes in body composition and function that may alter drug disposition. There is increase in the proportion of body fat to total body mass and decreased proportion of muscle mass and body water (150). Cardiac output and glomerular filtration rate are increased (151, 152), and liver function and protein binding may be altered (153). The effects of obesity on the pharmacokinetics and dynamics of neuromuscular blocking drugs are controversial (154, 155). Not surprisingly, larger dosages of pancuronium are required to maintain adequate relaxation in obese patients (154). However, the differences in pancuronium requirements decrease after correcting for body surface area (154). Other authors have reported prolonged duration of action in obese patients (156). Feingold (155) found that the cumulative dose of pancuronium correlated with the square root of the elapsed time, suggesting that the initial and repeat doses of pancuronium be determined from previously derived tables rather than by using body surface area (155). Soderberg and colleagues (157) found that the total dosage of pancuronium (per hour) in the obese was the same as in patients of normal weight. Therefore, they recommended that muscle relaxant dosage should be based on ideal body weight (157). If muscle relaxants are administered according to actual body weight, higher plasma concentrations may be obtained in obese patients (158). However, the volumes of distribution, plasma clearance, and distribution and elimination half-lives are similar for both obese and control patients (158). When the drug was administered on the basis of actual body weight, obese patients had slower recovery from vecuronium-induced neuromuscular blockade (158-160). The duration of neuromuscular blockade is significantly correlated with degree of obesity (159). Investigators have suggested that the use of percentage of ideal body weight (induction dose in μg/kg equals 162 μg/kg minus 0.62 μg/kg multiplied by percentage of ideal body weight) is a good predictor for duration of action of vecuronium-induced neuromuscular block (161). In obese patients, neuromuscular blocking drugs should be administered according to lean (ideal) body weight rather than according to actual body weight (158, 160).

Obstetric Patients

Neuromuscular blocking drugs do not readily cross the placenta because they are quaternary ammonium compounds with large molecules and are highly ionized in plasma. The transfer of these drugs through the placenta can be evaluated by measuring the concentrations of the drug in the umbilical vein, umbilical artery, and maternal vein. In addition, the effects of neuromuscular blocking drugs on the neonate may be evaluated using clinical tests (e.g., Apgar scores and neonatal neurologic and behavioral function tests). Placental transfer of pancuronium has been comprehensively reviewed by Agoston and colleagues (13). The fetal-maternal concentration ratios (i.e., umbilical venous-maternal venous ratio) for vecuronium and pancuronium are approximately 10 and 20%, respectively (162-164). Furthermore, the umbilical venous-maternal venous ratio is independent of the dose or time from injection to delivery. As 50% of the umbilical blood flow passes through the liver, the first-pass effect may be an important mechanism of elimination of steroidal neuromuscular blocking drugs. This results in a significant difference in the fetal arteriovenous concentrations. Predictably, investigators have no evidence of adverse neonatal effects with either pancuronium or vecuronium (163).

Maternal pancuronium and vecuronium pharmacokinetic studies found that clearance rates are significantly higher and elimination half-lives are shorter in women undergoing cesarean section compared with controls undergoing abdominal surgery (163, 164). However, no difference was observed in the steady-state volume of distribution and the distribution half-life values of these drugs. Furthermore, there was no difference in the pancuronium eliminated in the urine over 24 hours between the groups receiving the two muscle relaxants. The increased clearance during cesarean section may be due to acute blood loss, uptake of the relaxant drugs by the neonate and placenta, increased activity of the hepatic microsomal mixed function oxidase by progesterone, or deacetylation of these muscle relaxants by placental enzymes. Investigators have suggested that pregnant women are more sensitive to muscle relaxants, a sensitivity that leads to a faster onset and increased clinical duration of action (165, 166). Therefore, smaller doses of vecuronium are necessary for maintenance of relaxation during anesthesia in pregnant patients (167). Increased response to vecuronium has also been observed in the postpartum period within 1 to 4 days after delivery (166, 168).

Patients with Severe Renal Disease

Preexisting renal disease can decrease the elimination of nondepolarizing neuromuscular blocking drugs and their metabolites by the kidney. Therefore, the duration of action of these drugs may be increased in patients with renal failure. In addition, renal failure can cause significant physiologic changes including increase in volume of distribution, hypoalbuminemia, changes in protein structure, and accumulation of endogenous substances that may compete for drug-binding sites. The increase in distribution volume may be due to increases in extracellular fluid volumes or to decreased protein binding associated with renal failure (169). Affrime and associates (170) also found that hemodialysis affected plasma protein binding of drugs.

The duration of action of pancuronium is increased and recovery is prolonged in patients with renal failure (Table 15-4) (171-173). The elimination half-life is prolonged as much as fourfold in this patient population (39, 40, 172, 174) because biliary excretion does not compensate for the lack of renal elimination (174). In patients with renal failure, the infusion rates of pancuronium required to achieve a steady-state neuromuscular blockade are decreased by 62% (175), as compared with patients with normal renal function (176).

The principal route of elimination of pipecuronium is by the kidneys (accounting for 77% of the administered dose). In animals, the elimination of pipecuron-

TABLE 15-4. Pharmacokinetics of Steroidal Neuromuscular Blocking Drugs in Patients with Renal Dysfunction

Muscle Relaxant	Volume of Distribution at Steady State (ml/kg)	Plasma Clearance (ml/kg/min)	Elimination Half-life (min)	References
Pancuronium	240–300	0.3–0.75	260–490	39, 40, 172
Pipecuronium	442	1.6	263	46
Vecuronium	240–470	2.5–4.5	70–150	55, 67, 182, 183
Rocuronium	210–265	2.5–3.0	95–105	56, 73

ium was decreased if the kidneys were excluded from the circulation (42, 43). Similar observations have been reported in the studies on rats in which urinary excretion accounted for 45% of the administered dose (64). The biliary elimination of pipecuronium accounts for only 4.5% of the administered dose (43). Although a fourfold increase in hepatobiliary elimination occurs in the absence of renal function, this does not compensate for the loss of urinary excretion (43). However, humans are less dependent on the kidneys for elimination of pipecuronium than are animals.

Earlier studies using a colorimetric assay to measure the plasma concentrations determined that the plasma clearance of pipecuronium is reduced and its elimination half-life is increased in patients with renal failure (177, 178). In a more recent study using a more sensitive and specific capillary gas chromatographic assay, the investigators determined that patients with reduced renal function had a 34% reduction in clearance (46), and patients in renal failure had a larger volume of distribution at steady state. Only a small amount (4 to 10%) of the 3-hydroxy metabolite were recovered from the urine during the first 24 hours after surgery (45). Caldwell and colleagues (46) found that the duration of action (time to 25% recovery) of pipecuronium was not affected in patients undergoing renal transplantation, but there was increased variability in this patient population.

Compared with pancuronium or pipecuronium, vecuronium is less affected by renal impairment. The liver is the major route of excretion in animals with a maximum of 14% of the injected dose of vecuronium is excreted unchanged in the urine (19). In humans, 20 to 30% of vecuronium is dependent on the kidney for its elimination (47). However, the influence of renal failure on the dynamics and kinetics of vecuronium has been controversial. Initial studies reported that neither the onset, duration, and recovery rate times nor the pharmacokinetics of vecuronium is affected by renal impairment (67). Although the elimination half-life is increased in renal failure (97 to 150 minutes), this change does not significantly increase the duration of action. Hunter and associates (179) found no difference in the duration of action and evidence of accumulation of vecuronium in patients with or without renal failure. These authors described vecuronium as a suitable nondepolarizing relaxant for clinically or anatomically anephric patients. However, other investigators have observed an increased duration of action of supplemental doses of vecuronium, suggesting that accumulation occurs in anephric patients (180, 181). Importantly, cumulation may be seen if repeated doses are injected during the distributional phase of the previous dose. Despite differences in electrolyte and plasma protein concentrations and possible fluid volume shifts from recent hemodialysis, the potency of vecuronium is unchanged in the presence of chronic renal insufficiency (180).

Some investigators have found moderately decreased plasma clearance and increased duration of action and recovery rate of vecuronium in patients with renal failure (47, 55). On the other hand, Meistelman and colleagues (182) reported a prolonged spontaneous recovery rate, but no change in plasma clearance or duration of action of vecuronium in patients with renal impairment. Gramstad (175) demonstrated that the infusion requirements of vecuronium to achieve 90% block were decreased by 20% in patients with renal failure compared with normal controls. Lynam and associates (183) observed that the clearance of vecuronium was decreased by 42% and the clinical duration of action was significantly prolonged in patients undergoing renal transplantation. However, the steady-state volume of distribution of vecuronium was similar in the presence and absence of renal failure (183). These authors confirm that smaller supplemental doses of vecuronium should be administered to patients with renal dysfunction.

Because vecuronium can accumulate in patients with renal dysfunction, Lepage and colleagues (181) concluded that vecuronium may be less safe than atracurium in this patient population. However, other investigators found no difference in the recovery indices between vecuronium and atracurium (184). These authors suggest that, with proper neuromuscular monitoring, vecuronium can be administered safely in this patient population (184). In animal models, cyclosporine has potentiated vecuronium-induced neuromuscular blockade (185). Therefore, nondepolarizing muscle relaxants should be administered judiciously in patients with renal failure who are receiving cyclosporine. The principal metabolite of vecuronium, 3-hydroxy vecuronium, has 70% the neuromuscular blocking action of vecuronium in animals (63, 70) and 50 to 80% in humans. This metabolite may cause prolonged paralysis after long-term administration of vecuronium, particularly in critically ill patients with renal failure (186, 187). A meta-analysis of pharmacodynamics of vecuronium in patients with and without renal failure reported no difference in onset time or recovery index between the two groups (188); however, the duration of action was longer in the group with renal failure (188).

Rocuronium is primarily eliminated by hepatobiliary mechanisms (76%), and only 9% is excreted by kidney (53). Ligation of the renal pedicle in cats did not significantly change the elimination half-life, onset of neuromuscular block, or the duration of action of rocuronium (53). Szenohradszky and associates (73) examined the effect of end-stage renal disease on the pharmacokinetics of rocuronium and found that the clearance rate of rocuronium was similar in patients with normal renal function (2.89 ml/kg/min) and in those undergoing renal transplantation. However, the volume of distribution at steady state was increased by 28%, and the elimination half-life was prolonged by 22% in patients undergoing renal transplantation. Following administration of a bolus dose of rocuronium, 0.6 mg/kg, the clearance rates were decreased and the mean residence times were increased in patients with renal failure, compared with patients with normal renal function (56). However, no differences in the pharmacodynamic characteristics (e.g., onset time, clinical duration of action, and recovery index) were noted for patients with normal renal function and those in renal failure (56, 189).

Patients with Hepatobiliary Disease

The liver plays an important role in the metabolism and excretion of muscle relaxants. Hepatobiliary disease, like renal failure, can affect the kinetics and dynamics of neuromuscular blocking drugs in complex ways. Muscle relaxants that depend on the liver for their metabolism and elimination which are affected by alterations in hepatic blood flow and decreased function of the hepatocytes. Hepatic failure influences the volume of distribution and protein binding of the muscle relaxants, thereby increasing the volume of distribution (190).

Although pancuronium is primarily excreted in the urine (38), the mean elimination half-life is prolonged twofold in patients with liver disease (60, 191), probably because hepatic uptake is an important factor in the plasma clearance of pancuronium (38). The principal route of metabolism of pancuronium is deacetylation at the 3 position in the liver (59). Approximately 10 to 20% of pancuronium is found in the liver and bile as both the parent drug and its metabolite. In patients with cirrhosis, the initial dose to achieve adequate muscle relaxation is high, and the elimination half-life of the drug is increased (59), resulting in prolonged neuromuscular blockade (Table 15-5) (60, 191). The plasma clearance of pancuronium in patients with extrahepatic cholestasis was 16% lower than in the control group (1.47 versus 1.76 ml/min/kg) (60). The de-

TABLE 15-5. Pharmacokinetics of Steroidal Neuromuscular Blocking Drugs in Patients with Liver Disease

Muscle Relaxant	Volume of Distribution at Steady State (ml/kg)	Plasma Clearance (ml/kg/min)	Elimination Half-life (min)	References
Pancuronium	307–425	1.15–1.47	208–224	59, 60, 191
Pipecuronium	300–500	1.3–2.5	99–179	66, 192
Vecuronium	100–250	2.4–2.7	75–100	196, 199, 200
Rocuronium	235–320	2.4–3.0	100–170	203, 204

creased clearance of pancuronium in liver disease may be due to reduced hepatic uptake (62). In patients with liver disease, the increased resistance to initial doses of pancuronium may be due to the increase in volume of distribution rather than changes in the protein binding (13, 36, 59), because the binding of pancuronium in human plasma is low (37). However, because the duration of action is increased significantly, subsequent doses should be administered with caution.

Only 2% of a bolus dose of pipecuronium is excreted in the bile (66). In one study, the total plasma clearance of pipecuronium, 0.1 mg/kg, did not differ between controls and cirrhotic patients (2.96 versus 2.61 ml/kg/min); however, the terminal half-life was increased in cirrhotic patients (111 versus 143 minutes) (192). The volume of distribution at steady state did not differ between controls and cirrhotic patients. The onset of block was longer in cirrhotic patients, but the clinical duration of action was similar to that in the control group (192).

Unlike pancuronium, vecuronium is predominantly eliminated by the liver (58, 193, 194). Exclusion of the hepatic circulation intensifies the degree of vecuronium-induced blockade and increases its duration of action. In animals, 30 to 40% of vecuronium was recovered in the bile as compared with 8% in the urine (19, 70). Furthermore, the 3-hydroxy metabolite of vecuronium has neuromuscular blocking activity (195) that may prolong the duration of the neuromuscular blockade. Measurement of the plasma protein binding of vecuronium has shown that the protein binding of vecuronium is unaffected by liver disease (36). In addition, vecuronium is not highly protein bound (approximately 30%), and protein binding should have minimal effects. The onset of vecuronium (0.1 mg/kg) is delayed in patients with liver disease (196, 197), and plasma clearance is decreased, prolonging the elimination half-life (from 58 minutes in controls to 84 minutes) and the duration of action (51, 198-200). In contrast, Arden and associates (196) reported that the plasma clearance, volume of distribution at steady state, and elimination half-life of vecuronium, 0.1 mg/kg, were not affected by alcohol-induced liver disease. The absence of changes in the plasma clearance of vecuronium in the patients with alcohol-induced liver disease may be due to the drug's low liver extraction ratio (201) and the preservation of its biliary excretory capacity despite extensive hepatocellular disease (202).

Rocuronium is eliminated primarily by the liver, with 54% found in bile and 21% in liver homogenate (53). The clinical duration of action of rocuronium is increased threefold when the liver is excluded from the circulation (by a portal vein-to-inferior vena cava shunt) (53). Khalil and colleagues (203) observed prolonged onset time and recovery index following rocuronium, 0.6 mg/kg, in cirrhotic patients. However, the clinical duration was not different as compared with patients with normal liver function (203). The pharmacokinetic profile of these patients failed to show any increase in the initial volume of distribution in cirrhotic patients compared with patients with normal liver function (203).

Magorian and colleagues (204) demonstrated that hepatic dysfunction increased the volume of distribution of rocuronium but did not alter its clearance. The increase in initial and steady-state volumes of distribution may not be related to the hypoalbuminemia observed in cirrhotic patients because rocuronium is not significantly protein bound (25% bound to albumin) (96). In one study, although the onset of action was not affected by liver disease, its clinical duration was prolonged (204). The authors suggest that initial recovery after rocuronium, a result of distribution, is not affected in liver disease. Later recovery is prolonged in patients with liver disease because it is a function of elimination rather than distribution (204). One study demonstrated that the pharmacodynamic and pharmacokinetic profiles of repeated doses of rocuronium in cirrhotic patients are altered when compared with healthy patients (205). The investigators observed a reduction in the clinical efficacy of the initial dose, a trend toward prolongation of action during the maintenance period, and delayed spontaneous recovery. However, the large interindividual variability in this patient population suggested the need for monitoring neuromuscular function and titrating the dosage of muscle relaxant to meet patients' needs.

Patients in the Intensive Care Unit

Neuromuscular blocking drugs, particularly pancuronium and vecuronium, are frequently administered in the critically ill patients in the intensive care unit (ICU) (206-208). These drugs are administered in the ICU to facilitate management of mechanical ventilation and increased intracranial pressure, to reduce oxygen consumption (e.g., to decrease work of breathing and eliminate shivering), and to provide immobility for certain diagnostic procedures (209-211). However, their appropriate use is questioned because of the absence of any outcome data (206, 212). One of the complications of long-term use of muscle relaxants is prolonged residual paralysis after cessation (186, 208, 213, 214). Prolonged neuromuscular blockade after termination of long-term treatment with vecuronium in the ICU is associated with metabolic acidosis, elevated plasma magnesium concentrations, presence of renal failure, and high plasma concentrations of vecuronium's 3-hydroxy metabolite (187).

Despite the unpredictable effect and well-known complications, muscle relaxants are still frequently administered in large doses to critically ill patients (187, 213, 215, 216). Furthermore, with increasing stress on pharmacoeconomics, the use of less expensive, long-acting muscle relaxants such as pancuronium has been emphasized (217). However, the possibility of increased incidence of prolonged residual paralysis is an important consideration. Recently published practice parameters state that pancuronium is the preferred neuromuscular blocking drug for most critically ill patients; however, vecuronium is preferred for patients with cardiac disease or hemodynamic instability in whom tachycardia may be deleterious (218). In addition, patients receiving prolonged infusions of neuromuscular blocking drugs should be periodically assessed for the degree of blockade (218).

One prospective study demonstrated that, by monitoring the neuromuscular transmission and providing adequate sedation and analgesia, smaller doses of pancuronium or pipecuronium were adequate, and no prolonged paralysis occurred (219). Another study concluded that routine monitoring of neuromuscular transmission does not eliminate prolonged weakness and myopathy in ICU patients receiving muscle relaxants (220). The use of muscle relaxants in the ICU deserves careful considerations in terms of indication, selection of the relaxant, dose, and duration of administration (214, 221). In addition, monitoring of neuromuscular transmission is essential, particularly in critically ill patients in whom the pharmacodynamic and pharmacokinetics of muscle relaxants may be significantly altered (222). However, the goal of monitoring neuromuscular transmission is different in the ICU than in the operating room (220). In the operating room, monitoring is used to document a sufficient degree of neuromuscular blockade, whereas in the ICU, it is used to avoid excessive blockade.

MUSCLE RELAXANT INTERACTIONS

Interactions with Anesthetic Agents

Inhaled anesthetics potentiate the action of nondepolarizing muscle relaxants in a concentration-dependent fashion (223). Decrease in the train-of-four (TOF) ratio and a concentration-dependent fade of the response to tetanic stimulation have been reported with halothane, enflurane, isoflurane, and desflurane (224-226). In one study, the appearance to T_1 to T_4 was prolonged in the following rank order: sevoflurane (greatest), enflurane, isoflurane, and halothane (least) (227). This may be because halothane caused the least increase in the blood flow in the skeletal muscle compared with other inhaled anesthetics (228, 229).

The infusion requirements of vecuronium and rocuronium are reduced during inhalation anesthesia as compared with a nitrous oxide-narcotic anesthetic technique (230, 231). In contrast to halothane, isoflurane increases the clinical duration of action of pipecuronium (65). Similarly, the potency of pipecuronium is enhanced more by enflurane and isoflurane than by halothane (232). Although isoflurane potentiates rocuronium, there may be no need to alter the dose of rocuronium if the duration of anesthesia is less than 1 hour (233).

Desflurane depresses neuromuscular function and augments the action of pancuronium to a degree similar to that of isoflurane (225). The ED_{50} of pancuronium was less with 1.25 minimum alveolar concentration (MAC) desflurane than with 1.25 MAC isoflurane (225). Similarly, desflurane and isoflurane potentiate the neuromuscular effects of vecuronium equally (234). In contrast, Wright and associates (235) reported that, in an crossover study in volunteers, desflurane potentiated the effect of vecuronium (during both bolus and infusion administration) approximately 20% more than an equipotent dose of isoflurane. Sevoflurane potentiated vecuronium more than halothane; when compared with balanced anesthesia, the dose requirements of vecuronium were reduced by approximately 60 and 40% with sevoflurane and halothane, respectively (236). However, sevoflurane and isoflurane potentiated vecuronium-induced blockade and impaired the spontaneous recovery rate to a similar degree (237).

Following development of an inhaled anesthetic, the recovery of neuromuscular function is faster because of reversal of the potentiating effects. However, several studies suggest that the potentiating effect persists after termination of the inhaled agent (238, 239). Isoflurane impedes antagonism of neuromuscular block with anticholinesterase drugs, probably because of persistence of the inhaled anesthetic agent at the neuromuscular junction (238, 239). As compared with isoflurane, sevoflurane causes a greater impairment of neostigmine antagonism (240). However, the potentiation of neuromuscular blockade is reversed faster with the use of desflurane as compared with isoflurane (235).

Several mechanisms have been proposed for potentiation of neuromuscular blockade by inhaled anesthetics, including increased availability of relaxant at the neuromuscular junction because of increased muscle blood flow (228, 229), muscle relaxation resulting from depression of the central nervous system (241), and decreased availability of acetylcholine at the neuromuscular junction (242). In addition, inhaled anesthetics are reported to potentiate muscle relaxants primarily by acting at the postjunctional membrane (243). Furthermore, potentiation of neuromuscular blockade by inhaled anesthetics may be due to changes in the pharmacodynamics (i.e., increased neuromuscular sensitivity) rather than in the pharmacokinetics of the muscle relaxants (230).

Temperature

Unintentional or intentional hypothermia (during cardiac or neurosurgical procedures) may have significant effects on the pharmacodynamics and pharmacokinetics of muscle relaxants. Hypothermia causes fluid shifts from vascular space that may increase blood viscosity. In addition, metabolic processes are slowed and may thereby decrease elimination of these drugs. In animals, hypothermia decreases the release of acetylcholine and may enhance the sensitivity of the neuromuscular junction to the effects of muscle relaxants (244). One study found that the potencies of the steroidal neuromuscular blocking drugs (namely, rocuronium, pipecuronium, vecuronium, and pancuronium) are increased significantly during hypothermia (27°C) (245). Thus, the net result of hypothermia is enhancement and prolongation of neuromuscular blockade.

In the cat, decreased temperature decreases plasma clearance and the renal and hepatic excretion of pancuronium (246). Decreased requirement of steroidal neuromuscular blocking drugs has been reported during hypothermic cardiopulmonary bypass (247-249). However, depending on the relaxant, differences exist in the degree of prolongation of its action. Hypothermia augments the duration of action of both pancuronium and vecuronium such that their durations of action are similar during hypothermia (248). Hypothermia significantly increases the duration of action of and time for spontaneous recovery from vecuronium-induced neuromuscular blockade (250, 251). During a constant-rate infusion of vecuronium, the magnitude of neuromuscular block increases significantly when the temperature decreases by a mean of 2.6°C (252). However, these investigators failed to observe any change in the concentration-effect relationship with mild hypothermia (34.4°C) (252). Surface cooling (31°C) in neurosurgical patients prolonged the duration of action of rocuronium and delayed spontaneous recovery secondary to a decreased clearance of the relaxant (253). Hypothermic cardiopulmonary bypass prolongs the duration of action of maintenance doses and decreases the plasma concentration-response relationship of rocuronium (254). These authors suggest that the increased duration of action may be due to increased sensitivity at the neuromuscular junction to rocuronium, decreased plasma clearance, or diminished hepatic uptake and storage of rocuronium in the liver during hypothermia.

Change in temperature also affects the interpretation of monitoring of neuromuscular transmission, making it unreliable (255). Decreased temperature decreases the force of contraction of the adductor pollicis by 10 to 16% per degree Celsius decrease in muscle temperature below 35.2°C (256). Furthermore, localized hypothermia influences the assessment of recovery from neuromuscular blockade (257).

Interactions among Muscle Relaxants

Neuromuscular blocking drugs are often combined in clinical practice in an attempt to optimize the onset and duration of neuromuscular blockade. A rapid-acting muscle relaxant (rocuronium) is used during induction of anesthesia to facilitate tracheal intubation, and a short-acting relaxant (mivacurium) may be administered for subsequent maintenance of neuromuscular blockade. Combinations of structurally dissimilar neuromuscular blocking drugs may be synergistic, whereas combinations of neuromuscular blocking drugs with similar molecular structure may be simply additive (258-262). With consecutive administration of neuromuscular blocking drugs, the duration of action depends more on the kinetics of the initial neuromuscular blocking drug than on the subsequently administered relaxant drug (263).

The interactions of muscle relaxant drugs may result from multiple factors including effects at the receptor sites, as well as pharmacokinetic differences (264). Synergism between two muscle relaxants with dissimilar molecular structures is possibly related to their differential actions on the pre- and postsynaptic acetylcholine receptors (262) or differential sensitivity of the α-subunit acetylcholine recognition sites (258). The duration of the muscle relaxant action can be attributed to the relative concentrations of the two drugs at the receptor site (265). When different neuromuscular blocking drugs are administered for induction and maintenance of muscle relaxation, the acetylcholine receptors are still largely occupied by the first neuromuscular blocking drug, and the subsequent drug needs to occupy only a small fraction of the vacant receptors to increase the degree of blockade. Because most receptors remain occupied by the initially administered drug, the clinical duration depends more on the kinetics of the first neuromuscular blocking drug than on the subsequently administered drug. With each subsequent maintenance dose, a progressively smaller proportion of the receptor sites is occupied by the first neuromuscular blocking drug. Thus, the duration of action of each subsequent bolus dose more closely resembles the that of drug used for maintenance of neuromuscular blockade.

The interaction between rocuronium and vecuronium, and between pipecuronium and vecuronium or pancuronium, was found to be additive (77, 261, 266). When a "priming dose" of pancuronium was administered before mivacurium, its duration of action was significantly prolonged (267). Naguib (268) demonstrated a synergistic interaction between rocuronium and mivacurium when they were administered concomitantly. Kay and associates (269) observed similar interactions between vecuronium and pancuronium. However, the prolongation of vecuronium with prior administration of pancuronium was negligible by the third increment of vecuronium. Similarly, Smith and White (266) reported that pipecuronium prolonged the duration of action of subsequent doses of vecuronium such that standard maintenance doses of vecuronium and pipecuronium had a similar duration of action. These investigators observed a significant progressive decline in duration with each of the first three maintenance doses. However, even after four supplemental doses, the duration of action of the maintenance relaxant was still significantly prolonged. Prior administration of succinylcholine, 1 mg/kg, reduced the onset time of pipecuronium, 80 μg/kg; however, the clinical duration of action was not affected (270). However, prior administration of succinylcholine does not have any effect on the dynamics of rocuronium (271, 272).

Middleton and associates (264) examined the duration of incremental doses of vecuronium or atracurium during recovery from tubocurarine block. Their results indicate that the duration of action of the first maintenance bolus was the longest and decreased with successive increments until the response to further increments remained unchanged. The duration of action became constant after the third increment of atracurium, but 6 to 7 increments of vecuronium were required to achieve a constant duration (264). Thus, the clinical interaction between tubocurarine and vecuronium was greater than that between tubocurarine and atracurium. The duration of action of mivacurium was prolonged by prior administration of rocuronium or vecuronium, such that maintenance boluses of mivacurium resembled the duration of rocuronium and vecuronium, respectively (263). These authors concluded that there was no clinical advantage in combining nondepolarizing muscle relaxants with differing durations of action (263).

PHARMACOECONOMICS OF MUSCLE RELAXANTS

Reducing costs while maintaining quality has become a major goal in the delivery of health care. The newer neuromuscular blocking drugs have advantageous pharmacologic profiles and fewer side effects; however, their costs are predictably higher than the drugs they are designed to replace. Given the current emphasis on controlling health care costs, it is necessary to examine the impact of these drugs not only on the quality of anesthesia care, but also on the overall cost effectiveness of the care provided (273, 274).

Muscle relaxants constitute a major component (20 to 30%) of anesthesia-related drug expenses (275). Although costs of newer drugs have assumed increased importance, anesthesia-related costs represent only a small fraction (less than 6%) of the costs of a surgical procedure (276). However, the costs associated with the use of any muscle relaxant are not just for the acquisition of the drugs but also include indirect costs such as the cost of complications arising from the use of these drugs (277). Unfortunately, no prospective, randomized, controlled trials address the issue of cost effectiveness of neuromuscular blocking drugs.

In an effort to reduce costs, many anesthesiologists have switched from intermediate-acting muscle relaxants to less expensive longer-acting drugs (e.g., pancuronium). However, with the introduction of intermediate-acting muscle relaxants, the incidence of residual postoperative weakness was decreased (278, 279). The increase in the duration of stay in the operating room and the postanesthesia care unit (PACU) would significantly increase the overall anesthesia-related costs. The costs associated with the operating room and the PACU account for a significant portion of the perioperative costs because it is labor and equipment intensive (276). Therefore, the costs of postoperative complications related to the inappropriate use of muscle relaxants outweigh the costs of the drugs. More important, the costs associated with patient dissatisfaction as a result of myalgias, postoperative emesis, or prolonged tracheal intubation in the PACU are difficult to measure. Finally, attention to simple measures such as appropriate choice of the drug and avoiding "overtreatment" and waste could result in substantial savings (280).

PHARMACOLOGY OF INDIVIDUAL MUSCLE RELAXANT DRUGS

Pancuronium

Pancuronium is a long-acting muscle relaxant with a high potency. Following its introduction into clinical practice, pancuronium was an instant success because it does not cause histamine release and hypotension. However, it frequently increases heart rate and arterial blood pressure. The use pancuronium is increasing because of the current emphasis on cost containment. However, no prospective cost-effectiveness studies have been conducted to evaluate the costs and outcome when using pancuronium as an alternative to the intermediate-acting muscle relaxants.

The ED_{95} for pancuronium in healthy adults is 0.06 to 0.07 mg/kg (78). As for all nondepolarizing muscle relaxants, the onset time of pancuronium is dose dependent. The onset time for pancuronium, 0.08 and 0.04 mg/kg, is 1.6 and 2.9 minutes, respectively. The duration of action of an intubating dose (0.08 to 0.12 mg/kg) is 60 to 120 minutes. To achieve a steady-state pancuronium concentration of 0.2 μg/ml, Somogyi and colleagues (281) recommended a loading dose of 62.5 μg/kg and a constant-rate infusion of 0.35 μg/kg/min (21 μg/kg/h). On cessation of the pancuronium infusion, the twitch height increased by 1% per minute (281). Gramstad and Lilleaasen (176) reported that the maintenance doses of pancuronium and vecuronium for 90% blockade during nitrous oxide-narcotic anesthesia were 37 and 102 μg/kg/h, respectively.

Pancuronium has vagolytic (282) and sympathetic stimulatory effects (283, 284) that often increase heart rate, mean arterial blood pressure, and cardiac output (285, 286). The inhibitory effects of pancuronium on the muscarinic receptors located on the noradrenergic nerve terminals and the pacemaker cells of the right atria increase the evoked release of epinephrine and force of contraction of the electrically stimulated right atria (287). In one study, although pancuronium, 120 μg/kg, increased heart rate, mean arterial blood pressure, and cardiac output, it did not cause myocardial ischemia when assessed by electrocardiographic (ECG) ST-segment analysis or transesophageal echocardiography (288). Some investigators report that pancuronium administered after an adequate induction dose of fentanyl does not cause tachycardia and is similar to vecuronium and pipecuronium (289). Furthermore, no significant difference was noted in the need for hemodynamic interventions after pancuronium, pipecuronium, or doxacurium (290). In contrast, other investigators observed ECG signs of myocardial ischemia in 25% of patients receiving pancuronium during cardiac surgery, and the decay of plasma norepinephrine concentration was slower with pancuronium than with pipecuronium (291).

To achieve reliable antagonism of long-acting muscle relaxants, spontaneous recovery must be at least 25% (3 or 4 TOF responses) (279). The incidence of inadequate reversal (TOF ratios less than 0.7) in patients arriving in the PACU is greater in patients receiving pancuronium than in those receiving intermediate-acting muscle relaxants (278, 279). When neostigmine, 0.06 to 0.08 mg/kg, was administered with T_1 less than 10% of control in patients receiving pancuronium, 0.08 to 0.1 mg/kg, T_1 levels of 95% were achieved within 15 minutes. However, a TOF ratio of 0.7 was not achieved at 30 minutes in 50% of the patients studied.

Furthermore, increasing the dose of neostigmine did not enhance the degree of reversal (292).

Pipecuronium

Pipecuronium bromide is a steroid-base, bisquaternary neuromuscular blocking drug with a long duration of action. It is a pancuronium derivative in which the 2,16-substitutions of the steroid nucleus are piperazine rings, whereas pancuronium has piperidine rings. Pipecuronium has little or no inhibitory effect on the muscarinic receptors located on the noradrenergic nerve terminals and pacemaker cells of the right atria and consequently cause no elevation of heart rate or blood pressure (293). It has one-tenth the vagolytic activity of pancuronium. In addition, the absence of any ganglion-blocking potency makes pipecuronium free of any cardiovascular side effects with doses as high as four times ED_{95} (Fig. 15-10). Pipecuronium was found to be free of sympathomimetic or vagolytic activity in patients undergoing cardiac surgery (45, 288, 291, 294, 295).

Pipecuronium is approximately 20 to 30% more potent than pancuronium or vecuronium, with an ED_{95} of 40 to 45 μg/kg (20, 296, 297). The onset of pipecuronium neuromuscular relaxant effects is slow and dose dependent (298). The onset of maximum blockade after pipecuronium, 45 and 70 μg/kg, is 3.5 minutes and 2.5 minutes, respectively (298, 299). The clinical duration of action following a dose of 45 μg/kg is approximately 50 minutes, and after 70 to 85 μg/kg, it is 80 to 120 minutes (44, 125, 298). The time course of the neuromuscular effects of pipecuronium is similar to that of pancuronium (65, 297, 300). The recommended supplemental dose of pipecuronium for maintenance of relaxation is approximately 5 to 10 μg/kg, with an expected duration of 30 to 45 minutes.

As with other long-acting muscle relaxants, reversal of pipecuronium may be slow and incomplete. Patients with less than 20% recovery of T_1 before administration of neostigmine may require longer time to achieve full recovery of muscle function (299, 301). There was no difference between the reversibility of neuromuscular block produced by pipecuronium, 0.07 mg/kg, or pancuronium, 0.1 mg/kg, following administration of edrophonium (0.5 or 1 mg/kg), neostigmine (0.04 mg/kg), or pyridostigmine (0.3 mg/kg) (301). In addition, complete antagonism of the twitch response was produced within 15 minutes (301). However, other investigators report that neostigmine (0.06 mg/kg) is more effective than edrophonium (1 mg/kg), when administered at T_1 recovery of 20% (302). In addition, the TOF ratio was less than 0.7 (i.e., inadequate reversal) in 33% of the pipecuronium-treated patients receiving neostigmine and in 80% of the patients receiving edrophonium (302). Because edrophonium is unreliable in reversing the pipecuronium-induced blockade, neostigmine should be used for reversal of residual blockade at the end of the surgery (302). It may take more than 2 hours to reach 25% recovery without reversal drugs after standard doses of pipecuronium because of the clinical variability in response to neuromuscular blocking drugs (303). Therefore, pipecuronium is suited only for long operations (> 3 to 4 hours) in which early extubation is not mandatory and when cardiovascular stability is advantageous.

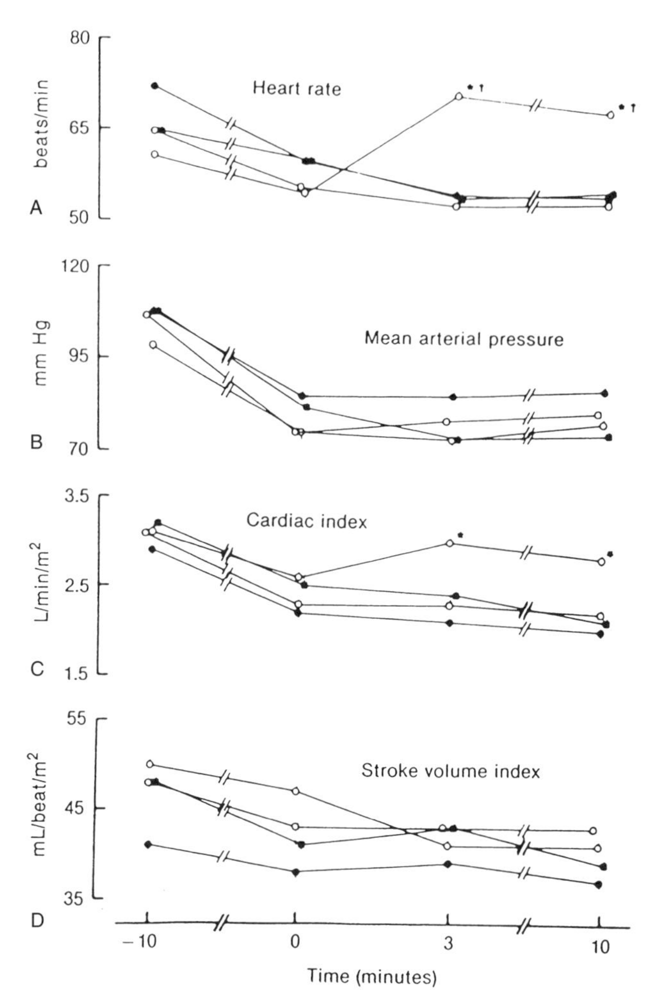

FIGURE 15-10. A to D, Hemodynamic changes following induction of anesthesia and muscle relaxant administration (T=0). The open circles represent the patient group receiving pancuronium, 0.15 mg/kg; the filled-in circles, pipecuronium, 0.05 mg/kg; the filled-in squares, pipecuronium, 0.01 mg/kg; and the open squares, 0.15 mg/kg of pipecuronium. (From Tassonyi E, Neihaid E, Pittet JF, et al. Cardiovascular effects of pipecuronium and pancuronium in patients undergoing coronary bypass grafting. Anesthesiology 1988;69:793–796.)

Vecuronium

Vecuronium is the monoquaternary analog of pancuronium that differs from pancuronium only in the deletion of a methyl group at the N-piperidino position of the steroid molecule, thereby eliminating the vagolytic effects observed with pancuronium (14). It is a white powder that is soluble but unstable in aqueous solutions over a wide range of pH, and the acetate groups at 3 and 17 are subject to hydrolysis. Vecuronium has minimal cardiovascular effects even at high doses (0.4 mg/kg) and does not release histamine (304).

The ED_{95} for vecuronium is 0.05 mg/kg. The onset of maximum block with vecuronium 0.1 mg/kg is approximately 3 minutes (305). The onset time for vecuronium is similar to that of pancuronium; however, the clinical duration of action and the recovery index from equipotent doses of vecuronium are one-half to one-third those of pancuronium (306). The usual duration of an intubating dose of vecuronium (0.1 to 0.2 mg/kg) is 45 to 90 minutes, whereas the typical duration of a supplemental dose (0.01 to 0.02 mg/kg) is 15 to 30 minutes. The onset of action can be reduced to 88 to 106 seconds by increasing the dose from 0.1 to 0.4 mg/kg (100, 304). However, the clinical duration of action increased significantly with increase in dose (100, 304). The clinical duration of vecuronium, 0.3 mg/kg, was longer than that of pancuronium, 0.08 mg/kg (111 versus 86 minutes) (304). No evidence indicates cumulation with incremental doses of vecuronium (307, 308).

Vecuronium infusion offers a stable degree of twitch depression for long surgical procedures, and the suggested infusion rate for vecuronium is 0.8 to 2 μg/kg/min (309, 310). The time required to achieve a steady state depends on the loading dose, on the time interval between the loading dose and the start of infusion, and on the rate of the infusion. Investigators have suggested that the loading dose should be 1.5 times ED_{90}, and the same dose should be infused per hour (311). Inhalation agents decrease the infusion requirements in a dose-dependent manner. In addition, a constant infusion of vecuronium adjusted to maintain T_1 suppression of 90 to 95% results in cumulation that is manifest after the second hour of administration (312). When titrated to the patient's response, an infusion of vecuronium is easy to use and can be readily reversed (312). The steady-state infusion of vecuronium was reversible in about half the time of intermittently administered bolus doses of pancuronium (310). In addition, the duration of vecuronium infusion also predicts the reversal time (310).

Antagonism of vecuronium-induced neuromuscular block is usually prompt following administration of neostigmine (308). Caldwell (313) measured the degree of residual neuromuscular block at different times after a single dose of vecuronium and evaluated the effectiveness of two different doses of neostigmine in antagonizing the residual block. He found that clinically significant residual neuromuscular block could be present for up to 4 hours after a single dose of vecuronium, 0.1 mg/kg. In addition, neostigmine, 40 μg/kg, but not 20 μg/kg, could facilitate recovery, and both doses of neostigmine (and glycopyrrolate) were associated with clinically significant cardiovascular effects (313). A study evaluating recovery from vecuronium-induced blockade reported that the incidence of inadequate reversal (as defined as TOF ratio <0.7) was greater in patients receiving bolus doses of vecuronium compared with those receiving a titrated vecuronium infusion (12% versus 24%) (314).

Rocuronium

Rocuronium (Org 9426), a structure analog of vecuronium that has been introduced into clinical practice, is one of several steroidal compounds (Org 9426, Org 7616, Org 9616) with low potency and an onset profile allegedly similar to that of succinylcholine. Rocuronium is the least potent nondepolarizing muscle relaxant currently available for clinical use. Although it has a rapid onset of action, its duration of action is similar to that of other intermediate-acting muscle relaxants. Rocuronium has minimal potential for clinically significant adverse hemodynamic effects (23, 29, 315, 316) or histamine release (81, 316) over a wide range of doses (2 to 4 $\times$ ED_{95}) (Fig. 15-11). However, rocuronium can cause significant pain during rapid injection (317) and can form a precipitate when mixed with intravenous induction drugs (e.g., thiopental) (318).

The ED_{95} of rocuronium is 0.3 mg/kg, making it approximately 7 to 8 times less potent than vecuronium. Doses of two to three times ED_{95} provide good-to-excellent intubation conditions within 1 minute in most patients (10, 24, 271, 319). Although earlier studies reported onset times of rocuronium similar to that of succinylcholine, a wide variation exists (58 to 172 seconds) (10, 24, 271, 272, 319, 320). Studies have shown that the onset times of rocuronium are slower than that of succinylcholine (271). Magorian and colleagues compared varying doses of rocuronium with succinylcholine and vecuronium for rapid-sequence induction of anesthesia (101). These authors found a dose-dependent decrease in onset times with rocuronium. The onset time of rocuronium, 0.9 and 1.2 mg/kg, is similar to that of succinylcholine; however, the clinical duration of action is significantly longer (Table 15-6). The clinical duration and recovery index of rocuronium is similar to that of vecuronium. Onset time, clinical duration, and recovery index after two times ED_{90} of rocuronium, vecuronium, and mivacurium were 172 seconds, 28 minutes, and 11 minutes; 192 seconds, 33 minutes, and 14 minutes; and 229 seconds, 13 minutes, and 6 minutes, respectively (321).

In an effort to reduce the duration of action, some investigators have evaluated the time course of lower doses of rocuronium. The onset time of rocuronium, 0.3 mg/kg, was 65 and 69 seconds for alfentanil-propofol and fentanyl-thiopental-enflurane tech-

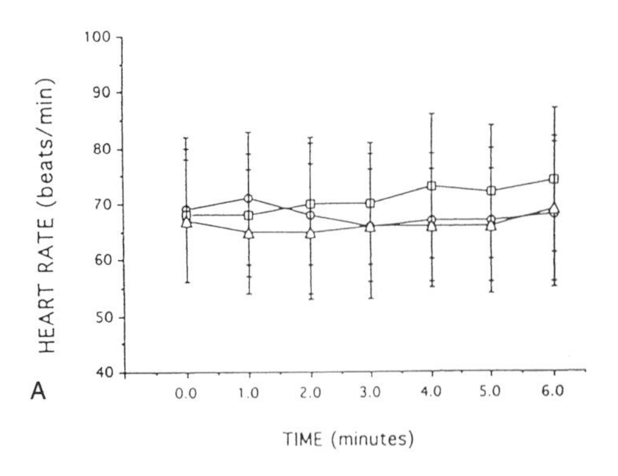

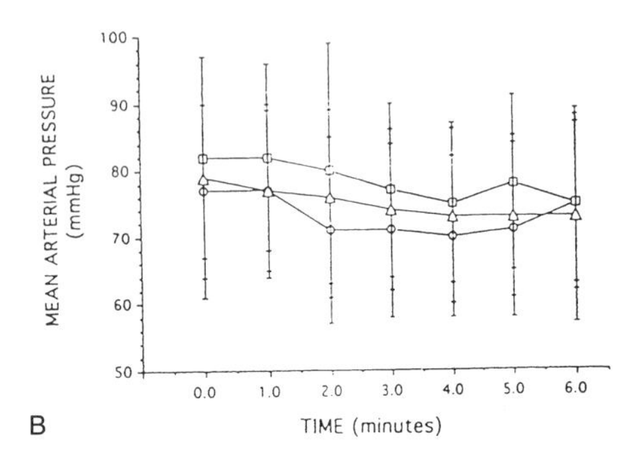

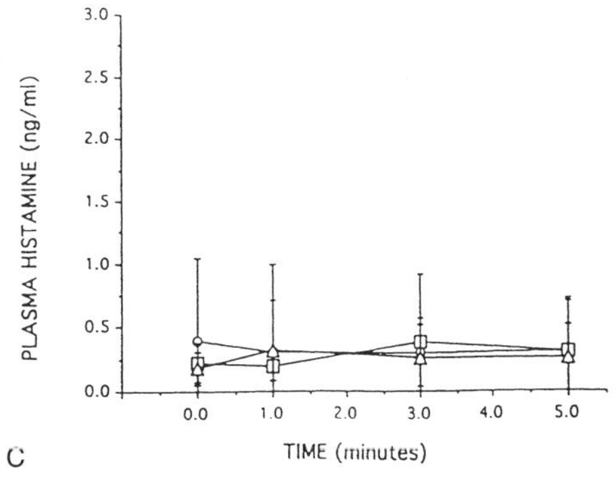

FIGURE 15-11. A to C, Changes in heart rate, mean arterial pressure, and plasma histamine concentrations after intravenous bolus administration of rocuronium. Data are expressed as mean ± SD. No significant differences in the heart rate, mean arterial pressure, or plasma histamine concentrations occurred after administration of rocuronium. Circles represent 600 μg/kg; squares represent 900 μg/kg; and triangles represent 1200 μg/kg. (From Levy JH, Davis GK, Duggan J, et al. Determination of the hemodynamics and histamine release of rocuronium [Org 9426] when administered in increased doses under N_2O/O_2 = sufentanil anesthesia. Anesth Analg 1994;78:318–321.)

niques, respectively (322). The intubating conditions with rocuronium, 0.45 mg/kg, were excellent compared with atracurium, 0.35 mg/kg, or vecuronium, 0.075 mg/kg. The mean clinical duration of blockade with rocuronium, 0.45 mg/kg, was 22 minutes. No correlation was noted between the intubation conditions and the degree of block at the adductor pollicis (323).

Use of a continuous infusion of rocuronium, 10 to 12 μg/kg/min, after early evidence of spontaneous recovery can provide adequate neuromuscular blockade (231). However, following a 1- to 2-hour infusion, the dose of rocuronium required to maintain 95% blockade during inhalation anesthesia may be reduced by as much as 30 to 50%. Antagonism of a profound rocuronium-induced neuromuscular blockade may be more reliable with neostigmine, 50 μg/kg, whereas edrophonium, 1 mg/kg, is advantageous when there is a greater spontaneous recovery (324). Like vecuronium, edrophonium is less effective than neostigmine at reversing rocuronium-induced neuromuscular blockade (325).

ORG 9487

The investigational muscle relaxant, Org 9487, an analog of vecuronium, is a steroidal neuromuscular blocking drug currently undergoing extensive clinical investigation. It is reported to have a rapid onset and a relatively short duration of action. Preliminary trials suggested that Org 9487 has a favorable profile with respect to time course of action, tracheal intubating conditions, and cardiovascular side effects. Org 9487 does not appear to have significant cardiovascular side effects; however, a transient decrease in arterial blood pressure and a concomitant increase in heart rate have been reported (31). The ED_{90} of Org 9487 is 1.15 mg/kg. The onset time for Org 9487, 1.5 mg/kg (1.3 × ED_{90}), is 83 to 90 seconds, slightly longer than that of succinylcholine (67 seconds) (11, 31). The tracheal intubation conditions at 1 minute were also similar with Org 9487 and succinylcholine (Table 15-7) (11).

In one report, the clinical duration of action following a 1.5 mg/kg dose of Org 9487 was 8.9 minutes (31), and the time to clinically sufficient recovery after neostigmine antagonism (11.6 minutes) was similar to that of succinylcholine (10.6) (11). However, the time to recovery to a TOF ratio of 0.7 was longer (approximately 25 minutes) than that of succinylcholine (11). In one study, Org 9487 was easy to administer as an infusion, with an initial infusion rate of 3.4 mg/kg/h required to maintain 80% block, and during the final 15 minutes of the infusion, the requirements were decreased to 2.5 mg/kg/h (54). The time to reach a TOF ratio of 0.7 when the block was allowed to recover spontaneously was approximately 40 minutes, compared with 15 minutes following reversal with neostigmine (54). The investigators concluded that, following an infusion of Org 9487, the time course characteristics changed gradually from those of a short-acting neuromuscular blocking drug to those of an intermediate-acting drug (54). Unlike the bolus injection of Org 9487 (a short-acting drug), in which the recovery of block occurs during the distribution phase, the recovery of block following a prolonged infusion of Org 9487 occurs during the elimination phase, which depends on the slower plasma clearance of the drug. In addition, the plasma concentration of the 3-hydroxy metabolite of

TABLE 15-6. Onset and Recovery Data for Rocuronium, Vecuronium, and Succinylcholine*

	Rocuronium (0.6 mg/kg)	Rocuronium (0.9 mg/kg)	Rocuronium (1.2 mg/kg)	Vecuronium (0.1 mg/kg)	Succinylcholine (1 mg/kg)
Onset (s)	89 ± 33	75 ± 28	55 ± 14	144 ± 39	50 ± 17
	(48–156)	(48–144)	(36–84)	(56–204)	(24–89)
Clinical Duration	37 ± 15	53 ± 21	73 ± 32	41 ± 19	9 ± 2
(min)	(23–75)	(25–88)	(38–150)	(17–82)	(5–14)
Recovery Index	14 ± 8	22 ± 14	24 ± 11	20 ± 18	2 ± 1
(min)	(6–27)	(8–29)	(8–29)	(6–57)	(1–3)

Values are mean ± SD (range).

Onset, The time interval between the completion of injection of muscle relaxant and the time to maximal depression T_1; clinical duration, the time interval between the completion of injection of muscle relaxant to recovery of T_1 to 25% of control; recovery index, recovery of T_1 from 25 to 75%. (From Magorian T, Flannery KB, Miller RD. Comparison of rocuronium, succinylcholine, and vecuronium for rapid-sequence induction of anesthesia in adult patients. Anesthesiology 1993;79:913–918.)

TABLE 15-7. Comparative Onset and Recovery Characteristics of Org 9487, a Short-acting Steroidal Muscle Relaxant, and Succinylcholine*

	Succinylcholine 1 mg/kg (control)	Org 9487 1.5 mg/kg (with reversal)	Org 9487 1.5 mg/kg (without reversal)
Onset (s)	67 ± 20	83 ± 38	83 ± 38
Recovery (min)			
T_1 = 25%	8.0 ± 2.5	5.7 ± 0.6	8.0 ± 1.9
T_1 = 90%	10.6 ± 3.3	10.8 ± 3.5	16.4 ± 5.8[†]
TOF > 0.7	NA	11.6 ± 1.4	24.1 ± 6.2[†]

Values are mean ± SD.

[†] *$p < 0.05$ versus control and neostigmine-reversed groups.*

T_1, First-twitch response; TOF, train-of-four. (From Wierda JM, van den Broek L, Proost JH, et al. Time course of action and endotracheal intubating conditions of Org 9487, a new short-acting steroidal muscle relaxant: a comparison with succinylcholine. Anesth Analg 1993;79:579–584.)

Org 9487 is increased during infusion, and it may contribute to the neuromuscular blockade and may prolong the recovery phase (54).

In summary, since the introduction of pancuronium, steroidal neuromuscular blocking drugs have assumed an increasingly important place in anesthetic practice. Pancuronium is a long-acting muscle relaxant that causes increases in heart rate and blood pressure but does not release histamine. Pipecuronium has a pharmacodynamic profile similar to that of pancuronium; however, unlike pancuronium, it is associated with excellent hemodynamic stability over a wide dose range. Vecuronium is an intermediate-acting muscle relaxant with a stable hemodynamic profile. Rocuronium is the first nondepolarizing muscle relaxant with a rapid onset; however, its duration of action is similar to that of vecuronium. Org 9487 reportedly has a pharmacodynamic profile more similar to that of succinylcholine.

During the last decade, much research has been directed toward designing and developing a nondepolarizing neuromuscular blocking drug with a time course more closely resembling that of succinylcholine but without side effects. Thus far, all attempts to develop a neuromuscular blocking drug with a time course similar to that of succinylcholine have been frustrated either by unwanted cardiovascular side effects or by the inability to confirm in humans the short recovery profile reported in experimental animals. With improved understanding of structural pharmacodynamic-pharmacokinetic relationships, it should be possible to design a nondepolarizing neuromuscular blocking drug with a pharmacologic profile similar to that of succinylcholine.

REFERENCES

1. Griffith HR, Johnson GE. The use of curare in general anesthesia. Anesthesiology 1942;3:418.
2. Gray TC, Holton J. Technique for the use of d-tubocurarine chloride with balanced anaesthesia. Br Med J 1946;2:293–5.
3. Mushin WW, Mapleson WW. Relaxant action in man of dipyrandium chloride (M & B 9105A) (a steroid bis-quaternary ammonium salt). Br J Anaesth 1964;36:761.
4. Baird WLM, Reid AM. Neuromuscular blocking properties of a new steroidal compound, pancuronium bromide: a pilot study in man. Br J Anaesth 1967;39:775.
5. Savarese JJ, Kitz RJ. Does clinical anesthesia need new neuromuscular blocking agents? Anesthesiology 1975;42:236.
6. Savage DS, Sleigh T, Carlyle I. The emergence of ORG NC 45, 1-[2 beta, 3 alpha, 5 alpha, 16 beta, 17 beta)-3, 17-bis(acetyloxy)-2-(1-piperidinyl)androstan-16-yl]-1-methylpiperidinium bromide, from the pancuronium series. Br J Anaesth 1980;52:3S–9S.
7. Durant NN, Savage DS, Nelson DN, et al. The neuromuscular and autonomic blocking activities of pancuronium, ORG NC 45, and other pancuronium analogues in the cat. J Pharm Pharmacol 1979;31:831.
8. Booji LHDJ, Edwards RP, Sohn YJ, et al. Cardiovascular and neuromuscular effects of ORG 45, pancuronium, metocurine and d-tubocurarine in dogs. Anesth Analg 1980;59:26.
9. Karpati E, Biro K. Pharmacological study of a new competitive neuromuscular blocking steroid, pipecuronium bromide. Arzneimittelforschung 1980;30:346.
10. Wierda JM, de Wit AP, Kuizenga K, et al. Clinical observations on the neuromuscular blocking action of Org 9426, a new steroidal non-depolarizing agent. Br J Anaesth 1990;64:521–523.
11. Wierda JM, van den Broek L, Proost JH, et al. Time course of action and endotracheal intubating conditions of Org 9487, a new short-acting steroidal muscle relaxant: a comparison with succinylcholine. Anesth Analg 1993;77:579–584.
12. Ramzan IM, Somogyi AA, Walker JS, et al. Clinical pharma-

cokinetics of nondepolarizing muscle relaxants. Clin Pharmacokinet 1981;6:25–60.
13. Agoston S, Vandenbrom RH, Wierda JM. Clinical pharmacokinetics of neuromuscular blocking drugs. Clin Pharmacokinet 1992;22:94–115.
14. Ducharme J, Donati F. Pharmacokinetics and pharmacodynamics of steroidal muscle relaxants. Anesthesiol Clin North Am 1993;11:283–307.
15. Bovet D. Some aspects of the relationship between chemical constitution and curare-like activity. Ann NY Acad Sci 1951; 54:107.
16. Riesz M, Karpati E, Szporny L. Steroid derivatives. Handb Exp Pharmacol 1986;79:301.
17. Durant NN, Houwertjes MC, Crul JF. Comparison of the neuromuscular blocking properties of ORG NC 45 and pancuronium in the rat, cat and rhesus monkey. Br J Anaesth 1980; 52:723–30.
18. Marshall IG, Agoston S, Booij LH, et al. Pharmacology of ORG NC 45 compared with other non-depolarizing neuromuscular blocking drugs. Br J Anaesth 1980;52:11S–19S.
19. Upton RA, Nguyen TL, Miller RD, et al. Renal and biliary elimination of vecuronium (ORG NC 45) and pancuronium in rats. Anesth Analg 1982;61:313–316.
20. Boros M, Szenohradszky J, Marosi G, et al. Comparative clinical study of pipecuronium bromide and pancuronium bromide. Arzneimittelforschung 1980;30:389–393.
21. Bowman WC, Rodger IW, Houston J, et al. Structure: action relationships among some desacetoxy analogues of pancuronium and vecuronium in the anesthetized cat. Anesthesiology 1988;69:57–62.
22. Kopman AF. Gallamine, pancuronium and d-tubocurarine compared: is onset time related to drug potency? Anesthesiology 1989;70:915–920.
23. Muir AW, Houston J, Green KL, et al. Effects of a new neuromuscular blocking agent (Org 9426) in anaesthetized cats and pigs and in isolated nerve-muscle preparations. Br J Anaesth 1989;63:400–410.
24. Foldes FF, Nagashima H, Nguyen HD, et al. The neuromuscular effects of ORG 9426 in patients receiving balanced anesthesia. Anesthesiology 1991;75:191.
25. Marshall RJ, Muir AW, Sleigh T, et al. Research and development of aminosteroid neuromuscular blocking agents: past and future. Eur J Anaesthesiol 1995;11:5–10.
26. Muir AW, Houston J, Marshall RJ, et al. A comparison of neuromuscular blocking and autonomic effects of two new short-acting muscle relaxants with those of succinylcholine in the anesthetized cat and pig. Anesthesiology 1989;70:533.
27. van den Broek L, Wierda JM, Proost JH, et al. Clinical pharmacology of ORG 7617, a short-acting non-depolarizing neuromuscular blocking agent. Eur J Clin Pharmacol 1994;46:225–229.
28. Muir AW, Anderson K, Marshall RJ, et al. The effects of a 16-N-homopiperidino analogue of vecuronium on neuromuscular transmission in anaesthetized cats, pigs, dogs and monkeys, and in isolated preparation. Acta Anaesthesiol Scand 1991; 35:85–90.
29. Cason B, Baker DG, Hickey RF, et al. Cardiovascular and neuromuscular effects of three steroidal neuromuscular blocking drugs in dogs (ORG 9616, ORG 9426, ORG 9991). Anesth Analg 1990;70:382–388.
30. van den Broek L, Lambalk LM, Richardson FJ, et al. Dose-response relation, neuromuscular blocking action, intubation conditions, and cardiovascular effects of Org 9273, a new neuromuscular blocking agent. Anesth Analg 1991;72:811–816.
31. Wierda JM, Beaufort AM, Kleef UW, et al. Preliminary investigations of the clinical pharmacology of three short-acting non-depolarizing neuromuscular blocking agents, Org 9453, Org 9489 and Org 9487. Can J Anaesth 1994;41:213–220.
32. Shanks CA. Pharmacokinetics of the nondepolarizing neuromuscular relaxants applied to calculation of bolus and infusion doasge regimens. Anesthesiology 1986;64:72–86.
33. Miller RD, Agoston S, Booij LDHJ, et al. Comparative potency and pharmacokinetics of pancuronium and its metabolites in anesthetized man. J Pharmacol Ther 1978;207:539–543.
34. Castognoli KP, Gruenke LD, Miller RD, et al. Quantitative estimation of quaternary ammonium neuromuscular blocking agents in serum by direct insertion probe chemical ionization mass spectrometry. Biomed Environ Mass Spectrometry 1986; 13:327–332.
35. Paanakker JE, Thio JM, Van den Wildenberg HM, et al. Assay of vecuronium in plasma using solid-phase extraction, high-performance liquid chromatography and post-column ion-pair extraction with fluorimetric detection. J Chromatogr 1987; 421:327–335.
36. Duvaldestin P, Henzel D. Binding of d-tubocurarine, fazadinium, pancuronium, and org NC 45 to serum proteins in normal man and in patients with cirrhosis. Br J Anaesth 1982; 54:513–516.
37. Wood M, Stone WJ, Wood AJJ. Plasma binding of pancuronium: effects of age, sex, and disease. Anesth Analg 1983;62:29–32.
38. Agoston S, Kersten UW, Meijer DKF. The fate of pancuronium bromide in man. Acta Anaesthesiol Scand 1973;17:267.
39. McLeod K, Watson MJ, Rawlins MD. Pharmacokinetics of pancuronium in patients with normal and impaired renal function. Br J Anaesth 1976;48:341.
40. Somogyi AA, Shanks CA, Triggs EJ. Clinical pharmacokinetics of pancuronium bromide. Eur J Clin Pharmacol 1976;10:367.
41. Bodrogi L, Feher T, Vairdi A, et al. Pharmacokinetics of pipecuronium bromide in the rat. Arzneimittelforschung 1980; 30:366–370.
42. Agoston S, Vandenbrom RHG, Wierda JMKH, et al. Pharmacokinetics and disposition of pipecuronium bromide in the cat. Eur J Anaesthesiol 1988;5:233–242.
43. Khuenl-Brady KS, Sharma M, Chung K, et al. Pharmacokinetics and disposition of pipecuronium bromide in dogs with or without ligated renal pedicles. Anesthesiology 1989;71:919–922.
44. Caldwell JE, Castagnoli KP, Canfell PC, et al. Pipecuronium and pancuronium: comparison of pharmacokinetics and duration of action. Br J Anaesth 1988;61:693–697.
45. Wierda JMKH, Karliczek GF, Vandenbrom RHG, et al. Pharmacokinetcs and cardiovascular dynamics of pipecuronium bromide during coronary artery surgery. Can J Anaesth 1990; 37:183–191.
46. Caldwell JE, Canfell PC, Castagnoli KP, et al. The influence of renal failure on the pharmacokinetics and duration of action of pipecuronium bromide in patients anesthetized with halothane and nitrous oxide. Anesthesiology 1989;70:7–12.
47. Bencini AF, Scaf AHJ, Sohn YJ, et al. Clinical pharmacokinetics of vecuronium: clinical experiences with Norcuron. In: Agoston S, et al, eds. Current clinical practice series. Amsterdam: Excerpta Medica, 1983:115–123.
48. Shanks CA, Avram MJ, Fragen RJ, et al. Pharmacokinetics and pharmacodynamics of vecuronium administered by bolus and infusion during halothane or balanced anesthesia. Clin Pharmacol Ther 1987;42:459–464.
49. Sohn YJ, Bencini AF, Scaf AHJ, et al. Comparative pharmacokinetics and dynamics of vecuronium and pancuronium in anesthetized patients. Anesth Analg 1986;65:233–239.
50. Cronnelly R, Fisher DM, Miller RD, et al. Pharmacokinetics and pharmacodynamics of vecuronium (ORG NC45) and pancuronium in anesthetized humans. Anesthesiology 1983;58:405–408.
51. Bencini AF, Scaf AH, Sohn YJ, et al. Hepatobiliary disposition of vecuronium bromide in man. Br J Anaesth 1986;58:988–995.
52. Fisher DM, Rosen JI. A pharmacokinetic explanation for in-

creasing recovery time following larger or repeated doses of nondepolarizing muscle relaxants. Anesthesiology 1986; 65:192–198.
53. Khuenl-Brady K, Castagnoli KP, Canfell PC, et al. The neuromuscular blocking effects and pharmacokinetics of ORG 9426 and ORG 9616 in the cat. Anesthesiology 1990;72:669–674.
54. van den Broek L, Wierda JM, Smeulers NJ, et al. Pharmacodynamics and pharmacokinetics of an infusion of Org 9487, a new short-acting steroidal neuromuscular blocking agent. Br J Anaesth 1994;73:331–335.
55. Bencini AF, Scaf AHJ, Sohn YJ, et al. Disposition and urinary excretion of vecuronium bromide in anaesthetized patients with normal renal function or renal failure. Anesth Analg 1986; 65:245–251.
56. Cooper RA, Maddineni VR, Mirakhur RK, et al. Time course of neuromuscular effects and pharmacokinetics of rocuronium bromide (Org 9426) during isoflurane anaesthesia in patients with and without renal failure. Br J Anaesth 1993;71:222–226.
57. Wierda JMKH, Kleef UW, Lambalk LM, et al. The pharmacodynamics and pharmacokinetics of ORG 9426, a new non-depolarizing neuromuscular blocking agent, in patients anaesthetized with nitrous oxide, halothane and fentanyl. Can J Anaesth 1991;38:430–435.
58. Bencini AF, Mol WEM, Scaf AHJ, et al. Uptake and excretion of vecuronium bromide and pancuronium bromide in the isolated perfused rat liver. Anesthesiology 1988;69:487–492.
59. Duvaldestin P, Agoston S, Henzel D, et al. Pancuronium pharmacokinetics in patients with liver cirrhosis. Br J Anaesth 1978; 50:1131–1136.
60. Westra P, Vermeer GA, De Lange AR, et al. Hepatic and renal disposition of pancuronium and gallamine in patients with extrahepatic cholestasis. Br J Anaesth 1981;53:331.
61. Duvaldestin P, Saada J, Berger JL, et al. Pharmacokinetics, pharmacodynamics, and dose-response relationships of pancuronium in control and elderly subjects. Anesthesiology 1982; 56:36–40.
62. Westra P, Houwertjes MC, De Lange AR, et al. Effect of experimental cholestasis on neuromuscular blocking drugs in cats. Br J Anaesth 1980;52:747–757.
63. Marshall IG, Gibb AJ, Durant NN. Neuromuscular and vagal blocking actions of pancuronium bromide, its metabolites, and vecuronium bromide (Org NC45) and its potential metabolites in the anaesthetized cat. Br J Anaesth 1983;55:703–714.
64. Vereczkey L, Szporny L. Disposition of pipecuronium bromide in rats. Arzneimittel-forschung 1980;30:364–366.
65. Wierda JMKH, Richardson FJ, Agoston S. Dose-response relationship and time-course of action of pipecuronium bromide under isoflurane, halothane and neurolept anaesthesia. Br J Anaesth 1989;62:194–198.
66. Wierda JM, Szenohradszky J, et al. The pharmacokinetics, urinary and biliary excretion of pipecuronium bromide. Eur J Anaesthesiol 1991;8:451–457.
67. Fahey MR, Morris RB, Miller RD, et al. Pharmacokinetics of Org NC45 (Norcuron) in patients with and without renal failure. Br J Anaesth 1981;53:1049–1053.
68. Bencini AF, Scaf AHF, Agoston S, et al. Disposition of vecuronium bromide in the cat. Br J Anaesth 1985;57:782–788.
69. Caldwell JE, Szenohradszky J, Segredo V, et al. The pharmacodynamics and pharmacokinetics of the metabolite 3-desacetylvecuronium (ORG 7268) and its parent compound, vecuronium, in human volunteers. J Pharmacol Exp Ther 1994; 270:1216–1222.
70. Bencini AF, Houwertjes MC, Agoston S. Effects of hepatic uptake of vecuronium bromide and its putative metabolites on their neuromuscular blocking actions in the cat. Br J Anaesth 1985;57:789.
71. Segredo V, Shin YS, Sharma ML, et al. Pharmacokinetics, neuromuscular effects, and biodisposition of 3-desacetylvecuronium (Org 7268) in cats. Anesthesiology 1991;74:1052.
72. Sandker GW, Weert B, Olinga P, et al. Characterization of transport in isolated human hepatocytes: a study with the bile acid taurocholic acid, the uncharged ouabain and the organic cations vecuronium and rocuronium. Biochem Pharmacol 1994; 47:2193–2200.
73. Szenohradszky J, Fisher DM, Segredo V, et al. Pharmacokinetics of rocuronium bromide (ORG 9426) in patients with normal renal function or patients undergoing cadaver renal transplantation. Anesthesiology 1992;77:899–904.
74. Ali HH, Saverese JJ. Stimulus frequency and dose-reponse curve to d-tubocurarine in man. Anesthesiology 1980;52:36–39.
75. Holford NH, Sheiner LB. Kinetics of pharmacologic response. Pharmacol Ther 1982;16:143.
76. Shanks CA, Somogyi AA, Triggs EJ. Dose-response and plasma concentration-response relationships of pancuronium in man. Anesthesiology 1979;51:111–118.
77. Naguib M, Samarkandi AH, Bakhamees HS, et al. Comparative potency of steroidal neuromuscular blocking drugs and isobolographic analysis of the interaction between rocuronium and other aminosteroids. Br J Anaesth 1995;75:37–42.
78. Gramstad L, Lilleaasen P. Dose-response relation for atracurium, ORG NC 45 and pancuronium. Br J Anaesth 1982;54:647–651.
79. McCarthy GJ, Cooper R, Stanley JC, et al. Dose-response relationships for neostigmine antagonism of vecuronium-induced neuromuscular block in adults and the elderly. Br J Anaesth 1992;69:281–283.
80. McCarthy GJ, Mirakhur RK, Maddineni VR, et al. Dose-responses for edrophonium during antagonism of vecuronium block in young and older adult patients. Anaesthesia 1995; 50:503–506.
81. Naguib M, Samarkandi AH, Bakhamees HS, et al. Histamine-release haemodynamic changes produced by rocuronium, vecuronium, mivacuronium, atracurium and d-tubocurarine. Br J Anaesth 1995;75:588–592.
82. Appadu BL, Lambert DG. Studies on the interaction of steroidal neuromuscular blocking drugs with cardiac muscarinic receptors. Br J Anaesth 1994;72:86–88.
83. Donati F. Onset of action of relaxants. Can J Anaesth 1988; 35:S52–S58.
84. Chauvin M, Lebreault C, Duvaldestin P. The neuromuscular effect of vecuronium on the human diaphragm. Anesth Analg 1987;66:117–122.
85. Donati F, Antzaka C, Bevan DR. Potency of pancuronium at the diaphragm and the adductor pollicis muscles in humans. Anesthesiology 1986;65:1–5.
86. Lebrault C, Chauvin M, Guirimand F, et al. Relative potency of vecuronium on the diaphragm and the adductor pollicis. Br J Anaesth 1989;63:389–392.
87. Cantineau JP, Porte F, d'Honneur G, et al. Neuromuscular effects of rocuronium on the diaphragm and adductor pollicis muscles in anesthetized patients. Anesthesiology 1994;81:585–590.
88. Donati F, Meistelman C, Plaud B. Vecuronium neuromuscular blockade at the diaphragm, the orbicularis oculi, and adductor pollicis muscles. Anesthesiology 1990;73:870–875.
89. Donati F, Meistelman C, Plaud B. Vecuronium neuromuscular blockade at the adductor muscles of the larynx and adductor pollicis. Anesthesiology 1991;74:833–837.
90. Meistelman C, Plaud B, Donati F. Rocuronium (ORG 9426) neuromuscular blockade at the adductor muscles of the larynx and adductor pollicis in humans. Can J Anaesth 1992;39:665–669.
91. Wright PM, Caldwell JE, Miller RD. Onset and duration of rocuronium and succinylcholine at the adductor pollicis and laryngeal adductor muscles in anesthetized humans. Anesthesiology 1994;81:1110–1115.
92. D'Honneur G, Guignard B, Slavov V, et al. Comparison of the

neuromuscular blocking effect of atracurium and vecuronium on the adductor pollicis and the geniohyoid muscle in humans. Anesthesiology 1995;82:649–654.
93. Paton WD, Waud DR. The margin of safety of neuromuscular transmission. J Physiol (Lond) 1967;191:59–90.
94. Min JC, Bekavac I, Glavinovic MI, et al. Iontophoretic study of speed of action of various muscle relaxants. Anesthesiology 1992;77:351–356.
95. Donati F, Meistelman C. A kinetic-dynamic model to explain the relationship between high potency and slow onset time for neuromuscular blocking drugs. J Pharmacokinet Biopharm 1991;19:537–552.
96. Wierda JMKH, Proost JH, Muir AW, et al. Design of drugs for rapid onset. Anaesth Pharmacol Rev 1993;1:57–68.
97. Hof RP, Hof A, Scholtysik G, et al. Effects of the new calcium antagonist PN-200-110 on the myocadium and the regional peripheral circulation in anesthetized cats and dogs. J Cardiovasc Pharmacol 1984;6:407–416.
98. Bowman WC. Prejunctional and postjunctional cholinoceptors at the neuromuscular junction. Anesth Analg 1980;59:935–943.
99. Iwasaki H, Igarashi M, Yamauchi M, et al. The effect of cardiac output on the onset of neuromuscular block by vecuronium. Anaesthesia 1995;50:361–362.
100. Ginsberg B, Glass PS, Quill T, et al. Onset and duration of neuromuscular blockade following high-dose vecuronium administration. Anesthesiology 1989;71:201–205.
101. Magorian T, Flannery KB, Miller RD. Comparison of rocuronium, succinylcholine, and vecuronium for rapid-sequence induction of anesthesia in adult patients. Anesthesiology 1993; 79:913–918.
102. Mehta MP, Choi WW, Gergis SD, et al. Facilitation of rapid endotracheal intubations with divided doses of nondepolarizing neuromuscular blocking drugs. Anesthesiology 1985; 62:392–395.
103. Schwartz S, Illias W, Lackner F, et al. Rapid tracheal intubation with vecuronium: the priming principle. Anesthesiology 1985; 62:388–391.
104. Taboda JA, Rupp SM, Miller RD. Refining the priming principle for vecuronium during rapid-sequence induction of anesthesia. Anesthesiology 1986;64:243–247.
105. Naguib M. Different priming techniques, including mivacurium, accelerate the onset of rocuronium [See comments]. Can J Anaesth 1994;41:902–907.
106. Huemer G, Schwarz S, Gilly H, et al. Pharmacodynamics, pharmacokinetics, and intubation conditions after priming with three different doses of vecuronium. Anesth Analg 1995; 80:538–542.
107. Miller RD. The priming principle [Editorial]. Anesthesiology 1985;54:381–382.
108. Silverman SM, Culling RD, Middaugh RE. Rapid-sequence orotracheal intubation:a comparison of three techniques. Anesthesiology 1990;73:244–248.
109. D'Honneur G, Gall O, Gerard A, et al. Priming doses of atracurium and vecuronium depress swallowing in humans. Anesthesiology 1992;77:1070–1073.
110. Baumgarten RK, Carter CE, Reynolds WJ, et al. Priming with nondepolarizing relaxants for rapid tracheal intubation: a double-blind evaluation. Can J Anaesth 1988;35:5–11.
111. Glass PS, Wilson W, Mace JA, et al. Is the priming principle both effective and safe? Anesth Analg 1989;68:127–134.
112. Motsch J, Fuchs W, Hoch P, et al. Side effects and changes in pulmonary function after fixed dose precurarization with alcuronium, pancuronium or vecuronium. Br J Anaesth 1987; 59:1528–1532.
113. Goudsouzian NG. Maturation of neuromuscular transmission in the infant. Br J Anaesth 1980;52:205.
114. Fisher DM, O'Keefe CO, Stanski DR, et al. Pharmacokinetics and pharmacodynamics of d-tubocurarine in infants, children and adults. Anesthesiology 1982;57:203.
115. Fisher DM, Miller RD. Neuromuscular effects of vecuronium (ORG NC45) in infants and children during N_2O, halothane anesthesia. Anesthesiology 1983;58:519–523.
116. Fisher DM, Castagnoli K, Miller RD. Vecuronium kinetics and dynamics in anesthetized infants and children. Clin Pharmacol Ther 1985;37:402.
117. Meistelman C, Loose JP, Saint-Maurice C, et al. Clinical pharmacology of vecuronium in children: studies during nitrous oxide and halothane in oxygen anaesthesia. Br J Anaesth 1986; 58:996–1000.
118. Woelfel SK, Dong ML, Brandom BW, et al. Vecuronium infusion requirements in children during halothane-narcotic-nitrous oxide, and narcotic-nitrous oxide anesthesia. Anesth Analg 1991;73:33.
119. Goudsouzian NA, Martyn JJA, Liu LMP, et al. The dose-response effect of long-acting nondepolarizing neuromuscular blocking agents in children. Can Anaesth Soc J 1984;31: 246.
120. Meretoja OA, Wirtavuori K, Neuvonen PJ. Age-dependence of the dose-response curve of vecuronium in pediatric patients during balanced anesthesia. Anesth Analg 1988;67:21–26.
121. Bevan JC, Donati F, Bevan DR. Attempted acceleration of the onset of action of pancuronium: effects of divided doses in infants and children. Br J Anaesth 1985;57:1204.
122. Koscielniak-Nielsen ZJ, Bevan JC, Popovic V, et al. Onset of maximum neuromuscular block following succinylcholine or vecuronium in four age groups. Anesthesiology 1993;79:229–234.
123. Meretoja OA. Is vecuronium a long-acting neuromuscular blocking agent in neonates and infants? Br J Anaesth 1989; 62:184–187.
124. Baxter MR, Bevan JC, Samuel J, et al. Postoperative neuromuscular function in pediatric day-care patients. Anesth Analg 1991;72:504–508.
125. Pittet JF, Tassonyi E, Morel DR, et al. Pipecuronium-induced neuromuscular blockade during nitrous oxide-fentanyl, isoflurane and halothane anesthesia in adults and children. Anesthesiology 1989;71:210–213.
126. Pittet J-F, Tassonyi E, Morel DR, et al. Neuromuscular effect of pipecuronium bromide in infants and children during nitrous oxide-alfentanil anesthesia. Anesthesiology 1990;72:432–435.
127. Sarner JB, Brandom BW, Cook DR, et al. Clinical pharmacology of pipecuronium in infants and children during halothane anesthesia. Anesth Analg 1990;71:362–366.
128. Woefel SK, Brandom B, McGowan F, et al. Neuromuscular effects of 600 $\mu g/kg$ of rocuronium in infants during nitrous oxide-halothane anesthesia. Paed Anaesth 1994;4:173–177.
129. Woefel SK, Brandom BW, Cook DR, et al. Effects of bolus administration of ORG 9426 in children during nitrous oxide-halothane anesthesia. Anesthesiology 1992;76:939–942.
130. Motsch J, Leuwer M, Bottiger BW, et al. Dose-response, time-course of action and recovery of rocuronium bromide in children during halothane anaesthesia. Eur J Anaesthesiol 1995; 11:73–78.
131. Vuksanaj D, Fisher DM. Pharmacokinetics of rocuronium in children aged 4-11 years. Anesthesiology 1995;82:1104–1110.
132. Tomonaga M. Histochemical and ultrastructural changes in senile human skeletal msucle. J Am Geriatr Soc 1977;25:125–131.
133. Crooks J, O'Malley K, Stevenson I. Pharmacokinetics in the elderly. Clin Pharmacokinet 1976;1:280.
134. Frolkis V, Martynenko O, Zamostyan V. Aging of the neuromuscular appratus. Gerontology 1976;22:244–279.
135. Matteo RS, Backus WW, McDaniel DD, et al. Pharmacokinetics and pharmacodynamics of d-tubocurarine and metocurine in the elderly. Anesth Analg 1985;64:23–29.

136. Bell PF, Mirakhur RK, Clarke RS. Dose-response studies of atracurium, vecuronium and pancuronium in the elderly. Anaesthesia 1989;44:925–927.
137. Boyd E. Normal variability in weight of the adult human liver and spleen. Arch Pathol 1933;16:350–372.
138. Schnegg M, Lauterburg BH. Quantitative liver function in the elderly assessed by galactose elimination capacity, aminopyrine demethylation and caffeine clearance. J Hepat 1986;3:164–171.
139. McLeod K, Hull CJ, Watson MJ. Effects of ageing on the pharmacokinetics of pancuronium. Br J Anaesth 1979;51:435–438.
140. O'Hara DA, Fragen RJ, Shanks CA. The effects of age on the dose-response curves for vecuronium in adults. Anesthesiology 1985;63:542–544.
141. Rupp SM, Castagnoli KP, Fisher DM, et al. Pancuronium and vecuronium pharmacokinetics and pharmacodynamics in younger and elderly adults. Anesthesiology 1987;67:45–49.
142. Triggs EJ, Nation RI. Pharmacokinetics in the aged: a review. J Pharmacokinet Biopharm 1975;3:387–418.
143. Azad SS, Larijani GE, Goldberg ME, et al. A dose-response evaluation of pipecuronium bromide in elderly patients under balanced anaesthesia. J Clin Pharmacol 1989;29:657–659.
144. Ornstein E, Matteo R, Schwartz A, et al. Pharmacokinetics and pharmacodynamics of pipecuronium bromide (Arduan) in elderly surgical patients. Anesth Analg 1992;74:841.
145. d'Hollander A, Massaux F, Nevelsteen M, et al. Age-dependent dose-response relationship of ORG NC 45 in anaesthetized patients. Br J Anaesth 1982;54:653–657.
146. Lien CA, Matteo RS, Ornstein E, et al. Distribution, elimination, and action of vecuronium in the elderly. Anesth Analg 1991; 73:39–42.
147. Lowry KG, Mirakhur RK, Lavery GG, et al. Vecuronium and atracurium in the elderly: a clinical comparison with pancuronium. Acta Anaesthesiol Scand 1985;29:405–408.
148. Matteo RS, Ornstein E, Schwartz AE, et al. Pharmacokinetics and pharmacodynamics of rocuronium (Org 9426) in elderly surgical patients. Anesth Analg 1993;77:1193–1197.
149. Bevan DR, Fiset P, Balendran P, et al. Pharmacodynamic behaviour of rocuronium in the elderly. Can J Anaesth 1993; 40:127–132.
150. Womersley J, Durnin J, Boddy K, et al. Influence of muscular development, obesity and age on the fat-free mass of adults. J Appl Physiol 1976;41:273–279.
151. Stokholm KH, Brochner-Mortensen J, Hoilund-Carlsen PF. Increased glomerular filtration rate and adrenocortical function in obese women. Int J Obes 1980;4:57–63.
152. Abernethy DR, Greenblatt DJ. Pharmacokinetics of drugs in obesity. Clin Pharmacokinet 1982;7:108–124.
153. Abernethy DR, Greenblatt DJ, Divoll M, et al. Alterations in drug distribution and clearance due to obesity. J Pharmacol Exp Ther 1981;217:681–685.
154. Tsueda K, Warren JE, McCafferty LA, et al. Pancuronium bromide requirement during anesthesia for the morbidly obese. Anesthesiology 1978;48:438.
155. Feingold A. Pancuronium requirements of the morbidly obese. Anesthesiology 1979;50:269–270.
156. Matteo RS, Schwartz AE, Ornstein E, et al. Pharmacokinetics and pharmacodynamics of pancuronium in the obese surgical patients. Anesthesiology 1989;71:A820.
157. Soderberg M, Thomson D, White T. Respiration, circulation and anaesthetic management in obesity: investigation before and after jejunoileal bypass. Acta Anaesthesiol Scand 1977;21:55–61.
158. Schwartz AE, Matteo RS, Ornstein E, et al. Pharmacokinetics and pharmacodynamics of vecuronium in the obese surgical patient. Anesth Analg 1992;74:515–518.
159. Weinstein JA, Matteo RS, Ornstein E, et al. Pharmacodynamics of vecuronium and atracurium in the obese surgical patient. Anesth Analg 1988;67:1149–1153.
160. Harrison MJ, Gunn K. Weight determined dosage of vecuronium bromide. Anaesthesia 1989;44:692.
161. Kirkegaard-Nielsen H, Helbo-Hansen HS, Toft P, et al. Anthropometric variables as predictors for duration of action of vecuronium-induced neuromuscular block. Anesth Analg 1994; 79:1003–1006.
162. Demetriou M, Depoix JP, Diakite B, et al. Placental transfer of Org NC 45 in women undergoing caesarean section. Br J Anaesth 1982;54:643–645.
163. Dailey PA, Fisher DM, Shnider SM, et al. Pharmacokinetics, placental transfer, and neonatal effects of vecuronium and pancuronium administered during cesarean section. Anesthesiology 1984;60:569.
164. Duvaldestin P, Demetriou M, Henzel D, et al. The placental transfer of pancuronium and its pharmacokinetics during Caesarean section. Acta Anaesthesiol Scand 1978;22:327.
165. Baraka A, Jabbour S, Tabboush Z, et al. Onset of vecuronium neuromuscular block is more rapid in patients undergoing caesarean section. Can J Anaesth 1992;39:135–138.
166. Camp CE, Tessem J, Adenwala J, et al. Vecuronium and prolonged neuromuscular blockade in postpartum patients. Anesthesiology 1987;67:1006–1008.
167. Baraka A, Noueihed R, Sinno H, et al. Succinylcholine-vecuronium (Org NC 45) sequence for cesarean section. Anesth Analg 1983;62:909–913.
168. Khuenl-Brady KS, Koller J, Mair P, et al. Comparison of vecuronium- and atracurium-induced neuromuscular blockade in postpartum and nonpregnant patients. Anesth Analg 1991; 72:110–113.
169. Reidenberg MM, Affrime M. Influence of disease on binding of drugs plasma proteins. Ann N Y Acad Sci 1973;226:115–126.
170. Affrime AB, Blecker DL, Lyons PJ, et al. The effect of renal transplantation on plasma protein binding. J Dialysis 1979; 3:207–218.
171. Miller RD, Stevens WC, Way WL. The effect of renal failure and hyperkalemia on the duration of pancuronium neuromuscular blockade in man. Anesth Analg 1973;52:661.
172. Somogyi AA, Shanks CA, Triggs EJ. The effect of renal failure on the disposition and neuromuscular blocking action of pancuronium bromide. Eur J Clin Pharmacol 1977;23.
173. Bertman L, Rosenburg B, Shweikh I, et al. Atracurium and pancuronium in renal insufficiency. Acta Anaesthesiol Scand 1989; 33:48.
174. Buzello W, Agoston S. Pharmacokinetics of pancuronium in patients with normal and impaired renal function. Anaesthetist 1978;27:291.
175. Gramstad L. Atracurium, vecuronium and pancuronium in end-stage renal failure: dose-response properties and interactions with azathioprine. Br J Anaesth 1987;59:995–1003.
176. Gramstad L, Lilleaasen P. Neuromuscular blocking effects of atracurium, vecuronium and pancuronium during bolus and infusion administration. Br J Anaesth 1985;57:1052.
177. Tassonyi E, Szabo G, Vereczkey L. Pharmacokinetics of pipecuronium bromide, a new non-depolarizing neuromusuclar blocking agent, in humans. Arzneimittel forschung 1981; 31:1754–1756.
178. Tassonyi E, Szabo G, Vimlati L. Pipecuronium bromide (Arduan). In: Kharkevich DA, ed. Handbook of experimental pharmacology. Berlin: Springer-Verlag, 1986:599–616.
179. Hunter JM, Jones RS, Utting JE. Comparison of vecuronium, atracurium and tubocurarine in normal patients and in patients with no renal function. Br J Anaesth 1984;56:941–951.
180. Bevan DR, Donati F, Gyasi H, et al. Vecuronium in renal failure. Can Anaesth Soc J 1984;31:491–496.
181. Lepage JY, Malinge M, Cozian A, et al. Vecuronium and atracurium in patients with end-stage renal failure: a comparative study. Br J Anaesth 1987;59:1004–1010.
182. Meistelman C, Lienhart A, Leveque C, et al. Pharmacology of

vecuronium in patients with end-stage renal failure. Eur J Anaesthsiol 1986;3:153–158.
183. Lynam DP, Cronnelly R, Castagnoli KP, et al. The pharmacodynamics and pharmacokinetics of vecuronium in patients anesthetized with isoflurane with normal renal function or with renal failure. Anesthesiology 1988;69:227–231.
184. Starsnic MA, Goldberg ME, Ritter DE, et al. Does vecuronium accumulate in the renal transplant patient? [See comments]. Can J Anaesth 1989;36:35–39.
185. Gramstad L, Gjerlow JA, Hysing ES, et al. Interaction of cyclosporin and its solvent, cremophor, with atracurium and vecuronium: studies in cat. Br J Anaesth 1986;58:1149–1155.
186. Segredo V, Matthay MA, Sharma ML, et al. Prolonged neuromuscular blockade after long-term administration of vecuronium in two critically ill patients. Anesthesiology 1990;72: 566.
187. Segredo V, Caldwell JE, Matthay MA, et al. Persistent paralysis in critically ill patients after long-term administration of vecuronium. N Engl J Med 1992;327:524.
188. Beauvoir C, Peray P, Daures JP, et al. Pharmacodynamics of vecuronium in patients with and without renal failure: a meta-analysis. Can J Anaesth 1993;40:696–702.
189. Khuenl-Brady KS, Pomaroli A, Puhringer F, et al. The use of rocuronium (ORG 9426) in patients with chronic renal failure. Anaesthesia 1993;48:873–875.
190. Wilkinson GR, Shand DG. A physiological approach to hepatic drug clearance. Clin Pharmacol Ther 1975;18:377–390.
191. Somogyi AA, Shanks CA, Triggs EJ. Disposition kinetics of pancuronium bromide in patients with total biliary obstruction. Br J Anaesth 1977;49:1103.
192. D'Honneur G, Khalil M, Dominique C, et al. Pharmacokinetics and pharmacokinetics of pipecuronium in patients with cirrhosis. Anesth Analg 1993;77:1203–1206.
193. Westra P, Keulemans GTP, Houwertjes MC, et al. Mechanisms underlying the prolonged duration of action of muscle relaxants caused by extrahepatic cholestasis. Br J Anaesth 1981; 53:217.
194. Westra P, Houwertjes MC, Wesseling H, et al. Bile salts and neuromuscular blocking agents. Br J Anaesth 1981;53:407–415.
195. Marshall IG, Agoston S, Booij LHD, et al. Pharmacology of Org NC 45 compared with other non-depolarizing neuromuscular blocking drugs. Br J Anaesth 1982;52:115.
196. Arden JR, Lynam DP, Castagnoli KP, et al. Vecuronium in alcoholic liver disease:a pharmacokinetic and pharmacodynamic analysis. Anesthesiology 1988;68:771–776.
197. Bell CF, Hunter JM, Jones RS, et al. Use of atracurium and vecuronium in patients with oesophageal varicies. Br J Anaesth 1985;57:160–168.
198. Hunter JM, Parker CJR, Bell CF, et al. The use of different doses of vecuronium in patients with liver dysfunction. Br J Anaesth 1985;57:758–764.
199. Lebrault C, Berger JL, D'Hollander AA, et al. Pharmacokinetics and pharmacodynamics of vecuronium (ORG NC 45) in patients with cirrhosis. Anesthesiology 1985;62:601–605.
200. Lebrault C, Duvaldestin P, Henzel D, et al. Pharmacokinetics and pharmacodynamics of vecuronium in patients with cholestasis. Br J Anaesth 1986;58:983–987.
201. Goldfarb G, Gaqnneau P, Ang ET, et al. Hepatic extraction and clearance of vecuronium in humans. Anesthesiology 1988; 69:A480.
202. Mol WEM, Fokkema GN, Meijer DKF, et al. Mechanisms for the hepatic uptake of organic cations: studies with the muscle relaxant vecuronium in isolated rat hepatocytes. J Pharmacol Exp Ther 1988;244:268–275.
203. Khalil M, D'Honneur G, Duvaldestin P, et al. Pharmacokinetics and pharmacodynamics of rocuronium in patients with cirrhosis. Anesthesiology 1994;80:1241–1247.
204. Magorian T, Wood P, Caldwell J, et al. The pharmacokinetics and neuromuscular effects of rocuronium bromide in patients with liver disease. Anesth Analg 1995;80:754–759.
205. Servin FS, Lavaut E, Kleef U, et al. Repeated doses of rocuronium bromide administered to cirrhotic and control patients receiving isoflurane. Anesthesiology 1996;84:1092–1100.
206. Hansen-Flaschen JH, Brazinsky S, Basile C, et al. Use of sedating drugs and neuromuscular blocking agents in patients requiring mechanical ventilation for respiratory failure. JAMA 1991;266:2870.
207. Klessig HT, Geiger HJ, Murray MJ, et al. national survey on the practice patterns of anesthesiologist intensivists in the use of muscle relaxants. Crit Care Med 1992;20:1341.
208. Hansen-Flaschen J, Cowen J, Raps EC. Neuromuscular blockade in the intensive care unit: more than we bargained for. Am Rev Respir Dis 1993;147:234.
209. Coursin DB, Kelly JS, Prielipp RC. Muscle relaxants in critical care. Curr Opin Anaesthiol 1993;6:341–365.
210. O'Connor MF, Roizen MF. Use of muscle relaxants in the intensive care unit. J Intensive Care Med 1993;8:34–46.
211. Agoston S, Seyr M, Khuenl-Brady K, et al. Use of neuromuscular blocking agents in the intensive care unit. Anesthesiol Clin North Am 1993;11:345–360.
212. Durbin CJ. Neuromuscular blocking agents and sedative drugs: clinical uses and toxic effects in the critical care unit. Crit Care Clin 1991;7:489.
213. Gooch JL, Suchyta MR, Balbierz JM, et al. Prolonged paralysis after treatment with neuromuscular junction blocking agents. Crit Care Med 1991;19:1125–1131.
214. Coursin DB. Neuromuscular blockade: should patients be relaxed in the ICU? Chest 1992;102:988–989.
215. Coakley JH. Muscle relaxants and neuromuscular disorders in the intensive care unit. Baillieres Clin Anesthesiol 1994;8:483–499.
216. Subramony SH, Carpenter DE, Raju S, et al. Myopathy and prolonged neuromuscular blockade after lung transplant. Crit Care Med 1991;19:1580–1582.
217. Tobias JD, Lynch A, McDuffee A, et al. Pancuronium infusion for neuromuscular block in children in the pediatric intensive care unit [See comments]. Anesth Analg 1995;81:13–16.
218. Shapiro BA, Warren J, Egol AB, et al. Practice parameters for sustained neuromuscular blockade in the adult critically ill patient: an executive summary. Crit Care Med 1995;23:1601–1605.
219. Khuenl-Brady KS, Reitstatter B, Schlager A, et al. Long-term administration of pancuronium and pipecuronium in the intensive care unit. Anesth Analg 1994;78:1082–1086.
220. Prielipp RC, Coursin DB, Scuderi PE, et al. Comparison of the infusion requirements and recovery profiles of vecuronium and cisatracurium 51W89 in intensive care unit patients. Anesth Analg 1995;81:3–12.
221. Flamengo SA, Savarese JJ. Use of muscle relaxants in intensive care units. Crit Care Med 1991;19:1457–1459.
222. Lee C. Intensive care unit neuromuscular syndrome? Anesthesiology 1995;83:237–240.
223. Rupp SM, Miller RD, Gencarelli PJ. Vecuronium-induced neuromuscular blockade during enflurane, isoflurane, and halothane anesthesia in humans. Anesthesiology 1984;60:102–105.
224. Lebowitz MH, Blitt CD, Walts LF. Depression of twitch response to stimulation of the ulnar nerve during Ethrane anesthesia in man. Anesthesiology 1970;33:52–57.
225. Caldwell JE, Laster MJ, Magorian T, et al. The neuromuscular effects of desflurane, alone and combined with pancuronium or succinylcholine in humans. Anesthesiology 1991;74:412–418.
226. Fogdall RP, Miller RD. Neuromuscular effects of enflurane, alone and combined with d-tubocurarine, pancuronium, and succinylcholine, in man. Anesthesiology 1975;42:173–178.
227. Saitoh Y, Toyooka H, Amaha K. Recoveries of post-tetanic

twitch and train-of-four responses after administration of vecuronium with different inhalation anaesthetics and neuroleptanaesthesia [See comments]. Br J Anaesth 1993;70:402–404.
228. Miller RD, Wat WL, Dolan WM, et al. Comparative neuromuscular effects of pancuronium, gallamine, and succinylcholine during forane and halothane anesthesia in man. Anesthesiology 1971;35:509–514.
229. Itagaki T, Tai K, Katsumata N, et al. A clinical and experimental study on potentiation with sevoflurane of neuromuscular blocking effects of vecuronium bromide. Masui 1988;37:943–948.
230. Cannon JE, Fahey MR, Castagnoli KP, et al. Continuous infusion of vecuronium:the effect of anesthetic agents. Anesthesiology 1987;67:503–506.
231. Shanks CA, Fragen RJ, Ling D. Continuous intravenous infusion of rocuronium (ORG 9426) in patients receiving balanced, enflurane, or isoflurane anesthesia. Anesthesiology 1993; 78:649–651.
232. Naguib M, Seraj M, Abdulrazik E. Pipecuronium-induced neuromuscular blockade during nitrous oxide-fentanyl, enflurane, isoflurane, and halothane anesthesia in surgical patients. Anesth Analg 1992;75:193–197.
233. Larijani GE, Gratz I, Afshar M, et al. The effect of isoflurane versus balanced anesthesia on rocuronium's pharmacokinetics and infusion requirement. Pharmacotherapy 1995;15:36–41.
234. Ghouri AF, White PF. Comparative effects of desflurane and isoflurane on vecuronium-induced neuromuscular blockade. J Clin Anesth 1992;4:34–38.
235. Wright PM, Hart P, Lau M, et al. The magnitude and time course of vecuronium potentiation by desflurane versus isoflurane. Anesthesiology 1995;82:404–411.
236. Taivainen T, Moretoja OA. the neuromuscular blocking effects of vecuronium during sevoflurane, halothane and balanced anaesthesia in children. Anaesthesia 1995;50:1046–1049.
237. Morita T, Tsukagoshi H, Sugaya T, et al. The effects of sevoflurane are similar to those of isoflurane on the neuromuscular block produced by vecuronium. Br J Anaesth 1994;72:465–467.
238. Dernovoi B, Agoston S, Barvais L, et al. Neostigmine antagonism of vecuronium paralysis during fentanyl, halothane, isoflurane, and enflurane anesthesia. Anesthesiology 1987;66:698–701.
239. Baurain MJ, d'Hollander AA, Melot C, et al. Effects of residual concentrations of isoflurane on the reversal of vecuronium-induced neuromuscular blockade. Anesthesiology 1991;74:474–478.
240. Morita T, Tsukagoshi H, Sugaya T, et al. Inadequate antagonism of vecuronium-induced neuromuscular block by neostigmine during sevoflurane or isoflurane anesthesia. Anesth Analg 1995;80:1175–1180.
241. Gergis SD, Dretchen KL, Sokoll MD, et al. Effect of anesthetics on acetylcholine release from myoneural junction. Proc Soc Biol Med 1972;141:629.
242. Waud BE, Waud DR. The effects of diethylether, enflurane, and isoflurane at the neuromuscular junction. Anesthesiology 1975; 42:275.
243. Gissen AJ, Karis JH, Nasuk WL. Effect of halothane on neuromuscular transmission. JAMA 1966;197:116–120.
244. Thornton RJ, Blakeney C, Feldman SA. the effect of hypothermia on neuromuscular conduction. Br J Anaesth 1976;48:264.
245. Aziz L, Ono K, Ohta Y, et al. Effect of hypothermia on the in vitro potencies of neuromuscular blocking agents and on their antagonism by neostigmine. Br J. Anaesth 1994;73:662–666.
246. Miller RD, Agoston S, van der Pol F. Hypothermia and pharmacokinetics and pharmacodynamics of pancuronium in cat. J Pharmacol Exp Ther 1978;207:532–538.
247. Denny NM, Kneeshaw JD. Vecuronium and atracurium infusions during hypothermic cardiopulmonary bypass. Anaesthesia 1986;41:919–922.
248. Buzello W, Schluermann D, Schindler M, et al. Hypothermic cardiopulmonary bypass and neuromuscular blockade by pancuronium and vecuronium. Anesthesiology 1985;62:201–204.
249. d'Hollander AA, Duvaldestin P, Henzel D, et al. Variations in pancuronium requirements, plasma concentration and urinary excretion induced by cardiopulmonary bypass with hypothermia. Anesthesiology 1983;58:505–509.
250. Wierda JMKH, Agoston S. Pharmacokinetics of vecuronium during hypothermic bypass. Br J Anaesth 1989;63:627–628.
251. Heier T, Caldwell JE, Sessler DI, et al. Mild intraoperative hypothermia increases duration of action and spontaneous recovery of vecuronium blockade during nitrous oxide-isoflurane anesthesia in humans. Anesthesiology 1991;74:815–819.
252. Heier T, Caldwell JE, Eriksson LI, et al. The effect of hypothermia on adductor pollicis twitch tension during continuous infusion of vecuronium in isoflurane-anesthetized humans. Anesth Analg 1994;78:312–317.
253. Beaufort AM, Wierda JM, Belopavlovic M, et al. The influence of hypothermia (surface cooling) on the time-course of action and on pharmacokinetics of rocuronium in humans. Eur J Anaesthesiol 1995;11:95–106.
254. Smeulers NJ, Wierda MKH, van den Broek L, et al. Effects of hypothermic cardioplumaonary bypass on the pharmacodynamics and pharmacokinetics of rocuronium. J Cardiothorac Vasc Anesth 1995;9:700–705.
255. Eriksson LI, Viby MJ, Lennmarken C. The effect of peripheral hypothermia on a vecuronium-induced neuromuscular block. Acta Anaesthesiol Scan 1991;35:387.
256. Heier T, Caldwell JE, Sessler DI, et al. The relationship between adductor pollicis twitch tension and core, skin, and muscle temperature during nitrous-oxide-isoflurane anesthesia in humans. Anesthesiology 1989;71:381.
257. Young ML, Hanson CWR, Bloom MJ, et al. Localized hypothermia influences assessment of recovery from vecuronium neuromuscular blockade. Can J Anaesth 1994;41:1172–1177.
258. Waud BE, Waud DR. Quantitative examination of interaction of competitive neuromuscular blocking agents on the indirectly elicited muscle twitch. Anesthesiology 1984;61:420–427.
259. Waud BE, Waud DR. Interaction among agents that block endplate depolarization competitively. Anesthesiology 1985;63:4–15.
260. Meretoja OA, Brandom BW, Taivainen T, et al. Synergism between atracurium and vecuronium in children. Br J Anaesth 1993;71:440–442.
261. Naguib M, Abdulatif M. Isobolographic and dose-response analysis of the interaction between pipecuronium and vecuronium. Br J Anaesth 1993;71:556–560.
262. Lebowitz PW, Ramsey FM, Savarese JJ, et al. Potentiation of neuromuscular blockade in man produced by combination of pancuronium and metocurine or pancuronium and d-tubocurarine. Anesth Analg 1980;59:604–609.
263. Kim DW, Joshi GP, White PF, et al. Interactions between mivacurium, rocuronium and vecuronium during general anesthesia. Anesth Analg (in press).
264. Middleton CM, Pollard BJ, Healy TE, et al. Use of atracurium or vecuronium to prolong the action of d-tubocurarine. Br J Anaesth 1989;62:659–663.
265. Rashkovsky OM, Agoston S, Ket JM. Interaction between pancuronium bromide and vecuronium bromide. Br J Anaesth 1985;57:1063–1066.
266. Smith I, White PF. Pipecuronium-induced prolongation of vecuronium neuromuscular block [See comments]. Br J Anaesth 1993;70:446–448.
267. Brandom BW, Meretoja OA, Taivainen T, et al. Accelerated onset and delayed recovery of neuromuscular block induced by mivacurium preceded by pancuronium in children. Anesth Analg 1993;76:998–1003.
268. Naguib M. Neuromuscular effects of rocuronium bromide and

mivacurium chloride administered alone and in combination. Anesthesiology 1994;81:388–395.
269. Kay B, Chestnut RJ, Sum Ping JS, et al. Economy in the use of muscle relaxants: vecuronium after pancuronium. Anaesthesia 1987;42:277–280.
270. Dubois MY, Fleming NW, Lea DE. Effects of succinylcholine on the pharmacodynamics of pipecuronium and pancuronium. Anesth Analg 1991;72:364–368.
271. Tang J, Joshi GP, White PF. Compariosn of rocuronium and mivacurium to succinylcholine during outpatient laparoscopic surgery. Anesth Analg 1996;82:994–998.
272. Dubois MY, Lea DE, Kataria B, et al. Pharmacodynamics of rocuronium with and without prior administration of succinylcholine. J Clin Anesth 1995;7:44–48.
273. White PF, Watcha MF. Are new drugs cost-effective for patients undergoing ambulatory surgery? Anesthesiology 1993;78:2–5.
274. White PF, White LD. Cost containment in the operating room: who is responsible? J Clin Anesth 1994;6:351–356.
275. DeMonaco HJ, Shah AS. Economic considerations in the use of neuromuscular blocking drugs. J Clin Anesth 1994;6:383–387.
276. Macario A, Vitez TS, Dunn B, et al. Where are the costs in perioperative care? Analysis of hospital costs and charges for inpatient surgical care. Anesthesiology 1995;83:1138–1144.
277. Detsky AS, Naglie IG. A clinician's guide of cost-effectiveness analysis. Ann Intern Med 1990;113:147–154.
278. Bevan DR, Smith CE, Donati F. Postoperative neuromuscular blockade: a comparison between atracurium, vecuronium, and pancuronium. Anesthesiology 1988;69:272–276.
279. Bevan DR, Donati F, Kopman AF. Reversal of neuromuscular blockade. Anesthesiology 1992;77:785–805.
280. Donati F. Cost-benefit analysis of neuromuscular blocking agents. Can J Anaesth 1994;41:R3–R7.
281. Somogyi AA, Shanks CA, Triggs EJ. Combined intravenous bolus and infusion of pancuronium bromide. Br J Anaesth 1978; 50:575–582.
282. Hughes R, Chapple DJ. Effects of non-depolarizing neuromuscular blocking agents on autonomic mechanisms in cats. Br J Anaesth 1976;48:59.
283. Ivankovich AD, Milevich DJ, Albrecht RF, et al. The effects of pancuronium on myocardial contraction and catecholamine metabolism. J Pharm Pharmacol 1975;27:837.
284. Docherty JR, McGrath JC. Sympathomimetic effects of pancuronium bromide on the cardiovacular system of the pithed rat. Br J Pharmacol 1978;64:589.
285. Stoeling RK. The hemodynamic effects of pancuronium and d-tubocurarine in anesthetized patients. Anesthesiology 1972; 36:612.
286. Miller RD, Eger EII, Stevens WC. Pancuronium induced tachycardia in relation to alveolar halothane, doe of pancuronium, and prior atropine. Anesthesiology 1975;42:352.
287. Foldes FF, Kobayashi O, Kinjo O, et al. Presynaptic effect of muscle relaxants on the release of 3H-norepinephrine controlled by endogenous acetycholine in guinea pig atrium. Neural Transm 1988;76:169–180.
288. Shorten CD, Sieber T, Maslow AD, et al. Left ventricular regional wall motion and haemodynamic changes following bolus administration of pipecuronium or pancuronium to adult patients undergoing coronary artery bypass grafting. Can J Anaesth 1995;42:695–700.
289. Manger D, Turnago WS, Connell CR, et al. Pancuronium, vecuronium, and heart rate during anesthesia for aortocoronary bypass operations. Eur J Cardiothorac Surg 1993;7:524–527.
290. Rathmell JP, Brooker RF, Prielipp RC, et al. Hemodynamic and pharmacodynamic comparison of doxacurium and pipecuronium with pancuronium during induction of cardiac anesthesia: does the benefit justify the cost? Anesth Analg 1993;76:513–519.
291. Neidhart PP, Champion P, Vogel J, et al. A comparison of pipecuronium with pancuronium on haemodynamic variables and plasma catecholamines in coronary artery bypass patients [See comments]. Can J Anaesth 1994;41:469–474.
292. Goldhill DR, Embree PB, Ali HH, et al. Reversal of pancuronium. Neuromuscular and cardiovascular effects of a mixture of neostigmine and glycopyrronium. Anaesthesia 1989;43:443–446.
293. Vizi ES, Kobayashi O, Torocsik O, et al. Heterogeneity of presynaptic muscarinic receptors involved in modulation of transmitter release. Neuroscience 1989;31:259–267.
294. Tassonyi E, Neidhard E, Pittet JF, et al. Cardiovascular effects of pipecuronium and pancuronium in patients undergoing coronary bypass grafting. Anesthesiology 1988;69:793–796.
295. Stanley JC, Carson IW, Gibson FM, et al. Comparison of the haemodynamic effects of pipecuronium and pancuronium during fentanyl anaesthesia. Acta Anaesthesiol Scand 1991;35:262–266.
296. Donlon JV, Savarese JJ, Ali HH, et al. Human dose-response curves for neuromuscular blocking drugs: a comparison of two methods of construction and analysis. Anesthesiology 1980; 53:161–166.
297. Foldes FF, Nagashima H, Nguyen HD, et al. Neuromuscular and cardiovascular effects of pipecuronium. Can J Anaesth 1990;37:549–555.
298. Stanley JC, Mirakhur RK, Bell PF, et al. Neuromuscular effects of pipecuronium bromide. Eur J Anaesthesiol 1991;8:151–156.
299. Larijani GE, Bartkowski RR, Azad SS, et al. Clinical pharmacology of pipecuronium bromide. Anesth Analg 1989;68:734–739.
300. Newton DEF, Richardson FJ, Agoston S. Preliminary studies in man with pipecuronium bromide (Arduan), a new steroid neuromuscular blocking agent. Br J Anaesth 1982;54:789–790.
301. Gyermek L, Cantley EM, Lee C. Antagonism of pancuronium- and pipecuronium-induced neuromuscular block. Br J Anaesth 1995;74:410–414.
302. Abdulatif M, Naguib M. Neostigmine and edrophonium for reversal of pipecuronium neuromuscular blockade. Can J Anaesth 1991;38:159–163.
303. Diefenbach C, Mellinghoff H, Buzello W. Neuromuscular effect of pipecuronium neuromuscular blockade. Acta Anaesthesiol Scand 1993;37:189–191.
304. Tullock WC, Diana P, Cook DR, et al. Neuromuscular and cardiovascular effects of high-dose vecuronium. Anesth Analg 1990;70:86–90.
305. Bencini A, Newton DEF. Rate of onset of good intubating conditions, respiratory depression and hand muscle paralysis after vecuronium. Br J Anaesth 1984;56:959–965.
306. Engbaek J, Ording H, Viby-Mogensen J. Neuromuscular blocking effects of vecuronium and pancuronium during halothane anaesthesia. Br J Anaesth 1983;55:497–500.
307. Kerr WJ, Baird WL. Clinical studies on Org NC 45: comparison with pancuronium. Br J Anaesth 1982;54:1159–1165.
308. Mirakhur RK, Ferres CJ, Clarke RS, et al. Clinical evaluation of Org NC 45. Br J Anaesth 1983;55:119–124.
309. Swen J, Gencarelli PJ, Koot HWJ. Vecuronium infusion dose requirements during fentanyl and halothane anesthesia in humnas. Anesth Analg 1985;64:411–414.
310. Beattie WS, Buckley DN, Forrest JB. Continuous infusions of atracurium and vecuronium, compared with intermittent boluses of pancuronium: dose requirements and reversal. Can J Anaesth 1992;39:925–931.
311. Noeldge G, Hinsken H, Buzello W. Comparison between the continuous infusion of vecuronium and the intermittent administration of pancuronium and vecuronium. Br J Anaesth 1984;56:473–478.
312. Martineau RJ, St.-Jean B, Kitts JB, et al. Cumulation and reversal with prolonged infusions of atracurium and vecuronium. Can J Anaesth 1992;39:670–676.
313. Caldwell JE. Reversal of residual neuromuscular block with

neostigmine at one to four hours after a single intubating dose of vecuronium. Anesth Analg 1995;80:1168–1174.
314. Fawcett WJ, Dash A, Francis GA, et al. Recovery from neuromuscular blockade: residual curarisation following atracurium or vecuronium by bolus dosing or infusions. Acta Anaesthesiol Scand 1995;39:288–293.
315. McCoy EP, Maddineni VR, Elliott P, et al. Haemodynamic effects of rocuronium during fentanyl anaesthesia: comparison with vecuronium. Can J Anaesth 1993;40:703–708.
316. Levy JH, Davis GK, Duggan J, et al. Determination of the hemodynamics and histamine release of rocuronium (Org 9426) when administered in increased doses under N_2O/O_2-sufentanil anesthesia. Anesth Analg 1994;78:318–321.
317. Moorthy SS, Dierdorf SF. Pain on injection of rocuronium bromide [Letter]. Anesth Analg 1995;80:1067.
318. Molbegott L. The precipitation of rocuronium in the needleless intravenous injection adaptor [Letter]. Anesthesiology 1995; 83:223.
319. Puhringer FK, Khuenl-Brady KS, Koller J, et al. Evaluation of the endotracheal intubating conditions of rocuronium (ORG 9426) and succinylcholine in outpatient surgery [See comments]. Anesth Analg 1992;75:37–40.
320. Cooper RA, Mirakhur RK, Maddineni VR. Neuromuscular effects of rocuronium bromide (Org 9426) during fentanyl and halothane anaesthesia. Anaesthesia 1993;48:103–105.
321. Wierda JM, Hommes FD, Nap HJ, et al. Time course of action and intubating conditions following vecuronium, rocuronium and mivacurium. Anaesthesia 1995;50:393–396.
322. Prien T, Zahn P, Menges M, et al. 1 × ED90 dose of rocuronium bromide: tracheal intubation conditions and time-course of action. Eur J Anaesthesiol 1995;11:85–90.
323. Pollard BJ, Chetty MS, Wilson A, et al. Intubation conditions and time-course of action of low dose rocuronium bromide in day-case dental surgery. Eur J Anaesthesiol 1995;11:81–83.
324. McCoy EP, Mirakhur RK, Maddineni VR, et al. Administration of rocuronium (Org 9426) by continuous infusion and its reversibility with anticholinesterases. Anaesthesia 1994;49:940–945.
325. Naguib M, Abdulatif M, al-Ghamdi A. Dose-response relationships for edrophonium and neostigmine antagonism of rocuronium bromide (ORG 9426)-induced neuromuscular blockade. Anesthesiology 1993;79:739–745.

16 Benzylisoquinoline Compounds

Cynthia A. Lien, Matthew R. Belmont, Lori Rubin, John J. Savarese

The classic muscle relaxant studies of Claude Bernard were done with a crude extract of *Chondodendron tomentosum* from the Amazon. More than 80 years later, Harold King proposed a chemical structure (Fig. 16-1) of the purified material, d-tubocurarine (1). The structure was widely accepted as indicating that neuromuscular blocking activity was associated with the presence of two quaternary nitrogen atoms spaced 1.2 to 1.4 nm apart. Daniel Bovet postulated that incorporation of the quaternary nitrogens into the rigid structure of heterocyclic ring systems would promote nondepolarizing blocking activity that could be antagonized by anticholinesterase agents (2).

These concepts guided drug developers in the design of new and improved neuromuscular blockers for the next 35 years. In 1970, Everett and associates (3) published a revised structure of d-tubocurarine (see Fig. 16-1) that contained only one quaternary nitrogen and revolutionized thinking regarding the design of neuromuscular blocking drugs. Currently, interquaternary distances are considered of minor importance. Structural factors considered fundamental to the properties of the nondepolarizing drugs include stereochemistry, functional groups that promote metabolism or degradation, modified lipophilic or hydrophilic relationships that alter distribution and elimination kinetics, and molecular design that avoids structural features known to be associated with undesirable side effects (4, 5). After the corrected structure of d-tubocurarine was published, Martin-Smith and Stenlake and colleagues (6-8) observed that a simple quaternary alkaloid called petaline underwent ring opening and conversion to an open-chain tertiary amine in the presence of alkaline pH by Hofmann elimination. This discovery led to further studies of structure-activity relationships by Stenlake and associates culminating in the development of atracurium (8), which is the first successful synthetic benzylisoquinolinium drug. Subsequently, doxacurium (a long-acting relaxant), mivacurium (a short-acting relaxant), and most recently cis-atracurium (an isomer of atracurium with fewer side effects) were introduced into clinical practice.

Enormous progress has been made in the development and clinical application of the benzylisoquinolinium class of neuromuscular blockers. New and improved relaxant drugs are certain to appear in the future as the chemistry and pharmacology of the benzylisoquinolinium compounds continue to be better understood and as clinical practice becomes more sophisticated.

GENERAL PHARMACOLOGY

Potency

The benzylisoquinolinium compounds are potent neuromuscular blocking agents. This is clinically relevant because autonomic side effects and, thus, cardiovascular effects tend to diminish with enhanced neuromuscular blocking potency and specificity for blockade of nicotinic receptors at the neuromuscular junction. d-Tubocurarine is the least potent of the available benzylisoquinolines (Table 16-1), with an ED_{95} of 0.5 mg/kg in patients receiving nitrous oxide-opioid-barbiturate anesthesia. All the newer benzylisoquinoliniums are more potent neuromuscular blocking compounds than d-tubocurarine. For example, atracurium, mivacurium, and doxacurium are approximately 4, 12, and 40 times more potent than d-tubocurarine on a molar basis. Doxacurium, with an ED_{95} of 0.025 mg/kg, is the most potent of all the available nondepolarizing muscle relaxants.

Mivacurium and atracurium consist of mixtures of stereoisomers with varying potencies, as well as pharmacokinetics. Mivacurium consists of a mixture of three stereoisomers, a *cis-trans*, a *trans-trans*, and a *cis-cis* isomer. The *cis-trans* isomer constitutes 34 to 40% of the mixture, the *trans-trans* isomer 52 to 62%, and the *cis-cis* isomer 4 to 8%. The *trans-trans* and *cis-trans* iso-

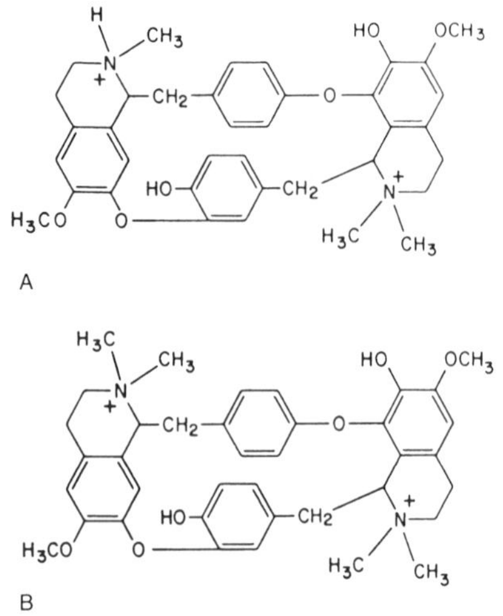

FIGURE 16-1. The chemical structure of d-tubocurarine. That originally proposed by King (1935) (A) was later revised by Everett (1970) (B) to the monoquaternary structure.

TABLE 16-1. Potency of Benzylisoquinoline Relaxant Drugs

Relaxant	ED_{95} (mg/kg)
d-Tubocurarine	0.50
Metocurine	0.28
Doxacurium	0.025
Atracurium	0.25
Cisatracurium	0.05
Mivacurium	0.08
BW 785U	0.9

mers are equally potent in terms of their neuromuscular blocking potentials, with ED_{95} values of 42±3 and 45±3 μg/kg, respectively. The *cis-cis* isomer is approximately 1/13th as potent in cats as the other two isomers, with an ED_{95} of 592 μg/kg (9, 10).

Atracurium consists of 10 stereoisomers. Six of these have been evaluated for neuromuscular blocking activity (11). Each of the six isomers differs in terms of neuromuscular blocking potency, as shown in Table 16-2. In patients receiving nitrous oxide-opioid-barbiturate anesthesia, the ED_{95} of cisatracurium, the 1R-*cis*, 1R′-*cis* isomer that comprises approximately 15% of atracurium, has an ED_{95} of 0.05 mg/kg (12). On a molar basis, this would make cisatracurium approximately three times more potent as a neuromuscular blocker than atracurium.

Autonomic Effects

Ganglionic Blockade

The autonomic blocking properties typical of many neuromuscular blocking drugs are caused by blockade of both nicotinic and muscarinic receptors. Nicotinic receptor blockade causes interruption of ganglionic transmission, and muscarinic receptor blockade inhibits the transmission of vagal impulses. Several reviews have been written on this topic (13-15). The benzylisoquinolinium relaxants are virtually free of vagolytic properties. This structural feature is inherent to this class of neuromuscular blockers. In general, they rarely cause ganglionic blockade. The only benzylisoquinolinium that causes blockade of ganglionic transmission at doses less than 10 times its ED_{95} for neuromuscular blockade is d-tubocurarine (16-18). The other benzylisoquinoliniums block ganglionic transmission only at substantially greater doses (17, 19). Therefore, this class of relaxant is unlikely to cause cardiovascular changes secondary to autonomic effects.

TABLE 16-2. Neuromuscular Blocking Potency of Atracurium and Five of Its Isomers

Compound	ED_{95} (μg/kg)
Atracurium	488±56
35 W89	162±6
36 W89	88±8
49 W89	79±6
50 W89	43±2
Cisatracurium (51W89)	62±8

TABLE 16-3. Effects of Stimulation of Histamine Receptors

H_1	H_2
Increased capillary permeability	Increased gastric acid production
Bronchoconstriction	Systemic and cerebral vasodilation
Intestinal contraction	Positive inotropic effects
Negative dromotropic effects	Positive chronotropic effects
Coronary artery spasm	

Histamine Release

The primary mechanism whereby the benzylisoquinolinium relaxants cause a cardiovascular response in patients is through the release of histamine. Histamine, a β-imidazolethyamine, is stored in the granules of mast cells, as are prostaglandins and other vasoactive substances. Three different mechanisms can result in the release of histamine. The release can be mediated by antigen, as in anaphylaxis, or by complement, by an immune complex of IgG or IgM and antigen attached to the surface of cells resulting in histamine release. Finally, the chemically mediated (nonimmunologic) serosal mast cell degranulation is associated with histamine release by muscle relaxants.

Histamine can have various effects because it stimulates H_1 and H_2 receptors (Table 16-3). The clinical picture of drug-induced histamine release is that of erythema, decreased blood pressure, and increased heart rate. In general, the hypotension and tachycardia are transient, lasting 1 to 5 minutes. Bronchospasm in this setting is rare (19). Normal plasma histamine concentrations are less than 500 pg/ml (20, 21). Two- to threefold increases in plasma histamine levels are generally associated with clinical symptoms (13, 21-25). The amount of histamine released in response to relaxant administration is related to both the dose of the relaxant and the rate of administration. As the dose of drug is increased, a greater percentage of patients will develop histamine release. As demonstrated in Figure 16-2, if the dose is administered over 30 to 60 seconds rather than as a rapid intravenous bolus, histamine release is decreased (23-25). Furthermore, subsequent doses of equal or smaller size cause decreasing amounts of histamine release, presumably because available histamine has previously been released from mast cells and subsequently has been metabolized by histamine N-methyltransferase and diamine oxidase. The final mediator of hypotension resulting from histamine release is likely to be a metabolite of prostaglandin $F_{1\alpha}$ ($PGF_{1\alpha}$) (26). Through its stimulation of H_1 receptors on vascular endothelium, histamine initiates the eicosanoid cascade. As part of this process, cyclooxygenase liberates $PGF_{1\alpha}$, a potent vasodilator.

Drug-mediated histamine release can be caused by tertiary or quaternary ammonium compounds (e.g., morphine sulfate and nondepolarizing relaxants). Among the relaxants, the benzylisoquinolines are most commonly associated with the release of histamine. Not all benzylisoquinoliniums, however, cause histamine release. The bisquaternary structures are less likely to cause histamine release (16, 17). The propensity of a benzylisoquinolinium to cause histamine release may be estimated by the ratio of the dose of relaxant required for histamine release (ED_{50}) divided by the dose of relaxant required for 95% neuromuscular block (ED_{95}). This ratio indicates the margin of safety for a compound's ability to create cardiovascular side effects secondary to histamine release. The ratio varies for each compound, and for some drugs it is many multiples of the ED_{95} for neuromuscular block. As is shown in Table 16-4, 0.5 to 1 times the ED_{95} of d-tubocurarine may cause histamine release (5). Metocurine, the synthetic derivative of d-tubocurarine, has an improved margin of safety and is less likely to cause histamine release; it requires a dose 1.5 to 2 times its ED_{95} (0.28 mg/kg) as a rapid intravenous bolus (27). Administration of two to three times the ED_{95} of atracurium (0.25 mg/kg) (28, 29) or mivacurium (0.08 mg/kg) (23) (see Fig. 16-2) produces clinically significant histamine release. Doses as large as 3.2 times the ED_{95} (0.025 mg/kg) of doxacurium are free of histamine-related cardiovascular side effects (30-32). Cisatracurium, the newest of the benzylisoquinolines, causes no histamine release when doses as large as eight times its ED_{95} (0.05 mg/kg) are administered as a rapid intravenous bolus (33). As shown in Figure 16-3, rapid administration of cisatracurium doses up to 0.4 mg/kg ($8 \times ED_{95}$) causes no histamine release and no hemodynamic changes even when large doses are ad-

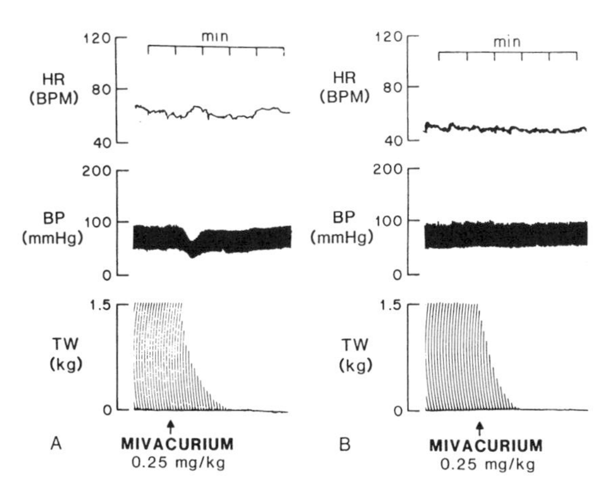

FIGURE 16-2. Effects of 0.25 mg/kg mivacurium in an individual patient on heart rate (HR), mean arterial pressure (MAP), and twitch response (TW). A, The transient decrease in blood pressure (BP) and increase in HR are typical of hemodynamic changes caused by the histamine release associated with rapid administration of 0.25 mg/kg mivacurium. B, Slower administration of the same dose has less of a tendency to cause histamine release and allows for more stable hemodynamics.

TABLE 16-4. Margin of Safety for Histamine Release

Muscle Relaxant	Multiples of the ED_{95} Causing Histamine Release
d-Tubocurarine	1
Metocurine	2
Doxacurium	>3.2
Atracurium	2
Cisatracurium	>8
Mivacurium	3

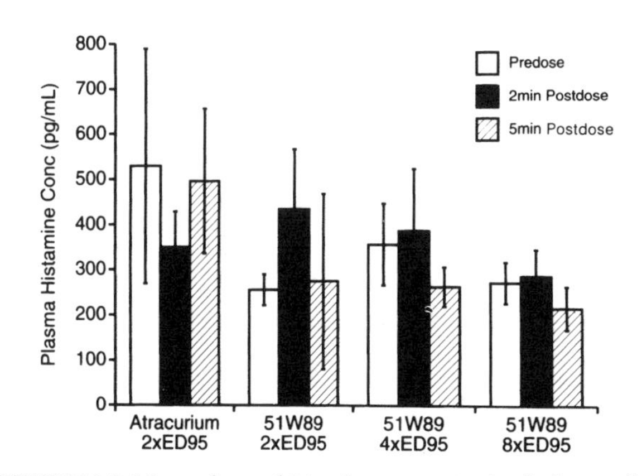

FIGURE 16-3. Mean plasma histamine concentration before and 2 and 5 minutes following the administration of 2 times ED_{95} of atracurium or two, four, or eight times ED_{95} of cisatracurium (51W89) as a rapid intravenous bolus. No dose-related changes in plasma histamine concentrations occurred in any of the groups.

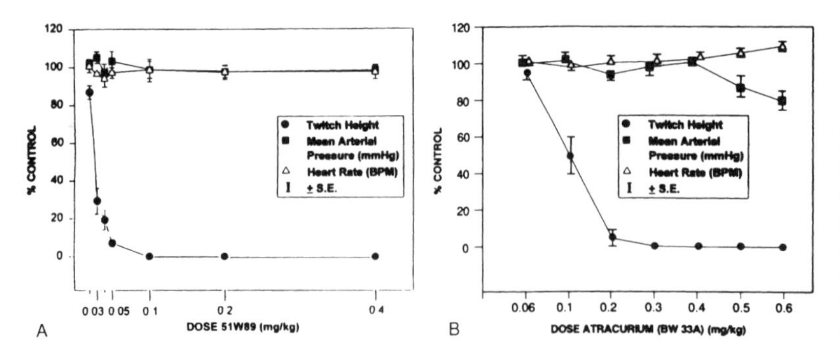

FIGURE 16-4. Mean neuromuscular, heart rate, and mean arterial pressure responses to various doses of cisatracurium (A) and atracurium (B). Although significant decreases in mean arterial pressure occurred following administration of two times ED_{95} or more of atracurium, no hemodynamic changes occurred following administration of doses up to eight times ED_{95} of cisatracurium (51W89).

ministered as a rapid bolus (Fig. 16-4). This finding is in marked contrast to atracurium, which not infrequently causes histamine release and a subsequent decrease in blood pressure and increase in heart rate (see Fig. 16-4).

Other benzylisoquinoliniums have been studied, and in spite of favorable pharmacodynamic profiles, these compounds have not been developed for marketing because of unacceptably low margins of safety with respect to histamine release. An example is BW 785U is an ultrashort-acting relaxant with a rapid onset of action (34). It is hydrolyzed by plasma cholinesterase at a rate greater than that of succinylcholine. In spite of its favorable pharmacodynamic profile, however, it does cause histamine release when doses less than its ED_{95} are administered, a property that limits its clinical usefulness. BW A444U is a benzylisoquinolinium ester neuromuscular blocking agent that, like atracurium, has an intermediate duration of action. Its margin of safety for histamine release is less than that of atracurium, with doses as low as 0.16 mg/kg (1.5 times its ED_{95}), causing histamine release (35, 36).

Histamine release from compounds such as mivacurium or atracurium can be attenuated in several ways. These include slower administration of the relaxant (over 30 to 60 seconds rather than as a rapid intravenous bolus) (23), use of smaller doses of the relaxant, or use of H_1 and H_2 blockers before the administration of the relaxant (13, 28). For example, rapid infusion of 0.2 mg/kg of mivacurium decreases blood pressure and increases heart rate secondary to histamine release; however, slower administration of this dose minimizes these cardiovascular side effects (Fig. 16-5). This slower administration of mivacurium doses 2 to 2.5 times its ED_{95} is associated with excellent hemodynamic stability. When doses of twice the ED_{95} of mivacurium were given to patients undergoing coronary artery bypass, despite their delicate hemodynamic status, their blood pressure and heart rate remained stable (37).

Because of the dose-response relationship for histamine release with some of the benzylisoquinoliniums, the administration of smaller doses of these relaxants results in less or no histamine release and improved hemodynamic stability. With both atracurium and mivacurium (23, 38, 39), the dose required to cause histamine release is two and one-half to three times its ED_{95} values. Rapid administration of smaller doses does not cause histamine release.

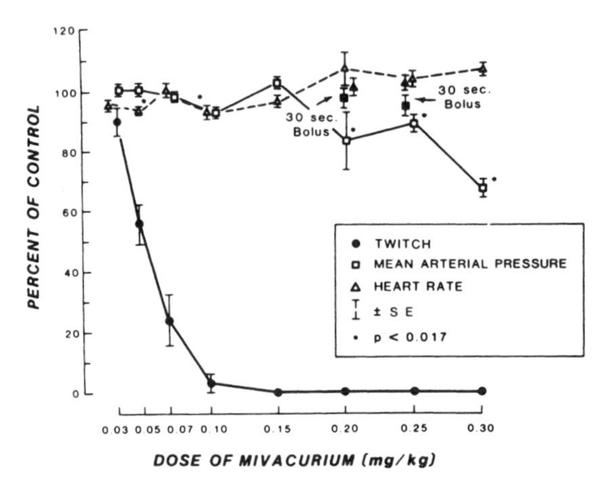

FIGURE 16-5. Changes in neuromuscular, heart rate, and mean arterial pressure in response to administration of various doses of mivacurium. The decrease in mean arterial pressure following rapid administration of doses of at least 0.2 mg/kg is minimized by administration of the relaxant over 30 seconds (squares) rather than as a rapid intravenous bolus.

At times, the effective use of a muscle relaxant requires larger doses. With the benzylisoquinoline compounds, this can be done safely by minimizing the hemodynamic side effects of histamine release by pharmacologically blocking both the H_1 and H_2 receptors. Vasodilation is mediated by both H_1 and H_2 receptors; it is therefore necessary to block both sites when attempting to attenuate the cardiovascular effects of histamine. Scott and colleagues (28, 36) used the H_1 blocker chlorpheniramine (0.1 mg/kg) and the H_2 blocker cimetidine (4 mg/kg), both administered intravenously 15 minutes before the administration of atracurium, 0.6 mg/kg, in an effort to attenuate the hemodynamic effects of histamine release. The hemodynamic response to two and one-half times the ED_{95} administered as a rapid bolus dose in patients receiving H_1 and H_2 receptor antagonists was significantly diminished compared with that in patients receiving no pretreatment. Similar results were obtained when

TABLE 16-5. Pharmacodynamic Profiles of Benzylisoquinoline Muscle Relaxants

Relaxant	Dose (mg/kg)	Multiples of the ED_{95}	Onset (min)	Clinical Duration of Action (min)	Time to 95% Twitch Recovery (min)	Time to Recovery of Train-of-Four Ratio = 0.70 (min)
d-Tubocurarine	0.60	1.2	3–4	80	—	—
Metocurine	0.40	1.4	3–4	100	—	—
Doxacurium	0.05	2	4–5	90	—	—
Atracurium	0.50	2	3.0	35–45	50–70	—
Cisatracurium	0.20	4	2.7	68	87	90
Cisatracurium	0.10	2	5.2	45	64	67
Mivacurium	0.25	3	2.3	18–22	26–32	32

even larger doses of atracurium (five times the ED_{95}) were administered 30 minutes following 1 mg/kg of diphenhydramine and 4 mg/kg of cimetidine. Despite a 10- to 19-fold increase in plasma histamine levels, no hemodynamic aberrations were attributable to relaxant administration.

$$OH^{-}\; H-{}_{\beta}\underset{\displaystyle X}{CH}-CH_2-{}^{+}NR_3 \xrightarrow[37^{\circ}C]{pH\,7.4} H_2O + \underset{\displaystyle X}{CH}=CH_2 + NR_3$$

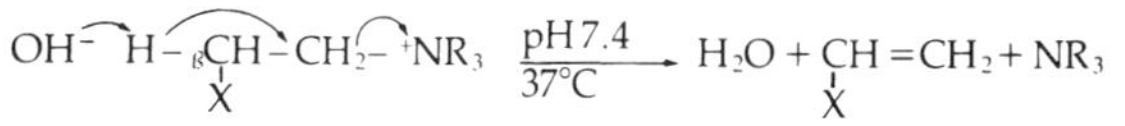

FIGURE 16-6. Hofmann elimination. The presence of an electron withdrawing substituent at the βC weakens the βC-H bond so the degradation of a quaternary ammonium to a tertiary base with the loss of water can occur under physiologic conditions.

METABOLISM AND ELIMINATION

The biodisposition of the benzylisoquinolinium group of relaxants is the most varied of any chemical class of neuromuscular blocking drugs because metabolism (i.e., biotransformation or degradation) of this group of drugs ranges from essentially none (e.g., d-tubocurarine and doxacurium) to rapid and extensive (e.g., mivacurium). Consequently, the duration of action of the different agents in clinical practice varies from long to short (Table 16-5). Unlike any other available nondepolarizing relaxant, mivacurium, with its short duration of action, is rapidly hydrolyzed by plasma cholinesterase.

In general, the longer-lasting members of this class (e.g., doxacurium) are primarily excreted unchanged in the urine, with the biliary tract being a secondary and much less important pathway. The compounds of intermediate duration (e.g., atracurium and cisatracurium) undergo Hofmann elimination, which is a base-catalyzed and temperature-dependent chemical process, as demonstrated in Figure 16-6. In 1851, Hofmann initially described the process as a chemical degradation of a quaternary ammonium salt to a tertiary base with the loss of water, requiring strong alkali and high temperatures. In the 1980s, Stenlake described the reaction as occurring under physiologic conditions in the presence of an electron-withdrawing substituent (e.g., an ester carbonyl group in atracurium, at the β carbon, which weakens the βC-H bond). Even with these chemical substitutions, the reaction depends on temperature and is catalyzed by alkali. In vitro decreases of temperature of 14°C, from 37°C to 23°C, increase the in vitro plasma half-life of atracurium from 18 to 49 minutes (40). Consistent with this finding, hypothermic patients undergoing cardiopulmonary bypass have a lower atracurium dose requirement (41). In animals, average increases of pH of 0.32 to 0.40, with either hyperventilation or an infusion of Na_2CO_3, decreased the depth of atracurium-induced neuromuscular block approximately twofold (42).

COMPARATIVE PHARMACOKINETICS

Young Adults

Doxacurium

The pharmacokinetics of doxacurium has been studied in patients undergoing elective surgical procedures under isoflurane anesthesia (43). In this study, patients received a dose of 0.015 mg/kg doxacurium, and blood samples were obtained for 6 hours after the administration of the relaxant. Noncompartmental methods were used for the analysis of the pharmacokinetic data. The investigators found that the clearance of the drug was 2.6±1.6 ml/kg/min, the volume of distribution at steady state was 220±110 ml/kg, and the elimination half-life was 99±54 minutes. Doxacurium is eliminated unchanged in the bile and the urine. From 30 to 40% of doxacurium is recovered in the urine within 12 hours, consistent with the elimination of unchanged drug primarily by the kidney (24, 43).

Doxacurium is a weak substrate for plasma cholinesterase. In vitro, at high substrate concentrations, it is hydrolyzed at only 6% the rate of succinylcholine (30, 44). In vivo, however, little or no metabolism of the relaxant occurs because sufficiently high plasma concentrations are never achieved.

d-Tubocurarine

The principal route of elimination for d-tubocurarine is the kidney, with approximately 80% of a dose renally excreted (45, 46). The liver is the secondary route of elimination for this relaxant because it undergoes little or no metabolism, with a clearance rate of 2.4 ml/kg/min, a volume of distribution of 250 ml/kg, and an elimination half-life value of is 84 minutes (47).

Metocurine

Like d-tubocurarine, metocurine is eliminated primarily through the kidney. It does not appear to have an alternative means of elimination through the liver (45, 48), and it is not metabolized. Its plasma clearance has been reported to be 1.2 ml/kg/min, with a volume of distribution of 472 ml/kg and an elimination half-life value of 80 to 100 minutes (45, 48).

Atracurium

Atracurium is eliminated from the plasma through Hofmann elimination (8) and ester hydrolysis (Fig. 16-7) (40, 49, 50). When incubated in an aqueous buffer at 37°C and pH 7.3 to 7.4, atracurium has an in vitro half-life value of 60 to 80 minutes (51). Hofmann elimination is a chemical process accelerated by an alkaline pH (42) and an increase in temperature (40). When atracurium is incubated in plasma at physiologic pH and temperature, the in vitro half-life is reduced by 50 to 65% of that in buffer alone (40) because of the compound's hydrolysis by esterases. The ester hydrolysis is unrelated to pseudocholinesterase, which has no effect on the degradation of atracurium (29). The extent to which Hofmann elimination versus ester hydrolysis contributes to the elimination of atracurium in humans has been investigated (52-54). Evidence suggests that both processes may be important in humans; however, ester hydrolysis probably plays the more dominant role in patients with a lower pH (42). Less that 10% of the relaxant is eliminated through the kidneys, and it undergoes no hepatic elimination. Although investigators have suggested that as much as 50% of atracurium undergoes organ-based elimination, (54) little direct evidence supports this position. Thus, clearance of atracurium occurs primarily in the plasma in both the central and peripheral compartments and is relatively independent of end-organ function.

In healthy adults, atracurium has a clearance of 5 to 6 ml/kg/min (55-60), and its elimination half-life of 20 minutes is similar to the in vitro value obtained in plasma or whole blood (55-61). As is shown in Figure 16-7, one of the by-products of Hofmann elimination is laudanosine, a tertiary amine that can enter the central nervous system (CNS), where it acts as a stimulant. Following administration of large doses of atracurium in animals, evidence of CNS excitement can be seen (62-65). No information is available as to the CNS effects of laudanosine at increasing plasma levels in humans. In spite of its elimination through the liver and kidney (66), no reports have been published of CNS stimulation even in patients with hepatic or renal failure (67, 68).

Cisatracurium

Like atracurium, cisatracurium undergoes Hofmann elimination (Fig. 16-8); however, it does not undergo ester hydrolysis (69). Organ-based clearance accounts for the elimination of only 16% of the compound (Kisor DF, Schmith VD, Wargin WA, et al. Importance of organ-independent elimination of cisatracurium [submitted for publication]). In healthy patients, the pharmacokinetics of cisatracurium is independent of dose following doses that are two to four times the ED_{95} (70). The *in vivo* elimination half-life of cisatracurium is 23 minutes, similar to its *in vitro* half-life (69, 70). The clearance of cisatracurium is 5 ml/kg/min,

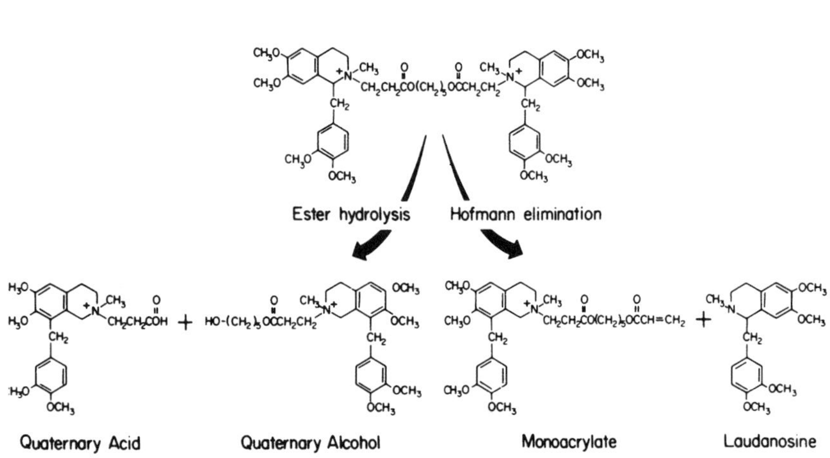

Ester hydrolysis
Hofmann elimination
Quaternary Acid
Quaternary Alcohol
Monoacrylate
Laudanosine

FIGURE 16-7. Means of elimination of atracurium. The compound undergoes both ester hydrolysis and Hofmann elimination as well as organ-based clearance.

similar to other intermediate-acting nondepolarizing relaxants.

Hofmann elimination of cisatracurium yields laudanosine and a monoquaternary metabolite, as illustrated in Figure 16-8. Following administration of twice the ED_{95} of cisatracurium, the maximum laudanosine concentration was 38 ng/ml (70), far less than the landanosine concentration (190 ng/ml) following administration of one and one-half times the ED_{95} of atracurium (59). The lower maximum plasma laudanosine concentration following cisatracurium may be explained in part by the greater relative potency of cisatracurium. The maximum plasma concentrations of laudanosine measured following administration of doses as large as four times the ED_{95} of cisatracurium are 30- to 100-fold greater than concentrations associated with cerebral excitation in animals (64, 65).

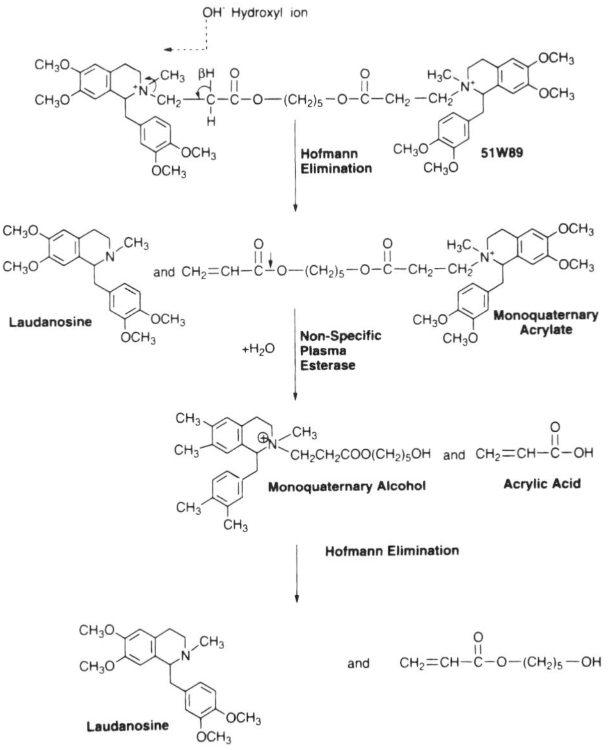

FIGURE 16-8. Like atracurium, cisatracurium undergoes Hofmann elimination to laudanosine and a monoquaternary acrylate. It does not undergo ester hydrolysis.

Mivacurium

The pharmaceutical preparation of mivacurium is supplied as a mixture of three isomers: a *trans-trans*, a *cis-trans*, and a *cis-cis* isomer. These isomers are distinct compounds that do not interconvert and comprise approximately 55, 40, and 5% of the mixture, respectively (Data on File, Burroughs Wellcome, Research Triangle Park, NC). As well as differing in potency (e.g., the *cis-trans* and *trans-trans* isomers are 13 times more potent than the *cis-cis* isomer) (10), the isomers have differing pharmacokinetics. In human plasma, the *trans-trans* and *cis-trans* isomers have elimination half-life values of 0.83 and 1.30 minutes, respectively. In contrast, the *cis-cis* isomer has an in vitro elimination half-life of 276 minutes (Croft-Harrelson J. Personal communication, 1993). *In vivo*, the *cis-trans* and *trans-trans* isomers have short elimination half-life values of 1.8 and 1.9 minutes, respectively. The clearance rate of the *cis-cis* isomer (4.6 ml/kg/min) is similar to that of the intermediate-acting nondepolarizing relaxants, resulting a half-life value of the *cis-cis* isomer of 53 minutes (71). The clearances of the more potent *cis-trans* and *trans-trans* isomers are substantially faster, 100 and 60 ml/kg/min, respectively, (71) because to their extensive metabolism in the plasma (Fig. 16-9). The pharmacokinetics of the two more potent isomers accounts for the neuromuscular blocking potency and unique pharmacodynamic properties of mivacurium (71). The presence of the *cis-cis* isomer appears to be clinically insignificant. In addition to its low neuromuscular blocking potential, the *cis-cis* isomer comprises a small portion of the mivacurium mixture. Furthermore, in spite of its slow clearance and prolonged elimination

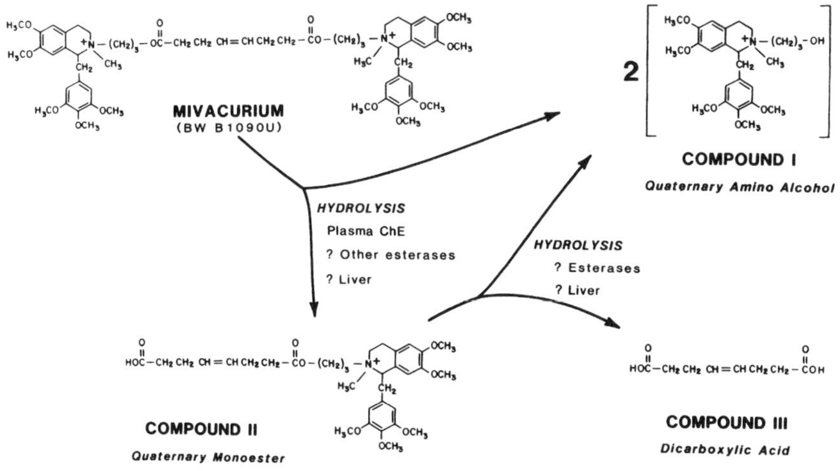

FIGURE 16-9. Metabolic pathways of mivacurium. Its primary route of elimination is through hydrolysis of its potent *cis-trans* and *trans-trans* isomers by plasma cholinesterase.

half-life relative to the other isomers, its plasma concentrations do not increase even during a prolonged infusion of mivacurium (72).

The pharmacokinetics of the potent isomers of mivacurium is independent of dose and infusion time when administered at a rate of 5 or 10 μg/kg/min (71). Mivacurium's short duration of action is due to the rapid hydrolysis of its potent isomers by plasma cholinesterase (see Fig. 16-9). Patient clearance of both *cis-trans* and *trans-trans* isomers is related to plasma cholinesterase activity (71). Mivacurium is metabolized to a quaternary amino alcohol, a dicarboxylic acid, and a quaternary monoester (see Fig. 16-9) by plasma cholinesterase at a rate 70 to 88% that of succinylcholine at comparable multiples of k_m (73, 74). These metabolites are free of CNS-stimulating effects and neuromuscular blocking properties at doses of 100 times the ED_{95} of mivacurium. Essentially all the drug is recovered as pharmacologically inactive metabolites (74). In phenotypically normal patients, an inverse relationship exists between plasma cholinesterase activity and recovery time; individuals with the greatest levels of plasma cholinesterase activity have the shortest duration of action of the relaxant (75). The wide range of "normal" values of plasma cholinesterase activity may account for some of the interpatient variability seen in response to the relaxant in healthy patients. When given by infusion, the rate of administration required to maintain a stable depth of neuromuscular block is proportional to the patient's plasma cholinesterase activity (76). The dose-dependent antagonism of mivacurium-induced block by the administration of plasma cholinesterase in phenotypically normal patients (77) is presumably due to increased hydrolysis of the relaxant in the plasma.

Pediatric Populations

In spite of an immature neuromuscular junction at birth (78, 79), muscle relaxants can be used safely and effectively in neonates.

d-Tubocurarine

An increased sensitivity to d-tubocurarine (80), coupled with an increased volume of distribution in neonates and infants, means that relaxant doses do not have to be decreased. The increased volume of distribution and decreased clearance of relaxant in infants prolongs the elimination half-life of this compound when compared with its pharmacokinetics in adults (80).

Doxacurium

Doxacurium has a higher ED_{95} in children than in adults (81). Its potency in children receiving halothane anesthesia is similar to its potency in adults receiving nitrous oxide-opioid anesthesia. In children, therefore, a larger dose of doxacurium is required to achieve the same level of neuromuscular block as in adults (82). The onset of neuromuscular block with doxacurium is faster in children than it is in adults, and its clinical duration of action is shorter. These pharmacodynamic alterations are most likely due to an increased cardiac output, resulting in more rapid redistribution in children (82). The recovery interval of doxacurium in children is significantly shorter than in adults (30 versus 60 minutes) (81, 82).

Atracurium

Atracurium is commonly administered to pediatric patients. In young children, its ED_{95} is higher than in adults (83). Its clinical duration of action is not different in children than it is in adult patients (84-86). At twice the ED_{95}, children rarely demonstrate flushing or elevation of heart rate, and significant decreases in blood pressure secondary to histamine release are rare. Comparing the pharmacokinetics of atracurium in the pediatric population with that in adults reveals similar elimination half-life values. The absence of age-related changes in elimination half-life values results from parallel changes in the volume of distribution and clearance with age (87).

When the agent is administered as an infusion to patients receiving either opioid or halothane anesthesia, a child's requirement to maintain a neuromuscular block between 90 and 99% of the baseline value is 9 μg/kg/min, similar to the requirement of adults receiving opioid anesthesia (88). Enflurane potentiates atracurium-induced neuromuscular block and decreases the infusion rate requirements to 5 μg/kg/min. Recovery of neuromuscular function after discontinuation of an atracurium infusion does not seem to be slowed by the presence of a volatile agent (88).

Cisatracurium

Cisatracurium is more potent in children than in adults. Its ED_{95} in children receiving halothane anesthesia is 40 μg/kg (89). The clinical duration of action of a dose equal to twice the ED_{95} is 30 minutes, and the 25 to 75% recovery interval is 11 minutes (89, 90), compared with 45 minutes and 14 minutes for the clinical duration of action and recovery interval, respectively, in adults. As with atracurium, the clearance of the relaxant is greater in children than in adults (90). Following administration of twice to two and one-half times the ED_{95} doses in children, no significant changes occur in either heart rate or blood pressure (89, 90).

Mivacurium

Mivacurium has a higher ED_{95} in children than in adult patients. Its ED_{95} in children receiving halothane anesthesia is 0.09 mg/kg and in those receiving opioid anesthesia is 0.10 mg/kg (91, 92). Following administration of twice the ED_{95} of mivacurium, maximal block is achieved in less than 2 minutes. Doubling the dose from 0.10 to 0.20 mg/kg results in a 20% prolongation in the duration of the block (91). With this larger dose of mivacurium, cardiovascular stability is maintained, although occasional facial flushing may be observed. Following administration of larger doses of mivacurium (0.25 mg/kg), transient hypotension may be seen in addition to facial flushing (92) in 10 to 15% of pediatric patients. In addition to being resistant to mivacurium-induced neuromuscular block (versus adults), children recover more quickly. The clinical duration of this relaxant is 12 minutes, compared with 20 minutes in adults (74). The 25 to 75% recovery interval is also shorter in children than in adults.

Halothane potentiates mivacurium-induced neuromuscular block and reduces the effective dose, but it does not affect recovery indices or the clinical duration of action (91, 92). As a result of the higher plasma cholinesterase activity in children, when the relaxant is administered as an infusion, the rates required (10 to 15 μg/kg/min) are approximately twice those required for adults (93, 94).

Geriatric Populations

Anatomic and physiologic changes occur at the neuromuscular junction as a result of aging, including an increase in the distance between the junctional axon and the motor end plate, a decreased concentration in acetylcholine receptors at the motor end plate, a flattening of the folds of the motor end plate, a decrease in the amount of acetylcholine stored in each vesicle in the prejunctional axon, and a decreased amount of acetylcholine released from the preterminal axon in response to a neural impulse (95). Acetylcholine receptor sensitivity to nondepolarizing muscle relaxants is unaltered with advancing age (Fig. 16-10) (95, 96). As a result of age-related changes in hepatic and renal blood flow and function, nondepolarizing muscle relaxants often have altered pharmacokinetics and pharmacodynamics in the elderly. Some of the benzylisoquinoliniums are unique among muscle relaxants in that neither the kidney nor the liver is necessary for their elimination. This results in a lack of age-related changes in the pharmacokinetics and pharmacodynamics of these relaxants in the elderly.

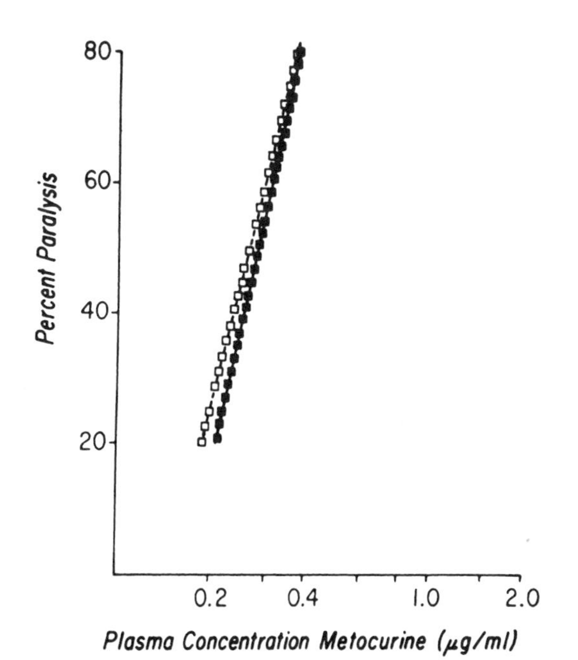

FIGURE 16-10. Relationship between plasma metocurine concentration and reduction in twitch height in young (open squares) and elderly (closed squares) patients.

d-Tubocurarine and Metocurine

Both d-tubocurarine and metocurine have altered pharmacokinetics and pharmacodynamics in the elderly (96). A decreased clearance from the plasma accounts for their prolonged duration of action in this patient population. These two relaxants depend largely on the kidney for their elimination from the plasma.

Doxacurium

The pharmacokinetics and pharmacodynamics of this long-acting relaxant are not significantly affected by advanced age because doxacurium depends almost exclusively on the kidney for its elimination from the plasma. Dresner and colleagues (97) examined the pharmacokinetic and dynamic behavior of doxacurium in young and elderly patients receiving isoflurane anesthesia and found that, although recovery from doxacurium-induced neuromuscular block tended to be slower and more variable in elderly patients, however, the times to 5 and 25% recovery were not significantly different in these two patient populations. Similarly, clearance and elimination half-life values of the relaxant were not different in the two patient populations. As a result of the drug's larger volume of distribution at steady state in the elderly, these patients have a prolonged recovery time. In this study, the elderly patients lost significantly more blood intraoperatively and received more intravenous fluids than the younger patients, a factor that may have influenced the results.

Atracurium

The pharmacokinetics and dynamics of atracurium appear to be largely unaffected by advanced age. D'Hollander and colleagues (98) studied the pharmacodynamics of atracurium in three patient populations: an older population (older than 60 years) and two younger populations (younger than 40 years and 40 to 60 years). All patients received an atracurium infusion to maintain 90% suppression of twitch response for at least 90 minutes. Once the infusion was discontinued, recovery indices of 10 to 25% and 25 to 75% twitch heights were determined, and the dose of atracurium required for maintenance of neuromuscular block was calculated. No difference was found in either the dose of atracurium required to maintain relaxation or the recovery indices among the three study groups. The lack of age-associated variation in the pharmacodynamics of atracurium is readily explained by the lack of dependence of this relaxant on either kidney or hepatic function for its inactivation or elimination from the plasma. Kitts and associates (99) studied atracurium infusions in six elderly patients to achieve approximately 70% twitch suppression. Although the pharmacodynamics of atracurium in the elderly was similar to that in the young adults and the clearance values of atracurium were the same in young and elderly patients, the elimination half-life value of atracurium was prolonged in the elderly (21.8±3.3 versus 15.7±2.5 minutes).

Cisatracurium

Because of its apparent lack of dependence on end-organ function for elimination from the plasma (100), one would expect the pharmacokinetics and dynamics of cisatracurium to be unaffected by advanced age. In a pharmacokinetic and pharmacodynamic study of cisatracurium in elderly patients receiving nitrous oxide-isoflurane anesthesia (101), a dose of twice the ED_{95} caused 99% twitch suppression in the older patients (ages 65 to 82 years) and 99.5% twitch suppression in younger adult patients (30 to 49 years). Maximal effect was achieved 1 minute later in elderly patients than in young patients (3.4±1.0 versus 2.5±0.6 minutes, respectively). Recovery was the same in the elderly and young adult patients following administration of a single dose of twice the ED_{95}. The 25 to 75% recovery interval following administration of this dose was not significantly different in the two study groups (19.0±4.5 minutes in the elderly versus 16.1±2.9 minutes in younger adult patients).

The elimination half-life value was prolonged by 19% in the elderly (4 minutes), and the steady-state volume of distribution (calculated assuming elimination only from the central compartment) was 17% larger in elderly patients. However, no difference was noted in plasma clearance between elderly and young patients (5.0±0.9 versus 4.6±0.8 ml/kg/min, respectively).

Mivacurium

The pharmacodynamics of mivacurium has been studied in the elderly. In comparing the dynamics of mivacurium 0.10 mg/kg, in young and elderly adults (102), both groups achieved similar degrees of neuromuscular block and durations of action (18.0±1.7 versus 19.9±1.2 minutes, respectively). In another study of the pharmacodynamics of mivacurium in the elderly (103), the onset of block was the same in young and elderly patients. However, recovery to a T_1 of 25%, a T_1 of 90%, and a train-of-four ratio of 0.7 occurred more slowly in the elderly than in the young, a finding suggesting that clearance of mivacurium may decrease with advancing age.

Renal Failure

Renal failure, like hepatic failure, can affect the pharmacokinetics and dynamics of muscle relaxants in many different ways. It can influence the elimination of the drug from the plasma and alter the drug's volume of distribution.

d-Tubocurarine

The long-acting benzylisoquinolone d-tubocurarine has a longer duration of action in patients with renal failure (104). Approximately 40% of a dose of this muscle relaxant is excreted in the urine within 24 hours of its administration (105). Miller and associates demonstrated that, in patients with renal failure, this decreases to about 15% of a dose (46). Because equal plasma concentrations of d-tubocurarine cause similar depression of neuromuscular function in patients with normal renal function and those with renal failure, the decrease in renal clearance, rather than electrolyte and acid-base abnormalities, accounts for its prolonged duration of action in this patient population (46).

Metocurine

Like d-tubocurarine, metocurine is extensively eliminated through renal mechanisms. Forty-eight percent of a single dose of this benzylisoquinoline muscle relaxant is found unchanged in the urine within 24 hours of its administration (106). As would be expected, its pharmacokinetics is altered in the presence of renal disease. Relative to patients with normal renal function, the volume of distribution is smaller, the elimination half-life is prolonged twofold, and the clearance is decreased fourfold in the presence of renal failure (48).

Doxacurium

Doxacurium is also eliminated primarily unchanged in the urine. Although its volume of distribution at steady state is not significantly altered in patients with renal failure, its clearance is reduced by 50%(to 1.2 ml/kg/min), and its elimination half-life is doubled to 221 minutes (43). The clinical duration of action of doxacurium in patients with renal failure is significantly prolonged (107). The 5 to 10% and 10 to 25% recovery intervals are similar in patients with and without renal failure. The time required for spontaneous recovery beyond 25% has not been studied in these compromised patients.

Atracurium
Atracurium is eliminated from the plasma by mechanisms discussed previously (8, 54). Fisher and associates, using a specific two-compartment model to estimate the clearance of atracurium due to both organ-dependent and nonorgan-dependent elimination, found that more than 50% of the clearance of atracurium occurred by pathways other than Hofmann elimination (54). Atracurium's volume of distribution, clearance, and elimination half-life values are unaffected by the presence of renal disease (56, 57). Therefore, the pharmacodynamics of atracurium is unchanged in patients with renal failure (57, 58). Even after infusions of atracurium lasting 14 to 219 minutes in patients with renal failure, spontaneous recovery proceeds rapidly (67, 108).

Cisatracurium
Cisatracurium, like atracurium, undergoes Hofmann elimination. Approximately 16% of the drug is eliminated through the kidney (109). Except for a slower onset of neuromuscular block in patients with renal failure, no differences were noted in the pharmacodynamics of cisatracurium-induced neuromuscular block when twice the ED_{95} of the relaxant was administered to otherwise healthy patients, compared with those with renal failure (110). Despite the lack of influence of renal failure on the pharmacodynamics of cisatracurium-induced neuromuscular block, the pharmacokinetics of the relaxant is different in this patient population when compared with patients with intact renal function. In the presence of renal failure, clearance is reduced by 13% (293 to 254 ml/min), and the elimination half-life is prolonged by 14% (from 30.0 to 34.2 minutes) (111).

Mivacurium
The short-acting muscle relaxant mivacurium does not depend directly on the kidney for its elimination; however, its duration of action is prolonged in patients with renal failure (112, 113). Although Cook and associates were unable to demonstrate any pharmacokinetic differences in patients with renal failure (114), these patients may have an acquired decrease in plasma cholinesterase activity (115). Decreases in plasma cholinesterase activity are not related to hemodialysis (116), but are most likely secondary to the uremia that accompanies renal failure. The clearance rates of the more potent *cis-trans* and *trans-trans* isomers of mivacurium are inversely related to plasma cholinesterase activity (71). The less potent *cis-cis* isomer depends on secondary routes of elimination, such as the kidney, for its elimination from the plasma. Cook and associates may have found neither pharmacokinetic nor dynamic differences in patients with renal failure and normal plasma cholinesterase activity.

Hepatic Failure

Hepatic failure can affect the pharmacokinetics and dynamics of nondepolarizing muscle relaxants in various ways. If a muscle relaxant depends on hepatic elimination, its kinetics and dynamics may be altered by changes in hepatic blood flow, by the capacity of hepatocytes to metabolize or excrete the drug, or by decreased synthesis of plasma cholinesterase by hepatocytes. Hepatic failure may also influence the distribution of drug into the various compartments and the degree to which muscle relaxants are protein bound.

Doxacurium
Doxacurium is eliminated unchanged through the urine and, to a lesser extent, through the bile. Although it is a benzylisoquinolinium and, therefore, a potential metabolite for plasma cholinesterase, it undergoes minimal (if any) metabolism in humans. Because of its almost exclusive dependence on the kidney for clearance from the plasma, its pharmacokinetics and dynamics are not significantly affected by the presence of liver disease (43). Interpatient variability is increased in this patient population, and doxacurium often has a prolonged duration of action.

Atracurium
Only with the introduction of the intermediate-acting benzylisoquinolones into clinical practice have hepatic blood flow and hepatocyte function become unimportant in terms of their impact on the pharmacokinetics and dynamics of relaxants. Atracurium's pharmacokinetics and dynamics remain unchanged in the presence of hepatic failure. Ward and Neill (117) found that, in patients with chronic renal failure and superimposed acute hepatic failure, the elimination half-life of atracurium was the same as in patients with normal hepatic and renal function. The patients with hepatic and renal failure did have larger volumes of distribution and slightly faster clearance rates. Because the clearance was increased, the elimination half-life was not prolonged in spite of an increased volume of distribution.

Cisatracurium
Tullock and associates (118) reported that the pharmacodynamics of cisatracurium-induced neuromus-

cular block was unaffected by the presence of liver disease. As with atracurium, the volume of distribution was larger in patients with hepatic failure, the clearance rate was greater, and there was no difference in the elimination half-life value compared with patients with normal hepatic function.

Mivacurium

Although the short-acting muscle relaxant mivacurium does not depend on the liver for its metabolism and elimination, it is extensively metabolized by plasma cholinesterase. The synthesis of this enzyme depends on hepatocyte synthetic function. The duration of action of mivacurium is inversely related to the plasma cholinesterase activity in phenotypically normal patients (75, 76). Plasma cholinesterase activity is decreased in patients with hepatic failure (114). The prolonged recovery from mivacurium-induced neuromuscular block in patients with hepatic failure is due to decreased plasma cholinesterase activity, (114) resulting in a decreased clearance of the potent isomers of mivacurium and prolonged elimination half-life values (119). Because of the decreased enzyme activity, clearance of mivacurium from the plasma of these patients is only 50% that of patients with normal hepatic function, and the mean residence time is twice that in healthy patients. The volume of distribution of the muscle relaxant is not significantly different in the two patient populations (114).

ANTAGONISM

The benzylisoquinolinium compounds are nondepolarizing relaxants, and residual neuromuscular blockade is readily antagonized by anticholinesterase drugs. Because the clearance of the relaxants varies widely, the speed of antagonism is related to the rate of drug clearance. The antagonism of mivacurium occurs more rapidly than that of atracurium or cisatracurium, whose effects, in turn, are antagonized more quickly than those of metocurine, d-tubocurarine, or doxacurium (12, 27, 30, 74). These differences are easily understood if one considers the dynamics of antagonism as a static process occurring at the same rate and by the same pharmacologic mechanisms irrespective of the relaxant drug. If this process is aided, as in the case of mivacurium, by a rapid clearance rate (74), the clinical picture of antagonism occurs on a shorter time scale than in the presence of a slow clearance drug (e.g., doxacurium or d-tubocurarine) (43, 46).

The pharmacokinetics of the intermediate- and short-acting relaxants is independent of dose (70, 71, 120), and their elimination is largely independent of end-organ function. The spontaneous recovery of neuromuscular function occurs over much the same time course following repeated dosing of the relaxant or an infusion of these relaxants as it does following their initial dosing. The 5 to 95% and 25 to 75% recovery intervals are shown in Table 16-6 and do not vary with the dose of relaxant.

Recovery from mivacurium-induced blockade can present some interesting dilemmas. Although the agent is a short-acting relaxant, marked interpatient variability occurs in response to a given dose of the relaxant because of the range of normal plasma cholinesterase activities. The time required for spontaneous recovery from 5 to 95% of muscle strength can be predicted on the basis of the time required for recovery from the 5 to 25%. Following administration of an initial dose of mivacurium, the time required for return of one and three twitches in response to a train-of-four stimulus is the 5 to 25% recovery index, according to the scheme of Lee (121). Thus, the final 5 to 95% recovery index can be predicted by multiplying the 5 to 25% recovery index by four (122). The ability to predict the final recovery from mivacurium is advantageous because it allows the clinician to dose the relaxant such that pharmacologically facilitated antagonism may not be required at the conclusion of the surgical procedure. This calculation is possible because recovery following one or more doses of mivacurium proceeds at the same rate in a given patient, regardless of the total amount of the relaxant administered.

The duration of action of mivacurium is directly related to the patient's plasma cholinesterase activity (75). As mentioned previously, the clearance of the more potent isomers depends on plasma cholinesterase activity (71). In patients homozygous for atypical plasma cholinesterase, mivacurium, 0.03 mg/kg, caused 100% neuromuscular block within 5 minutes (123), and return of response to a train-of-four stimulus

TABLE 16-6. Recovery Intervals Following Different Doses of Muscle Relaxants

Muscle Relaxant	Dose (mg/kg)	25–75% Recovery Interval (min)	5–95% Recovery Interval (min)
Atracurium	0.20	12	—
	0.30	10	—
	0.40	11	—
	0.50	12	—
	0.60	12	—
Cisatracurium	0.10	13	30
	0.20	14	32
	0.40	14	31
	Infusion	15	33
Mivacurium	0.10	7	13
	0.15	7	14
	0.20	7	15
	0.25	7	14
	0.30	7	15
	Infusion	7	14

ranged from 26 to 128 minutes. The time for 25% recovery of the first twitch in the train-of-four was a minimum of 57 minutes. The incidence of an atypical homozygous patient is 1 in 3000 (124).

Patients with a prolonged mivacurium-induced neuromuscular block can be managed in various ways (125-128). Both conservative therapy with mechanical ventilation and sedation during spontaneous recovery of neuromuscular function and aggressive therapy with anticholinesterase drugs have been described. Unlike with succinylcholine, when recovery begins, antagonism may be facilitated with the use of anticholinesterase drugs because mivacurium is a nondepolarizing blocker. Neostigmine, 0.05 to 0.06 mg/kg, may be administered and repeated in 30 minutes if neuromuscular function has not completely recovered. Whole-blood transfusions containing plasma cholinesterase have been given to patients homozygous for atypical plasma cholinesterase to shorten recovery time after succinylcholine (124); however, the risk of transfusion-acquired infection makes this alternative less desirable. Highly purified human plasma cholinesterase has also been used with success in patients with low plasma cholinesterase activity to accelerate recovery from succinylcholine-induced neuromuscular blockade (129). Östergaard and associates described the use of human plasma cholinesterase in patients with atypical plasma cholinesterase after receiving mivacurium (125). In patients with the atypical gene, treatment with human plasma cholinesterase significantly reduced recovery time compared with spontaneous recovery alone, even though it remained slower than in patients with normal plasma cholinesterase. The administration of neostigmine following treatment with human plasma cholinesterase further enhanced recovery (125).

Reversal of mivacurium in those patients requires more time before complete antagonism is achieved. The recovery process may be slower because there is no contribution of cholinesterase hydrolysis in promoting rapid reversal. In these cases, the elimination of mivacurium proceeds slowly through the kidney (in a manner analogous to that of pancuronium), and the reversal process should follow a slow pattern as customarily seen during antagonism of any long-acting relaxant from "deep" blockade.

In theory, antagonism of mivacurium-induced neuromuscular block in patients with a normal genotype for plasma cholinesterase presents some interesting issues. Anticholinesterase agents are typically administered to hasten the process of recovery from nondepolarizing neuromuscular block. Both in vitro and in vivo, however, neostigmine decreases plasma cholinesterase activity and can possibly slow the metabolism of mivacurium, resulting in a delayed plasma clearance and a prolonged effect (130, 131). Use of reversal drugs has been reported to prolong recovery from profound mivacurium-induced neuromuscular blockade (132) and has failed to antagonize neuromuscular block effectively during a mivacurium infusion (131). Other studies, however, have found neostigmine to be an effective antagonist of residual mivacurium-induced neuromuscular block (133-136). Although edrophonium does not decrease plasma cholinesterase activity (130, 137), it has been reported to increase the plasma concentration of mivacurium (137). Nevertheless, even small doses of edrophonium have been found effective in antagonizing residual mivacurium-induced neuromuscular blockade (138, 139). The pharmacodynamics of spontaneous, edrophonium-enhanced, or neostigmine-augmented recovery from a mivacurium infusion has been examined (140). A 3- to 5-minute decrease in recovery times was identified following administration of anticholinesterase drugs. No alteration in the clearance or elimination half-life of the isomers of mivacurium was found following administration of either anticholinesterase drug.

Because mivacurium is metabolized by plasma cholinesterase, administration of butyrylcholinesterase is available to hasten recovery from mivacurium-induced neuromuscular blockade. Bownes and associates (141) administered butyrylcholinesterase or neostigmine (0.05 mg/kg) 2 minutes following administration of a dose three times the ED_{95} of mivacurium. Acceleration of recovery time from profound neuromuscular block was achieved with butyrylcholinesterase, but not with neostigmine. The enzyme effectively antagonizes mivacurium-induced neuromuscular block in humans (77). Availability of purified butyrylcholinesterase may solve an infrequent but vexing clinical problem, namely, prolonged neuromuscular blockade following administration of either mivacurium or succinylcholine to patients homozygous for atypical plasma cholinesterase.

SYNERGISM

Although many synergistic interactions have been described and quantitated for similar and dissimilar classes of muscle relaxants, the exact mechanism underlying these interactions has only been hypothesized. Some investigators postulate the presence of multiple binding sites at the neuromuscular junction, both presynaptic and postsynaptic (142, 143). Other investigators state that the asymmetric azimuthal orientation of the subunits in the pentamer determines different contacts for the two α chains, causing nonequivalence of binding sites (144, 145). The alteration of the pharmacokinetic behavior of one drug by another drug is a theory disputed by still other investigators (146).

In some clinical situations, intubation of the patient is achieved with succinylcholine, and the relaxation is maintained with a nondepolarizing agent. The effect of succinylcholine preceding mivacurium has been studied in adult patients undergoing either a nitrous oxide-opioid anesthetic (147-149) or an inhalation anesthetic. In the study by Erkola et al (147), patients received either succinylcholine, 1 mg/kg, followed by mivacurium, 0.15 mg/kg, or the same dose of mivacurium alone. All patients had normal dibucaine values, with little variance in cholinesterase activity. The recovery index and the time to recovery of train-of-four ratio 0.7 were not different between groups. These authors concluded that, in a healthy population, the use of mivacurium following intubation with succinylcholine is not significantly different from that of mivacurium alone.

Synergism has been studied between mivacurium and multiple nondepolarizers, both between benzylisoquinoliniums and steroidal compounds (150, 151). The interactions between mivacurium and atracurium were studied in patients receiving nitrous oxide-fentanyl-isoflurane anesthesia (152). When equipotent doses of the two drugs in combination were studied, fractional analysis demonstrated zero (additive) interaction. The combination was precisely that expected from the dose-response relations of the individual agents. This supports a well-substantiated finding that combinations of structurally similar muscle relaxants produce an additive response. The investigators then followed either atracurium, 0.5 mg/kg, or mivacurium, 0.15 mg/kg, with additional maintenance doses of mivacurium (0.10 mg/kg) given when the first twitch recovered to 10% of control. These investigators found that the duration of this first maintenance dose of mivacurium to 10% recovery of the first twitch was greater after atracurium than mivacurium. When subsequent doses of mivacurium were given to either group, the duration was similar (152). This prolongation is due to the relative concentrations of the two drugs at the myoneural function receptor sites. The pharmacologic profile of the initial drug dominating the receptor sites is the pharmacokinetics that predominate, whereas the kinetics of the second drug becomes more evident as doses are repeated and time passes.

A subsequent study compared the synergism between atracurium and mivacurium with that of vecuronium and mivacurium (153), to assess the effect of structural differences among classes of nondepolarizing neuromuscular blockers. In this study, children anesthetized with a propofol-alfentanyl-nitrous oxide-oxygen anesthetic received either an ED_{50} dose of atracurium, vecuronium, or mivacurium or a single-dose combination of 0.5 times the ED_{50} of either atracurium plus mivacurium or vecuronium plus mivacurium. The maximum neuromuscular block established by either of the two-dose combinations was greater than the block produced by either atracurium or vecuronium alone. These authors concluded that molecular structure alone cannot account for the synergism observed. Other studies have demonstrated that synergism between atracurium and vecuronium is greatest when the drugs are administered on an equipotent basis (154). Goudsouzian and associates studied the use of mivacurium following atracurium in children (155). The children were intubated with atracurium, and mivacurium was administered either following an additional dose of atracurium or as an infusion of 4 μg/kg/min (to maintain the twitch height at 90% of T_1). A prolonged effect of mivacurium was noted, and the mivacurium infusion requirement was decreased following atracurium. Similarly, the residual neuromuscular effects of atracurium were prolonged. Jalkanen commented that the administration of halothane in Goudsouzian's study may have furthered the potentiation (153).

In another study, patients received combinations of rocuronium and mivacurium in equipotent doses. Rocuronium has a rapid onset but is intermediate in its duration of action. Naguib found that the interaction between rocuronium and mivacurium was synergistic (156), producing a shorter onset time and longer duration of neuromuscular blockade than expected by simple additivity. For example, a combination of rocuronium, 150 μg/kg, and mivacurium, 37.5 μg/kg, had a rapid onset time (114 seconds) and a short duration of action (14.7 minutes). As the doses of rocuronium and mivacurium were increased, the onset time decreased and the duration of block was prolonged. Rocuronium, 300 μg/kg, and mivacurium, 75 μg/kg, had a rapid onset (69 seconds) and an intermediate duration of action (34 minutes).

Synergism between atracurium and vecuronium was studied in infants, using a 5:1 ratio, and in children, using a 4:1 ratio (157). These investigators found the combinations to be more potent than either agent alone, especially in children. They postulated that this was the result of one competitive blocking agent attaching to the α subunit of the postsynaptic acetylcholine receptor and decreasing the likelihood of a second agent's attaching to another subunit. The authors believed the results could not be explained by differences in pharmacokinetics between the drugs, because no data indicate that one neuromuscular blocker affects the clearance or distribution half-life of another.

Other investigators have studied the use of intermediate-acting agents after blockade with longer-acting agents. Whalley and associates investigated the recovery of atracurium when administered following blockade with pancuronium in healthy adults (158). All patients were intubated with pancuronium, 0.1 mg/kg, and subsequently redosed when train-of-four returned to 25% of control with equipotent doses of either pancuronium or atracurium. The time from reversal with neostigmine, 0.07 mg/kg, and gycopyrrolate, 0.015 mg/kg, to a train-of-four ratio of 70% was similar in both groups. Following pancuronium, equipotent doses of atracurium and pancuronium were associated with similar recovery times. If the operations had lasted longer than 5 hours, the characteristics of the clinical duration and recovery probably would have been similar to the maintenance relaxant. In a case report, prolonged neuromuscular blockade was seen when 7 mg of mivacurium followed pancuronium, 3.5 mg, for pediatric surgery. Mivacurium had been given when the patient had four twitches without evidence of fade. Forty minutes after the mivacurium (7 mg) was given, the patient had no evidence of return of twitches (159). Similarly, Brandom and colleagues reported prolonged action of mivacurium in children given a priming dose of pancuronium before an intubating dose of mivacurium (160).

COST ISSUES

In our current economic climate, comparing the cost of the available relaxant drugs is useful. Obviously, other factors should be considered when a nondepolarizing muscle relaxant is chosen. When all other considerations are equal, the acquisition drug cost is a useful piece of information in the decision-making process. In calculating relative cost, several assumptions were used to generate the cost values in Tables 16-7 and 16-8. The hypothetical patient being anesthetized was considered to be a 70-kg healthy adult receiving a nitrous oxide-oxygen-opioid anesthetic and was intubated with the nondepolarizing drug. Because the anesthetic technique did not utilize a volatile agent, the dosages chosen for subsequent relaxation were at the upper end of the recommended doses (161, 162). Table 16-8 presents the cost per hour for intubation and maintenance of neuromuscular block for 5 hours.

SPECIFIC RELAXANTS

Long-Acting Drugs

d-Tubocurarine

BASIC PHARMACOLOGY. d-Tubocurarine (see Fig. 16-1) is the prototypic benzylisoquinolinium. It is a weak neuromuscular blocking compound with prominent cardiovascular side effects, including ganglionic blockade and histamine release, that occur within the clinical dose range (see Table 16-4) (16-18, 22, 163).

CLINICAL PHARMACOLOGY. d-Tubocurarine has an ED_{95} in humans of 0.5 mg/kg. ED_{95} doses have a clinical duration of action of 75 to 80 minutes (27). This relaxant is rarely used to facilitate endotracheal intubation because the large doses required to achieve profound neuromuscular blockade rapidly are associated with both ganglionic blockade and histamine release. Residual neuromuscular blockade is readily antagonized with anticholinesterases. Large doses of neostigmine (50 to 60 μg/kg) are generally recommended for antagonism of residual block because of the relaxant's long duration of action and slow clearance (45, 46).

CARDIOVASCULAR EFFECTS. Doses of 0.3 mg/kg or more of d-tubocurarine commonly cause a decrease in blood pressure (164, 165). When doses of 0.5 mg/kg or larger are administered as a rapid intravenous bolus, increases in heart rate and facial flushing are likely to

TABLE 16-7. Dosage Recommendations of the Benzylisoquinoline Muscle Relaxants

Relaxant	ED_{95}	Intubating Dose mg/kg	Redose mg/kg	Intubation Dose (min)	Maintenance Dose (min)
d-Tubocurarine	0.5	0.5–0.6	0.1–0.15	60–100	30–45
Metocurine	0.28	0.3–0.4	0.05–0.1	60–120	30–45
Doxacurium	0.025	0.05–0.08	0.005–0.01	90–150	30–60
Atracurium	0.25	0.5–0.6	0.1–0.15	30–45	15–20
Mivacurium	0.08	0.2–0.25	0.05	15–20	5–10
Cisatracurium (51 W89)	0.09	0.15–0.2	0.01–0.02	40–70	15–20

TABLE 16-8. Acquisition Cost per Hour for Intubation and Maintenance of Neuromuscular Blockade

Muscle Relaxant	Approximate cost/mg	Intubation Cost	1 h	2 h	3 h	4 h	5 h	Total Cost
d-Tubocurarine	$ .08	$ 3.36	—	$ .84	$ .84	$ 1.68	$ .84	$ 7.56
Metocurine	$ .56	$15.68	—	$ 3.92	$ 3.92	$ 3.92	$ 3.92	$31.36
Doxacurium	$2.88	$16.13	—	—	$ 2.02	$ 2.02	$ 2.02	$22.19
Atracurium	$ .42	$17.64	$4.41	$13.23	$13.23	$13.23	$13.23	$74.97
Mivacurium	$ .62	$10.85	$8.68	$13.02	$13.02	$13.02	$13.02	$71.61
Cisatracurium	$ .73	$19.60	—	$ 5.88	$ 5.88	$ 5.88	$ 5.88	$43.12

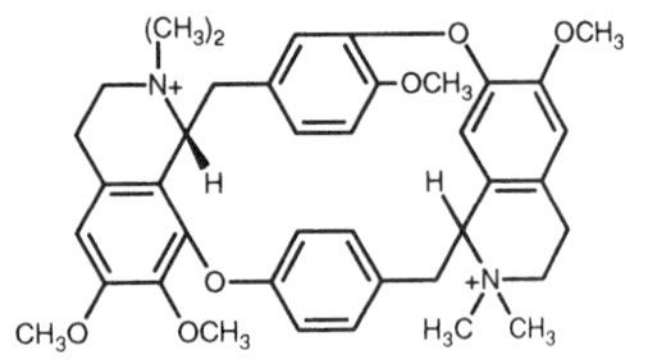

FIGURE 16-11. Chemical structure of metocurine.

occur as a result of histamine release (5, 21). The ganglion-blocking effect of d-tubocurarine can be demonstrated at doses of 0.8 to 1.6 mg/kg (17).

Metocurine

BASIC PHARMACOLOGY. Metocurine is the N,O,O-trimethylated derivative of d-tubocurarine (Fig. 16-11). Its major advantages over its parent compound are greater potency and a greater margin of safety with respect to histamine release and ganglion blockade (17, 18, 163). It was originally introduced into clinical practice as an alternative to d-tubocurarine with fewer side effects (166-168).

CLINICAL PHARMACOLOGY. The ED_{95} of metocurine is 0.28 mg/kg. Doses of 0.4 to 0.5 mg/kg allow endotracheal intubation within 3 minutes. Doses of this magnitude, however, should be injected over 30 to 60 seconds because histamine release can occur at doses of 1.5 times its ED_{95}. At equipotent doses, the duration of action of metocurine is similar to that of d-tubocurarine (18). Residual metocurine-induced neuromuscular block can be antagonized by anticholinesterases. Because of metocurine's long elimination half-life, large doses of neostigmine (0.05 to 0.06 mg/kg) should be used to antagonize profound levels of neuromuscular blockade (27, 45, 48).

CARDIOVASCULAR EFFECTS. The principal cardiovascular side effect of metocurine is histamine release. Its propensity to cause histamine release, however, is less than that of d-tubocurarine. Doses of 0.2 to 0.3 mg/kg, which produce adequate muscle relaxation, cause little or no change in heart rate or blood pressure (see Fig. 16-3) (27). Larger doses (0.4 mg/kg or more) should be injected more slowly because their rapid administration is associated with histamine release.

Doxacurium

BASIC PHARMACOLOGY. Doxacurium chloride (Fig. 16-12) is a bisquaternary benzylisoquinolinium diester. Like metocurine and d-tubocurarine, it is a long-acting muscle relaxant. Doxacurium's advantage over both these compounds is a lack of cardiovascular side effects in the clinical dosage range.

CLINICAL PHARMACOLOGY. The ED_{95} of doxacurium is 0.025 to 0.030 mg/kg, making it the most potent of the currently available nondepolarizing muscle relaxants (30, 31, 169). The onset of block with doxacurium is slower than that with other nondepolarizing muscle relaxants (170, 171). An ED_{95} dose has an onset time to maximal effect of approximately 10 minutes (31). The onset of block can be shortened to about 5 minutes by increasing the dose to 0.05 mg/kg (twice the ED_{95}). The clinical duration of action of doxacurium following a dose twice the ED_{95} is approximately 90 minutes. As with other long-acting muscle relaxants, significant interpatient variability exists in terms of response to a given dose of the relaxant (30, 31, 169). The time course of neuromuscular responses to repeated small maintenance doses of doxacurium administered at 25% recovery seems to remain constant in individual patients (31). The time course of recovery following antagonism of residual block with neostigmine is inversely proportional to the depth of block present at the time of administration of the reversal drug. When residual doxacurium block is antagonized at 10 to 15% recovery with 0.06 mg/kg of neostigmine, recovery to 95% twitch height occurs in 15 to 30 minutes during "balanced" anesthesia (30, 31, 169). Antagonism to train-of-four values greater than 70% requires 30 minutes or more in the presence of potent volatile anesthetics (172).

CARDIOVASCULAR EFFECTS. Although benzylisoquinolinium compounds often cause histamine release when large doses (two to three times the ED_{95}) are administered as rapid intravenous boluses, even when rapidly administered in doses as high as three times its ED_{95}, doxacurium does not cause changes in heart rate, blood pressure, or plasma histamine concentrations (30, 31). This lack of side effects is evident in patients undergoing cardiac surgery as well as in relatively healthy patients undergoing elective surgery (31, 32, 173).

Intermediate-acting Drugs

Atracurium

BASIC PHARMACOLOGY. Atracurium (Fig. 16-13) is a nondepolarizing relaxant of intermediate duration. It is chemically inactivated by decomposition through the well-known Hofmann elimination pathway, and it also undergoes ester hydrolysis.

CLINICAL PHARMACOLOGY. Atracurium has an intermediate duration secondary to its chemical inactivation by the Hofmann mechanism (see Figs. 16-6 and

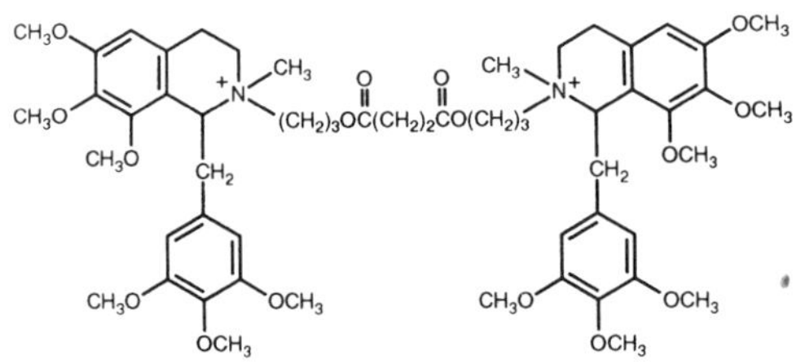

FIGURE 16-12. Chemical structure of doxacurium.

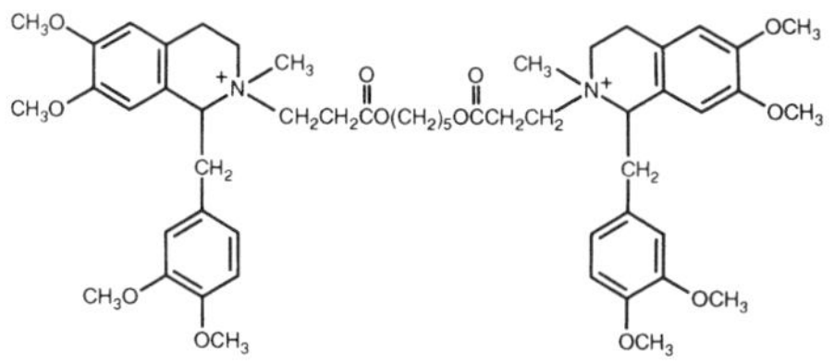

FIGURE 16-13. Chemical structure of atracurium.

16-7). It is less potent than mivacurium and cisatracurium, with an ED_{95} of 0.25 mg/kg. Onset to peak twitch suppression is achieved in about 2 to 3 minutes following administration of twice the ED_{95}, and its total duration of effect is 64 minutes (29). Repeat bolus doses of atracurium given at 25% twitch height yield a consistent recovery pattern with changes neither in the dose requirement nor in the duration of block, suggesting a lack of cumulative neuromuscular blocking effects (29). Because of this lack of accumulation and relatively short elimination half-life, atracurium-induced neuromuscular block may be maintained with a continuous infusion. Infusion rates of 5 to 10 μg/kg/min are generally necessary to maintain 95% twitch suppression under balanced anesthesia (139). Complete spontaneous recovery following infusions requires approximately 30 minutes. These recovery times are similar to recovery times noted following single or repeat bolus doses (29, 139). Atracurium block can be readily antagonized by either neostigmine or edrophonium. As with other nondepolarizers, the deeper the block, the longer the time to complete recovery (29, 174). However, blocks averaging 75% twitch inhibition are antagonized within 9 to 10 minutes.

CARDIOVASCULAR EFFECTS. Doses of atracurium up to twice the ED_{95} (0.4 to 0.5 mg/kg) produce little change in heart rate or blood pressure. At two and one-half to three times ED_{95}, decreases in arterial blood pressure of 15 to 20% and increases in heart rate of 5 to 8% may be seen following a rapid bolus injection of atracurium (see Fig. 16-4), owing to the release of histamine (22, 28). The phenomenon may be blunted and the hemodynamic response attenuated by either slow intravenous injection (30 to 75 seconds) or prophylaxis with H_1 and H_2 antagonists (175, 176).

Cisatracurium

BASIC PHARMACOLOGY. Cisatracurium (Fig. 16-14) is one of the 10 stereoisomers comprising atracurium and has been developed as a "new" relaxant because of its improved cardiovascular profile. Like atracurium, it is a neuromuscular blocker of intermediate duration.

CLINICAL PHARMACOLOGY. The ED_{95} of cisatracurium is 0.05 mg/kg (12), making it approximately three times more potent than atracurium. Doses of twice the ED_{95} produce maximum block in about 5 minutes and provide a clinical duration of 45 minutes. Faster onset times may be achieved by increasing the dose to four to eight times the ED_{95} with an onset of 2 to 3 minutes. Similar to other nondepolarizing neuromuscular blockers, the clinical duration increases as the dose of drug is increased. Doses of four and eight times the ED_{95} yield clinical durations of approximately 70 and 90 minutes, respectively. Infusion rates necessary to produce 95% block are 1 to 2 μg/kg/min and are independent of the duration of the infusion. The 25 to 75% recovery index is 14 minutes and, as with other benzylisoquinolinium neuromuscular blockers, it is independent of the dose or the duration of the infusion because of its noncumulative pharmacodynamics (12, 177). Cisatracurium is easily reversed with neostigmine, which shortens the 25 to 75% recovery index to approximately 3 minutes. Intubation studies performed using cisatracurium have suggested that intubation should be performed no earlier than 2 minutes following twice the ED_{95} or at 90 seconds following a dose to three to four times the ED_{95} (178-180). Cisatracurium's high potency compared with other intermediate-acting nondepolarizing neuromuscular blocking agents contributes to its slower onset (181). In children given cisatracurium during stable halothane anesthesia, the drug showed potency similar to that seen in adults; however, onset and recovery times were shorter. Children also required 1- to 2-μg/kg/min infusion rates to maintain stable neuromuscular block of more than 90% (89, 90). Geriatric surgical patients demonstrated slower onset times (attributed to slower circulation times), but recovery time were similar to those in younger adults (101).

The pharmacokinetics of cisatracurium is similar to that of atracurium. The elimination half-life is 23 minutes, with a clearance of 5 ml/min/kg, and these values are independent of dose in the range of two and four times the ED_{95} (182). Concentrations of laudanosine are lower than those found with atracurium at equipotent doses. Cisatracurium may also have distinct advantages in patients in the intensive care unit (ICU) because of its Hofmann elimination. In the ICU, infusion of cisatracurium was characterized by more rapid recovery compared with vecuronium in patients who received infusions averaging more than 65 hours (183).

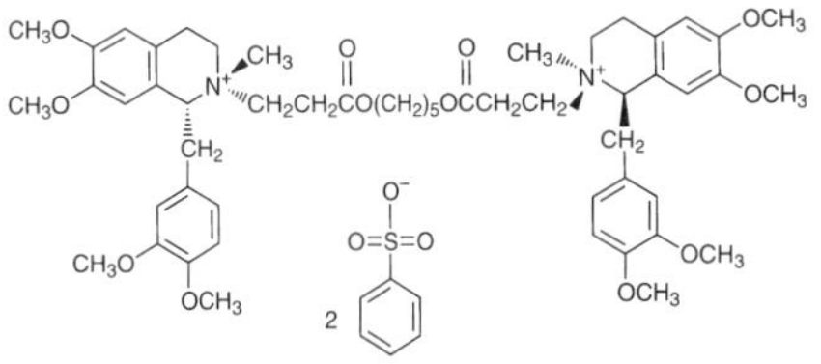

51W89 Besylate

FIGURE 16-14. Chemical structure of cisatracurium.

CARDIOVASCULAR EFFECTS. The most important advantage of cisatracurium is its lack of cardiovascular side effects. No dose-related changes in arterial pressure or heart rate are associated with the administration of doses of cisatracurium ranging from two to eight times the ED_{95} (Fig. 16-15) (33), nor do dose-related increases in plasma histamine levels occur at this range of doses, in contradistinction to atracurium (see Fig. 16-3). The hemodynamic changes observed in patients undergoing elective coronary artery revascularization who were given rapid bolus doses of two times the ED_{95} of cisatracurium were indistinguishable from those of a control group given vecuronium (184).

BW A444U

BASIC PHARMACOLOGY. BW A444U is an investigational benzylisoquinolinium ester (Fig. 16-16) that undergoes slow hydrolysis by human plasma cholinesterase at about 6% the rate of succinylcholine, at relatively high substrate concentrations (35, 185).

CLINICAL PHARMACOLOGY. In a clinical trial, the potency of BW A444U was four times greater than that of d-tubocurarine and twice that of atracurium. It had an ED_{95} of 0.11 mg/kg, and it produced a typical nondepolarizing block with train-of-four fade as block deepened. Because of its relatively slow hydrolysis, BW A44U has an intermediate duration of action. Like other metabolized benzylisoquinolinium esters, BW A444U demonstrates a lack of cumulative neuromuscular blocking properties with repeated dosing. Onset of maximal block at twice the ED_{95} (0.2 mg/kg) was 2.5 minutes, significantly shorter than 5 minutes for a single ED_{95} dose. However, the duration of blockade increased only 44% with a 100% increase in the dosage. As in the case of mivacurium, duration of block was inversely related to the individual's plasma cholinesterase activity (186, 187). However, residual blockade could be easily antagonized by neostigmine (35, 185).

CARDIOVASCULAR EFFECTS. A dose of BW A444U that caused 97% mean twitch inhibition (0.12 mg/kg) showed minimal cardiovascular side effects. Signs of histamine release, however, were evident at doses as low as one and one-half times the ED_{95} (0.16 mg/kg). These included brief decreases in arterial pressure, slight increases in heart rate (Fig. 16-17), increased serum histamine levels, and brief facial flushing (35, 185).

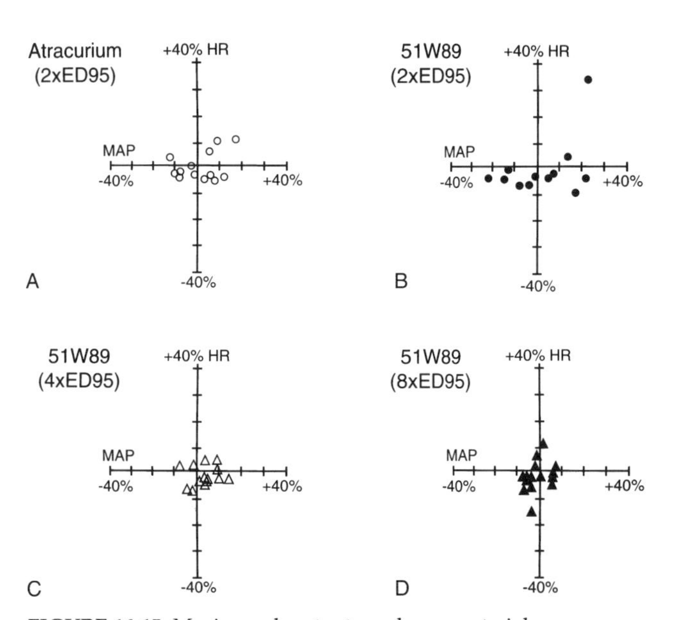

FIGURE 16-15. Maximum heart rate and mean arterial pressure changes in individual patients in the 5 minutes following administration of two times ED_{95} atracurium (A), two times ED_{95} cisatracurium (51W89) (B), four times ED_{95} cisatracurium (C), or eight times ED_{95} cisatracurium (D). No changes are attributable to histamine release.

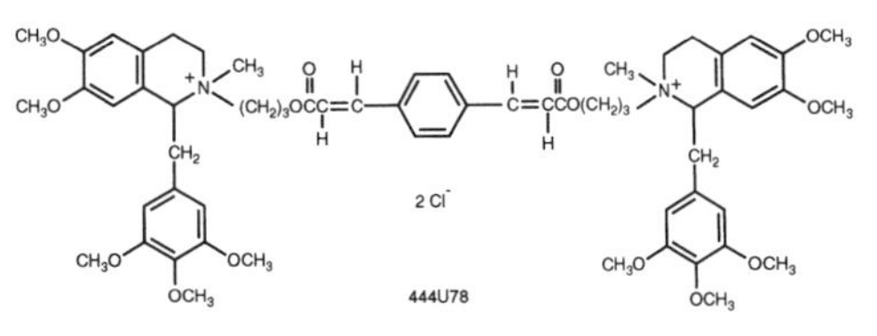

FIGURE 16-16. Chemical structure of BW A444U (444U78).

Short-acting Drugs

Mivacurium

BASIC PHARMACOLOGY. Mivacurium (Fig. 16-18) is a bis-benzylisoquinolinium disester and consists of a combination of three sterioisomers. It has a short duration of action and is a substrate for plasma cholinesterase.

CLINICAL PHARMACOLOGY. Mivacurium is a potent nondepolarizing muscle relaxant with an ED_{95} of 0.08 mg/kg in young adult patients receiving nitrous oxide-opioid anesthesia (74). Administration of 0.25 mg/kg of mivacurium, three times the ED_{95}, causes 100% neuromuscular block in 2 to 3 minutes (74), similar to the time required to develop maximal block with equipotent doses of atracurium and vecuronium. When mivacurium is used to facilitate endotracheal intubation, laryngoscopy should be started once fade is detectable in the train-of-four response. Because the onset of neuromuscular block occurs more rapidly in the muscles of the airway than in those of the extremities (188-193) (Fig. 16-19), one can expect good-to-excellent intubating conditions even in the presence of some response of the adductor pollicis to stimulation. The rapid metabolism of mivacurium may further shorten the time to peak effect at the diaphragm, making intubating conditions better than expected based on the adductor muscle twitch response (181). The ED_{95} of mivacurium is 0.08 mg/kg (74). In spite of its greater potency, however, its onset of action is fast because its rapid plasma clearance shortens the time to its maximal effect. Maximal twitch suppression in healthy persons receiving 0.15 to 0.25 mg/kg occurs within 3.3

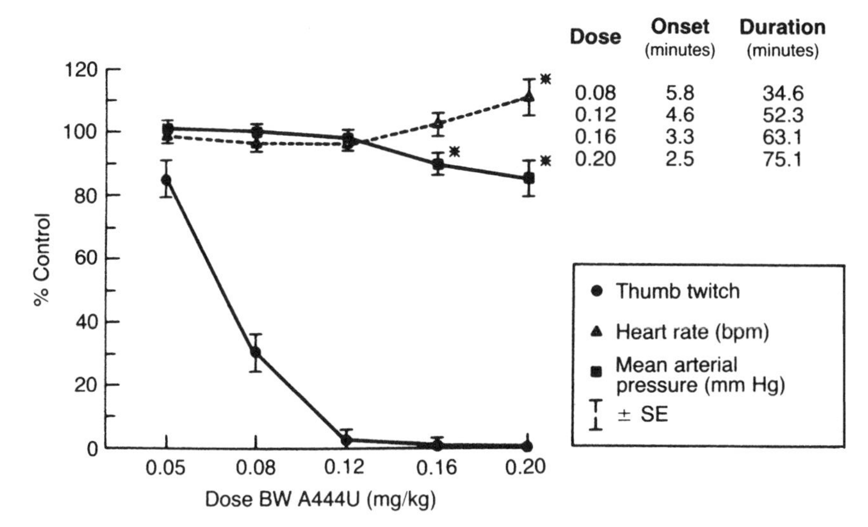

FIGURE 16-17. Effects of BW A444U on heart rate, mean arterial pressure, and twitch response of the adductor pollicis in patients. At 1.5 times ED_{95} (0.16 mg/kg), a significant decrease in mean arterial pressure and increase in heart rate occur, suggesting that histamine release is caused by this small dose of relaxant.

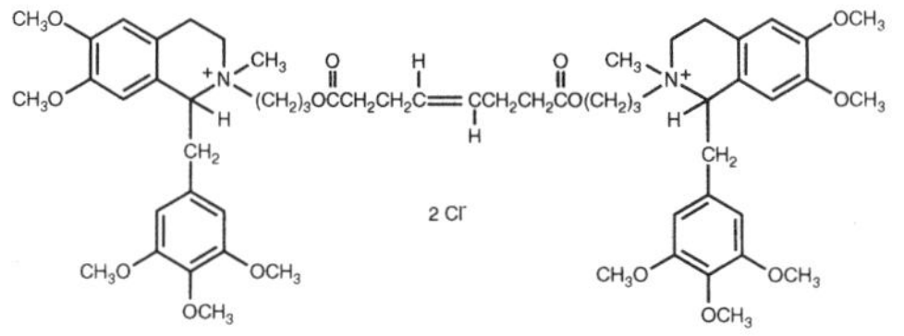

FIGURE 16-18. Chemical structure of mivacurium.

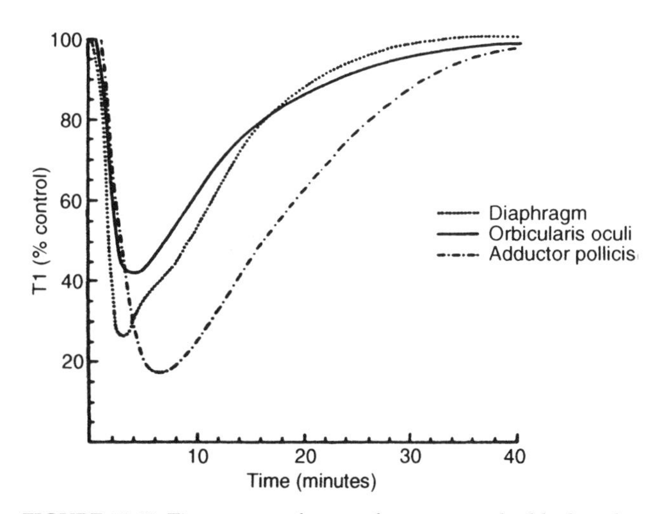

FIGURE 16-19. Time course of onset of neuromuscular block and recovery of neuromuscular function in the diaphragm, orbicularis oculi, and adductor pollicis as a function of time. The adductor pollicis lags behind both the diaphragm and the orbicularis oculi in terms of onset of block and spontaneous recovery of function. (19D) (Can J Anaesth 1988;35:552–558)

and 2.3 minutes (74). Administering the 0.25-mg/kg dose of mivacurium as a divided dose 30 seconds apart achieves good-to-excellent intubating conditions within 60 seconds (194). When the mivacurium dose is increased from 0.15 mg/kg (twice the ED_{95}) to 0.30 mg/kg (four times the ED_{95}), the onset time decreases from 3.3 to 1.9 minutes, with an increase in total duration of only 10 minutes (74). Following administration of three times the ED_{95} of mivacurium (0.25 mg/kg), 20 minutes are required for spontaneous recovery to 25% and 30 minutes for spontaneous recovery of 95% of baseline muscle strength (74). The slope of recovery from mivacurium-induced neuromuscular block is unaffected by either the total dose of drug administered or the duration of infusion of the relaxant. Once recovery begins, it follows the same pattern regardless of the number of bolus doses or the total dose infused (Fig. 16-20). The times required for recovery from 25 to 75% of baseline twitch response and 5 to 95% recovery baseline twitch response are 6.5 and 14 minutes, respectively, at all doses of the relaxant (74).

As a result of its short duration of action, mivacurium is well suited for administration as an infusion. Infusion rates of 5 to 15 μg/kg/min are required to maintain a stable 90 to 99% neuromuscular block. Because the drug is noncumulative, once the desired depth of neuromuscular block is achieved, further adjustments in the infusion rate should not be necessary. When mivacurium is administered by repeated boluses, doses of 0.05 to 0.1 mg/kg are required every 6 to 12 minutes. Recovery is slowed in the presence of volatile agents, as with other relaxants, especially after the long-term administration of mivacurium. Infusions of mivacurium, when titrated to maintain a 90% neuromuscular block, are potentiated by either isoflurane or halothane. One can expect that, over 90 minutes, at 1 MAC halothane, the mivacurium infusion rate will decrease by 37% and, at 1 MAC isoflurane, the mivacurium infusion rate will decrease 73% when a stable depth of neuromuscular block is maintained. This effect appears to be time dependent and is maximal at 90 minutes (139, 195).

CARDIOVASCULAR EFFECTS. Although mivacurium is free of autonomic effects, cardiovascular changes do occur following administration of large doses (23). Large doses of mivacurium administered rapidly

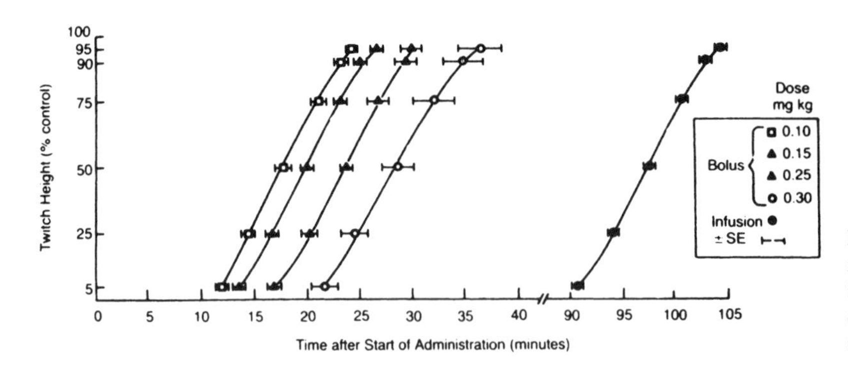

FIGURE 16-20. Spontaneous recovery curves following various doses of mivacurium. Recovery times of 5 to 95% are the same regardless of the dose of relaxant administered and average 13 to 14 minutes.

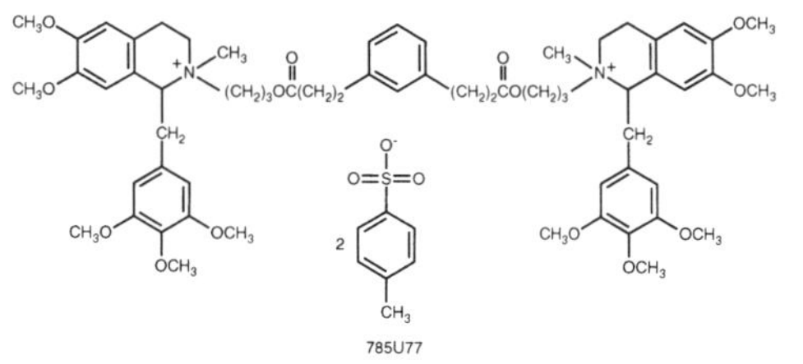

FIGURE 16-21. Chemical structure of BW 785U.

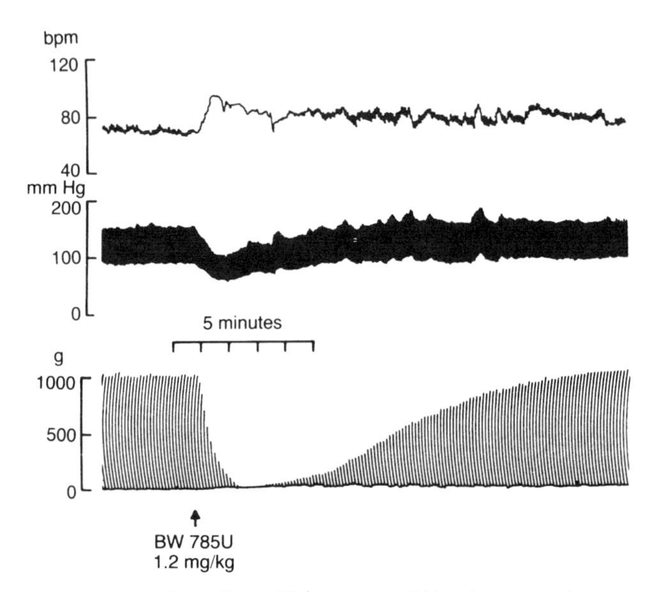

FIGURE 16-22. Recording of heart rate and blood pressure in a human subject receiving nitrous oxide-opioid-barbiturate anesthesia. The subject received 1.2 times ED_{95} of BW 785U, which caused a rapid onset of block (1.5 minutes) and recovery of neuromuscular function (12 minutes). This dose, however, also decreased arterial pressure and increased heart rate, probably because of histamine release.

cause hypotension and tachycardia secondary to histamine release (see Figs. 16-2 and 16-5). When three times the ED_{95} dose of mivacurium was given over 15 seconds, the plasma concentration of histamine increased 132% above baseline levels. However, when this same dose was injected over 1 minute, plasma histamine levels were unchanged (23). The histamine release response is dose related and occurs more frequently when the drug is given as a rapid intravenous bolus.

Ultrashort-acting Drugs

BW 785U

BASIC PHARMACOLOGY. BW 785U (Fig. 16-21) is an ultrashort-acting nondepolarizing muscle relaxant. It is a diester of m-phenylenedipropionic acid. Like mivacurium, it is metabolized by plasma cholinesterase (34). In animal studies, the duration of action of BW 785U was similar to that of succinylcholine. It is hydrolyzed by human plasma cholinesterase at 150% the rate of succinylcholine.

CLINICAL PHARMACOLOGY. The ED_{95} in humans is 0.8 to 1.0 mg/kg. In this dose range, the duration of action is short (10 to 15 minutes), and the onset is rapid (1 to 2 minutes). A similarly rapid recovery is observed when infusions of the drug are given. As with all nondepolarizing drugs, neuromuscular blockade produced by BW 785U can be antagonized by neostigmine. Detailed kinetic studies were not completed, other than the measurement of hydrolysis by plasma cholinesterase (34).

CARDIOVASCULAR EFFECTS. As promising as these characteristics appeared initially, further human studies were not completed because its cardiovascular side effects were too pronounced. This drug caused the most common side effect of the benzylisoquinoliniums, namely, histamine release (Fig. 16-22). At less than the ED_{95} for the drug, most subjects experienced elevations in heart rate, decreases in blood pressure, and facial erythema. Thus, a drug with exciting potential in terms of its kinetic profile was eliminated from clinical use (162).

In summary, benzylisoquinolinium-based neuromuscular blocking drugs are an established segment of our anesthetic practice. They are nondepolarizing relaxants that do not block the vagus nerve, nor do they cause blockade of sympathetic ganglia. Less potent and older compounds in the series, such as d-tubocurarine, readily cause histamine release at doses below the ED_{95} for neuromuscular blockade. Newer, more potent compounds, such as atracurium or mivacurium, may cause histamine release when doses larger than two or three times the ED_{95} are rapidly injected. Cisatracurium, the newest relaxant in this class, does not cause histamine release. The most striking feature of this class of blocking drugs is the opportunity to design short, intermediate, or long half-lives into the various compounds. This can be achieved by adjusting the rate of degradation or metabolism of the benzylisoquinolinium esters. Two routes of breakdown are available, namely, Hofmann elimination and plasma cholinesterase-catalyzed hydrolysis.

REFERENCES

1. King H. Curare alkaloids. I. Tubocurarine. J Chem Soc 1935; 1381–1387.
2. Bovet D. Some aspects of the relationship between chemical constitution and curare-like activity. Ann N Y Acad Sci 1951; 54:407–437.
3. Everett AJ, Lowe LA, Wilkinson A. Revision of the structures of (+)-tubocurarine chloride and (+)-chondrocurine. Chem Commun 1970;1020–1021.
4. Hughes R. Evaluation of the neuromuscular blocking properties and side-effects of the two new isoquinolinium bisquaternary compounds (BW252C64 and BW403C65). Br J Anaesth 1972;44:27–34.
5. Moss J, Rosow CE, Savarese JJ, et al. Role of histamine in the hypotensive action of d-tubocurarine in humans. Anesthesiology 1981;55:19–25.
6. Stenlake JB, Waigh RD, Dewar GH, et al. Biodegradable neuromuscular blocking agents. Part 4. Atracurium besylate and related polyalkylene di-esters. Eur J Med Chem 1981;16:515–521.
7. Martin-Smith M. Rational elements in the development of superior neuromuscular blocking agents. In: Ariens EJ, ed. Drug design. vol II. New York: Academic Press, 1971:453–540.
8. Stenlake JB. Atracurium: conception and inception. Br J Anaesth 1983;55:3S–10S.
9. Belmont MR, Wray DL, Maehr RB, et al. Comparative pharmacology of mivacurium isomers in cats [Abstract]. Anesthesiology 1991;75 (suppl):A773.
10. Maehr RB, Belmont MR, Wray DL, et al. Autonomic and neuromuscular effects of mivacurium and its isomers in cats [Abstract]. Anesthesiology 1991;75 (suppl):A772.
11. Maehr RB, Wastila WB. Comparative pharmacology of atracurium and six isomers in cats [Abstract]. Anesthesiology 1993; 79 (suppl):A950.
12. Belmont MR, Lien CA, Quessy S, et al. The clinical neuromuscular pharmacology of 51W89 in patients receiving nitrous oxide/opioid/barbiturate anesthesia. Anesthesiology 1995; 82:1139–1145.
13. Scott RPF. Autonomic and cardiovascular effects of neuromuscular blocking drugs. Curr Opin Anaesthesiol 1992;5:568–571.
14. Scott RPF, Belmont MR, Savarese JJ. Cardiovascular and autonomic effects of neuromuscular blocking drugs. In: Kaplan J, ed. Cardiac anesthesia. Philadelphia: Grune & Stratton, 1992.
15. Marshall RJ. Cardiovascular effects of neuromuscular blocking drugs. Curr Opin Anaesth 1991;4:599–602.
16. Hughes R, Chapple DJ. Cardiovascular and neuromuscular effects of dimethyl tubocurarine in anaesthetized cats and rhesus monkeys. Br J Anaesth 1976;48:847–852.
17. Hughes R, Chapple DJ. Effects of non-depolarizing neuromuscular blocking agents on peripheral autonomic mechanisms in cats. Br J Anaesth 1976;48:59–68.
18. Savarese JJ. The autonomic margins of safety of metocurine and d-tubocurarine in the cat. Anesthesiology 1979;50:40–46.
19. Basta SJ. Modulation of histamine release by neuromuscular-blocking drugs. Curr Opin Anaesth 1992, 5:572–576.
20. Dyer J, Warren K, Merlin S, et al. Measurement of plasma histamine: Description of an improved method and normal values. J Allergy Clin Immunol 1982;70:82–87.
21. Moss J, Rosow CE. Histamine release by narcotics and muscle relaxants in humans. Anesthesiology 1983;59:330–339.
22. Basta SJ, Savarese JJ, Ali HH, et al. Histamine-releasing potencies of atracurium, dimethyl-tubocurarine, and tubocurarine [Abstract]. Br J Anaesth 1983;55:105S.
23. Savarese JJ, Ali HH, Basta SJ, et al. The cardiovascular effects of mivacurium chloride (BW B1090U) in patients receiving nitrous oxide-opiate-barbiturate anesthesia. Anesthesiology 1989; 90:386–394.
24. Savarese JJ, Wastila WB. Current research in relaxant development. Semin Anaesth 1986;5:304–311.
25. Stoops CM, Curtis CA, Kovach DA, et al. Hemodynamic effects of mivacurium chloride administered to patients during oxygen-sufentanil anesthesia for coronary artery bypass grafting or valve replacement. Anesth Analg 1989;68:333.
26. Hatano Y, Arai T, Noda J, et al. Contribution of prostacyclin to d-tubocurarine-induced hypotension in humans. Anesthesiology 1990;72:28–32.
27. Savarese JJ, Ali HH, Antonio RP. The clinical pharmacology of metocurine: dimethyltubocurarine revisited. Anesthesiology 1977;47:277–284.
28. Scott RPF, Savarese JJ, Basta SJ, et al. Clinical pharmacology of atracurium given in high dose. Br J Anaesth 1986;58:834–838.
29. Basta SJ, Ali HH, Savarese JJ, et al. Clinical pharmacology of atracurium besylate (BW33A): a new non-depolarizing muscle relaxant. Anesth Analg 1982;61:723–729.
30. Basta SJ, Savarese JJ, Ali HH, et al. Clinical pharmacology of doxacurium chloride: a new long-acting nondepolarizing muscle relaxant. Anesthesiology 1988;69:478–486.
31. Murray DJ, Mehta MP, Choi WW, et al. The neuromuscular blocking and cardiovascular effects of doxacurium chloride in patients receiving nitrous oxide narcotic anesthesia. Anesthesiology 1988;69:472–477.
32. Stoops CM, Curtis CA, Kovach DA, et al. Hemodynamic effects of doxacurium chloride in patients receiving oxygen-sufentanil anesthesia for coronary artery bypass or valve replacement. Anesthesiology 1988;69:365–370.
33. Lien CA, Belmont MR, Abalos A, et al. The cardiovascular effects and histamine-releasing properties of 51W89 in patients receiving nitrous oxide/opioid/barbiturate anesthesia. Anesthesiology 1995;82:1131–1138.
34. Savarese JJ, Wastila WB. Pharmacology of BW 785U, a short-acting nondepolarizing ester neuromuscular blocking agent [Abstract]. Anesthesiology 1979;51 (suppl):S278.
35. Savarese JJ, Ali HH, Basta SJ, et al. The clinical pharmacology of BWA 444U: a nondepolarizing ester relaxant of intermediate duration. Anesthesiology 1983;58:333–341.
36. Scott RPF, Savarese JJ, Basta SJ, et al. Atracurium: clinical strategies for preventing histamine release and attenuating the hemodynamic response [Abstract]. Anesthesiology 1984; 61:A287.
37. Powers D, Simpson K, Morici M, et al. The hemodynamic effects of mivacurium chloride in patients undergoing coronary artery bypass graft during fentanyl/valium anesthesia [Abstract]. Anesthesiology 1988;69:A530.
38. Choi WW, Mehta MP, Murray DJ, et al. Neuromuscular and cardiovascular effects of mivacurium chloride in surgical patients receiving nitrous oxide-narcotic or nitrous oxide-isoflurane anaesthesia. Can J Anaesth 1989;36:641–650.
39. From RP, Pearson KS, Choi WW, et al. Neuromuscular and cardiovascular effects of mivacurium chloride (BW B1090U)

during nitrous oxide-fentanyl-thiopentane and, nitrous oxide-halothane anaesthesia. Br J Anaesth 1990;64:193–198.
40. Merrett RA, Thompson CW, Webb FW. In vitro degradation of atracurium in human plasma. Br J Anaesth 1983;55:61–66.
41. Flynn PJ, Hughes R, Walton B. Use of atracurium in cardiac surgery involving cardiopulmonary bypass with induced hypothermia. Br J Anaesth 1984;56:967–972.
42. Hughes R, Chapple DJ. The pharmacology of atracurium: a new competitive neuromuscular blocking agent. Br J Anaesth 1981; 53:31–44.
43. Cook DR, Freeman JA, Lai AA, et al. Pharmacokinetics and pharmacodynamics of doxacurium in normal patients and in those with hepatic or renal failure. Anesth Analg 1991;72:145–150.
44. Savarese JJ, Wastila WB, El-Sayad HA, et al. Some aspects of the basic and clinical pharmacology of mivacurium (BW B1090U) and doxacurium (BW A938U): a preliminary report. In: Jones RM, Payne JP, eds. Recent development in muscle relaxation: atracurium in perspective. London: Royal Society of Medicine Services International Congress and Symposium Series No. 131, 1988.
45. Matteo RS, Brotherton WP, Nishitateno K, et al. Pharmacodynamics and pharmacokinetics of metocurine in humans: comparison to d-tubocurarine. Anesthesiology 1982;57:183–190.
46. Miller RD, Matteo RS, Benet LZ, Sohn YJ. The pharmacokinetics of tubocurarine in man with and without renal failure. J Pharmacol Exp Ther 1977;202:1–7.
47. Sheiner LB, Stanski DR, Vozeh S, et al. Simultaneous modeling of pharmacokinetics and pharmacodynamics: application to d-tubocurarine. Clin Pharmacol Ther 1979;25:358.
48. Brotherton WP, Matteo RS. Pharmacokinetics and pharmacodynamics of metocurine in humans with and without renal failure. Anesthesiology 1981;55:273.
49. Chapple DJ, Clark JS. Pharmacologic action of breakdown products of atracurium and related substances. Br J Anaesth 1983;55:115.
50. Stiller RL, Cook DR, Chakravorti S. In vitro degradation of atracurium in human plasma. Anesth Analg 1985;64:289.
51. Stiller RL, Cook DR, Chakravorti S. In vitro degradation of atracurium in human plasma. Br J Anaesthesia 1985;57:1085–1088.
52. Cook DR, Stiller R, Ingram M. In vitro degradation of atracurium. Anesth Analg 1986;65:543.
53. Nigrovic V, Pandya JB, Auen M, et al. Inactivation of atracurium in human and rat plasma. Anesth Analg 1985;64:1047–1052.
54. Fisher DM, Canfell PC, Fahey MR, et al. Elimination of atracurium in humans: contributions of Hofmann elimination and ester hydrolysis versus organ-based elimination. Anesthesiology 1985;65:6–12.
55. Ward S, Weatherley BC. Pharmacokinetics of atracurium and its metabolites. Br J Anaesth 1986;58:6S–10S.
56. Ward S, Boheimer N, Weatherley BC, et al. Pharmacokinetics of atracurium and its metabolites in patients with normal renal function, and in patients with renal failure. Br J Anaesth 1987; 59:697–706.
57. deBros FM, Lai A, Scott R, et al. Pharmacokinetics and pharmacodynamics of atracurium during isoflurane anesthesia in normal and anephric patients. Anesth Analg 1986;65:743–746.
58. Fahey MR, Rupp SM, Fisher DM, et al. The pharmacokinetics and pharmacodynamics of atracurium in patients with and without renal failure. Anesthesiology 1984;61:699–702.
59. Ward S, Neill EAM, Weatherly BC, Corall IM. Pharmacokinetics of atracurium besylate in healthy patients (after a single IV bolus dose). Br J Anaesth 1983;55:113–117.
60. Donati F, Gill SS, Bevan DR, et al. Pharmacokinetics and pharmacodynamics of atracurium with and without previous suxamethonium administration. Br J Anaesth 1991;66:557–561.
61. Tsui D, Graham GG, Torda TA. The pharmacokinetics of atracurium isomers in vitro and in humans. Anesthesiology 1987; 67:722–728.
62. Lanier WL, Milde JH, Michenfelder JD. The cerebral effects of pancuronium and atracurium in halothane anesthetized dogs. Anesthesiology 1985;63:589–597.
63. Shi W, Fahey MR, Fisher DM, et al. Laudanosine (a metabolite of atracurium) increases the MAC of halothane in rabbits Anesthesiology 1985;63:584–588.
64. Chapple DJ, Miller AA, Ward JB, Wheatley PL. Cardiovascular and neurological effects of laudanosine. Br J Anesth 1987; 59:218–225.
65. Shi WZ, Fahey MR, Fisher DM, Miller RD. Modification of central nervous system effects of laudanosine by inhalational anaesthetics. Br J Anaesth 1989;63:598–600.
66. Canfell PC, Castagnoli N, Fahey MR, et al. The metabolic disposition of laudanosine in dog, rabbit, and man. Drug Metab Dispos Biol Fate Chem 1986;14:703.
67. Yate PM, Flynn PJ, Arnold RW, et al. Clinical experience and plasma laudanosine concentrations during the infusion of atracurium in the intensive therapy unit. Br J Anaesth 1987;59:211.
68. Beemer GH, Bjorksten AR, Dawson PJ, et al. Production of laudanosine following infusion of atracurium in man and its effect on awakening. Br J Anaesth 1989;63:26.
69. Welch R, Brown A, Dahl R. In vitro degradation of cisatracurium in Sorensen buffer, rat, and human plasma. Clin Pharmacol Ther 1995;58:132–134.
70. Lien CA, Schmith VD, Belmont MR, et al. Pharmacokinetics of cisatracurium in patients receiving nitrous oxide/opioid/barbiturate anesthesia. Anesthesiology 1996;84:300–308.
71. Lien CA, Schmith VD, Embree PB, et al. The pharmacokinetics and pharmacodynamics of the stereoisomers of mivacurium in patients receiving nitrous oxide/opioid/barbiturate anesthesia. Anesthesiology 1994;80:1296–1302.
72. deBros F, Goudsouzian N, Chakravorty S, et al. Pharmacokinetic evaluation of the *cis-cis* isomer, alcohol and ester metabolites of mivacurium during prolonged infusions in neurosurgical patients [Abstract]. Anesthesiology 1994;81:A1085.
73. Cook RD, Stiller RL, Weakly JN, et al. In vitro metabolism of mivacurium chloride (BW B1090U) and succinylcholine. Anesth Analg 1989;68:452–456.
74. Savarese JJ, Ali HH, Basta SJ, et al. The clinical neuromuscular pharmacology of mivacurium chloride (BW B1090U): a short acting nondepolarizing ester neuromuscular blocking drug. Anesthesiology 1988;68:723–732.
75. Östergaard D, Jensen FS, Jensen E, et al. Influence of plasma cholinesterase activity on recovery from mivacurium-induced neuromuscular blockade in phenotypically normal patients. Acta Anaesth Scand 1992;36:702–706.
76. Hart PS, McCarthy GJ, Brown R, et al. The effect of plasma cholinesterase activity on mivacurium infusion rates. Anesth Analg 1995;80:760–763.
77. Naguib M, Daoud W, El-Gammal M, et al. Enzymatic antagonism of mivacurium-induced neuromuscular blockade by human plasma cholinesterase. Anesthesiology 1995;83:694–701.
78. Kelly SS, Robert DV. The effect of age on the safety factor in neuromuscular transmission in the isolated rat diaphragm. Br J Anaesth 1977;149:271.
79. Goudsouzian NG. Maturation of neuromuscular transmission in the infant. Br J Anaesth 1980;52:205.
80. Fisher DM, O'Keefe C, Stanski DR, et al. Pharmacokinetics and pharmacodynamics of d-tubocurarine in infants, children and adults. Anesthesiology 1982;57:203.
81. Goudsouzian NG, Alifimoff JK, Liu LM, et al. Neuromuscular and cardiovascular effects of doxacurium in children anesthetized with halothane. Br. J Anaesth 1989;62:263–268.
82. Sarner JB, Brandom BW, Cook DR, et al. Clinical pharmacology of doxacurium chloride (BWA938U) in children. Anesth Analg 1988;67:303–306.

83. Brandom BW, Rudd GD, Cook DR. Clinical pharmacology of atracurium in paediatric patients. Br J Anaesth 1983;55:117S–121S.
84. Brandom BW, Woelfel SK, Cook DR, et al. Clinical pharmacology of atracurium in infants. Anesth Analg 1984;63:309.
85. Goudsouzian NG, Liu LMP, Gionfriddo M, Rudd GD. Safety and efficacy of atracurium in adolescents and children anesthetized with halothane. Anesthesiology 1985;62:75.
86. Meretoja OA, Kalli I. Spontaneous recovery of neuromuscular function after atracurium in infants. Anesth Analg 1986; 65:1042.
87. Fisher DM, Canfell PC, Spellman MJ, Miller RD. Pharmacokinetics and pharmacodynamics of atracurium in infants and children. Anesthesiology 1990;73:33–37.
88. Goudsouzian NG, Martyn J, Rudd GD, et al. Continuous infusion of atracurium in children. Anesthesiology 1986;64:171–174.
89. Meretoja OA, Taivainen T, Wirtavouri K. Pharmacodynamic effects of 51W89, an isomer of atracurium, in children during halothane anaesthesia. Br J Anaesth 1995;74:6–11.
90. Brandom BW, Woelfel SK, Gronert BJ, et al. Effects of 51W89 (cisatracurium) in children during halothane nitrous oxide anesthesia. Anesthesiology 1995;83:A921.
91. Goudsouzian NG, Alifimoff JK, Eberly D, et al. Neuromuscular and cardiovascular effects of mivacurium in children. Anesthesiology 1989;70:237–42.
92. Sarner JB, Brandom BW, Woelfel SK, et al. Clinical pharmacology of mivacurium chloride (BW1090U) in children during nitrous oxide-halothane and nitrous oxide-narcotic anesthesia. Anesth Analg 1989;68:116–121.
93. Alifimoff JK, Goudsouzian NG. Continuous infusion of mivacurium in children. Br J Anaesth 1989;63:520–524.
94. Brandom BW, Sarner JB, Woelfel SK, et al. Mivacurium infusion requirements in pediatric surgical patients during nitrous oxide-halothane and during nitrous oxide-narcotic anesthesia. Anesth Analg 1990;71:16–22.
95. Frolkis VV, Martynenko OA, Zamostyan VP. Aging of the neuromuscular apparatus. Gerontology 1976;22:244–279.
96. Matteo RS, Backus WW, McDaniel DD, et al. Pharmacokinetics and pharmacodynamics of d-tubocurarine and metocurine in the elderly. Anesth Analg 1985;64:23–29.
97. Dresner DL, Basta SJ, Ali HH, et al. Pharmacokinetics and pharmacodynamics of doxacurium in young and elderly patients during isoflurane anesthesia. Anesth Analg 1990;71;498.
98. D'Hollander AA, Luyckx C, Barvais L, et al. Clinical evaluation of atracurium besylate requirement for a stable muscle relaxation during surgery: Lack of age-related effects. Anesthesiology 1983;59:237–240.
99. Kitts JB, Fisher DM, Canfell PC, et al. Pharmacokinetics and pharmacodynamics of atracurium in the elderly. Anesthesiology 1990;72:272–275.
100. Kisor D, Wargin W, Weatherly B, et al. Organ-independent Hofmann elimination is the major clearance pathway of the neuromuscular blocking agent 51W89 in man. Pharm Res 1994; 11:S335.
101. Ornstein E, Lien CA, Matteo RS, et al. Pharmacodynamics and pharmacokinetics of 51W89 in geriatric surgical patients. Anesthesiology 1994;81:A1075.
102. Basta SJ, Dresner DL, Schaff LP, et al. Neuromuscular effects and pharmacokinetics of mivacurium in elderly patients under isoflurane anesthesia. Anesth Analg 1989;68:S18.
103. Maddineni VR, Mirakhur RK, McCoy EP, Sharpe TDE. Neuromuscular and haemodynamic effects of mivacurium in elderly and young adult patients. Br J Anaesth 1994;73:608–612.
104. Rierdan DD, Gilbertson AA. Prolonged curarization in a patient with renal failure. Br J Anaesth 1971;43:506–508.
105. Matteo RS, Pau EK, Horowitz PE, Spector S. Urinary excretion of *d*-tubocurarine in man: effect of osmotic diuretic. In: Abstracts of Scientific Papers, American Society of Anesthesia, 1975:211–212.
106. Meijer DKF, Weitering JG, Vermeer GA, et al. Comparative pharmacokinetics of *d*-tubocurarine and metocurine in man. Anesthesiology 1979;51:402–407.
107. Cashman JN, Luke JJ, Jones RM. Neuromuscular block with doxacurium (BWA938U) in patients with normal or absent renal function. Br J Anaesth 1990;64:186–192.
108. Griffiths RB, Hunter JM, Jones RS. Atracurium infusions in patients with renal failure on an ITU. Anaesthesia 1986;41:375–381.
109. Kisor DF, Schmith VD, Wargin WA, et al. Importance of organ-independent elimination of cisatracurium. Anesth Analg (in press).
110. Boyd AH, Eastwood NB, Parker CJR, Hunter JM. Pharmacodynamics of the 1R*cis*-1'R*cis* isomer of atracurium (51W89) in health and chronic renal failure. Br J Anaesth 1995;74:400–404.
111. Eastwood NB, Boyd AH, Parker CJR, Hunter JM. Pharmacokinetics of 1R*cis*-1'R*cis* atracurium besylate (51W89) and plasma laudanosine concentrations in health and chronic renal failure. Br J Anaesth 1995;75:431–435.
112. Phillips BJ, Hunter JM. Use of mivacurium chloride by constant infusion in the anephric patient. Br J Anaesth 1992;68:492–498.
113. Mangar D, Kirchhoff GT, Rose PL, Castellano FC. Prolonged neuromuscular block after mivacurium in a patient with end-stage renal disease. Anesth Analg 1993;76:866–867.
114. Cook DR, Freeman JA, Lai AA, et al. Pharmacokinetics of mivacurium in normal patients and in those with hepatic or renal failure. Br J Anaesth 1992;69:580–585.
115. Ryan DW. Preoperative serum cholinesterase concentration in chronic renal failure: clinical experience of suxamethonium in 81 patients undergoing renal transplant. Br J Anaesth 1977; 49:945–949.
116. Thomas JL, Holmes JH. Effect of hemodialysis on plasma cholinesterase. Anesth Analg 1970;49:323–325.
117. Ward S, Neill EAM. Pharmacokinetics of atracurium in acute hepatic failure (with acute renal failure). Br J Anaesth 1983; 55:1169–1172.
118. Tullock W, Scott V, Smith DA, et al. Kinetics/dynamics of 51W89 in liver transplant patients and in healthy patients. Anesthesiology 1994;81:A1076.
119. Head-Rapson AG, Devlin JC, Parker JCR, Hunter JM. Pharmacokinetics of the three isomers of mivacurium and pharmacodynamics of the chiral mixture in hepatic cirrhosis. Br J Anaesth 1994;73:613–618.
120. Weatherly BC, Williams SG, Niell EAM. Pharmacokinetics, pharmacodynamics and dose-response relationships of atracurium administered I.V. Br J Anaesth 1983:55;39S–45S.
121. Lee C. Train-of-four quantitation of competitive neuromuscular block. Anesth Analg 1975;54:649–653.
122. Belmont M, Lien C, Abalos A, Savarese J. The accuracy of the 10-25% (T_2-T_4) twitch recovery interval in predicting the speed of spontaneous recovery from mivacurium-induced neuromuscular blockade. Anesthesiology 1995;83:A889.
123. Östergaard D, Jensen FS, Jensen E, et al. Mivacurium-induced neuromuscular blockade in patients with atypical plasma cholinesterase. Acta Anaesthesiol Scand 1993;37:314–318.
124. Bevan DR. Prolonged mivacurium-induced neuromuscular block. Anesth Analg 1993;77:4–6.
125. Östergaard D, Jensen FS, Viby-Mogensen J. Reversal of intense mivacurium block with human plasma cholinesterase in patients with atypical plasma cholinesterase. Anesthesiology 1995;82:1295–1298.
126. Maddineni VR, Mirakhur RK. Prolonged neuromuscular block following mivacurium. Anesthesiology 1993;78:1181–1184.
127. Petersen RS, Bailey PL, Kalameghan R, Ashwood ER. Prolonged neuromuscular block after mivacurium. Anesth Analg 1993;76:194–196.

128. Goudsouzian NG, d'Hollander AA, Viby-Mogensen J. Prolonged neuromuscular block from mivacurium in two patients with cholinesterase deficiency. Anesth Analg 1993;77:183–185.
129. Viby-Mogensen J. Succinylcholine neuromuscular blockade in subjects homozygous for atypical plasma cholinesterase. Anesthesiology 1981;55:429–434.
130. Cook DR, Chakravorti S, Brandom BW, Stiller RL. Effects of neostigmine, edrophonium and succinylcholine on the in vitro metabolism of mivacurium: clinical correlates. Anesthesiology 1992;77:A948.
131. Szenohradszky J, Lau M, Brown R, et al. The effect of neostigmine on twitch tension and muscle relaxant concentration during infusion of mivacurium or vecuronium. Anesthesiology 1995;83:83–87.
132. Kao YJ, Le N, Barker SJ. Neostigmine prolongs profound neuromuscular blockade induced by mivacurium in surgical patients [Abstract]. Anesthesiology 1993;79 (suppl):A929.
133. Naguib M, Abdulatif M, Al-Ghamdi A, et al. Dose-response relationships for edrophonium and neostigmine antagonism of mivacurium-induced neuromuscular block. Br J Anaesth 1993; 71:709–714.
134. Bryson GL, Kitts LB, Miller DR, et al. Edrophonium requirements for reversal of neuromuscular block following infusion of mivacurium [Abstract]. Can J Anaesth 1994;41:A4B.
135. Goldhill DR, Whitehead JP, Emmot RS, et al. Neuromuscular and clinical effects of mivacurium chloride in healthy adult patients during nitrous oxide-enflurane anaesthesia. Br J Anaesth 1991;67:289–295.
136. Caldwell JE, Heier T, Kitts JB, et al. Comparison of the neuromuscular block induced by mivacurium, suxamethonium or atracurium during nitrous oxide-fentanyl anaesthesia. Br J Anaesth 1989;63:393–399.
137. Hart PS, Wright PMC, Brown R, et al. Edrophonium increases mivacurium concentrations during constant mivacurium infusion, and large doses minimally antagonize paralysis. Anesthesiology 1995;82:912–918.
138. Kopman AF, Mallhi MU, Justo MD, et al. Antagonism of mivacurium-induced neuromuscular blockade in humans: edrophonium dose requirements at threshold train-of-four count of 4. Anesthesiology 1994;81:1394–1400.
139. Ali HH, Savarese JJ, Embree PB, et al. Clinical pharmacology of mivacurium chloride (BW B1090U) infusion: comparison with vecuronium and atracurium. Br J Anaesth 1988;61:541–546.
140. Lien CA, Belmont MR, Wray DL, et al. Pharmacokinetics and dynamics of mivacurium during spontaneous and anticholinesterase-facilitated recovery. Anesthesiology 83:1995;A896.
141. Bownes PB, Hartman GS, Chiscolm D, et al. Antagonism of mivacurium blockade by purified human butyryl cholinesterase in cats. Anesthesiology 1992;77:A909.
142. Lebowitz PW, Ramsey FM, Savarese JJ, Ali HH. Potentiation of neuromuscular blockade in man produced by combinations of pancuronium and metocurine or pancuronium and d-tubocurarine. Anesth Analg 1980;59:604–609.
143. Bowman WC, Prior C, Marshall IG. Presynaptic receptors in the neuromuscular junction. Ann N Y Acad Sci 1990;604:69–81.
144. Waud BE, Waud DR. Interaction among agents that block endplate depolarization competitively. Anesthesiology 1985;63: 4–15.
145. Sine SM. Molecular dissection of subunit interfaces in acetylcholine receptor: identification of residues that determine curare selectivity. Proc Natl Acad Sci U S A 1993;90:9436–9440.
146. Martyn JAJ, Leibel WS, Matteo RS. Competitive nonspecific binding does not explain the potentiating effects of muscle relaxants combinations. Anesth Analg 1983;63:160–163.
147. Erkola O, Rautoma P, Meretoja OA. Interaction between mivacurium and succinylcholine. Anesth Analg 1995;80:534–537.
148. Poler SM, Watcha MF, White PF. Use of mivacurium as an alternative to succinylcholine during outpatient laparoscopy. J Clin Anesth 1992;4:127–133.
149. Tang J, Joshi GP, White PF. Comparison of rocuronium and mivacurium to succinylcholine during outpatient laparoscopic surgery. Anesth Analg 1996;82:994–998.
150. Kim DW, Joshi G, Johnson E, White PF. Interactions between mivacurium, rocuronium and vecuronium during balanced anesthesia. Anesth Analg 1996.
151. Smith I, White PF. Pipecuronium-induced potentiation of vecuronium. Anesth Analg 1992;74:S299.
152. Naguib M, Abdulatif M, Al-Ghamdi A, et al. Interactions between mivacurium and atracurium. Br J Anaesth 1994;73:484–489.
153. Jalkanen L, Meretoja OA, Taivainen T, et al. Synergism between atracurium and mivacurium compared with that between vecuronium and mivacurium. Anesth Analg 1994;79:998–1002.
154. Meretoja OA, Brandom BW, Taivainen T, Jalkanen L. Synergism between atracurium and vecuronium in children. Br J Anaesth 1993;71:440–442.
155. Goudsouzian NG, Denman W, Matta E. Mivacurium after atracurium in children. Anesth Analg 1994;79:345–349.
156. Naguib M. Neuromuscular effects of rocuronium bromide and mivacurium chloride administered alone and in combination. Anesth Analg 1994;81:388–395.
157. Meretoja OA, Taivainen T, Jalkanen L, Wirtavuori K. Synergism between atracurium and vecuronium in infants and children during nitrous oxide-oxygen-alfentanil anaesthesia. Br J Anaesth 1994;73:605–607.
158. Whalley DG, Lewis B, Bedocs NM. Recovery of neuromuscular function after atracurium and pancuronium maintenance of pancuronium block. Can J Anaesth 1994;41:31–35.
159. Herschman Z, Pamaar CG. Prolonged neuromuscular blockade when mivacurium and pancuronium were administered in series. Clin Toxicol 1995;33:271–272.
160. Brandom BW, Meretoja OA, Taivainen T, Wirtavuori K. Accelerated onset and delayed recovery of neuromuscular block induced by mivacurium preceded by pancuronium in children. Anesth Analg 1993;76:998–1003.
161. Belmont MR, Maehr RB, Wastila WB, Savarese JJ. Pharmacodynamics and pharmacokinetics of benzylisoquinolinium (curare-like) neuromuscular blocking drugs. Anesth Clin North Am 1993;11:251–281.
162. Savarese JJ, Miller RD, Lien CA, Caldwell JE. Pharmacology of muscle relaxants and their antagonism. In: Miller RD, ed. Anesthesia. 4th ed. New York: Churchill Livingstone,1994:417–487.
163. Durant NN, Bowman WC, Marshall IG. A comparison of the neuromuscular and autonomic blocking activities of (+)-tubocurarine and its N-methyl and O, O, N-trimethyl analogues. Eur J Pharmacol 1977;46:297–302.
164. Stoelting RK. Hemodynamic effects of dimethyltubocurarine during nitrous oxide-halothane anesthesia. Anesth Analg 1974; 53:513–515.
165. Stoelting RK. The hemodynamic effects of pancuronium and *d*-tubocurarine in anesthetized patients. Anesthesiology 1972; 36:612–615.
166. Collier HOJ, Hall RA. Pharmacology of d-o-o-dimethyl tubocurarine iodide in relation to its clinical use. Br Med J 1950; 1:1293–1295.
167. Stoelting VK, Graf JP, Vieira Z. Dimethyl ether of *d*-tubocurarine iodide as an adjunct to anesthesia. Proc Soc Exp Biol Med 1948;69:565–566.
168. Wilson HB, Gordon HE, Raffan AW. Dimethyl ether of *d*-tubocurarine iodide as a curarising agent in anaesthesia for thoracic surgery. Br Med J 1950;1:1296–1301.

169. Basta SJ, Savarese JJ, Ali HH, et al. Neuromuscular and cardiovascular effects in patients of BW A938U: a new long-acting neuromuscular blocking agent. Anesthesiology 1986;65:A281.
170. Bowman WC, Rodger IW, Houston J, et al. Structure: action relationships among some desacetoxy analogues of pancuronium and vecuronium in the anesthetized cat. Anesthesiology 1988;69:57–86.
171. Kopman AF. Gallamine, pancuronium and d-tubocurarine compared: is onset time related to drug potency? Anesthesiology 1989;70:915–520.
172. Lien CA, Matteo RS, Ornstein E, et al. Neostigmine antagonism of doxacurium or pancuronium blockade under isoflurane [Abstract]. Anesthesiology 1992;77:A959.
173. Emmot RS, Bracey BJ, Goldhill DR, et al. Cardiovascular effects of doxacurium, pancuronium, and vecuronium in anesthetized patients presenting for coronary artery bypass surgery. Br J Anaesth 1990;65:480–486.
174. Engback J, Östergaard D, Skovgaard LT, Viby-Mogensen J. Reversal of intense neuromuscular blockade following infusion of atracurium. Anesthesiology 1990;72:803–806.
175. Hosking MP, Lennon RL, Gronert GA. Combined H_1 and H_2 receptor blockade attenuates the cardiovascular effects of high-dose atracurium for rapid sequence endotracheal intubation. Anesth Analg 1988;67:1089–1093.
176. Scott RPF, Savarese JJ, Basta SJ, et al. Atracurium: clinical strategies for preventing histamine release and attenuating the hemodynamic response. Br J Anaesth 1985;57:550–555.
177. Fisher DM, Rosen JI. A pharmacokinetic explanation for increasing recovery time following larger or repeated doses of nondepolarizing muscle relaxants. Anesth Analg 1986;65:286–291.
178. Lien CA, Pavlin EG, Belmont MR, et al. A two-center study to evaluate cisatracurium (51W89) for tracheal intubation in patients receiving propofol or thiopental anesthesia. Anesth Analg 1995;83:A925.
179. Schmautz E, Deriaz M, Vrillon A, Lienhart A. Evaluation of 51W89 for endotracheal intubation in surgical patients during N_2O/O_2/propofol anesthesia. Anesth Analg 1994;81:A1081.
180. Stout RG, Belmont MR, Pavlin EG, et al. Evaluation of intubation at 90 and 120 seconds following 51W89 administration. Anesth Analg 1994;81:A1078.
181. Kopman A. Nondepolarizing relaxants: new concepts and new drugs. J Clin Anesth 1993;5 (suppl 1):395–455.
182. Lien CA, Schmith VD, Belmont MR, et al. Pharmacokinetics of 51W89 in patients receiving nitrous oxide-opioid-barbiturate anesthesia. Anesthesiology 1995;83:300–308.
183. Prielipp RC, Coursin DB, Scuderi PE, et al. Comparison of the infusion requirements and recovery profiles of vecuronium and cisatracurium 51W89 in intensive care unit patients. Anesth Analg 1995;81:3–12.
184. Reich DL, Konstadt SN, Stanley TE, et al. A two-center study of the cardiovascular effects of 51W89 in patients with coronary artery disease. Anesth Analg 1995;80:S393.
185. Savarese JJ, Basta SJ, Ali HH, et al. Clinical neuromuscular pharmacology of BW A444U. Anesthesiology 1981;55:A197.
186. Östergaard D, Jensen E, Jensen FS, Viby-Mogensen J. The duration of action of mivacurium-induced neuromuscular block in patients homozygous for the atypical plasma cholinesterase gene. Anesthesiology 1991;75:A774.
187. Östergaard D, Jensen E, Jensen FS, Viby-Mogensen J. Mivacurium-induced neuromuscular blockade in patients heterozygous for the atypical gene for plasma cholinesterase. Anesthesiology 1989;71:A782.
188. Plaud B, Legueau F, Debaene B, et al. Mivacurium neuromuscular blockade at the adductor muscles of the larynx and adductor pollicis in man. Anesthesiology 1992;77:A908.
189. Cantineau JP, Parte F, Horns JB, et al. Neuromuscular blocking effect of ORG 9426 on human diaphragm. Anesthesiology 1991; 75:A785.
190. Donati F. Onset of action of relaxants. Can J Anaesth 1988; 35:S52–S58.
191. Donati F, Antzaka C, Bevan DR. Potency of pancuronium at the diaphragm and adductor pollicis muscles in humans. Anesthesiology 1986;65:1–5.
192. Donati F, Plaud B, Meistleman D. Vecuronium neuromuscular blockade at the adductor muscles of the larynx and at the adductor pollicis. Anesthesiology 1991;74:833–837.
193. Plaud B, Meistleman C, Donati F. Organon 9426 neuromuscular blockade at the adductor muscles of the larynx and adductor pollicis in man. Anesthesiology 1991;75:A784.
194. Ali HH, Brull SJ, Witkowski T, et al. Efficacy and safety of divided-dose administration for rapid tracheal intubation. Anesthesiology 1993;79:A934.
195. Wirtavuori K, Meretoja OA, Taivainen T, Olkkola KT. Time course of potentiation of halothane and isoflurane on mivacurium infusion. Anesthesiology 1993;79:A939.

V BASIC INTRAVENOUS ANESTHETIC TECHNIQUES

17 Balanced Anesthesia

Tong J. Gan and Peter S. A. Glass

Balanced anesthesia describes most anesthetic administration in today's clinical practice. Modern anesthetic management involves the simultaneous use of several drugs, including combinations of intravenous and inhaled anesthetics. A survey of mortality in 100,000 anesthetic administrations revealed that the practice of combining several drugs to administer anesthesia may be safer than the use of only one or two drugs (1). For example, the relative odds of dying within 7 days were 2.9 times greater when one or two anesthetic drugs were used, compared with the odds when three or more drugs were used. Hence, the skillful use of multiple intravenous anesthetics is preferable in maintaining smooth anesthesia and optimal patient care. The purpose of this chapter is to provide information on the rationale of combining different intravenous drugs during anesthesia as a practical guide to achieving an optimal state of balanced anesthesia.

HISTORY

In the early days, anesthesia was conducted with a single anesthetic drug (e.g., nitrous oxide, ether, or chloroform). These early drugs were used as sole anesthetic agents for most of the first hundred years of anesthesia, with the exception of "gas-oxygen-ether" (GOE) in combinations of nitrous oxide and ether, used by Clover in 1873. GOE was a rudimentary form of balanced anesthesia. The concept of combining various drugs was probably first suggested by George Washington Crile of Cleveland, who proposed that more than one anesthetic drug could be administered simultaneously to produce the ideal anesthetic state. His concept was termed "anoci-association" and was the forerunner of what others have termed balanced anesthesia (2, 3). Crile believed that psychic stimuli (auditory, visual, olfactory) associated with surgery could be prevented by light anesthesia, whereas associated painful stimuli could be ablated by local anesthetics. In 1915, Dennis Jackson described a method for the production and maintenance of prolonged anesthesia using nitrous oxide, ethyl chloride, ether, chloroform, ethyl bromide, and somnoform (4).

John Lundy in 1926 first used the term "balanced anesthesia" to describe the use of a combination of anesthetic drugs during a single operation (5), leading to greater flexibility and patient safety. The rationale of this practice related to the use of small amounts of each drug, thereby avoiding the side effects caused by a large single dose of a given drug. Lundy used a combination of premedication, regional, and general anesthesia such that unconsciousness and pain relief were obtained by a balanced technique.

In 1938, Organe and Broad combined thiopental with nitrous oxide and oxygen (6). This combination resulted in anesthesia superior to that obtained with thiopental alone. The analgesic action of nitrous oxide permitted a marked reduction in the barbiturate dose, resulting in a faster return of consciousness. The synergism between the two drugs was further demonstrated in 1952 by Paulson, who studied the combination of thiopental, ether, and nitrous oxide. The total dose of thiopental required was markedly reduced, laryngeal spasm was avoided, tracheal intubation was easily accomplished, and levels of patient safety and satisfaction were high (7).

The introduction of the muscle relaxant curare by Griffith and Johnson in 1942 (8) resulted in a significant advance in the practice of balanced anesthesia. For the first time, anesthesiologists were able to achieve relative control of muscle relaxation without having to resort to excessively deep levels of general anesthesia. Muscle relaxation was one of the essential components of the anesthetic state, defined as "narcosis, analgesia and muscle relaxation" by Gray and Rees (9). Several techniques of balanced anesthesia were described involving anesthetic induction with thiopental, maintenance with nitrous oxide and oxygen supplemented with small additional doses of thiopental, and muscle relaxation with d-tubocurarine (10, 11).

This "triad of anesthesia" was further expanded by Woodbridge in 1957 to include abolition of autonomic reflexes (12). The combination of thiopental and nitrous oxide provided insufficient analgesia to prevent unwanted sympathetic stimulation reliably during surgery. Hence, not all the components of balanced anesthesia were achieved. In an attempt to obtain additional analgesia, Neff and colleagues introduced meperidine as a supplement during thiopental, d-tubocurarine, and nitrous oxide anesthesia in the United States (13). Two years later, a similar technique was introduced in England by Mushin and Rendell-Baker (14). These techniques rapidly achieved widespread popularity, and many individual variations were described using other opioid analgesics.

Despite the firm establishment of the concept of multiple intravenous anesthetics as an integral part of balanced anesthesia, groups of anesthesiologists who practiced cardiac anesthesia (Lowenstein and colleagues in 1969 and Stanley and Webster in 1979) suggested that the use of high-dose opioid anesthesia in critically ill patients having major operations could improve outcome in this high-risk population. With the subsequent commercial development of many synthetic opioids, "anesthesia" was achieved with the administration of one of the potent opioids (e.g., fentanyl and its new analogue), together with oxygen and a muscle relaxant. Potential problems became apparent, including intraoperative and chest wall rigidity, especially during induction of anesthesia. Prolonged postoperative respiratory depression was not uncommon and increased the length of time patients required assisted ventilation in the hospital intensive care unit. Hence, high-dose opioid techniques as originally described had only limited application in modern practice. The practice of balanced anesthesia with the use of a combination of intravenous drugs to produce hypnosis, amnesia, and analgesia while avoiding cardiopulmonary depression and providing for a rapid emergence from anesthesia has reestablished itself as a key concept in modern clinical anesthetic practice (i.e., "fast tracking").

PREMEDICATION

The objectives of premedication as defined by Mushin (15) were as follows: 1) to prevent side effects; 2) to assist anesthesia; 3) to prevent unwanted autonomic reflexes; and 4) to reduce preoperative anxiety. Claude Bernard first observed, in 1869, that if morphine were given to a dog before chloroform, anesthesia was achieved more rapidly, more smoothly, and with a smaller dose of chloroform (16). In 1937, Guedel postulated that anesthetic requirements were increased by any state that resulted in an increased metabolic rate, such as pain, fever, and excitement (17). Combinations of a sedative, barbiturate, and opioid given as premedication are effective in reducing pain and excitement and have been shown to reduce the anesthetic requirements. Eger demonstrated that premedication with morphine or diazepam decreased the minimum alveolar concentration (MAC) for halothane in humans. The influence of premedication on induction of anesthesia with intravenous agents has been clearly demonstrated for many agents and is not a simple summation of the actions of two sedative drugs. The excitatory side effects associated with methohexital are decreased by opioids and can be increased by premedication with hyoscine or the phenothiazines (18). Although these drugs did influence the induction characteristics, no clear evidence indicated a reduction in their dosage requirements. The principle that opioid premedication improves the quality of the induction of anesthesia is generally true. This observation is significant only when potent opioids are given intravenously, however, such that adequate plasma concentrations are still present at the time of induction.

The role of premedication in facilitating anesthesia has not been accepted by all practitioners. For example, Cohen and Beecher (19) and Eckenhoff and Helrich (20) were unable to demonstrate that the course of anesthesia with nitrous oxide and ether was any smoother after heavy premedication, although induction with cyclopropane was made easier with respect to premedication. Beecher remarked over 45 years ago, that "empirical procedures firmly entrenched in habits of good doctors seem to have a vigor and life, not to say an immortality of their own" (21). The practice of premedication over the past decade has changed because of changing clinical practice. Most surgical patients are admitted to hospital on the day of the surgical procedure and generally receive no premedication before arriving in the preoperative holding area. The use of a benzodiazepine as premedication shortly before induction of anesthesia has thus increased in popularity in recent years. The choice of premedication varies and depends on the individual clinician.

Benzodiazepines

The benzodiazepines are the most commonly used premedication in North America. Benzodiazepines have become the sedative and anxiolytic drugs of choice and are much more widely used than opioid premedication. The advantages of benzodiazepines are as follows: 1) excellent anxiolysis and sedation compared with morphine (22); 2) reliable effects following oral, intranasal, or parenteral administration; 3) no emetic action; 4) wide therapeutic margin; 5) antegrade amnesia; 6) antihallucinatory effect; and 7) spinally mediated muscle relaxation. The commonly used benzodiazepines are shown in Table 17-1.

The oral route of administration has been popular; however, absorption is variable and may be influenced by concomitant intravenous drugs. The opioids and anticholinergics delay gastric emptying and delay peak plasma concentration of the benzodiazepines. Prior administration of metoclopramide allows the peak effect of oral diazepam to be reached in approximately 20 minutes (23). When lorazepam is given orally, however, its peak effect may not be achieved until 2 to 4 hours later. Intravenous administration of lorazepam results in a faster onset of action, with peak concentration achieved in 30 to 40 minutes (24). Its long duration of action means that the time of administration is not critical, and changes in the order of the operating list are of less consequence. Lorazepam's prolonged duration of action may also be advantagous in patients who may require long a postoperative period of sedation (e.g., cardiac surgery). On the other hand, lorazepam may not be useful in outpatients undergoing ambulatory surgery and other short procedures (25).

Diazepam is insoluble in water and must be dissolved in organic solvents. Pain and phlebitis may result from intravenous injection (26). More recently, diazepam has been dissolved in soybean oil and phospholipids (Dizac), with markedly reduced side effects. Complete absorption of diazepam occurs in 30 to 60 minutes following an oral dose and in less than 30 minutes in children. Because of its effects on cardiorespiratory function, the benzodiazepine dose needs to be adjusted according to the general condition of the patient. Benzodiazepine premedication also ameliorates the unpleasant dreams associated with ketamine and reduces the incidence and severity of opioid-related rigidity and the dysphoria associated with the agonist-antagonist drugs.

Temazepam, 10 to 40 mg orally, must be given 1 to 2 hours before surgery to allow sufficient time for absorption, with clinical effects lasting 4 to 5 hours. Triazolam is a short-acting benzodiazepine with good anxiolytic and amnesic properties. The usual adult dose of triazolam, 0.25 to 0.5 mg orally, produces a peak plasma concentration in 1 hour, and the elimination half-life is 2 to 5 hours. When triazolam was compared with diazepam in outpatients undergoing ambulatory surgery, however, no difference was seen in recovery times (27).

TABLE 17-1. Doses of Benzodiazepines Commonly Used for Premedication

Generic Name	Trade Name	Doses
Diazepam	Valium, Diazemuls, Stesoild,	5–20 mg PO
	Dizac	1–3 mg IV
Triazolam	Halcion	0.25–0.50 mg PO
Lorazepam	Ativan	0.5–4 mg PO or IV
Midazolam	Hypnovel, Dormicum,	2–5 mg IM
	Dobralam, Versed	1–2 mg IV
Temazepam	Restoril	10–30 mg PO

Midazolam is water soluble, and its use is not associated with pain on injection or venous irritation. Midazolam has become an extremely popular benzodiazepine for premedication. Nevertheless, large doses (or rapid injection) of midazolam may result in apnea when the drug is combined with an opioid analgesic, especially in elderly and debilitated patients. When compared with equipotent doses of diazepam, midazolam has a slower onset of action, more predictable absorption, and a more rapid recovery. Hence, midazolam is ideal for short procedures and day-case surgery. The elimination half-life of midazolam is about 1 to 4 hours, although this may be prolonged in the elderly (28). Consistent with other benzodiazepines, it has sedative, anxiolytic, and amnesic effects (Fig. 17-1) (29). The lack of recall with midazolam is augmented by concomitant administration of hyoscine (30). Pretreatment with ranitidine has also been associated with a greater degree of drowsiness after midazolam than in a nonpretreated group. Midazolam is commonly given shortly before induction of anesthesia in doses of 1 to 5 mg (32). Within this dosage range, midazolam reduces the induction dose of thiopental (32) or propofol (33) without signifcantly prolonging recovery.

Opioids

The opioids are analgesics with sedative rather than anxiolytic properties and are associated with occasional dysphoria as well as a high incidence of perioperative nausea and vomiting. Nevertheless, for patients in acute pain, opioids can provide effective analgesia and even euphoria. Preoperative administration of opioids reduces the subsequent anesthetic requirements (34, 35) and provides for smooth inhalational induction.

Premedication with opioids produces respiratory depression as a result of the depressed carbon dioxide response at the medullary respiratory center, and the responsiveness to hypoxia is decreased at the carotid body. Opioid compounds should be avoided in patients with increased intracranial pressure. Spasm of the sphincter of Oddi has also been reported after opioid premedication (36, 37).

Anticholinergics

Anticholinergics possess vagolytic, sedative, amnesic, and antisialogogue actions. Their use in premedication

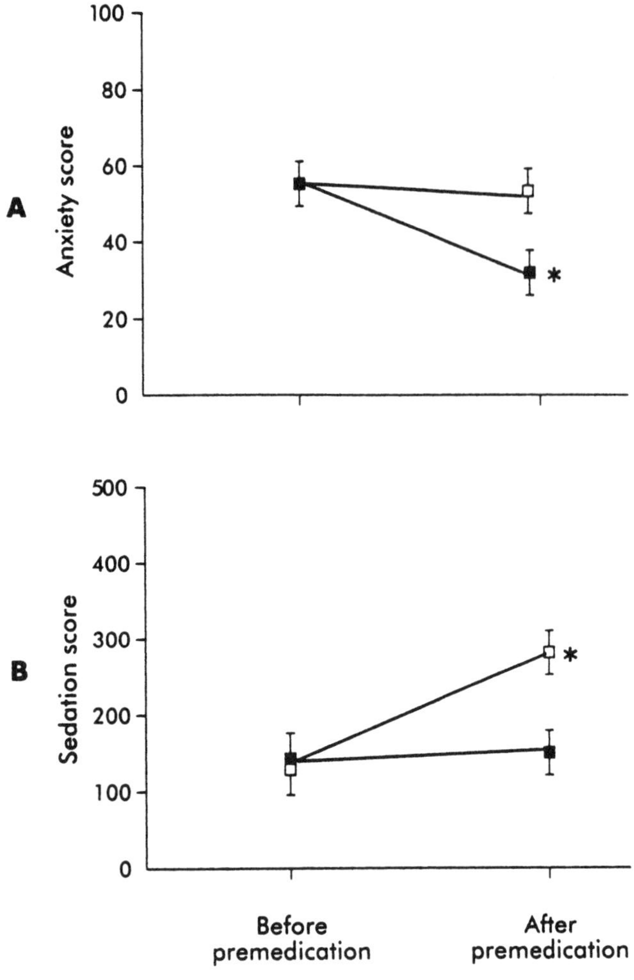

FIGURE 17-1. Anxiety scores (A) and sedation scores (B) before and after premedication for patients who received saline placebo or midazolam. Values are mean ± SEM. The asterisk indicates a significant difference between groups, $p < 0.05$. (From Shafer A, White PF, Urquhart ML, Doze VA. Outpatient premedication: use of midazolam and opioid analgesics. Anesthesiology 1989;71:49–501.)

was more popular in the days of ether anesthesia when excessive salivation and bradycardia were problematic. As safer and more effective anesthetic agents have become available, the routine use of anticholinergics has fallen out of favor. Anticholinergics can cause patient discomfort because of drying of the mouth and difficulty in clearing viscid secretions, and when given to the elderly, scopolamine (and even atropine) may cause postoperative mental confusion. Anticholinergics can be useful, however, in achieving a smooth intraoperative course during balanced anesthesia by preventing bradycardia during surgery from stimulation of the carotid sinus or traction on abdominal viscera or extraocular muscles. The antisialogogue effect may also be important before awake fiberoptic intubation to enhance the efficacy of the topical anesthetic and to improve visibility during the procedure. Anticholinergics are also useful for procedures that require extensive instrumentation of the pharynx and airway. Glycopyrrolate is more effective as an antisialogogue than atropine. Scopolamine is less likely to increase heart rate and more likely to produce amnesia and sedation. Atropine or glycopyrrolate given intravenously just before the surgical stimulus is more reliable in preventing the anticipated bradycardia than if given before the patient's arrival in the operating room.

Histamine Receptor Antagonists

Histamine type–2 (H_2) blocking drugs raise gastric fluid pH by reducing secretion of gastric hydrogen ion. The commonly used H_2 receptor antagonists include cimetidine and ranitidine. Although these drugs reduce acidity, they should not be expected to decrease gastric volume or emptying time. As with benzodiazepines, the H_2 blockers have relatively few side effects. Cimetidine can interfere with the hepatic mixed function oxidase enzyme system, however, and it may prolong the actions of benzodiazepines, lidocaine, theophylline, warfarin, and other drugs metabolized by this enzyme system.

Antiemetics

Patients undergoing operations with a high emetic potential (Table 17-2), obese patients, women during their menses, and patients with a previous history of postoperative nausea and vomiting can benefit from the prophylactic use of an antiemetic drug. Anesthesiologists generally believe that an antiemetic is best given as a premedication before induction of anesthesia when various drugs with emetogenic potential (e.g., opioids, nitrous oxide, inhalation agents) are given. Nevertheless, some studies have demonstrated the superior antiemetic efficacy of both droperidol and ondansetron when these agents are given toward the end of surgery than at the beginning of anesthesia (38, 39). Droperidol, 0.625 to 1.25 mg intravenously, has been found effective in adults (40-44). Higher doses of droperidol are associated with side effects such as sedation, restlessness, and extrapyramidal reactions, al-

TABLE 17-2. Surgical Procedures Associated with a High Incidence of Postoperative Nausea and Vomiting

Surgical Subspecialty	Type of Procedure
Ophthalmic surgery	Strabismus correction Retinal detachment repair
Gynecologic surgery	Laparoscopy Ovum retrieval
Breast surgery	Mastectomy Breast implant
Ear, nose, and throat surgery	Tonsillectomy Middle ear surgery
Intra-abdominal surgery	Gastric manipulation

though small doses are not be completely devoid of these unwanted effects (45). In addition to its gastrokinetic properties, metoclopramide, 0.25 mg/kg intravenously, possesses antiemetic properties through antidopaminergic actions at the chemoreceptor trigger zone.

Ondansetron, a serotonin antagonist, is effective in the prevention and treatment of postoperative nausea and vomiting (46, 47). It has relatively few side effects and has rapidly gained popularity (40, 48–50). Investigators have also postulated that ondansetron may possess mood-elevating properties that may have clinical relevance during recovery from balanced anesthesia (40). Other serotonin antagonists include granisetron, dolasetron, and tropisetron.

β-Adrenergic Blockers

Interest has increased in the use of β blockers to control sympathetic responses and to prevent adverse myocardial effects resulting from perioperative stress. Stone and associates (51) found that a premedicant dose of a β-adrenergic blocking agent significantly reduced the risks of myocardial ischemia. The patients receiving the β blocker were less likely to develop tachycardia and myocardial ischemia during tracheal intubation and emergence from balanced anesthesia.

Alpha-2 Agonists

In 1979, Kaukinen and associates found that clonidine was able to "smooth out" the perioperative hemodynamic profile and prevent postoperative hypertensive crises (52). The perioperative use of clonidine and other α_2 agonists has gained popularity. In a placebo-controlled study, Flacke and associates studied the hemodynamic and anesthetic effects of preoperative and intraoperative administration of clonidine, 0.2 to 0.3 mg (53). The clonidine-treated patients were more sedated on arrival in the operating room, and the total sufentanil requirement was reduced by 40% (Fig. 17-2). Despite the lower dose of opiate used, heart rate and blood pressure were significantly lower in the clonidine-treated group. Cardiac output was consistently higher and systemic vascular resistance was consistently lower in the clonidine-treated group after cardiopulmonary bypass. Plasma catecholamine levels remained lower, and time to extubation was significantly shorter in the clonidine-treated group. α_2 Agonists have also been found to reduce anesthetic and analgesic drug doses in both normotensive and hypertensive patients undergoing noncardiovascular surgery (54-56). Ghignone and colleagues found that patients pretreated with clonidine, 5 μg/kg orally, required 40% less isoflurane and 75% less fentanyl than a matched control group (54). In another study, elderly patients having ophthalmic surgery required

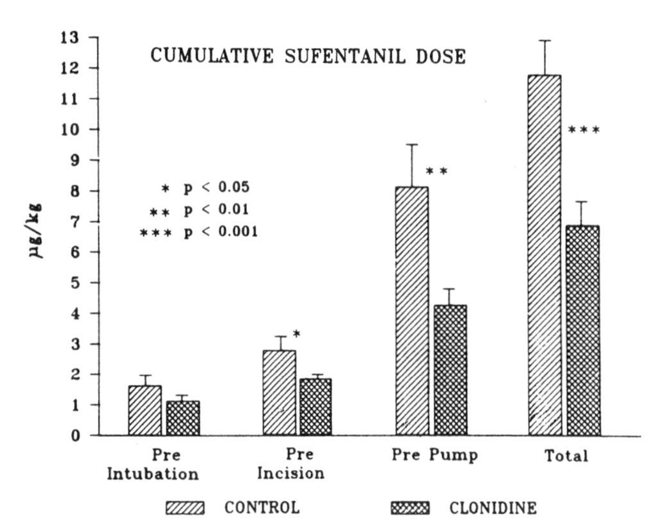

FIGURE 17-2. Mean cumulative sufentanil doses are shown for the periods before intubation, before incision, before cardiopulmonary bypass, and for the entire anesthetic period. (From Flacke JW, Bloor BC, Flacke WE, et al. Reduced narcotic requirement by clonidine with improved hemodynamic and adrenergic stability in patients undergoing coronary bypass surgery. Anesthesiology 1987;67:11–19.)

50% less fentanyl and 30% less isoflurane (55). In a study involving oral and transdermally administered clonidine, two different doses were administered to achieve steady-state perioperative plasma clonidine levels of 1.0 or 1.5 ng/ml. Both clonidine-treated groups were more sedated at the time of arrival in the operating room, had lower volatile anesthetic requirements to achieve hemodynamic end points, and had greater intraoperative hemodynamic stability and more rapid emergence from anesthesia following radical prostatectomy procedures. Patients in the high-dose clonidine-treated group also required 50% less patient-controlled morphine (56). Oral clonidine premedication has also been shown to reduce propofol requirements during surgery, but it has prolonged recovery times (57).

Dexmedetomidine has highly selective α_2-agonist properties (58). Its potential therapeutic benefit is especially evident in the postsurgical period (i.e., during the emergence and recovery phases), with improved hemodynamic and metabolic stability resulting from its sympatholytic effects, improved patient comfort with less shivering, antagonized opioid-induced muscle rigidity, decreased nausea and vomiting, and reduced the requirement for opiates in the postoperative period with decreased respiratory depression (59–67). Preliminary studies involving dexmedetomidine given as an infusion suggest that the drug may decrease the risk of adverse cardiac events including myocardial ischemia. The preliminary results from studies involving the use of α_2 agonists as a premedicant and adjuvant to anesthesia are extremely promising. These compounds are expected to play a significant role in balanced anesthesia in the future.

Pediatric Patients

The use of premedication is particularly important in children, to allay the anxieties of surgery, separation, pain, and body disfigurement. Premedication allows for smoother and safer induction and maintenance of anesthesia. Although the importance of a carefully conducted preoperative visit to foster trust and proper psychologic preparation cannot be overemphasized (68-70), a pharmacologic adjunct often makes the transition to the operating room less traumatic and more psychologically acceptable. The issue of which child benefits most from premedication and the specific pharmacologic agent chosen should be based on the needs of each child.

Benzodiazepines

Sedative and hypnotic premedication is used in pediatric patients, to reduce apprehension and to produce sedation and amnesia. Anesthesiologists tend to avoid intramuscular injections because of a child's fear of needles and pain of association with the injection. Diazepam, temazepam, and midazolam given orally are the most popular techniques. Intranasal and transmucosal midazolam has also been investigated for premedication in children. These "nonthreatening" routes of administration have provided highly effective sedation, allowing atraumatic separation from parents and smoother induction of anesthesia. Oral and intranasal absorption are rapid, with peak concentration at 5 to 10 minutes and peak effect at 10 to 15 minutes. The midazolam dose for oral premedication is 0.5 to 1 mg/kg, whereas the intranasal and transmucosal dosage is only 0.1 to 0.2 mg/kg. Because the midazolam solution has a bitter taste, it is usually mixed with a sweetener. Rita and colleagues noted that midazolam with atropine was more effective in allaying anxiety and in promoting smooth anesthetic induction than morphine and atropine (71).

Anticholinergics

Anticholinergic drugs have always had a special place in pediatric premedication. As alluded to earlier, increased vagal tone and bradycardia may occur during an inhalation induction, following laryngoscopy and other intraoperative manipulations, and after the use of succinylcholine to facilitate tracheal intubation (72-74). To administer atropine or glycopyrrolate intravenously immediately before induction of anesthesia is generally more effective; however, the potential side effects of anticholinergics must be borne in mind, and their use must be avoided in children with fevers.

Opioids

Opioids are an important component of pediatric premedication, except in children with a history of apnea and those younger than 1 year old because of the increased sensitivity of these patients to opioid-induced respiratory depression (75, 76). Narcotic premedication can also result in dysphoria and nausea and vomiting. These effects are attenuated by anticholinergics and barbiturates, however (77). In an attempt to avoid parenteral injections, intranasal sufentanil has been introduced. Its pharmacokinetic profile following intranasal administration is similar to that of the intravenous route of administration (78). In addition to the unpleasantness of nose drops and increased nausea and vomiting, a decrease in lung compliance has been reported. Other studies have evaluated the safety and efficacy of oral transmucosal fentanyl citrate (OTFC) as a premedicant in the pediatric population (79–83). These studies have demonstrated that OTFC is effective in producing preoperative sedation and anxiolysis in children. High-dose OTFC (20 to 25 μg/kg) produced significantly more side effects than a conventional premedicant combination consisting of oral meperidine, diazepam, and atropine (84). An OTFC dosage of 10 to 15 μg/kg was determined to be as effective as the higher dosage for sedation and anxiolysis (79, 81). Nonetheless, the incidence of side effects was similar with the various dosage forms. The most common side effect was preoperative pruritus, with an incidence of 60 to 100% (83-85). Only rarely was the pruritus troublesome, however. Unfortunately, nausea and vomiting were also common, with an incidence of 22 to 65% (83-85). One study using a high dosage of OTFC reported a 30% incidence of vomiting before induction of anesthesia. Residual gastric volumes have also been reported to be increased in children receiving OTFC preoperatively, compared with children receiving no premedication (85). Unfortunately, prophylactic droperidol (50 μg/kg intravenously) does not significantly decrease postoperative nausea and vomiting following OTFC administration (81). Although respiratory depression is a serious adverse effect of opioid administration, the incidence of clinically important ventilatory impairment is minimized when the fentanyl dosage is less than 15 μg/kg. Hence OTFC is a safe and effective premedicant for children; however, its use is associated with an increased incidence of pruritus, nausea, and vomiting.

Ketamine

Ketamine has been used for premedication in children when it is administered orally, nasally, or rectally. Studies comparing oral ketamine (5 to 6 mg/kg) with midazolam (0.5 to 1 mg/kg) as premedication suggest that both drugs provide good sedation. Ketamine resulted in slightly more prolonged recovery (86), increased secretions, (87) and a higher incidence of postoperative vomiting (88), however.

INDUCTION AND MAINTENANCE

Pharmacodynamic Principles

Characterizing Drug Interactions

To achieve balanced anesthesia, two or more drugs are usually combined to provide hypnosis, analgesia, and muscle relaxation. The interaction between two volatile agents has been shown to be simply additive (i.e., their combined effect is the result of adding their individual effects). Hence, 30% of the MAC of an agent combined with 40% of the MAC of another agent will produce the same effect as 70% of the MAC of either agent alone. The apparent additivity of MAC can be used to determine the appropriate target concentration of one of the gases based on the concentration of the other. This simple additivity is likely due to a uniform mechanism of action. On the other hand, the intravenous anesthetic technique involves the use of a variety of drugs including hypnotics, opioids and nonopioid analgesics, anxiolytics, and local anesthetics with different receptors and mechanisms of action within the central nervous system (CNS). The interactions among intravenous drugs and between inhalational and intravenous anesthetics result in complex drug interactions that may not be easily predicted because of pharmacokinetic and pharmacodynamic actions.

The induction of anesthesia can be achieved either with a single agent or with a combination of several drugs. Kissin and colleagues were the first investigators systematically to study the interaction of drugs during the induction of anesthesia (89-93). They and other investigators used the concept of isobolograms (94, 95) to analyze these interactions. A dose-response curve for loss of consciousness is obtained, and for each drug a line is drawn between the ED_{50} values (i.e., dose required to produce the desired effect in 50% of patients). If the interactions between the two drugs are simply additive, a straight line would represent the combination of the two drugs that would result in loss of consciousness in 50% of patients. The combinations of drugs that would be estimated from this line to produce loss of consciousness in 50% of patients are then tested. If the combination results in greater than the predicted 50% response (i.e., below and to the left of the line), then the drugs appear to be acting synergistically. On the other hand, if the interactions are less than the predicted 50% response (i.e., above and to the right of the line), the drugs are considered to be acting antagonistically (Fig. 17-3).

Numerous studies have now characterized the drug interactions of two or three different drug combinations for induction of anesthesia. The interaction between opiates and hypnotics is clearly synergistic. An even greater degree of synergy occurs between the benzodiazepines and other hypnotic and opioid combinations, however. Some interactions are additive or even antagonistic. For example, thiopental can partially antagonize the opioid-benzodiazepine synergism (91). Drugs may be combined at the induction of anesthesia not only to reduce the doses necessary to provide loss of consciousness, but also to ablate the sympathetic responses to laryngoscopy and endotracheal intubation as well as to the skin incision. Several studies have demonstrated that fentanyl, 2 to 6 μg/kg, attenuates the hypertensive response associated with laryngoscopy and intubation (96–98). The β-blocking drugs labetalol (99–103) and esmolol (104-107) have also been shown effective in ablating this hypertensive response. The synergistic action of commonly used drug combinations can also result in undesirable side effects, however, such as enhanced hypotension when benzodiazepines are combined with opiates (108). In clinical practice, the use of a small dose of a benzodiazepine (e.g., midazolam, 1 to 3 mg) and an opiate (fentanyl, 50 to 150 g) in combination with an induction dose of the chosen hypnotic compound can provide a smooth induction devoid of these side effects.

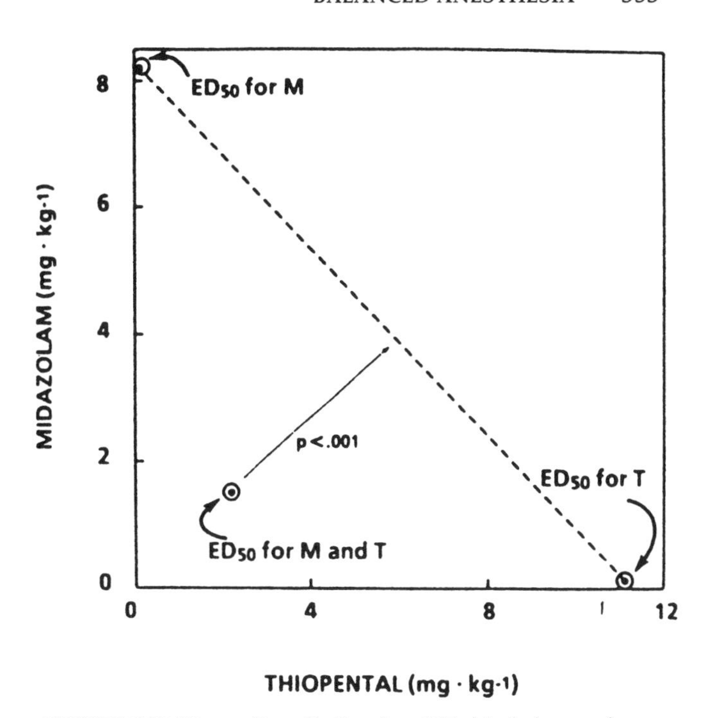

FIGURE 17-3. The median effective dose (ED_{50}) isobologram for the interaction between two drugs, e.g., midazolam (M) and thiopental (T), as characterized by the righting reflex. Points shown are ED_{50} values for midazolam and thiopental alone, and the ED_{50} value for their combination. (From Kissin I, Mason JOD, Bradley EL Jr. Pentobarbital and thiopental anesthetic interactions with midazolam. Anesthesiology 1987;67:26–31.)

Whereas isobolograms are useful in the assessment

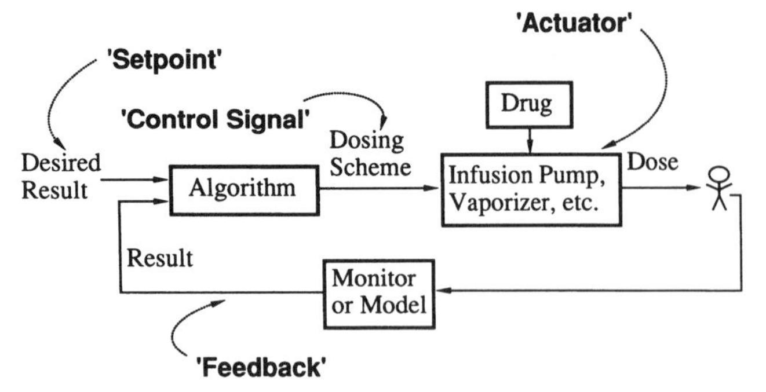

FIGURE 17-4. Schematic illustration of our approach to a pharmacokinetic model-driven drug delivery system. In this computer-assisted continuous infusion device, the physician enters the desired plasma drug concentration. An infusion device control algorithm uses a pharmacokinetic model for the drug being infused to determine what the infusion rate should be for the next infusion interval (e.g., 10 seconds). The infusion device delivers drug to the patient, and the infusion rate is fed into a simulation of the pharmacokinetic model to compute the current predicted plasma drug concentration. The stated variables computed in the simulation are available to the algorithm. On the basis of monitored and anticipated patient response and knowledge of approximate therapeutic and current predicted plasma drug concentrations, the physician can titrate the desired plasma drug concentration as necessary. (From Reves JG, Jacobs JR, Glass PSA. Automated drug delivery in anesthesia. ASA refresher course in anesthesiology. Philadelphia: JB Lippincott, 1991:19.)

of interactions between two different drugs, it is not possible to discern whether the synergistic-antagonistic interaction is due to an effect on the drug's pharmacokinetic profile (i.e., resulting in higher than expected CNS concentrations) or to a pharmacodynamic effect (i.e., greater sensitivity resulting from central effects of the combination). Because of their pharmacokinetic properties, all drugs demonstrate some delay between the dosing interval, and peak effect (i.e., hysteresis). This delay is different for each drug, and thus possibly many of the interactions are not measured at the "peak" effect of both drugs. A different approach to evaluating the interaction of the intravenous anesthetics is to administer both drugs to a constant concentration and then assess their effects when the plasma and biophase (effect) concentrations have equilibrated. For intravenous drugs, this has been made possible with the advent of pharmacokinetic model-driven drug delivery systems in which biophase concentrations can be rapidly achieved and maintained (Fig. 17-4). This method ensures that pharmacokinetic differences are accounted for by evaluating the concentration response of the drug, and thus only the pharmacodynamic interaction is assessed. Utilizing this type of system, anesthesiologists can determine the concentration-effect relationship of intravenous anesthetics for induction and maintenance of anesthesia, as well as the interaction of adjunctive drugs used to achieve similar end points of anesthesia.

Inhalation anesthetic depth has been classically characterized by the MAC concept as developed by Eger and associates (109). The measurement of MAC has several important elements. A constant partial pressure of volatile anesthetic at the central site of action must be achieved before measurement of the re-

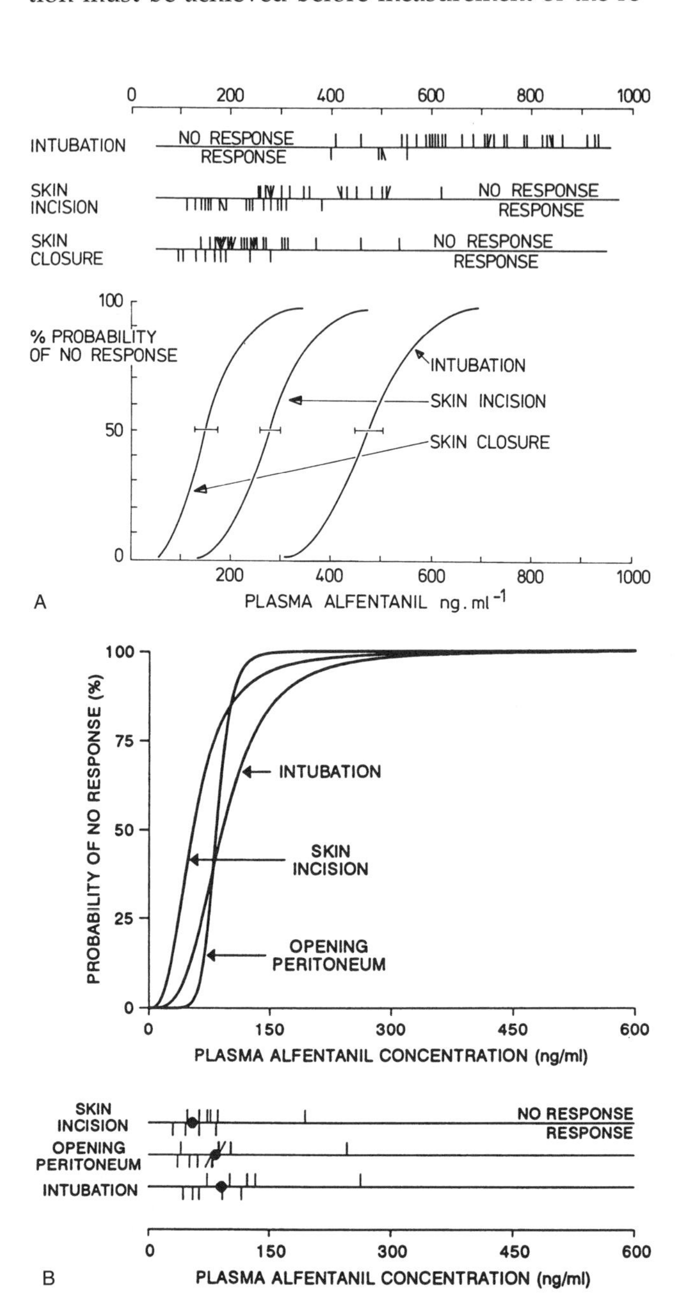

FIGURE 17-5. Relationship between the alfentanil plasma concentrations (with 66% nitrous oxide) and their effects for three specific events of short duration (intubation, skin incision, and skin closure). A, The alfentanil plasma concentrations of every patient associated with (downward deflection) or without (upward deflection) a response to each of these three stimuli. B, The plasma concentration-effect curves for these stimuli were defined from the quantal data shown in A using logistic regression. (From Ausems ME, Hug CC Jr, Stanski DR, Burm AG. Plasma concentrations of alfentanil required to supplement nitrous oxide anesthesia for general surgery. Anesthesiology 1986;65:362–373.)

sponse. A specific, noxious stimuli (e.g., initial skin incision in humans) is applied, and a positive clinical response is a purposeful movement. A similar quantifiable measure of the concentration-effect responses for intravenous anesthetics is needed. The Cp_{50} represents the steady-state plasma concentration after equilibration with the biophase that prevents a predefined response (e.g., movement, hypertension, catecholamine release) to a given stimulus (e.g., skin incision, intubation, sternal spreading, skin closure) in 50% of patients. Ausems and colleagues (110) defined Cp_{50} for several noxious stimuli for alfentanil in the presence of 66% nitrous oxide (Fig. 17-5). Smith and Glass and their colleagues used computer-controlled infusions to provide more rapid equilibration between plasma and the effect site concentration (111, 112). Using this technique, the Cp_{50} value for skin incision for fentanyl in the presence of 70% nitrous oxide was determined to be 4.2 ng/ml (113). The Cp_{50} value for sufentanil at skin incision has also been defined (114). The steady-state concentrations of various intravenous anesthetic drugs when combined with nitrous oxide for predefined effects are summarized in Table 17-3.

To define the interaction between volatile anesthetics and opiates, target-controlled infusions of opioid analgesics have been used to define their MAC-reducing effects. Isoflurane MAC reduction studies have been performed with fentanyl (113) (Fig. 17-6), alfentanil (115) (Fig. 17-7), sufentanil (Fig. 17-8) (116), and remifentanil (117).

As shown in Figure 17A-6, fentanyl, 1 ng/ml, resulted in a 39% MAC reduction. Increasing the fentanyl plasma concentration to 3 ng/ml resulted in a further MAC reduction to 63%; however, further increases in fentanyl concentration (greater than 3 ng/ml) produced a similar reduction in MAC. A 50% reduction in isoflurane MAC was achieved at a fentanyl concentration of 1.67 ng/ml (113). These data suggest that a substantial reduction in the isoflurane requirement (40 to 60%) can be achieved at low (1 to 3 ng/ml) plasma concentrations of fentanyl (see Fig. 17A-6). In clinical practice, fentanyl given as an initial bolus dose of 3 μg/kg over 5 minutes followed by an infusion of 1 μg/kg/h will achieve a 1-ng/ml fentanyl concentration. Doubling these loading-maintenance dosages will result in a doubling of the fentanyl plasma concentration. In addition, little can be gained by further increasing the plasma concentration of fentanyl.

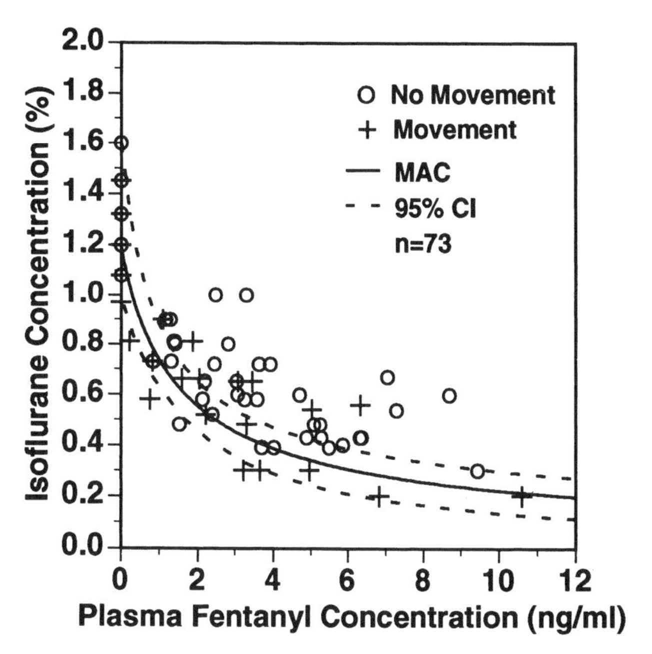

FIGURE 17-6. Maximum likelihood (logistic regression) solution for the minimum alveolar concentration (MAC) reduction of isoflurane by increasing concentrations of fentanyl is represented by the solid line. The 95% confidence intervals of the isoflurane MAC are also plotted as dashed lines. (From McEwan AI, Smith C, Dyar O, et al. Isoflurane MAC reduction by fentanyl. Anesthesiology 1993;78:864–869.)

TABLE 17-3. Steady-State Plasma Concentrations of Intravenous Anesthetics and Analgesics

Drug	IC50 (± SD)	Cp_{50} Incision or Painful Stimulus (± SD)	Cp_{50} LOC (± SD)	Cp_{50} Spont Vent (± SD)	50% Reduction in Isoflurane MAC	MEAC
Alfentanil (ng/ml)	520 ± 123	241 ± 16	—	226 ± 10	50	10
Fentanyl (ng/ml)	6.9 ± 1.9	4.2	—	(3–4)	1.67	0.7
Sufentanil (ng/ml)	0.68 ± 0.31	(0.3–0.4)	—	(0.3–0.4)	0.145	0.04
Remifentanil (ng/ml)	14.7	(3–4)	12	(2–3)	1.37	(0.6)
Thiopental	17.9	39.8 ± 3.3	15.6 ± 1.1	—	—	—
Propofol	—	15.8	3.4	—	—	—

IC_{50}, The steady-state serum concentration in equilibration with the effect compartment that causes a 50% slowing of maximal electrosencephalogram; Cp_{50} skin incision, the steady-state plasma concentration in equilibration with the effect compartment that prevents a somatic or autonomic response in 50% of patients; Cp_{50} LOC, the steady-state plasma concentration in equilibration with the effect compartment that provides absence of a response to a verbal command in 50% of patients; Cp_{50} Spont Vent, the steady-state plasma concentration in equilibration with the effect compartment associated with adequate spontaneous ventilation in 50% of patients; MEAC; the minimum effective plasma concentration providing postoperative analgesia.

From Glass PSA, Shafer S, Jacobs J, Reves JG. Intravenous drug delivery systems. In: Miller RD, ed. Anesthesia. vol. 1. 4th ed. New York: Churchill Livingstone, 1994:389–416.)

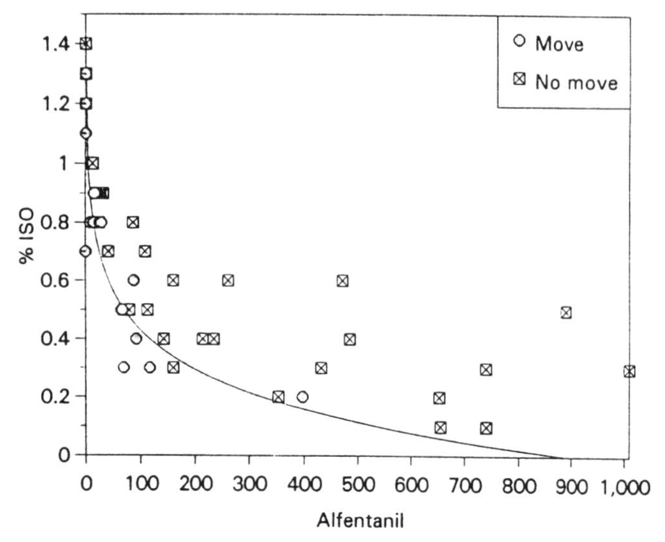

FIGURE 17-7. Graph of end-tidal isoflurane (ISO) concentration against mean alfentanil concentration for each patient. Each point represents the move-no move response for an individual patient. The line represents the 50% likelihood of movement to skin incision. (From Westmoreland CL, Sebel PS, Gropper A. Fentanyl or alfentanil decreases the minimum alveolar anesthetic concentration of isoflurane in surgical patients. Anesth Analg 1994; 78:23–28.)

Plasma fentanyl concentrations above 2 ng/ml have been associated with significant respiratory depression (118), and no additional MAC reduction is achieved at higher opiate concentrations.

Similarly sufentanil, 0.1 to 0.5 ng/ml, produced a substantial reduction of the MAC of isoflurane (116). Increasing the plasma concentrations of sufentanil beyond 0.5 ng/ml results in little further reduction in isoflurane MAC (see Fig. 17A-8). A sufentanil plasma concentration of 0.15 ng/ml can be achieved with a manual infusion consisting of an initial loading dose of 0.15 μg/kg, followed by an infusion of 0.003 μg/kg/min. A 0.5-μg/kg loading dose followed by a continuous infusion of 0.008 μg/kg/min would achieve a sufentanil plasma concentration of 0.5 ng/ml (Table 17-4).

The decrease in the Cp_{50} value of propofol by fentanyl (111) (Fig. 17-9) or alfentanil (119) (Fig. 17-10) has also been described. The opioid-propofol interaction is similar to that seen with volatile anesthetics and opiates. The steep decrease in propofol requirements with low concentrations of opioid compounds seen initially is followed by a "ceiling" effect at concentrations above 3 to 4 ng/ml for fentanyl or 100 to 150 ng/ml for alfentanil. Similarly, this plateau effect occurred at a Cp_{50} of 3.5 μg/ml of propofol.

Choice and Timing of Intravenous Drug Administration

To select drugs for induction more rationally and to determine the optimal timing of their administration, it is important to know the time to their peak effect and their k_{e0} values. The k_{e0} represents the rate of equilibration of a drug between the plasma and the biophase. The $t_{1/2}$ k_{e0} is the time it takes for half the equilibration to occur between the biophase and the plasma concentration. If the $t_{1/2}$ k_{e0} for fentanyl is 4.7 minutes, this means that if the plasma concentration of fentanyl was maintained at a constant level of 4 ng/ml, the effect compartment fentanyl concentration would be 2 ng/ml at 4.7 minutes after the infusion was initiated. Because it takes about four half-lives to achieve equilibrium, about 18.8 minutes will elapse before when equilibrium is achieved between plasma and effect compartment. The $t_{1/2}$ k_{e0} of commonly used intravenous anesthetic is summarized in Table 17-5.

The time required to achieve a peak effect of a drug following a bolus injection is a function of the drug's k_{e0} and its disposition (120). A drug with a short $t_{1/2}$ k_{e0} has a rapid onset to peak effect. For example, with rapid-sequence induction, it is desirable to use drugs with short $t_{1/2}$ k_{e0} values (e.g., thiopental, 100 seconds, and alfentanil, 82 seconds) such that loss of consciousness is rapid and both drugs achieve their peak effect at about the same time, thus minimizing the hemodynamic response to laryngoscopy and endotracheal intubation. If fentanyl (216 seconds) is administered at the same time as thiopental and succinylcholine, its peak effect will not be achieved at the time of greatest stimulus (intubation). As a result, hypertension and

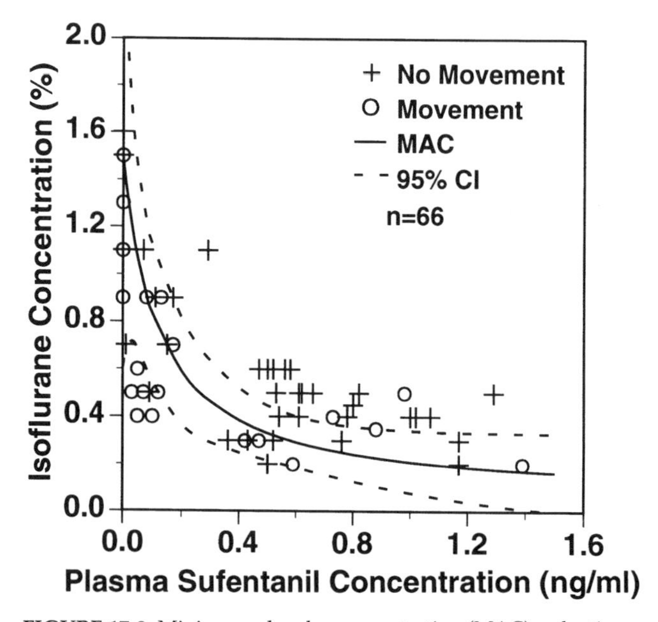

FIGURE 17-8. Minimum alveolar concentration (MAC) reduction of isoflurane by increasing concentrations of sufentanil: solid line, maximum likelihood (logistic regression) solution; dashed lines, 95% confidence interval of isoflurane MAC. The plus sign represents no movement; the minus sign represents movement. (From Brunner MD, Braithwaite P, Jhaveri R, et al. MAC reduction of isoflurane by sufentanil. Br J Anaesth 1994;72:42–46.)

TABLE 17-4. Manual Infusion Dosage Regimens for Intravenous Anesthetics and analgesics*

Drug	Anesthesia (with 66% Nitrous Oxide) Loading Dose (μg•kg•$^{-1}$)	Anesthesia (with 66% Nitrous Oxide) Maintenance Infusion (μg•kg•$^{-1}$•min^{-1})	Sedation or Analgesia Loading Dose (μg•kg•$^{-1}$•min^{-1})	Sedation or Analgesia Maintenance Infusion (μg•kg•$^{-1}$•min^{-1})
Alfentanil	50–150	0.5–3	10–25	0.25–1
Fentanyl	5–15	0.03–0.1	1.5–3	0.01–0.03
Sufentanil	1–2	0.006–0.02	0.15–0.3	0.002–0.007
Remifentanil	1–2	0.1–0.4	—	0.025–0.1
Methohexital	1000–2000	50–150	500–1000	10–50
Ketamine	1000–2000	10–50	500–1000	10–20
Propofol	1000–2000	80–150	250–1000	10–50
Midázolam	50–150	0.25–1.0	20–100	0.25–1

**Following the loading dose, an initially high infusion rate to account for redistribution should be used and then titrated to the lowest infusion rate that will maintain adequate anesthesia or sedation. For sedation, the loading dose is given over 5 to 10 minutes and is adjusted according to the patient's response. For anesthesia, midazolam must be administered combined with an opiate. For nonanesthetized patients, it is recommended that no loading dose of remifentanil be given. With an infusion alone, a steady-state concentration is rapidly achieved (i.e., 10 to 15 minutes).*

(From Glass PSA, Shafer S, Jacobs J, Reves JG. Intravenous drug delivery systems. In: Miller RD, ed. Anesthesia. vol 1. 4th ed. New York: Churchill Livingstone, 1994:389–416.)

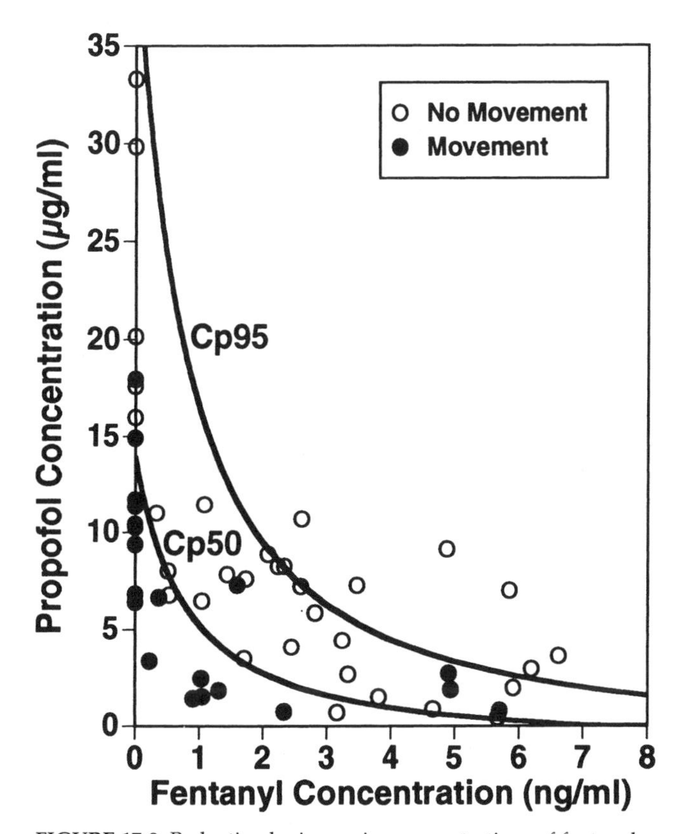

FIGURE 17-9. Reduction by increasing concentrations of fentanyl of propofol concentration at which 50% or 95% of patients did not move at skin incision ($Cp_{50}i$ and $Cp_{95}i$, respectively). Solid lines represent logistic regression solution. (From Smith C, McEwan AI, Jhaveri R, et al. The interaction of fentanyl on the Cp_{50} of propofol for loss of consciousness and skin incision [Discussion 26A]. Anesthesiology 1994;81:820–828.)

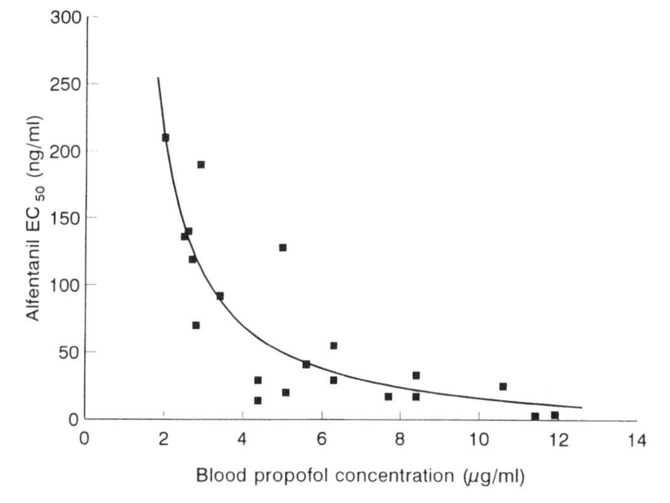

FIGURE 17-10. Plasma alfentanil concentrations versus blood propofol concentrations associated with a 50% probability of no response to intra-abdominal surgical stimuli. Squares represent the median effective dose (EC_{50}) of alfentanil at corresponding mean blood propofol concentration for suppression of responses to intra-abdominal surgical stimuli as determined in the individual patients by logistic regression. (From Vuyk J, Lim T, Engbers FH, et al. Pharmacodynamics of alfentanil as a supplement to propofol or nitrous oxide for lower abdominal surgery in female patients. Anesthesiology 1993;78:1036–1045.)

tachycardia may occur with laryngoscopy and intubation, followed by hypotension, because the fentanyl will achieve its peak effect when the stimuli are minimal. Thus, fentanyl needs to be given 3 to 5 minutes before an anticipated noxious stimulus. Alfentanil has a rapid onset of peak effect and only needs to be given 1 to 2 minutes before the anticipated noxious stimulus. When intravenous drugs are given by intermittent bolus, the interval between doses should be of sufficient duration that the peak effect of the drug is observed before the subsequent dose of the drug is administered. For example, if two bolus doses of midazolam are given 1 minute apart (i.e., before observing the peak effect of the drug), the effect continues to increase, resulting in the second dose's producing greater sedation than anticipated from the first dose (Fig. 17-11). A knowledge of the k_{e0} values allows for

TABLE 17.5. The Values for the Time Taken for Half the Equilibration to Occur Between Biophase and Plasma Concentrates ($T_{1/2}$ k_{e0}) and the Times to Peak Effect of Various Intravenous Anesthetic Drugs

Drug	Time to Peak Effect (min)	$T_{1/2}$ k_{e0} (min)
Fentanyl	3.6	4.7
Alfentanil	1.4	0.9
Sufentanil	5.6	3.0
Remifentanil	1.1	1.2
Propofol	2.2	2.4
Thiopental	1.7	1.5
Midazolam	2.8	4.0
Etomidate	2.0	1.5

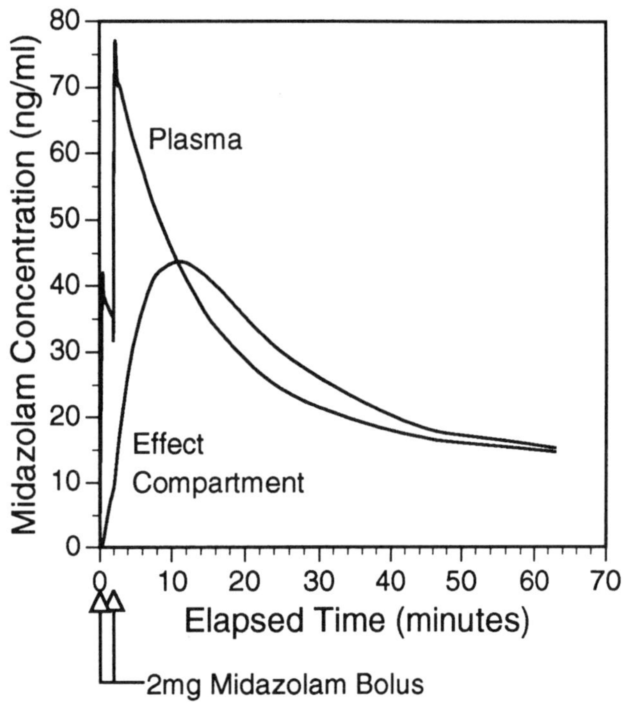

FIGURE 17-11. Simulation of the resultant midazolam plasma and effect site concentration after two bolus doses of 1 mg of midazolam spaced 1 minute apart. Note that although the plasma concentration has peaked, the effect site concentration and thus effect is still rising at the time of the second dose.

the more rational choice of intravenous anesthetic drugs as well as the most appropriate timing of their administration. The time to peak effect of intravenous anesthetic drugs is also summarized in Table 17A-5.

Specific Drugs

Propofol

Propofol was first introduced as an induction agent (126-129) and was subsequently used to maintain anesthesia (130-132). A few years later, propofol was shown to be highly suitable for sedation during local and regional anesthesia (126-129), as well as for sedation in the intensive care unit (130-132). At extremely low doses, propofol was found to possess direct antiemetic properties (133) and to be effective against pruritus secondary to liver disease (134) as well as opioid-induced pruritus (135).

Propofol has a unique pharmacokinetic profile relative to other intravenous induction agents. The metabolic clearance of propofol has been estimated to be 10 times higher than that of thiopental, exceeding the hepatic blood flow. Hence, its concentration declines faster than thiopental after the initial period of redistribution (136) (Fig. 17-12). In a simulation based on pharmacokinetics of each drug, the time required for a 50% decrease in propofol concentration was shorter than for thiopental following an initial bolus dose, and the difference in recovery time became more pronounced over time as the propofol infusion time was prolonged (136, 137) (Fig. 17-13).

Despite propofol's anticonvulsant properties, it can produce excitatory activity (e.g., movement, myoclonic twitching, muscle tremor, and hiccuping) during induction of anesthesia. Although the incidence of these excitatory effects is higher than with thiopental, it is less than that with either methohexital or etomidate. The administration of small doses of potent, rapidly acting opioid analgesics (e.g., fentanyl or alfentanil) decreases the incidence of excitatory activity. On the other hand, the addition of opioid analgesics increases the incidence and duration of apnea following propofol induction. When a bolus dose of propofol (2 to 2.5 mg/kg) is administered rapidly for induction of anesthesia, transient apnea (30 to 90 seconds) occurs in 30 to 60% of unpremedicated patients. If an opioid is

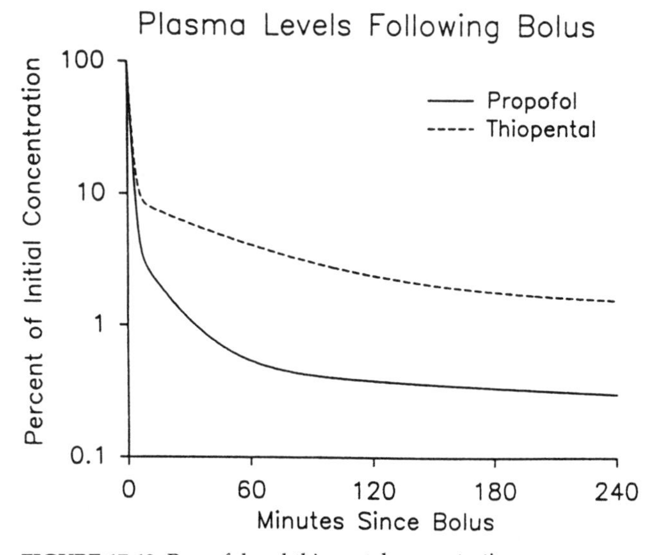

FIGURE 17-12. Propofol and thiopental concentrations, as a percentage of the initial concentration, following bolus injection. (From Shafer SL. Advances in propofol phramacokinetics and phramacodynamics. J. Clin. Anesth 1993;5 [suppl 1]:14S–21S.)

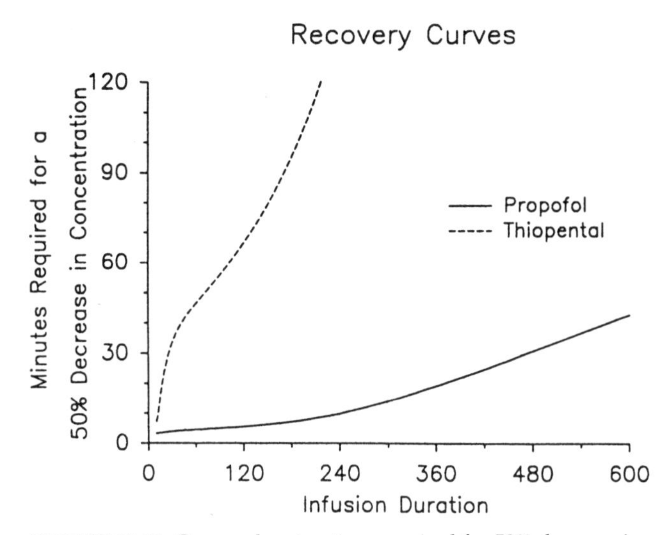

FIGURE 17-13. Curves showing time required for 50% decrease in propofol and thiopental concentration following discontinuation of a continuous infusion. (From Shafer SL. Advances in propofol phramacokinetics and phramacodynamics. J. Clin. Anesth 1993;5 [suppl 1]:14S–21S.)

administered as premedication or as an adjuvant during the induction period, apnea occurs in virtually all patients unless the propofol dose is carefully titrated to achieve loss of consciousness (e.g., 20 to 40 mg every 10 to 20 seconds). The addition of an opioid also significantly decreases ventilatory drive during the maintenance period (138). The addition of an opioid analgesic only modestly reduces the induction dose of propofol, in contrast to the marked reduction in the propofol dose required for loss of consciousness when combined with midazolam. For example, midazolam, 0.05 mg/kg, reduces the induction dose of propofol from 1.3 mg/kg to 0.7 mg/kg (139). Commonly, an opioid and a benzodiazepine are both given before induction of anesthesia with propofol, thereby reducing the propofol induction dose requirement. When using a triple combination, anesthesiologists must carefully titrate the propofol dose to avoid hypotension.

The propofol Cp_{50} for loss of response to verbal command is 3.5 μg/ml (111, 140), and the Cp_{50} to prevent movement on skin incision is 16 μg/ml (111) (see Table 17-3). The latter value is markedly reduced by the presence of fentanyl or alfentanil. The propofol Cp_{50} for skin incision when combined with benzodiazepine premedication (lorazepam 1 to 2 mg) and 66% nitrous oxide is 2.5 μg/ml (141) and is reduced to 1.7 μg/ml when morphine (0.15 mg/kg) is used for premedication (142). The plasma concentration of propofol when combined with 66% nitrous oxide required during minor surgery varies from 1.5 to 4.5 μg/ml (143, 144) and for major surgery varies from 2.5 to 6 μg/ml (145). Awakening usually occurs below a concentration of 1.6 μg/ml and orientation below 1.2 μg/ml (143, 146, 147).

Although opioids potentiate propofol, it has been difficult to demonstrate that the propofol-sparing effect is actually associated with improvement in recovery. Thomas and associates found that, in short outpatient cases, premedication with fentanyl (100 μg) decreases the requirement for propofol and shortens induction time, but it does not result in an improvement in recovery time or subjective assessment of the quality of anesthesia (148). These patients underwent procedures that were extremely brief (8 to 9 minutes), however, and the total amount of propofol administered was small. The use of propofol in combination with fentanyl in longer cases, when compared with propofol alone, provides for a significantly smoother intraoperative course and a shorter recovery period (149). When propofol is combined with nitrous oxide, recovery is faster and more predictable (150). When small doses of opiate (fentanyl, less than 1 μg/kg/h) are added to propofol and nitrous oxide, a further small reduction in propofol requirements can be achieved. When propofol is administered as part of a true total intravenous anesthesia (TIVA) technique with an opioid, the interaction is complex, as illustrated in Figure 17-14. Vuyk and colleagues (151) demonstrated that high concentrations of both opiate and propofol are required to ablate a response to tracheal intubation. These high concentrations are provided by the initial opiate loading dose and the propofol induction dose. During the maintenance period, small concentrations of opiate reduce the propofol concentration required for adequate anesthesia until a plateau is reached at a fentanyl concentration of 3 to 4 ng/ml or an alfentanil concentration of 180 to 240 ng/ml. Using an opiate infusion designed to achieve a concentration equivalent to fentanyl, 0.5 to 1 ng/ml, alfentanil, 75 to 150 ng/ml, and acute hemodynamic responses occur, it is more appropriate to adjust the opiate concentration (152). Adjustments in the propofol infusion should be performed if patients display signs of inadequate anesthesia not responding to additional opioid medication. Other factors also influence rational choices about which drug to titrate to achieve adequate anesthesia. For example, the choice of the supplemental drug may depend on which has a shorter k_{e0}. Hence, when using low-dose alfentanil and propofol, a bolus of alfentanil may be the fastest means of achieving an adequate anesthesia in response to increasing surgical stimulus (152).

Another consideration when administering a propofol-opioid combination is the time to recovery. In the study by Vuyk and colleagues (151), the effect of drug interaction on the recovery profile was examined. Using pharmacokinetic simulations, the ideal combination of propofol and alfentanil that provides both adequate intraoperative anesthesia and the fastest recovery was determined (see Fig. 17-14). In the editorial by Stanski and Shafer (153), the loading and in-

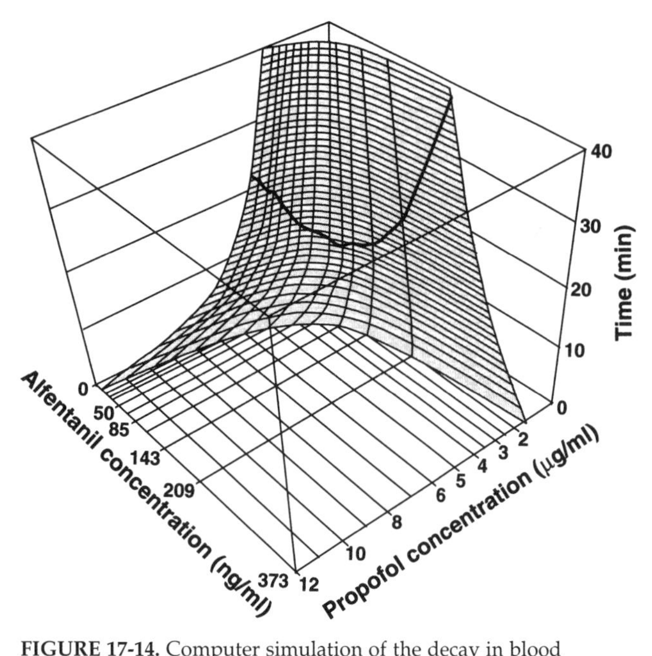

FIGURE 17-14. Computer simulation of the decay in blood propofol and plasma alfentanil concentrations, showing the first 40 minutes after the termination of a computer-controlled infusion that had been given for 180 minutes, with target propofol and alfentanil concentrations equal to the alfentanil concentration associated with 50% probability of no response determined for intra-abdominal surgery. The bold line represents the blood propofol and plasma alfentanil concentration at which 50% of patients regain consciousness. The interval between the termination of the infusion of propofol and alfentanil and the time that the propofol and alfentanil concentrations had decreased to concentrations equal to those at which 50% of patients regain consciousness was found to be shortest (10 minutes) after a 180-minute infusion of propofol and alfentanil at concentrations of 3.5 µg/ml and 85 ng/ml, respectively. (From Vuyk J, Lim T, Engbers FH, et al. The pharmacodynamic interaction of propofol and alfentanil during lower abdominal surgery in women. Anesthesiology 1995;83:8–22.)

Does the same relationship hold true when propofol is combined with other opiates? The interaction appears similar, but the recovery profiles of alfentanil, sufentanil, and fentanyl may differ. Because the context-sensitive half-time for a fentanyl infusion longer than 1 hour is longer than that of alfentanil, recovery occurs most rapidly when relatively higher concentrations of propofol and lower concentrations of fentanyl are used. In contrast, as the context-sensitive half-times following sufentanil infusions lasting up to 9 hours are shorter than those of alfentanil, lower concentrations of propofol and relatively higher concentrations of sufentanil may give the ideal maintenance and recovery profile. If the opiate concentration is maintained above an equivalent of 3 ng/ml fentanyl, 180 ng/ml alfentanil, or 0.45 ng/ml sufentanil to achieve adequate analgesia during maintenance of propofol anesthesia, infusion rates required to provide this ideal combination for TIVA were simulated (Fig. 17-15). Recommendations were that an initial loading dose of propofol of 0.7 mg/kg be administered 2.3 minutes before intubation and that alfentanil, 30 µg/kg, be administered 1.4 minutes before intubation. A maintenance infusion of propofol, 180 µg/kg/min, was recommended after intubation for 10 minutes, decreasing to 140 µg/kg/min from 10 to 30 minutes after induction, and then further decreased to approximately 100 µg/kg/min. The alfentanil infusion should be started 10 minutes after intubation at a rate of 0.35 µg/kg/min, and subsequently decreased to 0.275 to 0.24 µg/kg/min. Increasing the induction dose of propofol to 1 mg/kg only prolongs recovery by an additional minute. The propofol and alfentanil concentrations during maintenance and on emergence after termination of infusions lasting 10 to 600 minutes using the recommended dosing guidelines are illustrated in Figure 17A-15.

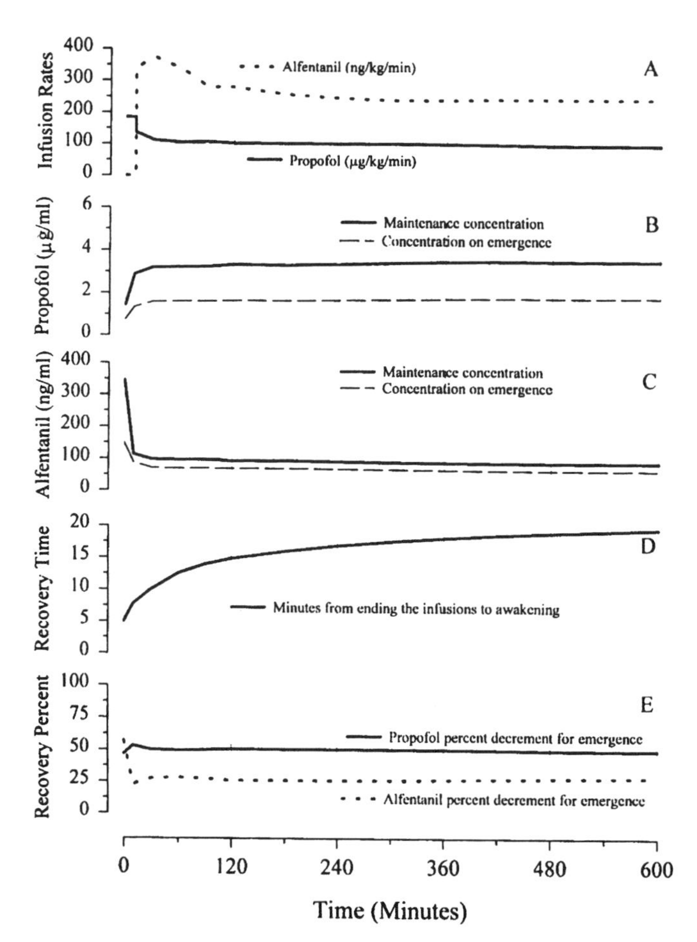

FIGURE 17-15. The propofol and alfentanil infusion rates (A), propofol and alfentanil concentrations (B and C, respectively), time for recovery from anesthesia (D), and percentage decrease required for recovery (E) for an anesthetic regimen that provides 50% probability of response to intra-abdominal surgery and the most rapid emergence from anesthesia, based on the interaction models of Vuyk and colleagues. The regimen assumes intubation at time 0, after a 0.7-mg/kg propofol bolus 2.3 minutes before intubation and a 30-µg/kg alfentanil bolus 1.4 minutes before intubation. (From Stanski D, Shafer S. Quantifying anesthetic drug interaction: implications for drug dosing. Anesthesiology 1995;83:1–5.)

covery to an awake state with adequate breathing is prolonged.

Another common dose regimen for alfentanil when used in combination with propofol consists of a loading dose of fentanyl, 50 μg/kg, followed by an infusion of 50 μg/kg/h (57). A constant blood concentration of alfentanil is achieved within 20 minutes and provides satisfactory conditions for body surface surgery, while allowing for a rapid return to an adequate breathing pattern when the alfentanil infusion rate is decreased to 20 μg/kg/h. A 20% decrease in blood pressure and heart rate when compared with the preinduction rate is commonly seen, and these changes may be minimized by premedicating with glycopyrrolate, 5 μg/kg intravenously (154). This infusion scheme is equivalent to the combined effects of morphine 10 mg and 67% nitrous oxide (142).

Barbiturates

The usual induction dose of thiopental is 2.5 to 5 mg/kg, with slightly higher doses recommended in children and infants and lower dosages in the elderly. In certain situations, it may be advisable to titrate the thiopental to loss of consciousness by injecting 50% of the calculated dose and observing the patient's level of consciousness, following with additional 50-mg bolus doses until the desired response is obtained. Premedicated geriatric patients require 30 to 35% less thiopental on a milligram-per-kilogram basis compared with a younger population. The blood-brain equilibration half-life for thiopental is 1.2 minutes (k_{e0} = 0.238/min), compared with 2.9 minutes for propofol (155). This difference in effect-site equilibration time affects the induction characteristics and allows for a slightly more rapid loss of consciousness with thiopental compared with propofol following equipotent doses. This difference makes it easier to titrate thiopental to reach a desired effect (i.e., loss of consciousness) while minimizing the overshoot in the effect-site compartment. Following bolus administration, the time to peak drug concentration in the effect site is 1.7 minutes for thiopental, 2.2 minutes for propofol, and 2.8 minutes for midazolam (see Table 17-5). When thiopental is used to maintain anesthesia, the time for drug concentration in the effect compartment to decline is significantly longer with thiopental than with propofol and midazolam (Fig. 17-16). In addition, the metabolism of thiopental results in active metabolites that may further prolong recovery. Thus, thiopental is an excellent drug to provide loss of consciousness; however, it is an inappropriate drug to maintain prolonged anesthesia.

The barbiturates and benzodiazepines work by similar mechanisms and produce greater than additive effects when combined. Benzodiazepines increase chloride conductance in postsynaptic membranes by potentiating the effects of τ-aminobutyric acid, whereas barbiturates bind at or near chloride channels to produce similar chloride hyperpolarization (156). Midazolam and barbiturates have synergistic hypnotic effects (92, 157). In human patients, the combination of midazolam and thiopental has 1.8 times the expected potency of the individual agents. Midazolam, 0.02 mg/kg mg, reduces the thiopental induction dose from 6 mg/kg to 2.5 mg/kg (32).

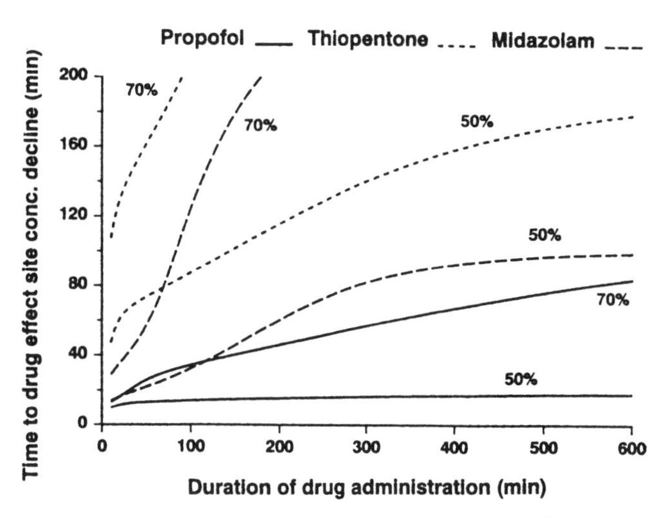

FIGURE 17-16. The time for drug concentration in the effect compartment to decline by 50% and by 70% following infusions of increasing duration of propofol (solid lines) thiopental (short dashed lines) and midazolam (long dashed lines) using computer simulation. Computer simulation is based on the methods described in reference 115. (From Shafer A, Doze VA, Shafer SL, White PF. Pharmacokinetics and pharmacodynamics of propofol infusions during general anesthesia. Anesthesiology 1988;69:348–356.)

Methohexital infusions have also been used successfully as part of a balanced anesthetic technique with nitrous oxide, an opiate, and a muscle relaxant. The infusion rates for methohexital are similar to those used for propofol (i.e., loading dose of 1 to 2 mg/kg is needed for induction and 100 to 140 μg/kg/min for maintenance when combined with nitrous oxide or an opiate) (Fig. 17-17) (158). Methohexital infusions (20 to 40 mg/kg/min) have also been titrated to produce sedation (159) and have been used in conjunction with regional anesthesia (160-162). In comparison with midazolam, methohexital has been found to have a more rapid recovery (162).

Opioids

The use of high doses of opioid analgesics as anesthetics achieved popularity in the 1970s, especially for patients with preexisting cardiovascular diseases. The use of an opioid as the primary anesthetic component was first described at the turn of the century, however. In 1900, Schneiderlein described the administration of scopolamine, 2.5 mg, and morphine, 70 mg intramuscularly (163), to render patients oblivious to pain and without any recollection of the surgical procedure.

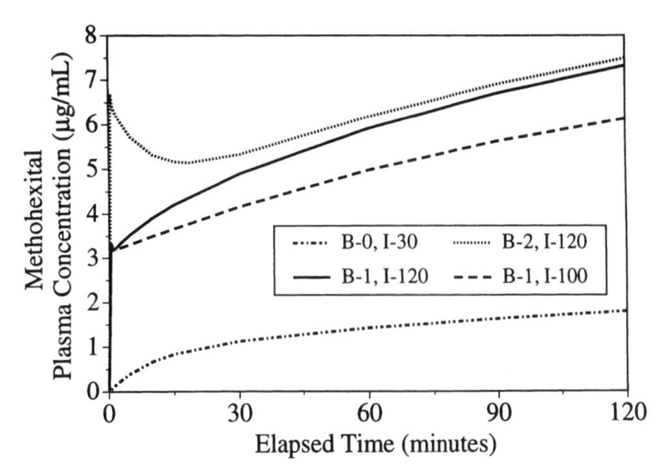

FIGURE 17-17. A simulation of methohexital plasma concentrations after initial boluses followed by continuous infusions for sedation and general anesthesia. B, Bolus (mg/kg); I, infusion (μg/kg/min).

However, 70% of patients required some restraint during surgery (164), and perioperative deaths led to an abandonment of this technique (165). With the introduction of the newer synthetic opiates (fentanyl and its analogues) and the advent of controlled ventilation, high-dose opiate techniques again become popular. In high-risk patients, induction of anesthesia can be readily achieved with fentanyl; however, the use of high doses of fentanyl has been associated with profund bradycardia and trunkal rigidity. When this drug is used for induction of anesthesia, the incidence of bradycardia is higher when patients breathe pure oxygen than when nitrous oxide is used with oxygen because of the increase in sympathetic nervous system activity associated with nitrous oxide. Bradycardia can be minimized by premedication with atropine and small-to-moderate doses of intravenous pancuronium (0.5 to 2 mg) before induction of anesthesia with fentanyl or other potent narcotics.

Induction of anesthesia with opioids may cause muscle rigidity to a degree that makes ventilation of the lungs difficult. Problems with muscle rigidity associated with the use of opioids during anesthesia was noted as far back as 1953 (166), but it did not gain widespread attention until the introduction of neuroleptanesthesia (167, 168). Chest wall rigidity is associated with the use of droperidol and fentanyl as well as high-dose (0.5 to 0.8 mg) fentanyl. Opioid-induced muscle rigidity is characterized by increased muscle tone progressing to severe stiffness. It usually occurs as the patient is losing consciousness, although it may be felt by the conscious patient. Rigidity is more common with older patients (older than 60 years) and is related to the speed of injection and the presence of nitrous oxide (169-174). Benzodiazepines, nondepolarizing neuromuscular blockers, and the α_2 agonist dexmedetomidine have been shown to reduce opioid-related muscle rigidity (59).

During the maintenance of anesthesia, the Cp_{50} of opiates (e.g., alfentanil) for various surgical stimuli is different in the presence of 66% nitrous oxide. For example, in one study, the Cp_{50} concentration of alfentanil with nitrous oxide for tracheal intubation was 475 $\pm$ 28 ng/ml, for skin incision it was 279 $\pm$ 20 ng/ml, and for skin closure it was 150 $\pm$ 23 ng/ml. The Cp_{50} for spontaneous ventilation after the discontinuation of nitrous oxide was higher (223 $\pm$ 13 ng/ml) than for skin closure when nitrous oxide was maintained. Different surgical procedures with varying intensity of surgical stimuli were associated with different Cp_{50} values. The alfentanil Cp_{50} for breast surgery (with 66% nitrous oxide) was 270 $\pm$ 63 ng/ml, for lower abdominal surgery it was 309 $\pm$ 44 ng/ml, and for upper abdominal surgery it was 412 $\pm$ 135 ng/ (110). The Cp_{50} value for skin incision for fentanyl in the presence of 70% nitrous oxide was 4.2 ng/ml. Because of the pharmacokinetics of fentanyl, it is difficult to titrate the concentration of fentanyl to determine the Cp_{50} for all the other stimuli within the same patient. Utilizing the Cp_{50} for skin incision (alfentanil, 279 ng/ml, versus fentanyl, 4.2 ng/ml), however, the relative potency can be calculated (i.e., alfentanil is 66 times less potent than fentanyl). Thus, the Cp_{50} of fentanyl for tracheal intubation would be estimated to be 7 to 8 ng/ml, and that for spontaneous ventilation would be 3 ng/ml. The Cp_{50} for tracheal intubation with sufentanil has been determined to be 2.08 $\pm$ 0.62 ng/ml. Based on the depression of the spectral edge of the electroencephalogram (EEG) and the reduction in isoflurane MAC, sufentanil is estimated to be 12 times more potent than fentanyl. Hence, the predicted Cp_{50} for spontaneous ventilation with sufentanil would be 0.3 to 0.4 ng/ml (see Table 17-3), which is less than values established in clinical studies (175). Because these values are simply guidelines, opiate administration must be titrated to the individual needs of the patient. The recommended infusion rates to reach the Cp_{50} values for fentanyl and its analogues are summarized in Table 17-4.

The combination of opioids with other anesthetic agents may profoundly alter the concentration-effect relationship. As mentioned previously, the induction dose of propofol is reduced by alfentanil (176, 177). For a fentanyl and propofol combination, an additive effect for hypnosis has been demonstrated (178); however, for a fentanyl and midazolam combination, a synergistic hypnotic effect has been observed (179). Kissin and colleagues demonstrated that a small dose of alfentanil (3 μg/kg) potentiates the hypnotic effect of midazolam, reducing the ED_{50} from 270 μg/kg to 142 μg/kg (180). During induction of anesthesia, an opioid is often used in combination with a hypnotic to suppress the hypertensive response to intubation. Addition of an opioid may result in hypotension in the time interval between induction and intubation, however. Propofol, 2 to 3.5 mg/kg, caused a decrease in systolic blood pressure of 28 mm Hg. Combination of propofol with fentanyl, 2 to 4 μg/kg, caused a further decrease in systolic blood pressure (181). Propofol at the same dose was associated with an increase of 65 mm Hg in systolic pressure from the preinduction value after intubation. The increase was less marked at 50 mm Hg when propofol was used in combination with fentanyl, 2 μg/kg, and only 37 mm Hg when propofol was combined with fentanyl at 4 μg/kg (181). The administration of opioids also decreases the dose of thiopental required for loss of consciousness (97, 182, 183). The addition of fentanyl (3 to 7 μg/kg) or sufentanil (0.4 to 1 μg/kg) before anesthetic induction can attenuate changes in heart rate, blood pressure, pulmonary capillary wedge pressure, and the neuroendocrine stress response during laryngoscopy and intubation (184-186).

The interaction between opiates and intravenous anesthetics during the maintenance period to prevent response to a noxious stimulus differs from the interaction needed to provide hypnosis. Smith and associates (111) showed that increasing concentrations of fentanyl decreased the induction concentration of propofol by a maximum of 30 to 40%. In preventing the response to skin incision, however, increasing the opiate concentration reduced the propofol concentration by nearly 90%. Alfentanil requirements in patients undergoing surgery are significantly higher when the drug is used as a supplement to 66% nitrous oxide compared with propofol (4 μg/ml) (119). In one study, the Cp_{50} values of alfentanil during nitrous oxide anesthesia were 429 ng/ml for intubation, 101 ng/ml for skin incision, and 206 ng/ml for intra-abdominal surgery, and the values for alfentanil when combined with propofol (3 μg/ml) were considerably lower at 92 ng/ml for intubation, 55 ng/ml for skin incision, and 66 ng/ml for intra-abdominal surgery. The interaction between propofol and alfentanil was similar to the interaction between propofol and fentanyl. Interactions between isoflurane and fentanyl (113), sufentanil (116), alfentanil (115), and remifentanil have also been established. These studies have demonstrated that interactions for the prevention of responses to skin incision are similar among opiates and vary only according to their different potencies.

Remifentanil is a novel synthetic μ-opioid agonist that possesses potent analgesic activity. It is the first ultrashort-acting opioid and is unique in that recovery from its effect does not seem to depend on the duration of the infusion (Fig. 17-18) or the total dose (187-189). Remifentanil has an elimination half-life of 8 minutes in humans and is 30 times more potent than alfentanil after an intravenous bolus (190). Hence, its use will be most helpful when an intense opioid effect with rapid recovery is required (e.g., outpatient surgery and painful diagnostic procedures). In preliminary studies, remifentanil has been administered as an infusion (0.0125 to 2.0 μg/kg/min) during propofol-nitrous oxide-vecuronium anesthesia, with the time to sponta-

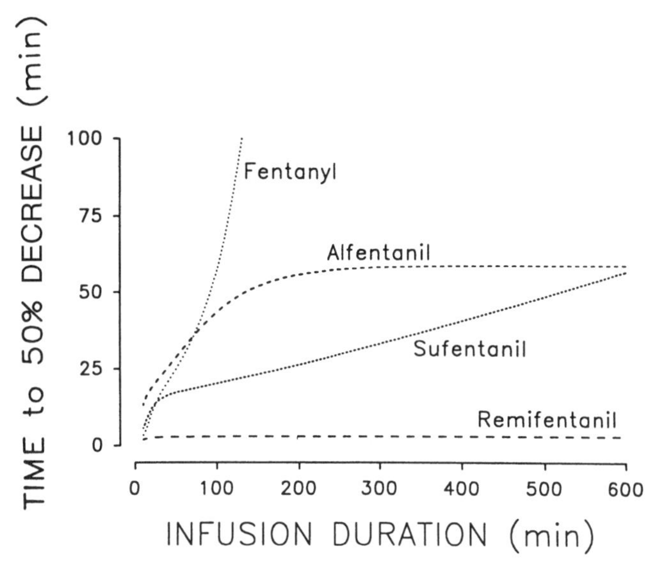

FIGURE 17-18. A simulation of the time necessary to achieve a 50% decrease in drug concentration in the blood (or plasma) after variable-length intravenous infusions of remifentanil, fentanyl, alfentanil, and sufentanil. The simulation for remifentanil was done using the NONMEM three-compartment model parameters. (From Westmoreland CL, Hoke JF, Sebel PS, et al. Pharmacokinetics of remifentanil (GI87084B) and its major metabolite (GI90291) in patients undergoing elective inpatient surgery [See comments]. Anesthesiology 1993;79:893–903.)

neous respiration differing by only 1 to 3 minutes between the groups despite a 20-fold difference in the final infusion rate, and most patients were breathing spontaneously within 5 minutes (191). A constant rate of infusion of remifentanil rapidly achieves steady-state conditions, and therefore small loading doses are sufficient in most cases. Because of remifentanil's extremely short context-sensitive half-time, recovery is still rapid even if remifentanil is maintained at concentrations providing maximal MAC reduction, and isoflurane or propofol is maintained at concentrations close to their MAC awake or Cp_{50} asleep values, respectively.

Ketamine

Ketamine is a dissociative anesthetic agent that has acquired a unique place in clinical practice. The ketamine anesthetic state has been described as a functional and electrophysiologic dissociation between the thalamoneocortical and limbic systems. The drug possesses analgesic, anesthetic, and amnesic properties. To achieve these effects, ketamine interacts with several pharmacologic receptors. The analgesic effects of ketamine are mediated by opioid receptors located in the brain, spinal cord, and peripheral sites (192, 193). Ketamine is a potent noncompetitive N-methyl-D-aspartate (NMDA) receptor antagonist and also interacts with σ receptors. The initial experience with ketamine as a sole anesthetic agent led to the recognition of unpleasant emergence reactions (i.e., illusions and delirium) and cardiovascular stimulant properties. Supplementation with other centrally active drugs (e.g., benzodiazepines thiopental, propofol) has reduced these side effects, however.

Ketamine has been used during major surgery in critically ill and elderly patients in whom periods of hemodynamic instability and ventilatory depression must be avoided. The drug is also regarded as advantageous for patients in a hypovolemic state. Typically, ketamine is administered as a continuous intravenous infusion (25 to 50 μg/kg/min) in combination with a volatile agent, an intravenous hypnotic, or nitrous oxide. With increasing interest in TIVA techniques, ketamine is being used in combination with other intravenous anesthetic agents. For example, the combination of ketamine with midazolam, thiopental, or propofol has been used for induction (194) or as a TIVA technique (195–197). The combination of the two hypnotic drugs is usually additive rather than synergistic. Ketamine has been used with thiopental (198), midazolam (199), diazepam (200), or a midazolam-sufentanil combination for intravenous anesthesia (201).

TIVA for minor gynecologic surgery with ketamine (1 mg/kg) and midazolam (0.1 mg/kg) has been described (202). All patients were spontaneously breathing room air, no incidents of airway obstruction or desaturation were observed, and the patients' acceptance of the technique was high. When a TIVA technique based on a combination of either propofol-ketamine or propofol-fentanyl was compared with respect to their hemodynamics, stability, and analgesia (195), both groups of patients showed a fall in mean arterial blood pressure and heart rate following induction of anesthesia, but cardiovascular parameters were more stable during the maintenance phase in the propofol-ketamine group. In the postoperative period, the patients receiving ketamine showed superior vigilance and experienced better pain relief. Some mild emergence phenomena were reported in the ketamine-treated group, however. In another study evaluating a similar combination, a prolonged recovery phase and an increased incidence of dizziness was found in the ketamine-propofol group. All patients in this group judged the anesthesia as pleasant, however, compared with 89% of the patients in the propofol-fentanyl group (197). Ketamine-benzodiazepine based anesthesia has also been shown to result in a shorter gastrocecal transit time compared with an opioid-benzodiazepine-based anesthesia technique. Hence, the advantages of using a combination of a benzodiazepine with ketamine include better hemodynamic stability, attenuation of intraoperative tachycardia and hypertension intraoperatively, superior analgesia with less respiratory depression during the early recovery phase, and fewer unpleasant emergence phenomena.

Ketamine has also been successfully used in a variety of clinical settings (203). In dressing changes in patients who have burns, the drug is used in subanesthetic intravenous doses (<1.0 mg/kg), often in combination with premedication of a barbiturate, propofol, or a benzodiazepine and an antisialagogue. The sedative-hypnotic drug reduces the dose requirement of ketamine, and the antisialagogue reduces troublesome salivation. In adults and children, ketamine has been used as a supplement to regional anesthesia. For example, ketamine has been used before the application of painful blocks (204), but more commonly it is used for sedation during local anesthesia (205) or supplemental anesthesia during long or uncomfortable procedures. When used for supplementation of regional anesthesia, ketamine (0.5 mg/kg), combined with diazepam (0.15 mg/kg) or midazolam (0.05), is better accepted by patients and reduces ketamine-induced side effects (206). Ketamine in low doses can also be combined with nitrous oxide for the supplementation of conduction or local anesthesia.

Benzodiazepines

Benzodiazepines have been used extensively for sedation as preoperative premedication, intraoperatively during regional and local anesthesia, and postoperatively in the intensive care setting. Midazolam has become the primary benzodiazepine used in the perioperative period. The time to peak effect with midazolam is about 3 minutes, and this benzodiazepine should be titrated in incremental doses to achieve the desired end point (Table 17-6). Despite the wide margin of safety with benzodiazepines, respiratory function must be monitored when these agents are used for sedation, to prevent serious respiratory depression. An apparent synergistic action occurs between midazolam and spinal anesthesia, with resulting respiratory depression. Marked synergism occurs when benzodiazepines and opioids are combined, and hence a high degree of vigilance must be exercised when this combination is used for sedation during local or regional anesthesia.

Benzodiazepines have also been used as induction and maintenance agents. Both diazepam and lorazepam have been used for induction of anesthesia. With

TABLE 17-6. Dosages of Intravenous Benzodiazepines for Induction and Maintenance of Anesthesia, as well as for Sedation

Use	Midazolam	Diazepam	Lorazepam
Induction	0.1–0.2 mg/kg	0.3–0.5 mg/kg	0.1 mg/kg
Maintenance	0.05 mg/kg PRN 1.0 mg/kg/min	0.1 mg/kg PRN	0.02 mg/kg PRN
Sedation*	0.5–1 mg repeated 0.07 mg/kg IM	2 mg repeated	0.25 mg repeated

*Incremental doses given until desired degree of sedation obtained

PRN, As required to keep patient hypnotic and amnestic.

(From Glass PSA, Shafer S, Jacobs J, Reves JG. Intravenous drug delivery systems. In: Miller RD, ed. Anesthesia. vol 1. 4th ed. New York: Churchill Livingstone, 1994:247–289.)

its faster onset compared with lorazepam and its lack of venous complications compared with diazepam, midazolam is the benzodiazepine of choice for induction of anesthesia. With midazolam, 0.1 to 0.2 mg/kg, induction occurs less rapidly than with thiopental, but amnesia is more reliable (207). Although midazolam (0.2 to 0.6 mg/kg) lowers the halothane MAC by 30% (208), the sedative effects of midazolam in the presence of morphine are only additive (i.e., the requirement of one agent to produce a certain degree of sedation is decreased by another agent, but only to a degree equivalent to the sedative dose of the latter) (209). Midazolam and alfentanil are both relatively short-acting agents commonly used in combination. The interaction between these two intravenous drugs is synergistic (210) even in subanalgesic doses of the opioid (180). Vinik and colleagues (177) demonstrated that the combination of midazolam, alfentanil, and propofol produces marked synergism (Fig. 17-19). This combination may be advantagous for induction and maintenance of general anesthesia; however, this triple combination has to be employed cautiously if the anesthetic plan is only sedation and hypnosis during monitored anesthetic care. Experience indicates that a mild-to-moderate level of sedation is required from the benzodiazepine for the maintenance of anesthesia when the drug is combined with a opiate. Thus, a desired plasma level of midazolam of 100 to 150 ng/ml is required when it is used in combination with opioids or nitrous oxide. This concentration of midazolam can be achieved with a bolus of 0.1 to 0.15 mg/kg followed by a continuous infusion of 0.5 to 1.5 μg/kg/min. Because the currently available opioids have relatively long context-sensitive half-time values, nitrous oxide is useful in combination with midazolam-based technique because it allows one to administer lower concentrations of both midazolam and the opioid analgesic and thus provides for a more rapid recovery.

Neuroleptanesthesia

In the 1950s, the major tranquilizers were introduced into clinical practice. Laborit and Huguenard proposed that a combination of a major tranquilizer (chlorpromazine), a short-acting barbiturate, and an opioid would induce a state they termed "ganglioplegia" or artificial hibernation (211). This combination of different compounds was novel and represented an exciting approach to providing balanced intravenous anesthesia. This technique blocked not only cerebral cortical responses, but also cellular, endocrine, and autonomic mechanisms usually activated by surgical stimulation and led to the concept of neuroleptanesthesia as proposed by DeCastro and Mundeleer in 1959 (212). These investigators used a combination of a butyrophenone (e.g., droperidol), a potent opioid, and nitrous oxide to produce general anesthesia. The butyrophenone produced hypnosis, the opioid produced analgesia, and nitrous oxide contributed to both effects. This form of balanced anesthesia technique has limited popularity in Europe and the United States. When fentanyl is used in combination with droperidol for neuroleptanesthesia, the droperidol can have a du-

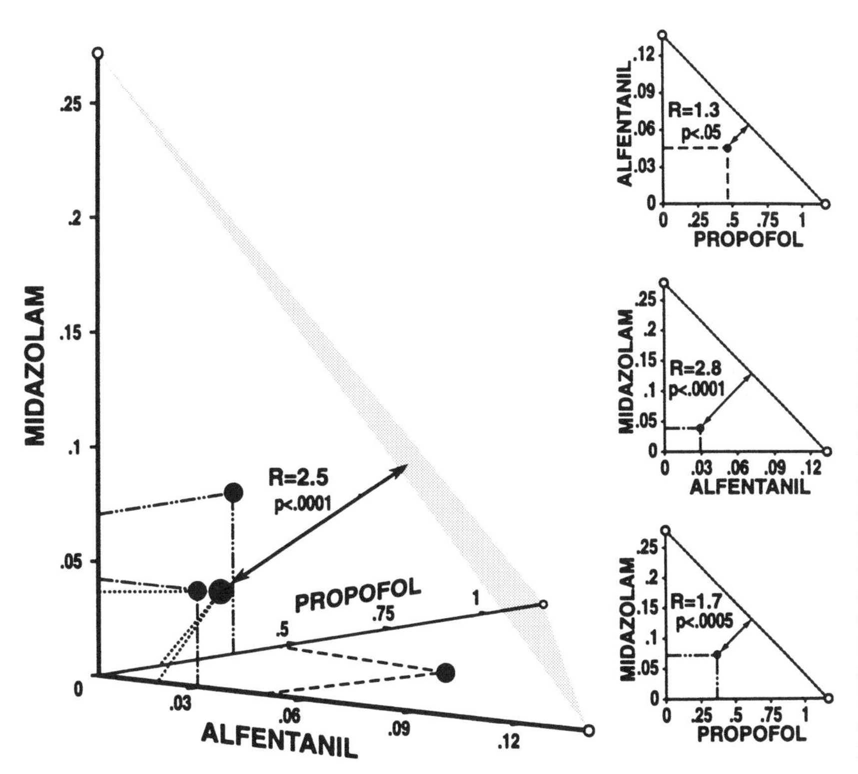

FIGURE 17-19. Median effective dose (ED_{50}) isobologram for the hypnotic interactions among midazolam, alfentanil, and propofol. Shown on the left are triple interaction, and along the axes, doses of the drugs in milligrams per kilogram. The dotted area shows an additive plane passing through three single-drug ED_{50} points (small open circles); the closed circle is the ED_{50} point for the triple combination, and the large open circles are ED_{50} points for the binary combinations. The R-ratio of the single-drug dose (ED_{50} = 1) to combined fractional dose (in fractions of single-drug ED_{50} values) reflects the degree of synergism. (From Vinik HR, Bradley Jr EL, Kissin I. Triple anesthetic combination: propofol-midazolam-alfentanil. Anesth Analg 1994;78:354–358.)

ration of action of up to 24 hours, even though its pharmacokinetic profile appears to be short. Hence, the effect of the tranquilizer may last much longer than that of the analgesic and may result in a patient who appears calm but who is restless and mentally agitated (213). Morgan and colleagues (214) used this technique for major surgery and found that doses of droperidol (5 to 20 mg) and fentanyl (0.1 to 0.8 mg) were necessary for induction of anesthesia in combination with muscle relaxant. This anesthetic technique has been reported for cardiac surgery (215) and neurosurgery (216) in which it has resulted in a fall in cerebral spinal fluid pressure in patients with and without space-occupying lesions (216). One of the advantages of droperidol as part of a balanced technique is its potent antiemetic action; however, this effect is present at much lower doses (e.g., 0.3 to 0.6 mg). Droperidol doses of less than 1.25 mg provide effective antiemetic action without significant sedation (40-42, 217).

RECOVERY PROFILE

Anesthesiologists can use the synergistic interaction of hypnotics and volatile anesthetics to design the optimal combination of both drugs to provide the most rapid recovery. Vuyk and associates (151) demonstrated that when propofol and alfentanil are combined, target propofol concentrations of 3.5 μg/ml and alfentanil of 85 ng/ml provide adequate anesthesia intraoperatively and the most rapid recovery (see Fig. 17-14). Obviously, the exact target concentration for each drug combination that provides the most rapid recovery is a result of both the interaction and the recovery profile (context-sensitive time) of the individual drugs. For example, in the propofol-alfentanil combination, it is preferable to keep the alfentanil concentration low (i.e., analgesic levels) and to provide relatively higher propofol concentrations as the context-sensitive half-time of propofol is much shorter than that of alfentanil. In contrast, with the opioid remifentanil, which has a context-sensitive half-time of 3 to 5 minutes, it is preferable to administer the minimal dose of propofol to ensure hypnosis while administering remifentanil at concentrations needed to provide adequate anesthesia. When both drugs have long context-sensitive half-times, the addition of nitrous oxide is particularly useful because it both reduces the dosage of the other drugs used and has an extremely short elimination time.

Propofol

The use of propofol as an alternative to thiopental for induction results in faster initial and intermediate recovery (218-220). Compared with induction and maintenance of anesthesia with a methohexitol-nitrous oxide combination (221), propofol-nitrous oxide has provided a better recovery profile. Although this effect is most prominent following procedures lasting less than 1 hour, it may also be true for even more prolonged surgery. When propofol is used for maintenance of anesthesia, it provides a more rapid recovery than isoflurane in procedures lasting less than 1 hour. When compared with sevoflurane (221) or desflurane (222) in similar procedures, recovery is equally rapid for all three techniques. Emergence from anesthesia following brief outpatient procedures and recovery of cognitive function has been faster after TIVA with alfentanil and propofol than with an alfentanil-methohexital combination. The duration of postoperative drowsiness and the time to resumption of normal activities have also been significantly shorter (223, 224). The use of nitrous oxide-propofol-alfentanil has been alleged to be associated with longer postoperative recovery after day-case surgery compared with a similar group without nitrous oxide (225).

The incidence of postoperative nausea and vomiting is decreased when propofol is administered in an anesthetic combination (221). Doze and colleagues observed a 50% reduction of this complication in a group of patients who underwent major and minor surgical procedures under general anesthesia when propofol-nitrous oxide was used compared with a thiopental-isoflurane-nitrous oxide combination (138). Similarly, Best and Traugott noted an incidence of postoperative nausea and vomiting of 5% (versus 35%) in patients receiving propofol (versus methohexitone) as the sole anesthetic for microlaryngeal surgery (226). Raftery and Sherry assessed the incidence of this complication and requirements for antiemetic medication in day-case patients undergoing laparoscopy for assisted conception therapy (227). The group that received TIVA with a propofol-alfentanil combination had less postoperative nausea and vomiting, a decreased requirement for rescue antiemetic, and a lower probability of unplanned admission to the hospital compared with the group receiving a nitrous oxide-enflurane anesthetic combination. More recently, the use of propofol intraoperatively was shown as effective as ondansetron in the prevention of nausea and vomiting in the early postoperative period (228). A study by Ding and colleagues suggested that for propofol to protect against postoperative nausea and vomiting, the drug should be given throughout the procedure (229).

Opioids

The duration of action of opioids after anesthesia is not necessarily predicted by elimination half-life values (230). The rate of decline in plasma concentration after administration depends on the complex combination of pharmacokinetic parameters. A small central volume of distribution and a high elimination clearance result in a rapid decrease in plasma concentration. Computer simulations of the recovery of fentanyl, alfentanil, and sufentanil after intravenous administration by bolus injection, brief infusion, or prolonged infusion have provided information on the recovery profiles of the various opioids. When one uses a nitrous oxide-narcotic technique, the concentration of the opioid needs to decrease by approximately 50% to permit adequate spontaneous respiration and awakening. Investigators have estimated that for a patient to become "street ready," the concentration must decrease by 80% or greater. The order in which the opioids fentanyl, alfentanil, and sufentanil decrease by 50% may not be the same as the order in which they reach an 80% decline in their plasma concentrations. For procedures lasting approximately 1 hour, the time for 50% recovery is similar for all three opioids; however, for an 80% decline this is reached most rapidly by sufentanil followed by alfentanil and finally by fentanyl. Following a 6-hour infusion, the time to reach a 50% decrease is most rapid with sufentanil, followed by alfentanil and then by fentanyl. For an 80% decrease, alfentanil is the most rapid, followed by sufentanil and finally by fentanyl. For a 20 to 30% decrease in drug concentration, the rate of decline is similar for all three opioids for infusions of up to 4 hours. The esterase-metabolized opioid remifentanil has a shorter duration of action than fentanyl, alfentanil, or sufentanil, and the termination of its effects is independent of redistribution. When remifentanil and alfentanil were titrated to provide an equal degree of respiratory depression, recovery following a 3-hour infusion was significantly faster for remifentanil (4 minutes) than for alfentanil (45 minutes) (231). The rapid termination of remifentanil's analgesic effect implies that postoperative analgesia must be instituted even before remifentanil is terminated.

ANESTHETIC ANTAGONISTS

Flumazenil

Flumazenil was synthetized in 1981 by Hunkeler and colleagues (232, 233). Flumazenil has high affinity for the benzodiazepine receptor, but it is virtually devoid of intrinsic agonist activity. In clinically relevant doses (0.5 to 2 mg), flumazenil appears to act as a competitive antagonist. It can antagonize all the effects of the benzodiazepines, including sedation, amnesia, muscle relaxation, and their anticonvulsant action. Flumazenil has no effect on centrally active drugs that do not act at the central benzodiazepine receptor (e.g., barbiturates, propofol, opioids, and alcohol), however. It has a rapid onset (1 to 3 minutes), and the peak effect occurs in 5 to 8 minutes (234). It also has a relatively short duration of action because of its rapid redistribution coupled with high liver extraction rate (60%), contributing to an elimination half-life of 60 to 90 minutes. The pharmacokinetics of flumazenil is not significantly altered by coadministration of another benzodiazepine (235).

In addition to its antagonistic properties, flumazenil possesses weak generalized central arousal and anticonvulsant activities. Hart and associates (236) demonstrated, in a single-blind crossover study of epileptic patients, that flumazenil (3 mg) was as effective as diazepam (10 mg) in reducing the number of "epileptic transients" as measured by the EEG. Savic and associates (237) also found that flumazenil (0.75 mg) significantly reduced epileptic discharges in patients with partial seizures, but this dose had no effect in patients with generalized seizures. Flumazenil and benzodiazepines given in therapeutic doses demonstrate dose-dependent effects (234). Reversal of benzodiazepine effects occurs in a sequence opposite to their appearance (i.e., hypnosis, sedation, amnesia, and finally anxiolysis). In addition, the dose of antagonist needed to reverse benzodiazepine effect is reciprocal to the dose of benzodiazepines (Table 17-7). For example, high doses of flumazenil are needed to reverse anxiolysis, and low doses of flumazenil are needed to reverse the hypnotic effect of benzodiazepines (238). Thus, flumazenil doses that reverse sedation and amnesia (0.5 to 1 mg) do not increase anxiety or stress hormone levels (239).

Flumazenil may be used to reverse residual sedation after general anesthesia when a benzodiazepine is used for induction. Mandema and colleagues (240) used aperiodic EEG analysis to characterize the interaction between flumazenil and midazolam. No evi-

Table 17-7. Reciprocal Dose-Dependent Effects of Benzodiazepine Agonists (Midazolam) and Antagonists (Flumazenil)

Midazolam (Agonist)	Clinical Effects	Flumazenil (Antagonist)
Low dose ↑	Anxiolysis	High dose ↑
	Anticonvulsion	
	Slight sedation	
	Reduced attention	
	Amnesia	
	Intense sedation	
↓	Muscle relaxation	↓
High dose	Hypnosis	Low dose

(Modified from Amrein R, Hetzel W, Bonetti EP, et al. Clinical pharmacology of Dormicum (midazolam) and Anexate (flumazenil). Resuscitation 1988;16:S5.)

dence of hysteresis was noted between the flumazenil plasma concentration and its CNS effects. The rapid equilibration between the blood and effect site accounts for the observed rapid onset of clinical effects. The degree of reversal achieved with flumazenil should be carefully titrated by adminstering 0.2-mg increments every 1 to 2 minutes. In a study involving patients who underwent induction of anesthesia with midazolam, flumazenil was titrated in 0.2-mg increments to a total dose of 0.83 ± 0.04 mg (range, 0.6 to 1.0 mg). The patients showed significant subjective and objective improvement in their levels of sedation and psychomotor coordination. By 2 hours after surgery, the psychomotor scores of the flumazenil-treated group were no longer different from those of the placebo-treated group (241).

Numerous studies have examined the reversal effects of flumazenil following benzodiazepine administration for day-case endoscopy (242), dental procedures (243), and ophthalmologic (244), urologic (245), bronchoscopic (246), nonsurgical cardiac procedures (247), as well as surgical procedures under local anesthesia (248). The largest trial involved 700 patients sedated for up to 3 hours with diazepam, midazolam, or a midazolam-opioid combination; 5-minute complete reversal of sedation was observed in 80% of patients after administration of flumazenil, 0.7 mg intravenously. Psychomotor performance also returned to normal in 80 to 92% of patients. Flumazenil was well tolerated, with dizziness (2 to 13%) and nausea (2 to 12%) the most frequently reported adverse events (249). Flumazenil reversal after midazolam sedation also compares favorably with recovery after propofol sedation (250). Even in studies involving midazolam, resedation has been reported. Other concerns include the rare occurrence of arrhythmias and convulsions. Arrhythmias including complete heart block, ventricular tachycardia, and asystole have been associated with the use of flumazenil in "overdose" situations. These complications have occurred in the setting of an acute overdose with a combination of sedative and proarrhythmic drugs (e.g., tricyclic antidepressants, chloral hydrate) (251). Nearly 50% of the patients who had convulsions had ingested an overdose of proconvulsant drugs, and some patients had a history of an epileptic disorder. Nevertheless, flumazenil should be avoided in patients who are predisposed to seizure activity.

In summary, flumazenil provides the ability to antagonize iatrogenic overdose of a benzodiazepine. Benzodiazepines are commonly given during the perioperative period, and residual sedation and amnesia can be effectively reversed with flumazenil. The clinical and economic advantages of routine use of flumazenil after benzodiazepine sedation have not been clearly demonstrated, however.

Opioid Antagonists

Opioid antagonists are occasionally used to restore spontaneous respiration in patients who are breathing inadequately after receiving intraoperative opioids. Opioid antagonists have also been reported to reverse opioid-induced nausea and vomiting, pruritus, urinary retention, rigidity, and biliary spasm. In addition to pain, other side effects related to their use include hypertension, pulmonary edema, and even ventricular tachycardia and fibrillation. The mechanism producing increases in arterial blood pressure and heart rate after naloxone reversal are not well defined; however, an increase in pain, rapid awakening, and sympathetic activation are possible explanations. Oxygen consumption and minute ventilation can increase two- to threefold following administration of an opioid antagonist (252). Naloxone can also produce nonspecific analeptic effects through activation of the CNS arousal system (253, 254). Hence, opioid reversal should be avoided in patients in whom increases in arterial blood pressure and heart rate would be detrimental (e.g., patients with pheochromocytoma, chromaffin tissue tumors, or compromised myocardial function).

The most commonly used opioid antagonist is naloxone. Its onset of action after intravenous administration is rapid (1 to 2 minutes), and its duration of action is relatively short (30 to 60 minutes). Naloxone, titrated in 0.5 to 1.0 μg/kg boluses every 2 to 3 minutes (to a total dose of 2 μg/kg), rapidly restores adequate spontaneous ventilation (86, 255). However, renarcotization may occur with longer-acting opioids. Naloxone infusions in the dosage range of 1 to 10 μg/kg/h are used to prevent respiratory depression in the postoperative period in patients receiving large doses of epidural (256, 257) or intrathecal opioid analgesics (258). Low-dose naloxone infusions (0.25 to 1 μg/kg/h) have been used in conjunction with morphine administered by a patient-controlled analgesia device to decrease opioid-related side effects in the postoperative period (259). Longer-acting opioid antagonists such as naltrexone (elimination half-life of 8 to 12 hours) and nalmefene (elimination half-life of 8 to 10 hours) may avoid the problem of renarcotization. In addition, these longer-acting opioid antagonists can be taken orally because they are not subjected to exensive first-pass hepatic metabolism, in contrast to naloxone.

In conclusion, balanced anesthesia was first popularized because it resulted in greater flexibility and safety. We have come a long way since John Lundy first embraced the concept of balanced anesthesia 80 years ago. Nevertheless, with the increasing choices of drugs and greater understanding of pharmacokinetic and pharmacodynamic principles, modifications and improvements have occurred in the techniques for administering intravenous anesthetics. The art of "balanced" anesthesia is considered to be the cornerstone of anesthesia practice in the foreseeable future.

REFERENCES

1. Cohen MM, Duncan PG, Tate RB. Does anesthesia contribute to operative mortality? JAMA 1988;260:2859–2863.
2. Crile GW. An experimental and clinical research into certain problems relating to surgical operations. Philadelphia: JB Lippincott, 1901.
3. Crile GW. Phylogenetic association in relation to certain medical problems. Boston Med Surg J 1910;163:893–984.
4. Jackson DE. A new method for the production of general analgesia and anesthesia with a description of the apparatus used. J Lab Clin Med 1915;1:1–12.
5. Lundy JS. Balanced anesthesia. Minn Med 1926;9:399.
6. Organe GSW, Broad RJB. Pentothal with nitrous oxide and oxygen. Lancet 1938;2:1170–1172.
7. Paulson JA. Thiopental sodium and ether anesthesia. JAMA 1952;150:983–987.
8. Griffith HR, Johnson GE. The use of curare in general anesthesia. Anesthesiology 1942;3:418–420.
9. Gray TC, Rees GJ. The role of apnoea in general anethesia. Br Med J 1952;2:891–892.
10. Chadwick TH, Swerdlow M. Thiopentone-curare in abdominal surgery. Anesthesia 1949;4:76–78.
11. Gray TC, Halton J. A milestone in anesthesia (d-tubocurarine hydrochloride). Proc R Soc Med 1946;34:400–406.
12. Woodbridge PD. Changing concepts concerning depth of anesthesia. Anesthesiology 1957;18:536–550.
13. Neff W, Mayer EC, de la Luz Perales M. Nitrous oxide and oxygen anesthesia with curare relaxation. Calif Med 1947; 66:67–69.
14. Mushin WW, Rendell-Baker L. Pethidine as a supplement to nitrous oxide anesthesia. Br Med J 1949;2:472.
15. Mushin W. Administration of drugs before anesthesia. Br Med J 1960;1:1558–1560.
16. Bernard C. The combined action of morphia and chloroform. Claude Bernard's lecture at the College De France. Lancet 1869; 2:789.
17. Guedel AE. Inhalation anesthesia. New York: Macmillan, 1937.
18. Dundee JW, Riding JE, Barron DW, Nicholl RM. Some factors influencing the induction characteristics of methohexitone anesthesia. Br J Anaesth 1961;33:296–301.
19. Cohen EN, Beecher HK. Narcotics in preanesthetic medication: a controlled study. JAMA 1951;147:1664.
20. Eckenhoff JE, Helrich M. The effect of narcotics, thiopental and nitrous oxide upon respiration and respiratory response to hypercapnia. Anesthesiology 1958;19:240.
21. Beecher H. Measurement of subjective responses: quantitative effects of drugs. New York: Oxford University Press, 1959.
22. Haslett WHK, Dundee JW. Studies of drugs given before anaesthesia. XIV. Two benzodiazepine derivatives, chlordiazepoxide and diazepam. Br J Anaesth 1968;40:250–258.
23. Gamble JAS, Gaston JH, Nair SG, Dundee JW. Some pharmacological factors influencing the absorption of diazepam following oral administration. Br J Anaesth 1976;48:1181–1185.
24. Dundee JW, Lilburn JK, Nair SG, George KA. Studies of drugs given before anaesthesia. XXVI. Lorazepam. Br J Anaesth 1977; 49:1047–1056.
25. George KA, Dundee JW. Relative amnesia actions of diazepam, flunitrazepam and lorazepam in man. Br J Clin Pharmacol 1977; 4:45.
26. Kawar P, Dundee JW. Frequency of pain on injection and venous sequelae following the I.V. administration of certain anaesthetics and sedatives. Br J Anaesth 1982;54:935–939.
27. Pinnock CA, Fell D, Hunt PC, et al. A comparison of triazolam and diazepam as premedication for minor gynaecologic surgery. Anaesthesia 1985;40:324.
28. Greenblatt DJ, Abernethy DR, Locniskar A, et al. Effect of age, gender and obesity on midazolam kinetics. Anesthesiology 1984;61:27–35.
29. Shafer A, White PF, Urquhart ML, Doze VA. Outpatient premedication: use of midazolam and opioid analgesics. Anesthesiology 1989;71:495–501.
30. Fragen RJ, Funk DI, Avram MJ, et al. Midazolam versus hyroxyzine as intramuscular premedicants. Can Anaesth Soc J 1983; 30:136.
31. Kissin I, Vinik HR, Bradley EL Jr. Midazolam potentiates thiopental sodium anesthetic induction in patients. J Clin Anesth 1991;3:367–370.
32. DeLucia JA, White PF. Effect of midazolam on induction and recovery characteristics of propofol. Anesth Analg 1992;74:S63.
33. Short TG, Chui PT. Propofol and midazolam act synergistically in combination. Br J Anaesth 1991;67:539–545.
34. Saidman LJ, Eger EI. Effect of nitrous oxide and of narcotic premedication on the alveolar concentration of halothane required for anesthesia. Anesthesiology 1964;26:302–306.
35. Tsunoda Y, Hattori Y, Takasuka E, et al. Effects of hydroxyzine, diazepam and pentazocine on halothane minimum alveolar anesthetic concentration. Anesth Analg 1973;52:390.
36. Radnay PA, Brodman E, Mankikor D, et al. The effect of equianalgesic doses of fentanyl, morphine, meperidine and pentazocine on common bile duct pressure. Anesthetist 1980;29:26.
37. Economou G, Ward-McQuaid JN. A cross-over comparison of the effect of morphine, pethidine and pentazocine on biliary pressure. Gut 1971;12:218.
38. Rowbotham DJ. Current management of postoperative nausea and vomiting [Review]. Br J Anaesth 1992;69 (suppl 1):46S–59S.
39. Sun R, Wang B, Klein K, White PF: The effect of timing of ondansetron administration on efficacy in outpatients undergoing ENT surgery. Anesth Analg (submitted for publication).
40. Gan TJ, Collis R, Hetreed M. Double-blind comparison of ondansetron, droperidol and saline in the prevention of postoperative nausea and vomiting. Br J Anaesth 1994;72:544–547.
41. Kauste A, Tuominen M, Heikkinen H, et al. Droperidol, alizapride and metoclopramide in the prevention and treatment of post-operative emetic sequelae. Eur J Anaesthesiol 1986;3:1–9.
42. Madej TH, Simpson KH. Comparison of the use of domperidone, droperidol and metoclopramide in the prevention of nausea and vomiting following major gynaecological surgery. Br J Anaesth 1986;58:884–887.
43. Watcha MF, White PF. Postoperative nausea and vomiting: its etiology, treatment, and prevention [Review]. Anesthesiology 1992;77:162–184.
44. Tang J, Sun R, White PF. Clinical efficacy of prophylactic antiemetics for outpatients at high-risk of postoperative emesis. Anesthesiology 1995;83:A9.
45. Melnick BM. Extrapyramidal reactions to low-dose droperidol. Anesthesiology 1988;69:424–426.
46. McKenzie R, Kovac A, O'Connor T, et al. Comparison of ondansetron versus placebo to prevent postoperative nausea and vomiting in women undergoing ambulatory gynecology surgery. Anesthesiology 1993;78:21–28.
47. Bodner M, White PF. Antiemetic efficacy of ondansetron after ambulatory surgery. Anesth Analg 1991;73:250–254.
48. Helmers JH, Briggs L, Abrahamsson J, et al. A single i.v. dose of ondansetron 8 mg prior to induction of anaesthesia reduces postoperative nausea and vomiting in gynaecological patients. Can J Anaesth 1993;40:1155–1161.

49. McKenzie R, Sharifi-Azad S, Dershwitz M, et al. A randomized, double-blind pilot study examining the use of intravenous ondansetron in the prevention of postoperative nausea and vomiting in female inpatients. J Clin Anesth 1993;5:30–36.
50. Scuderi P, Wetchler B, Sung YF, et al. Treatment of postoperative nausea and vomiting after outpatient surgery with the 5-HT3 antagonist ondansetron [See comments]. Anesthesiology 1993;78:15–20.
51. Stone JG, Foex P, Sear JW, et al. Myocardial ischemia in untreated hypertensive patients: effect of a single small oral dose of beta-adrenergic blocking agent. Anesthesiology 1988;68:495.
52. Kaukinen S, Kaukinen L, Eerola R. Postoperative use of clonidine with neuroleptanaesthesia. Acta Anaesthesiol Scand 1979; 23:113–120.
53. Flacke JW, Bloor BC, Flacke WE, et al. Reduced narcotic requirement by clonidine with improved hemodynamic and adrenergic stability in patients undergoing coronary bypass surgery. Anesthesiology 1987;67:11–19.
54. Ghignone M, Quintin L, Duke PC, et al. Effects of clonidine on narcotic requirements and hemodynamic endothracheal intubation. Anesthesiology 1986;64:36–42.
55. Ghignone M, Noe C, Calvillo O, Quintin L. Anesthesia for ophthalmic surgery in the elderly: the effects of clonidine on intraocular pressure, perioperative hemodynamics, and anesthetic requirement. Anesthesiology 1988;68:707–716.
56. Segal IS, Jarvis DA, Duncan SR, et al. Clinical efficacy of oral-transdermal clonidine combinations during the perioperative period. Anesthesiology 1991;74:220–225.
57. Richards MJ, Skues MA, Jarvis AP, Prys-Roberts C. Total i.v. anaesthesia with propofol and alfentanil: dose requirements for propofol and the effect of premedication with clonidine. Br J Anaesth 1990;65:157–163.
58. Jaakola ML, Salonen M, Lehtinen R, Scheinin H. The analgesic action of dexmedetomidine--a novel alpha 2-adrenoceptor agonist--in healthy volunteers. Pain 1991;46:281–285.
59. Weinger MB, Segal IS, Maze M. Dexmedetomidine, acting through central alpha-2 adrenoceptors, prevents opiate-induced muscle rigidity in rat. Anesthesiology 1989;71:242–249.
60. Aho M, Erkola O, Kallio A, et al. Comparison of dexmedetomidine and midazolam sedation and antagonism of dexmedetomidine with atipamezole. J Clin Anesth 1993;5:194–203.
61. Jaakola ML. Dexmedetomidine premedication before intravenous regional anesthesia in minor outpatient hand surgery. J Clin Anesth 1994;6:204–211.
62. Aantaa R, Jaakola ML, Kallio A, et al. A comparison of dexmedetomidine, and alpha 2-adrenoceptor agonist, and midazolam as i.m. premedication for minor gynaecological surgery. Br J Anaesth 1991;67:402–409.
63. Jaakola ML, Ali-Melkkila T, Kanto J, et al. Dexmedetomidine reduces intraocular pressure, intubation responses and anaesthetic requirements in patients undergoing ophthalmic surgery. Br J Anaesth 1992;68:570–575.
64. Aho M, Lehtinen AM, Erkola O, et al. The effect of intravenously administered dexmedetomidine on perioperative hemodynamics and isoflurane requirements in patients undergoing abdominal hysterectomy. Anesthesiology 1991;74:997–1002.
65. Aho MS, Erkola OA, Scheinin H, et al. Effect of intravenously administered dexmedetomidine on pain after laparoscopic tubal ligation. Anesth Analg 1991;73:112–118.
66. Scheinin H, Jaakola ML, Sjovall S, et al. Intramuscular dexmedetomidine as premedication for general anesthesia: a comparative multicenter study. Anesthesiology 1993;78:1065–1075.
67. Aho M, Scheinin M, Lehtinen AM, et al. Intramuscularly administered dexmedetomidine attenuates hemodynamic and stress hormone responses to gynecologic laparoscopy. Anesth Analg 1992;75:932–939.
68. Visintainer MA, Wolfer JA. Psychological preparation for surgical prediatric patients: the effect on chilren's parents' stress responses and adjustment. Pediatrics 1975;56:187.
69. Jackson K. Psychological preparation as a method of reducing the emotional trauma of anesthesia in children. Anesthesiology 1981;12:293.
70. Booker PD, Chapman DH. Premedication in children undergoing day-care surgery. Br J Anaesth 1979;51:1083.
71. Rita L, Seleny FL, Mazurek A, Rabins Sf. Intramuscular midazolam for pediatric preanesthetic sedation: a double-blind controlled study with morphine. Anesthesiology 1985;63:528.
72. Kessel J. Atropine premedication. Anaesth Intensive Care 1974; 32:77.
73. Rackow H, Salanitre E. Modern concepts in pediatric anesthesiology. Anesthesiology 1969;30:324.
74. Steward DJ. Psychological preparation and premedication. In: Gergory GA, ed. Pediatric anesthesia. New York: Churchill-Livingstone, 1989.
75. Way WL, Costley EC, Way EL. Respiratory sensitivity of the newborn infant to meperidine and morphine. Clin Pharmacol Ther 1965;6:454.
76. Kupferberg HJ, Way EL. Pharmacologic basis for the increased sensitivity of the newborn rat to morphine. J Pharmacol Exp Ther 1963;141:105.
77. Nicolson SC, Betts EK, Jobes DR, et al. Comparison of oral and intramuscular preanesthetic medication for pediatric surgery. Anesthesiology 1989;71:8–10.
78. Helmers JH, Noordiun H, Van Peer A, et al. Comparison IV and intranasal sufentanil. Can J Anaesth 1989;36:494.
79. Ashburn MA, Streisand JB, Tarver SD, et al. Oral transmucosal fentanyl citrate for premedication in pediatric outpatients. Can J Anaesth 1990;37:857–866.
80. Feld LH, Champeau MW, van Steennis CA, Scott JC. Preanesthetic medication in children: a comparison of oral transmucosal fentanyl citrate versus placebo. Anesthesiology 1989; 71:374–377.
81. Friesen RH, Lockhart CH. Oral transmucosal fentanyl citrate for preanesthetic medication of pediatric day surgery patients with and without droperidol as a prophylactic anti-emetic. Anesthesiology 1992;76:46–51.
82. Goldstein-Dresner MC, Davis PJ, Kretchman E, et al. Double-blind comparison of oral transmucosal fentanyl citrate with oral meperidine, diazepam, and atropine as preanesthetic medication in children with congenital heart disease. Anesthesiology 1991;74:28–33.
83. Streisand JB, Stanley TH, Hague B, et al. Oral transmucosal fentanyl citrate premedication in children. Anesth Analg 1989; 69:28–34.
84. Nelson PS, Streisand JB, Mulder SM, et al. Comparison of oral transmucosal fentanyl citrate and an oral solution of meperidine, diazepam, and atropine for premedication in children. Anesthesiology 1989;70:616–621.
85. Stanley TH, Leiman BC, Rawal N, et al. The effects of oral transmucosal fentanyl citrate premedication on preoperative behavioral responses and gastric volume and acidity in children. Anesth Analg 1989;69:328–335.
86. Alderson PJ, Lerman J. Oral premedication for paediatric ambulatory anaesthesia: a comparison of midazolam and ketamine. Can J Anaesth 1994;41:221–226.
87. Gingrich BK. Difficulties encountered in a comparative study of orally administered midazolam and ketamine. Anesthesiology 1994;80:1414–1415.
88. Alfonzo-Echeverri EC, Berg JH, Wild TW, Glass N. Oral ketamine for pediatric outpatient dental surgery sedation. Pediatr Dent 1993;15:192–185.
89. Kissin I, Mason JOD, Bradley EL Jr. Morphine and fentanyl interactions with thiopental in relation to movement response to noxious stimulation. Anesth Analg 1986;65:1149–1154.

90. Kissin I. Morphine-halothane interaction controversy [Letter]. Anesth Analg 1986;65:319–321.
91. Kissin I, Mason JOD, Bradley EL Jr. Morphine and fentanyl hypnotic interactions with thiopental. Anesthesiology 1987; 67:331–335.
92. Kissin I, Mason JOD, Bradley EL Jr. Pentobarbital and thiopental anesthetic interactions with midazolam. Anesthesiology 1987;67:26–31.
93. Kissin I, Brown PT, Bradley EL Jr. Morphine and fentanyl anesthetic interactions with diazepam: relative antagonism in rats. Anesth Analg 1990;71:236–241.
94. Loewe S, Aldous RA, Fox SR, et al. Isobols of dose-effect relations in the combination of trimethadione and pentylenetetrazole. J Pharmacol Exp Ther 1955;113:475–480.
95. Loewe S, Muischnek H. Ueber Konbinationswirjungen. I. Mitteilung: Hilfsmittel der Fragestellung. Naunyn Schmiedebergs Arch Pharmacol 1926;114:313–326.
96. Billard V, Moulla F, Bourgain JL, et al. Hemodynamic response to induction and intubation: propofol/fentanyl interaction. Anesthesiology 1994;81:1384–1393.
97. Martin DE, Rosenberg H, Aukburg SJ, et al. Low-dose fentanyl blunts circulatory responses to tracheal intubation. Anesth Analg 1982;61:680–684.
98. Gaubatz CL, Wehner RJ. Evaluation of esmolol and fentanyl in controlling increases in heart rate and blood pressure during endotracheal intubation. Am Assoc Nurs Anesth J 1991;59:91–96.
99. Leslie JB, Kalayjian RW, McLoughlin TM, Plachetka JR. Attenuation of the hemodynamic responses to endotracheal intubation with preinduction intravenous labetalol. J Clin Anesth 1989;1:194–200.
100. Bernstein JS, Ebert TJ, Stowe DF, et al. Partial attenuation of hemodynamic responses to rapid sequence induction and intubation with labetalol. J Clin Anesth 1989;1:444–451.
101. Inada E, Cullen DJ, Nemeskal AR, Teplick R. Effect of labetalol or lidocaine on the hemodynamic response to intubation: a controlled randomized double-blind study. J Clin Anesth 1989; 1:207–213.
102. Chung KS, Sinatra RS, Chung JH. The effect of an intermediate dose of labetalol on heart rate and blood pressure responses to laryngoscopy and intubation. J Clin Anesth 1992;4:11–15.
103. Ramanathan J, Sibai BM, Mabie WC, et al. The use of labetalol for attenuation of the hypertensive response to endotracheal intubation in preeclampsia. Am J Obstet Gynecol 1988;159:650–654.
104. Yuan L, Chia YY, Jan KT, et al. The effect of single bolus dose of esmolol for controlling the tachycardia and hypertension during laryngoscopy and tracheal intubation. Acta Anaesthesiol Sin 1994;32:147–152.
105. Wang SC, Wu CC, Lin MS, Chang CF. Use of esmolol to prevent hemodynamic changes during intubation in general anesthesia. Acta Anaesthesiol Sin 1994;32:141–146.
106. Helfman SM, Gold MI, DeLisser EA, Herrington CA. Which drug prevents tachycardia and hypertension associated with tracheal intubation: lidocaine, fentanyl, or esmolol? [See comments]. Anesth Analg 1991;72:482–486.
107. Parnass SM, Rothenberg DM, Kerchberger JP, Ivankovich AD. A single bolus dose of esmolol in the prevention of intubation-induced tachycardia and hypertension in an ambulatory surgery unit. J Clin Anesth 1990;2:232–237.
108. Reves JG, Kissin I, Fournier SE, Smith LR. Additive negative inotropic effect of a combination of diazepam and fentanyl. Anesth Analg 1984;63:97–100.
109. Eger EI, Saidman LJ, Brandstater B. Minimal alveolar anesthetic concentration: a standard of anesthetic potency. Anesthesiology 1965;26:756–763.
110. Ausems ME, Hug CC Jr, Stanski DR, Burm AG. Plasma concentrations of alfentanil required to supplement nitrous oxide anesthesia for general surgery. Anesthesiology 1986;65:362–373.
111. Smith C, McEwan AI, Jhaveri R, et al. The interaction of fentanyl on the Cp_{50} of propofol for loss of consciousness and skin incision. Anesthesiology 1994;81:820–828.
112. Glass PS, Doherty M, Jacobs JR, et al. Plasma concentration of fentanyl, with 70% nitrous oxide, to prevent movement at skin incision. Anesthesiology 1993;78:842–847.
113. McEwan AI, Smith C, Dyar O, et al. Isoflurane MAC reduction by fentanyl. Anesthesiology 1993;78:864–869.
114. Bailey JM, Schwieger IM, Hug CC Jr. Evaluation of sufentanil anesthesia obtained by a computer-controlled infusion for cardiac surgery. Anesth Analg 1993;76:247–252.
115. Westmoreland CL, Sebel PS, Gropper A. Fentanyl or alfentanil decreases the minimum alveolar anesthetic concentration of isoflurane in surgical patients. Anesth Analg 1994;78:23–28.
116. Brunner MD, Braithwaite P, Jhaveri R, et al. MAC reduction of isoflurane by sufentanil. Br J Anaesth 1994;72:42–46.
117. Kapila A, Lang E, Glass PSA, et al. Minimum alveolar concentration reduction of isoflurane by remifentanil. Anesthesiology 1994;81:A378.
118. McClain DA, Hug CC Jr. Intravenous fentanyl kinetics. Clin Pharmacol Ther 1980;28:106–114.
119. Vuyk J, Lim T, Engbers FH, et al. Pharmacodynamics of alfentanil as a supplement to propofol or nitrous oxide for lower abdominal surgery in female patients. Anesthesiology 1993; 78:1036–1045.
120. Shafer SL, Varvel JR. Pharmacokinetics, pharmacodynamics, and rational opioid selection. Anesthesiology 1991;74:53–63.
121. Fahy LT, Van Mourik GA, Utting JE. A comparison of the induction characteristics of thiopentone and propofol (2,6 di-isopropyl phenol). Anaesthesia 1985;40:939–944.
122. Prys-Roberts C, Davis JR, Calverley RK, Goodwin NW. Haemodynamic effects of infusion of di-isopropyl phenol (ICI 35868) during nitrous oxide anaesthesia. Br J Anaesth 1983; 55:105–111.
123. Coates DP, Prys-Roberts C, Speline KR, et al. Propofol ("Diprivan") by intravenous infusion with nitrous oxide: Dose requirements and haemodynamic effects. Postgrad Med J 1985;61 (suppl):76–79.
124. Cockshott JD, Briggs LP, Douglas EJ, White M. Pharmacokinetics of propofol in female patients. Br J Anaesth 1987;59:1103–1110.
125. Price ML, Walmsley A, Ponte J. Comparision of a total intravenous anaesthetic technique using a propofol infusion, with an inhalational technique using enflurane for day case surgery. Anaesthesia 1988;43 (suppl):84–87.
126. Mackenzie N, Grant IS. Comparison of propofol with methohexitone in the provision of anaesthesia for surgery under regional blockade. Br J Anaesth 1985;57:1167–1172.
127. White PF, Negus JB. Sedative infusions during local or regional anesthesia: a comparison of midazolam and propofol. J Clin Anesth 1991;3:32–39.
128. Taylor E, Ghouri AF, White PF. Midazolam in combination with propofol for sedation during local anesthesia. J Clin Anesth 1992;4:213–216.
129. Jessop E, Grounds RM, Morgan M, Lumley J. Comparison of infusions of propofol and methohexitone to provide light general anaesthesia during surgery with regional blockade. Br J Anaesth 1985;57:1173–1177.
130. Gounds RM, Lalor JM, Lumley J, et al. Propofol infusion for sedation in the intensive care unit. Br Med J 1987;294:397–400.
131. Newman LH, McDonald JC, Wallace PGM, Ledingham IMA. Propofol infusion for sedation in intensive care. Anaesthesia 1987;42:929–937.
132. Snellen F, Lauwers P, Demeyere R, et al. The use of midazolam

versus propofol for short-term sedation following coronary artery bypass grafting. Intensive Care Med 1990;16:312–316.
133. Borgeat A, Wilder-Smith OHG, Mentha G, Herbert O. Subhypnotic doses of propofol possess direct antiemetic properties. Anesth Analg 1993;74:539–541.
134. Borgeat A, Wilder-Smith OHG, Mentha G. Propofol and cholestatic pruritus. Am J Gastroenterol 1992;87:672–674.
135. Borgeat A, Wilder-Smith OHG, Mentha G. Subhypnotic doses of propofol relieve pruritus associated with liver disease. Gastroenterology 1993;104:244–257.
136. Shafer SL. Advances in propofol phramacokinetics and pharmacodynamics. J. Clin. Anesth 1993;5 (suppl 1):14S–21S.
137. Hughes MA, Glass PSA, Jacobs JR. Context-sensitive half-time in multicompartment pharmacokinetic models for intravenous anesthetic drugs. Anesthesiology 1992;76:334–341.
138. Doze VA, Shafer A, White PF. Propofol-nitrous oxide versus thiopental-isoflurane-nitrous oxide for general anesthesia. Anesthesiology 1988;69:63–71.
139. McClune S, McKay AC, Wright PM, et al. Synergistic interaction between midazolam and propofol. Br J Anaesth 1992; 69:240–245.
140. Vuyk J, Engers FHM, Lemmens HJM, et al. Pharmacodynamics of propofol in female patients. Anesthesiology 1992;77:3.
141. Turtle MJ, Cullen P, Prys-Roberts C, et al. Dose requirements of propofol by infusion during nitrous oxide anaesthesia in man. II. Patients premedicated with lorazepam. Br J Anaesth 1987;59:283.
142. Spelina KR, Coates DP, Monk CR, et al. Dose requirements of propofol by infusion during nitrous oxide anaesthesia in man. Br J Anaesth 1986;58:1080–1084.
143. Shafer A, Doze VA, Shafer SL, White PF. Pharmacokinetics and pharmacodynamics of propofol infusions during general anesthesia. Anesthesiology 1988;69:348–356.
144. Schuttler J, Kloos S, Schwilden H, Stoeckel H. Total intravenous anaesthesia with propofol and alfentanil by computer-assisted infusion. Anaesthesia 1988;43 (suppl):2S–7S.
145. Sanderson JH, Blades JF. Multicentre study of propofol in day case surgery. Anaesthesia 1988;43:70.
146. Schuttler J, Stoeckel H, Schwilden H. Pharmacokinetic and pharmacodynamic modeling of propofol (Diprivan) in volunteers and surgical patients. Postgrad Med J 1985;61:53.
147. Adam HK, Kay B, Douglas EJ. Blood disoprofol levels in anesthetized patients: correlation of concentration after single or repeated doses with hypnotic activity. Anaesthesia 1982;37:536.
148. Thomas VL, Sutton DN, Saunders DA. The effect of fentanyl on propofol requirements for day case anesthesia. Anaesthesia 1988;43 (suppl):73–75.
149. Dyar O, Glass PSA, Jhaveri R, et al. TIVA-Propofol and combinations of propofol with fentanyl. Anesthesiology 1991; 75:A44.
150. Sukhani R, Lurie J, Jabamoni R: Propofol for ambulatory gynecologic laparoscopy: does omission of nitrous oxide after postoperative emetic sequelaee and recovery? Anesth Analg 1994;78:831–835.
151. Vuyk J, Lim T, Engbers FH, et al. The pharmacodynamic interaction of propofol and alfentanil during lower abdominal surgery in women. Anesthesiology 1995;83:8–22.
152. Monk TG, Ding Y, White PF. Total intravenous anesthesia: effects of opioid versus hypnotic supplementation on autonomic responses and recovery. Anesth Analg 1992;75:798–804.
153. Stanski D, Shafer S. Quantifying anesthetic drug interaction: implications for drug dosing. Anesthesiology 1995;83:1–5.
154. Skues MA, Richards MJ, Jarvis AP, Pry-Roberts C. Pre-induction atropine or glycopyrrolate and hemodynamic anesthesia with propofol and alfentanil. Anesth Analg 1989;69:386–390.
155. Schuttler J, Schwilden H, Stoeckel H. Pharmacokinetic-dynamic modeling of Diprivan. Anesthesiology 1986;65:A549.
156. Haefely W, Polc P. Physiology of GABA enhancement by benzodiazepines and barbiturates, benzodiazepine-GABA receptors and chloride channels: structure and function properties. In: Olsen RW, Venter JC, eds. New York: Alan R Liss, 1986:97–133.
157. Tverskoy M, Fleyshman G, Bradley EL Jr, Kissin I. Midazolam-thiopental anesthetic interaction in patients. Anesth Analg 1988;67:342–345.
158. Breimer DD. Pharmacokinetics of methohexitone following intravenous infusion in humans. Br J Anaesth 1976;48:643–649.
159. Meyers CJ, Eisig SB, Kraut RA. Comparison of propofol and methohexital for deep sedation. J Oral Maxillofac Surg 1994; 52:448–452.
160. Dorman BH, Conroy JM, Duc TA Jr, et al. Postoperative analgesia after major shoulder surgery with interscalene brachial plexus blockade: etidocaine versus bupivacaine. South Med J 1994;87:502–505.
161. Ferrari LR, Donlon JV. A comparison of propofol, midazolam, and methohexital for sedation during retrobulbar and peribulbar block. J Clin Anesth 1992;4:93–96.
162. Urquhart ML, White PF. Comparison of sedative infusions during regional anesthesia: methohexital, etomidate, and midazolam. Anesth Analg 1989;68:249–254.
163. Schneiderlein HD. Eine neue Narkose. Aerztl Mittheil Baden 1900;54:101.
164. Babcock WW. A new method of surgical anesthesia. Proc Phila County Med Soc 1905;26:347–349.
165. Kochman N. Zur Frage der Morphinoscopolamin Narkose. Munchen Med Wochenschr 1905;52:810.
166. Hamilton WK, Cullen SC. Effect of levalorphan tartrate upon opiate induced respiratory depression. Anesthesiology 1953; 14:550–554.
167. Corssen G, Domino EF, Sweet RB. Neuroleptanalgesia and anesthesia. Anesth Analg 1964;43:748–762.
168. Janis KM. Acute rigidity with small intravenous doses of innovar: A case report. Anesth Analg 1972;51:375–376.
169. Bailey PL, Pace NL, Stanley TH. Rigidity and hemodynamics during fentanyl induction: pretreatment with diazepam and pancuronium. Anesthesiology 1983;59:A316.
170. Coe V, Shafer A, White PF. Technique for administering alfentanil during outpatient anesthesia: a comparison with fentanyl. Anesthesiology 1983;59:A347.
171. Freund FG, Martin WE, Wong KC, Hornbein TF. Abdominal muscle rigidity induced by morphine and nitrous oxide. Anesthesiology 1973;38:358–362.
172. Holderness MC, Chase PE, Drips Rd. A narcotic analgesic and butyrophenone with nitrous oxide for general anesthesia. Anesthesiology 1963;24:336–340.
173. Georgis SD, Hoyt JLO, Sokoll MD. Effects of innovar and innovar plus nitrous oxide on muscle tone and H-reflex. Anesth Analg 1971;50:743–747.
174. Sokoll MD, Hoyt JL, Georgis SD. Studies in muscle rigidity, nitrous oxide, and narcotic analgesic agents. Anesth Analg 1972;51:16–20.
175. Glass PSA, Doherty MA, Jacobs JR, et al. Cp_{50} for sufentanil. Anesthesiology 1990;73:A378.
176. Short TG, Plummer JL, Chui PT. Hypnotic and anaesthetic interactions between midazolam, propofol and alfentanil. Br J Anaesth 1992;69:162–167.
177. Vinik HR, Bradley Jr EL, Kissin I. Triple anesthetic combination: propofol-midazolam-alfentanil. Anesth Analg 1994;78:354–358.
178. Ben-Shlomo I, Finger J, Bar-Av E, et al. Propofol and fentanyl act additively for induction of anaesthesia. Anaesthesia 1993; 48:111–113.
179. Ben-Shlomo I, abd-el-Khalim H, Ezry J, et al. Midazolam acts synergistically with fentanyl for induction of anaesthesia. Br J Anaesth 1990;64:45–47.

180. Kissin I, Vinik HR, Castillo R, Bradley EL Jr. Alfentanil potentiates midazolam-induced unconsciousness in subanalgesic doses. Anesth Analg 1990;71:65–69.
181. Billard V, Moulla F, Bourgain JL, et al. Hemodynamic responses to induction and intubation: propofol/fentanyl interaction. Anesthesiology 1994;18:1384–1393.
182. Lawes EG, Downing JW, Duncan PW, et al. Fentanyl-droperidol supplementation of rapid sequence induction in the presence of severe pregnancy-induced and pregnancy-aggravated hypertension. Br J Anaesth 1987;59:1381–1391.
183. Cahalan MK, Lurz FW, Eger EI II, et al. Narcotics decrease heart rate during inhalational anesthesia. Anesth Analg 1987;66:166–170.
184. Glenski JA, Friesen RH, Lane GA, et al. Low-dose sufentanil as a supplement to halothane/N_2O anaesthesia in infants and children. Can J Anaesth 1988;35:379–384.
185. O'Connor M, Sear JW. Sufentanil to supplement nitrous oxide in oxygen during balanced anaesthesia. Anaesthesia 1988; 43:749–752.
186. Murkin JM. Sufentanil anaesthesia for major surgery: the multicentre Canadian clinical trial. Can J Anaesth 1989;36:343–349.
187. Rosow C. Remifentanil: a unique opioid analgesic. Anesthesiology 1993;79:875–876.
188. Egan TD, Lemmens HJ, Fiset P, et al. The pharmacokinetics of the new short-acting opioid remifentanil (GI87084B) in healthy adult male volunteers. Anesthesiology 1993;79:881–892.
189. Westmoreland CL, Hoke JF, Sebel PS, et al. Pharmacokinetics of remifentanil (GI87084B) and its major metabolite (GI90291) in patients undergoing elective inpatient surgery. Anesthesiology 1993;79:893–903.
190. Glass PSA, Hardman D, Kamiyama Y, et al. Preliminary pharmacokinetics and pharmacodynamics of an ultra-short-acting opioid: remifentanil (GI87084B). Anesth Analg 1993;77:1031–1040.
191. Dershwitz M, Randel G, Rosow EE, et al. Initial clinical experience with remifentanil, a new opioid metabolized by esterases. Anesth Analg 1995;81:619-623.
192. Smith DJ, Bouchal RL, deSanctis CA, et al. Properties of the interaction between ketamine and opiate binding sites in vivo and in vitro. Neuropharmacology 1987;26:1253–1260.
193. White PF. Comparative evaluation of intravenous agents for rapid sequence induction: thiopental, ketamine, and midazolam. Anesthesiology 1982;57:279–284.
194. Hui TW, Short TG, Hong W, et al. Additive interactions between propofol and ketamine when used for anesthesia induction in female patients. Anesthesiology 1995;82:641–648.
195. Mayer M, Ochmann O, Doenicke A, et al. The effect of propofol-ketamine anesthesia on hemodynamics and analgesia in comparison with propofol-fentanyl. Anaesthesist 1990;39:609–616.
196. Schuttler J, Schuttler M, Kloos S, et al. Optimal dosage strategies in total intravenous anesthesia using propofol and ketamine. Anaesthesist 1991;40:199–204.
197. Guit JB, Koning HM, Coster ML, et al. Ketamine as analgesic for total intravenous anaesthesia with propofol. Anaesthesia 1991;46:24–27.
198. Roytblat L, Katz J, Rozentsveig V, et al. Anaesthetic interaction between thiopentone and ketamine. Eur J Anaesthesiol 1992; 9:307–312.
199. Hong W, Short TG, Hui TW. Hypnotic and anesthetic interactions between ketamine and midazolam in female patients. Anesthesiology 1993;79:1227–1232.
200. Hatano S, Keane DM, Boggs RE, et al. Diazepam-ketamine anaesthesia for open heart surgery a "micro-mini" drip administration technique. Can Anaesth Soc J 1976;23:648–656.
201. Raza SM, Masters RW, Zsigmond EK. Haemodynamic stability with midazolam-ketamine-sufentanil analgesia in cardiac surgical patients. Can J Anaesth 1989;36:617–623.
202. Wegmann FJ, Jensen TH, Valentin N. Universelle intravenose Anaesthesie mit Ketamin und Midazolam: eine einfache Technik. Anaesthesist 1990;39:367–370.
203. Tsai SK, Mok MS, Lee C. Ketamine potentiates pancuronium-induced neuromuscular block. Anesth Analg 1987;66:S179.
204. Thompson GE, Moore DC. Ketamine, diazepam, and Innovar: a computerized comparative study. Anesth Analg 1971;50:458–463.
205. White PF, Vasconez LO, Mathes S, et al. Comparison of midazolam and diazepam for sedation during plastic surgery. J Plast Reconstr Surg 1988;81:703–710.
206. Korttila K, Levanen J. Untoward effects of ketamine combined with diazepam for supplementing conduction anaesthesia in young and middle-aged adults. Acta Anaesthesiol Scand 1978; 22:640–648.
207. Reves JG, Fragen RJ, Vinik HR, Greenblatt DJ. Midazolam: pharmacology and uses. Anesthesiology 1985;62:310.
208. Melvin MA, Johnson BH, Quasha AL, Eger EI II. Induction of anesthesia with midazolam decreases halothane MAC in humans. Anesthesiology 1982;57:238.
209. Tverskoy M, Fleyshman G, Ezry J, et al. Midazolam-morphine sedative interaction in patients. Anesth Analg 1989;68:282–285.
210. Vinik HR, Bradley EL Jr, Kissin I. Midazolam-alfentanil synergism for anesthetic induction in patients. Anesth Analg 1989; 69:213–217.
211. Laborit H, Hugyenard P. Practique de l'hibernothérapie en chirurgie et en medicine. Paris: Masson, 1954.
212. De Castro J, Mundeleer R. Anesthésie sans barbituratiques: la neuroleptanalgésie. Anaesth Analg (Paris) 1959;16:1022–1056.
213. Edmonds-Seal J, Prys-Roberts C. Pharmacology of drugs used in neurolept-analgesia. Br J Anaesth 1970;42:207–216.
214. Morgan M, Lumley J, Gillies DS. Neuroleptanalgesia for major surgery: experience with 500 cases. Br J Anaesth 1974;46:288–293.
215. Crossen G, Cjodoff P, Domino EF, Khan DR. Neuroleptanalgesia and anesthesia for open heart surgery. J Thorac Cardiovasc Surg 1965;49:901–920.
216. Fitch W, Barker J, Jennett WB, McDowall DG. The influence of neurolept-analgesic drugs on cerebralspinal fluid pressure. Br J Anaesth 1969;41:800–806.
217. Gan TJ, Alexander R, Fennelly M, Rubin AP. Comparison of different methods of administering droperidol in patient-controlled analgesia in the prevention of postoperative nausea and vomiting. Anesth Analg 1995;80:81–85.
218. Mackenzie N, Grant IS. Comparison of propofol with methohexitone in the provision of anaesthesia for surgery under regional blockade. Br J Anaesth 1985;57:1167–1172.
219. Gupta A, Larsen LE, Sjoberg F, et al. Thiopentone or propofol for induction of isoflurane-based anaesthesia for ambulatory surgery? Acta Anaesthesiol Scand 1992;36:670–674.
220. de Grood PM, Harbers JB, van Egmond J, Crul JF. Anaesthesia for laparoscopy: a comparison of five techniques including propofol, etomidate, thiopentone and isoflurane. Anaesthesia 1987; 42:815–823.
221. Smith I, Ding Y, White PF. Comparison of induction, maintenance, and recovery characteristics of sevoflurane-N_2O and propofol-sevoflurane-N_2O with propofol-isoflurane-N_2O anesthesia. Anesth Analg 1992;74:253–259.
222. Van Hemelrijck J, Smith I, White PF. Use of desflurane for outpatient anesthesia: a comparison with propofol and nitrous oxide. Anesthesiology 1991;75:197–203.
223. Doze VA, Westphal LM, White PF. Comparison of propofol with methohexital for outpatient anesthesia. Anesth Analg 1986;65:1189–1195.
224. Kay B, Healy TE. Propofol ("Diprivan") for outpatient cystoscopy: efficacy and recovery compared with althesin and methohexitone. Postgrad Med J 1985;61 (suppl 3):108–114.

225. Lindekaer AL, Skielboe H, Guldager H, Jensen EW. The influence of nitrous oxide on propofol dosage and recovery after total intravenous anaesthesia for day-case surgery. Anaesthesia 1995;50:397–399.
226. Best N, Traugott F. Comparative evaluation of propofol or methohexitone as the sole anaesthetic agent for microlaryngeal surgery. Anesth Intensive Care 1991;19:50–56.
227. Raftery S, Sherry E. Total intravenous anaesthesia with propofol and alfentanil protects against postoperative nausea and vomiting. Can J Anaesth 1992;39:37–40.
228. Gan TJ, Glass PSA, Ginsberg B, et al. Randomized comparison of ondansetron and intraoperative propofol in the prevention of postoperative nausea and vomiting. Anesthesiology 1995; 83:A286.
229. Ding Y, Fredman B, White PF. Recovery following outpatient anesthesia: use of enflurane versus propofol. J Clin Anesth 1993;5:447–450.
230. Shafer SL, Stanski DR. Improving the clinical utility of anesthetic drug pharmacokinetics. Anesthesiology 1992;76:327–330.
231. Kapila A, Glass PSA, Jacobs JR, et al. Measured context-sensitive half-times of remifentanil and alfentanil. Anesthesiology 1995;83:968–975.
232. Hunkeler W, Mohler H, Pieri L, et al. Selective antagonists of benzodiazepines. Nature 1981;290:514–516.
233. Haefely W, Hunkeler W. The story of flumazenil. Eur J Anaesthesiol Suppl 1988;2:3–14.
234. Amrein R, Hetzel W, Bonetti EP, Gerecke M. Clinical pharmacology of dormicum (midazolam) and anexate (flumazenil). Resuscitation 1988;16 (Suppl):S5-S27.
235. Klotz U, Ziegler G, Ludwig L, Reimann IW. Pharmacodynamic interaction between midazolam and a specific benzodiazepine antagonist in humans. J Clin Pharmacol 1985;25:400–406.
236. Hart YM, Hermilejm M, Sander JWAS, et al. The effect of intravenous flumazenil in interictal electroencephalographic epileptic activity:results of placebo-controlled study. J Neurol Neurosurg Psychiatry 1991;54:305–309.
237. Savic I, Widen L, Stone-Elander S. Feasibility of reversing benzodiazepine tolerance with flumazenil. Lancet 1991;337:133–137.
238. Amrein R, Hetzel W, Hartmann D, Lorscheid T. Clinical pharmacology of flumazenil. Eur J Anaesthesiol Suppl 1988;2:65–80.
239. White PF, Shafer A, Boyle WA, et al. Benzodiazepine antagonism does not provoke a stress response. Anesthesiology 1989; 70:636–639.
240. Mandema JW, Tukker E, Danhof M. In vivo characterization of the pharmacodynamic interaction of a benzodiazepine agonist and antagonist: midazolam and flumazenil. J Pharmacol Exp Ther 1992;260:36–44.
241. Philip BK, Simpson TH, Hauch MA, et al. Flumazenil reverses sedation after midazolam-induced general anesthesia in ambulatory surgery patients: selective antagonists of benzodiazepines. Anesth Analg 1990;71:371–376.
242. Pearson RC, McCloy RF, Morris P, Bardhan KD. Midazolam and flumazenil in gastroenterology. Acta Anaesthesiol Scand Suppl 1990;92:21–24.
243. Thomson PJ, Coulthard P, Snowdon AT, Mitchell K. Recovery from intravenous sedation with midazolam: the value of flumazenil. Br J Oral Maxillofac Surg 1993;31:101–103.
244. Gobeaux D, Sardnal F. Midazolam and flumazenil in ophthalmology. Acta Anaesthesiol Scand Suppl 1990;92:35–38.
245. Birch BR, Anson K, Gelister J, et al. The role of midazolam and flumazenil in urology. Acta Anaesthesiol Scand Suppl 1990; 92:25–32.
246. Geller E, Silbiger A, Niv D, et al. The reversal of benzodiazepine sedation with Ro15–1788 in brief procedures. Anesthesiology 1986;65:A357.
247. Geller E, Halperin P, Silbiger A, et al. The use of anexate (Ro15–1788) for the reversal of benzodiazepine sedation in cardiac patients. In: Proceedings of the World Federation of Anaesthesiologists Association Congress, Washington DC, 1988.
248. Brogden RN, Goa KL. Flumazenil: a reappraisal of its pharmacological properties and therapeutic efficacy as a benzodiazepine antagonist. Drugs 1991;42:1061–1089.
249. Miller RD. U.S. clinical trials of flumazenil, a benzodiazepine antagonist. Clin Ther 1992;14:860–924.
250. Ghouri AF, Ruiz MA, White PF. Effect of flumazenil on recovery after midazolam and propofol sedation. Anesthesiology 1994;81:333–339.
251. Weinbroum A, Halpern P, Geller E. The use of flumazenil in the management of acute drug poisoning: a review. Intensive Care Med 1991;17 (Suppl 1):S32-S38.
252. Just B, Delva E, Camus Y, Lienhart A. Oxygen uptake during recovery following naloxone. Anesthesiology 1992;76:60.
253. Kraynack BJ, Gintautas JG. Naloxone: analeptic action unrelated to opiate receptor antagonism? Anesthesiology 1982; 56:251.
254. Aldrete JA, Goldman E. Is naloxone a nonspecific analeptic? Anesthesiology 1979;50:270.
255. Bailey PL, Clark NJ, Pace NL, et al. Antagonism of postoperative opoid induced respiratory depression: nalbuphine vs. naloxone. Anesth Analg 1987;66:1109.
256. Gueneron JP, Ecoffey C, Carli P, et al. Effect of naloxone infusion on analgesia and respiratory depression after epidural fentanyl. Anesth Analg 1988;67:35–38.
257. Rawal N, Schott U, Dahlstrom B, et al. Influence of naloxone infusion on analgesia and respiratory depression following epidural morphine. Anesthesiology 1986;64:194–201.
258. Johnson A, Bengtsson M, Lofstrom JB, et al. Influence of postoperative naloxone infusion on respiration and pain relief after intrathecal morphine. Reg Anesth 1988;13:146–151.
259. Gan TJ, Ginsberg B, Fortney J, et al. Double-blind comparison of two doses of naloxone infusions on the incidence of side effects and quality of analgesia in patients receiving patient-controlled morphine after major gynecological procedures. Anesthesiology 1995;83:A788.

18 Total Intravenous Anesthesia

Frederic Camu, Marilyn Lauwers, and Caroline Vanlersberghe

Total intravenous anesthesia (TIVA) is by definition a technique involving the induction and maintenance of the anesthetic state with intravenous drugs alone, avoiding both volatile agents and nitrous oxide. Independent regulation of each component of anesthesia (namely, unconsciousness, amnesia, analgesia, control of the sympathetic nervous system, and muscle relaxation) is achieved by selecting specific intravenous agents. Early attempts at TIVA were hampered by the cumulative effects of intravenous agents (e.g., thiopental, diazepam, and neuroleptics), inevitably resulting in long recovery times, and by inadequate methods of administration, with intermittent-bolus administration resulting in unstable anesthetic conditions. More recently, the fear of intraoperative awareness has contributed to the slow acceptance of TIVA, although this complication is entirely avoidable if adequate doses of hypnotic drugs are given. The development of hypnotic and analgesic drugs with short and predictable durations of action and better insights into their clinical pharmacology have improved future prospects for TIVA. In particular, propofol and the newer rapid and short-acting opioids and muscle relaxants allow enhanced control of the state of anesthesia for the entire duration of the surgical procedure. Advances in pharmacokinetic knowledge have further improved the delivery systems by targeting appropriate effect site concentrations in relation to the nature and intensity of the surgical stimulation.

This chapter reviews the advantages and limitations of TIVA, the selection of drugs, and methods of administration for different surgical procedures. Because the choice of muscle relaxants is dictated by the type and duration of surgery, this review focuses on the hypnotic and analgesic drugs used in TIVA.

ADVANTAGES AND LIMITATIONS

In certain clinical situations, TIVA offers significant advantages because of the high concentrations of oxygen that can be administered (one-lung anesthesia, bronchoscopy, high-frequency jet ventilation, patients at risk of hypoxemia, or brain ischemia), and the minimal cardiovascular depression induced by the intravenous drugs. These anesthetic techniques are increasingly popular for laparoscopy, cardiac operations, and neurosurgery, as well as in situations where anesthesia with volatile agents is difficult (war zones or lack of delivery equipment or appropriate drugs). Moreover, TIVA is appropriate for surgical procedures in which the use of nitrous oxide may be contraindicated (e.g., ear surgery, treatment of air embolism, emphysematous bullae, and pneumothorax, and bowel surgery of long duration), or when the deleterious organ effects of volatile anesthetics (e.g., hepatotoxicity, increased cerebral blood flow (CBF) with preexisting intracranial hypertension, and coronary blood flow steal phenomenon) must be avoided. Other claimed advantages of TIVA include a decreased incidence of postoperative nausea and vomiting, a lesser neurohumoral response to surgery, the lack of trigger effect for malignant hyperthermia, and a reduction in atmospheric pollution. To compensate for the omission of nitrous oxide, however, larger doses of intravenous agents are required than during balanced anesthesia techniques.

To achieve an adequate state of anesthesia, the method of administration of the drugs is important. Intermittent injections of the drugs result in high peak plasma concentrations with possible side effects and unstable plasma levels with peaks and troughs influencing the kinetics of the drugs at the receptor sites. Moreover, significant accumulation of drug may result if the dosing intervals are short. With shorter-acting drugs given as an intravenous infusion, tighter control of the clinical effects can be maintained with a higher degree of precision, reliability, and predictability. Fixed-rate infusions are not useful in the context of TIVA because stable anesthetic conditions are not rapidly achieved. Indeed, steady-state plasma concentrations of drugs are reached only after four to five elimination half-lives. Therefore, in clinical anesthesia, more complex administration regimens are needed to attain the drug concentration in the blood quickly, at the site of action in the central nervous system (CNS), and for maintenance of the desired effect site (biophase) concentration.

The next difficulty relates to the definition of the therapeutic window for drug effect. Patients display a moderate variation in dosing needed for a defined response, thereby reducing the predictability of the dose-response relationship. The interpretation of dose-effect relationships in many studies is further confounded by the use of premedication and bolus dosing, which results in unstable plasma concentrations because of rapid initial distribution and redistribution of the drug in the body. Because drug effects are generally more closely related to concentrations than to dose, the best approach to define a therapeutic window is to use the concept of target plasma or effect site drug concentrations. Few data are available on concentration-effect relationships during TIVA in the absence of nitrous oxide or premedications. Anesthetic requirements are further affected by aging, as shown by the increased sensitivity of the brain to fentanyl and alfentanil (1). A dosage scheme designed to maintain the anesthetic concentration at the low end of the therapeutic window in the absence of stimulation and to raise the concentration to the upper end rapidly and only for as long as necessary should result in a more stable anesthetic state, a reduction of the total amount of drug administered, and a faster recovery from its effects.

Other problems may arise with TIVA at the end of anesthesia. The disappearance of a pharmacologic effect depends on the redistribution of the drug and its metabolic clearance. Several studies have demonstrated that the distribution and elimination kinetics of intravenous drugs vary with age, gender, and other nonphysiologic factors. Thus, recovery from anesthesia and postanesthetic side effects are not easily predicted. Furthermore, because of interindividual variability in the relationship between plasma concentration and the CNS effect, techniques to shorten recovery time, such as stopping the infusion before wound closure, are not entirely reliable. Finally, many drugs show cumulative properties that also prolong recovery with TIVA techniques, difficulties of administration, drug interactions, adequate definition of the clinical end points of anesthesia, and potential delays in awakening from anesthesia.

ANESTHESIA AND AWARENESS

Intraoperative awareness is a major concern with intravenous anesthetic techniques. At present, no accepted standard exists by which to assess adequacy of anesthesia. A satisfactory degree of anesthesia requires adequate cardiovascular and respiratory stability, no or minimal patient movement, and no awareness or recall of events during the procedure. The most sensitive clinical signs of depth of anesthesia appear to be changes in muscle tone and pattern of respiration (2). In patients given muscle relaxants, these signs are lost, and one must rely primarily on signs of autonomic hyperactivity. Blood pressure changes are a less sensitive end point for judging depth of anesthesia when intravenous agents are used (3), and signs mediated by the autonomic nervous system are unreliable indicators of anesthetic adequacy when potent opioids or adrenergic blocking agents are used. In addition, many drugs used during anesthesia directly interfere with autonomic responses independent of their anesthetic effect. Scoring has been developed for the clinician as an index of anesthetic adequacy (4).

The noxious stimulation produced by surgery induces a variety of reflex responses. Pain is the conscious perception of such a noxious stimulus. Several factors influence this conscious perception and include the stimulus intensity and the level of arousal. If patients are given appropriate doses of opioids for antinociception and of hypnotics for maintaining unconsciousness, awareness and recall will be unlikely. Awareness is the quality of being vigilant or conscious and does not necessarily result in memory or recall. Patients may respond to commands under anesthesia without recall postoperatively, but they may also show evidence of implicit memory without being aware and without showing explicit recall (5). Convincing evidence of retention of memory during anesthesia has been questioned, however (6). Benzodiazepines affect memory processes by impairing both explicit and implicit memory (7).

An inadequate depth of anesthesia is likely to occur when blood or biophase concentrations are widely fluctuating. As with all physiologic functions, awareness is a threshold phenomenon, and thus, its appearance is expected to be related to insufficient concentrations of the intravenous drugs at the brain site. When appropriate concentrations for unconsciousness of these agents are maintained, awareness is as unlikely as with inhalation agents. With the exception of propofol, the dose-response relationship for consciousness and unconsciousness under stable infusion conditions is not known for most intravenous drugs. Surprisingly, the effect of opioids on the dose requirements to ensure unconsciousness of the hypnotic agents is not known. For propofol, blood concentrations of 3.3 to 5.4 μg/ml should be maintained even in the presence of analgesic concentrations of fentanyl (8). To prevent awareness, one must remain vigilant for signs of light anesthesia. When signs of light anesthesia are present, administration of intravenous hypnotics allows rapid deepening of the state of anesthesia. Intermittent boluses of propofol are much more suitable for briefly extending and deepening the anesthetic state than thiopental. Because several minutes are required before the patient is sufficiently aware that recall is possible, prompt treatment with a bolus of propofol prevents postoperative recall.

PHARMACODYNAMIC ASPECTS

Efficacy and safety are important factors that influence the selection of an intravenous drug. Intravenous agents are specific because they act at receptor sites rather than having more widespread cellular effects, which appear to be produced by volatile anesthetics. Aside from their effects on consciousness and nociception, intravenous agents affect the function of different vital organs.

Cardiovascular System

One of the advantages of TIVA is its ability to provide optimal hemodynamic control; however, each agent has specific dose-related hemodynamic effects that may be additive if several drugs are administered concurrently. Etomidate is probably the drug with the least disturbing effects on hemodynamics, although a decrease in the cardiac index and a small increase in systemic vascular resistance do occur (9). The benzodiazepines cause venodilatation and a decrease in systemic vascular resistance. Because both preload and afterload are reduced, cardiac output may transiently fall. Compensatory mechanisms, if intact, respond to the decreased blood pressure by increasing heart rate, by splanchnic blood mobilization through increased autonomic activity, and by a slight increase of myocardial contractility. Barbiturates induce concentration-related decreases in blood pressure, stroke volume, and systemic vascular resistance, as well as marked venodilatation (10, 11). With propofol, the hemodynamic changes are pronounced because the arteriolar and venous vasodilatation (12) are accompanied by a mild negative inotropic effect. Although the baroreceptor reflex is not affected, tachycardia in response to reduction in blood pressure does not occur (13, 14). Propofol must be judiciously administered in elderly and hypovolemic patients and in those with cardiac disease. In patients with coronary artery disease and hypertension, TIVA is often utilized because the myocardial oxygen supply-demand ratio is better maintained than with volatile agents, thereby reducing the risk of myocardial ischemia.

Respiratory System

Most intravenous drugs induce dose-related decreases in tidal volume, progressing to apneic episodes and extensive changes in respiratory rate and expired minute volume. A rise in the end-tidal carbon dioxide tension is expected because of the quantitative changes consequent to changes in ventilatory mode. Indeed, many hypnotic drugs disturb the relative contribution of thoracic rib cage and diaphragmatic and abdominal wall movements to tidal ventilation, thus inducing mismatching of the ventilation and perfusion. Propofol, fentanyl, and ketamine do not impair the pulmonary hypoxic vasoconstrictive reflex, however (15-17).

The quality of ventilation is also measured by the chemoreceptor response of the brain stem to hypercapnia, hypoxia, and inspiratory load. These adaptive mechanisms are of the utmost importance to the anesthetized patient during spontaneous breathing and recovery from anesthesia. Of all the agents that impair central carbon dioxide chemosensitivity, the opioids have the greatest influence. Noteworthy is the maintenance of chemosensitivity to oxygen with the barbiturates and etomidate.

Visceral Organ Systems

During general anesthesia, the hepatic blood flow is decreased by 20 to 25% as a result of a reduction in perfusion pressure and changes in splanchnic vascular resistance. If cardiac output is maintained, the decrease in hepatic blood flow is likely mediated by the autonomous nervous system and controlled ventilation. Adequate liver perfusion in particular is of importance because the liver is the main organ for metabolic breakdown and elimination of intravenous anesthetics. If liver perfusion is decreased, the oxidative pathways for drug metabolism will be impaired. The glucuronide detoxification process is less sensitive to decreases in hepatic blood flow, however.

Liver blood flow, assessed with indocyanine green (ICG), was adequately maintained during prolonged infusions of propofol (10 hours) for reconstructive surgery, and no impairment of hepatic function was observed (18). Factors affecting hepatic blood flow are unlikely to be important for alfentanil pharmacokinetics because no correlation was found between ICG clearance and that of alfentanil (19). TIVA techniques also have fewer effects on renal perfusion and renal function than volatile anesthetics. No evidence suggests that any of the intravenous anesthetics induce nephrotoxicity.

Central Nervous System

Intravenous anesthetics provide stable intracranial homeostasis and better control of cerebral metabolism. Except for ketamine, the intravenous drugs are cerebral vasoconstrictors, depress cerebral metabolism, and do not adversely influence cerebrovascular autoregulation, flow-metabolism coupling, or carbon dioxide reactivity of the vascular bed. The decreased swelling of the brain provides for better operating conditions. The improved oxygen supply-demand relationship and the intact flow-metabolism coupling observed with TIVA may be preferable for neuroprotection of the ischemic brain (20).

PHARMACOKINETIC CONCEPTS

The interindividual pharmacokinetic and pharmacodynamic variability of intravenous drugs is known, but it should not be a reason for withholding the use of TIVA. A similar degree of variability may exist for inhalation agents, however, and it is dealt with by changing the inspired concentration of the volatile anesthetics. For intravenous agents, changing the drug infusion rate (with manual infusion methods) or the "target" concentration (with computer-controlled infusion pumps) is used to manage differing patient sensitivity to anesthetic effects. The pharmacokinetic properties of anesthetic drugs (i.e., concentration-time relationship) are altered by acute physiologic changes during anesthesia, including the acute hemodynamic changes associated with induction of anesthesia itself, intraoperative blood loss, coexisting pathologic processes, and the acute stress response to surgery. Anesthetic drugs may affect the disposition of other drugs (21) as well as their own disposition if they produce marked cardiovascular effects (22).

The mathematical description of the pharmacokinetics with a two- or three-compartment model has been extended to include an effect compartment where the measurable effect can be related to the theoretic concentration of the drug within such a compartment (i.e., effect site). This effect compartment is characterized by k_{e0}, the elimination rate constant from the effect compartment. If k_{e0} is large, the drug will rapidly equilibrate between blood and the effect site or biophase. Conversely, if the k_{e0} is small, this equilibration will be slow. Modeling concepts are useful for predicting the speed of onset of effect of the drug at the biophase. Following intravenous administration, the onset of clinical effect is governed by the rate of rise in the concentration at the effect site. The $t_{1/2}\,k_{e0}$ (the half-time for equilibration between blood and effect site concentrations) is the time delay between peak plasma concentration and maximum effect at the site of action.

The disappearance of clinical effect is conditioned by the redistribution of the drug from the biophase. The distribution clearance is a measure of the movement of drug from the central compartment (i.e., highly perfused vessel-rich tissues) into tissues with lower blood flow. A high distribution clearance indicates that the drug distribution is governed by cardiac output and regional blood flow. The steady-state volume of distribution (V_{dss}) is a measure of how extensively the drug distributes into tissues and is a function of the drug's lipid solubility (Table 18-1).

TABLE 18-1. Pharmacokinetic Parameters of Intravenous Agents

Drug	V_c (L)	V_{dss} (L)	Cl_m (L/min)	Cl_{df} (L/min)	Cl_{ds} (L/min)
Hypnotic agents					
Thiopental	16.8	88	0.2	2.1	0.3
Propofol	16.9	345	1.8	1.9	0.9
Eltanolone	22.2	182	1.8	8.6	0.8
Opioid agents					
Fentanyl	13	366	0.6	4.9	2.3
Alfentanil	4.1	34.1	0.36	2.52	0.3
Sufentanil	14.3	339	0.92	1.55	0.33
Remifentanil	7.6	21.8	2.9	1.95	0.1

V_c, Central volume of distribution; V_{dss}, volume of distribution at steady state; Cl_m, metabolic clearance; Cl_{df}, rapid distribution clearance; Cl_{ds}, slow distribution clearance. (Data from references 43, 93, 102, 123, and 153).

The rate of recovery from the anesthetic effect depends on the speed of decline in the biophase (or brain) concentration. If the rate of blood-brain (or biophase) equilibration is rapid, changes in blood concentration can swiftly translate into changes in the brain concentration. The decrease in the blood and the biophase concentration are mainly conditioned by the intercompartmental clearances as long as the drug concentrations are not in equilibrium with all the different compartments (i.e., the V_{dss} is not saturated). In this situation, the metabolic clearance is not the major determinant of the decrease of the blood drug levels. This is clearly evident from the context-sensitive half-time of the drug (23), which reflects the importance of drug distribution to other tissues. Only when drug distribution is complete (i.e., V_{dss} is saturated) during infusions of long duration, or when the metabolic clearance is extremely high (e.g., remifentanil, esmolol, and mivacurium) is the decline in the drug concentrations influenced by the metabolic clearance.

Therefore, the time required for a 50% decline in the plasma concentration increases far less with increasing duration of infusion for propofol and etomidate than for midazolam and thiopental (Fig. 18-1). The same principles apply to sufentanil and alfentanil as compared with fentanyl. Thus, the selection of a drug for TIVA should not be based on the elimination half-life of the drug, which is of no value for dosing or predicting the plasma concentration of the drug in short-term therapy such as anesthesia.

The design of a drug infusion regimen for intravenous agents must take into account the desired target biophase concentration for the desired clinical end point and the time to peak effect (Table 18-2). To achieve an effective plasma concentration, and thus the desired effect of a drug, a loading dose must be given before a continuous infusion is administered. The loading dose required to produce the desired effect is selected to ensure that apparent biophase concentration at the time of peak effect equals the concentration necessary for achieving that effect and, thus, is calculated using the volume of distribution that incorporates the biophase. Because the plasma and apparent biophase concentrations should be equal at the time of the peak drug effect, the loading dose is the dose necessary to reach that plasma concentration at the time of peak effect. The size of the volume of distribution at the time of the peak effect (i.e., $V_{d\ peak\ effect}$) is the central volume of distribution (V_c) divided by the percentage of concentration still remaining at the time of peak effect (24). To maintain stable biophase concentrations, thereby producing a constant drug effect, the maintenance infusion rate requires more complex calculations. Indeed, for multicompartmental models, the infusion rate changes over time ultimately to reach the desired

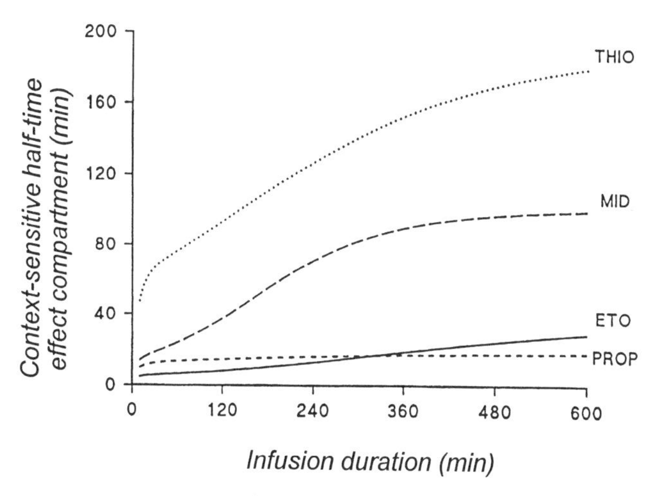

FIGURE 18-1. The context-sensitive half-time of the effect compartment of different hypnotic agents as related to the duration of infusion. THIO, Thiopental; MID, midazolam; ETO, etomidate; PROP, propofol.

plasma concentration when the distribution phase is complete, according to the classic formula:

maintenance infusion rate

$$= \text{desired plasma concentration} \times \text{clearance rate}$$

A more appropriate formula is the following, however:

$$\text{Rate (t)} = \text{desired plasma concentration} \times V_c \, [k_{10} + k_{12} \times e(-k_{21} \times t) + k_{13} \times e(-k_{31} \times t)]$$

where k_{10}, k_{12}, k_{21}, k_{13}, and k_{31} represent the intercompartmental transfer rate constants. The maintenance infusion rate constantly changes because it depends on an exponential function of time that reflects the drug disposition into peripheral tissues. The decreasing infusion rate is necessary because distribution from the plasma to peripheral compartments decreases over time as drug accumulates in the peripheral compartments. In clinical practice, one can calculate the infusion rate necessary to maintain a high and a low concentration in the biophase over different time intervals, so only minimal adjustments in rate are required to maintain a stable concentration (25).

Future developments of TIVA will likely rely on the pharmacokinetic modeling of anesthesia techniques with fast recovery using combinations of drugs to reduce individual drugs doses and to use the pharmacokinetic advantages of each intravenous drug more effectively.

METHODS OF ADMINISTRATION

Drugs with short blood-biophase equilibration times and fast "onset and offset" of clinical effects are required for rapidly adapting the state of anesthesia. In recent years, TIVA has benefited from drugs with more appropriate pharmacokinetic profiles. These newer in-

TABLE 18-2. Pharmacodynamic Parameters for Intravenous Hypnotics and Opioid Analgesics in Total Intravenous Anesthesia

Drug	k_{e0} (L/min)	$t_{1/2}\ k_{e0}$ (min)	Time to Peak C_E (min)	Peak C_E as % of Initial Plasma Cp	V_d at Peak Effect (L)
Hypnotics					
Thiopental	0.577	1.2	3.4	64	26
Propofol	0.238	2.9	4	35	48
Eltanolone	0.100	6.9	10	17	130
Etomidate	0.478	1.6	3	50	44
Opioid analgesics					
Fentanyl	0.147	4.7	3.8	17	76
Alfentanil	1.41	0.96	1.0	49	8
Sufentanil	0.227	3.05	4.8	40	36
Remifentanil	1.14	0.76	1.2	48	16

Cp, Plasma concentration; C_E, effect site concentration; V_d, volume of distribution; K_{e0}, elimination rate constant from the effect compartment; $t_{1/2}\ k_{e0}$, half-time for equilibration between blood and effect site concentrations. (Data from references 43, 93, 103, 106, 124, 152, and 153 using the methods described by Shafer and Varvel [102].)

travenous agents have large distribution volumes with dose-independent disposition kinetics and high clearance rates, and they are metabolized to inactive compounds. In addition, they also have a short delay for equalization of the drug concentration in the biophase with that in the blood. These properties have allowed significant improvements in the infusion techniques of the intravenous agents, to avoid peaks and troughs in effect site concentrations and therefore to provide better control of the pharmacologic effects. Moreover, because dosing is easily adjusted to the individual patient's requirements, these infusion techniques offer improved intraoperative hemodynamic and respiratory stability with fewer side effects.

Several different infusion strategies are possible for TIVA. The infusion rates of the hypnotic and analgesic drugs can be varied, or one can be held constant for the major part of the surgical procedure. Each of these approaches has potential drawbacks, however. For example, fixing the opioid at an analgesic effect site concentration seems, logical but the intensity of the surgical nociceptive stimulation varies with time, and thus this technique may lead to "overdosing" the opioid and delaying spontaneous ventilation at the end of anesthesia. This technique offers better control of side effects, however, provided the opioid infusion can be designed to permit spontaneous respiration postoperatively with adequate analgesia. An example is the combination of propofol and sufentanil infusions during anesthesia. Because propofol concentrations decline much faster than sufentanil concentrations, maintaining a constant opioid concentration and titrating the propofol concentration are pharmacokinetically sound. As a result of the faster blood-brain equilibration time for propofol (1 to 2 minutes) (26), deepening or lightening anesthesia is more rapidly achieved by altering the propofol infusion rate than by titrating the opioid (27).

The alternative of maintaining a constant hypnotic infusion throughout surgery and varying the opioid concentration in response to the changing surgical stimuli may jeopardize the fast recovery from these drugs after ending the infusion unless these agents have rapid offsets of effect. This technique may be considered with agents such as propofol and alfentanil. Because the level of unconsciousness does not change during the course of surgery, in contrast to the required level of analgesia, and because the blood-brain equilibration half-time of alfentanil is shorter than that of propofol, periods of inadequate anesthesia are better treated by increasing the plasma alfentanil concentration. For example, Monk and associates (28) showed that the time required for obtunding acute hypertensive responses was significantly shorter for alfentanil-treated patients (6.3 minutes) compared with patients treated with propofol (10.1 minutes). For prolonged infusions, the context-sensitive half-time of the drugs should be taken into consideration because the decline of plasma concentrations of propofol should be faster than that of alfentanil concentrations. Similar reasoning applies to the combination of propofol and remifentanil infusions. With remifentanil, however, this technique remains applicable whatever the duration of the infusion.

TABLE 18-3. Recommended Dosing Guidelines for Hypnotics and Opioid Analgesics during Total Intravenous Anesthesia (29) (Modified from White, 1989)

Drug	Loading (or priming) Dose (μg/kg)	Maintenance Infusion Rates (μg/kg/h)
Hypnotic agents		
Thiopental	2000–4000	9000–18,000
Methohexital	1000–2000	3000–24,000
Midazolam	100–420	125–250
Propofol	1000–2000	6000–12,000
Ketamine	500–1000	1500–4500
Opioid agents		
Alfentanil	10–50	30–120
Fentanyl	2–4	1.2–5
Remifentanil	1–3	30–150
Sufentanil	0.5–1	0.3–1.2

A third technique is to titrate both the hypnotic and the analgesic drug infusions to the desired clinical effect, with adjustments in the infusion rate of the opioid based on sympathetic hyperactivity, or to the intensity of the expected surgical stimulation, with adjustments in the hypnotic drug infusion rate based on movements or other clinical signs of an inadequate state of anesthesia. To exploit these clinical signs fully, patients should not be completely paralyzed.

What are the recommended dosing guidelines for drugs used as part of a TIVA technique? Aside from interindividual variability in pharmacokinetics and pharmacodynamics, the therapeutic window itself changes with the nature of the stimulation and the type of surgery (Table 18-3). The wide range of recommended doses emphasizes the need to adjust dosing to the individual patient's response to surgical stimuli.

RATIONAL CHOICE OF THE HYPNOTIC DRUG

No single agent possesses all the properties of the ideal agent (29). TIVA-induced unconsciousness is usually maintained by continuous infusion of the hypnotic agent during the surgical procedure. Drugs such as thiopental, diazepam, and even midazolam show evidence of accumulation during prolonged administration, however, and they are therefore unsuitable for continuous infusion. Propofol, methohexital, and ketamine are more appropriate, but they may prolong recovery.

Knowledge of the therapeutic concentrations of the anesthetics for producing loss of consciousness (LOC) and those required to suppress the various stimuli associated with anesthesia and surgery, as well as an understanding of the pharmacokinetic behavior of the drugs and their metabolism, is necessary if these agents are used for maintenance of anesthesia. Some metabolites indeed have clinical effects and delayed elimination from the body (e.g., desmethyldiazepam). The index of potency of hypnotic agents has been defined as the "pseudosteady-state" blood or plasma concentration equilibrated with the biophase that will prevent a response to a given stimulus in 50% of patients (Cp_{50}).

Barbiturates

Barbiturates produce dose-dependent depression of the CNS with LOC and have a rapid distribution profile; however, full recovery from the central depressant effects is delayed for thiopental, compared with methohexital. Administration by continuous infusion decreases the anesthetic requirement, improves cardiovascular stability with less myocardial depression and venous dilatation, and provides a faster recovery with fewer side effects.

Thiopental has a time to peak effect of about 100 seconds, and the k_{e0} for its cerebral effects is 0.58 per minute (see Table 18-2). The dose requirements for thiopental's hypnotic effect on induction are influenced by body weight or lean body mass (30). The dose-response relationship is altered in elderly patients because of a different initial volume of distribution (31) and because of age-related decreases of intercompartmental clearances (32). Cardiac output, which is an important determinant of initial intravascular drug mixing and drug distribution, contributes only to a minor extent in determining thiopental dosage requirement (30).

Minimal data are available on concentration-response relationships for barbiturates. For thiopental, a plasma concentration of 42.2 μg/ml prevented movement in response to surgery in the presence of nitrous oxide (33). Using computer-controlled infusion pumps to maintain stable target concentrations, Hung and associates (34) reported Cp_{50} values for movement in response to laryngoscopy and intubation of 50.7 and 78.8 μg/ml respectively, much higher than the concentrations for LOC (15.6 μg/ml). No blood level-response data are available for maintenance of anesthesia during TIVA.

A thiopental infusion (18 mg/kg/h) in combination with alfentanil was compared with propofol (12 mg/kg/h) for TIVA with jet ventilation for endolaryngeal procedures (35). The acute hemodynamic response to insertion of the laryngoscope was more pronounced than with propofol. Thiopental was also less effective than propofol in blocking the catecholamine response to endolaryngeal surgery. The recovery time following thiopental was also longer (100 minutes) than for propofol infusions (41 minutes).

Methohexital produced loss of corneal reflex at concentrations of 5 to 6 μg/ml (36). When used by continuous infusion (5 to 10 mg/kg/h) with fentanyl (2 μg/kg), in comparison with an equianesthetic dose of propofol (6 to 12 mg/kg/h) for microlaryngoscopy, the lower methohexital infusion rate was unable to control the blood pressure response to laryngoscopy. The lower infusion rate yielded plasma methohexital concentrations of about 3 μg/ml, compared with 8 μg/ml in the higher infusion rate group. Use of a methohexital infusion decreased mean arterial pressure and increased heart rate, and the lower infusion rate was associated with a significant increase in the plasma catecholamine level, whereas only plasma norepinephrine increased during the higher infusion rate group (37). Extremely high infusion rates of methohexital (24 mg/kg/h) used during neurosurgical procedures had marked effects on systemic vascular resistance (−24%), but they did not affect cardiac output (11).

Etomidate

Etomidate has a rapid onset of effect and recovery time with excellent cardiovascular and respiratory stability. Its short duration of action is related to rapid redistribution of the drug from the brain to less-well perfused tissues. Etomidate's metabolic clearance rate is five times greater than that of thiopental, and its pharmacokinetics is not influenced by the mode of administration, such as bolus versus infusion (38). Etomidate decreases CBF, cerebral metabolic rate for oxygen ($CMRO_2$), and intracranial pressure (ICP), without producing significant changes in cerebral perfusion pressure (CPP). It does not decrease the hepatic or renal perfusion, contrary to most other intravenous drugs. Adjunctive administration of opioid analgesics markedly attenuates the myoclonic activity. Etomidate anesthesia is associated with a high incidence of postoperative nausea and vomiting, however, and it transiently suppresses adrenal steroidogenesis (39, 40).

In volunteer studies, an etomidate concentration of at least 0.65 μg/ml was required to achieve loss of corneal reflex, whereas LOC was attained at plasma concentrations between 0.3 and 0.5 μg/ml (38). Using the median electroencephalographic (EEG) frequency, the ratios of the concentration inducing half-maximal slowing of the EEG (IC_{50}) of thiopental, propofol, and etomidate are 1:6.7:50 (41-43). With benzodiazepine premedication, etomidate infusions (e.g., a loading infusion of 0.1 mg/kg followed by 0.6 to 1 mg/kg/h) combined with alfentanil or fentanyl provided good hemodynamic and ventilatory control during upper airway endoscopy and abdominal hysterectomy procedures, with recovery times varying between 18 and 25 minutes (44). Postoperative nausea and vomiting were frequent, however, and some patients complained of difficulty in concentrating (45).

Benzodiazepines

Benzodiazepines have anxiolytic, sedative, hypnotic, amnestic, anticonvulsant, and muscle relaxant properties. Anterograde amnesia (or lack of recall) is a consistent component of their CNS action. Benzodiazepines exhibit minimal cardiovascular depressant effects, decrease peripheral vascular resistance, dilate the venous capacitance vessels, and do not alter the baroreflex mechanism. Benzodiazepine-induced ventilatory depression is more prolonged than that induced by thiopental and is significantly enhanced by the use of opioids. Benzodiazepines produce minimal changes in CPP and ICP and dose-dependent decrease in CBF and $CMRO_2$. With the exception of midazolam, most benzodiazepines have low hepatic clearance rates and are metabolized to less active compounds with a similar spectrum of CNS activity. The primary metabolite of midazolam, (α-hydroxymidazolam, is a benzodiazepine agonist with effects similar to those of midazolam on the EEG (46).

Benzodiazepines have a slow onset of effect, with a time to peak EEG effect of 9.5 minutes (47). The rate of blood-brain equilibration is actually slower for midazolam than for diazepam (48), with midazolam $t_{1/2}$ k_{e0} values ranging from 0.9 to 5.6 minutes (46, 49). Recovery of psychomotor and cognitive functions is slower with midazolam compared with thiopental, methohexital, propofol, or etomidate.

The Cp_{50} for LOC with midazolam decreased significantly with increasing age from 595 ng/ml at 40 years to 135 ng/ml at 80 years; this finding demonstrates increased pharmacodynamic sensitivity to the hypnotic effect of midazolam in the elderly (50). Intraoperative plasma midazolam concentrations of 250 to 350 ng/ml are required to ensure LOC during TIVA for abdominal and superficial surgery (51). In combination with alfentanil and fentanyl, midazolam concentrations are reduced to 200 to 250 ng/ml (52). Although awakening occurs at plasma concentrations of 50 to 80 ng/ml, arousal from midazolam anesthesia and awareness can occur at concentrations below 200 ng/ml (53, 54). The simultaneous administration of alfentanil and midazolam did not affect the kinetics of alfentanil, but shifted the midazolam concentration-hypnotic effect relationship to the left with a greater interindividual variation compared with midazolam alone (55).

Following an infusion of midazolam, 0.6 mg/kg/h, in the presence of alfentanil (60 μg/kg/h), recovery was prolonged to 36 minutes for eye opening, with residual ventilatory depression lasting 48 minutes after terminating the infusion. This prolonged recovery was shortened to 11 minutes by administering the benzodiazepine antagonist flumazenil (56). Vuyk and associates (57) reported recovery times of 17 minutes following a midazolam infusion, 0.125 mg/kg/h, in combination with a variable-rate infusion of alfentanil (avg. 68 μg/kg/h); however, normalization of psychomotor function required an additional 3 to 4 hours. The use of a midazolam-alfentanil infusion combination was also associated with a high incidence of postoperative respiratory depression (58). When compared with a propofol-alfentanil combination, infusions of midazolam and alfentanil provided greater hemodynamic stability for ambulatory ear, nose, and throat endoscopic procedures in patients with cardiovascular disease. Reversal of midazolam effects with flumazenil provided a faster recovery than with propofol; however, full reversal of the residual sedative effects of midazolam required an infusion of flumazenil and significantly delayed the recovery and discharge of these patients (59).

The combination of diazepam and ketamine has been used for cardiac surgery (60, 61). The benzodiazepine is administered to attenuate the acute cardiovascular stimulation and psychomimetic emergence reactions associated with ketamine (62). Ketamine-midazolam infusions provided improved hemodynamic stability compared with a high-dose fentanyl technique (63). Use of a flunitrazepam and ketamine anesthetic technique showed a lower incidence of postoperative nausea and vomiting compared with neuroleptanalgesia (64).

Propofol

Dose-dependent cardiovascular and respiratory depression has been reported with propofol. The hypotensive effects of propofol are related to both the dose and the rate of infusion (12, 65, 66). Propofol does not impair baroreflex sensitivity, but central sympatholytic mechanisms result in a stable heart rate despite decreases of blood pressure (13, 14). Propofol decreases intraocular pressure by 20 to 50%, reduces CBF, $CMRO_2$, and ICP and may have a neuroprotective effect (67). Variable-rate infusions of propofol are associated with recovery times comparable to those seen with methohexital, with fast recovery of psychomotor and cognitive skills (67). In contrast to the barbiturates, propofol causes less residual postoperative sedation and psychomotor impairment. The incidence of postoperative side effects (e.g., nausea and vomiting) is low (47).

Propofol's rapid onset of effect and recovery time compares favorably with those of the barbiturates and etomidate. The k_{e0} of propofol is slightly smaller than those of thiopental and etomidate, and thus, the onset of effect is slower (see Table 18-2). Propofol has a $t_{1/2}$

k_{e0} of 2.9 minutes and a large V_{dss} (345 L), with a total distribution clearance of 2.8 L/min (see Table 18-1). The metabolic clearance rate for propofol exceeds hepatic blood flow, a most important pharmacokinetic difference from thiopental. Although many studies have reported "therapeutic" blood concentrations, the interpretation of these data is hampered by the concomitant use of other adjunctive drugs that are likely to influence the clinical end point, the use of venous blood sampling, or determinations made before equilibration of blood concentrations with the biophase. Propofol blood concentrations of 3 to 5 μg/ml resulted in lack of response to various surgical stimuli (68). When combined with alfentanil (50 μg/kg/h), the ED_{50} of propofol required to suppress movement was 2.94 mg/kg/h, and the ED_{95} was 4.98 mg/kg/h (69). Despite the presence of larger alfentanil doses, significantly higher infusion rates of propofol are required in children than in adults. Browne and associates (70) reported a propofol ED_{50} infusion rate of 6 mg/kg/h and an ED_{95} of 8.7 mg/kg/h following alfentanil (85 μg/kg followed by an infusion of 65 μg/kg/h).

Studies involving computer-controlled infusion pumps with arterial blood sampling allow a more reliable determination of potency because they maintain a constant target blood concentration. Smith and associates (8) determined Cp_{50} and Cp_{95} values of propofol for LOC and skin incision in unpremedicated healthy patients using logistic regression. The LOC Cp_{50} and Cp_{95} for propofol were 3.3 μg/ml and 5.4 μg/ml, respectively, and the Cp_{50} and Cp_{95} for skin incision were 15.2 and 27.4 μg/ml, respectively. The Cp_{50} value required for LOC was decreased almost 20% per decade of age. Other investigators have reported LOC Cp_{50} and Cp_{90} values for propofol of 3.4 and 4.3 μg/ml, respectively (71). Based on these data, an effect compartment concentration of 4.5 to 6.5 μg/ml of propofol was recommended for achieving LOC. Using various sampling techniques, propofol concentrations at awakening are 1.6 to 2.9 μg/ml (72-74). In contrast, a Cp_{50} awake concentration of 3.5 μg/ml has been determined (8). During TIVA with propofol, the propofol concentration should be maintained above 3.5 μg/ml to avoid awareness. To achieve this concentration rapidly requires an infusion rate of 11 mg/kg/h following a loading dose of 1.5 mg/kg.

Acute autonomic responses to surgical stimulation can be suppressed at mean blood propofol concentrations of 2.97 μg/ml for minor surgery and at 4.05 μg/ml when propofol is administered in combination with meperidine for major surgical procedures (72). When administered in combination with alfentanil (loading dose of 100 μg/kg followed by 60 μg/kg/h), propofol infusions of 3 to 4 mg/kg/h were required to achieve satisfactory anesthetic conditions for orthopedic surgery (75). Lower propofol infusion rates (2 mg/kg/h) require frequent supplemental bolus doses of propofol and alfentanil for suppression of sympathetic responses. Recovery occurred 13 to 15 minutes after discontinuing the propofol infusion irrespective of the infusion rate.

Propofol has also been combined with ketamine for TIVA (76). The use of propofol-ketamine provided superior hemodynamic stability with less postoperative respiratory depression than a propofol-fentanyl combination (77, 78). The sedative effects of ketamine and propofol are additive (79).

The use of propofol-opioid combinations for TIVA in cardiac surgery is controversial. In patients with ischemic heart disease and good left ventricular function, the combination of propofol and fentanyl produced a negative inotropic effect with decreased left ventricular stroke work (80). Other investigators, however, reported reduced end-diastolic volume with unchanged end-systolic volume and ejection fraction (81). More recently, Vermeyen and associates (82) reported that propofol infusions did not affect myocardial oxygen consumption or myocardial lactate extraction. In patients with low cardiac output, moderate doses of propofol (8 mg/kg/h followed by 4 mg/kg/h) and fentanyl did not affect the right ventricular ejection fraction or myocardial contractility (83). The combination of propofol and alfentanil had hypotensive effects similar to those of the propofol-fentanyl combination (84). Unfortunately, many of the clinical studies have reported inconsistent results because of the use of single-dose regimens, the lack of equipotency between anesthetic techniques, and a lack of proper control groups. Mora and associates (85) reported that a TIVA technique consisting of fentanyl (25 μg/kg) and propofol (50 to 250 μg/kg/min) provided excellent hemodynamic stability and a prompt recovery profile in patients premedicated with diazepam and morphine.

Although propofol produces vasodilatation, decreases in CPP were not observed in normovolemic patients with intracranial mass lesions (86). The $CMRO_2$ was reduced to the same extent as with barbiturates (87), and the cerebral vasomotor responsiveness to carbon dioxide was not altered (88). In studies comparing recovery in patients undergoing intracranial surgery, use of propofol-alfentanil provided for a faster recovery of cerebral function during the postoperative period than a thiopental-isoflurane-fentanyl technique (89, 90). In studies to date, the anesthetic technique has not had a significant effect on perioperative outcome (91). The use of a propofol-based TIVA has been recommended for stereotaxic craniotomy and induction of burst suppression during cerebral aneurysm clipping when temporary vessel occlusion is required (92).

Eltanolone

Eltanolone (pregnanolone) is a steroid anesthetic with a large therapeutic margin with respect to hemodynamic stability and a low incidence of apnea when administered for induction of anesthesia. Eltanolone decreases arterial pressure mainly through peripheral vasodilatation combined with a limited depression of cardiac function. The drug has a high metabolic clearance rate (26 to 38 ml/kg/min) and a V_{dss} of 4.2 L/kg (93). The eltanolone concentration-effect relationship for hypnosis shows a marked hysteresis effect (k_{e0} 0.1/min), with a steep response curve (94). Therefore, the $t_{1/2}$ k_{e0} of eltanolone is 6.9 minutes, consistent with its slower onset of effect compared with those of thiopental and propofol. It has a hypnotic potency comparable to that of etomidate and is six times more potent than thiopental and three times more potent than propofol when used for induction of anesthesia (95). The ED_{50} induction dose of eltanolone was 0.33 mg/kg and 0.44 mg/kg in benzodiazepine- and opioid-premedicated patients, respectively (96, 97). In elderly patients, the induction doses for LOC have varied from 0.59 to 0.89 mg/kg, depending on the infusion rate (98). The EC_{50} and EC_{95} for loss of consciousness were 664 and 887 μg/L, respectively, whereas EC_{50} and EC_{95} for abolishing response to laryngoscopy were 2120 and 3207 μg/L, respectively (99). Recovery from eltanolone is initially slower than with propofol (100). Following infusions of 1 to 3 hours' duration, etlanolone's context-sensitive half-time is 20 to 30 minutes. The role of eltanolone in TIVA is yet to be defined.

RATIONAL CHOICE OF THE OPIOID

Opioid analgesics are essential for the suppression of reflex responses to noxious anesthetic and surgical stimuli during TIVA. These compounds provide profound analgesia and hemodynamic stability with minimal effects on myocardial contractility. Opioids are not complete anesthetics, however, and beyond certain concentrations greater anesthetic effect is not possible. Even after large doses of fentanyl (resulting in concentrations greater than 20 ng/ml), significant hemodynamic responses have been reported in patients with good ventricular function who are undergoing coronary surgery (101).

The intensity of the opioid effect depends on the intrinsic activity of the drug at the CNS receptor site as well as its concentration at the site of drug effect. The former depends on the drug selection, and the latter depends on the dosing scheme and the pharmacokinetics of the opioid compound. Onset, peak intensity, and duration of effect evolve in parallel, depending on the rise and fall of the opioid concentration in the biophase (i.e., the site of drug effect), and are proportional to the dose administered. Optimal clinical practice aims at rapidly achieving the desired drug effect, maintaining that effect as long as necessary, and allowing prompt recovery after surgery. Thus, optimal dose sizing and timing of administration are key issues. The opioid concentration required to suppress reflex responses to noxious stimuli depends on the nature and intensity of the stimulation and is influenced by pharmacodynamic variables, including drug interactions, aging, and the development of tolerance. Preference is usually given to opioids that rapidly equilibrate between plasma and neuronal tissue, whereby changes in plasma levels more closely reflect changes within the CNS.

The ability of opioid analgesics to enter the CNS is primarily dependent on the free (nonprotein-bound) un-ionized fraction and their lipophilicity at physiologic pH. Drugs with a long $t_{1/2}$ k_{e0} have a delayed onset of effect. Slow equilibration between drug concentrations in the blood and biophase allows more drug to be redistributed to nonactive tissues, resulting in a less intense drug effect. Larger doses of opioids are required to obtain the expected therapeutic effect, but they do not affect the actual time to achieve peak drug concentration in the biophase. The equilibration between the blood and biophase is rapid for alfentanil and intermediate for fentanyl and sufentanil. Drugs that rapidly equilibrate between the plasma and their site of action in the CNS demonstrate close relationships between the plasma concentration and the intensity of opioid effect. Thus, to sustain a given intensity of opioid activity, one must maintain the plasma concentration of the opioid. Failure to maintain therapeutic levels of the opioid compound results in failure to suppress the sympathetic and hemodynamic responses to noxious stimuli and may elicit arousal, awareness, and recall. The usual titration methods (e.g., intermittent bolus injections or a variable-rate infusion) rely extensively on the use of clinical criteria for assessing the adequacy of the anesthetic state and on the pharmacologic characteristics of the drugs used. The absence of hemodynamic changes in association with intense noxious stimuli does not guarantee an adequate depth of anesthesia in all patients, however, particularly in patients treated on a long-term basis with drugs interfering with the hemodynamic responses (e.g., β blockers, calcium channel blockers, and angiotensin-converting enzyme inhibitors).

The therapeutic window for an opioid effect can vary by 30 to 60% depending on the operative stimuli, significantly higher than the levels associated with adequate postoperative ventilation. As the intensity of noxious stimuli decreases toward the end of surgery, the opioid concentration at the site of effect can be progressively reduced to approach that associated with minimal respiratory depression at the end of anesthesia. In clinical practice, the opioid concentration must decrease by 80 to 90% for adequate ventilation in the early postoperative period when an opioid-based technique is used. Shafer and Varvel (102) suggested that fentanyl is a poor choice for infusions lasting longer than 1 hour because it requires at least 40 minutes and 8 hours to decrease the effect site concentration by 50% and 70%, respectively. Sufentanil displays a better recovery profile because of its rapid and extensive distribution and higher hepatic clearance rate, resulting in a 50% decrease in effect site concentration in 18 and 50 minutes, respectively, for infusions of 1 and 10 hours. This advantage is reduced if a 70% decrease in effect site concentration is required to reestablish adequate spontaneous ventilation, however. Based on effect site calculations, sufentanil is the drug of choice for infusions lasting less than 12 hours, whereas alfentanil allows a more rapid recovery for infusions lasting longer than 12 hours (Fig. 18-2).

Alfentanil

Alfentanil has appropriate pharmacokinetic and pharmacodynamic properties for use as a variable-rate infusion during TIVA (see Tables 18-1 and 18-2). It has a short blood-brain equilibration half-time (1 minute), providing for a rapid onset of effect and a relatively short terminal elimination half-life (90 minutes) (103). Alfentanil has a definable therapeutic window that varies depending on the intensity of the surgical stimulation (104). As a supplement to propofol infusions, the EC_{50} alfentanil for tracheal intubation was 92 ng/ml, the EC_{50} for skin incision was 55 ng/ml, and the EC_{50} for opening the peritoneal cavity was 84 ng/ml. Alfentanil requirements during propofol anesthesia were lower than during nitrous oxide anesthesia, a finding indicating a greater synergistic effect of alfentanil when combined with propofol (105). The potency ratio values of alfentanil to fentanyl and sufentanil based on the IC_{50} are 765:12:1 (106). Based on the EEG surrogate end point, alfentanil is approximately 60 times less potent than fentanyl. In clinical situations, the potency ratio of alfentanil to fentanyl for achieving hemodynamic stability during surgery was 16:1 (107); lower ratios showed marked cardiovascular effects with alfentanil (108). When used as a maintenance infusion during balanced anesthesia (109), however, the alfentanil-fentanyl potency ratio is 7:1. Plasma alfentanil concentrations of at least 1 μg/ml were required to block adrenergic activation in response to noxious stimuli during cardiac surgery (110, 111). During ambulatory surgery, alfentanil concentrations of 5 to 150 ng/ml provided adequate analgesia as part of a balanced anesthetic technique (109).

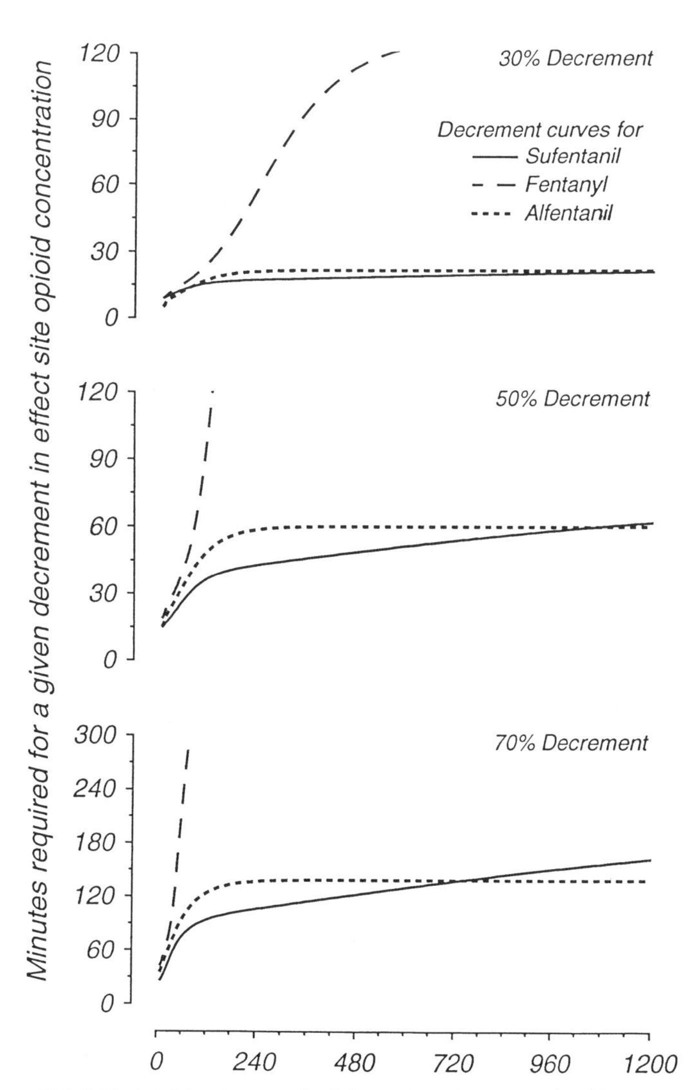

FIGURE 18-2. The time required for a given decrement in effect-site concentration of sufentanil, fentanyl, and alfentanil in relation to the duration of their infusion (102). (from Schaker and Varvel.)

Fentanyl and Sufentanil

Opioid-based TIVA techniques are often utilized during cardiac surgery. High doses of sufentanil (20 μg/kg) and fentanyl (100 μg/kg) have provided good cardiovascular stability during the intraoperative period (112-114). These high doses of sufentanil have significant vasodilatory effects, however, contributing to an increase in cardiac index and heart rate compared with fentanyl (115). Both fentanyl and sufentanil have suppressed metabolic and endocrine responses to surgery, but have failed to prevent increases in catecholamines during cardiopulmonary bypass and in the early postoperative period (115-117). Sufentanil has maintained a lasting analgesic effect longer than fentanyl with less residual respiratory depression during the postoperative period (118). When fentanyl infusions (9 to 18 μg/kg/h) were compared with alfentanil infusions (180 to 360 μg/kg/h), they provided comparable cardiovascular stability during cardiac surgery with similar hemodynamic responses to sternotomy, cardiopulmonary bypass, and awakening (111). As reported in several other cardiac studies (119-121), even plasma fentanyl concentrations exceeding 30 ng/ml were unable to prevent acute hemodynamic responses to intense surgical stimuli. In addition, high opioid concentrations prolong the return to consciousness and extubation for several hours after cessation of the infusion.

Crozier and associates studied the combination of sufentanil or fentanyl with midazolam for TIVA during major abdominal surgery. For similar plasma concentrations of midazolam (500 to 600 ng/ml), the dose potency ratio for fentanyl and sufentanil was 5.4:1. During induction of anesthesia, the combination of midazolam and opioid analgesia produced a significant decrease in blood pressure with frequent vagotonic actions, possibly enhanced by the use of vecuronium for muscle relaxation. During maintenance of anesthesia, similar hemodynamic effects were noted with both sufentanil, 1.7 ± 0.5 μg/kg/h, and fentanyl, 9.3 ± 3.3 μg/kg/h, but neither opioid suppressed the catecholamine response to surgery even though benzodiazepines reduce sympathetic outflow and adrenal medullary catecholamine secretion (122).

Remifentanil

The availability of a rapid-acting and enzymatically metabolized opioid analgesic should further enhance the application of TIVA techniques. With an analgesic potency slightly less than that of fentanyl, remifentanil can produce intense analgesia with an extremely rapid onset (k_{e0} 1.14/min and $t_{1/2}$ k_{e0} 0.76 minute). Because the terminal elimination half-life of remifentanil is only 10 to 20 minutes, a constant rate of infusion rapidly achieves steady-state conditions. The drug is hydrolyzed by circulating and nonspecific tissue esterases with a metabolic clearance of 3 L/min, allowing a fast return of spontaneous respiration even with high-dose infusions. With remifentanil, the context-sensitive half-time (3 to 5 minutes) is independent of the duration of the opioid infusion (123). In addition, the time required to decrease blood concentration by 80% is less than 15 minutes regardless of the duration of the infusion.

A bolus dose of remifentanil is approximately 20 times more potent than that of alfentanil on a milligrams-per-kilogram basis and is 30 to 40 times greater in terms of the measured plasma concentration (ng/ml). The IC_{50} for half-maximal EEG slowing is 20 ng/ml, indicating that remifentanil is 35 times more potent than alfentanil (IC_{50} of 376 ng/ml), almost half as potent as fentanyl (IC_{50} 8.1 ng/ml), and approximately one-twentieth (1/20) as potent as sufentanil (IC_{50} 0.68 ng/ml using this surrogate endpoint) (99, 103, 106, 124).

RECOVERY FROM ANESTHESIA

Modern anesthetic techniques strive for a fast recovery with minimal side effects (e.g., postoperative nausea and vomiting). The increased acceptance of TIVA relates to the ability to achieve improved recovery profiles compared with traditional inhalation techniques. Anesthesiologists generally agree that recovery from anesthesia is faster when propofol infusions are used as the hypnotic agent, rather than thiopental (125) or midazolam infusions (56, 57). Moreover, the combination of midazolam with alfentanil can prolong respiratory depression (58).

The choice of the opioid analgesic can also influence the recovery from anesthesia. In a comparison of fentanyl and alfentanil for supplementation of a propofol infusion during TIVA, alfentanil produced a longer impairment of cognitive and psychomotor function than fentanyl (107), even though the pharmacokinetic profile of alfentanil suggests that it should be superior to fentanyl. No differences in recovery profiles were seen between fentanyl and sufentanil infusions when they were combined with propofol infusions for TIVA in patients undergoing craniotomy for tumor (126).

DRUG INTERACTIONS

When a single drug is administered for TIVA, rapidly achieving adequate surgical anesthesia is difficult without producing significant cardiovascular and respiratory changes or disturbing side effects. Therefore, combining hypnotic and analgesic drugs with similar pharmacokinetic and pharmacodynamic profiles is a logical approach. These combinations can rapidly achieve and smooth induction, maintenance, and emergence from anesthesia without untoward side effects.

The quantification of the interactions among hypnotic agents has rarely been performed. Only after the anesthetic potency of these drugs has been defined can their interaction with other anesthetic drugs and opioids be quantified. Synergism was demonstrated for the hypnotic interaction of opioids with etomidate (127), midazolam (128), and thiopental (129) and for the interaction of midazolam with methohexital (130) and propofol (131), as well as for the interaction of thiopental with propofol (132) and midazolam (133). Additivity was also demonstrated for the hypnotic and anesthetic effects of ketamine with propofol (79), midazolam (134), and thiopental (135). If these interactions relate to the cerebral effects, synergism (or additivity) may not be demonstrable for other physiologic effects. For example, the reduction in arterial blood pressure was the same for the combination of propofol and midazolam as for the individual drugs alone (136).

Interactions among drugs can also have a pharmacokinetic basis. Gepts and associates (21) demonstrated that alfentanil infusions did not modify the pharmacokinetic profile of propofol; however, propofol induced higher plasma alfentanil concentrations than expected because of an alteration in the disposition kinetics of the opioid analgesic. For fentanyl, a pharmacokinetic interaction with propofol has not been demonstrated (137), but such an interaction appears to exist with etomidate (38). Finally, genetic factors may contribute to variability in drug metabolism, as demonstrated with the benzodiazepines.

Only by simultaneously assessing the pharmacokinetics and pharmacodynamics for each drug can one determine whether the synergisms are purely a pharmacodynamic phenomenon. The interaction between fentanyl and propofol for LOC and skin incision was investigated with computer-controlled infusion pumps after equilibration between blood and biophase concentrations (8). Under pseudosteady-state conditions, increasing concentrations of fentanyl up to 3 ng/ml reduced the LOC Cp_{50} of propofol by 40% and the skin incision Cp_{50} by 89%. This interaction was not linear; a ceiling effect appeared for concentrations of fentanyl greater than 3 ng/ml.

The interaction of opioids with hypnotic agents is not uniform. Indeed, the interaction of alfentanil with propofol on LOC is controversial (138, 139). Furthermore, the plasma concentrations of thiopental needed for LOC were not significantly reduced by fentanyl even at concentrations of 2 ng/ml (140). Opioid effects on other organ systems may further be influenced by preanesthetic medication and muscle relaxants. Following scopolamine premedication, a hyperdynamic circulatory response was described during induction of anesthesia with sufentanil or fentanyl (141); however, these sympathomimetic effects were reduced by premedication with lorazepam. Significant bradycardia and decreases in arterial blood pressure may occur in benzodiazepine-premedicated patients when opioids are combined with vecuronium during the induction period.

Information on the interactions of α_2-adrenergic agonists with intravenous anesthetics during TIVA is limited. These agents may prove clinically useful as adjuncts to anesthesia, but their acute hemodynamic effects (e.g., hypotension and bradycardia) may limit their routine clinical use. Clonidine potentiated the effect of opioids, improved hemodynamic stability by attenuating sympathoadrenal stimulation during anesthesia (142), and displayed a beneficial effect on hemodynamics during emergence from anesthesia, a period associated with increased sympathetic activity (143). Dexmedetomidine markedly reduced the induction dose of thiopental, the cardiovascular responses to laryngoscopy and intubation, the fentanyl requirements during the operation, and the need for postoperative analgesics (144). α_2-Adrenergic agonists (e.g., dexmedetomidine) can interfere with the human liver alfentanil oxidation (145), however, resulting in higher than expected plasma alfentanil concentrations.

TARGET-CONTROLLED INFUSIONS

Any infusion scheme for TIVA should be simple, reliable, and accurate in rapidly achieving the desired blood and biophase concentrations within reasonable limits, while avoiding "overshoots" (with potential toxic effects) and "undershoots" (with subtherapeutic concentrations). In clinical practicing, infusion regimens are generally based on the patient's lean body weight. Given the poor correlation between systemic clearance and body weight for some intravenous anesthetics, this calculation may result in significant differences between predicted and measured blood concentrations. Infusion schemes with manual adjustments in the infusion rate (i.e., staged infusions) have been proposed (146). Multistepped infusions are appropriate to maintain steady-state concentrations of drugs, but they cannot respond accurately to changing surgical and anesthetic requirements. Computer-controlled infusion schemes based on a pharmacokinetic model that describes the elimination and redistribution of the drug (e.g., the Bolus, Elimination, and Transfer or BET scheme) were introduced to achieve stable blood concentrations of intravenous anesthetics rapidly (42, 147). This evolved into techniques that titrate the predicted blood concentration to the patient's response to stimulation (target-controlled infusion systems). With this system, the anesthesiologist controls the state of anesthesia by choosing a desired theoretic target blood concentration instead of an infusion rate.

These techniques based on pharmacokinetic principles provide infusion schemes to attain and maintain a predefined blood concentration of the anesthetic drugs rapidly (147, 148). The currently available systems are based on open mamillary two- or three-compartment models, with the computer calculating the drug concentrations in the various compartments and the infusion rates required to achieve the desired target blood concentration within a defined time interval. The performance of these systems is affected by the choice of the pharmacokinetic parameters, tissue uptake of the drugs, and altered hemodynamics resulting from the drug itself. If most of these delivery systems perform remarkably well during clinical anesthesia in comparison with manual systems, the major problem related to clinical use is the appropriate choice of the target concentration for achieving the desired clinical end point. The required blood concentration depends on the desired pharmacologic effect, the presence of other central and peripheral acting drugs, the type of operation, and the individual patient's sensitivity to the drug. These delivery systems also require changes in the target blood concentration depending on the patient's response to a given surgical stimulus. As a result of the continuous mode of drug administration, increasing the target blood concentration rapidly achieves the desired clinical effect. In addition, careful attention to titration at the end of surgery improves the rate of recovery.

To achieve a stable state of anesthesia with these target-controlled infusion systems, the anesthesiologist must know the concentration-response relationship for

TABLE 18-4. Target Plasma Concentrations (μg/ml) for Hypnotic Drugs

Drug	Cp_{50} LOC	Cp_{95} LOC	Cp_{50} Incision	Cp_{95} Incision	Reference
Propofol	3.3	5.4	15.2	27.4	8
with fentanyl, 1 ng/ml	—	—	5.2	—	8
with fentanyl, 2 ng/ml	—	—	2.7	—	8
	3.4	4.3 (Cp_{90})	—	—	71
	2.4	4.2	4.0	7.8	79
Thiopental	15.6	—	39.8	—	34
Midazolam	0.14–0.6	0.25–0.35	—	—	50, 53
Ketamine	0.6	1.2	1.0	1.6	79
Etomidate	—	0.31–0.5	—	—	41

Cp_{50}, Plasma concentration that prevents a response to a given stimulus in 50% of patients; LOC, loss of consciousness; Cp_{95}, plasma concentration that prevents a response to a given stimulus in 95% of patients.

each drug used relative to the desired clinical end point. When sufficient time was allowed for equilibration of drug concentrations between blood and biophase (approximately four times the $t_{1/2}$ k_{e0}), several studies were able to predict the ED_{50}, EC_{50}, ED_{95}, and EC_{95} for suppression of somatic and visceral stimuli in adults using different anesthetic agents (Tables 18-4 and 18-5). These data are clinically more useful than the minimum infusion rate (149), which does not specifically relate to the blood concentration. The minimal infusion rate, which is the infusion rate necessary to prevent bodily movement in response to surgical skin incision in 50% of patients, is indeed a measure of adequacy of anesthesia, but it depends on both the pharmacokinetics and pharmacodynamics of the drug as related to the patient.

The value of targeting either the plasma concentration or the effect site concentration depends on the drug and the desired effect. To date, little information indicates which is the optimal target of control. For drugs with a short $t_{1/2}$ k_{e0} (alfentanil, remifentanil, and propofol), targeting the plasma concentration is sufficient to provide adequate control of anesthesia. If the $t_{1/2}$ k_{e0} of the drug is long, it is more reasonable to target the effect site concentration. If the concentrations at the effect site lag behind those in the plasma, a faster infusion rate can be utilized to achieve the necessary effect site drug concentrations more rapidly. The fallacy of targeting the plasma drug concentration when designing optimal dosage regimens for drugs with significant delays in equilibrating with the effect site (e.g., fentanyl) has been emphasized by Shafer (150). The k_{e0} value is different for each physiologic function, however. If a drug can produce profound changes in hemodynamics and has a large $t_{1/2}$ k_{e0}, targeting the brain effect site concentration may result in an "overdose" for the cardiovascular system and may thereby produce hypotension or bradycardia. For such drugs, it is better to target the plasma concentration and to allow the cerebral effects to be achieved more slowly.

Many target-controlled infusion systems have been used for induction and maintenance of intravenous anesthesia. A target propofol concentration of 5 μg/ml successfully induced anesthesia in patients premedicated with temazepam without major hemodynamic or respiratory effects (151). Mean target propofol concentrations to maintain anesthesia during cardiac surgery were 3.6 μg/ml in combination with a continuous infusion of alfentanil of 60 μg/kg/h (L. Barvais, unpublished data).

TABLE 18-5. Target Plasma Concentrations for Opioid Analgesics during Intravenous Anesthesia

	Sufentanil (ng/ml)	Remifentanil (ng/ml)	Fentanyl (ng/ml)	Alfentanil (ng/ml)
Induction/intubation				
Thiopental	0.5	11	4	325
O_2	1.0	22	9	575
Maintenance				
O_2 only	5.0	100	37.5	2500
Spontaneous ventilation	0.3	4–5	1.5	125
EEG IC_{50}	0.7	20	8.1	376

EEG IC_{50}, Concentration of drug causing half-maximal slowing of the electroencephalogram.

In summary, the successful provision of TIVA requires an appreciation of pharmacokinetic and pharmacodynamic principles. Pharmacokinetic modelling concepts offer a rational basis for the selection and administration of hypnotic and analgesic drugs during TIVA. The choice of anesthetic drug also depends on the intended mode of administration. The rational application of pharmacokinetic and pharmacodynamic principles to the design and assessment of drug dosage regimens should enhance the clinicians' ability to titrate intravenous anesthetics based on clinical signs. The newer hypnotic and analgesic drugs with their faster onsets of action and improved recovery profiles should permit more precise control of the anesthetic state. The use of drug combinations will greatly reduce the amount of each drug needed to achieve the desired clinical endpoint. The safety and reliability of TIVA techniques have also been enhanced by improvements in drug delivery systems for intravenous anesthetics.

REFERENCES

1. Scott JC, Stanski DR. Decreased fentanyl and alfentanil dose requirements with increasing age: a simultaneous pharmacokinetic and pharmacodynamic evaluation. J Pharmacol Exp Ther 1987;240:159–166.
2. Chang T-L, Dworsky WA, White PF. Use of continuous electromyography for monitoring depth of anesthesia. Anesth Analg 67:521–525, 1988.
3. White PF, Boyle WA. Relationship between hemodynamic and electroencephalographic changes during general anesthesia. Anesth Analg 1989;68:177–181.
4. Evans JM, Davies WL. Monitoring anaesthesia. Clin Anaesthesiol 1984;2:242–262.
5. Ghoneim MM, Block RI. Learning and consciousness during general anesthesia. Anesthesiology 1992;76:279–305.
6. Eich E, Reaves JL, Katz RL. Anesthesia, awareness and the memory/awareness distinction. Anesth Analg 1985;64:1143–1148.
7. De Roode A, Jelicic M, Bonke B, Bovill JG. The effect of midazolam premedication on implicit memory activation during alfentanil-nitrous oxide anaesthesia. Anaesthesia 1995;50:191–194.
8. Smith C, McEwan AI, Jhaveri R, et al. The interaction of fentanyl on the Cp_{50} of propofol for loss of consciousness and skin incision. Anesthesiology 1994;81:820–828.
9. Price ML, Millar B, Grounds M, Cashman J. Changes in cardiac index and estimated systemic vascular resistance during induction of anaesthesia with thiopentone, methohexitone, propofol and etomidate. Br J Anaesth 1992;69:172–176.
10. Todd MM, Drummond JC, U HS. The hemodynamic consequences of high-dose thiopental anesthesia. Anesth Analg 1985; 64:681–687.
11. Todd MM, Drummond JC, U HS. The hemodynamic consequences of high-dose methohexital anesthesia in humans. Anesthesiology 1984;61:495–501.
12. Claeys MA, Gepts E, Camu F. Haemodynamic changes during anaesthesia induced and maintained with propofol. Br J Anaesth 1988;60:3–9.
13. Cullen PM, Turtle M, Prys Roberts C, et al. Effect of propofol anesthesia on baroreflex activity in humans. Anesth Analg 1987;66:1115–1120.
14. Samain E, Marty J, Gauzit R, et al. Effects of propofol on baroreflex control of heart rate and on plasma noradrenaline levels. Eur J Anaesthesiol 1989;6:321–326.
15. Van Keer L, Van Aken H, Vandermeersch E, et al. Propofol does not inhibit hypoxic pulmonary vasoconstriction in humans. J Clin Anesth 1989;1:284–289.
16. Steegers PA, Backx PJ. Propofol and alfentanil anesthesia during one-lung ventilation. J Cardiothorac Anesth 1990;4:194–199.
17. Bjertnaes LJ, Hauge A, Kriz M. Hypoxia-induced pulmonary vasoconstriction: effects of fentanyl following different routes of administration. Acta Anaesthesiol Scand 1980;24:53–57.
18. Murray JM, Trinick TR. Hepatic function and indocyanine green clearance during and after prolonged anaesthesia with propofol. Br J Anaesth 1992;69:643–644.
19. Henthorn TK, Avram MJ, Krejcie TC. Alfentanil clearance is independent of the polymorphic debrisoquin hydroxylase. Anesthesiology 1989;71:635–639.
20. Ravussin P, De Tribolet N, Wilder-Smith OH. Total intravenous anesthesia is best for neurological surgery. J Neurosurg Anesthesiol 1994;6:285–289.
21. Gepts E, Jonckheer K, Maes V, et al. Disposition kinetics of propofol during alfentanil anaesthesia. Anaesthesia 1988;43 (suppl):8–13.
22. Henthorn TK, Krejcie TC, Avram MJ. The relationship between alfentanil distribution kinetics and cardiac output. Clin Pharmacol Ther 1989;45:56–65.
23. Hughes MA, Glass PSA, Jacobs JR. Context-sensitive half-time in multicompartment pharmacokinetic models for intravenous anesthetic drugs. Anesthesiology 1992;76:334–341.
24. Shafer SL, Gregg K. Algorithms to rapidly achieve and maintain stable drug concentrations at the site of drug effect with a computer controlled infusion pump. J Pharmacokinet Biopharm 1992;20:147–169.
25. Stanski DR, Shafer SL, Kern SE. The scientific basis of infusion techniques in anesthesia. North Reading, MA: Bard MedSystems Division, 1990:16–17.
26. Dyck JB, Shafer SL. Effects of age on propofol pharmacokinetics. Semin Anesth 1992;11 (suppl 1):2–4.
27. Shafer SL. Advances in propofol pharmacokinetics and pharmacodynamics. J Clin Anesth 1993;5 (suppl 1):14S–21S.
28. Monk TG, Ding Y, White PF. Total intravenous anesthesia: effects of opioid versus hypnotic supplementation on autonomic responses and recovery. Anesth Analg 1992;75:798–804.
29. White PF. Clinical uses of intravenous anesthetic and analgesic infusions. Anesth Analg 1989;68:161–171.
30. Avram MJ, Sanghvi R, Henthorn TK, et al. Determinants of thiopental induction dose requirements. Anesth Analg 1993; 76:10–17.
31. Homer TD, Stanski DR. The effect of increasing age on thiopental disposition and anesthetic requirement. Anesthesiology 1985;62:714–724.
32. Stanski DR, Maitre PO. Population pharmacokinetics and pharmacodynamics of thiopental: the effects of age revisited. Anesthesiology 1990;72:412–422.
33. Becker KE. Plasma levels of thiopental necessary for anesthesia. Anesthesiology 1978;49:192–196.
34. Hung OR, Varvel JR, et al. Thiopental pharmacodynamics. II. Quantitation of clinical and electroencephalographic depth of anesthesia. Anesthesiology 1992;77:237–244.
35. Mustola ST, Baer GA, Metsä-Ketelä T, Laippala P. Haemodynamic and plasma catecholamine responses during total intravenous anaesthesia for laryngomicroscopy. Anaesthesia 1995; 50:108–113.
36. Schwilden H, Schüttler J, Stoeckel H. Closed loop feedback control of methohexital anesthesia by quantitative EEG analysis in humans. Anesthesiology 1987;67:341–347.
37. Sellgren J, Ejnell H, Ponten J, Sonander HG. Anesthetic modulation of the cardiovascular response to microlaryngoscopy: a comparison of propofol and methohexital with special reference to leg blood flow, catecholamines and recovery. Acta Anaesthesiol Scand 1995;39:384–389.
38. Schüttler J, Wilms M, Lauven PM, et al. Pharmakokinetische Untersuchungen über Etomidat beim Menschen. Anaesthesist 1980;29:658–661.
39. Wagner RL, White PF. Etomidate inhibits adrenocortical function in surgical patients. Anesthesiology 1984;61:647–651.
40. Wagner RL, White PF, Kan PB, et al. Inhibition of adrenal steroidogenesis by the anesthetic etomidate. N Engl J Med 1984; 310:1415–1421.
41. Schwilden H, Schüttler J, Stoeckel H. Quantitation of the EEG and pharmacodynamic modelling of hypnotic drugs: etomidate as an example. Eur J Anaesthesiol 1985;2:121–131.
42. Schwilden H, Stoeckel H, Schüttler J, Lauven PM. Pharmacological models and their use in clinical anaesthesia. Eur J Anaesthesiol 1986;3:175–208.
43. Hudson RJ, Stanski DR, Saidman LJ, Meathe E. A model for studying depth of anesthesia and acute tolerance to thiopental. Anesthesiology 1983;59:301–308.

44. Boisson-Bertrand D, Taron F, Laxenaire MC. Etomidate vs. propofol to carry out suspension laryngoscopies. Eur J Anaesthesiol 1991;8:141–144.
45. Fruergaard K, Jenstrup M, Schierbeck J, Wiberg-Jorgensen F. Total intravenous anaesthesia with propofol or etomidate. Eur J Anaesthesiol 1991;8:385–391.
46. Mandema JW, Tuk B, Van Steveninck AL, et al. Pharmacokinetic-pharmacodynamic modelling of the central nervous system effects of midazolam and its main metabolite alpha-hydroxymidazolam in healthy volunteers. Clin Pharmacol Ther 1992;51:715–728.
47. Gepts E, Trenchant A. Propofol. Anaesth Pharmacol Rev 1995; 3:46–56.
48. Greenblatt DJ, Ehrenberg BL, Gunderman J, et al. Pharmacokinetic and electroencephalographic study of intravenous diazepam, midazolam and placebo. Clin Pharmacol Ther 1989; 45:356–365.
49. Bührer M, Maitre PO, Crevoisier C, Stanski DR. Electroencephalographic effects of benzodiazepines. II. Pharmacodynamic modelling of the electroencephalographic effects of midazolam and diazepam. Clin Pharmacol Ther 1990;48:555–567.
50. Jacobs JR, Reves JG, Marty J, et al. Aging increases pharmacodynamic sensitivity to the hypnotic affects of midazolam. Anesth Analg 1995;80:143–148.
51. Persson MP, Nilsson A, Hartvig P, Tamsen A. Pharmacokinetics of midazolam in total IV anaesthesia. Br J Anaesth 1987; 59:548–556.
52. Nilsson A, Tamsen A, Persson MP. Midazolam/fentanyl anaesthesia for major surgery: plasma levels of midazolam during prolonged total intravenous anaesthesia. Acta Anaesthesiol Scand 1986;30:66–69.
53. Persson MP, Nilsson A, Hartvig P. Relation of sedation and amnesia to plasma concentrations of midazolam in surgical patients. Clin Pharmacol Ther 1988;43:324–331.
54. Klausen NO, Juhl O, Sörensen J, et al. Flumazenil in total intravenous anaesthesia using midazolam and fentanyl. Acta Anaesthesiol Scand 1988;32:409–412.
55. Persson MP, Nilsson A, Hartvig P. Pharmacokinetics of alfentanil in total IV anaesthesia. Br J Anaesth 1988;60:755–761.
56. Steib A, Freys G, Jochum D, et al. Recovery from total intravenous anesthesia: propofol versus midazolam-flumazenil. Acta Anaesthesiol Scand 1990;34:632–635.
57. Vuyk J, Hennis PJ, Burm AGL, et al. Comparison of midazolam and propofol in combination with alfentanil for total intravenous anesthesia. Anesth Analg 1990;71:645–650.
58. Jensen AG, Moller JT, Lybecker H, Hansen PA. A random trial comparing recovery after midazolam-alfentanil anesthesia with and without reversal with flumazenil and standardised neuroleptanesthesia for major gynecologic surgery. J Clin Anesth 1995;7:63–70.
59. Chollet-Rivier M, Ravussin P. Midazolam-flumazenil vs. propofol in ambulatory ENT endoscopic procedures. Eur J Anaesthesiol 1992;9:377–385.
60. Dhadphale PR, Jackson APF, Alseri S. Comparison of anesthesia with diazepam and ketamine vs morphine in patients undergoing heart valve replacement. Anesthesiology 1979;51:200–203.
61. Hatano S, Keane DM, Boggs RE, et al. Diazepam-ketamine anesthesia for open heart surgery: a micro-mini drip administration technique. Can Anaesth Soc J 1976;23:648–656.
62. White PF. Comparative evaluation of intravenous agents for rapid sequence induction: thiopental, ketamine, and midazolam. Anesthesiology 1982;57:279–284.
63. Chai M, Thanga D, Morgan E, Viljoen J. Ketamine-midazolam continuous infusion in cardiac surgical patients. Anaesthesia 1989;44:364.
64. Freuchen I, Ostergaard J, Mikkelsen BO. Anaesthesia with flunitrazepam and ketamine. Br J Anaesth 1981;53:827–830.
65. Peacock JE, Lewis RP, Reilly CS, Nimmo WS. Effect of different rates of infusion of propofol for induction of anaesthesia in elderly patients. Br J Anaesth 1990;65:346–352.
66. Stokes DN, Hutton P. Rate dependent induction phenomena with propofol: implications for the relative potency of intravenous anaesthetics. Anesth Analg 1991;72:578–583.
67. Weir DL, Goodchild CS, Graham DI. Propofol: effects on indices of cerebral ischemia. J Neurosurg Anesthesiol 1989;1:284–289.
68. Monk CR, Coates DP, Prys Roberts C, et al. Haemodynamic effects of prolonged infusion of propofol as a supplement to nitrous oxide anaesthesia: studies in association with peripheral arterial surgery. Br J Anaesth 1987;59:954–960.
69. Richards MJ, Skues MA, Jarvis AP, Prys Roberts C. Total IV anaesthesia with propofol and alfentanil: dose requirements for propofol and the effects of premedication with clonidine. Br J Anaesth 1990;65:157–163.
70. Browne BL, Wolf AR, Prys Roberts C. Dose requirements of propofol in children during total IV anaesthesia. Br J Anaesth 1990;64:396P.
71. Vuyk J, Engbers FHM, Lemmens HJM, et al. Pharmacodynamics of propofol in female patients. Anesthesiology 1992;77:3–9.
72. Shafer A, Doze VA, Shafer SL, White PF. Pharmacokinetics and pharmacodynamics of propofol infusions during general anesthesia. Anesthesiology 1988;69:348–356.
73. Doze VA, Westphal LM, White PF. Comparison of propofol with methohexital for outpatient anesthesia. Anesth Analg 1986;65:1189–1195.
74. Adam HK, Kay B, Douglas EJ. Blood disoprofol levels in anaesthetised patients: correlation of concentration after single or repeated doses with hypnotic activity. Anaesthesia 1982; 37:536–540.
75. Van Leeuwen L, Zuurmond WWA, Deen L, Helmers HJH. Total intravenous anaesthesia with propofol, alfentanil and oxygen-air: three different dosing schemes. Can J Anaesth 1990; 37:282–286.
76. Schüttler J, Schüttler M, Kloos S, et al. Optimal dosing strategies in total intravenous anaesthesia using propofol and ketamine. Anaesthesist 1991;40:199–204.
77. Mayer M, Ochmann O, Doenicke A, et al. Influence of propofol-ketamine vs. propofol-fentanyl anaesthesia on haemodynamics and analgesia. Anaesthesist 1990;39:609–616.
78. Guit JBM, Koning HM, Coster ML, et al. Ketamine as analgesic for total intravenous anaesthesia with propofol. Anaesthesia 1991;46:24–27.
79. Hui TW, Short TG, Hong W, et al. Additive interactions between propofol and ketamine when used for anesthesia induction in female patients. Anesthesiology 1995;82:641–648.
80. Vermeyen KM, Erpels FA, Janssen LA, et al. Propofol-fentanyl anaesthesia for coronary bypass surgery in patients with good left ventricular function. Br J Anaesth 1987;59:1115–1120.
81. Lepage JYM, Pinaud ML, Helias JH, et al. Left ventricular function during propofol and fentanyl anesthesia in patients with coronary artery disease: assessment with a radionuclide approach. Anesth Analg 1988;67:949–955.
82. Vermeyen KM, De Hert SG, Erpels FA, Adriaensen HF. Myocardial metabolism during anaesthesia with propofol-low dose fentanyl for coronary artery bypass surgery. Br J Anaesth 1991; 66:504–508.
83. Bell J, Sartain J, Wilkinson GAL, Sherry KM. Propofol and fentanyl anaesthesia for patients with low cardiac output state undergoing cardiac surgery: comparison with high-dose fentanyl anaesthesia. Br J Anaesth 1994;73:162–166.
84. Manara AR, Monk CR, Bolsin SN, Prys Roberts C. Total i.v. anaesthesia with propofol and alfentanil for coronary artery bypass grafting. Br J Anaesth 1991;66:716–718.
85. Mora CT, Duke C, Torjman MC, White PF. Effect of anesthetic

technique on the hemodynamic response and recovery profile after coronary revascularization. Anesth Analg 1995;81:900–910.

86. Muzzi D, Losasso T, Weglinski M, et al. The effect of propofol on cerebrospinal fluid pressure in patients with supratentorial mass lesions [Abstract]. Anesthesiology 1992;77:A216.
87. Vandesteene A, Trempont V, Engelman E, et al. Effect of propofol on cerebral blood flow and metabolism in man. Anaesthesia 1988;43 (suppl):42–43.
88. Strebel S, Kaufmann M, Guardiola PM, Schaefer HG. Cerebral vasomotor responsiveness to carbon dioxide is preserved during propofol and midazolam anesthesia in humans. Anesth Analg 1994;78:884–888.
89. Van Hemelrijck J, Van Aken H, Merckx L,Mulier J. Anesthesia for craniotomy: total intravenous anesthesia with propofol and alfentanil compared to anesthesia with thiopental sodium, fentanyl and nitrous oxide. J Clin Anesth 1991;3:131–136.
90. Ravussin P, Tempelhoff R, Modica PA, Bayer-Berger MM. Propofol vs. thiopental-isoflurane for neurosurgical anesthesia: comparison of hemodynamics, CSF pressure and recovery. J Neurosurg Anesthesiol 1991;3:85–95.
91. Todd MM, Warner DS, Sokoll MD, et al. A prospective comparative trial of three anaesthetics for elective supratentorial craniotomy: propofol/fentanyl, isoflurane/nitrous oxide and fentanyl/nitrous oxide. Anesthesiology 1993;78:1005–1020.
92. Ravussin P, de Tribolet N. Total intravenous anesthesia with propofol for burst suppression in cerebral aneurysm surgery: preliminary report of 42 patients. Neurosurgery 1993;32:236–240.
93. Carl P, Hogskilde S, Lang-Jensen T, et al. Pharmacokinetics and pharmacodynamics of eltanolone (pregnanolone), a new steroid intravenous anaesthestic, in humans. Acta Anaesthesiol Scand 1994;38:734–741.
94. Schüttler J, Hering W, Ihmsen I, et al. Pharmacokinetic-dynamic modelling of the new intravenous anesthetic eltanolone [Abstract]. Anesthesiology 1994;81:A409.
95. Van Hemelrijck J, Mulier P, Van Aken H, White PF. Relative potency of eltanolone, propofol and thiopental for induction of anesthesia. Anesthesiology 1994;80:36–41.
96. Powell H, Morgan M, Sear JW. Pregnanolone: a new steroid intravenous anaesthetic: dose finding study. Anaesthesia 1992; 47:287–290.
97. Hering W, Biburger G, Rugheimer E. Induction of anaesthesia with the new steroid intravenous anaesthetic eltanolone (pregnanolone): dose finding and pharmacodynamics. Anaesthesist 1993;42:74–80.
98. Myint Y, Peacock JE, Reilly CS. Induction of anaesthesia with eltanolone at different rates of infusion in elderly patients. Br J Anaesth 1994;73:771–774.
99. Gepts E, Parivar K, Vägerö M. Concentration-effect relationship of eltanolone in patients undergoing laparoscopic surgery. Personal communication.
100. Kallela H, Haasio J, Korttila K. Comparison of eltanolone and propofol in anesthesia for termination of pregnancy. Anesth Analg 1994;79:512–516.
101. Wynands JE, Wong P, Townsend GE, et al. Narcotic requirements for intravenous anesthesia. Anesth Analg 1984;63:101–105.
102. Shafer SL, Varvel JR. Pharmacokinetics, pharmacodynamics and rational opioid selection. Anesthesiology 1991;74:53–63.
103. Scott JC, Ponganis KV, Stanski DR. EEG quantitation of narcotic effect: the comparative pharmacodynamics of fentanyl and alfentanil. Anesthesiology 1985;62:234–241.
104. Ausems ME, Hug CC, Stanski DR, Burm AGL. Plasma concentrations of alfentanil required to supplement nitrous oxide for general surgery. Anesthesiology 1986;65:362–373.
105. Vuyk J, Lim T, Engbers FHM, et al. Pharmacodynamics of alfentanil as a supplement to propofol and nitrous oxide for lower abdominal surgery in female patients. Anesthesiology 1993;78:1036–1045.
106. Scott JC, Cooke JE, Stanski DR. Electroencephalographic quantitation of opioid effect: comparative pharmacodynamics of fentanyl and sufentanil. Anesthesiology 1991;74:34–42.
107. Jenstrup M, Nielsen J, Fruergard K, et al. Total IV anaesthesia with propofol-alfentanil or propofol-fentanyl. Br J Anaesth 1990;64:717–722.
108. Rucquoi M, Camu F. Cardiovascular responses to large doses of alfentanil and fentanyl. Br J Anaesth 1983;55 (suppl 2):223–230.
109. White PF, Coe V, Shafer A, Sung M-L. Comparison of alfentanil with fentanyl as adjuvants during outpatient surgery. Anesthesiology 1986;64:99–106.
110. De Lange S, de Bruyn NP. Alfentanil-oxygen anaesthesia: plasma concentrations and clinical effects during variable rate continuous infusion for coronary artery surgery. Br J Anaesth 1983;55 (suppl 2):183S–190S.
111. Hynynen M, Takkunen O, Salmenperä M, et al. Continuous infusion of fentanyl or alfentanil for coronary artery surgery: plasma opiate concentrations, haemodynamics and postoperative course. Br J Anaesth 1986;58:1252–1259.
112. Sebel PS, Bovill JG. Cardiovascular effects of sufentanil anesthesia: a study in patients undergoing cardiac surgery. Anesth Analg 1982;61:115–119.
113. De Lange S, Boscoe MJ, Stanley TH, Pace N. Comparison of sufentanil-O_2 and fentanyl-O_2 for coronary artery surgery. Anesthesiology 1982;56:112–118.
114. Raza SMA, Masters RW, Vasireddy AR, Zsigmond EK. Haemodynamic stability with midazolam-sufentanil analgesia in cardiac surgical patients. Can J Anaesth 1988;35:518–525.
115. Howie MB, McSweeney TD, Lingam RP, Maschke SP. A comparison of fentanyl-O_2 and sufentanil-O_2 for cardiac anesthesia. Anesth Analg 1985;64:877–887.
116. Sebel PS, Bovill JG, Fiolet JWT, et al. Hormonal effects of sufentanil anesthesia. Anesth Analg 1982;61:214–215.
117. Bovill JG, Sebel PS, Fiolet JWT, et al. The influence of sufentanil on endocrine and metabolic responses to cardiac surgery. Anesth Analg 1983;62:391–397.
118. Bailey PL, Streisand JB, East KA, et al. Differences in magnitude and duration of opioid induced respiratory depression and analgesia with fentanyl and sufentanil. Anesth Analg 1990;70:8–15.
119. Moldenhauer CC, Hug CC. Continuous infusion of fentanyl for cardiac surgery [Abstract]. Anesth Analg 1982;61:S206.
120. Sprigge JS, Wynands JE, Whalley DG, et al. Fentanyl infusion anesthesia for aortocoronary bypass surgery: plasma levels and hemodynamic response. Anesth Analg 1982;61:972–978.
121. Wynands JE, Townsend GE, Wong P, et al. Blood pressure response and plasma fentanyl concentrations during high-dose and very high-dose fentanyl anesthesia for coronary artery surgery. Anesth Analg 1983;62:661.
122. Crozier TA, Langenbeck M, Müller J, et al. Total intravenous anaesthesia with sufentanil-midazolam for major abdominal surgery. Eur J Anaesthesiol 1994;11:449–459.
123. Egan TD, Lemmens HJM, Fiset P, et al. The pharmacokinetics of the new short-acting opioid remifentanil (GI87084B) in healthy adult male volunteers. Anesthesiology 1993;79:881–892.
124. Egan TD, Minto CF, Hermann DJ, et al. Remifentanil versus alfentanil: comparative pharmacokinetics and pharmacodynamics in healthy adult male volunteers. Anesthesiology 1996; 84:821-833.
125. Kashtan H, Edelist G, Mallon J, Kapala D. Comparative evaluation of propofol and thiopentone for total intravenous anaesthesia. Can J Anaesth 1990;37:170–176.
126. Jansen GF, Kedaria M, Zuurmond WWA. Total intravenous anaesthesia during intracranial surgery: continuous propofol in-

fusion in combination with either fentanyl or sufentanil [Abstract]. Can J Anaesth 1990:37:S128.
127. Kissin I, Brown PT, Bradley EL. Morphine and fentanyl interactions with etomidate [Abstract]. Anesthesiology 1987; 67:A383.
128. Kissin I, Brown PT, Bradley EL. Sedative and hypnotic midazolam-morphine interactions in rats. Anesth Analg 1990; 71:137–143.
129. Kissin I, Mason EL. Morphine and fentanyl hypnotic interactions with thiopental. Anesthesiology 1987;67:331–335.
130. Tverskoy M, Ben-Shlomo J, Ezry J, et al. Midazolam acts synergistically with methohexitone for induction of anaesthesia. Br J Anaesth 1989;63:109–112.
131. McClune S, McKay AC, Wright PMC, et al. Synergistic interaction between midazolam and propofol. Br J Anaesth 1992; 69:240–245.
132. Naguib M, Sari-Kouzel A. Thiopentone-propofol hypnotic synergism in patients. Br J Anaesth 1991;67:4–6.
133. Tverskoy M, Fleyshman G, Bradley EL, Kissin I. Midazolam-thiopental anesthetic interaction in patients. Anesth Analg 1988;67:342–345.
134. Hong W, Short TG, Hui TW. Hypnotic and anesthetic interactions between ketamine and midazolam in female patients. Anesthesiology 1993;79:1227–1232.
135. Royblat L, Katz J, Rozentsveig V, et al. Anaesthetic interaction between thiopentone and ketamine. Eur J Anaesthesiol 1992; 9:307–312.
136. Short TG, Chui PT. Propofol and midazolam act synergistically in combination. Br J Anaesth 1991;67:539–545.
137. Gill SS, Wright EM, Reilly CS. Pharmacokinetic interaction of propofol and fentanyl: single bolus injection study. Br J Anaesth 1990;65:760–765.
138. Short TG, Plummer JL, Chui PT. Hypnotic and anaesthetic interactions between midazolam, propofol and alfentanil. Br J Anaesth 1992;69:162–167.
139. Vinik HR, Bradley EL, Kissin I. Triple anesthetic combination: propofol-midazolam-alfentanil. Anesth Analg 1994;78:354–358.
140. Telford RJ, Glass PSA, Goodman D, Jacobs JR. Fentanyl does not alter the "sleep" plasma concentration of thiopental. Anesth Analg 1992;75:523–529.
141. Thomson IR, MacAdams CL, Hudson RJ, Rosenbloom M. Drug interactions with sufentanil: hemodynamic effects of premedication and muscle relaxants. Anesthesiology 1992;76:922–929.
142. Ghignone M, Quintin L, Duke PC, et al. Effects of clonidine on narcotic requirements and hemodynamic responses during induction of fentanyl anesthesia and endotracheal intubation. Anesthesiology 1986;64:36–42.
143. Bernard JM, Bourrelli B, Hommeril JL, Pinaud M. Effects of oral clonidine premedication and postoperative iv infusion on haemodynamic and adrenergic responses during recovery of anaesthesia. Acta Anaesthesiol Scand 1991;35:54–59.
144. Scheinin B, Lindgren L, Randell T, et al. Dexmedetomidine attenuates sympathoadrenal responses to tracheal intubation and reduces the need for thiopentone and perioperative fentanyl. Br J Anaesth 1992;68:126–131.
145. Karasch E. Hill H, Eddy C. Influence of dexmedetomidine and clonidine on human liver microsomal alfentanil metabolism. Anesthesiology 1991;75:520–524.
146. Roberts FL, Dixon J, Lewis GT, et al. Induction and maintenance of propofol anaesthesia, a manual infusion scheme. Anaesthesia 1988;43 (suppl):14–17.
147. Schüttler J, Kloos S, Schwilden H, Stoeckel H. Total intravenous anaesthesia with propofol and alfentanil by computer assisted infusions. Anaesthesia 1988;43 (suppl):2–7.
148. White M, Kenny GNC. Intravenous propofol anaesthesia using a computerized infusion system. Anaesthesia 1990;45:204–209.
149. Sear JW. Pharmacokinetic and pharmacodynamic aspects of continuous infusion anaesthesia: concept of minimum infusion rate as an index of equipotency for intravenous agents. Clin Anesthesiol 1984;2:223–242.
150. Shafer SL. Targeting the effect site with a computer controlled infusion pump. In: D'Argento DZ, ed. Advanced methods of pharmacokinetic and pharmacodynamic systems analysis. New York: Plenum, 1991:185–195.
151. Chaudhri S, White M, Kenny GNC. Induction of anaesthesia with propofol using a target-controlled infusion system. Anaesthesia 1992;47:551–553.
152. Van Hamme M, Ghoneim MM, Ambre JJ. Pharmacokinetics of etomidate, a new intravenous anesthetic. Anesthesiology 1978; 49:274–277.
153. Gepts E, Shafer SL, Camu F, et al. Linearity of pharmacokinetics and model estimation of sufentanil. Anesthesiology 1995; 83:1194-1204.

19 Neurolept and Dissociative Anesthesia

Elemer K. Zsigmond

Since the introduction of thiopental by Lundy (1), many millions of patients have experienced a rapid and pleasant loss of consciousness before the administration of an inhalation anesthetic. However, sudden death occurred in soldiers during World War II when intravenous thiopental was administered to hypovolemic patients by inexperienced practitioners (2). Soon after the Second World War, a French navy surgeon, Henry Laborit, observed in the operating room that some of his surgical patients developed side effects that looked almost like an acute illness, so he named it "post-aggressive disease," in keeping with Selye's stress theory (3). Laborit tried to attenuate this adverse response through control of the "neurovegetative" system by attenuating the sympathetic overactivity using phenergan, a drug with antiadrenergic, antihistaminic, and antiemetic properties. Because phenergan does not induce unconsciousness and provides no analgesia, it was necessary to combine this agent with meperidine, an opioid analgesic with spasmolytic and vagolytic action. To obtain more detachment from the surrounding environment, Laborit added chlorpromazine, a "neuroleptic" agent, and he named this new mixture a "lytic cocktail" (4).

The most commonly used neuroleptic mixture consisted of chlorpromazine, 50 mg, phenergan, 50 mg, and meperidine, 100 mg, administered as a slow intravenous infusion or in intermittent bolus doses (4). At present, 12 neuroleptic compounds (3 congeners of phenothiazine, 5 butyrophenones, 3 benzamides, and thioxanthene) are used in various formulations of the original lytic cocktail. Inappropriate dosing of neuroleptic agents resulted in serious complications that led to the virtual abandonment of the use of lytic cocktail techniques. Despite improper use and incorrect dosages, no fatalities were reported during the first 10-year period (5). On the other hand, many fatalities occurred with the available inhalation anesthetics during the same period. The early neuroleptic technique was then taken a step further by introducing hypothermia with the lytic cocktail, a so-called state of "artificial hibernation" (6). Because hypothermia and hypometabolism provide additional cellular protection, inadvertent hypoxemia is less likely to cause serious tissue hypoxia during hypothermia than during normothermia, and this technique also diminishes adrenergic responsiveness. The availability of this technique facilitated the early advancement of both cardiothoracic surgery and neurosurgery.

One of the shortcomings of the lytic cocktail was the limited analgesic potency of meperidine. Subsequently, Janssen and colleagues succeeded in the synthesis of meperidine congeners with a 500 to 10,000-fold greater analgesia potency and a 260 to 26,000-fold higher safety profile in animals. DeCastro and Mundeleer (7) introduced an anesthetic technique involving the use of a combination of neuroleptic (haloperidol or droperidol) and analgesic agents, the so-called neuroleptanalgesia (NLA) technique. Later, hydroxyzine was added for analgesic potentiation. This new mixture provided stable hemodynamics in poor-risk and critically ill patients. Unfortunately, the manufacturer discontinued the intravenous formulation of hydroxyzine because of malpractice suits related to the inappropriate intra-arterial injection of the drug (with a pH of 4.2), which led to gangrene of the extremities.

A few years later, the benzodiazepine diazepam became available for premedication, cardioversion, and cardiac catheterization (8). Diazepam was also combined with analgesics to produce neuroleptanesthesia (NLAN). When Innovar (a 50:50 mixture of fentanyl, 50 μg/ml, and droperidol 2.5 mg/ml) became available in the United States, it was combined with diazepam as a premedicant and coinduction agent during general, regional, and local anesthesia. The Innovar dosage requirements were markedly reduced by diazepam, and hemodynamic stability during induction and intubation was comparable to that seen with Innovar alone. A few years later, when ketamine was introduced into clinical practice (9, 10), diazepam was used to attenuate ketamine's adverse central nervous system (CNS) effects, namely, sympathetic hyperactivity and psychotomimetic side effects (11, 12). This technique became known as dissociative anesthesia.

NEUROLEPTANESTHESIA AND ANALGESIA

NLA is a state of apathy, immobility, and analgesia produced by the combination of a neuroleptic drug, droperidol, and fentanyl, or one of its newer analogs (i.e., sufentanil, alfentanil, or remifentanil). When diazepam and nitrous oxide (N_2O) or an inhalation anesthetic was added to NLA, it became NLAN. DeCastro and others devised many variations of NLAN (Table 19-1). More recently, ketamine (a so-called dissociative anesthetic) was introduced as a component of NLAN (10).

NEUROLEPTIC DRUGS

Neurolepsis is a clinical syndrome first observed in human patients receiving haloperidol (13), a butyrophenone synthesized by Janssen (14). This syndrome involves the inhibition of various vegetative, psychic, and motor functions with suppression of emetic symptoms after modest doses and catalepsy after higher doses (Table 19-2). DeCastro and Mundeleer (7) combined this haloperidol with phenoperidine for NLA (15). Janssen synthesized a more powerful butyrophenone, droperidol (16), after synthesizing fentanyl (17). The combination of droperidol and fentanyl by DeCastro and Mundeleer induced analgesia more rapidly with less respiratory depression and fewer extrapyramidal side effects than the haloperidol-phenoperidine combination (7).

Neuroleptic drugs can be classified into two categories, phenothiazines and butyrophenones. Droperidol is the most popular butyrophenone because its use is associated with a lower incidence of side effects than many of the other neuroleptic drugs. However, after high doses of droperidol, side effects including, dyskinesia, restlessness, hyperactivity, chills and shivering, dysphoria with inner anxiety, hallucinations, loss of body image, and a sensation of weightlessness have been reported (18, 19). Phenothiazines, on the other hand, produce orthostatic hypotension, hypothermia, hypnotic, antiemetic effects, and sympatholytic activity.

TABLE 19-1. Variants of neuroleptanesthesia (NLAN) and neuroleptanalgesia (NLA)

Pure analgesic anesthesia
Potentiated analgesic anesthesia
Ataractanalgesia
Sympatholeptanalgesia
Antiserotonin analgesia
Stress-free NLAN and NLA
Dissociative anesthesia

TABLE 19-2. Physiologic Effects of Neuroleptic Anesthetic and Analgesic Techniques

Neuroleptic behavior (i.e., mineralization)
Quiescence
Indifference to surroundings
Reduced motor activity
Anxiolysis
Antiaggressivity
Arousability
Autonomic nervous system inhibition
Peripheral and central effects
α-Adrenergic blockade
Dopaminergic blockade
Serotoninergic blockade
Histaminergic blockade

The neuroleptic potency of the butyrophenones is related to their binding affinity to the specific membranes in the CNS where dopamine, serotonin, and norepinephrine function as neurotransmitters (20-23). As a result of their structural similarity to γ-aminobutyric acid (GABA), neuroleptics agents can occupy GABA receptors on the postsynaptic membrane, reducing synaptic transmission and increasing the concentration of dopamine in the intersynaptic cleft. In addition, they also inhibit the reuptake of dopamine and norepinephrine into the storage granules at the presynaptic nerve terminals. The normal balance of acetylcholine and dopamine in certain areas of the brain is altered and leads to the inhibition of the "operant behavior" by neuroleptic drugs. The antiemetic effect of neuroleptic drugs is probably related to their binding affinity to the GABA receptors in the chemoreceptor trigger zone (24). Droperidol is approximately 200 times more effective as an antiemetic than chlorpromazine and is about 20 to 50 times more efficacious than prochlorperazine (25).

Haloperidol

Haloperidol is a potent and long-acting neuroleptic drug. Its onset of action is within 5 to 10 minutes, and its duration of action is 24 to 48 hours (26). Haloperidol is primarily used to treat psychotic disease states (27). Droperidol has completely replaced the use of haloperidol in clinical anesthesia.

Droperidol

Droperidol is similar in its actions to the phenothiazines, but it is more potent and more specific (25). The neuroleptic syndrome in humans is manifested by psychomotor slowing, emotional quieting, and affective indifference (Table 19-3). Patients tend to fall asleep but are readily arousable. Because of the indifference of patients to their surroundings and the semicon-

TABLE 19-3. Pharmacologic Properties and Side Effects of Droperidol

- Neuroleptic behavior
- Antiemetic activity
- Potentiation of CNS depressants
- Potentiation of analgesic agonists
- Autonomic nervous system inhibition
- Anticonvulsant activity
- Long duration of action
- Antifibrillatory effects
- Minimal cardiovascular depression (except in hypovolemic states)
- Side effects
  - Extrapyramidal symptoms (e.g., dystonia, tremor, rigidity)
  - Adverse psychomotor effects (e.g., anxiety, akathisia, dysphoria, insomnia, restlessness)

scious state, this condition was termed "mineralization" in Europe by the pioneers of NLA. Droperidol provides no analgesia and fails to potentiate the analgesic effects of opioid drugs (28), although it may prolong their duration of action (29).

Droperidol possesses a moderate α-adrenergic blocking effect, thereby reducing peripheral and pulmonary vascular resistance and inducing moderate hypotension (30, 31). This effect may be of benefit in avoiding hypertension during cross-clamping of the aorta (32). In routinely used doses, droperidol does not produce significant depression of myocardial contractility (33, 34). It provides protection against epinephrine-induced arrhythmias, which may be related to a quinidine-like effect in lengthening of the refractory period (35, 36). Hypotension may occur with droperidol doses exceeding 150 $\mu g \cdot kg^{-1}$, but it is usually mild and of short duration (37). If the reduction in blood pressure is marked, the possibility of hypovolemia should be considered. Extrapyramidal symptoms occur with higher doses and can be managed using antiparkinsonian and anticholinergic drugs (24). Dystonia, hyperkinetic movements, akathisia, and uncontrolled restlessness also occur after higher doses of droperidol. Excessive dopaminergic activity in the basal ganglia region may be responsible for the occurrence of these side effects.

Droperidol causes neither respiratory depression nor potentiation of the respiratory depression induced by fentanyl (38, 39). One of the advantage of droperidol is its protective effect against histamine, serotonin, and acetylcholine-induced bronchospasm (40). Because bis-quinoline muscle relaxants and airway manipulation may induce bronchospasm, droperidol may prove useful during anesthetic induction or anesthesia in patients with reactive airway disease. Droperidol has no effect on the gastrointestinal tract and does not cause even transient changes in liver function (41). Oxygen consumption is reduced by 20 to 30% (21) as a result of droperidol's ability to reduce sympathetic and motor activity.

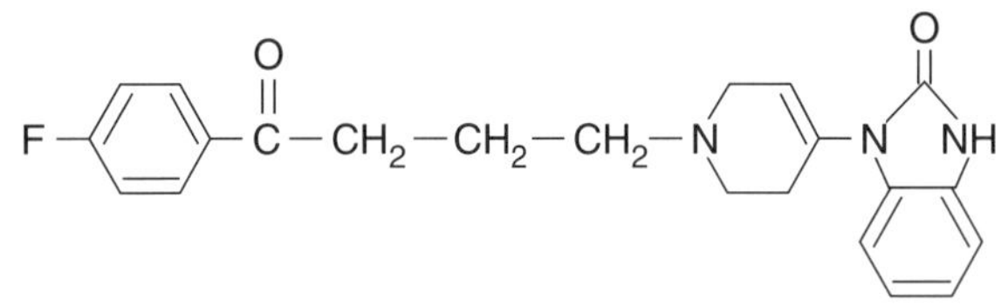

F—C$_6$H$_4$—C(=O)—CH_2—CH_2—CH_2—N(tetrahydropyridyl)—N(benzimidazolone)NH

Mol. weight (dalton)	379
pKa	7.68
Plasma $t_{1/2}\beta$ (min)	140

FIGURE 19-1. Physiochemical and pharmacokinetic characteristics of droperidol.

Droperidol was reported to have a short elimination half life (about 104 minutes), however, its duration of clinical effect is 3 to 6 hours (Fig. 19-1). The mean total body clearance is 14 $ml \cdot min^{-1} \cdot kg^{-1}$, and the total apparent volume of distribution is 2 L/kg. The extensive uptake of droperidol by the tissues is related to its high lipid solubility (42). The drug is primarily metabolized in the liver (42).

STANDARD NEUROLEPTANESTHESIA TECHNIQUE: FENTANYL

Originally, fentanyl was marketed in an ampule mixed with droperidol in a 1:50 ratio. It was recommended that the combination be given in a dose of 1 ml per 10 kg of body weight in a single injection to "speed up" induction (10, 15, 43). On a clinical pharmacologic basis, this practice was not logical because the onset of effect of droperidol is slower and its duration of action is much longer than those of fentanyl. When this combination is used, droperidol should be administered before fentanyl, which should be administered in either small incremental doses (25 to 50 μg) or by a continuous infusion.

Because a "ceiling" effect has been observed with respect to the anesthetic-sparing effects of fentanyl and its newer analogs, it is rational to administer a small dose of fentanyl, 1 to 2 $\mu g/kg$ intravenously, before induction and 0.25- to 0.5-$\mu g/kg$ incremental doses 3 to 5 minutes before an anticipated painful surgical stimulus (44, 45). Children and neonates have differing opioid dose requirements (46, 47). Careful titration of the fentanyl dose is important because the resultant blood levels of fentanyl can differ after identical dosages (48-50). In addition, the required dose of fentanyl may vary from patient to patient, depending on the intensity of the surgical stimulus (Fig. 19-2). To minimize the adverse hemodynamic changes in response to extubation, fentanyl, 1 to 2 $\mu g/kg$ intravenously, can be given at the time of peritoneal closure without producing excessive respiratory depression in the

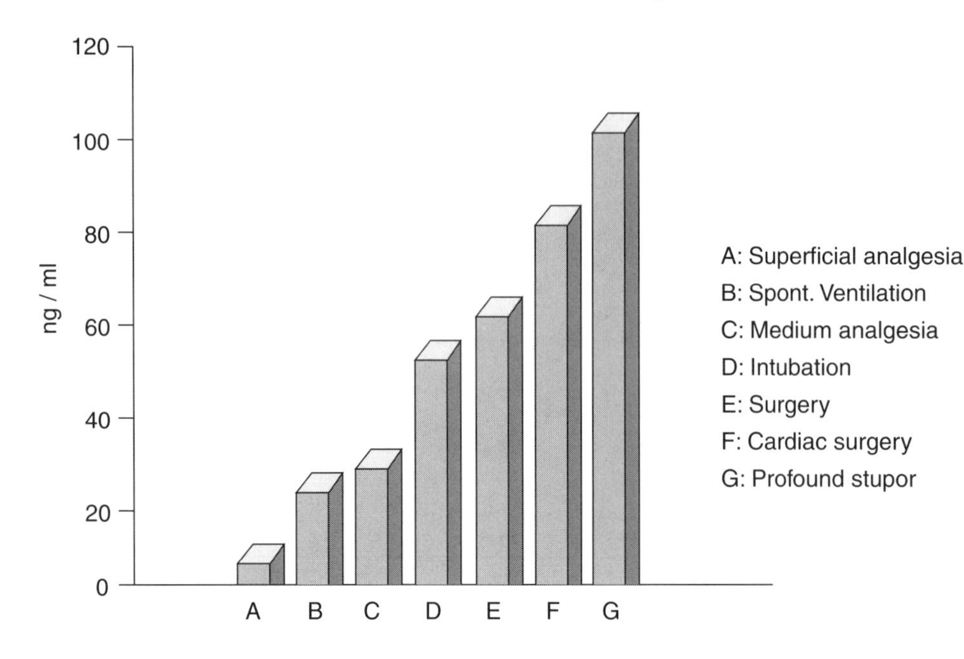

FIGURE 19-2. Plasma fentanyl concentrations required to prevent acute hemmodynamic responses to stimuli during cardiac surgery. (Adapted from Hug CC, Chaffman M: Alfentanil Pharmacology and Uses in Anesthesia. Camu F, Spierdyk J, eds. Aukland, New Zealand, ADIS Press, 1984.)

postoperative period (51). Supplemental analgesia at the end of surgery also helps to maintain adequate postoperative analgesia.

The patient recovering from NLAN is usually sedated but cooperative and responsive. However, respiratory depression is always a potential problem in the postoperative period when an opioid-based technique is used (52, 53). Prevention of respiratory depression with naltrexone, 50 mg orally every 12 hours, was demonstrated in human volunteers receiving a fentanyl infusion of 50 μg/h for 48 hours, 150 μg/h for 0.33 hours every 4 hours, or 150 μg/h for 0.33 hours every hour (54).

Studies by Dundee and associates (55)* suggested that premedication with analgesics reduces the induction doses of intravenous anesthetics and diminishes side effects. Hydroxyzine and diazepam have been used for premedication with NLA and NLAN techniques. The optimal dose of hydroxyzine, 1.5 mg/kg orally 60 to 90 minutes before surgery, produced no clinically significant respiratory depression or potentiation of opioid-induced respiratory depression (56-58). In patients with severe chronic obstructive pulmonary disease (COPD), hydroxyzine produces bronchodilation (59, 60). Similar observations have been made with diazepam (61, 62). The additional benefit of diazepam (versus hydroxyzine) is anterograde amnesia, which potentiates the sedative-amnestic effects of fentanyl as part of a NLAN technique. The most commonly used drugs for potentiation of fentanyl are lorazepam, diazepam, and midazolam. In 75 patients undergoing coronary artery revascularization, neither diazepam nor midazolam caused adverse hemodynamic changes (Table 19-4). Although significant reductions in systolic blood pressure, systemic vascular resistance, and heart rate were observed, cardiac index, stroke volume index, and left ventricular stroke work index were unchanged. Catecholamines were reduced to baseline levels after both drugs (63). Even in patients with valvular heart disease and a reduced cardiac index, Schulte-Sasse and associates (64)* and Gob and associates (65)* observed no adverse hemodynamic effects.

For over two decades, high doses of fentanyl (50 to 150 μg/kg) and, more recently, of sufentanil have been used for cardiac anesthesia. Stanley and associates were the first to suggest that profound anesthesia with protection against acute stress responses could be provided with high-dose narcotic techniques (66, 67). However, the usual tests of unconsciousness (e.g., loss of verbalization, loss of response to verbal commands) were present in 75% of patients even after a 30-μg/kg dose of fentanyl (68). Awareness during "opioid anesthesia" has been reported after 100- to 150-μg/kg doses of fentanyl (69, 70). Hypertension, tachycardia, and increased catecholamine levels have also been reported with this technique (71-74). In defense of the high-dose narcotic techniques, Lowenstein (75)* suggested that the hypertensive episodes were caused by inadequate "anesthetic" depth even though the electroencephalographic (EEG) changes were consistent with deep depression of cerebral activity (76). Waller and associates (77)* also reported increases in arterial pressure and systemic vascular resistance after intubation, skin incision, and sternotomy despite a total fentanyl dose of 162 ± 6 μg/kg (mean ± S.D.). Hall and associates (78)* observed marked increases in vasopressin and antidiuretic hormone levels after 75 μg/kg doses of fentanyl. Fentanyl alone, even in high doses, is clearly inferior to the combination of droperidol-fentanyl or benzodiazepine-fentanyl-ketamine for NLAN.

TABLE 19-4. Fentanyl and Sufentanil Dose Requirements During Cardiac Surgery Following Premedication with Either Diazepam or Midazolam

Anesthetic Drugs	Total Dose ($\mu \cdot kg^{-1}$)	Before CPB ($\mu \cdot kg^{-1}$)	After CPB ($\mu \cdot kg^{-1}$)
D-F-P	55.8 ± 11.8	28.0 ± 5.3	27.8 ± 5.6
D-S-P	11.9 ± 0.9	7.5 ± 1.1	4.4 ± 0.6
M-S-P	13.9 ± 1.3	9.5 ± 0.4	4.4 ± 0.5
M-S-K-P	9.1 ± 0.9	6.5 ± 0.6	2.6 ± 0.4
M-S-K-V	8.0 ± 0.8	5.5 ± 0.5	2.5 ± 0.3

D, Diazepam; M, midazolam; F, fentanyl; S, sufentanil; K, ketamine; P, pancuronium; V, vecuronium; CPB, cardiopulmonary bypass.

The traditional fentanyl-droperidol (Innovar) NLAN technique is still practiced in many parts of the world. The United States Food and Drug Administration (FDA) considered the fentanyl-droperidol combination a safeguard against illicit use of the opioid analgesic (79), because the mixture was known to cause dysphoria rather than euphoria. However, the combination of the long-acting neuroleptic, droperidol, with a relatively short-acting opioid, fentanyl, adversely affected the popularity of NLA in the United States. More frequent fentanyl dosing was necessary for longer procedures. With this combination, frequent dosing results in an overdosage of droperidol and its resultant adverse hemodynamic and psychologic sequelae.

Innovar is still used for premedication before NLA. It is recommended for analgesia in patients in pain and for relief of pain-induced anxiety, as well as to facilitate anesthetic induction or supplementation of local or regional anesthesia. Moreover, the droperidol component is effective in the prevention of opioid-induced nausea and vomiting. The usual recommended dose of Innovar in adults is 2 ml (containing 5.0 mg droperidol and 100 μg of fentanyl) intramuscularly 45 to 90 minutes before anesthetic induction. It should be used with caution in patients with COPD, in the elderly, in debilitated patients, and in patients receiving multiple drug treatments, because it may make them prone to hypotension or respiratory depression. In high-risk patients, the combination of hydroxyzine with meperidine may be preferable because it is less likely to produce adverse respiratory or circulatory side effects (61, 62).

When the clinical effects of droperidol and fentanyl were studied alone and as a combination in healthy volunteers, those who received droperidol experienced dysphoria rather than euphoria. Although fentanyl alone caused euphoria and the expected respiratory depression, droperidol neither antagonized nor potentiated the respiratory depression produced by fentanyl (80). Kallos and associates (81) observed a reduction in the functional residual capacity of the lung even in the absence of chest wall rigidity with Innovar, and the ventilatory depressant effects of Innovar can be enhanced by both benzodiazepines and barbiturates.

NLA is commonly used for operations in which the maintenance of a conscious state facilitates the conduct of surgery (e.g., endoscopic, diagnostic short procedures, arthroscopic, and laparoscopic procedures, as well as breast biopsy and dental procedures under local anesthesia). Combinations of midazolam (or propofol) and fentanyl (or alfentanil) have become more popular than the classic droperidol and fentanyl technique (so-called "dope and drope," a term popularized by Dr. Edward R. Johnson of the University of Texas Southwestern Medical Center in Dallas) because of the higher incidence of side effects with the latter technique. Extrapyramidal side effects (e.g., dystonic contractions of facial, neck, and pharyngeal muscles, grimacing, torticollis, trismus, and speech and swallowing difficulties) are disturbing to the patient and the recovery room nurses and may delay discharge home or cause the patient to return to the emergency room. Therefore, modifications in the classic NLA and NLAN techniques have been introduced in an attempt to enhance its clinical utility.

MODIFIED NEUROLEPTANESTHESIA TECHNIQUES

When NLAN was initially introduced, few agents could safely be added to NLAN, except N_2O. The two major advantages of supplementing NLAN with N_2O are a reduction in "awareness" (e.g., intraoperative recall) and a decrease in the neuroleptic drug dose requirements. Unfortunately, the incidence of nausea and vomiting increased with the addition of N_2O (82-85). Use of N_2O activates the medullary dopaminergic systems (86), which may increase nausea and vomiting, as well as the extrapyramidal side effects of NLAN. Indeed, a meta-analysis by Tramer and associates (87) demonstrated that omitting N_2O from general anesthesia significantly decreased vomiting in patients at high-risk of developing postoperative nausea and vomiting (PONV). However, elimination of N_2O in patients at low risk of emetic sequalae was associated with an increased risk of awareness. The decision to use N_2O must be made on an individual basis, after weighing the expected risk of PONV and the potential of intraoperative awareness.

Crile described the so-called anociassociation theory (88), which involved local infiltration of the surgical wound and operative area with local anesthetics to reduce the anesthetic and analgesic requirements, as well as to ensure better hemodynamic and autonomic control. Indeed, several investigators have demonstrated that the concomitant administration of local and regional anesthetic techniques reduces NLAN requirements and improves hemodynamic stability. Supplementation of NLA or NLAN with local and regional anesthetic techniques is also feasible in clinical practice (89-92).

Sufentanil

Sufentanil is the most potent fentanyl analog in clinical use (700 to 1000 times more potent than morphine and 5 to 10 times more potent than fentanyl). When this agent is used as part of a neurolept technique, the stress reaction may be more effectively blocked with sufentanil than with fentanyl (93-95). Sufentanil appears to blunt more effectively the centrally mediated hemodynamic responses to painful stimuli (e.g., laryngeal manipulations, surgical incision, organ retraction) than fentanyl (96). Sufentanil produces minimal cardiac depression (96-98) and minimal depression of the baro- and chemoreceptor reflexes (99). Sufentanil also produces more marked bradycardia than fentanyl, especially when it is administered in combination with vecuronium (100-102).

Recovery from anesthesia is faster after sufentanil-based NLAN than after isoflurane (103). Compared with fentanyl, recovery of normal ventilatory function is allegedly faster with sufentanil (104-105a), even though its duration of analgesia is longer (94, 102). However, sufentanil produces more bradycardia (100-102) and hypotension than fentanyl. Chest wall rigidity, myoclonus, renarcotization, and nausea and vomiting are similar after both sufentanil and fentanyl.

Because sufentanil has anesthetic-sparing effects, it is commonly used in combination with other anesthetic agents as an alternative to fentanyl (106, 107). Geriatric patients appear to tolerate sufentanil better than fentanyl (105, 108, 109). Both Ghoneim and associates (110) and Komatsu and associates (111) reported that sufentanil had an advantage over fentanyl as an adjuvant during balanced anesthesia. In attenuating the stress response during rapid sequence intubation, Kleiman and associates (112) reported more favorable results with sufentanil than fentanyl. In ambulatory surgery, Kuperwasser and associates (113) found sufentanil superior to alfentanil because it provided better postoperative sedation and analgesia, whereas overall recovery times and side effects were similar.

When sufentanil was introduced into clinical practice, DeCastro and associates (93) utilized droperidol with sufentanil. The rationale for the use of droperidol was to potentiate the CNS effects of sufentanil, to reduce the opioid dosage requirements, to provide effective anxiolysis (or ataraxia), to reduce excess sympathetic activity, to enhance amnesia, and to improve the recovery profile. The initial loading doses of sufentanil range from 0.5 to 2 $\mu g/kg$ in combination with N_2O for procedures lasting less than 2 hours. Ideally, 50 to 70% of the loading dose is given before intubation, and the remainder is administered during the preparation period before skin incision. For major intracavitary procedures with an expected duration exceeding 2 hours, the initial loading dose of sufentanil ranges from 2 to 4 $\mu g/kg$. For maintenance of anesthesia, sufentanil, 10 to 50 μg (0.2 to 1.0 ml), can be given by incremental (bolus) injection, depending on the patient's response. A common approach is to give small bolus doses (5 to 10 μg) until unresponsiveness occurs and then to give the same dose before surgical incision by a continuous intravenous infusion. The induction time with sufentanil is faster than with fentanyl (3 *versus* 6 minutes) (104). Fahmy (103) demonstrated that sufentanil-N_2O maintains hemodynamic stability despite marked changes in intraoperative stimuli. During thiopental-sufentanil-N_2O anesthesia utilizing meperidine, morphine, fentanyl, or sufentanil, hemodynamic values were more stable and catecholamine levels were lower with sufentanil (114, 114a). Early recovery and extubation times were also faster with sufentanil compared with isoflurane (103, 115).

Alfentanil

Alfentanil has about one-third the peak analgesic potency of fentanyl and about one-third of its duration of action (116). Before the availability of remifentanil, alfentanil had the fastest onset of effect and the shortest duration of action among the fentanyl congeners. Its pharmacokinetic profile facilitates a rapid onset of its analgesic effect and a rapid recovery (117). A practical induction method was suggested by DeCastro (118). It consisted of a three-step technique: 1) a loading dose of 40 to 80 $\mu g/kg$; 2) an infusion of 1.0 to 1.5 $\mu g/kg/min$; and 3) incremental bolus doses from 5 to 10 $\mu g/kg$. Use of a continuous variable-rate infusion of alfentanil after a loading dose is another reasonable approach (119). A loading dose of alfentanil, 16 $\mu g/kg$, was reported to be effective in attenuating the adverse hemodynamic responses to intubation (120). One important practical point is that alfentanil plasma levels rapidly decrease below "therapeutic" plasma levels ($<$400 ng/ml) unless the maintenance infusion is initiated immediately after the initial loading dose. Obesity reduces alfentanil's clearance (45%) from 321 to 179 ml/min and leads to an increase in its elimination half-life value (121). Interindividual variability in clearance rates is greater than sixfold (122). In addition, the drug's pharmacodynamics may be altered in the aged (123, 123a). Therefore, alfentanil must be carefully titrated to an individual patient's clinical response in this high-risk patient population.

Alfentanil has advantages including fast onset of its clinical effect, minimal cardiovascular depression, absence of systemic toxicity, and a short and predictable duration of action and recovery. Therefore, it is amenable for supplementation of volatile and intravenous anesthetics for ambulatory surgery and for any painful procedures. It is commonly supplemented with droperidol, midazolam, and propofol. Droperidol is given in small doses (7 to 20 μg/kg) before induction or on termination of surgery as a prophylactic antiemetic drug.

For short ambulatory surgical procedures, Brown and associates (124) did not find marked advantages of alfentanil over fentanyl in a double-blind study. Rosow and associates (125) administered alfentanil, 10 or 20 μg/kg, or fentanyl, 1 or 2 μg/kg, in a placebo-controlled double-blind study involving urologic surgical patients. No patient required supplemental medication in the alfentanil groups, in contrast to 82% in the placebo group. Many patients in the alfentanil group required only one injection for the entire procedure. However, investigators noted a 40% overall incidence of PONV. Alfentanil was easier to titrate than fentanyl, and 20 μg/kg alfentanil was frequently sufficient for a 15 to 20 minute procedure. White and associates (126) demonstrated that the incidence of PONV did not differ between alfentanil and fentanyl, whereas recovery times were consistently shorter with alfentanil.

The two common approaches to administration of alfentanil infusions are fixed-rate and variable-rate infusions. The fixed-rate infusion technique utilizes a loading dose of 25 to 50 μg/kg followed by an infusion of 0.5 to 1.5 μg/kg/min (127). The infusion should be stopped 15 to 20 minutes before the anticipated end of surgery to ensure prompt recovery of consciousness and spontaneous ventilation. Continuous infusion is probably the most reliable technique of alfentanil administration; one uses either a manual or a computer-controlled infusion pump (128-130). White and associates (126) found that more precise titration of alfentanil, minimizing the dosage requirement and the incidence of adverse effects, could be accomplished by the use of continuous variable-rate infusion.

Alfentanil is a suitable alternative to fentanyl for neurosurgical anesthesia using a loading dose of 15 to 30 μg/kg, infused over a 5-minute period, followed by a maintenance infusion of 0.5 μg/kg/min. When given in combination with midazolam to patients with raised intracranial pressure (ICP), alfentanil produced a greater reduction in ICP than fentanyl (131). Alfentanil in combination with droperidol has also been used for NLA for patients undergoing awake craniotomy in which intraoperative cooperation is vital (132). Regional blocks may also be supplemented by small doses of alfentanil. For postoperative analgesia, infusion rates of alfentanil, ranging from 0.25 to 0.50 μg/kg/min in ventilated patients and from 0.1 to 0.2 μg/kg/min in spontaneously breathing patients, have been recommended by Yate and associates (131) and by Andrews and colleagues (133).

Remifentanil

A comparative study by Glass and associates (134) suggested that remifentanil was 20 to 30 times more potent than alfentanil. When remifentanil, 0.05 μg/kg/min, was infused over a 4-hour period, it produced respiratory depression equal to that induced by alfentanil, 0.5 to 1.0 μg/kg/min. The recovery of normal ventilation took 8.3 minutes after discontinuation of remifentanil, in contrast to 61 minutes after alfentanil. When the EEG spectral edge was used for comparing remifentanil and alfentanil (135), remifentanil appeared to be 16 times more potent than alfentanil. The potency of remifentanil in reducing the volatile anesthetic requirement is 80 times greater than fentanyl's, and it has one-tenth the potency of sufentanil.

Remifentanil, 3 to 5 μg/kg intravenously, reduced the induction dose of thiopental to 200 mg (136). Single bolus doses of remifentanil are not practical except for transient painful stimuli because the effect is short-lasting and dissipates within minutes. Hence, an infusion of remifentanil should be started after the initial injection of a hypnotic drug. When a hypnotic dose of propofol (1 to 2 mg/kg) was administered with remifentanil, 1 μg/kg, followed by an infusion of 0.4 μg/kg/min, only 33% of patients responded to intubation (137). When the same induction scheme was combined with N_2O, remifentanil, 0.5 μg/kg/min, prevented the somatic and autonomic response to skin incision in 80% of patients (137). Thus, after an initial remifentanil loading dose combined with a hypnotic agent for induction, a remifentanil infusion of 0.4 to 0.8 μg/kg/min should be started and decreased to 0.1 to 0.25 μg/kg/min following intubation when supplemented by propofol 100 μg/kg/min or N_2O in combination with a volatile agent. For monitored anesthesia care, small incremental doses of remifentanil (25 μg intravenously) or an infusion of 0.025 to 0.15 μg/kg/min may be utilized after premedication with midazolam, 1 to 3 mg intravenously (138).

Remifentanil can be used for induction and maintenance of anesthesia for many different surgical procedures, particularly when the agent is combined with hypnotics, tranquilizers, N_2O and inhalation anesthetics. An initial dose of remifentanil, 3 to 5 μg/kg intravenously, and a remifentanil infusion of 0.5 $\mu g \cdot kg^{-1} \cdot min^{-1}$ intravenously in combination with 66% N_2O in oxygen, prevents a response to skin incision in virtually all patients (139). Other investigators have reported good hemodynamic stability during the maintenance period and prompt recovery following a remifentanil-N_2O combination (139-140). Remifentanil plasma concentrations of 2 $ng \cdot ml^{-1}$ can be achieved using an intravenous infusion of 0.1 $\mu g \cdot kg^{-1} \cdot min^{-1}$ and have been reported to decrease the anesthetic requirement for isoflurane by 50%. After a hypnotic dose of propofol, a loading dose of remifentanil,

1 μg/kg, followed by an infusion of 0.4 $\mu g \cdot kg^{-1} \cdot min^{-1}$ prevented 67% of patients from developing acute hyperdynamic responses to tracheal intubation. After intubation, the remifentanil infusion rate was reduced to 0.1 to 0.25 μg/kg/min.

Avramov and associates (141) determined the optimal remifentanil infusion rate to provide adequate patient comfort and respiratory function during breast biopsy procedures under local anesthesia as part of a monitored anesthesia care technique. An initial infusion of 0.1 μg/kg/min remifentanil was started 5 minutes after 2, 4, or 8 mg intravenous midazolam (or saline), and the infusion rate was varied as necessary to optimize patient comfort. A low dose of midazolam (2 mg intravenously) assured easy titratability and predictability of remifentanil infusion and provided patient comfort and intraoperative satisfaction (142). Based on this study, it appears that incremental adjustments in the remifentanil infusion rate of 0.025 μg/kg/min would be practical for ambulatory anesthesia, and the average remifentanil infusion rate was 0.06 μg/kg/min (141).

Use of propofol for induction of anesthesia, followed by remifentanil, has been extensively studied in both inpatients and outpatients, as well as in patients undergoing local and regional anesthesia (143-146). Fragen and associates (147) found the combination of remifentanil with propofol as part of a total intravenous anesthetic (TIVA) technique to be advantageous in preventing hyperdynamic responses to intubation and skin incision in outpatients undergoing knee arthroscopic surgery.

During hepatic transplantation, remifentanil seems to be the ideal agent for intraoperative analgesia because of its unique esterase metabolism. Remifentanil's rapid clearance rate is unchanged even in patients with clinically significant liver disease (148, 149). In geriatric patients (older than 70 years of age), remifentanil causes minimal hemodynamic changes. Like other opioids, remifentanil appears to cause no significant changes in intraocular pressure, a potential advantage in elderly patients undergoing ophthalmologic surgery.

For neurosurgical procedures, remifentanil may become the opioid of choice because of its rapid onset and recovery and its high degree of titratability. As a result of its short context-sensitive half-time, remifentanil has a predictable recovery profile after terminating an infusion that allows the neurosurgeon to evaluate the patient immediately after surgery.

As an intravenous adjuvant during regional anesthesia, remifentanil was found safe and effective by Camu and associates (150). "Fast-track" recovery can be ensured by the use of remifentanil in combination with local anesthetics as part of a monitored anesthesia care technique (151). Early extubation and discharge from the intensive care unit, critical for successful "fast-tracking" after open-heart surgery, also appear to be facilitated in patients receiving remifentanil as part of a "balanced" neurolept or TIVA (152).

Clinical evidence of an increase in histamine levels has not been demonstrated after remifentanil administration. Sebel and associates (153) investigated hemodynamic changes and histamine release when a large bolus dose of remifentanil (30 μg/kg) was given intravenously over 1 minute. Although this large dose of remifentanil produced significant reductions in blood pressure and heart rate, these investigators saw no evidence of histamine release.

As a result of its favorable pharmacokinetic profile, remifentanil is also popular in pediatric anesthesia. The pharmacokinetics of remifentanil in anesthetized children between 2 to 12 years of age has been extensively studied by Davis and associates (154). If intravenous access has been established, remifentanil can be given in combination with propofol and midazolam as part of a TIVA or neurolept technique. A newer method of induction of anesthesia in children involving the jet injection of midazolam and ketamine may make it possible to more rapidly insert an intravenous catheter (155, 156) and thereby to facilitate the use of remifentanil-based anesthetic techniques.

A remifentanil infusion of 1 to 3 μg/kg/min was reported by Howie and associates (149, 150) to prevent increases in catecholamine levels during induction, intubation, sternotomy, and the prebypass period in patients undergoing coronary revascularization procedures. Isoflurane was required for supplementation in most of these cardiac patients, specifically 92%, 61%, and 67% of the patients receiving remifentanil 1-, 2-, and 3-$\mu g \cdot kg^{-1} \cdot min^{-1}$ intravenous infusions, respectively. Respiratory depression may occur after remifentanil-based anesthesia, although in most instances it is self-limited and does not require reversal by opioid antagonists. Yarmush and associates (159) found that a remifentanil infusion of 0.23 μg/kg/min provided significantly better analgesia than morphine, 0.15 mg/kg, in the 25-minute period after extubation. Although analgesia was increased with increasing doses of remifentanil, respiratory depression did not parallel these changes. However, "analgesic" doses of remifentanil can produce muscle rigidity, as well as opioid-related side effects (e.g., PONV) (160).

USE OF OPIOID AGONIST-ANTAGONISTS DURING NEUROLEPTANESTHESIA

Pentazocine

Pentazocine is alleged to be one-fourth as potent as morphine (i.e., 30 to 60 mg is equivalent to 10 mg morphine). It has moderate affinity for the μ receptor, in contrast to its high affinity for the κ receptor. Pentazocine's bioavailabilty is similar to that of morphine; however, it is more highly protein bound, (i.e., 60 to 70% versus 23 to 26% for morphine). It also has a pharmacokinetic profile similar to that of morphine, with an elimination half-life of 2 to 4 hours. There appears to be a ceiling effect with respect to its ability to potentiate the minimum alveolar concentration of inhalation anesthetics (161). Clinically, pentazocine is no longer used alone for anesthetic induction or maintenance because of its limited analgesic potency and because of the marked increases in systemic and pulmonary artery (as well as left ventricular diastolic) pressures when this agent is used as the primary analgesic component of a NLAN technique. Furthermore, pentazocine induces dysphoria, psychotomimetic reactions, and even hallucinations during the early postoperative recovery period.

As of its "ceiling effect" with respect to analgesia, it has only been used as part of a balanced anesthetic technique in combination with N_2O after preanesthetic medication. Indeed, Keeri-Szanto and Pomeroy reported that adequate hemodynamic stability could be achieved with pentazocine when it was administered in combination with N_2O and other adjunctive drugs (162). When Schoenfeld, Aldrete, and Jourde and their colleagues administered pentazocine in combination with diazepam, it was referred to as "pentazepam somnoanalgesia (163)." This NLA technique provided good operative conditions for gynecologic and oral surgery (164, 165). Although no muscle rigidity or histamine release was reported, protracted recovery with nausea, vomiting, and dizziness was problematic. DeCastro and associates (166, 166a) and White and colleagues observed pre-epileptic seizure-type activity on the EEG when doses of pentazocine exceeded 200 mg intravenously. Given the limited analgesic potency of pentazocine, many patients undergoing cardiac anesthesia manifest pupillary signs of inadequate analgesia with elevated blood pressure, heart rate, and catecholamine levels during diazepam-pentazocine-N_2O anesthesia. Fentanyl and its newer congeners offer a better alternative to pentazocine as the analgesic component of an NLAN technique.

Butorphanol

Butorphanol is approximately five times more potent than morphine (e.g., 2 mg is equivalent to 10 mg of morphine). It is primarily an agonist at the κ receptors and at the σ opioid receptors, with only weak μ-antagonist activity. Butorphanol's bioavailabilty and protein binding are similar to those of pentazocine. Its terminal elimination half-life and volumes of distribution are also similar to those of pentazocine; however, its clearance is about two to four times faster (40 to 68 ml/kg/min *versus* 15 to 20 ml/kg/min). Analogous to pentazocine, butorphanol only reduces the volatile anesthetic requirement by 10 to 20%, with analgesia lasting approximately 4 hours (167, 168). When the agent was administered to volunteers, the respiratory depression produced by 4 mg of butorphanol was equal to that caused by 10 mg morphine (169). A ceiling effect (170) with respect to ventilatory depression was observed by Nagashima and associates (171). Plasma histamine levels are not increased by pentazocine (172), and increases in biliary duct pressure are less after butorphanol than after equianalgesic doses of morphine (173). During enflurane-N_2O anesthesia, butorphanol caused no changes in biliary duct caliber, whereas morphine caused severe biliary constriction (174).

Even extremely large doses of burtophanol, 0.3 to 1.0 mg/kg intravenously, do not induce a state of profound analgesia characteristic of the pure opioid agonists (175, 176). In doses of 0.025 to 0.1 mg/kg, however, butorphanol can suppress the autonomic responses to intubation (177). With butorphanol, a ceiling effect exists for analgesia, as well as for respiratory depression (170, 178). Given the absence of chest wall rigidity and the ceiling effect with respect to respiratory depression, Dobkin and associates (179) suggested that butorphanol would be a useful adjuvant during balanced anesthesia. Butorphanol, 1.5 to 4.0 mg intravenously, was administered before thiopental, 2 to 4 mg/kg intravenously, and supplemental doses of butorphanol, 0.5 to 1.0 mg, and 65% N_2O were administered after intubation. Only 1 patient in 53 required chlorpromazine to control acute hemodynamic reactions during the surgical procedure. In a double-blind study, Del Pizzo (180) could not differentiate between morphine and butorphanol used during a balanced anesthetic technique with N_2O. The incidences of nausea and vomiting were 26 and 13%, respectively.

In another double-blind study, Stehling and Zauder (167) failed to find any advantages of butorphanol over fentanyl. Furthermore, these authors encountered patients who remained hypertensive despite additional bolus doses of butorphanol during surgery, a finding confirming the ceiling effect with respect to intraoperative analgesia. Stanley and associates (175) also found that butorphanol was unable to block the acute hemodynamic responses to painful stimuli during cardiac surgery. Because a marked increase in pulmonary artery pressure has been observed after intravenous administration (177), butorphanol should not be used in patients in whom an increase in right ventricular work may be deleterious. Although psychotomimetic effects of butorphanol are less frequent and severe than with pentazocine, they can delay discharge from the recovery room. In view of these adverse effects, fentanyl derivatives are also considered preferable to butorphanol for NLAN.

Nalbuphine

Nalbuphine appears to be less potent than morphine when it is used for relief of acute postoperative pain despite the 1:1 potency ratio reported by Beaver and Feise (182). Nalbuphine is also reported to be equipotent to morphine in children (183). Although nalbuphine comes closer to the "ideal" analgesic agent than other agonist-antagonists with respect to side effects, its potency is too low, and it has to be supplemented with N_2O and other adjuvants. It produces its analgesic effect at the κ receptors and its antagonistic effects at the μ receptor. However, Bluhm and associates (184) reported a μ-agonist effect potentiated by antihistaminic compounds (e.g., hydroxyzine, diphenhydramine). Its activity at the σ receptor is significantly less than that of pentazocine and butorphanol; therefore, even extremely large doses (1 to 2 g intravenously) do not produce psychotomimetic side effects. Nalbuphine has almost identical pharmacokinetics to morphine, including its bioavailability and protein binding. DiFazio and associates (185) demonstrated a reduction in the inhalation anesthetic requirement with nalbuphine.

As with other agonist-antagonists, a ceiling effect with respect to respiratory depression was observed by Romagnoli and Keats (186). At a nalbuphine dose exceeding 50 mg, the carbon dioxide response curve is flat (170). Magruder and associates (187) succeeded in reversing the respiratory depression produced by fentanyl with a 0.1 mg/kg dose of nalbuphine. In patients who received NLA with fentanyl, hemodynamic stability was maintained following nalbuphine reversal, and no increase in catecholamine levels was observed (188). Analgesia was not reversed despite complete and prompt reversal of respiratory depression. The antagonist profile of nalbuphine is useful in clinical practice because naloxone can cause adverse hemodynamic changes as well as increases in pain and emesis in the early postoperative period. Even after extremely large doses of nalbuphine, 7.0 mg/kg (500 mg intravenously), histamine release is clinically unimportant (189). Nalbuphine, like butorphanol, causes no constriction of the common bile duct (174).

The cardiovascular profile of nalbuphine appears to be favorable because it caused no adverse effects in patients with a history of an acute myocardial infarction before surgery (190). Mean arterial pressure fell significantly after morphine, but not after nalbuphine. Both drugs decreased cardiac index, whereas nalbuphine caused a significant increases in systemic vascular resistance without elevating left ventricular filling pressure. The stroke work index was unchanged after both drugs; however, the mean velocity of left ventricular fiber shortening was reduced more by nalbuphine than by morphine. This oxygen-sparing effect of nalbuphine may be beneficial in cardiac patients with reduced oxygen supply. Lake and associates (191) further confirmed the hemodynamic stability associated with the use of nalbuphine, 0.5 to 3.0 mg/kg, in patients with coronary disease. Unfortunately, even the highest nalbuphine dose, 3.0 mg/kg, could not provide sufficient analgesia for cardiac surgery.

Using diazepam premedication (0.4 mg/kg) before 3.0 mg/kg nalbuphine and 66% N_2O supplementation provides adequate cardiac anesthesia for coronary bypass surgery (188). In one study, the total nalbuphine dose requirements for the surgical procedure were 18.3 mg/kg, with a range of 10 to 30 mg/kg, and the total diazepam dosage requirement for the procedure was 0.78 mg/kg, with a range of 0.4 to 1.1 mg/kg. Nalbuphine levels peaked before sternotomy with a mean value of 7.8 μg/ml, and a blood level exceeding 1.5 μg/ml was necessary to maintain adequate analgesia. Hemodynamic stability was excellent, and patients had no increases in catecholamine, cortisol, or histamine levels. The advantages of a nalbuphine-based NLAN technique were minimal hemodynamic changes, absence of chest wall rigidity, lack of catecholamine response to intubation, skin incision, and sternotomy, no histamine release, and no postoperative respiratory depression. Studies in patients undergoing cardiac surgery suggest that κ agonists with limited μ-agonist activity (nalbuphine) can be effective when administered in combination with an amnesiac (diazepam), an analgesic (N_2O), and a muscle relaxant (188). Fahmy (192) also confirmed that nalbuphine was an acceptable analgesic component for balanced anesthesia.

Buprenorphine

Buprenorphine is 25 to 50 times more potent than morphine and produces analgesia and other CNS effects that are qualitatively similar to those induced by other opioid agonist-antagonist compounds. Thus, 0.4 mg of buprenorphine is equivalent to 10 mg of morphine. Buprenorphine is a partial μ agonist that is highly lipophilic; the drug can be given intravenously, intramuscularly, and sublingually. It has the highest protein binding among the opioid compounds (96%); however, its bioavailability is the same as that of other agonist-antagonists. Buprenorphine's clearance rate is 19 $ml \cdot kg^{-1} \cdot min^{-1}$, with a volume of distribution at steady state of 2.8 ml/kg, and an elimination half-life of 3 hours. Although a ceiling effect exists with respect to ventilatory depression, the respiratory depressant effects of buprenorphine are difficult to reverse even after repeated doses of naloxone (193, 194).

Buprenorphine is not suitable as the sole anesthetic for any procedure, but it has been successfully used as an analgesic component of balanced or NLAN (194). It causes decreases in heart rate and mean arterial pressure after intravenous administration, but it does not cause hemodynamic instability even in patients with reduced cardiovascular reserve. The incidence of psychotomimetic emergence reactions is low, and the drug can antagonize the analgesic effects of morphine when it is given for postoperative pain control.

Dezocine

Dezocine is as potent as morphine, but it has a more rapid onset and slightly shorter duration of action.

Large doses of dezocine have been reported to reduce the minimum alveolar concentration of enflurane by 50% (195). In a double-blind study, Ding and associates (196) compared ketolorac and dezocine as alternatives to fentanyl during outpatient laparoscopic procedures. Hemodynamic changes during induction and maintenance of anesthesia, as well as early recovery times, were similar. Although less postoperative fentanyl was required in the dezocine-treated group than in the control group, dezocine caused a higher incidence of PONV (62%) than fentanyl or ketolorac (0%). One-third of the dezocine-treated patients required antiemetic therapy in the recovery room, and this contributed to delayed discharge following these ambulatory procedures. In a study by Ding and White (197) involving women undergoing minor gynecologic procedures, dezocine had no advantages over either fentanyl or ketorolac. Postoperative emesis was again more common with dezocine. Even when used as the analgesic component of a monitored anesthesia care technique (198), dezocine failed to offer any advantages over other commonly used opioid and nonopioid analgesic drugs. The advantages and disadvantages of dezocine in modified NLAN have to be further investigated.

DISSOCIATIVE ANESTHESIA

Ketamine, a racemic mixture of the S(+) and R(−) isomers, was introduced in the mid-1960s by Corssen and colleagues at the University of Michigan. From the early published reports (199, 200), it was evident that ketamine was a unique intravenous anesthetic that would have limited application in anesthesiology unless its side effects could be "tamed." Because ketamine caused limbic stimulation, diazepam was a logical choice to antagonize ketamine's CNS and cardiovascular side effects. Diazepam, 0.2 mg/kg intravenously, was reported by Zsigmond and colleagues to reduce the sympathetic stimulation, the increase in catecholamine levels, and the psychotomimetic emergence reactions produced by ketamine (201, 202). Even in burn patients, asthmatics, patients with pericardial tamponade, and children undergoing cardiac surgery, the coadministration of diazepam and ketamine proved to be a highly effective anesthetic technique with an acceptable recovery profile (200). The coadministration of diazepam and ketamine, so-called ataract-analgesia, became a new form of NLAN. The pharmacokinetics and pharmacodynamics of ketamine have been extensively studied with and without diazepam pretreatment (201, 202). In 1982, White and associates (203) reviewed the clinical pharmacology of ketamine and its stereoisomers. More recently, its pharmacokinetics (204) and pharmacodynamics (205) were extensively described.

The anesthetic state produced by ketamine was characterized by an unusual form of catalepsy, which was termed "dissociative anesthesia," a variant of NLAN. Although an induction dose of 2 to 2.5 mg/kg was recommended in the early publications, a ketamine dose of 0.5 to 1.0 mg/kg is adequate for induction of anesthesia when ketamine is administered in combination with other sedative-hypnotic drugs (206, 207). The use of lower dosages of ketamine is associated with a lower incidence of adverse side effects.

Because of its favorable physicochemical properties, ketamine can be given by oral, nasal, rectal, intramuscular, and intravenous routes of administration (Table 19-5). Ketamine hydrochloride dissolved in water to produce a stable, colorless solution with a pH of 3.5 to 5.5 is marketed in three different concentrations of 10 mg/ml, 50 mg/ml, and 100 mg/ml containing a benzethonium preservative. The lower concentrations of ketamine are primarily used for intravenous administration, whereas the high concentration is for intramuscular use.

In diazepam-premedicated patients, anesthesia is induced with a ketamine loading dose of 0.5 to 1.0 mg/kg intravenously and is maintained with a ketamine infusion of 1.0 to 2.0 mg/kg/h (202, 203). In one study, diazepam significantly elevated ketamine blood levels when it was given for coinduction before ketamine (201). Awareness was not a problem with this bolus-infusion technique, and the incidence of psychotomimetic effects was reduced from 92% to below 12%. A multicenter trial with the diazepam-ketamine induction sequence followed by ketamine infusion also showed a favorable outcome (207). It is essential to allow 5 to 8 minutes for diazepam to equilibrate at the effector site because its plasma-effect site equilibrium half-life (k_{e0}) is about 1.6 minutes (208). With midazolam, an even longer waiting period may be necessary because it has an even longer k_{e0} than diazepam. When benzodiazepine pretreatment is used, even a lower loading dose of ketamine (e.g., 0.5 to 1.0 mg/kg) was sufficient for outpatient anesthesia (209). The lower dose of ketamine produced less cardiovascular stimulation than that observed with the "standard" 2.0-mg/kg dose (209).

The commercially available racemic mixture of ketamine contains equal amounts of the two optical iso-

TABLE 19-5. Ketamine Dosage Recommendations When Used as Part of a "Balanced" Anesthetic or Sedation Technique

Induction in adults:	1.0 mg/kg IV over 30–60 s
Maintenance of anesthesia:	1.0–2.0 mg/kg/h IV infusion
Intraoperative analgesia:	0.2–0.4 mg/kg IV when needed
Postoperative sedation-analgesia:	0.25–1.0 mg/kg/h IV infusion
Induction in children:	3–8 mg/kg IM
	6–8 mg/kg PO
	8–15 mg/kg rectally
	6–8 mg/kg intranasally
	2.5–5.0 mg/kg by jet injection

mers, S(+) and R(−) ketamine. The comparative pharmacology of the isomers of ketamine has been studied by White and associates in healthy volunteers and in patients (210-213). These investigators found that the S(+) isomer of ketamine is three to five times more potent than the R(−) isomer (210). In animal experiments, the S(+) isomer of ketamine had a higher therapeutic index and produced greater sedation, better analgesia, and less CNS stimulation. When administered during surgery, the S(+) isomer was associated with less cardiovascular stimulation than R(−) ketamine (211). In healthy young volunteers, the cardiocirculatory stimulation was similar with the individual isomers to that produced by racemic ketamine (210) (Fig. 19-3). In this study, White and associates also observed a lower incidence of agitation and psychic emergence reactions with S(+) ketamine than with the racemic mixture or the R(−) ketamine isomer. The R(−) ketamine isomer also caused less EEG slowing than the S(+) or racemic ketamine (213). Even if S(+) ketamine becomes commercially available, benzodiazepine pretreatment and other intravenous adjuvants (e.g., droperidol, 0.625 to 1.25 mg intravenously) are recommended with S(+) ketamine to ensure hemodynamic stability and an acceptably low incidence of adverse side effects in clinical practice.

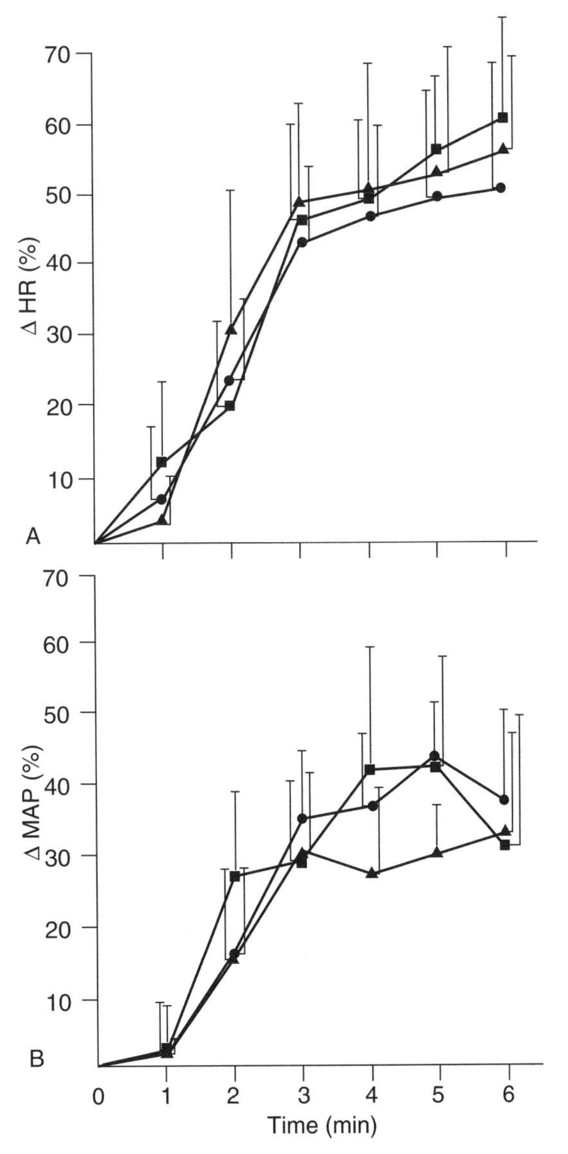

FIGURE 19-3. Acute changes in mean arterial pressure (MAP) and heart rate (HR) following infusion of either racemic ketamine (●—●), S (+) ketamine (■—■) or R (−) ketamine (▲—▲). (From White PF, Schuttler J, Shafer A, et al. Comparative pharmacology of ketamine isomers: studies in volunteers. Br J Anaesth 1985; 57:197–203.)

Use of Ketamine as Part of a Neuroleptanesthesia Technique

Ketamine is an effective anesthetic in clinical situations in which other intravenous anesthetic agents may be contraindicated. However, use of ketamine as a "sole" anesthetic may be problematic. Benzodiazepine pretreatment has made ketamine a far more acceptable anesthetic for induction and maintenance of anesthesia, leading to the concept "ataractanalgesia," a variant of NLAN. Diazepam pretreatment before ketamine administration has made hemodynamically stable inductions possible even in unstable cardiac patients (202, 214).

To evaluate the effects of diazepam pretreatment on ketamine and intubation-induced sympathetic hyperactivity, Zsigmond and his colleagues (202) conducted a double-blind study in healthy volunteers and in patients with preexisting cardiac disease. In the double-blind crossover study in volunteers, diazepam, 0.3 mg/kg/3 min, or saline was administered 8 minutes earlier, followed by ketamine, 2.2 mg/kg intravenously. Diazepam significantly prolonged ketamine-induced unconsciousness, with the time to following simple commands and to verbalizing coherently increasing from a mean duration of 15 minutes to 22 minutes (214, 215). Diazepam pretreatment significantly reduced the acute hypertensive effects of ketamine (Table 19-6). The ejection fraction was minimally reduced by the diazepam-ketamine combination, and the tabletile response was not altered by either ketamine or diazepam-ketamine. Ketamine alone caused a significant decrease in $PaCO_2$ and pH, and an increase in PCO_2, which was further enhanced by diazepam. In double-blind study conducted in 56 healthy gynecologic patients, diazepam, 0.2 mg/kg intravenously, produced a highly significant reduction in the mean arterial pressure, heart rate, and plasma catecholamine levels when given 10 minutes before ketamine, 2.2 mg/kg (216).

In cardiac patients, the effects of diazepam, 0.3 mg/kg, and midazolam, 0.15 mg/kg intravenously, on hemodynamic variables and catecholamines were comparable (217, 218). When administered as part of a ketamine induction sequence, both diazepam and midazolam effectively prevented increases in mean arterial pressure, heart rate, and catecholamine levels fol-

TABLE 19-6. Effect of Pretreatment with Saline or Diazepam, 0.3 mg/kg, on the Hemodynamic response to Ketamine, 2.2 mg/kg IV

Treatment	Maximum BP (mm Hg) (mean ± SEM) Baseline	2 min	p-value
Saline (0.9% NaCl)	124.0 ± 9.9	166.7 ± 7.4	< 0.002
Diazepam (0.3 mg/kg)	122.9 ± 8.0	118.0 ± 11.0	< 0.70
p-value	< 0.90	< 0.01	

(From Zsigmond EK, Domino EF: Ketamine: clinical pharmacology, pharmokinetics and current clinical use. Anesthesiology Rev 1980;7:13–33.)

lowing ketamine, 1 mg/kg intravenously (217-219). Thus, midazolam appears to be as effective as diazepam for protection against ketamine-induced cardiostimulatory and CNS stimulant effects. Similarly, no major differences were found between the cardiocirculatory effects of midazolam and thiopental when administered in combination with ketamine (206). The combination of midazolam with fentanyl (or sufentanil) also proved to be safe in cardiac patients (219). In patients undergoing cardiac surgery, midazolam, 0.12 mg/kg intravenously, followed by ketamine, 1.0 mg/kg intravenously, did not produce significant changes in cardiac output, cardiac index, stroke volume, or stroke index; however, systemic vascular resistance and left ventricular stroke work index were reduced by midazolam and were further decreased by the midazolam-ketamine sequence (219). Pretreatment with pancuronium decreased the ketamine-induced hyperdynamic response (220). When pancuronium was given before or simultaneously with ketamine, the increase in mean arterial pressure and heart rate was blocked by pancuronium. Similar observations were made by Kumar and associates (218) in cardiac surgical patients. Raza and associates (219) also reported stable hemodynamic variables and catecholamine levels following a midazolam-ketamine-sufentanil-pancuronium induction sequence when maintenance of anesthesia included incremental doses of sufentanil and an infusion of ketamine.

Induction combinations of benzodiazepines and ketamine were comparable to benzodiazepine combinations with fentanyl or sufentanil (221). Furthermore, Dhadphale and associates (222) reported no significant differences between diazepam-ketamine-N_2O and morphine-N_2O techniques. However, when ketamine was utilized for cardiac anesthesia without diazepam pretreatment, Reves and associates (223) found greater cardiovascular stability with diazepam-morphine-N_2O sequence than with ketamine-N_2O anesthesia. Improved hemodynamic stability can be achieved if anesthesia is maintained with a diazepam-ketamine-N_2O sequence, as reported by Kumar and associates (217, 218), Dadphale and colleagues (222), and Raza and associates (219).

For cardiac transplantation, the diazepam-ketamine combination appears to offer the best hemodynamic stability in patients with cardiomyopathies (224). Newsome and associates (225) also found that moderate doses of fentanyl (15 to 30 μg/kg) made ketamine a highly acceptable cardiac anesthetic.

NEUROLEPT "BALANCED" ANESTHESIA

Anesthesia has four primary components (namely, analgesia, amnesia, ataraxia, and atonia), which can be represented by a tetrahydron, as shown in Figure 19-4. When all the essential components are provided, a "balanced" state of CNS activity and autonomic stability is analogous to the stability in the center of a stereogeometric crystal configuration. Ideally, somatic and autonomic stability is achieved using a combination of drugs, which provide all the necessary components of anesthesia.

To assess autonomic stability during intravenous anesthesia, Wynands (226) proposed the concept of MIC-BAR, similar to MAC-BAR for inhalation anesthetics. MIC-BAR was defined as the minimal concentration of an opioid analgesic that prevented acute hypertensive responses to noxious stimuli in 50% of a study population, reflecting the potency of an analgesic in protecting against autonomic hyperactivity (227-229). Unfortunately, attempts to determine the MIC-BAR concentrations for the commonly used opioid analgesics have failed because of the intrinsic pharmacokinetic and dynamic variability in the responses of individual patients. Even arterial plasma fentanyl levels exceeding 30 ng/ml failed to block acute adrenergic responses in some patients. Despite the transient popularity of high-dose fentanyl for cardiac anesthesia, DeCastro (230, 231) realized that it was difficult to achieve autonomic balance with an analgesic alone, and he recommended a combined approach rather

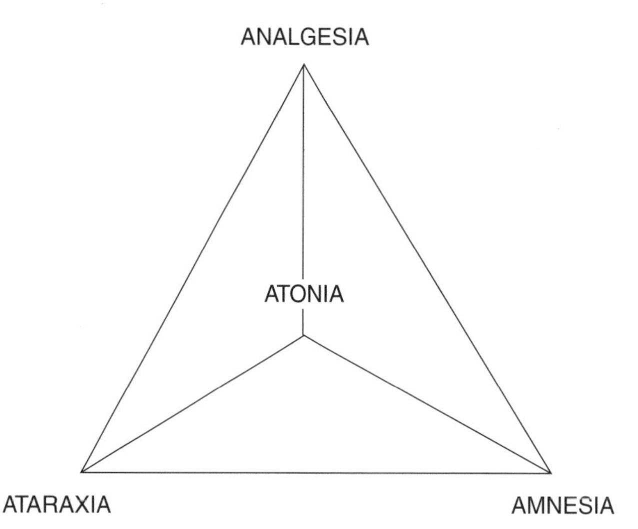

FIGURE 19-4. The essential components of an "ideal balanced" neurolept anesthetic are illustrated with a tetrahedron, the symbol of the Society of Intravenous Anesthesia (SIVA).

than "l'anesthésie analgésique pure" (i.e., the sole use of large doses of potent opioids).

When ether and N_2O were introduced 150 years ago, anesthesiologists were able to provide freedom from pain and fear during surgery. Indeed, a single agent, ether, provided analgesia and amnesia at "light" levels of anesthesia and atonia and ataraxia at "deeper" planes. Unfortunately, using ether to achieve deeper surgical levels of anesthesia was associated with increased morbidity and mortality. Because N_2O was even less potent than ether, it required supplementation with an opiate to achieve adequate intraoperative analgesia. Following the introduction of barbiturates, the concept of "balanced" anesthesia with thiopental-N_2O-meperidine began to increase in popularity.

Clinical Applications

Ophthalmologic Surgery

Droperidol employed in NLA reduces intraocular pressure and decreases the incidence of PONV, which itself may pose a serious risk after cataract operation (232-234). This technique also facilitates the conduct of peri- and retrobulbar block procedures (233, 234).

Otorhinologic Surgery

NLA reduces the chances of nausea and vomiting following operations on the middle ear (235-237). For stapedectomy operations, NLA allows the use of vasoconstrictor drugs (236). When the patient is seated or is in the semirecumbent position, there is little likelihood of hypotension with NLA, and it can be easily converted into NLAN (235, 237). For tonsillectomy and adenoidectomy procedures in children, NLA techniques allows retention of airway reflexes, and the endotracheal tube is well-tolerated at the end of the procedure. For short, painful procedures and in patients at risk of postoperative respiratory depression (e.g., COPD, elderly), droperidol in combination with a remifentanil infusion may be the safest regimen.

Oral Surgery

Local anesthesia or peripheral nerve blocks can be performed and supplemented with NLA (238). Major reconstructive oral surgical procedures lasting 4 to 6 hours have been performed using modified NLAN techniques (237).

Endoscopic Procedures

Patients remain cooperative and follow commands with NLA techniques (239, 240). For bronchoscopy (or laryngoscopy) procedures, spontaneous ventilation may facilitate the diagnostic process. For upper alimentary endoscopy, the prevention of nausea and vomiting is a major advantage of NLA (241). For short endoscopic procedures, remifentanil may offer advantages over other fentanyl congeners as part of an NLA technique.

Awake Intubation

NLA facilitates patient cooperation during intubation of the trachea, while the patient remains semiconscious and cooperative with spontaneous ventilation. Droperidol is also alleged to reduce the occurrence of nausea and vomiting in patients with a full stomach.

Neurosurgical Radiologic Procedures

NLA may also be used for angiography, pneumoencephalography, ventriculography, and myelography (242-245). Headaches, vomiting, and acute hypertensive responses to intraventricular injections are reduced by NLA (244, 245). Postural hypotension occurs less frequently with Innovar or ketamine than with the inhalation agents. For awake stereotactic neurosurgery, NLA offers advantages over other general anesthetic techniques (244). Diazepam-nalbuphine-N_2O followed by a small dose of droperidol (0.625 to 1.25 mg intravenously) is also a suitable technique for intracranial procedures because the patients awaken promptly with minimal pain or respiratory depression after the procedure, and they are communicative with the surgeons during the postoperative neurologic evaluation (246). When hypothermia is used during neurosurgery, NLAN facilitates cooling and rewarming (247), compared with the inhalational agents.

Cardiac Surgery

NLAN provides cardiac patients with a rapid induction of unconsciousness without cardiovascular instability, unaltered response of the heart to vasoactive drugs, moderate α-adrenergic blockade, good perioperative analgesia, and minimal depression of airway reflexes and central respiratory drive. In comparing droperidol-diazepam-fentanyl-N_2O anesthesia with thiopental-halothane-N_2O anesthesia in cardiac patients, the incidence of hypotension and hypertension was higher in the halothane-treated group than in the NLAN group (248). Corssen and associates (249) made similar observations when comparing Innovar-based NLAN with halothane-based anesthesia. The introduction of diazepam as part of the NLAN technique greatly facilitated the use of this technique because the benzodiazepine decreased the dose of fentanyl required and improved hemodynamic stability by reducing the excess sympathetic activity following tracheal intubation. Catecholamine levels were reduced by diazepam, and norepinephrine overflow was prevented during the stressful phases of induction, intubation, and sternotomy. It is useful to administer diazepam before initiating a fentanyl or sufentanil infusion to ensure that the peak effect of the benzodiazepine has been achieved during the stressful periods. For maintenance of analgesia, an intravenous infusion of fentanyl or sufentanil maintains a more stable hemodynamic state than intermittent bolus injections (250, 250a). No significant differences were noted between fentanyl and sufentanil when these agents were used after diazepam or midazolam. Similarly, no differences were found among pancuronium, vecuronium, and pipecuronium as the primary muscle relaxant during NLA (219, 251, 252). Use of nalbuphine as the analgesic component of an NLA technique has also been reported to maintain good hemodynamic stability during the perioperative period (188). However, Lake and associates (191) could not achieve an adequate depth of anesthesia even with nalbuphine, 3.0 mg/kg intravenously.

Hemorrhagic Shock

Investigators have claimed (253, 254) that NLAN has particular advantages in hypovolemic patients and in the management of hemorrhagic shock because the droperidol component reduces pulmonary vascular resistance, improves tissue perfusion (by α-adrenergic blockade), and reduces left ventricular stroke work index. The droperidol dose should be limited to less than 0.15 mg/kg, and fentanyl (or sufentanil) should be titrated using a variable-rate intravenous infusion until verbal contact with the patient is lost, rather than giving a large bolus dose. Ketamine may provide an additional margin of safety when combined with NLAN for induction and maintenance of anesthesia in unstable patients.

Obstetric Anesthesia

During vaginal delivery, NLA allows the practitioner to maintain verbal contact with the patient and is preferable to NLAN. Peripheral nerve block (i.e., pudendal) can be added, if necessary, to provide analgesia for the episiotomy (255). For cesarean section and complicated obstetric manipulations, the combination of low-dose fentanyl-thiopental-ketamine for induction and a ketamine infusion with a bolus of fentanyl and midazolam after delivery is useful (256, 257).

Urologic Procedures

NLA without loss of consciousness may make the patient comfortable and cooperative during diagnostic and minor therapeutic procedures. For renal transplant patients, NLAN techniques have been used because the minimal cardiovascular depression leads to improved kidney perfusion. For immersion lithotripsy, NLA involving benzodiazepine-propofol and opioid-sedative combinations have been used (258-260). Although a midazolam-ketamine combination can provide excellent cardiorespiratory stability, spontaneous movements prolong the procedure (258).

In summary, modern concepts of "balanced" anesthesia and TIVA arose from the early experience with NLA and NLAN techniques. The introduction of ketamine represented an alternative form of NLA and NLAN, which was characterized as "dissociative" anesthesia and analgesia. To date, ketamine remains the only intravenous drug capable of functioning as a sole intravenous anesthetic without adjuvant drugs. Unfortunately, the high incidence of perioperative side effects has limited the clinical acceptance of neurolept and dissociative anesthetic techniques. Use of lower doses of these novel anesthetic drugs in combination with other intravenous anesthetic, analgesic, and muscle relaxant drugs has led to renewed interest in NLA and NLAN techniques. In the future, the challenge will be to find shorter-acting derivatives of the currently available neuroleptic and dissociative drugs to facilitate a more rapid recovery from NLAN techniques without side effects.

REFERENCES

1. Lundy JS, Tovell RM. Thiopenthal, a new anesthetic agent, North West Med 1935;33:308.
2. Beecher, HK, Todd DP. A study of the death associated with anesthesia and surgery based on a study of 599,548 anesthesias at 10 institutions 1948–1952. Ann Surg 1954;140:2.
3. Selye H. The alarm reaction. In Piersol GM and Bortz EL Eds. The Cyclopedia of Medicine, Surgery and Specialities, Philadelphia, F A Davis, 1940; Vol. 15, pp 15–38.
4. Laborit H, Huguenard P, Alluaume P. A new drug to stabilize the neurovegetative system, 4560 RP. Presse Med 1952; 10:206–207.
5. Huguenard P. A historical view: Neuroleptanalgesia. In: Wilder-Smith OHG, Tassonyi E: Intravenous Anesthesia and Antinociception: A New Philosophy of Anesthetic Control. Editions Medecine et Hygiene, SA, Geneve. 1995. pp 19–21.
6. Huguenard P. Essais de vasoplegie par association de drogues. Anesth Analg Reanim 1952;9:427–430.
7. DeCastro J, Mundeleer R. Anesthesie sans barbituriques: la neurolept analgesie. Anest Analg Reanim; 1959;16:1022–26.
8. Randall LO, Heise GA, Schallek W, Bagdon RE, Banziger R, Boris A, Moe R, Abrams WB. Pharmacological and clinical studies on Valium, a new psychotherapeutic agent of the benzodiazepine class. Curr Ther Res 1961;3:405.
9. McCarthy DA, Chen G, Kaump DH, Ensor C. General anesthetic and other pharmacologic properites of 2-(o-chlorophenyl)-2-methylamino cyclohexanone HC1 (CI 581). J New Drugs 1965;5:21.
10. Domino EF, Chodoff P, Corssen G. Pharmacologic effect of CI-581, a new dissociative anesthetic in man. Clin Pharmacol Ther 1965; 6:279.
11. Zsigmond EK. Theoretical basis for the use of droperidol in neuroleptanalgesia Communications in Anesthesiology 1971;1:12–14.
12. Zsigmond EK. Invited comment on Corssen GC: Ketamine in the anesthetic management of asthmatic patients. Anesth Analg 1972; 51:595–596.
13. Delay J. Psychopharmacology Frontiers 1959. Boston, Little Brown & Co.
14. Janssen P. The pharmacology of haloperidol. International J Neuropsychiatry 1967;3:10.
15. DeCastro J. Twenty-five years of neuroleptanalgesia-concepts, evolution, actual trends. Proc. First Internat Symposium of History of Modern Anesthesia, 1982, Rotterdam.
16. Janssen PAJ, Niemegeers CJE, Schellekens KHL, Verbruggen FJ, Van Heuten JM. The pharmacology of dihydrobenzperidol (R 4749), a new potent and short-acting neuroleptic agent chemically related to haloperidol. Anesth Analg 1959;16:1022.
17. Janssen PAJ, Eddy N. Compounds related to pethidine IV: New general chemical methods of increasing the analgesic activity of pethidine. J Med Chem 1960;2:32.
18. DeJong R. Neurologic complications of drugs with primary action on the nervous system. N Y State J Med 1980;70:1857.
19. Patton CM. Rapid induction of dyskinesia by droperidol. Anesthesiology 1975;43:126.

20. Edmonds-Seal J, Prys-Roberts C. Pharmacology of drugs used in neuroleptanalgesia. Brit J Anaesth 1970;42:207.
21. MacDonald HR. Clinical and circulatory effects of neuroleptanalgesia. Br Heart J 1966;28:654.
22. Janssen PAJ, et al. Vergleichende pharmakologische daten uber sechs neue basiche-4-fluorobutyrophenone-derivative Arzneim Forsch 1961;11:819.
23. Roos BE. Effects of certain tranquilizers on the level of homovanillic acid in the corpus striatum. J Pharm Pharmacol 1965;17:280.
24. Patton CM, Moon MR, Dannemiller FJ. The prophylactic antiemetic effect of droperidol. Anesth Analg 1974;53:361.
25. Janssen PAJ. Droperidol; Pharmacologic aspects. In: Bente D and Bradley P: Neuropsychopharmacology 1965 Amsterdam, Elsevier.
26. Soudijn W, Van Wijngaarden I, Allewijn F. Distribution and excretion of tritiated haloperidol in man. Int J Neuropsychiatry 1967; 3(Suppl 1):24.
27. Goldstein BJ. Haloperidol in controlling symptoms of acute psychoses. Curr Psychiatr Ther 1966;8:232.
28. Morrison JD, Loan WB, Dundee JW. Controlled comparison of the efficacy of fourteen preparations in the relief of postoperative pain. Brit Med J 1971;3:287.
29. Morrison JD. Alterations in response to somatic pain associated with anaesthesia XIX Studies with the drugs used in neuroleptanaesthesia. Brit J Anaesth 1970;43:838.
30. Schaper WKA, Jagenequ AHM, Bogaard JM. Haemodynamic and respiratory responses to dihydrobenzperidol (R4749), a potent neuroleptic compound in intact anaesthetized dogs. Arzneimittelforschung 1963;13:316.
31. Stanley TH. Cardiovascular effects of droperidol during enflurane and enflurane-nitrous oxide anaesthesia in man. Canad Anaesth Soc J 1978;25:26.
32. Au ASW, Evans D, Graco R, Jones WM. Blood pressure effects of lower abdominal aorta surgery with particular to the use of morphine and droperidol in modifying the responses. Canad Anaesth Soc J 1977:24:293.
33. Kreuscher H. The action of dihydrobenzperidol on the cardiovascular system in man. Acta Anaesth Scand 1965;9:155.
34. Yelonsky J, Katz R, Dietrich E. A study of some of the pharmacologic actions of droperidol. Toxicol Appl Pharmacol 1964;6:37.
35. Long G, Dripps RD, Price HL. Measurements of anti-arrhythmic potency of drugs in man: effects of dihydrobenzperidol. Anesthesiology 1967;28:318.
36. Bertolo L, Novakovic L, Penna M. Antiarrythmic effects of droperidol. Anesthesiology 1972;37:529.
37. Zauder HL, Delguercio LRM, Feins N, Barton N, Wollman S. Hemodynamics during neuroleptanalgesia. Anesthesiology 1965; 26:266.
38. Prys-Roberts C, Kelman GR. The influence of drugs used in neuroleptanalgesia on cardiovascular and ventilatory function. Brit J Anaesth 1967;39:134.
39. Corssen G, DeKornfeld TJ. Comparison of the respiratory depressant effects of phentanyl, phentanyl and droperidol, and morphine. Anesthesiology 1966;27:213.
40. Sato T, Hirota K, Matsuki A, Zsigmond EK, Rabito SF. Droperidol inhibits tracheal contractions induced by serotonin, histamine or carbachol in guinea pigs. Can J Anaesth 1996;43:1–7.
41. Tornetta FJ, Boger WP. Liver function studies in droperidol-fentanyl anesthesia. Anesth Analg 1964;43:544.
42. Cressman WA, Plostnieks J, Johnson PC. Absorption, metabolism and excretion of droperidol by human subjects following intramuscular and intravenous administration. Anesthesiology 1973;38:363.
43. Corssen G, Domino EF, Sweet RB. Neuroleptanalgesia and anesthesia: Pharmacological and anesthetic considerations. Anesth Analg 1964;43:748.
44. Murphy MR, Olson WA, Hug CC. Pharmacokinetics of 3-H-fentanyl in the dog anesthetized with enflurane. Anesthesiology 1979;50:13.
45. Murphy MR, Hug CC. The anesthetic potency of fentanyl in terms of its reduction of enflurane MAC. Anesthesiology 1982;57:485.
46. Friis-Hansen B. Body composition during growth. In vivo measurements and biochemical data correlated to differential anatomical growth. Pediatrics 1971;47:264.
47. Johnson KL et al. Fentanyl pharmacokinetics in the pediatric population. Anesthesiology 1984;61:A441.
48. Hess R, Stibler G, Herz A. Pharmacokinetics of fentanyl in man. J Clin Pharmacol Ther 1972;4:137.
49. McClain DA, Hug CC. Intravenous fentanyl kinetics. Clin Pharmacol Ther 1980;28:106.
50. Schleimer R et al. Pharmacokinetics of fentanyl as determined by radioimmuneassay. Clin Pharamcol Ther 1970;23:188.
51. Nishina K, Mikawa K, Maekawa N, Obara H. Fentanyl attenuates cardiovascular reponses to tracheal intubation. Acta Anaesth Scand 1995;39:85–89.
52. Stoeckel H, Hengstamm JH, Schuttler J. Pharmacokinetics of fentanyl as an explanation for recurrence of respiratory depression. Br J Anaesth 1979;51:741.
53. Murphy MR. Clinical pharmacology of fentanyl and alfentanil. Anesthesiol Rev 1984;11:17.
54. Gupta S, Southam MA, Hwang SS. Evaluation of diurnal variation in fentanyl clearance. J Clin Pharmacol 1995;35:159–162.
55. Dundee JW, Brown SS, Hamilton RC, McDowell SA. Analgesic supplementation of light general anesthesia using sequential analysis. Arzneimittelforschung 1969;24:52–61.
56. Matsuki A, Zsigmond EK. Objective evaluation of hydroxyzine as preanesthetic medication. Agressologie 1973;14:67–78.
57. Zsigmond EK, Flynn K, Shively JG. Effect of hydroxyzine and meperidine on arterial blood gases in healthy human volunteers. J Clin Pharmacol 1988;29:85–90.
58. Zsigmond EK, Patterson RL. Double blind evaluation of hydroxyzine hydrochloride in obstetrical anesthesia. Anesth Analg 1967; 46:275–280.
59. Zsigmond EK, Flynn K, Shively JG. Effect of hydroxyzine and meperidine on arterial blood gases in patients with chronic obstructive pulmonary disease. Intl J Clin Pharmacol Therap Toxicol 1993; 31:124–129.
60. Steen SN, Crane R, Thomas SJ. Effect of intramuscular hydroxyzine on specific airway conductance of patients with chronic bronchospastic disease (asthma). In: Abstract of scientific papers. Am Soc Anesthesiologists, Annual Meeting, Atlanta, GA, 16–20 Oct 1971. pp 85–86.
61. Zsigmond EK, Flynn K, Martinez OA. Diazepam and meperidine on arterial blood gases in healthy volunteers. J Clin Pharmacol 1974; 14:377–381.
62. Zsigmond EK, Shively JG, Flynn K. Diazepam and meperidine on arterial blood gases in patients with chronic obstructive lung disease. J Clin Pharmacol 1975;15:464–469.
63. Raza SMA, Masters RW, Zsigmond EK. Comparison of the hemodynamic effects of midazolam and diazepam in patients with coronary occlusion. Intl J Clin Pharmacol Ther Toxic 1989;27:1–6.
64. Schulte-Sasse U, Hess W, Tarnow J. Haemodinamische Analyse 6 verschiedener Anaesthesie-Einleitungverfahren bei koronarchirurgischen Patienten Anesth Intensivther Notfallmed 1982;17:195.
65. Gob E, Barankay A, Spath P, Richter JA. Induction and maintenance of anesthesia with midazolam-fentanyl-ketamine in patients with coronary artery disease—study on haemodynamics and myocardial oxygen demand. Proc. 6th European Congr Anaesth, 1982; Anaesthesia, Sep. pg. 289.
66. Stanley TH, Webster LR. Anesthetic requirements and cardiovascular effects of fentanyl-oxygen and fentanyl-diazepam-oxygen anesthesia in man. Anesth Analg 1978;57:411.
67. Stanley TH, Philbin DM, Coggins CH. Fentanyl-oxygen anesthesia for coronary artery surgery; cardiovascular and hormonal responses. Canad Anaesth Soc J 1979;26:168–172.
68. Bailey PL, Wilbrink J, Zwanikken P, Pace NL, Stanley TH. Anesthetic induction with fentanyl. Anesth Analg 1985;64:48.
68. Hilgenberg JC. Intraoperative awareness during high dose fentanyl oxygen anesthesia. Anesthesiology, 1981;54:341–343.
70. Mummaneni N, Rao TLK, Montoya A. Awareness and recall with high dose fentanyl-oxygen anesthesia. Anesth Analg 1980;5:948–949.
71. Kono K, Philbin DM, Coggins CH, Moss J, Rosow CE, Schneider RC, Slater EE. Renal function and stress response during halothane or fentanyl anesthesia. Anesth Analg 1981;60:552–556.
72. Lunn JK, Stanely TH, Eisele J, Webster L, Woodward A. High-dose

fentanyl anesthesia for coronary artery surgery: plasma fentanyl concentrations and influence of nitrous oxide on cardiovascular responses. Anesth Analg, 1979;56:390–395.
73. Quintin L, Whalley DG, Wynands JE, Morin JE, Mayer R. Oxygen high-dose fentanyl-droperidol anesthesia for aortocoronary bypass surgery. Anesth Analg, 1981;60:412–416.
74. Sprigge JS, Wynands JE, Whalley DG, Bevan DR, Townsend GE, Nathan H, Patel YC, Srikant CB. Fentanyl infusion anesthesia for aortocoronary bypass surgery: plasma levels and hemodynamic response. Anesth Analg, 1982;61:972–978.
75. Lowenstein E. Morphine "anesthesia", a perspective Editorial. Anesthesiology 1971;35:563–565.
76. Sebel PS, Bovill JG, Wauquier A, Rog P. Effects of high dose fentanyl anesthesia on the electroencephalogram. Anesthesiology. 1981; 55:203–211.
77. Waller JL, Hug C, Nagle DN, Craver JM. Hemodynamic changes during fentanyl-oxygen anesthesia for aortocoronary bypass operation. Anesthesiology 1981;55:212–217.
78. Hall GM, Young C, Holdcroft A, Alaghband-Zadeh J. Substrate mobilization during surgery; a comparison between halothane and fentanyl anesthesia. Anaesthesia, 1978;33:924.
79. Janssen P. Zur Chemie morphinartiger Korper Anaesthetist 1962; 11:1–7.
80. Becker LD et al. Biphasic respiratory depression of fentanyl-droperidol or fentanyl alone used to supplement nitrous oxide anesthesia. Anesthesiology 1976;44:291–296.
81. Kallos T, Wyche MQ, Garman JK. The effects of Innovar on functional residual capacity and total chest wall compliance in man. Anesthesiology 1973;39:558.
82. Scheinin B, Lindgren L, Scheinin TM. Preoperative nitrous oxide delays bowel function after colonic surgery. Brit J Anaesth 1990; 64:154–158.
83. Giuffre M, Gross JB. The effects of nitrous oxide on postoperative bowel motility. Anesthesiology, 1986;65:699–700.
84. Blackstock D, Gettes MA. Negative pressure in the middle ear in children after nitrous oxide anesthesia. Canad Anaesth Soc J, 1986; 33:32–35.
85. Montgomery CJ, Vaghadia H, Blackstock D. Negative middle ear pressure and postoperative vomiting in pediatric outpatients. Anesthesiology, 1988;68:288–291.
86. Murakawa M, Adachi T, Nakao S, Seo N, Shingu K, Mori K. Activation of the cortical and medullary dopaminergic systems by nitrous oxide in rats: a possible neurochemical basis for psychotropic effects and postanesthetic nausea and vomiting. Anesth Analg 1994; 78:376–381.
87. Tramer M, Moore A, McQuay H. Omitting nitrous oxide in general anesthesia: meta-analysis of intraoperative awareness and postoperative emesis in randomized controlled trials. Brit J Anaesth 1996; 76:186–193.
88. Crile GW. Psychogenic association in relation to certain medical problems. Boston Med J 1910;163:893–984.
89. Bridenbough LD, Moore DC, Bridenbough PO. Clinical experiences with Innovar as post-nerve block sedation: report of 100 patients. Bull Mason Clin 1969;23:86.
90. Kennedy WF. Innovar as a supplement to regional anesthesia. Anesthesiology 1969;31:574.
91. McNabb TG, Goldwyn RM. Blood gas and hemodynamic effects of sedatives and analgesics when used to supplement to regional anesthesia in plastic surgery. Plast Reconstr Surg 1976;58:37.
92. Schara J. Zur Kombination von Neuroleptanalgesia und Lokalanesthesie. In: Gemperle M: Fortschritte der Neuroleptanalgesie 1966; Berlin, Springer Verlag.
93. DeCastro J, Mundeleer P. La neuroleptanalgesia; Auswahl der Preparate; Bedeutung der Analgesie und der Nuerolepsie Anaesthesist 1982;11:1–10.
94. Clark NJ, Meuleman T, Liu WS, Zwanikken P, Pace NL, Stanley TH. Comparison of sufentanil-N_2O and fentanyl-N_2O in patients without cardiac disease undergoing general surgery. Anesthesiology 1987;66:130.
95. Flacke JW, et al. Intraoperative effectiveness of sufentanil, fentanyl, meperidine or morphine in balanced anesthesia: a double blind study. Anesth Analg 1983;62:259.
96. Smith NT, Dec-Silver, Harrison WK, Sanford TJ, Gillig J. A comparion among morphine, fentanyl and sufentanil anesthesia for open heart surgery. Induction, emergence and extubation. Anesthesiology 1982;57:A291.
97. Rosow CE, et al. Sufentanil vs fentanyl. Supression of hemodynamic response. Anesthesiology 1983;59:A323.
98. Sebel PS, Bovill JG. Cardiovascular effects of sufentanil anesthesia: A study in patients undergoing cardiac surgery. Anesth Analg 1982; 61:115.
98a. Parratt JR. Opioid receptors in the cardiovascular system. In: van Zwielen P, Schonebaum E, eds. Progress in pharamcology. Stuttgart: Gustav Fischer Verlag, 1978.
99. Ebert TJ, Kotrly KJ, Madsen KE, Bernstein JS, et al. Fentanyl-diazepam anesthesia with or without N_2O does not attenuate cardiopulmonary baroreflex-mediated vasoconstrictor responses to controlled hypovolemia in humans. Anesth Analg 1988;67:548–554.
100. Starr NJ, Sethna DH, Estefanous FG. Bradycardia and asystole following rapid administration of sufentanil with vecuronium. Anesthesiology 1986;64:521.
101. Inoue K, El-Banayosy A, Stolarki L, et al. Vecuronium induced bradycardia following induction of anesthesia with etomidate or thiopentone with or without fentanyl. Brit J Anaesth 1988;60:10.
102. Cayton D. Asystole associated with vecuronium. Brit J Anaesth 1986;58:937.
103. Fahmy NH. Sufentanil as an analgesic supplement in general surgical anesthesia. In: Estefanous FG, Ed: Opioids in Anesthesia. Proc Symp. held at the Cleveland Clinic Foundation, May 1983.
104. Clark N, Liu WS, Meuleman T, Zwanniken P, Pace NL, Stanley TH. Sufentanil versus fentanyl as a supplement to N_2O anesthesia during general surgery. Anesth Analg 1984;63:175.
105. Clark N, Meuleman T, Liu WS, Zwanniken P, Pace NL, Stanley TH. Comparison of sufentanil-N_2O and fentanyl-N_2O in patients without cardiac disease undergoing general surgery. Anesthesiology 1987;66:130.
105a. Bailey PL, Steisand JB, Pace NL, et al. Sufentanil produces shorter lasting respiratory depression and longer lasting analgesia than equipotent doses of fentanyl in human volunteers. Anesthesiology 1986;65:3.
106. Kay B, Nolan D, Mayall R, Healy TEJ. The effect of sufentanil on the cardiovascular responses to tracheal intubation. Anaesthesia 1987;42:382.
107. Licina MG, Newsome LR, Reeder DA, Hug CC, Moldenhauer CC. Sufentanil and succinylcholine for rapid sequence induction and tracheal intubation: hemodynamic and hormonal responses. J Cardiovascular Anesth 1990;4:318–322.
108. Keitzmann D, Larsen R, Rathgeber J, Bolte M, Kettler D. Comparison of sufentanil-nitrous oxide anesthesia with fentanyl-nitrous oxide anesthesia in geriatric patients undergoing major abdominal surgery. Brit J Anaesth 1991;67:269–276.
109. Thomson JR, Hudson RJ, Rosenbloom M, Meatherall RC. A randomized double-blind comparison of fentanyl and sufentanil anesthesia for coronary artery surgery. Can J Anaesth 1987;34:227–232.
110. Ghoneim MM, Dhanaraj, Choi WW. Comparison of four opioid analgesics as supplements to nitrous oxide anesthesia. Anesth Analg 1984:63:405.
111. Komatsu T, Shibutani K, Okamoto K, Kumar V, Kubal K, Sanchala V. Comparison of sufentanil-diazepam with fentanyl-diazepam anesthesia for induction. Anesth Analg 1986;65:82.
112. Kleiman J, Marlar K, Silva DA, Miller R, Kaplan JA. Sufentanil attenuation of stress response during raid sequence induction. Anesthesiology 1985;63:3.
113. Kuperwasser B, Dahl M, McSweeney TD, Howie MB. Comparison of alfentanil and sufentanil in ambulatory surgery procedures when used in balanced anesthesia technique. Anesth Analg 1988;67:1.
114. Fahmy NH. Sufentanil: A review in: Estefanous FG, Ed. Opioids in Anesthesia 1984; Butterworth Publ, Boston, London, Sydney, Wellington, Durban, Toronto.
114a. Flacke JW, Bloor BC, Kripke BJ, et al. Comparison of morphine, meperidine, fentanyl and sufentanil in balanced anesthesia: a double-blind study. Anesth Analg 1985;64:897.
115. de Lange S, Stanley TH, Boscoe MJ, Pace NL. Comparison of sufen-

tanil-O_2 and fentanyl-O_2 for coronary surgery. Anesthesiology 1982; 56:112–118.
116. Kay B, Pleuvry B. Human volunteers studies of alfentanil (R 39209), a new short acting narcotic analgesic. Anaesthesia 1980;35:952–956.
117. Bower S, Hull CJ. Comparative pharmacokinetics of fentanyl and alfentanil. Br J Anaesth 1982;54:871–877.
118. De Castro J. Analgesic anesthesia with alfentanil; a new short-acting of morphinomimetic. First clinical trials. In: New compounds in and new supplements for anesthesia. In: Stanley TH, and Petty, eds. Anesthesiology Today and Tommorow 1985; Martinus Nijhoff Publ Boston, Dordrecht/Lancaster.
119. de Lange S, deBriujin N, Stanley TH, Boscoe MJ. Alfentanil-oxygen anesthesia; comparison of continuous infusion and frequent bolus techniques for coronary artery surgery. Anesthesiology 1981; 55:A42.
120. Smith I, Jan Hemelrijck J, White PF. Effect of esmolol versus alfentanil as a supplement to propofol-nitrous oxide anesthesia. Anesth Analg 1991;73:540–546.
121. Bentley JB, Finley JH, Humphrey LR, et al. Obesity and alfentanil pharmacokinetics. Anesth Analg 1983;62:251.
122. Shafer A, Sun ML, White PF. Pharmacokinetics and pharmacodynamics of alfentanil infusions during general anesthesia. Anesth Analg 1986;65:1021.
123. Lemmens HJM, Bovill JG, Hennis PJ, Burm AGL. Influence of age on the pharmacokinetics of alfentanil. Anesthesiology 1988;69:A629.
123a. Goresky GV, Koren G, Sabourin MA, et al. The pharmacokinetics of alfentanil in children. Anesthesiology 1987;67:654.
124. Brown EM, Kunjappan VE, Alexander CD. Fentanyl/alfentanil for pelvic laparoscopy. Can Anaesth Soc J 1984;31:251–254.
125. Rosow CE, Latta WB, Keegan CR, Nozik DL, Murphy AL, Kimball WR, Philbin DM. Alfentanil and fentanyl in short surgical procedures. Anesthesiology 1983;59:A345.
126. White PF, Coe V, Shafer A, Sung M-L. Comparison of alfentanil and fentanil for outpatient anesthesia. Anesthesiology 1986;64:99–106.
127. van Leeuwen L, Zuurmond WWA, Helmers JHJH. Alfentanil-dauerinfusion fur chirurgische Eingriffe mittlerer und langerer Dauer, Anesthetist 1984;33:173–176.
128. Ausems ME, Stanski DR, Hug CC. An evaluation of the accuracy of pharmacokinetic data for the computer assisted infusion of alfentanil. Br J Anaesth 1985;57:1217.
129. Ausems, ME, Vuyk J, Hug CC, Stanski DR. Comparison of a computer-assisted infusion versus intermittent bolus administration of alfentanil as a supplement to nitrous oxide for lower abdominal surgery. Anesthesiology 1988;68:851.
130. Lemmens HJM, Bovill JG, Hennis PJ, Burm AGL. Age has no effect on the pharmacodynamics of alfentanil. Anesth Analg 1988;67:956–960.
131. Yate PM, Short SM, Sebel PS, Morton J. Comparisons of infusions of alfentanil or pethidine of ventilated patients in the ITU. Br J Anaesth 1986;58:1091–1099.
132. Welling EC, Donegan J. Neuroleptanalgesia using alfentanil for awake craniotomy. Anesth Analg 1989;68:57–60.
133. Andrews CHJ, Robertson JA, Chapman JM. Postoperative analgesia with intravenous infusions of alfentanil. Lancet 1985;2:671.
134. Glass PS, Hardman HD, Kamiyama Y, Donn KH, Hermann DJ. Pharmacodynamic comparison of GI87084B, a novel ultrashort acting opioid and alfentanil. Anesth Analg 1992;74:S113.
135. Glass PS, Kapila A, Muir KT, Hermann DJ, Shiraishi M. A model to determine the relative potency of mu opioids: alfentanil versus remifentanil. Anesthesiology 1993;79:A378.
136. Joshi P, Jhaveri R, Bauman V, McNeal S, Batenhorst RL, Glass PS. Comparative trial of remifentanil and alfetanil for anesthesia induction. Anesthesiology 1993;79:A379.
137. Avramov M, Smith I, White PF. Use of midazolam and remifentanil during monitored anesthesia care (MAC). Anesth Analg 1995; 80:S24.
138. Monk TG, Rater JM, White PF. Comparison of alfentanil and ketamine infusion in combination with midazolam for outpatient lithotripsy. Anesthesiology 74:1991;1023–1028.
139. Dershwitz M, Randel G, Rosow CE, Fragen R, Di Biase PM, Librojo ES, Jamerson B, Shaw DL, Batenhorst R. Dose-response relationship of GI87084B, a new ultra-short acting opioid. Anesthesiology 1992; 77:A396.
140. Monk TG, Batenhorst RL, Folger WH, Kirkham AJT, Lemon DJ, Martin KJ, Venker DC. A comparison of remifentanil and alfentanil during nitrous-narcotic anesthesia. Anesth Analg 1994;78:S293.
141. Avramov M, Smith I, White PF. Use of midazolam and remifentanil during monitored anesthesia care (MAC). Anesth Analg 1995:80–S24.
142. Reese PR, White PF, Lee JT, Avramov MN, Rhoney DH, Roland CL, Jamerson BD, Batenhorst RL. Remifentanil vs midazolam-remifentanil for monitored anesthesia care: Anesthesiologists assessment and patient satisfaction. Anesth Analg 1996;82:S374.
143. Hogue C, Camporesi E, Duncalf D, Miguel R, Pitts M, Streisand J, Batenhorst, Jamerson B, McNeal S. Total intravenous anesthesia with remifentanil and propofol in patients undergoing elective inpatient surgery. Anesthesiology 1995;83:A386.
144. Desmonts JM, Aitkenhead AR, Camu F, Duvaldestin P, Hanson A, Martisson S, Marty J, Raeder J, Reite K, Wattwil M, Wostyn L, Ertzbischoff O. Comparison of remifentanil and propofol as adjunct therapy during regional anesthesia. Anesthesiology 1995; 83:A857.
145. Peacock J, Reilly C, Luntley J, O'Connor B, Ogg T, Watson B, Shaikh S. Remifentanil in combination with propofol for spontaneous ventilation anesthesia. Anesthesiology 1995;83:A35.
146. Pitts MC, Palmore MM, Salmenpara MT, Kirkhart BA, Hug CC. Pilot study on hemodynamic effects of intravenous GI87084B in patients. Anesthesiology 1992;77:A101.
147. Fragen RJ, Randel GI, Librojo ES, Clarke MY, Jamerson BD. The interaction of remifentanil and propofol to prevent response to tracheal intubation and the start of surgery for outpatient knee. Anesthesiology 1994;81:A376.
148. Dershwitz M, Rosow CE, Michalowski P, Connors PM, Hoke JF, Muir KT, Dienstag JL. Pharmacokinetics an pharmacodynamics of remifentanil in volunteer subjects with severe liver disease compared with normal subjects. Anesthesiology 1994;81:A377.
149. Schlugman D, Dufore S, Dershwitz M, Michalowski, P, Hoke J, Muir KT, Rosow C, Glass PSA. Respiratory effects remifentanil in subjects with severe liver impairment compared to matched controls. Anesthesiology 1994;81:A1417.
150. Camu F, Breivik H, Hagelberg A, Rosen M, Sneyd R, Viby-Mogensen J, Noronha D, Shaikh S. A double-blind, placebo-controlled study on the safety and efficacy of remifentanil used as an adjunct sedative in patients receiving regional anesthesia. Anesthesiology 1995;83:A847.
151. Glass PSA. Pharmacokinetic and pharmacokinetic principles in providing "fast-track" recovery. J Cardiothorac Vascular Anesth 1995; 9/5 Suppl 1:16–20.
152. Bacon R, Chandrasekan V, Haigh A, Royston BD, Sundt T. Early extubation after open heart surgery with total intravenous anesthetic technique. Lancet 1995;345:133–134.
153. Sebel PS, Hoke JF, Westmoreland C, Hug CC, Muir KT, Szlam F. Histamine concentrations and hemodynamic responses to remifentanil. Anesth Analg 1995;80:990–993.
154. Davis PJ, Ross A, Stiller RL, et al. Pharmacokinetics of remifentanil in anesthetized children 2–12 years of age. Anesth Analg, 1995; 80:S93.
155. Zsigmond EK, Kovacs V, Fekete G. A new route, jet-injection for anesthetic induction in children. I. Midazolam dose-range finding studies. Internat J Clin Pharmacol Therap 1995;33:580–584.
156. Zsigmond EK, Kovacs, Fekete G. A new route, jet-injection for anesthetic induction in children. II. Ketamine dose-range finding studies. J Clin Pharmacol Therap 1996;34:84–88.
157. Howie MB, Michelsen LG, Porembka DT, Jopling MW, Kirkhart BA, Hug CC. Anesthesia induction with remifentanil for patients undergoing CABG. Anesth Analg 1996;82:S190.
158. Howie MB, Kelly WB, Porembka DT, Warren SA, Cain SR, Kirkhart BA. Catecholamine response during CABG with remifentanil anesthesia. Anesth Analg 1996;82:S189.
159. Yarmush J, D'Angelo R, O'Leary C, Pitts M, Graf G, Sebel P, Watkins WD, Miguel R, Streisand J, Maysick L, Vujic D, Kirkhart B. Remifentanil vs morphine for acute postoperative analgesia. Anesth Analg 1966;82:S504.
160. Sung YF, Stulting RD, Beatie CD, et al. Intraocular pressure (IOP) effects of remifentanil (R) (GI87074B) and alfentanil (A). Anesthesiology 1994;81:A35.

161. Bailey P, Stanley TH. Intravenous Opioid Anesthesia: In Miller R: Anaesthesia 1994; pp 291–387.
162. Keeri-Szanto M, Pomeroy JR. Atmospheric pollution and pentazocine metabolism. Lancet 1971;1:947.
163. Aldrete JA, Tan ST, Carrow DJ, Watts MK. "Pentazepam" (pentazocine-diazepam) supplementing local analgesia for laparoscopic sterilization. Anesth Analg 1976;55:177.
164. Schoenfeld A, Goldman JA, Levy E. Pentazocine and diazepam analgesia for minor gynaecological operations. Br J Anaesth 1974; 46:385.
165. Jourde J, Peri G, Menes H, et al. The value of associating diazepam and pentazocine in an anesthetic combination in maxillo-facial surgery. Ann Anesthesiol Fr 1972;13:173.
166. De Castro J. Les analgesiques centraux et l'anesthesie analgesique 1978; Elsevier B Press, S A Bruxelles, Belgium p 97.
167. Murphy Mr, Hug CC. The enflurane sparing effect of morphine, butorphanol and nalbuphine. Anesthesiology 1982;57:489–492.
168. Del Pizzo A. Butorphanol, a new intravenous analgesic: Double-blind comparison with morphine sulfate in postoperative patients with moderate or severe pain. Curr Ther Res 1976;20:221.
169. Zeedick JF. Efficacy and safety evaluation of butorphanol in postoperative pain. Curr Ther Res 1977;22:707.
170. Gal TJ, DiFazio CA, Mosicki J. Analgesic and respiratory depressant activity of nalbuphine: a comparison with morphine. Anesthesiology 1982;57:367.
171. Nagashima H, Karamanian A, Malovany R, Radnay P, Ang M, Koerner S, Foldes FF. Respiratory and circulatory effects of intravenous butorphanol and morphine. Clin Pharmacol Ther 1976; 19:738.
172. Schurig JE, Cavanaugh RL, Buyniski JP. The effects of butorphanol and morphine on pulmonary mechanics, arterial blood pressure and venous plasma histamine levels in anesthetized dogs. Fed Proc 1976;35:546.
173. Roebel LE, Cavanagh RL, Buyinski JP. Comparative gastrointestinal and biliary tract effects of morphine and butorphanol. J Med 1979; 10:225.
174. Vieira ZEG, Zsigmond EK, Duarte B, Renigers SA, Hirota K. Double-blind evaluation of nalbuphine and butorphanol on the common bile-duct by ultrasonography in man. Intl J Clin Pharmacol Therap Toxicol 1993;31:564–567.
175. Stanley TH, Reddy P, Gilmore S, Bennett G. The cardiovascular effects of high dose butorphanol-nitrous oxide anesthesia before and during operation. Can Anaesth Soc J 1983;30:337–341.
176. Rosow CE, Keegan CR. Butorphanol vs. morphine: Dose-related suppression of the response to intubation (abstract). Anesth Analg 1984;63:270.
177. Popio KA, Jackson DH, Ross AM, et al. Hemodynamic and respiratory effects of morphine and butorphanol. Clin Pharamacol Ther 1978;23:281.
178. Kallos T, Caruso FS. Respiratory effects of butorphanol and pethidine. Anaesthesia 1979;34:633–637.
179. Dobkin AB, Arandia HY, Byles PH, et al. Butorphanol tartarate 2. Safety and efficacy in balanced anesthesia. Can Anaesth Soc J 1976; 23:601.
180. Del Pizzo A. A double-blind study of the effect of butorphanol compared with morphine in balanced anaesthesia. Can Anaesth Soc J 1978;25:392.
181. Stehling LC, Zauder HL. Double-blind comparison of butorphanol tartarate and meperidine hydrochloride in balanced anesthesia. J Int Med Res 1978;6:384.
182. Beaver WT, Feise GA. A comparison of the analgesic effect of intramuscular nalbuphine and morphine in patients with postoperative pain. J Clin Pharmacol Exper Ther 1978;204:487.
183. Bikhazi GB. Comparison of morphine and nalbuphine in postoperative pediatric patients. Anesthesiology Rev 1978;5:34.
184. Bluhm R, Zsigmond EK, Winnie AP. Potentiation of opioid analgesia by H1 and H2 antagonists. Life Sci 1982;31:1229–1232.
185. Di Fazio CA, Moscicki JC, Magruder MR. Anesthetic potency of nalbuphine and interaction with morphine in rats. Anesth Analg 1981;60:629.
186. Romagnoli A, Keats AS. Ceiling effect for respiratory depressant activity of nalbuphine. Clin Pharmacol Ther 1980;27:478.
187. Magruder MR, Delaney RD, DiFazio CA. Reversal of narcotic-induced respiratory depression by nalbuphine hydrochloride. Anesthesiol Rev 1982;9:34.
188. Zsigmond EK, Winnie AP, Raza SMA, Wang XY, Barabas E. Nalbuphine as an analgesic component of balanced anesthesia for cardiac surgery. Anesth Analg 1987;66:1155–1164.
189. Doenicke A, Moss J, Lorenz W, Hoernecke R. Intravenous morphine and nalbuphine increase histamine and catecholamine release wihtout accompanying hemodynamic changes. Clin Pharmacol Ther 1995;58:81–89.
190. Lee G, Low RI, Amsterdam EA, DeMaria AN, Huber PW, Mason DT. Hemodynamic effects of morphine and nalbuphine in acute myocardial infarction. Clin Pharmacol Ther 1981;29:576–578.
191. Lake CL, Duckworth EN, DiFazio CA, Durbin CG, Magruder MR. Cardiovascular effects of nalbuphine in patients with coronary or valvular disease. Anesthesiology 1982;57:498.
192. Fahmy NR. Nalbuphine in "balanced" anesthesia; its analgesic efficacy and hemodynamic effects. Anesthesiology 1980;53:S66.
193. Heel RC, Brigden RN, Speight TM, et al. Buprenorphine: A review of its pharmacologic properties and therapeutic efficacy. Drugs 1979;17:81.
194. Cook PJ, James IM, Hobbs KEF, et al. Controlled comparison of im morphine and buprenorphine for analgesia after abdominal surgery. Brit J Anaesth 1982;54:285.
195. Rowlingson JC, Moscicki JC, DiFazio CA. Anesthetic potency of dezocine and its interaction with morphine in rats. Anesth Analg 1983; 62:899–902.
196. Ding Y, Terkonda R, White PF. Use of ketolorac and dezocine as alternatives to fentanyl during outpatient laparoscopy. Anesth Analg 1992;74:S67.
197. Ding Y, White PF. Comparative effects of ketolorac, dezocine and fentanyl during outpatient laparoscopy. Anesth Analg 1992;75:566–571.
198. Ramirez-Ruiz M, Smith I, White PF. Use of analgesics during propofol sedation: A comparison of ketolorac, dezocine and fentanyl. J Clin Anesth 1995;7:481–485.
199. Corssen G, Domino EF. Dissociative anesthesia; further pharmacologic studies and first clinical experience with the phencyclidine derivative CI-581. Anesth Analg 1966;45:29.
200. Corssen G, Miyasaka M, Domino EF. Changing concepts in pain control during surgery: dissociative anesthesia with CI-581: a progress report. Anesth Analg 1968;47:746.
201. Domino EF, Zsigmond EK, Domino LE, Domino KE, Kothary SP, Domino SE. Plasma levels of ketamine and two of its metabolites in surgical patients using a gas chromatographic-mass fragmentographic assay. Anesth Analg 1982;61:87–92.
202. Zsigmond EK, Domino EF. Ketamine: Clinical Pharmacology, Pharmacokinetics and Current Clinical Use. Anesthesiology Rev 1980; 7:13–33.
203. White PF, Way WL, Trevor AJ. Ketamine—Its pharmacology and therapeutic uses. Anesthesiology 1982;56:119–136.
204. Kharasch ED. Pharmacokinetics of ketamine. In: Pharmacologic Basis of Anesthesiology. Churchill Livingstone, New York, 1994, pp. 357–373.
205. Gajraj N, White PF. Clinical pharmacology and applications of ketamine. In: The Pharmacologic Basis of Anesthesiology (Bowdel et al, Eds.). Churchill Livingstone, New York, 1994, pp. 375–392.
206. White PF. Comparative evaluation of intravenous agents for rapid sequence induction-Thiopenthal, ketamine and midazolam. Anesthesiology 1982;57:279–284.
207. Fontenot J, Wilson RD, Domino EF, Zsigmond EK, Steen SN, Aldrete JA, McDonald JS, Fox GS. Efficacy and safety of low-dose intravenous (mini-drip) ketamine hydrochloride and concurrent intravenous diazepam in the induction and maintenance of balanced anesthesia. Clin Pharmacol Ther 1982;31:225.
208. Mould DR, DeFeo TM, Reele S, Milla G, Limjuco R, Crews T, Choma R, Patel IH. Simultaneous modeling of the pharmacokinetics and pharmacodynamics of midazolam and diazepam. Clin Pharmacol Ther 1995;58:35–43.
209. Zsigmond EK, Vieira ZEG, Dadabhoy Z, Golembiewski J, Ugarte B, Castillo R. Midazolam-ketamine co-induction on hemodynamics and catecholamines 1992; World Congr Anesth, The Hague, Netherlands. Excerp Med Intl Congr Series. ISBN 90-800899-2-3: p. 303.
210. White PF, Schuttler J, Shafer A, et al. Comparative pharmacology

of ketamine isomers. Studies in volunteers. Br J Anaesth 1985; 57:197–203.
211. Ryder S, Way WL, Trevor AJ. Comparative pharmacology of the optical isomers of ketamine in mice. Eur J Pharmacol 1978;49:15.
212. White PF, Ham J, Way WL, Trevor AJ. Pharmacology of ketamine isomers in surgical patients. Anesthesiology 1980;52:231.
213. Schuttler J, Stanski DR, White PF, et al. Pharmacodynamic modeling of the EEG effects of ketamine and its enantiomers in man. J Pharmacokinet Biopharm 1987;15:241.
214. Zsigmond EK, Domino EF. Clinical Pharmacology of Ketamine. In: Domino EF: Status of Ketamine in Anesthesiology 1990 NPP Books, Ann Arbor MI pp 68–69.
215. Zsigmond EK, Kothary SP, Martinez OA, Kelsch RO: Diazepam for the prevention of the rise in plasma catecholamines caused by ketamine. Clin Pharamacol Ther 1974;15:223.
216. Kothary SP, Zsigmond EK, Matsuki A. Antagonism of the ketamine induced rise in plasma free norepinephrine, blood pressure and pulse rate by intravenous diazepam. Clin Pharmacol Ther 1975; 17:238.
217. Kumar SM, Kothary SP, Zsigmond EK. Plasma free-norepinephrine and epinephrine concentrations following diazepam-ketamine induction in patients undergoing cardiac surgery. Acta Anaesth Scand 1978;22:593–600.
218. Kumar SM, Kothary SP, Zsigmond EK. The effect of pancuronium on plasma free-norepinephrine and epinephrine in adult cardiac surgical patients 1978;22:423–429.
219. Raza SMA, Masters RW, Zsigmond EK. Midazolam-ketamine-sufentanil analgesia in cardiac surgical patients. Can J Anaesth 1989; 36:617–623.
220. Zsigmond EK, Matsuki A, Kelsch RC, Kothary SP, Vadnay L. The effects of pancuronium bromide on plasma norepinephrine concentration during ketamine induction. Canad Anaesth Soc J 1974; 21:315–230.
221. Zsigmond EK, Raza SM, Barabas E. Comparison of four fentanyl-based neuroleptanalgesic technics on hemodynamics in cardiac surgical patients 1988: Proc 5th Intl Congr Belgian Soc Anesth, Brussels, Belgium, Sep 14–17. p 19.
222. Dhadphale R, Jackson APF, Alseri S. Comparison of anesthesia with diazepam-ketamine vs morphine in patients undergoing heart-valve replacement. Anesthesiology 1979;51:200.
223. Reves JG, Lell WA, McCracken LE, et al. Comparison of morphine and ketamine. Anesthetic techniques for coronary surgery; a randomized study. South Med J 1978;71:33–36.
224. Gutzke GE, Shah K, Glisson SN, et al. Sufentanil or ketamine: Induction in cardiomyopathic patients. Anesthesiology 1987;67:64.
225. Newsome LR, Moldenhauer CC, Hug CC, et al. Hemodynamnic interactions of moderate doses of fentanyl with etomidate and ketamine. Anesth Analg 1985;64:A260.
226. Wynands JE, Ping W, Towsend GE, Sprigge JS, Whalley DG. Narcotic requirements for intravenous anesthesia. Anesth Analg 1984; 63:101–105.
227. Hardy JF, et al. Influence of narcotics on hypertension after coronary bypass graft surgery. Can Anaesth Soc J 1983;30:370.
228. Lehtinen AM, Fyhrquist F, Kivalo I. The effect of fentanyl on arginine vasopressin and cortisol secretion during anesthesia. Anesth Analg 1984;63:25.
229. Wynands JE, Townsend GE, Wong P, Whalley DG, Srikant CB, Patel YC. Blood pressure response and plasma fentanyl concentrations of high and very high dose fentanyl anesthesia for coronary surgery. Anesth Analg 1983;62:665.
230. De Castro J. Practical applications and limitations of analgesic anesthesia. Acta Anaesthesiol Belg 1976;3:107–128.
231. DeCastro J. Neuroleptanalgesia: Yesterday, today and tomorrow. In: Stanley TH, Petty WC: Anesthesia: Today and Tomorrow; Martinus Nijhoff Publ, Boston, Dordrecht, Lancaster, 1985.
232. Tait EC, Tornetta FJ, Neuroleptanalgesia as adjunct to local anesthesia in intraocular surgery. Am J Ophtalmol 1965;59:412.
233. Jones WM, Samis WD, McDonald DA, Boyes HW. Neuroleptanalgesia for intraocular surgery. Can J Ophtalmol 1969;4:163.
234. Sarmany J. Further investigations on the effect of anesthetics on the intraocular pressure with special reference to neuroleptic analgesia. Anaesthetist 1969;18:72.
235. Hutschenreuter K, Beerhalter E, Beerhalter H. Erfahrungen mit der Neuroleptanalgesie in der Hals-Nasenohren Heilkunde. In: Gemperle M, ed. Fortschritte der Neuroleptanalgesie, 1966; Springer Verlag, Berlin.
236. Jones WM, Fee GA, Bell RD, Boyes HW. Neuroleptanalgesia for stapes surgery. Arch Otolaryngol 1968;88:491.
237. Leslie NH, Dontinon PJ. Neuroleptanalgesia in ear, nose, throat surgery. N Z Med J 1964;63:660.
238. Nyberg CD, Samartano JG, Terry RN. Use of Innovar as an anesthetic adjunct in oral surgery. J Oral Maxillofac Surg 1970;28:175.
239. Berenyi KJ, Sakarya I, Snow JC. Innovar-nitrous oxide anesthesia in otolaryngology. Laryngoscope 1966;76:772.
240. Keller R, Waldvogel H, Herzog H. Neuroleptanalgesia for brochoscopic examinations. Chest 1975;67:315.
241. Lebrun HI. Neuroleptanalgesia in upper alimentary endoscopy. Gut 1976;17:655.
242. Brindle GF. The use of neuroleptic agents in neurosurgical units. Clin Neurosurg 1969;16:234.
243. Hill ME, Wortzman G, Marshall MB. Clinical use of droperidol in pneumoencephalography. Can Med Assoc J 1968;98:359.
244. Brown AS. Neuroleptanalgesia: the present position for neurosurgery. Ir J Med Sci 1963;6:535.
245. Wolfson B, Siker ES, Wible I, Dubnansky J. Pneumoencephalography using neuroleptanalgesia. Anesth Analg 1968;47:14.
246. Neto OA, Zsigmond EK. The advantages of nalbuphine in the practice of anesthesia. Rev Brasil Anest 1984;34:203–205.
247. Shinozaki M. Clinical study on NLA in hypothermia for intracranial surgery with special consideration of comparison with halothane and methoxyflurane. Masui 1973;22:45.
248. Zsigmond EK. Atara-analgesic mixtures: Diazepam-ketamine. Excerp Med Intl Congr Series, 1974;330:39.
249. Corsen G, Chodoff P, Domino EF, Kahn DR. Neuroleptanalgesia and anesthesia for open heart surgery. Pharmacologic rationale and clinical experience. J Thorac Cardiovasc Surg 1965;49:901.
250. White PF. Use of continuous infusion versus intermittent bolus administration of fentanyl or ketamine during outpatient anesthesia. Anesthesiology 1983;59:294–300.
250a. White PF, Dworsky WA, Horai Y, Trevor AJ. Comparison of continuous infusion fentanyl or ketamine versus thiopental: determining the mean effective serum concentrations for outpatient surgery. Anesthesiology 1983;59:564–569.
251. Raza SMA, Masters RW, Vasireddy AR, Zsigmond EK. Hemodynamic stability with midazolam-sufentanil analgesia in cardiac surgical patients. Can J Anaesth 1988;35:518–525.
252. Neidhart PP, Campion P, Vogel J, Zsigmond EK, Tassonyi E. A comparison of pipecuronium with pancuroniumon hemodynamic variables and plasma catecholamines in coronary artery bypass surgery. Can J Anaesth 1994;41:469–474.
253. Corssen G, Chodoff P. Clinical management of the patient in shock: neuroleptanalgesia. Clin Anesth 1965;2:137.
254. de Bruijn NP, Christian C II, Fagreus L, Freedman B, Davis G, Hamm D, Everson C, Pellom G, Wechsler A. The effect of alfentanil on global ventricular mechanism. Anesthesiology 1983;59:A33.
255. Corssen G. Neuroleptanalgesia in obstetrics. Clin Obstet Gynecol 1974;17:241.
256. Marx GF, Hwang HS, Chandra P. Postpartum uterine pressure with different doses of ketamine. Anesthesiology 1979;50:163.
257. Oats JN, Vasey OP, Waldren BA. Effects of ketamine on the pregnant uterus. Brit J Anaesth 1979;51:1163.
258. Monk TG, Rader JM, White PF. A comparison of alfentanil and ketamine infusions for outpatient lithotripsy. Anesthesiology 1991; 74:1023–1028.
259. Monk TG, Bouré B, White PF, Meretyk S, Clayman RV. Comparison of intravenous sedative-analgesic techniques for outpatient immersion lithotripsy. Anesth Analg 1991;72:616–621.
260. Avramov M, Smith I, White PF. Use of midazolam and remifentanil during monitored anesthesia care (MAC). Anesth Analg 1995; 80:S24.

20A Adenosine Compounds

Atsuo F. Fukunaga

Since the potent extracellular effects of purine nucleosides and nucleotides were first described by Drury and Szent-Gyorgyi in 1929 (1), considerable research has been conducted in the field of adenosine compounds. The nature of the physiologic and pharmacologic actions of these agents and the receptor-effector coupling mechanisms involved have been reported in many scientific publications and are extensively reviewed elsewhere (2-9). However, only in the past decade has the molecular basis for the actions of adenosine been defined (10-12). Advances in cloning and pharmacologic characterization of numerous purinoceptors are revealing new physiopathologic roles of nucleosides and nucleotides and will further enhance understanding of these compounds and result in the development of new therapeutic modalities. The adenosine compounds play a multiplicity of roles in various biologic systems (13-17), particularly in the cardiovascular and central nervous systems (CNS). Adenosine is important in the regulation and neuromodulation (18-20) of both somatic and autonomic nervous systems (21-23), so vital for controlling homeostatic mechanisms (24-26) attributed to these purines. This overview discusses a potential clinical role of adenosine compounds in the practice of intravenous anesthesia.

BASIC PHARMACOLOGY

Chemically, adenosine consists of the purine base adenine linked to ribose; hence it is designated a nucleoside (Fig. 20A-1). Adenosine is a physiologic substance, one of the most ubiquitous metabolic intermediates in the body. It is also vital to the formation of adenosine triphosphate (ATP) and cyclic adenosine monophosphate (cAMP). Adenosine functions in nucleic acid biosynthesis and plays an important role in the disposition of the major methyl donor, S-adenosylmethionine. S-adenosylhomocysteine, a product of transmethylation reactions, is then converted to adenosine by S-adenosylhomocysteine hydrolase (Fig. 20A-2). Adenosine, as both a phosphorylated nucleotide and an enzyme cofactor, is involved in nearly every aspect of cell function (16, 25, 27). As a normal constituent of the body, adenosine exists both intra- and extracellularly. Levels of adenosine and ATP vary, depending on the physiologic state of the organism. Stimuli that lower cellular energy (e.g., hypoxia or ischemia) significantly decrease the level of ATP and augment the production of adenosine (28-32). Thus, the importance of adenosine as a metabolic regulator of cellular activity and its involvement in homeostatic regulation of tissue activity in various physiologic systems has become increasingly evident.

Adenosine presumably acts as a local hormone rather than a circulating hormone or neurotransmitter. Unlike classic neurotransmitters, adenosine can be produced by virtually all cells (analogous to the prostaglandins and leukotrienes) and is produced in direct proportion to the metabolic demand (33). The intracellular concentration of adenosine is closely regulated by a series of enzymatic steps. The extracellular concentration is closely matched to the intracellular concentration by transmembrane adenosine transporters. In addition, adenosine can be formed extracellularly from adenine nucleotides that are rapidly broken down by effective ectoenzymes.

Purine Receptors

Purine receptors mediate the important physiologic and pharmacologic actions of the purines (namely, adenosine and adenine nucleotides). Attempts to classify purinoceptors were made by several investigative groups in the late 1970s. In 1978, Burnstock (34) proposed a classification of purinoceptors into two types: P_1 and P_2, the former being more sensitive to adenosine and the latter to the nucleotide ATP (Table 20A-1). Other independent groups provided evidence for a distinction between the receptors mediating stimulatory and inhibitory effects of adenosine on adenylate cyclase (35-38). Two distinctive adenosine receptor subtypes were identified: A_1 and A_2.

The two extracellular receptor subtypes were originally defined in terms of effects on adenylate cyclase and cAMP levels. A_1 receptor activation caused enzyme inhibition, lowering of cAMP, and A_2 activation producing stimulation and raising cAMP production. However, considerable evidence suggests that some of the responses to adenosine are independent of cAMP (39), including closing calcium (Ca^{2+}) channels (40), opening potassium (K^+) channels (41, 42), and inhibiting (43) or stimulating (44) phosphatidylinositol turnover. Therefore, the receptors are now defined in terms of structure-activity requirements (45). Both the signal transduction processes linking A_1 and A_2 receptors to changes in adenylate cyclase activity and the structural aspects of the A_1 receptor have been extensively studied (see Fig. 20A-2). Analogous to other receptors coupled to adenylate cyclase, guanosine triphosphate (GTP) is required to observe stimulatory or inhibitory effects of adenosine on adenylate cyclase activity in purified membrane preparations. This GTP requirement translates into the involvement of distinct GTP regulatory proteins (G_i and G_s) that mediate these effects. Thus, the A_1 receptor inhibits adenylyl cyclase by interacting with GTP-binding protein G_i, whereas the A_2 receptor acts by G_s to activate the enzyme.

FIGURE 20A-1. Chemical structure of adenosine.

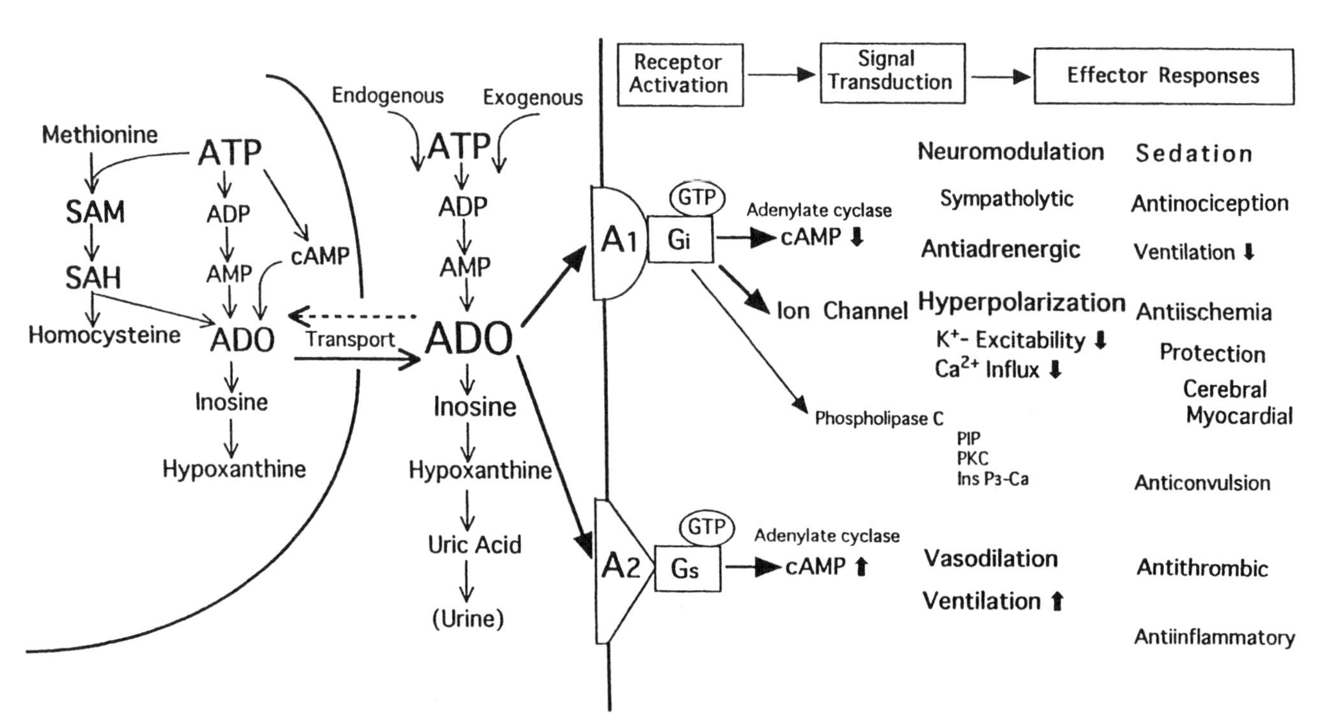

FIGURE 20A-2. Diagrammatic representation of intracellular or extracellular adenosine formation and the receptor-effector coupling mechanism. Activation of the A_1 or A_2 receptor inhibits or stimulates adenylate cyclase activity by inhibitory (G_i) or stimulatory (G_s) guanine nucleotide binding regulatory proteins and decreases or increases cyclic adenosine monophosphate (cAMP) production. The A_1 receptor can also influence ion channels without cAMP participation. Calcium (Ca^{2+}) channels are closed (decrease Ca^{2+} influx) and potassium (K^+) channels are opened, resulting in hyperpolarization of the plasma membrane, which produces various effects. ADO, Adenosine; AMP, adenosine monophosphate; ADP, adenosine diphosphate; ATP, adenosine triphosphate; SAM, S-adenosylmethionine; SAH, S-adenosylhomcysteine; GTP, guanosine triphosphate; PIP, phosphatidylinositol 4,5-bisphosphate; PKC, protein kinase C; $InsP_3$-Ca, inositol 1,4,5-trisphosphate.

TABLE 20A-1. Subtypes of Purinoceptors

Purinoceptor	Subclass	Rank Order of Agonist Potency	Antagonists	Adenylate Cyclase Activity	Prostaglandin Synthesis
P_1	A_1 (R_i)	L-PIA, CHA > CADO > NECA, D-PIA > adenosine	Non-selective: Caffeine, Theophylline, 8-PT, PACPX	↓	—
	A_2 (R_s)	NECA > CADO > L-PIA, CHA > adenosine	8-SPT, 9-MeA, DPSPX; Selective: CGS 15943A (A_1)	↑	—
	A_3 ?	L-PIA, CHA, NECA > CADO	DPCPX (A_1), PD 116,948 (A_2)	—	—
P_2	P_{2X}	α, β-meATP, β, γ-meATP > ATP = 2Me.S.ATP	ANAPP$_3$; Desensitization by α, β-meATP	—	↑
	P_{2Y}	2-Me.S.ATP ≫ ATP > α, β-meATP, β, γ-meATP	Reactive blue 2 (an anthraquinone sulphonic acid derivative)	—	↑
	P_{2Z}	ATP^4—> ATP		—	?
	P_{2T}	2-Me.S.ADP > ADP > α, β-meADP	ATP, AMP, adenosine (non-competitively)	↓	?

Abbreviations: CADO, 2-chloroadenosine; CHA, N^6-cyclohexyladenosine; DPCPX, 1,3-dipropyl-8-cyclopentylxanthine; DPSPX, 1,3-dipropyl-8-p-sulphophenylxanthine; 9-MeA, N^6-substituted 9-methyladenines; meADP, methylene ADP; meATP, methylene ATP; 2-Me.S.ADP, 2-methylthio-ADP; 2-Me.S.ATP, 2-methylthio-ATP; NECA, 5'-N-ethylcarboxamidoadenosine; PACPX, 1,3-dipropyl-8-(2-amino-4-chlorophenyl)xanthine; PIA, N^6-phenylisopropyladenosine; 8-PT, 8-phenyltheophylline; 8-SPT, 8-(p-sulphophenyl)theophylline.

(From Burnstock G. Purine Receptors. In: Adenosine Receptors in the Nervous System *(J.A. Ribeiro, ed.), Taylor & Francis, London, 1989, with permission)*

Adenosine Receptor Antagonists

Previously, the effects of the methylxanthines were believed to be based solely on the inhibition of cytoplasmic phosphodiesterase. However, investigators have shown that caffeine and theophylline act also at the plasma membrane level, inhibiting adenosine receptors in a competitive manner (46). Sattin and Rall (47) observed that caffeine and theophylline prevented cAMP formation and suggested that the xanthines were adenosine antagonists. Subsequent electrophysiologic, biochemical, and pharmacologic studies have supported this hypothesis. The behavioral stimulant effects of methylxanthines involve blockade of adenosine receptors and correlate with their potencies in competitively blocking the adenosine receptor sites (48, 49). These antagonistic effects of xanthines at adenosine receptors correlate with the central stimulant actions of caffeine. However, caffeine and theophylline are weak antagonists with varied spectrums of activity. Currently, there are more potent xanthines with more selective activities as adenosine antagonists, such as 8-phenyltheophylline (8-PT), which is A_1 selective and 100-fold more active at this receptor than theophylline (50). Numerous xanthines and nonxanthine adenosine antagonists have been synthetized (50, 51).

Activity of Adenosine

Adenosine, a ubiquitous biologic compound, influences numerous physiologic activities on tissues and organs under both physiologic and pathophysiologic conditions. In general, activation of adenosine receptors appears to protect against inadequate tissue oxygenation by maintaining a favorable tissue oxygen supply-demand balance. Hence, adenosine is an important metabolic and homeostatic modulator. Adenosine receptors have been found in many different tissues including the cardiovascular system and the CNS (52). Adenosine is a potent CNS depressant; it inhibits the spontaneous firing of neurons in many different regions of the CNS (2, 53). Adenosine can modulate the efficacy of synaptic transmission by altering transmitter release in both neuronal and nonneuronal cells, and it regulates the cellular transmembrane activity of ion channels (54, 55).

Adenosine receptor activation occurs at both presynaptic and postsynaptic sites. The effects of adenosine may be *indirect*, inhibiting the release of various conventional neurotransmitters from presynaptic terminals, or *direct*, by affecting postsynaptic process. Adenosine inhibits the release of many diverse classes of neurotransmitters, including norepinephrine (NE), acetylcholine, glutamate, γ-aminobutyric acid (GABA), dopamine, serotonin, and aspartate (20, 25, 56).

Behavioral Actions of Adenosine

Many behavioral responses following administration of adenosine and its analogs have been reported (2-4,

8, 12, 25, 57), including sedative-hypnotic, anticonvulsant, antinociceptive, analgesic, and hypothermic effects, depression of locomotor activity, inhibition of aggressive behaviors, and suppression of food intake.

Adenosine Interaction with Other Anesthetic Drugs
Several drugs commonly used in clinical anesthesia have been linked with adenosine receptors. Adenosine analogs have marked inhibitory locomotor activity (58-60), sedative effects (61,62), and hypnotic effects (63-65) after intracerebral or systemic administration. Investigators have suggested that drugs used as anxiolytic, hypnotic, and anticonvulsant agents including barbiturates, opioids, ethanol, and benzodiazepines may be mediated in part by central purine-linked mechanisms (66-68).

Phillis and colleagues have extensively studied the relationship between adenosine and benzodiazepine actions and have shown that some of the actions of benzodiazepines may be mediated by adenosine receptors (69, 70). Evidence suggests that the central actions of the benzodiazepines cannot be fully accounted for exclusively by the $GABA_A$-chloride (Cl^-) channel supramolecular complex. The interactions of benzodiazepine with adenosine helps to explain some of the anomalies that exist between the benzodiazepine-GABA hypothesis (71, 72). Because benzodiazepines do not act at adenosine receptors (67), investigators have suggested that the interaction of benzodiazepines with the purinergic system may be exerted by enhancing the effects of locally released adenosine (i.e., inhibiting adenosine uptake) (73). Diazepam has potentiated the depressant actions of adenosine on the spontaneous firing of cerebral cortical neurons (74); the concept is further supported by the inhibition of the depressant actions of flurazepam on the firing of cerebral cortical neurons by theophylline, an adenosine antagonist, (75). Indeed, a study of the effects of diazepam on purine and acetylcholine release from rat cerebral cortex demonstrated that benzodiazepines enhanced the rate of efflux of [^{3}H] adenosine. In addition, diazepam depressed the release of acetylcholine, which was blocked by a prior administration of theophylline, indicating that it was secondary to the increase in extracellular adenosine levels (76). After direct topical application of flurazepam and diazepam onto rat cerebral cortex, these agents enhanced the release of labeled purine (77). Numerous other studies have supported this hypotensis.

Benzodiazepines appeared to have the potential to inhibit adenosine transport by interaction with the transport-inhibitory site (78). In behavioral studies, concurrent intraperitoneal injection of diazepam and intracerebroventricular adenosine at doses with no significant effect on locomotor activity when given alone acted synergistically to produce a marked depression of locomotor activity (79). Investigations of adenosine on sleep (63, 64) confirmed the connection of adenosine with the benzodiazepines. In studies of long-term administration of diazepam (80), investigators found that A_1 receptors in different regions of the brain were significantly decreased, as demonstrated by adenosine receptor binding. Similar results were obtained with the long-term administration of triazolam, a benzodiazepine with a shorter duration of action (81). The adenosine receptor antagonists caffeine and theophylline reversed the benzodiazepine-induced sedation and anesthesia not only in animals, but also in humans (82-86).

Adenosine receptors have been implicated in the central actions of barbiturates. Lohse and associates found that barbiturates inhibit the binding of both agonist and antagonist radioligands to A_1 adenosine receptors (87). Among several barbiturates studied, investigators found that barbiturates were competitive antagonists at A_1 receptors, with pentobarbital more potent than phenobarbital at membrane-bound A_1 receptors (88). In addition, blockade of A_1 adenosine receptors is suggested for the basis of the excitatory effects of barbiturates, which can enhance the release of neurotransmitters in the hippocampus by blocking presynaptic A_1 receptors (89). Thus, investigators proposed that the excitatory actions of barbiturates were mediated, at least in part, by adenosine A_1 receptor blockade, and their inhibitory effects were mediated through the GABA-receptor system (90).

Analgesic Effects

Purines play an important role in antinociception. Numerous biochemical, physiologic, and pharmacologic studies have demonstrated the involvement of adenosine in analgesia. The vast amount of literature on the actions and mechanisms involving adenosine and pain has been comprehensively reviewed by Sawynok and associates (91, 92). Adenosine and adenosine analogs have had analgesic activity in various paradigms, including somatic (hot plate, tail-flick), visceral (writhing), and neurogenic (strychnine) assays following both systemic and central administration (93-102). Moreover, adenosine involvement has been demonstrated in the suppression of spinal dorsal horn wide dynamic range (WDR) neurons in response to somatic (103) and visceral (104) stimulation.

In addition to the central antinociceptive effects, adenosine stimulates peripheral nociceptive sensory nerve endings (e.g., adenosine has been reported to produce pain when applied to human blister preparation) (105). Intravenous administration of adenosine produces epigastric discomfort, and in patients with coronary insufficiency, adenosine has produced chest pain (106). However, adenosine's direct stimulating actions on the peripheral sensory system, including carotid chemoreceptors and cardiac sensory fibers, are transient and are mediated by different mechanisms from the central effects in which adenosine inhibits the transmission of nociceptive information (107). Investigators have proposed that adenosine, which is produced from the breakdown of ATP under ischemic conditions, may activate sensory nerve endings as a means of protecting tissue in a precarious metabolic state (108).

Mechanisms of Antinociceptive Action

Adenosine's mechanism of action in antinociception (analgesia) is complex. Like other neurotransmitters, adenosine has been implicated in the signaling and inhibition of pain at central and peripheral nerve endings. Adenosine receptors are located not only in the brain, but also in the dorsal horn region of the spinal cord (109-115), a finding that suggests a physiologic role in the regulation of sensory neurotransmission, including painful stimulation. However, adenosine's major role in analgesia may be as a neuromodulator (116), because adenosine appears to be involved in many of the systems related to pain.

The pre- and postsynaptic actions of adenosine are related to its indirect action on the release of other neurotransmitters and to its direct actions on cellular excitable membranes. Adenosine receptor activation is associated with modulation of the adenylate cyclase system, resulting in altered levels of cAMP and ions in the effector systems. Transmembrane cellular ionic mechanisms reflect changes in Ca^{2+} influx, increase in K^+ conductance, and possibly regulation of sodium movement. The receptor appears to be coupled to the K^+ channel by a pertussis toxin-sensitive G protein. A_1 adenosine receptors act through inhibitory G proteins and perhaps ultimately act by increasing transmembrane K^+ conductance followed by hyperpolarization (41, 117), in a way similar to that of α_2 adrenoceptors and opioids on their antinociceptive effects, because they have similar transduction pathways in their postreceptor mechanisms (118-120). Antinociception produced by R-phenylisopropyladenosine (R-PIA), an adenosine A_1 receptor agonist, was modulated by ATP-sensitive K^+ channels. K_{ATP} channel blockers antagonized, whereas a K_{ATP} channel opener enhanced, the antinociception of R-PIA (121).

Adenosine, Opioids, and Norepinephrine

Accumulating evidence indicates that the antinociceptive effects of opioids is in part mediated by endogenous adenosine. Interest in the involvement of adenosine in morphine's analgesic activity on the brain was aroused when Ho and colleagues reported that cyclic adenosine monophosphate antagonized morphine analgesia (122). The central actions of morphine and the involvement of adenosine have been further evidenced by the demonstration that morphine or opioid peptides induce cerebral release of adenosine. Therefore, opioids may conceivably exert some of their actions by enhancing extracellular levels of adenosine in the brain. Morphine enhances veratridine-induced release of adenosine (123); likewise, electrically stimulated neurons and KCl-evoked release of other purines have been observed in animal experiments (124, 125). In rat experiments, morphine (1.0 and 5 mg/kg intravenously) increased the rate of release of labeled purines from cortical tissue that had been preincubated with [^{3}H] adenosine (126, 127). In addition, the central neuronal depressant effects of morphine were blocked by the adenosine antagonist, aminophylline (128, 129).

The inhibitory effect of morphine on acetylcholine release was also antagonized by methylxanthines (130, 131). Further *in vitro* studies have confirmed that caffeine can reverse opiate effects on the gastrointestinal track. This antagonism seems to be greater for the μ-related than for the κ-related opioid interaction (132). A biphasic response of caffeine inhibition of the morphine analgesic action depended on the dose of caffeine administered (133). Dipyridamole, an adenosine uptake inhibitor, potentiated the analgesic effect of morphine in a dose-related manner in both the hot plate and tail-immersion tests (134). Long-term administration of caffeine increased the sensitivity of mice to the analgesic actions of morphine and decreased morphine-induced tolerance and dependence (135). Investigators have also reported that some of the opiate withdrawal syndrome can be associated with the adenylate cyclase system, and in behavioral studies, opiate withdrawal signs have been blocked by adenosine triphosphate (136) and adenosine analogs (137). Furthermore, the hypotensive effect of morphine has been related to released adenosine acting at A_2 vascular smooth muscle receptors (138).

At the spinal level, Sawynok and colleagues determined that the spinal adenosine release from primary afferent nerve terminals and subsequent activation of adenosine receptors mediated, at least in part, opioid-induced antinociception (139, 140). The authors demonstrated that morphine released adenosine from synaptosomes prepared from the dorsal half of the spinal cord (141) and the superfused spinal cord in vivo (142). Sweeney and associates demonstrated that a component of morphine antinociception could be mediated by spinal release of adenosine by demonstrating that intracerebroventricular administration of morphine released adenosine and cAMP from the spinal cord (143). The appearance time of adenosine was similar to the time required for morphine induction of antinociception. Furthermore, the methylxanthines, theophylline and 8-phenyltheophylline, reversed the spinal antinociceptive effect of intrathecal morphine in both the tail-flick and hot plate tests (141, 144). Further studies have shown that morphine can stimulate adenosine release from the spinal cord synaptosomes by activation of Ca^{2+} channels (145). In accordance with the foregoing hypothesis, other investigators found that a complex functional interaction between adenosine and opioid receptors existed in the modulation of nociceptive transmission in spinal system (146, 147). These findings are in agreement with the concept that adenosine plays a role in opioid-induced analgesia, a hypothesis strengthened by studies showing that inhibition of adenosine reuptake can enhance opioid actions at the spinal level (148).

Although investigators have reported that adenosine is not involved in the anesthetic-sparing effect of dexmedetomidine, an α_2-adrenergic agonist, based on results that pretreatment with an adenosine antagonist did not prevent the halothane minimum alveolar concentration (MAC)-reducing effect (149), evidence supports a role for adenosine in the spinal antinociception produced by NE and α-adrenergic agonists. In agreement with other investigators, Jones suggested that adenosine may play a role in neuronal adaptation at the cellular level by altering the pharmacologic characteristics of neurotransmitter receptor-effector complex. Adenosine has stimulated, in a dose-dependent manner, the formation of cAMP in spinal cord tissues (150). When adenosine was combined with NE, a synergistic increase in accumulation of cAMP occurred; this potentiated effect was blocked by theophylline, isobutylmethyxantine, and α-adrenergic antagonist (150).

Spinal administration of NE has released adenosine from dorsal spinal cord synaptosomes in vitro (141). This release is dose dependent and is reduced by phentolamine, a nonselective α-adrenoceptor antagonist, as well as by yohimbine, a selective α_2-adrenoceptor antagonist. Furthermore, intrathecal administration of Ca^{2+} releases adenosine (or a nucleotide, which is metabolized to adenosine), and subsequent activation of adenosine receptors potentiates the action of NE (151). Consistent with the foregoing hypothesis, other investigators reported a supra-additive antinociception produced by intrathecal coadministration of NE or clonidine (α_2 agonist) and N-ethylcarboxamide-adenosine (NECA), an adenosine agonist (152). This was attenuated by pretreatment with the adenosine antagonist, theophylline (153). Aran and Proudfit, therefore, suggested that purinergic and noradrenergic systems interact synergistically to modify nociceptive transmission in the spinal cord. The proposal that adenosine receptors may modulate the action of noradrenergic analgesia has been repeatedly observed using both the tail-flick and hot plate tests (141, 144, 151-154). Given the findings demonstrating that the antinociceptive effect of intrathecally administered NE was directly antagonized by aminophylline in rats (144), sufficient evidence supports adenosine involvement in NE-induced analgesia. Interactions between adenosine and 5-hydroxytryptamine (143,154), as well as adenosine and GABA systems, have also been reported (155, 156).

The evidence of the analgesic effects of purines has led many researchers to consider the use of adenosine analogs and adenosine-regulating agents to modulate pain (157). The notion that adenosine compounds may be used in analgesia has evolved into attempts for practical (clinical) demonstrations. Indeed, the intrathecal (spinal) administration of R-PIA and NECA has been systematically evaluated for pain control (158-162). Clinically, R-PIA has been reported to have potent analgesic effects in a patient suffering for more than 10 years with a well-characterized intractable neurogenic pain and allodynia (163).

The analgesic effects of ATP and adenosine have also been evaluated in studies of volunteers. The antinociceptive actions of ATP were determined using tooth pulp electrical stimulation (164). In a double-blind placebo-controlled study (165), a continuous intravenous infusion of ATP (100 μg/kg/min for 30 to 60 minutes) significantly elevated the pain thresholds of tooth pulp electrical stimulation in human volunteers without signs of hypotension. The subjects tolerated this dosage of ATP and did not complain of side effects during or after ATP administration.

On the other hand, investigators in Sweden have been evaluating the analgesic effects of intravenous administration of adenosine in various types of nociceptive stimuli. Segerdahl and colleagues, in a randomized, single-blind, and placebo-controlled study, found that intravenous adenosine, 70 μg/kg/min, significantly reduced pain in the ischemic muscle pain model. The adenosine infusion produced analgesia without causing significant changes in blood pressure, similar to the analgesic effects produced by morphine (0.1 mg/kg) and ketamine (0.1 mg/kg). Furthermore, significant potentiation of analgesia was observed when a combination of adenosine infusion and morphine was used (166). In a study assessing cutaneous heat pain threshold, neither morphine (0.1 mg/kg) nor ketamine (0.1 mg/kg) had any significant effects, but intravenous adenosine infusion (50 μg/kg/min) significantly increased the heat pain threshold (167). Further, to assess tactile allodynia, and skin injury pain, sensitivity was assessed using the von Frey filaments. This stimulation caused hyperalgesia resulting from peripheral sensitization of nociceptive afferent fibers. In a double-blind, placebo-controlled study in volunteers, intravenous adenosine infusion (50 μg/kg/min) attenuated touch-evoked allodynia produced by mustard oil (168). Low doses of intravenous adenosine (50 μg/kg/min) alleviated pain, tactile allodynia, and pinprick hyperalgesia in patients with peripheral neuropathic pain (169, 170).

USE OF ADENOSINE IN ANESTHESIA

Unlike therapeutics for a specific disease, perioperative care must deal with multiple variables on an acute basis. From the physiopathologic perspective, the concept of adenosine's retaliatory role (31), [that is, a global homeostatic role for the purine (171)], in response to chaotic physiologic changes is an attractive characteristic for acute therapies. The purine's ubiquity of actions as a homeostatic modulatory agent can be beneficial to accomplish the ultimate goal of anesthesia in protecting the patient from the pain and stress of surgical intervention, while maintaining global homeostasis during the perioperative period.

Since the early 1970s, the sedative and antinociceptive actions of adenosine and ATP were observed during studies of deliberate hypotension using adenosine as vasodilators. However, adenosine's ubiquity of effects has been considered a major hindrance to therapeutic targeting of these compounds. Indeed, adenosine's peripheral cardiovascular actions are so potent that, unless special provisions are taken into consideration, it is difficult to dissociate hypotension from centrally mediated sedation or antinociception. Therefore, regardless of the sedative and analgesic properties, this practical consideration would render the use of adenosine as an anesthetic agent untenable unless the questions regarding its side effects could be resolved.

An important discovery related to the finding that, despite its extremely short plasma half-life (less than 10 seconds), adenosine can exert long-lasting and potent sympatholytic-analgesic effects. In addition, adenosine's rapid action at the putative A_2 receptor can be advantageous with respect to hemodynamic control of sympathetic responses to noxious stimuli. Most important, adenosine can render effective analgesia without cardiorespiratory or metabolic decompensation, including significant decrease in blood pressure, respiratory depression, or metabolic acidosis. Therefore, because the analgesic activity can be effectively achieved without opioid-related side effects, it follows that clinical application of adenosine may be beneficial in anesthesiology and pain management. In light of this agent's many pharmacologic actions, the characteristics of adenosine have to be better defined for therapeutic targeting.

Characteristic of the Antinociceptive Effects of Adenosine and Adenosine Triphosphate

Halothane MAC was decreased by L-phenylisopropyladenosine (L-PIA, an adenosine analog) in rats (172), and by adenosine or ATP in dogs and rabbits (173, 174). However, in these studies, the standard tail clamp stimulation (175) was used, and the inhibitory responses were noted at the expense of severe hypotension. Because the effects of the purines do not appear to modify tactile sensation, a more discriminative and quantifiable stimulus is required to assess the antinociceptive activity of the purines properly. Electrical stimulation, although not a selective stimulation, was useful for this purpose and mimicked surgical stimulation. Motor behavior and touch stimulation remained unaffected by adenosine, although the animals were unresponsive to painful stimulation (176). The hypnotic-anesthetic and the analgesic responses of inhaled anesthetics (halothane, enflurane, isoflurane), intravenous opioids (morphine, fentanyl, and sufentanil), and intravenous adenosine, ATP, and R-PIA were assessed using electrical tail stimulation (ETS) with graded degree of electrical intensities. The two distinct behavioral responses were recognizable depending on whether the predominant drug action was sedative-hypnotic or analgesic. For example, isoflurane, a hypnotic-anesthetic, almost equally and concomitantly elevated both the sedative-hypnotic (arousal, head lift, HL), and analgesic (escape movement, EM) indices in a dose related manner (Fig. 20A-3), whereas with opioids, the EM response curve diverges (177). Likewise, with the purines (R-PIA, an

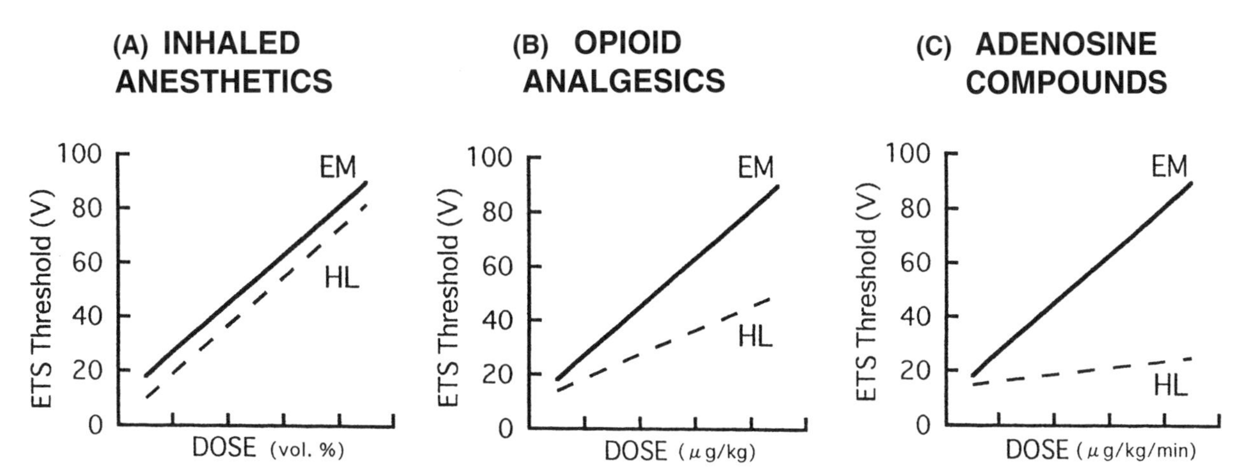

FIGURE 20A-3. Characterization of sedative-hypnotic and analgesic agents. Dose-response curves of inhaled anesthetics (A), opioid analgesics (B), and adenosine compounds (C). ETS, Electrical tail stimulation (1 ms, 5 Hz, square wave pulse, 0 to 100 V). ETS is gradually increased. Two distinctive behavioral responses are assessed: head lift (HL, sedative-hypnotic index) and escape movement (EM, analgesic index). Note that the inhaled anesthetics cause parallel elevation of both HL and EM thresholds. The curves for the opioid analgesics and adenosine compounds diverge, indicating a predominantly analgesic effect compared with the hypnotic effect.

adenosine agonist, adenosine, and ATP), the EM and HL response curves diverged even more widely than with the opioids, suggesting that the purines are characterized as having predominantly an analgesic profile as compared with the hypnotic-anesthetic profile of the volatile agents (178). Thus, in combination with sedative-hypnotic agents, it was reasonable that purines could enhance the anesthetic effectiveness of inhalational agents or intravenous sedative-hypnotic drugs (e.g., benzodiazepines, barbiturates, propofol).

Sustained Analgesic Effect of Intravenous Adenosine

A most impressive action of adenosine is its apparent prolonged analgesic action. Although adenosine rapidly disappears from the circulation, it was surprising to learn that intravenously administered adenosine could produce profound and sustained analgesia after its administration had been discontinued (179, 180).

In rabbits, 100 mg/kg intravenously of either adenosine (n = 12) or ATP (n = 12) consistently produced analgesia comparable to that induced by morphine (10 mg/kg intravenously). During infusion of adenosine or ATP alone, 1600 μg/kg/min for over a 1-hour period produced marked hypotension; however, heart rate and blood pressure returned to control levels without rebound hypertension. In half the experiments, adenosine (n = 6) or ATP (n = 6) was coadministered with NE to maintain a stable blood pressure during the infusion period (181) (Table 20A-2). The profound sedative and analgesic effects of adenosine and ATP were again sustained for over 5 hours after discontinuing the infusion with stable blood pressure and heart rate values, without evidence of respiratory depression, hypothermia, or metabolic acidosis (Figs. 20A-4 and 20A-5 and Table 20A-2). The purine's analgesic effects were antagonized by intravenous 8-phenyltheophylline, a specific adenosine-receptor antagonist. In addition, yohimbine, an α_2-adrenoceptor antagonist, was able to reverse the residual sedative effect in the group receiving purines and NE. These data suggested that intravenous adenosine or ATP could produce profound and sustained analgesia per se and not due to a decrease in blood pressure. The antinociceptive properties of adenosine or ATP are most likely mediated by adenosine receptors because these actions were almost completely antagonized by the specific adenosine receptor antagonist 8-phenyltheophylline.

Adenosine Triphosphate Reduces Inhaled Anesthetic Requirements

ATP combined with nitrous oxide (N_2O) produced anesthetic effects comparable to those of enflurane combined with N_2O (182). To assess the anesthetic activity of ATP, abolition of movement in response to tail clamp stimulation was used as the end point. Concurrently, antinociception was tested using ETS for a graded and quantitative measurement. As shown in Figure 20A-6, addition of enflurane to N_2O indeed increased the antinociceptive responses in a dose-related manner, but blood pressure decreased concomitantly in a dose-related fashion. Complete abolition of movement in response to tail clamp in all animals was achieved with 2.5% enflurane and N_2O (stage II). Although somatic responses were inhibited at these high doses of enflurane, blood pressure and heart rate were not inhibited at noxious stimulation.

To determine ATP's antinociceptive effects, doses of enflurane were decreased in a stepwise fashion. After positive movement response to tail clamp and decrease of ETS threshold were first confirmed, the infusion rates of ATP were gradually increased until movement in response to tail clamp was abolished. ATP was able to replace enflurane completely and yet resulted in no movement response to tail clamp stimulation (stage III in Fig. 20A-6), comparable to the anesthetic effect achieved with 2.5% enflurane. Blood

TABLE 20A-2. Cardiovascular, Respiratory and Blood Gas Data of Adenosine-Norepinephrine Coadministration (During and After Administration), and Following Antagonism

	Control	During ADO+NE	Post ADO Infusion (hours) 1	3	5	Antagonism 8-PT+Yohimbine
HR (bpm)	260 ± 19	243 ± 9	253 ± 14	237 ± 15	253 ± 13	240 ± 18
SBP (mm Hg)	109 ± 9	94 ± 4	98 ± 6	111 ± 5	119 ± 13	123 ± 10
DBP (mm Hg)	67 ± 4	39 ± 2*	65 ± 3	70 ± 4	75 ± 7	78 ± 5
pH	7.52 ± 0.03	7.43 ± 0.03	7.43 ± 0.02	7.42 ± 0.03	7.40 ± 0.03	7.31 ± 0.03
$PaCO_2$ (mm Hg)	28 ± 1	30 ± 2	28 ± 6	31 ± 3	34 ± 4	35 ± 3
PaO_2 (mm Hg)	532 ± 6	523 ± 9	507 ± 18	487 ± 26	502 ± 18	514 ± 13
HCO_3 (mEq/l)	23 ± 1	19 ± 1	18 ± 1	19 ± 1	20 ± 2	17 ± 2
BE	1 ± 1	−3 ± 3	−4 ± 2	−4 ± 1	−3 ± 3	−8 ± 2*
RR (bpm)	97 ± 6	128 ± 5*	104 ± 7	130 ± 8*	127 ± 16*	130 ± 11*
Urine (ml)	9 ± 4	10 ± 4	28 ± 11	38 ± 13	43 ± 15	106 ± 8
Temp (°C)	39.3 ± 0.2	38.7 ± 0.4	38.7 ± 0.4	38.2 ± 0.3	38.5 ± 0.2	37.6 ± 0.4

*ADO, Adenosine (100 mg/kg IV); NE, Norepinephrine (0.1 mg/kg IV); 8-PT, 8-phenyltheophylline (3 mg/kg IV); Yohimbine (30 μg/kg IV). Mean ± SD; (n=6); Statistical Analysis vs. Control, * p < 0.05 was considered significant.*

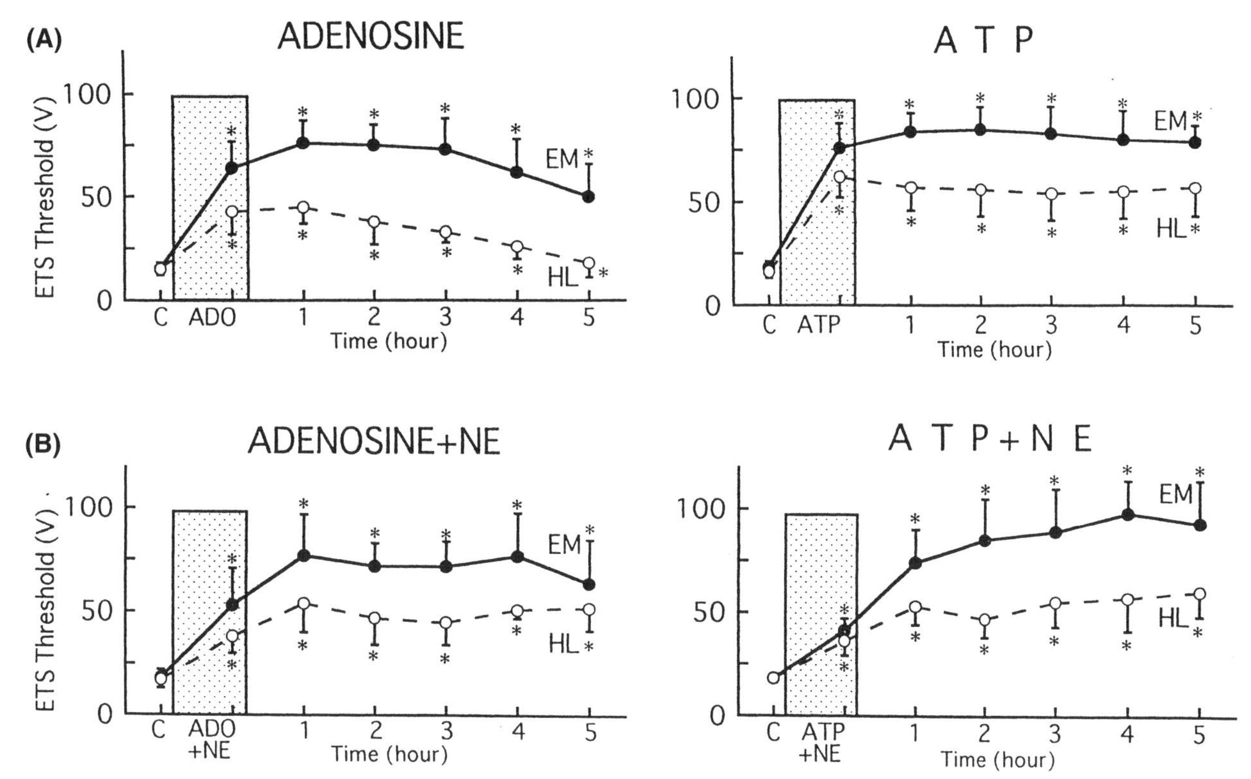

FIGURE 20A-4. Time course of changes in nociceptive thresholds during and after intravenous infusion of adenosine (n = 6) or adenosine triphosphate (ATP) (n = 6) alone (A), or coadministered with norepinephrine (NE, n = 12 [B]). Total administration dose of approximately 100 mg/kg of either adenosine or ATP. The coadministered dose of NE: 0.1 mg/kg + adenosine, and 0.33 mg/kg + ATP, respectively; infusion rate: 1600 μg/kg/min over 60-minute periods (dotted area). Rabbits were unmedicated and spontaneously breathing. Behavioral responses to electrical tail stimulation (ETS; 2 Hz, 1 ms, 1 to 100 V). EM, Escape movement (analgesic index); HL, head lift (sedative-hypnotic index). Measurements at control (C), almost at end of infusion and every 60 minutes after stopping infusion. Note that both EM and HL responses elevated significantly after adenosine or ATP infusions. The responses remained elevated for over 5 hours after stopping the infusion. Mean ± SEM, statistical comparison versus C was determined in each group using ANOVA followed by Dunnett's test. *$p < 0.05$ was considered significant.

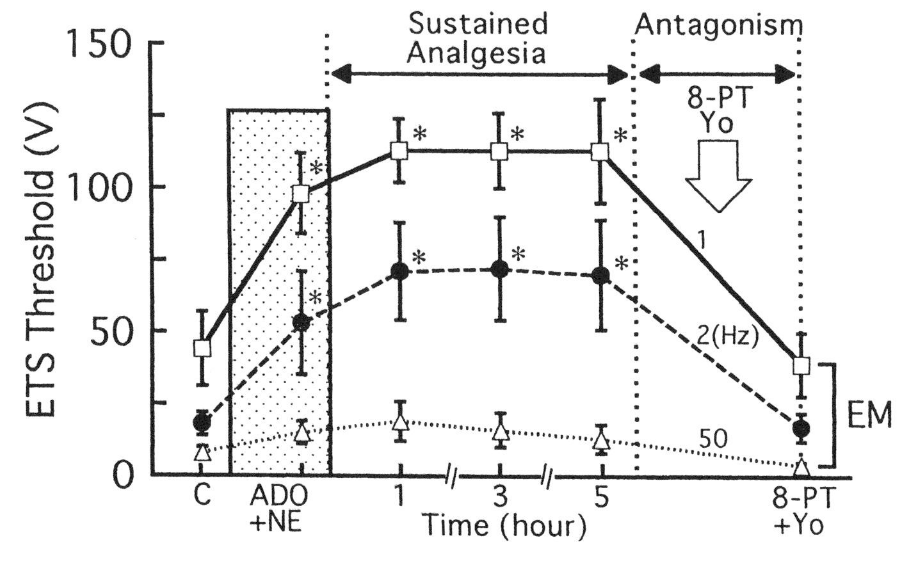

FIGURE 20A-5. Coadministration of adenosine (ADO) and norepinephrine (NE) produced sustained analgesia in spontaneously breathing rabbits (n = 6): ADO (100 mg/kg) + NE (0.1 mg/kg). The analgesic effect was antagonized by 8-phenyltheophylline (8-PT: 3 mg/kg) and yohimbine (Yo: 30 mg/kg). ETS, Electrical tail stimulation (1 ms, 1 to 150 V with three different frequencies: 1, 2, 50 Hz); EM, escape movement (analgesic index). Mean ± SEM, statistical comparison versus control (C) was determined using ANOVA followed by Dunnett's test. *$p < 0.05$ was considered significant.

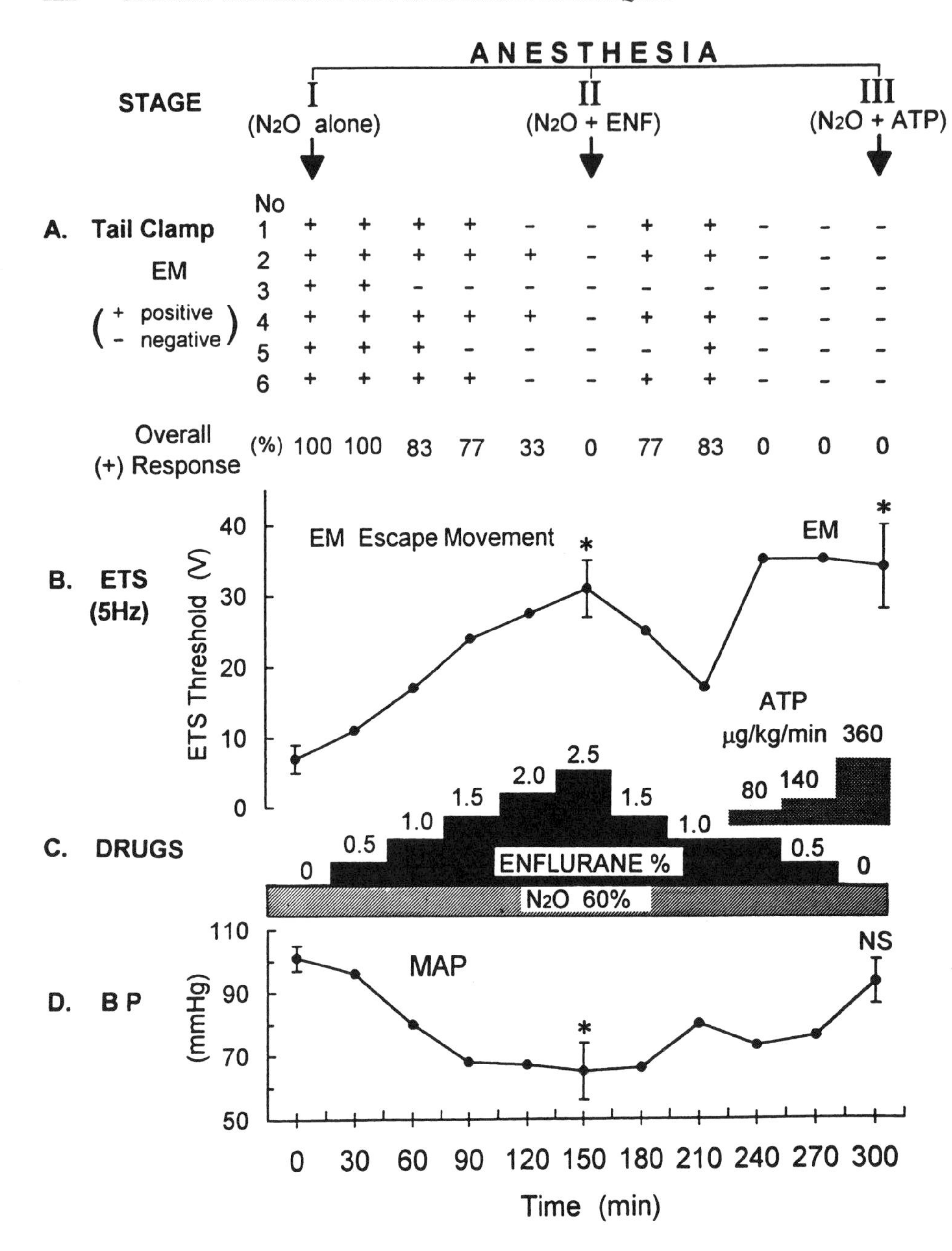

FIGURE 20A-6. A to D, Escape movement (EM) and blood pressure (BP) responses determined at three stages: I, N_2O; II, N_2O + enflurane (ENF); and III, N_2O + ATP with two anesthetic tests: tail clamp and electrical tail stimulation (ETS). Note that ATP completely replaced enflurane. ATP infusion rate: 83±67, 142±117, and 363±165 μg/kg/min at enflurane 1%, 0.5%, and 0% respectively. In contrast to the significant hypotensive effect observed with enflurane (2.5%, stage II), ATP at stage III did not cause significant BP decrease. Mean ± SEM of the results obtained from 6 rabbits. Statistical comparison versus stage I, using ANOVA followed by Dunnett's test. *$p < 0.05$ considered significant; NS, not significant. *(From Fukunaga AF. Purines in Anesthesia. In: Purinergic Approaches in Experimental Therapeutics. (K.A. Jacobson, M.F. Jarvis eds.), Wiley, New York, in press, with permission)*

pressure returned to near control, with normal values at the highest dose of ATP combined with N_2O (see Fig. 20A-6), contrasting with the significantly decreased blood pressure produced by the combination of N_2O and enflurane (2.5%). Moreover, other circulatory and respiratory variables remained unchanged during ATP infusion (Table 20A-3).

Inhibition of Cardiovascular Responses to Noxious Stimulation by Intravenous Adenosine: An Indication of a Sympatholytic Analgesic Effect

Noxious stimulation of various somatic sensory afferent nerves results in significant changes in autonomic-cardiovascular responses including blood pressure and heart rate. These reflex mediated responses have been termed the somatosympathetic reflex (SSR), mediated at spinal and supraspinal sites, and SSR may represent a nociceptive response.

In clinical practice, maintenance of hemodynamic stability during surgical stimulation is considered an indication of adequacy of anesthesia. Measurements of blood pressure and heart rate have been used as indirect indices of the level of sympathetic activity to assess "depth" of anesthesia. During general anesthesia, a principal concern of the anesthesiologist is to manage the acute hemodynamic changes that accompany interventions such as induction of anesthesia, tracheal intubation, painful surgical stimulation (e.g., entering cavitary spaces), and postoperative pain.

Continuous infusion of adenosine (170 to 190 μg/kg/min) titrated according to blood pressure responses during continuous ETS can effectively inhibit behavioral movement, as well as cardiovascular (blood pressure and heart rate) responses to noxious stimuli. In animals receiving 0.5% halothane and a purine infusion, movement was effectively inhibited and hemodynamic stability was maintained throughout the study period. After aminophylline administration, the animals responded with vigorous blood pressure and movement responses to the noxious stimuli (Fig. 20A-7). Cardiovascular and behavioral responses to painful stimuli appeared consistent with increased sympathetic activity. Thus, both adenosine and ATP effectively inhibited both sympathetic and somatic responses caused by noxious stimulation while maintaining circulatory and respiratory functions within normal levels, as confirmed by continuous monitoring (Tables 20A-4 and 20A-5). In another study, the effects of intravenous ATP and sodium nitroprusside (SNP) on the responses to SSR evoked by ETS revealed that increasing doses of intravenous ATP, but not SNP, effectively inhibited all SSR responses to electrical stimuli in a dose-dependent manner. This indicated that inhibition of sympathetic responses was related in part to the sympatholytic and analgesic property of the purines.

TABLE 20A-3. Cardiovascular, Respiratory and Blood Gas Data During Nitrous Oxide Alone, Enflurane/Nitrous Oxide and ATP/Nitrous Oxide in Spontaneously Breathing Rabbits

Stage Drugs	I N_2O Alone	II Enflurane + N_2O	III ATP + N_2O
BP (mmHg)			
systolic	120 ± 15	69 ± 22*	112 ± 20
diastolic	91 ± 11	49 ± 18*	83 ± 16
HR (beats/min)	267 ± 15	255 ± 33*	278 ± 26
Blood Gas			
pH	7.43 ± 0.02	7.42 ± 0.04*	7.45 ± 0.08
$PaCO_2$ (mmHg)	22 ± 2	25 ± 1*	22 ± 3
PaO_2 (mmHg)	147 ± 11	148 ± 16	154 ± 19
BE (mEq/L)	−7 ± 1	−7 ± 2	−7 ± 4
Respiratory Rate (breath/min)	85 ± 5	72 ± 19*	81 ± 14
Rectal Temperature (°C)	38.7 ± 0.3	38.8 ± 0.7	38.6 ± 0.4

*Nitrous oxide (N_2O): 60% in O_2; Enflurane: 2.5 vol %; ATP: 363 ± 165 (μg/kg/min, IV). Mean ± SD; (n=6); Statistical analysis vs. Stage I; * $p < 0.05$ was considered significant.*
(From Fukunaga AF. Purines in Anesthesia. In: Purinergic Approaches in Experimental Therapeutics. (K.A. Jacobson, M.F. Jarvis eds.), Wiley, New York, in press, with permission)

Clinical Considerations

Adenosine compounds do not appear to be readily absorbed by oral administration. ATP administered intravenously is converted rapidly into adenosine in the blood (183). Intravascular adenosine is then rapidly eliminated from vascular spaces, with a half-life of less than 10 seconds (estimated between 0.6 and 9.3 seconds) (184, 185). Therefore, standard pharmacokinetic

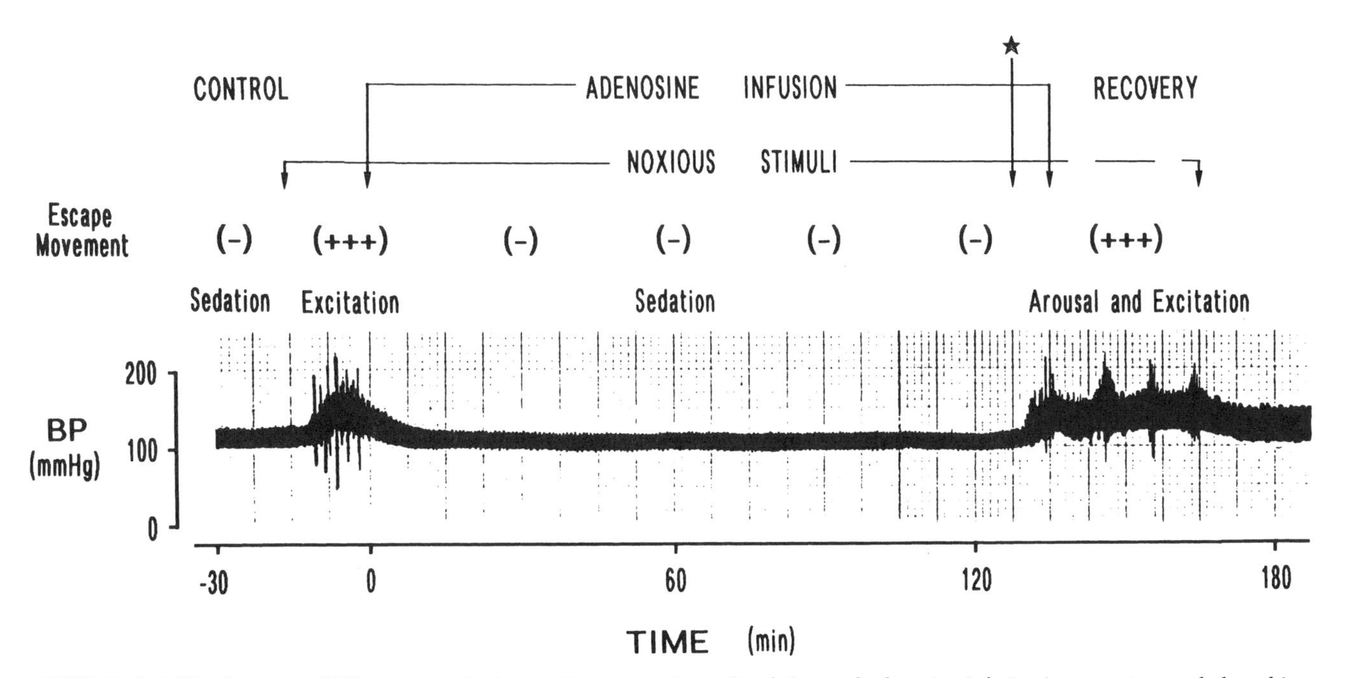

FIGURE 20A-7. Blood pressure (BP) responses during continuous noxious stimulation and adenosine infusion in a spontaneously breathing rabbit sedated with halothane (0.5%). Note the remarkably stable BP (sympatholytic action) during adenosine infusion (170 to 190 μg/kg/min). In contrast, sympathetic excitation caused by noxious stimulation is evidenced before adenosine and after aminophylline ★ (1 mg, injected intrathecally at the high spinal cervical level). Noxious stimulation was induced by electrical tail stimulation (15 V, 50 Hz, 1 ms, square pulse wave). *(From Fukunaga AF. Purines in Anesthesia. In: Purinergic Approaches in Experimental Therapeutics. (K.A. Jacobson, M.F. Jarvis eds.), Wiley, New York, in press, with permission)*

TABLE 20A-4. Cardiovascular, Respiratory and Blood Gas Data During Continuous Electrical Tail Stimulation and Adenosine Infusion in Rabbits Spontaneously Breathing Halothane (0.5%)

		Adenosine Infusion					
Continuous ETS	Control	ETS Onset	30 min	60 min	90 min	120 min	Aminophylline
Infusion Dose							
(μg/kg/min)		0	192 ± 66	176 ± 73	172 ± 76	176 ± 74	176 ± 74
BP (mmHg)							
Systolic	93 ± 13	101 ± 12	82 ± 8	87 ± 10	88 ± 7	88 ± 5	96 ± 24
Diastolic	68 ± 6	72 ± 4	53 ± 12	56 ± 15	54 ± 10	55 ± 13	68 ± 17
Mean	78 ± 9	83 ± 7	65 ± 14	66 ± 13	66 ± 8	66 ± 10	77 ± 19
Heart Rate							
(beat/min)	262 ± 19	282 ± 34	294 ± 22	295 ± 21	295 ± 23	294 ± 20	292 ± 48
Respiratory Rate							
(breath/min)	97 ± 25	109 ± 23	90 ± 14	87 ± 12	89 ± 15	89 ± 16	119 ± 44
Blood Gas							
pH	7.51 ± 0.06	7.51 ± 0.07	7.51 ± 0.09	7.51 ± 0.08	7.52 ± 0.10	7.50 ± 0.10	7.45 ± 0.08
$PaCO_2$ (mmHg)	29 ± 3	28 ± 6	26 ± 6	26 ± 4	24 ± 6	24 ± 5	27 ± 6
PaO_2 (mmHg)	499 ± 32	472 ± 35	479 ± 34	481 ± 41	485 ± 57	492 ± 77	516 ± 37
HCO_3 (mEq/L)	24 ± 4	22 ± 3	21 ± 2	20 ± 1	19 ± 3	19 ± 2	19 ± 2*
BE (mEq/L)	−2 ± 4	−1 ± 4	−1 ± 2	−1 ± 3	−2 ± 3	−2 ± 3	−4 ± 2
Rectal Temperature (°C)	37.6 ± 0.9	38.0 ± 1.4	38.3 ± 1.0	38.5 ± 0.6	38.8 ± 0.7	39.1 ± 0.5	39.3 ± 0.7

*ETS = Electrical Tail Stimulation (square pulse wave, 50Hz, 1ms, 10–20 V); Aminophylline (10 mg/kg IV). Mean ± SD; (n=5); Statistical analysis vs. control; * $p < 0.05$ was considered significant.*
(From Fukunaga AF. Purines in Anesthesia. In: Purinergic Approaches in Experimental Therapeutics. (K.A. Jacobson, M.F. Jarvis eds.), Wiley, New York, in press, with permission)

TABLE 20A-5. Cardiovascular, Respiratory and Blood Gas Data During Continuous Electrical Tail Stimulation and ATP Infusion in Rabbits Spontaneously Breathing Halothane (0.5%)

		ATP Infusion					
Continuous ETS	Control	ETS Onset	30 min	60 min	90 min	120 min	Aminophylline
Infusion Dose							
(μg/kg/min)		0	190 ± 90	150 ± 68	140 ± 69	130 ± 76	130 ± 76
BP (mmHg)							
Systolic	95 ± 22	104 ± 21	87 ± 10	81 ± 9	82 ± 11	82 ± 9	97 ± 10
Diastolic	72 ± 11	74 ± 12	60 ± 7	56 ± 4	58 ± 3	55 ± 6	72 ± 9
Mean	81 ± 15	86 ± 17	71 ± 7	66 ± 5	67 ± 6	67 ± 7	80 ± 9
Heart Rate							
(beat/min)	259 ± 19	270 ± 53	273 ± 41	265 ± 16	262 ± 23	264 ± 16	315 ± 35
Respiratory Rate							
(breath/min)	109 ± 36	122 ± 41	111 ± 36	105 ± 35	106 ± 33	99 ± 29	96 ± 20
Blood Gas							
pH	7.51 ± 0.03	7.51 ± 0.05	7.54 ± 0.05	7.54 ± 0.03	7.55 ± 0.03	7.56 ± 0.03	7.52 ± 0.05
$PaCO_2$ (mmHg)	22 ± 4	21 ± 3	19 ± 4	19 ± 4	18 ± 2	18 ± 2	17 ± 2
PaO_2 (mmHg)	512 ± 39	517 ± 23	502 ± 30	529 ± 29	536 ± 39	555 ± 9	533 ± 17
HCO_3 (mEq/L)	18 ± 3	17 ± 4	16 ± 2	16 ± 3	16 ± 2	16 ± 3	14 ± 3
BE (mEq/L)	−3 ± 3	−4 ± 4	−4 ± 1	−4 ± 3	−4 ± 2	−4 ± 3	−6 ± 4
Rectal Temperature (°C)	39.2 ± 0.6	39.6 ± 0.9	39.9 ± 0.9	39.8 ± 0.8	39.8 ± 0.7	39.8 ± 0.4	39.6 ± 0.2

*ETS = Electrical Tail Stimulation (square pulse wave, 50Hz, 1ms, 10–20 V); Aminophylline (10 mg/kg IV). Mean ± SD; (n=5); Statistical analysis vs. control; * $p < 0.05$ was considered significant.*
(From Fukunaga AF. Purines in Anesthesia. In: Purinergic Approaches in Experimental Therapeutics. (K.A. Jacobson, M.F. Jarvis eds.), Wiley, New York, in press, with permission)

descriptors are difficult to define (186). Adenosine's primary routes of elimination are cellular uptake by simple or facilitated diffusion by a nucleoside transport system and metabolism to inosine by adenosine deaminase, with further degradation of inosine to hypoxanthine, xanthine, and eventually to uric acid (see Fig. 20A-2).

A marked difference occurs in the clinical responses when adenosine (or ATP) is administered as a bolus injection versus as a continuous infusion. When injected as a bolus, these agents produce dose-related negative chronotropic and dromotropic effects (6). However, during continuous infusion even at high doses (187, 188), these effects are unusual and are rapidly reversed by lowering or discontinuing the infusion. Because of their short plasma half-life, these purines must be continuously infused to achieve the desired pharmacologic responses. The rapid responses to adenosine-induced hemodynamic changes, which allow easy titration of an effective dose in response to changing surgical stimuli, can be advantageous during the perioperative period. Further, the absence of accumulation and toxic effects during intravenous adenosine administration may be highly useful when this agent is given as an adjuvant during clinical anesthesia.

Studies in Volunteers

Intravenous ATP (100 μg/kg/min) administered in a peripheral vein of the forearm in volunteers potentiated the sedative and hypnogenic effects of midazolam in a double-blind placebo-controlled study (189). The degree of sedation, amnesia, anxiolysis, sleepiness, and impairment of psychomotor function (Romberg test) were assessed in this study (190). Coadministration of ATP and midazolam significantly increased the sedation scores as compared with midazolam alone, without producing side effects such as hypotension, or respiratory depression, which was in agreement with laboratory data (190).

Adenosine or Adenosine Triphosphate as Anesthetic Adjuvant

In most anesthetic practices, combinations of drugs are used to fulfill the requirements of general anesthesia. Often, small doses of a combination of intravenous and inhaled drugs are used to avoid the adverse effects of using a large dose of any single agent (191). Indeed, the low safety ratio (toxic/therapeutic doses) and the inherent dangers of the commonly used anesthetics are well recognized. Accordingly, a drug with rapid antiadrenergic sympatholytic and analgesic properties, which is devoid of respiratory depression, is capable of reducing the requirement of inhaled anesthetics, intravenous hypnotics, and/or opioids, and is easily titratable, appears to have potential advantages as an anesthetic adjuvant. Indeed, intravenous infusion of ATP could effectively reduce up to 50% of the anesthetic requirement for inhaled agents in patients undergoing major surgical procedures such as maxillofacial orthognathic surgery and surgery of the abdomen and extremities (192). Other investigators have found that ATP infusion combined with low doses of inhaled anesthetics (isoflurane and N_2O) was useful for surgery requiring intraoperative somatosensory evoked potential monitoring (193). In agreement with the purines' sympatholytic-analgesic activity, ATP attenuated the autonomic responses to stressful surgical stimulation. In operations involving painful intra-abdominal manipulations (e.g., resection and retraction of visceral organs) in which acute hypertensive responses accompanied by tachyarrhytmias are common, ATP in combination with N_2O and midazolam (194) maintained hemodynamic stability intraoperatively. Moreover, investigators observed that hypertension, a common occurrence during the early postoperative period, was attenuated even after ATP had been discontinued.

Maintenance of hemodynamic stability is a challenge during cardiac surgery as a result of the stress responses associated with sympathetic activation and concomitant increases in catecholamines (195). The use of ATP in combination with fentanyl effectively inhibited the cardiovascular responses to sternotomy and sternal spread and improved myocardial oxygen balance in patients undergoing coronary artery bypass surgery (196). The potent vasodilating, antiadrenergic (counteracting circulating catecholamine effects), sympatholytic (presynaptic inhibition of NE release), and analgesic properties of ATP contributed to inhibiting the responses to intense surgical stimulation. Indeed, Hashimoto and colleagues (197) demonstrated that, in patients undergoing cardiopulmonary bypass who had high blood perfusion pressure, serum catecholamines were significantly reduced in patients receiving ATP infusions, whereas no significant changes were noted in other vasoactive mediators (e.g., eicosanoid, angiotensin II, and endothelin). Thus, ATP has been found to be a safe and effective agent for stabilizing the perfusion pressure during stressful surgical procedures.

Other investigators demonstrated that adenosine infusions (70 to 130 μg/kg/min) could replace perioperative opioid administration during isoflurane-N_2O anesthesia (198). Segerdahl and colleagues reported that adenosine, 80 μg/kg/min, could significantly reduce the requirement of isoflurane in patients undergoing breast surgery (199), as well as in patients undergoing hysterectomy (200). In agreement with earlier studies (192), these authors confirmed that more stable hemodynamics was achieved in the adenosine-treated group. Moreover, additional benefits (e.g., reduction of blood loss) have been reported during the perioperative period.

Intraoperative Control of Blood Pressure Using Adenosine and Adenosine Triphosphate

Intravenous administration of adenosine compounds induces potent vasodilation by A_2 receptor activation. The hypotensive actions of adenosine and ATP are rapid in onset and dissipate rapidly following discontinuation of the infusion. Hypotension can be easily maintained during deliberate hypotensive anesthesia without tachycardia, tachyphylaxis, or rebound hypertension (187, 201-203). The vasodilatory action of adenosine is reversible within a few minutes (2 to 5 minutes) after the infusion is discontinued. The decrease in blood pressure is characterized by a decrease in peripheral vascular resistance (afterload reduction) and an increase in cardiac output and stroke volume, without significant tachycardia. In addition, one sees an increase in coronary blood flow, a reduction in myocardial and whole-body oxygen consumption, and avoidance of anerboic metabolism, as indicated by low plasma lactate levels (204). Systemic arterial pressure is decreased in a dose-dependent manner, with well-maintained right and left heart filling pressures and a stable heart rate (202).

Prevention or Attenuation of Hypertensive Crisis During Anesthesia

LARYNGOSCOPY AND TRACHEAL INTUBATION. Laryngoscopy and tracheal intubation cause acute hemodynamic responses such as hypertension, tachycardia, and arrhythmias that may be of concern in patients with compromised cerebrovascular and cardiovascular disease. Increases in blood pressure of 115 mm Hg systolic and 54 mm Hg diastolic parallel the increases in plasma NE levels (205). Acute hemodynamic responses have traditionally been treated with opioid analgesics or drugs that act peripherally to reduce the cardiovascular responses (e.g., α- or β-adrenergic blockers or vasodilators). The use of purines reduces the sympathetic outflow (i.e., central sympatholysis), counteracts the effects of circulating catecholamines (antiadrenergic action), and dilates peripheral vessels (direct arteriolar dilatation). ATP effectively inhibits the pressor response to laryngoscopy while attenuating the rate pressure product after tracheal intubation (206).

TUMOR REMOVAL OF PHEOCHROMOCYTOMA AND NEUROBLASTOMA. Prevention of acute hypertensive crisis is important in the anesthetic management of patients undergoing pheochromocytoma removal. Severe hypertension and cardiac arrhythmias occur as a result of massive release of catecholamine during resection of the tumor. Perioperative administration of α-adrenergic and β-adrenoceptor blocking agents (e.g., phentolamine, phenoxybenzamine, and propranolol) is essential. However, adenosine or ATP is more effective in controlling blood pressure and preventing hypertensive crisis and ventricular arrhythmias during the intraoperative period because of the potent antiadrenergic and vasodilating properties of these agents. The effectiveness of both ATP and adenosine has been demonstrated in patients during anesthesia maintained with halothane-N_2O or enflurane-N_2O (207), sevoflurane-N_2O (208), isoflurane-fentanyl (209), and isoflurane-N_2O (210).

In a 1-month-old infant who experienced severe hypertension and elevated plasma NE levels, blood pressure was effectively controlled by intravenous adenosine during dissection and manipulation of pelvic neuroblastoma (211).

Adenosine in Postoperative Care

Surgical Stress Inflammatory Responses and Wound Healing

Postoperative immunologic and inflammatory responses are a progression of complex interrelated events that occur in response to stress and tissue injury induced by surgical trauma. Potential inflammatory mediators such as increased polymorphonuclear leukocytes and cytokines can be released by activated monocytes-macrophages that may lead to considerable cell damage in tissues (212). Investigators have reported that purines are involved in modulation of inflammation (213), and adenosine release may be a cellular response to tissue stimulation or injury. Adenosine exhibits various anti-inflammatory activities including reduced cytokine production and inhibition of activated neutrophil-mediated oxygen free radicals generation (214). In patients with sepsis, endogenous adenosine may counteract inflammatory tissue damage by inhibiting the release by polymorphonuclear leukocytes of toxic superoxide anions and granular enzymes, and by inhibiting tumor necrosis factor-α production, which has been shown to be inhibited by 2-chloroadenosine (215). Adenosine and ATP have been reported to prevent joint tissue injury (216), and adenosine receptor agonists have anti-inflammatory effects in acute models of carrageenan-induced pleural inflammation (217).

In wound healing, progression of neovascularity is evident. Capillaries normally proliferate during inflammation and tissue repair. Adenosine has been suggested to play a role in angiogenesis (218). In addition to increased blood flow implicated as a physical factor involving capillary growth, direct chemical stimulation from locally increased concentrations of adenosine is believed to influence in part the neovascularization process because of its ability to stimulate endothelial cell proliferation and migration. Long-term administration of adenosine has increased capillary growth in the heart and skeletal muscle (219).

Delivery of oxygen to tissues is probably the most important determinant for wound healing and resistance to infection. Impaired oxygen supply contributes to infection and defective repair in surgical patients. Increasing blood supply permits more rapid accumulation of collagen, enhances the angiogenic response, and accelerates wound healing. Because systemic administration of purines decreases peripheral vascular resistance and increases regional blood flow, adenosine may conceivably improve tissue oxygenation in the extracellular environment and thereby promote wound healing.

Postoperative Pain and Stress

Postoperatively, vasoconstriction and thromboembolism are major causes of morbidity and mortality. Surgical trauma and subsequent postoperative pain and stress accompanied by increased sympathetic activity and high plasma catecholamines can affect platelet functions (i.e., increase platelet aggregation, decrease platelet survival) and promote thrombus formation (220), predisposing postoperative patients to vasospasm and thromboembolization. In addition to their sympatholytic, antiadrenergic and direct peripheral vasodilating effects, the purines are reported to regulate human platelet function. Adenosine- and ATP-mediated inhibition of platelet aggregation appears to be antithrombogenic and has been implicated in reducing the risk of thrombosis (221).

Providing adequate pain control is important following surgery. Opioid analgesics remain the most important component of modern pain management. However, these compounds produce respiratory depression, pruritus, nausea, vomiting, and urinary retention, among other opioid-related side-effects. Delayed respiratory depression has occurred 3 to 24 hours after injection (222, 223). Hence, aggressive use of opioid analgesics is restricted to intensive care settings, where constant vigilance can diminish the potential for serious adverse sequelae (224). Intraoperative analgesia produced by the purine compounds may permit more effective analgesia during the postoperative period. Adenosine's analgesic activity has been reported well beyond the time that their infusion has been discontinued (199). Continuing the infusion of purines into the postoperative period may provide additional benefits in attenuating sympathoadrenal responses (225, 226).

In summary, intravenous adenosine can enhance the retaliatory and protective property of the endogenous purine to inhibit surgical pain, as well as the autonomic and cardiovascular responses during the perioperative period. Adenosine's rapid cardiovascular action, which can respond to hemodynamic changes induced by acute and varied surgical stimuli, may be advantageous for ease of titration. The ability to achieve hemodynamic stability rapidly during the operation would minimize the therapeutic requirement for conventional anesthetics and during the perioperative period provide for prompt emergence from anesthesia while decreasing the risk of overdosage and other side effects. The sympatholytic analgesic effects of a "physiologic" substance, without increasing cardiorespiratory depression, appear to be highly desirable attributes in clinical for intravenous anesthesia.

NOTE AND ADDENDUM

The subtypes of adenosine/P_1 purinoceptors are designated as A_1, A_2, A_3 receptors and are further divided into A_{2a}, A_{2b} receptors. A rapid growing number of P_2 purinoceptor subtypes, sensitive to ATP and other purine nucleotides, have been described recently. The original criteria for distinguishing the purinoceptors have been continuously updated and modified with the availability of new information (227).

REFERENCES

1. Drury AN, Szent-Gyorgyi A. The physiological activity of adenine compounds with special reference to their action upon the mammalian heart. J Physiol 1929;68:213–237.
2. Phillis JW, Wu PH. The role of adenosine and its nucleotides in central synaptic transmission. Prog Neurobiol 1981;16:187–239.
3. Stone TW. Physiological roles for adenosine and adenosine 5'-triphosphate in the nervous system. Neuroscience 1981;6:523–555.
4. Dunwiddie TV. The physiological role of adenosine in the central nervous system. Int Rev Neurobiol 1985;27:63–139.
5. Gordon JL. Extracellular ATP: effects, sources and fate. Biochem J 1986;233:309–319.
6. Belardinelli L, Linden J, Berne RM. The cardiac effects of adenosine. Prog Cardiovasc Dis 1989;32:73–97.
7. Olsson RA, Pearson JD. Cardiovascular purinoceptors. Physiol Rev 1990; 70:761–845.
8. Daval JL, Nehlig A, Nicolas F. Physiological and pharmacological properties of adenosine: therapeutic implications. Life Sci 1991;49:1435–1453.
9. Gatell JA, Barner HB, Shevde K. Adenosine and myocardial protection. J Cardiothorac Vasc Anesth 1993;7:466–480.
10. Daly JW, Kuroda, Y, Phillis JW, eds. Physiology and pharmacology of adenosine derivatives. New York: Raven Press, 1983.
11. Bruns RF, Davis RE, Ninteman FW, et al. Adenosine antagonists as pharmacological tools. In: Paton DM, ed. Adenosine and adenine nucleotides: physiology and pharmacology. London: Taylor & Francis, 1988:39–49.
12. Williams M, ed. Adenosine and adenosine receptors. Clifton, NJ: Humana Press, 1990.
13. Ribeiro JA, ed. Adenosine receptors in the nervous system. London: Taylor & Francis, 1989.
14. Dubyak GR, Fedan JS eds. Biological actions of extracellular ATP. New York: New York Academy of Sciences, 1990.
15. Imai S, Nakazawa M, eds. Role of adenosine and adenine nucleotides in the biological system. Amsterdam: Elsevier, 1991.
16. Phillis JW, ed. Adenosine and adenine nucleotides as regulators of cellular function. Boca Raton, FL: CRC Press, 1991.
17. Belardinelli L, Pelleg A, eds. Adenosine and adenine nucleotides: from molecular biology to integrative physiology. Boston: Kluwer Academic, 1995.
18. Fredholm BB, Hedqvist P. Modulation of neurotransmission by purine nucleotides and nucleosides. Biochem Pharmacol 1980; 29:1635–1643.
19. Williams M. Adenosine: a selective neuromodulator in the mammalian CNS? Trends Neurosci 1984;7:164–168.
20. Snyder SH. Adenosine as a neuromodulator. Annu Rev Neurosci 1985;8:103–124.
21. Burnstock G. Purinergic nerves. Pharmacol Rev 1972;24:509–581.
22. White, TD. Role of adenine compounds in autonomic *neuro*transmission. Pharmacol Ther 1988;38:129–168.
23. Silinsky EM. Purinergic effects in autonomic ganglia. In: Phillis JW, ed. Adenosine and adenine nucleotides as regulators of cellular function. Boca Raton, FL: CRC Press, 1991:319–327.
24. McIlwain H, Poll JD. Adenosine in cerebral homeostatic role: appraisal through actions of homocysteine, colchicine, and dipyridamole. J Neurobiol 1986;17:39–49.

25. Williams M. Adenosine: the prototypic neuromodulator. Neurochem Int 1989; 14:249–264.
26. Schrader J. Adenosine: a homeostatic metabolite in cardiac energy metabolism. Circulation 1990;81:389–391.
27. Arch JRS, Newsholme EA. The control of the metabolism and the hormonal role of adenosine. Essays Biochem 1978;14:88–123.
28. Berne RM. Cardiac nucleotides in hypoxia: possible role in regulation of coronary blood flow. Am J Physiol 1963;204:317–322.
29. Kleihues P, Kobayashi K, Hossmann KA. Purine nucleotide metabolism in the cat brain after one hour of complete ischemia. J Neurochem 1974;23:417–425.
30. Berne RM, Rubio R, Curnish RR. Release of adenosine from ischemic brain. Circ Res 1974; 35:262–271.
31. Newby AC. Adenosine and the concept of "retaliatory metabolites." Trends Biochem Sci 1984;9:42–44.
32. Sparks HV Jr, Bardenheuer H. Regulation of adenosine formation by the heart. Circ Res 1986;58:193–201.
33. Bruns RF. Adenosine receptors: roles and pharmacology. Ann N Y Acad Sci 1990;603:211–226.
34. Burnstock G. A basis for distinguishing two types of purinergic receptor. In: Straub RW, Bolis L, eds. Cell membrane receptors for drugs and hormones: a multidisciplinary approach. New York: Raven Press, 1978:107–118.
35. Londos C, Wolff J. Two distinct adenosine-sensitive sites on adenylate cyclase. Proc Natl Acad Sci U S A 1977;74:5482–5486.
36. Van Calker D, Muller M, Hamprecht B. Adenosine inhibits the accumulation of cyclic AMP in cultured brain cells. Nature 1978;276:839–841.
37. Van Calker D, Muller M, Hamprecht B. Adenosine regulates via two different types of receptors, the accumulation of cyclic AMP in cultured brain cells. J Neurochem 1979;33:999–1005.
38. Londos C, Cooper DMF, Wolff J. Subclasses of external adenosine receptors. Proc Natl Acad Sci U S A 1980;77:2551–2554.
39. Dunwiddie TV, Proctor WR. Mechanisms underlying physiological responses to adenosine in the central nervous system. In: Gerlach E, Becker BF, eds. Topics and perspectives in adenosine research. Berlin: Springer-Verlag, 1987:499–508.
40. Ribeiro JA, Sebastiao AM. Adenosine receptors and calcium: basis for proposing a third (A_3) adenosine receptor. Prog Neurobiol 1986;26:179–209.
41. Trussell LO, Jackson MB. Dependence of an adenosine-activated potassium current on a GTP-binding protein in mammalian central neurons. J Neurosci 1987;7:3306–3316.
42. Dart C, Standen NB. Adenosine-activated potassium current in smooth muscle cells isolated from the pig coronary artery. J Physiol 1993;471:767–786.
43. Delahunty TM, Cronin MJ, Linden J. Regulation of GH_3-cell function via adenosine A_1 receptors: inhibition of prolactin release, cyclic AMP production and inositol phosphate generation. Biochem J 1988;255:69–77.
44. Arend LJ, Handler JS, Rhim JS, et al. Adenosine-sensitive phosphoinositide turnover in a newly established renal cell line. Am J Physiol 1989;256:F1067–F1074.
45. Hamprecht B, van Calker D. Nomenclature of adenosine receptors. Trends Pharmacol Sci 1985;6:153–154.
46. Daly JW, Bruns RF, Snyder SH. Adenosine receptors in the central nervous system: relationship to the central actions of methylxanthines. Life Sci 1981;28:2083–2097.
47. Sattin A, Rall TW. The effect of adenosine and adenine nucleotides on the cyclic adenosine 3′,5′-phosphate content of guinea pig cerebral cortex slices. Mol Pharmacol 1970;6:13–23.
48. Snyder SH, Katims JJ, Annau Z, et al. Adenosine receptors and behavioral actions of methylxanthines. Proc Natl Acad Sci U S A 1981;78:3260–3264.
49. Katims JJ, Annau Z, Snyder SH. Interactions in the behavioral effects of methylxanthines and adenosine derivatives. J Pharmacol Exp Ther 1983;227:167–173.
50. Williams M. Adenosine antagonists. Med Res Rev 1989;9:219–243.
51. Trivedi BK, Bridges AJ, Bruns RF. Structure-activity relationships of adenosine A_1 and A_2 receptors. In: Williams M, ed. Adenosine and adenosine receptors. Clifton, NJ: Humana Press, 1990:57–103.
52. Jarvis MF, Williams M. Adenosine in central nervous system function. In: Williams M, ed. Adenosine and adenosine receptors. Clifton, NJ: Humana Press, 1990:423–474.
53. Phillis JW, Edstrom JP, Kostopoulos GK, Kirkpatrick JR. Effects of adenosine and adenine nucleotides on synaptic transmission in the cerebral cortex. Can J Physiol Pharmacol 1979;57:1289–1312.
54. Dunwiddie TV. Electrophysiological aspects of adenosine receptor function. In: Williams M, ed. Adenosine and adenosine receptors. Clifton, NJ: Humana Press, 1990:143–172.
55. Greene RW, Haas HL. The electrophysiology of adenosine in the mammalian central nervous system. Prog Neurobiol 1991; 36:329–341.
56. Fredholm BB, Dunwiddie TV. How does adenosine inhibit transmitter release? Trends Pharmacol Sci 1988;9:130–134.
57. Barraco RA. Behavioral actions of adenosine and related substances. In: Phillis JW, ed. Adenosine and adenine nucleotides as regulators of cellular function. Boca Raton, FL: CRC Press, 1991:339–366.
58. Barraco RA, Coffin VL, Altman HJ, Phillis JW. Central effects of adenosine analogs on locomotor activity in mice and antagonism of caffeine. Brain Res 1983;272:392–395.
59. Barraco RA, Bryant SD. Depression of locomotor activity following bilateral injections of adenosine analogs into the striatum of mice. Med Sci Res 1987;15:421–422.
60. Barraco RA, Martens KA, Parizon M, Normile HJ. Adenosine A_{2a} receptors in the nucleus accumbens mediate locomotor depression. Brain Res Bull 1993;31:397–404.
61. Dunwiddie TV, Worth T. Sedative and anticonvulsant effects of adenosine analogs in mouse and rat. J Pharmacol Exp Ther 1982;220:70–76.
62. Crawley JN, Patel J, Marangos PJ. Behavioral characterization of two long-lasting adenosine analogs: sedative properties and interaction with diazepam. Life Sci 1981;29:2623–2630.
63. Radulovacki M, Miletich RS, Green RD. N^6 (L-phenylisopropyl)adenosine (L-PIA) increases slow-wave sleep (S_2) and decreases wakefulness in rats. Brain Res 1982;246:178–180.
64. Radulovacki M, Virus RM, Djuricic-Nedelson M, Green RD. Adenosine analogs and sleep in rats. J Pharmacol Exp Ther 1984;228:268–274.
65. Martin JV, Berman KF, Skolnick P, Mendelson WB. Behavioral and electroencephalographic effects of the $adenosine_1$ agonist, L-PIA. Pharmacol Biochem Behav 1989;34:507–510.
66. Phillis JW, Wu PH. Adenosine mediates sedative action of various centrally active drugs. Med Hypotheses 1982;9:361–367.
67. Williams M, Risley EA. Interaction of putative anxiolytic agents with central adenosine receptors. Can J Physiol Pharmacol 1981;59:897–900.
68. Bruns RF, Katims JJ, Annau Z, et al. Adenosine receptor interactions and anxiolytics. Neuropharmacology 1983;22:1523–1529.
69. Phillis JW, Wu PH, Bender AS. Inhibition of adenosine uptake into rat brain synaptosomes by the benzodiazepines. Gen Pharmacol 1981;12:67–70.
70. Phillis JW. Adenosine's role in the central actions of the benzodiazepines. Prog Neuropsychopharmacol Biol Psychiatry 1984;8:495–502.
71. Phillis JW, O'Regan MH. Benzodiazepines interaction with adenosine systems explains some anomalies in GABA hypothesis. Trends Pharmacol Sci 1988;9:153–154.

72. Phillis JW, O'Regan MH. The role of adenosine in the central actions of the benzodiazepines. Prog Neuropsychopharmacol Biol Psychiatry 1988;12:389–404.
73. Phillis JW, Bender AS, Wu PH. Benzodiazepine inhibit adenosine uptake into rat brain synaptosomes. Brain Res 1980; 195:494–498.
74. Phillis JW. Diazepam potentiation of purinergic depression of central neurons. Can J Physiol Pharmacol 1979;57:432–435.
75. Phillis JW, Edstrom JP, Ellis SW, Kirkpatrick JR. Theophylline antagonizes flurazepam-induced depression of cerebral cortical neurons. Can J Physiol Pharmacol 1979;57:917–920.
76. Phillis JW, Siemens RK, Wu PH. Effects of diazepam on adenosine and acetylcholine release from rat cerebral cortex: further evidence for a purinergic mechanism in action of diazepam. Br J Pharmacol 1980;70:341–348.
77. Jhamandas K, Dumbrille A. Regional release of [^{3}H] adenosine derivatives from rat brain in vivo: effect of excitatory amino acids, opiate agonists, and benzodiazepines. Can J Physiol Pharmacol 1980;58:1262–1278.
78. Hammond JR, Paterson ARP, Clanachan AS. Benzodiazepine inhibition of site-specific binding of nitrobenzylthioinosine, an inhibitor of adenosine transport. Life Sci 1981;29:2207–2214.
79. Barraco RA, Phillis JW, DeLong RE. Behavioral interaction of adenosine and diazepam in mice. Brain Res 1984;323:159–163.
80. Hawkins M, Pravica M, Radulovacki M. Chronic administration of diazepam downregulates adenosine receptors in the rat brain. Pharmacol Biochem Behav 1988;30:303–308.
81. Hawkins M, Hajduk P, O'Connor S, et al. Effects of prolonged administration of triazolam on adenosine A_1 and A_2 receptors in the brain of rats. Brain Res 1989;505:141–144.
82. Polc P, Bonetti EP, Pieri L, et al. Caffeine antagonizes several central effects of diazepam. Life Sci 1981;28:2265–2275.
83. Mattila MJ, Nuotto E. Caffeine and theophylline counteract diazepam effects in man. Med Biol 1983;61:337–343.
84. Marrosu F, Marchi A, De Martino MR, et al. Aminophylline antagonizes diazepam-induced anesthesia and EEG changes in humans. Psychopharmacology 1985;69–70.
85. Roache JD, Griffiths RR. Interactions of diazepam and caffeine: behavioral and subjective dose effects in humans. Pharmacol Biochem Behav 1987;26:801–812.
86. Gurel A, Elevli M, Hamulu A. Aminophylline reversal of flunitrazepam sedation. Anesth Analg 1987;66:333–336.
87. Lohse MJ, Lenschow V, Schwabe U. Interaction of barbiturates with adenosine receptors in rat brain. Naunyn Schmiedebergs Arch Pharmacol 1984;326:69–74.
88. Lohse MJ, Klotz KN, Jakobs KH, Schwabe U. Barbiturates are selective antagonists at A_1 adenosine receptors. J Neurochem 1985;45:1761–1770.
89. Lohse MJ, Brenner AS, Jackisch R. Pentobarbital antagonizes the A_1 adenosine receptor-mediated inhibition of hippocampal neurotransmitter release. J Neurochem 1987;49:189–194.
90. Lohse MJ, Boser S, Klotz KN, Schwabe U. Affinities of barbiturates for the GABA-receptor complex and A_1 adenosine receptors: a possible explanation of their excitatory effects. Naunyn Schmiedebergs Arch Pharmacol 1987;336:211–217.
91. Sawynok J, Sweeney MI. The role of purines in nociception. Neuroscience 1989;32:557–569.
92. Sawynok J. Adenosine and pain. In: Phillis JW, ed. Adenosine and adenine nucleotides as regulators of cellular function. Boca Raton, FL: CRC Press, 1991:391–400.
93. Vapaatalo H, Onken D, Neuvonen PJ, Westermann E. Stereospecificity in some central and circulatory effects of phenylisopropyl-adenosine (PIA). Arzneimittelforschung 1975;25:407–410.
94. Yarbrough GG, McGuffin-Clineschmidt JC. In vivo behavioral assessment of central nervous system purinergic receptors. Eur J Pharmacol 1981;76:137–144.
95. Holmgren M, Hednar T, Nordberg G, Mellstrand T. Antinociceptive effects in the rat of an adenosine analogue, N^6-phenylisopropyladenosine. J Pharm Pharmacol 1983;35:679–680.
96. Holmgren M, Hedner J, Mellstrand T, et al. Characterization of the antinociceptive effects of some adenosine analogues in the rat. Naunyn Schmiedebergs Arch Pharmacol 1986;334:290–293.
97. Post C. Antinociceptive effects in mice after intrathecal injection of 5′-N-ethylcarboxamide adenosine. Neurosci Lett 1984; 51:325–330.
98. Sawynok J, Sweeney MI, White TD. Classification of adenosine receptors mediating antinociception in the rat spinal cord. Br J Pharmacol 1986;88:923–930.
99. Doi T, Kuzuna S, Maki Y. Spinal antinociceptive effects of adenosine compounds in mice. Eur J Pharmacol 1987;137:227–231.
100. Herrick-Davis K, Chippari S, Luttinger D, Ward SJ. Evaluation of adenosine agonists as potential analgesics. Eur J Pharmacol 1989;162:365–369.
101. Sosnowski M, Yaksh TL. Role of spinal adenosine receptors in modulating the hyperesthesia produced by spinal glycine receptor antagonism. Anesth Analg 1989;69:587–592.
102. Sosnowski M, Stevens CW, Yaksh TL. Assessment of the role of A_1/A_2 adenosine receptors mediating the purine antinociception, motor and autonomic function in the rat spinal cord. J Pharmacol Exp Ther 1989;250:915–921.
103. Salter MW, Henry JL. Physiological characteristics of responses of wide dynamic range spinal neurones to cutaneously applied vibration in the cat. Brain Res 1989;507:69–84.
104. Smith MA, Maehara Y, Ide Y, et al. Suppression of rat spinal WDR neuronal responses to visceral stimulation by the adenosine receptor agonist L-phenyl-isopropyl adenosine. Anesth Analg 1996;82:S420.
105. Bleehen T, Keele CA. Observations on the algogenic actions of adenosine compounds on the human blister base preparation. Pain 1977;3:367–377.
106. Sylven C, Beermann B, Edlund A, et al. Provocation of chest pain in patients with coronary insufficiency using the vasodilator adenosine. Eur Heart J 1988;9 (suppl):6–10.
107. Biaggioni I. Contrasting excitatory and inhibitory effects of adenosine in blood pressure regulation. Hypertension 1992; 20:457–465.
108. Sylven C, Jonzon B, Fredholm BB, Kaijser L. Adenosine injection into the brachial artery produces ischamia-like pain or discomfort in the forearm. Cardiovasc Res 1988;22:674–678.
109. Geiger JD, LaBella FS, Nagy JI. Characterization and localization of adenosine receptors in rat spinal cord. J Neurosci 1984; 4:2303–2310.
110. Salter MW, Henry JL. Effects of adenosine 5′-monophosphate and adenosine 5′-triphosphate on functionally identified units in the cat spinal dorsal horn: evidence for a differential effect of adenosine 5′-triphosphate on nociceptive vs non-nociceptive units. Neuroscience 1985;15:815–825.
111. Geiger JD, Nagy JI. Localization of [^{3}H] nitrobenzylthioinosine binding sites in rat spinal cord and primary afferent neurons. Brain Res 1985;347:321–327.
112. Geiger JD, Nagy JI. Distribution of adenosine deaminase activity in rat brain and spinal cord. J Neurosci 1986;6:2707–2714.
113. Salter MW, Henry JL. Evidence that adenosine mediates the depression of spinal dorsal horn neurons induced by peripheral vibration in the cat. Neuroscience 1987;22:631–650.
114. Choca JI, Proudfit HK, Green RD. Identification of A_1 and A_2 adenosine receptors in the rat spinal cord. J Pharmacol Exp Ther 1987;242:905–910.
115. Choca JI, Green RD, Proudfit HK. Adenosine A_1 and A_2 receptors of the substantia gelatinosa are located predominantly on intrinsic neurons: an autoradiography study. J Pharmacol Exp Ther 1988;247:757–764.
116. Fredholm BB. Adenosine receptors in the central nervous system. News Physiol Sci 1995;10:122–128.

117. Trussell LO, Jackson MB. Adenosine-activated potassium conductance in cultured striatal neurons. Proc Natl Acad Sci U S A 1985;82:4857–4861.
118. Ocana M, Del Pozo E, Barrios M, et al. An ATP-dependent potassium channel blocker antagonizes morphine analgesia. Eur J Pharmacol 1990;186:377–378.
119. Ocana M, Baeyens JM. Differential effects of K^+ channel blockers on antinociception induced by α_2-adrenoceptor, $GABA_B$ and K-opioid receptor agonists. Br J Pharmacol 1993;110:1049–1054.
120. Narita M, Suzuki T, Misawa M, et al. Role of central ATP-sensitive potassium channels in the analgesic effect and spinal noradrenaline turnover-enhancing effect of intracerebroventricularly injected morphine in mice. Brain Res 1992;596:209–214.
121. Ocana M, Baeyens JM. Role of ATP-sensitive K^+ channels in antinociception induced by R-PIA, an adenosine A_1 receptor agonist. Naunyn Schmiedebergs Arch Pharmacol 1994;350: 57–62.
122. Ho IK, Loh HH, Way EL. Cyclic adenosine monophosphate antagonism of morphine analgesia. J Pharmacol Exp Ther 1973; 185:336–346.
123. Fredholm BB, Vernet L. Morphine increases depolarization induced purine release from rat cortical slices. Acta Physiol Scand 1978;104:502–504.
124. Stone TW. The effects of morphine and methionine-enkephalin on the release of purines from cerebral cortex slices of rats and mice. Br J Pharmacol 1981;74:171–176.
125. Wu PH, Phillis JW, Yuen H. Morphine enhances the release of ^{3}H-purines from rat brain cerebral cortical prisms. Pharmacol Biochem Behav 1982;17:749–755.
126. Phillis JW, Jiang ZG, Chelack BJ, Wu PH. Morphine enhances adenosine release from the in vivo rat cerebral cortex. Eur J Pharmacol 1979;65:97–100.
127. Jiang ZG, Chelack BJ, Phillis JW. Effects of morphine and caffeine on adenosine release from rat cerebral cortex: is caffeine a morphine antagonist. Can J Physiol Pharmacol 1980;58:1513–1515.
128. Stone TW, Perkins MN. Is adenosine the mediator of opiate action on neuronal firing rate? Nature 1979;281:227–228.
129. Perkins MN, Stone TW. Blockade of striatal neurone responses to morphine by aminophylline: evidence for adenosine mediation of opiate action. Br J Pharmacol 1980;69:131–137.
130. Jhamandas K, Sawynok J. Methyxanthine antagonism of opiate and purine effects on the release of acetylcholine. In: Kosterlitz HW, ed. Opiates and endogenous opioid peptides. Amsterdam: Elsevier North-Holland, 1976:161–168.
131. Jhamandas K, Sawynok J, Sutak M. Antagonism of morphine action on brain acetylcholine release by methylxanthines and calcium. Eur J Pharmacol 1978;49:309–312.
132. Ahlijanian MK, Takemori AE. Effects of caffeine on 8-phenyltheophylline on the actions of purines and opiates in the guinea-pig ileum. J Pharmacol Exp Ther 1986;236:171–176.
133. Malec D, Michalska E. The effect of methyxanthines on morphine analgesia in mice and rats. Pol J Pharmacol Pharm 1988; 40:223–232.
134. Malec D, Michalska E. The effect of adenosine receptor agonists on analgesic effects of morphine. Pol J Pharmacol Pharm 1990; 42:1–11.
135. Ahlijanian MK, Takemori AE. The effect of chronic administration of caffeine on morphine-induced analgesia, tolerance and dependence in mice. Eur J Pharmacol 1986;120:25–32.
136. Gomaa AA, Moustafa SA, Farghali AA. Adenosine triphosphate blocks opiate withdrawal symptoms in rats and mice. Pharmacol Toxicol 1989;64:111–115.
137. Dionyssopoulos T, Hope W, Coupar IM. Effect of adenosine analogues on the expression of opiate withdrawal in rats. Pharmacol Biochem Behav 1992;42:201–206.
138. Calignano A, Persico P, Mancuso F, Sorrentino L. Adenosine release in morphine-induced hypotension in rats. Gen Pharmacol 1992;23:7–10.
139. Sawynok J, Sweeney MI, White TD. Adenosine release may mediate spinal analgesia by morphine. Trends Pharmacol Sci 1989; 10:186–189.
140. Sawynok J, Nicholson DJ, Sweeney MI, White TD. Adenosine release by morphine and spinal antinociception: role of G-proteins and cyclic AMP. NIDA Res Monogr 1991;105:40–46.
141. Sweeney MI, White TD, Sawynok J. Involvement of adenosine in the spinal antinociceptive effects of morphine and noradrenaline. J Pharmacol Exp Ther 1987;243:657–665.
142. Sweeney MI, White TD, Sawynok J. Morphine, capsaicin and K^+ release purines from capsaicin-sensitive primary afferent nerve terminals in the spinal cord. J Pharmacol Exp Ther 1989; 248:447–454.
143. Sweeney MI, White TD, Sawynok J. Intracerebroventricular morphine releases adenosine and adenosine 3′,5′-cyclic monophosphate from the spinal cord via a serotonergic mechanism. J Pharmacol Exp Ther 1991;259:1013–1018.
144. Yang SW, Zhang ZH, Chen JY, et al. Morphine and norepinephrine-induced antinociception at the spinal level is mediated by adenosine. NeuroReport 1994;5:1441–1444.
145. Cahill CM, White TD, Sawynok J. Morphine activates ω-conotoxin-sensitive Ca^{2+} channels to release adenosine from spinal cord synaptosomes. J Neurochem 1993;60:894–901.
146. DeLander GE, Mosberg HI, Porreca F. Involvement of adenosine in antinociception produced by spinal or supraspinal receptor-selective opioid agonists: dissociation from gastrointestinal effects in mice. J Pharmacol Exp Ther 1992;263:1097–1104
147. DeLander GE, Keil II GJ. Antinociception induced by intrathecal coadministration of selective adenosine receptor and selective opioid receptor agonists in mice. J Pharmacol Exp Ther 1994;268:943–951.
148. Keil II GJ, DeLander GE. Time-dependent antinociceptive interactions between opioids and nucleoside transport inhibitors. J Pharmacol Exp Ther 1995;274:1387–1392.
149. Segal IS, Vickery RG, Walton JK, et al. Dexmedetomidine diminishes halothane anesthetic requirements in rats through a postsynaptic $alpha_2$ adrenergic receptor. Anesthesiology 1988; 69:818–823.
150. Jones DJ. Adenosine regulation of cyclic 3′,5′-adenosine monophosphate formation in rat spinal cord. J Pharmacol Exp Ther 1981;219:370–376.
151. Sawynok J, Reid A, Isbrucker R. Adenosine mediates calcium-induced antinociception and potentiation of noradrenergic antinociception in the spinal cord. Brain Res 1990; 524:187–195.
152. Aran S, Proudfit HK. Antinociceptive interactions between intrathecally administered α noradrenergic agonists and 5′-N-ethylcarboxamide adenosine. Brain Res 1990;519:287–293.
153. Aran S, Proudfit HK. Antinociception produced by interactions between intrathecally administered adenosine agonists and norepinephrine. Brain Res 1990;513:255–263.
154. Sawynok J, Reid A. Desipramine potentiates spinal antinociception by 5-hydroxytryptamine, morphine and adenosine. Pain 1992;50:113–118.
155. Sabetkasai M, Zarrindast MR. Antinociception: interaction between adenosine and GABA systems. Arch Int Pharmacodyn 1993;322:14–22.
156. Sierralta F, Miranda HF. Adenosine modulates the antinociceptive action of benzodiazepines. Gen Pharmacol 1993;24:891–894.
157. Gungor T, Malabre P, Teulon JM, et al. N^6-substituted adenosine receptor agonists: synthesis and pharmacological activity as potent antinociceptive agents. J Med Chem 1994;37:4307–4316.
158. Karlsten R, Gordh T Jr, Hartvig P, Post C. Effects of intrathecal injection of the adenosine receptor agonists R-phenylisopropyl-

adenosine and N-ethylcarboxamide-adenosine on nociception and motor function in the rat. Anesth Analg 1990;71:60–64.
159. Karlsten R, Post C, Hide I, Daly JW. The antinociceptive effect of intrathecally administered adenosine analogs in mice correlates with the affinity for the A_1-adenosine receptor. Neurosci Lett 1991;121:267–270.
160. Karlsten R, Kristensen JD, Gordh T Jr. R-phenylisopropyl-adenosine increases spinal cord blood flow after intrathecal injection in the rat. Anesth Analg 1992;75:972–976.
161. Karlsten R, Gordh T Jr, Svensson BA. A neurotoxicologic evaluation of the spinal cord after chronic intrathecal injection of R-phenylisopropyl adenosine (R-PIA) in the rat. Anesth Analg 1993;77:731–736.
162. Kristensen JD, Karlsten R, Gordh T Jr, Holtz A. Spinal cord blood flow after intrathecal injection of an N-methyl-D-aspartate receptor antagonist or an adenosine receptor agonist in rats. Anesth Analg 1993;76:1279–1283.
163. Karlsten R, Gordh T Jr. An A_1-selective adenosine agonist abolishes allodynia elicited by vibration and touch after intrathecal injection. Anesth Analg 1995;80:844–847.
164. Gracely RH. Methods of testing pain mechanisms in normal man. In: Wall PD, Melzack R, eds. Textbook of Pain. New York: Churchill Livingstone, 1989:257–268.
165. Fukunaga A, Aida H, Fukunaga B, et al. Intravenous infusion of adenosine triphosphate elevates the pain threshold of electrical tooth pulp stimulation. Drug Dev Res 1994;31:272.
166. Segerdahl M, Ekblom A, Sollevi A. The influence of adenosine, ketamine, and morphine on experimentally induced ischemic pain in healthy volunteers. Anesth Analg 1994;79:787–791.
167. Ekblom A, Segerdahl M, Sollevi A. Adenosine increases the cutaneous heat pain threshold in healthy volunteers. Acta Anaesthesiol Scand 1995;39:717–722.
168. Segerdahl M, Ekblom A, Sjolund KF, et al. Systemic adenosine attenuates touch evoked allodynia induced by mustard oil in humans. NeuroReport 1995;6:753–756.
169. Sollevi A, Belfrage M, Lundeberg T, et al. Systemic adenosine infusion: a new treatment modality to alleviate neuropathic pain. Pain 1995;61:155–158.
170. Belfrage M, Sollevi A, Segerdahl M, et al. Systemic adenosine infusion alleviates spontaneous and stimulus evoked pain in patients with peripheral neuropathic pain. Anesth Analg 1995; 81:713–717.
171. Williams M. Purine receptors in mammalian tissues: pharmacology and functional significance. Annu Rev Pharmacol Toxicol 1987;27:315–345.
172. Birch BD, Louie GL, Vickery RG, et al. L-Phenylisopropyladenosine (L-PIA) diminishes halothane anesthetic requirements and decreases noradrenergic neurotransmission in rats. Life Sci 1988;42:1355–1360.
173. Seitz PA, ter Riet M, Rush W, Merrell WJ. Adenosine decreases the minimum alveolar concentration of halothane in dogs. Anesthesiology 1990;73:990–994.
174. Fukunaga AF, Taniguchi Y, Kikuta Y. Effects of intravenously administered adenosine and ATP on halothane MAC and its reversal by aminophylline in rabbits. Anesthesiolology 1989; 71:A260.
175. Quasha AL. Eger EI II, Tinker JH. Determination and applications of MAC. Anesthesiology 1980;53:315–334.
176. Ginsburg R, Fukunaga BM, Sasaki S, et al. Analgesic activity of intravenous adenosine: a comparison of potency with morphine sulphate. Anesthesiology 1990;73:A362.
177. Fukunaga AF, Fukunaga B, Kikuta Y. Assessing and characterizing the hypnotic and analgesic effects of anesthetic drugs. Anesthesiology 1991;75:A45.
178. Fukunaga AF, Fukunaga BM, Kikuta Y. Assessment and characterization of the anesthetic effects of intravenous adenosine in the rabbit. Anesth Analg 1992;74:S103.
179. Fukunaga AF, Fukunaga B, Ichinohe T. Intravenous adenosine produces profound and sustained analagesia in spontaneously breathing rabbits. Anesthesiology 1993;79:A423.
180. Fukunaga AF, Fukunaga B, Sakurai M. Co-administration of intravenous adenosine and norepinephrine produces both adenosine and α-2 adrenoceptor medited profound sedative analgesia. Anesthesiology 1995;83:A316.
181. Fukunaga AF. Intravenous administration of large dosages of adenosine or adenosine triphosphate with minimal blood pressure fluctuation. Life Sci 1995;56:PL209–PL218.
182. Kikuta Y, Fukunaga AF, Ginsburg R, et al. Effect of intravenous ATP on enflurane-N_2O MAC in spontaneously breathing rabbits: assessment of cardiorespiratory effects. Anesthesiology 1990;73:A401.
183. Sollevi A, Lagerkranser M, Andreen M, Irestedt L. Relationship between arterial and venous adenosine levels and vasodilation during ATP- and adenosine-infusion in dogs. Acta Physiol Scand 1984;120:171–176.
184. Moser GH, Schrader J, Deussen A. Turnover of adenosine in plasma of human and dog blood. Am J Physiol 1989;256:C799–C806.
185. Klabunde RE. Dipyridamole inhibition of adenosine metabolism in human blood. Eur J Pharmacol 1983;93:21–26.
186. Pelleg A, Porter RS. The pharmacology of adenosine. Pharmacotherapy 1990;10:157–174.
187. Fukunaga AF, Flacke WE, Bloor BC. Hypotensive effects of adenosine and adenosine triphosphate compared with sodium nitroprusside. Anesth Analg 1982;61:273–278.
188. Sollevi A. Effects of adenosine infusion on the conscious man. In: Phillis JW ed. Adenosine and adenine nucleotides as regulators of cellular function. Boca Raton, FL: CRC Press, 1991:283–291.
189. Kaneko Y, Fukunaga AF, Suzuki M, et al. Intravenous ATP potentiates the sedative and hypogenic effects of midazolam in man. Anesthesiology 1992;77:A9.
190. Fukunaga A, Fukunaga B, Kikuta Y. Adenosine potentiates the sedative effect of midazolam without respiratory depression in rabbits [Abstract 223]. The Hague: 10th World Congress on Anaesthesiology, 1992.
191. Warner MA, Dubbink DA. Parenteral anesthetic agents. In: Liu PL, ed. Principles and procedures in anesthesiology. Philadelphia: JB Lippincott, 1992:175–190.
192. Fukunaga AF, Miyamoto TA, Kikuta Y, et al. Role of adenosine and adenosine triphosphate as anesthetic adjuvants. In: Belardinelli L, Pelleg A, eds. Adenosine and adenine nucleotides: from molecular biology to integrative physiology. Boston; Kluwer Academic, 1995:511–523.
193. Andoh T, Ohtsuka T, Okazaki K, et al. Effects of adenosine triphosphate (ATP) on somatosensory evoked potentials in humans anesthetized with isoflurane and nitrous oxide. Acta Anaesthesiol Scand 1993;37:590–593.
194. Kikuta Y, Okada K, Fukunaga AF. Hemodynamic stability during ATP and midazolam-N_2O balanced anesthesia in surgical patients [Abstract 397]. The Hague: 10th World Congress on Anaesthesiology, 1992.
195. Sonntag H, Stephan H, Lange H, et al. Sufentanil does not block sympathetic responses to surgical stimuli in patients having coronary artery revascularization surgery. Anesth Analg 1989; 68:584–592.
196. Taniguchi Y, Fukunaga AF, Harano K, et al. ATP attenuates the cardiovascular responses to sternotomy during fentanyl anesthesia in CABG surgery. Anesthesiology 1993;79:A147.
197. Hashimoto K, Kurosawa H, Horikoshi S, et al. Perfusion pressure control by adenosine triphosphate given during cardiopulmonary bypass. Ann Thorac Surg 1993;55:123–126.
198. Sollevi A. Adenosine infusion during isoflurane-nitrous oxide anaesthesia: indications of perioperative analgesic effect. Acta Anaesthesiol Scand 1992;36:595–599.
199. Segerdahl M, Ekblom A, Sandelin K, et al. Perioperative aden-

osine infusion reduceds the requirements for isoflurane and postoperative analgesics. Anesth Analg 1995;80:1145–1149.
200. Segerdahl M, Irestedt L, Sollevi A. Adenosine reduces perioperative isoflurane and postoperative opioid requirements in hysterectomy. Anesthesiology 1995;83:A848.
201. Fukunaga AF, Ikeda K, Matsuda I. ATP-induced hypotensive anesthesia during surgery. Anesthesiology 1982;57:A65.
202. Sollevi A, Lagerkranser M, Irestedt L, et al. Controlled hypotension with adenosine in cerebral aneurysm surgery. Anesthesiology 1984:61:400–405.
203. Owall A, Lagerkranser M, Sollevi A. Effects of adenosine-induced hypotension on myocardial hemodynamics and metabolism during cerebral aneurysm surgery. Anesth Analg 1988; 67:228–232.
204. Bloor BC, Fukunaga AF, Ma CC, et al. Myocardial hemodynamics during induced hypotension: a comparison between sodium nitroprusside and adenosine triphosphate. Anesthesiology 1985;63:517–525.
205. Russell WJ, Morris RG, Frewin DB, Drew SE. Changes in plasma catecholamine concentrations during endotracheal intubation. Br J Anaesth 1981;53:837–839.
206. Mikawa K, Maekawa N, Kaetsu H, et al. Effects of adenosine triphosphate on the cardiovascular response to tracheal intubation. Br J Anaesth 1991;67:410–415.
207. Murata K, Sodeyama O, Ikeda K, Fukunaga AF. Prevention of hypertensive crisis with ATP during anesthesia for pheochromocytoma. J Anesth 1987;1:162–167.
208. Doi M, Ikeda K. Sevoflurane anesthesia with adenosine triphosphate for resection of pheochromocytoma. Anesthesiology 1989;70:360–363.
209. Mora A, Cortes C, Lopez G, et al. Adenosine triphosphate in the management of hypertensive crises and abnormal heart rhythm during surgery to remove pheochromocytoma. Rev Esp Anestesiol Reanim 1994;41:262–267.
210. Grondal S, Bindslev L, Sollevi A, Hamberger B. Adenosine: a new antihypertensive agent during pheochromocytoma removal. World J Surg 1988;12:581–585.
211. Sellden H, Kogner P, Sollevi A. Adenosine for perioperative blood pressure control in an infant with neuroblastoma. Acta Anaesthesiol Scand 1995;39:705–708.
212. Weissman C. The metabolic response to stress: an overview and update. Anesthesiology 1990;73:308–327.
213. Cronstein BN, Hirschhorn R. Adenosine and host defense. In: Williams M, ed. Adenosine and adenosine receptors. Clifton, NJ: Humana Press, 1990:475–500.
214. Cronstein BN. Adenosine, an endogenous anti-inflammatory agent. J Appl Physiol 1994;76:5–13.
215. Thiel M, Chouker A. Acting via A_2 receptors, adenosine inhibits the production of tumor necrosis factor-α of endotoxin-stimulated human polymorphonuclear leukocytes. J Lab Clin Med 1995;126:275–282.
216. Green PG, Basbaum AI, Helms C, Levine JD. Purinergic regulation of bradykinin-induced plasma extravasation and adjuvant-induced arthritis in the rat. Proc Natl Acad Sci U S A 1991; 88:4162–4165.
217. Schrier DJ, Lesch ME, Wright CD, Gilbertsen RB. The antiinflammatory effects of adenosine receptor agonists on the carrageenan-induced pleural inflammatory response in rats. J Immunol 1990;145:1874–1879.
218. Meninger CJ, Granger HJ. Role of adenosine in angiogenesis. In: Phillis JW, ed. Adenosinde and adenine nucleotides as regulators of cellular function. Boca Raton, FL: CRC Press, 1991:241–246.
219. Ziada AMAR, Hudlicka O, Tyler KR, Wright AJA. The effect of long-term vasodilatation on capillary growth and performance in rabbit heart and skeletal muscle. Cardiovasc Res 1984; 18:724–732.
220. Vlachakis ND, Pratilas V, Pratila M. Raised plasma catecholamines. Possible consequences following major surgery. N Y State J Med 1981;81:27–35.
221. Cusak NJ, Hourani MO. Adenosine, adenine nucleotides and platelet function. In: Phillis JW, ed. Adenosinde and adenine nucleotides as regulators of cellular function. Boca Raton, FL: CRC Press, 1991:121–131.
222. Knill RL, Clement JL, Thompson WR. Epidural morphine causes delayed and prolonged ventilatory depression. Can Anaesth Soc J 1981;28:537–543.
223. Rauck RL. Postoperative analgesia. In: Brown DL, ed. Risk and outcome in anesthesia. 2nd ed. Philadelphia: JB Lippincott, 1992:450–487.
224. Gilbert HC. Postoperative pain management. In: Vender JS, Spiess BD, eds. Post anesthesia care. Philadelphia: WB Saunders, 1992:292–314.
225. Halter JB, Pflug AE, Porte D Jr. Mechanism of plasma catecholamine increases during surgical stress in man. J Clin Endocrinol Metab 1977;45:936–944.
226. Derbyshire DR, Smith G. Sympathoadrenal responses to anaesthesia and surgery. Br J Anaesth 1984;565:725–739.
227. Fredholm BB, Abbracchio MP, Burnstock G et al. VI. Nomenclature and classification of purinoceptors. Pharmacol Rev 1994;46:143–156.

20B Alpha-2 Adrenergic Agonists

Mervyn Maze, Ann E. Buttermann, Takahiko Kamibayashi and Toshiki Mizobe

Although veterinary anesthesiologists have used α_2-adrenergic agonists for nearly two decades, no drugs in this class have been marketed for clinical anesthetic practice. More recently, anesthesia practitioners have administered clonidine, an α_2-adrenoceptor agonist, in the clinical setting and have demonstrated beneficial effects during the perioperative period. Clinical interest in these compounds is likely to be further aroused by the development and clinical introduction of more highly selective α_2 agonists such as dexmedetomidine. In this chapter, the basic and applied pharmacology of α_2-adrenergic agonists are reviewed, using practical examples of their use in the clinical setting.

BASIC PHARMACOLOGY

Classification of Adrenergic Receptors

Adrenergic receptors have been differentiated into α and β based on the rank order of potency of various natural and synthetic catecholamines in different physiologic preparations (1). The α adrenoceptors have since been separated into two subtypes, α_2 and α_1, depending on their sensitivity to the α_2-selective antagonist yohimbine or the α_1-selective antagonist prazosin (2). Activation of α_1 adrenoceptors can functionally antagonize α_2-mediated central nervous system (CNS) responses, so it is critical to use compounds with high selectivity for the α_2 adrenoceptor.

Classification of α_2-Adrenergic Receptors

Two separate nomenclatures, based on either pharmacologic (α_2A, α_2B, or α_2C) or molecular genetic studies, are reconciled to the existence of at least three different α_2-receptor subtypes (3). According to the molecular biologic classification, these subtypes are defined by the chromosomal location of the gene for the receptor subtype: α_2C2 on chromosome 2, α_2C4 on chromosome 4, or α_2C10 on chromosome 10. Different regions of the brain, like most other tissues in the body, are usually populated by more than one receptor subtype, but not necessarily. A species homologue for the α_2A receptor subtype is referred to as the α_2D subtype in rodents. It appears likely that the α_2A/D receptor subtype mediates the anesthetic and analgesic properties of the non-selective agonists.

Structure of the α_2 Adrenoceptor

Several predictive techniques have been developed to derive secondary structures of proteins from their amino acid sequence. Among these methods is the analysis of hydrophobicity of the different regions (4). Such analysis of adrenergic receptors has shown that they, together with several hundred other G protein-coupled receptors, are characterized by 7 hydrophobic domains, each composed of 20 to 30 amino acids, of sufficient length to span the lipid bilayer. In these putative transmembrane domains the endogenous ligands epinephrine and norepinephrine bind to the adrenoceptors. The tertiary structure of adrenoceptors has proved insoluble because of the difficulty in extracting large amounts of pure protein from the natural membranes for crystallography studies. In the absence of biophysical analysis, structural models have been devised, based largely on the folding pattern of the ancient retinal-linked visual pigment bacteriorhodopsin, which has 7 α helices arranged in a bundle perpendicular to the plane of the lipid bilayer (5). Although high sequence homology exists in the transmembrane domains for all the adrenoceptors, considerable differences in structure are found at the cytoplasmic side. The characteristic adrenergic responses are conferred by these cytosolic features, especially in the manner in which they provide "contact points" for the effector mechanism starting with the guanine nucleotide binding proteins (G proteins).

G Proteins

These "coupling proteins" promote transmembrane signaling to a discrete effector mechanism, which may be a transmembrane ion channel or an intracellular second messenger cascade (6). The more than 20 species of G proteins are characterized by differences in the amino acid sequence of one (a) of the three subunits. These discrete differences in the a subunit of the G protein provide the unique response mediated by each of the adrenergic receptors. G proteins can be classified according to their sensitivity to the bacterial toxins, cholera toxin and pertussis toxin. At least 4 different pertussis toxin-sensitive G proteins are capable of coupling the α_2 adrenoceptors to their effector mechanisms.

Effector Mechanisms

All α_2-adrenergic receptors, when activated, are able to inhibit adenylate cyclase. The resulting decrease in the accumulation of cyclic adenosine monophosphate (cAMP) reduces the stimulation of cAMP-dependent protein kinase and hence the phosphorylation of target regulatory proteins. However, in most cases, a decrease in cAMP production is insufficient to mediate the α_2-adrenoceptor effects, and they appear to be executing a permissive rather than a mediatory role. Another effector mechanism is efflux of potassium through the inward rectifier or calcium-activated potassium channels. This alteration in membrane ion conductance can hyperpolarize the excitable membrane and can provide an effective means of suppressing neuronal firing. Activation of α_2 adrenoceptors can also suppress calcium entry through voltage-operated calcium channels into the nerve terminals. This action may be responsible for the inhibitory effect that α_2 agonists exert on exocytotic release of neurotransmitters.

APPLIED PHARMACOLOGY

Clonidine, an imidazole compound, is a selective partial agonist for α_2 adrenoceptors with a ratio of approximately 200:1 (α_2:α_1). Clonidine is rapidly and almost completely absorbed after oral administration and reaches a peak plasma level within 60 to 90 minutes by this route. Clonidine can also be delivered through a time-release transdermal patch, although it takes a minimum of 2 days for therapeutic levels to be achieved by this route (7). The elimination half-life of clonidine is between 9 and 12 hours, with $\approx$50% of the drug being metabolized in the liver to inactive metabolites, whereas the rest is excreted unchanged in the kidney. Clonidine is now administered rectally in children, with 95% bioavailability and unchanged pharmacokinetic parameters (8). This form of administration may be especially appropriate for children.

α-Methyldopa is metabolized to α-methylnorepinephrine, which is a full agonist at the α_2 receptor and has a 10-fold selectivity for the α_2 over the α_1 adrenoceptor. Because transformation into the active compound is necessary, effects are slow to develop (4 to 6 hours) and are unpredictable. This agent is the only parenteral α_2 agonist formulation available for clinical use in the United States. Guanabenz is similar to clonidine in its clinical effects, but it is less potent and is shorter acting, with a terminal elimination half-life of 6 hours. Guanfacine has the longest half-life (14 to 18 hours) of all the clinically available α_2 agonists.

Medetomidine, 4(5)-[1-2,3-dimethylphenyl[ethyl] imidazole, is the prototype of the novel superselective α_2 agonists. It is an order of magnitude more selective than clonidine and is a full agonist at this class of receptor (9). Medetomidine is extremely potent and is active at low nanomolar concentrations. It has been widely used in veterinary practice in Europe. Because the D-enantiomer of this racemate is the active ingredient, dexmedetomidine has been developed for clinical use. Phase III studies with this compound are currently being conducted to investigate its perioperative use.

Some of the ligands have an imidazole ring that facilitates binding to nonadrenergic imidazole-preferring receptors (10, 11) as well as to the α_2 adrenoceptor. The cardiovascular properties of α_2 ligands may vary depending on whether the imidazole-preferring receptor is also activated (12).

CLINICAL APPLICATION OF α_2 AGONISTS

Pharmacologic Responses in Different Organ Systems

Central Nervous System

SEDATIVE EFFECT. Sedation is one of the most consistent effects mediated by central α_2 receptors. Although this property is an undesirable side effect when clonidine is administered to patients with hypertension, it has been used to great advantage for premedication in anesthesia. This effect of α_2 agonists is significantly potentiated when these agents administered together with a benzodiazepine in rats (13); appropriate studies to determine whether this synergy extends to humans are pending. The locus coeruleus has been shown to be a principal region responsible for the sedative effect (14, 15). The molecular components that participate in the signal transduction of the hypnotic response to α_2 agonists include a postsynaptic α_2 adrenoceptor and a pertussis toxin-sensitive G protein coupled to specific ion channels (16-19). Whether inhibition of adenylate cyclase plays a permissive or obligatory role in this response has not been determined.

ANXIOLYTIC EFFECT. Another characteristic effect of α_2 agonists in clinical situations is anxiolysis, which is comparable to that produced by benzodiazepine compounds (20-22). Clonidine can also depress panic disorder in humans (23, 24). However, higher doses of α_2 agonists may produce anxiogenic responses through the nonselective activation of α_1 receptors (25).

ANALGESIC EFFECT. The most difficult CNS effect to assess is the putative analgesic effect of α_2 agonists. Part of this difficulty stems from an inability to double-blind subjects in analgesic tests because of the supervention of other CNS effects, especially sedation. Thus, the subjects are "alerted" to the knowledge that they are receiving an active ingredient. Furthermore, in many of the animal pain paradigms, it may not be possible to separate the sedative from the analgesic properties of the drug. To circumvent this problem in animals, studies that examine spinal reflexive nociceptive effects (e.g., the tail-flick latency response) may be more likely to demonstrate an unequivocal analgesic effect than studies of responses that involve some element of supraspinal processing (e.g., hot plate latency response).

Given these caveats, α_2-adrenergic receptor activation produces an analgesic response involving both supraspinal and spinal sites (26-28). In animal experiments, clonidine exerts a more potent analgesic effect than that of morphine when compared on a molar basis (29). Furthermore, the analgesic potency of α_2 agonists is synergistically enhanced with concomitant treatment with opioids (30-34). Combining clonidine with opiate narcotics leads to a lower dose requirement for each drug while reducing the incidence and severity of side effects. Ossipov and associates studied the interaction between clonidine and opioids in rats (31). The type of interaction depended on the administration route (systemic or intrathecal), the combination ratio of these two kinds of drugs, and the nociceptive pathways involved (spinal or supraspinal). The synergistic effect was observed only when the drugs were administered intrathecally and only in the tail-flick test, which reflects a spinal reflex (31, 35). Eisenach and colleagues performed the clinical study to determine whether epidurally administered clonidine and fentanyl interact additively or synergistically for postoperative analgesia. Although their isobolographic analysis revealed a simple additive interaction, their patient groups were too small to detect a synergistic interaction (36).

In human volunteers, dexmedetomidine was reported to suppress ischemic pain (37) and to attenuate the affective component of ischemic pain (38). However, intravenous dexmedetomidine, in the dose range of 0.25 to 0.50 μg/kg, did not affect the experimental pain threshold (37).

Clonidine has a potent analgesic action that cannot be reversed by naloxone, an opioid antagonist, a finding indicating that clonidine and opioids mediate analgesia through independent receptor mechanisms (33), although these two classes of drugs have a similar transduction pathway in their postreceptor effector mechanisms (39). Some animal paradigms show a partial reversal by opiate antagonists of the analgesic effect of α_2 agonists (40). This similarity in their post-transduction pathways may be the mechanism for the development of cross tolerance between these two agents (41). α_2-agonists suppress the undesirable physiologic and psychologic symptoms following withdrawal from opiates (42, 43). The use of α_2 agonists has been extended to other withdrawal states, such as alcohol, benzodiazepine, and even nicotine "craving" (44-47).

Two groups of investigators have reported the possible involvement of spinal cholinergic mechanisms in the antinociceptive effects of α_2 agonists. Clonidine antinociception in sheep correlated with an increase in the concentration of acetylcholine in the cerebrospinal fluid. Moreover, the antinociceptive effect was enhanced when neostigmine, a cholinesterase inhibitor, was administered intrathecally (48). The interaction between the cholinesterase inhibitor and clonidine was shown to be synergistic and to involve muscarinic receptors (49). Subsequently, the combination of neostigmine and clonidine was found to be nontoxic when tested in the spinal cord of sheep (50).

A most impressive action of α_2 agonists in the CNS is their ability to reduce anesthetic requirements. A modest reduction (15%) of halothane minimum alveolar concentration (MAC) follows subacute administration of clonidine in rabbits (51). Acutely administered clonidine reduced halothane MAC by 50% in a dose-dependent fashion; this MAC-reducing effect was antagonized by an α_2 antagonists (52). The MAC-reducing properties of clonidine have a ceiling, either because of its partial agonist properties or because of the drug's affinity for, and activation of, α_1 adrenoceptors at higher concentrations (activation of α_1 adrenoceptors functionally antagonizes α_2 agonist action in the CNS). More selective α_2 agonists are able to reduce the MAC of volatile anesthetics to a much greater extent. Azepexole was shown to reduce isoflurane MAC by 85% in dogs (53), whereas dexmedetomidine, the most selective α_2 agonist, decreased halothane MAC by more than 95% in rats and dogs, indicating that it alone may produce an anesthetic state (54, 55). Neither the opiate nor the adenosine receptors are involved in the anesthetic-sparing action of α_2 agonists (54). This reduction in anesthetic requirement can also be demonstrated in humans and is not limited to volatile anesthetics.

Intraocular pressure can be reduced by α_2 agonists, and these agents can also attenuate the rise in intraocular pressure elevation associated with laryngoscopy and endotracheal intubation (56-58). This feature has been used clinically in patients with glaucoma. Whether through the same or different mechanisms, raised intracranial pressure is decreased by α_2 agonists in an animal model of subarachnoid hemorrhage. Experimental application of α_2 agonists and antagonists in the study of neuroprotection from cerebral ischemia has resulted in conflicting data. Hoffman and associates (59, 60) reported that the α_2 agonists clonidine and dexmedetomidine improved the outcome of incomplete global ischemia. The neuroprotective effect of dexmedetomidine has been reported in a rabbit model of focal ischemia in which a beneficial effect was demonstrated even when the α_2 agonist was administered *after* the onset of ischemia (61). On the other hand, idazoxan, an α_2 antagonist, also protects against global ischemia (62). This apparent paradox may be reconciled by the finding that both idazoxan and rilmenidine, α_2 antagonist and agonist with affinity for the imidazole-preferring receptor, are able to exert a protective against cerebral ischemia. These investigators hypothesized that the imidazoline-preferring receptor, and not α_2 adrenoceptors, is involved in the neuroprotective mechanism. Whichever receptor mediates the neuroprotective effect, it is unlikely to be due to a vascular action because dexmedetomidine has been shown to decrease cerebral blood velocity in humans in a dose-dependent manner (63).

Studies suggest that α_2 agonists may be effective in the treatment of autonomic dysreflexia. In an animal model of spinal cord transection resulting in autonomic hyperreflexia, clonidine was shown to decrease this response (64), suggesting a mediating role of α_2 adrenoceptors in this ameliorative action.

Cardiovascular System

The α_2 agonists exert their action on the cardiovascular system at both peripheral and central levels. α_2 Agonists inhibit norepinephrine release from peripheral prejunctional nerve endings, and this property, in part, contributes to the bradycardiac effect of α_2 agonists (65). No firm evidence supports the existence of postsynaptic α_2 receptors in the myocardium; therefore, it is unlikely that the α_2 agonists exert a direct effect on the heart (66, 67). Postjunctional α_2 receptors are present in both arterial and venous vasculature, where they produce vasoconstriction (68). Among the different vascular beds, the effect of α_2 agonists in the coronary circulation is important from the clinical standpoint. A putative vasoconstrictive action of α_2 agonists on the coronary vasculature may promote ischemia (69, 70); however, these agonists can ameliorate any direct constriction by reducing sympathetic outflow (71). Furthermore, α_2 agonists also have been documented to release endothelial-derived relaxant factor (nitric oxide) in coronary arteries (72) and to enhance coronary blood flow induced by endogenous and exogenous adenosine in an in vivo model (73). Thus, the effect on coronary arteries may be too complicated to distinguish clear changes in coronary blood flow in an in vivo model (74). Intrathecal administration of clonidine shows a biphasic effect on blood pressure. A small dose (150 μg) induces hypotension, whereas a larger dose (450 μg) causes hypertension, presumably because of peripheral vasoconstriction (75). An intermediate dose (300 μg) has little effect on blood pressure, presumably by offsetting peripheral and central effects.

Clonidine can produce hypotensive and bradycardic effects through the CNS. The mechanism of these actions may involve inhibition of sympathetic outflow and potentiation of parasympathetic nervous activity. However, the precise mechanism involved in these actions is not well understood. Although the nucleus solitarius (a site known to modulate autonomic control including vagal activity) is an important central site for the action of α_2 agonists (76), other nuclei including the locus coeruleus (77), the dorsal motor nucleus of vagus (78, 79), and the nucleus reticularis lateralis (80, 81) may also mediate hypotension or bradycardia. Bradycardia is especially likely to occur in patients with little counteracting sympathetic stimulation (82). The imidazoline-preferring receptors have been shown to play an important role in the hypotensive effect of α_2 agonists (83, 84). Investigators have also suggested that the α_2 agonists exert their hypotensive and sedative effects in different receptor-effector mechanisms, respectively.

Another cardiovascular property of α_2 agonists is their anti-arrhythmic effect. Dexmedetomidine attenuates epinephrine-induced arrhythmias during halothane anesthesia and also the arrhythmias that result from bupivacaine toxicity (85). The antiarrhythmic action in halothane-epinephrine arrhythmias is abolished in animals that have undergone vagotomy; this finding suggests that enhanced vagal activity mediates this action (86).

The effect of α_2 agonist on the cerebral circulation during anesthesia has been studied. Dexmedetomidine decreases cerebral blood flow in awake human volunteers (87). This characteristic may be favorable in protecting the brain from an abrupt increase in blood flow. This idea has been supported by the finding that dexmedetomidine blunts the cerebrovascular response to hypoxia during isoflurane anesthesia (88, 89).

Respiratory System

The respiratory depressant effects of clonidine are not remarkable unless massive doses are given (90, 91). Although intravenous clonidine induces a hypoxic effect in animals, this effect is not found in humans (92). Although α_2 agonists may cause mild respiratory depression (93), the effect of clonidine is less than that of opioid analgesics (94). In clinically appropriate doses, mild respiratory depression can be detected by hypercarbic ventilatory response studies (95). This appears to be equivalent to the respiratory depression that can be detected during physiologic sleep. Opioid-induced respiratory depression is not potentiated by clonidine (96, 97). Nebulized clonidine has been demonstrated to attenuate bronchoconstriction in asthmatic patients (98) and has also been prescribed to patients with obstructive sleep apnea syndrome (99).

Endocrine System

The α_2 agonists potentiate the secretion of growth hormone (100). Although a precise mechanism for this action has not been elucidated, α_2-receptor activation is coupled to growth hormone releasing factor (101, 102). α_2 Agonists that possess the imidazole ring inhibit steroidogenesis. However, at clinical doses, this mild effect is not likely to have serious consequences (103). The α_2 agonists decrease sympathoadrenal outflow, and these agents can suppress the stress response following surgical stimulation (104). Although in vitro studies indicate that α_2 agonists regulate catecholamine secretion in the adrenal medulla (105, 106), this effect has been questioned by other investigators (107, 108). The α_2 agonists also inhibit the release of insulin from the pancreatic β cells directly (109); however, this action does not result in severe hyperglycemia in clinical settings (110).

Gastrointestinal System

The α_2 agonists exert a prominent antisialogogue effect, which is a useful feature in their use as premedication agents (111). The α_2 agonists can modulate release of gastric acid by a presynaptic mechanism (112), yet no significant change in gastric pH is observed in humans (113). The α_2 agonists also may prevent intestinal ion and water secretion in the large bowel, a finding that indicates an effective treatment for watery diarrhea (114).

Renal System

The α_2 agonists induce a diuretic response both in animals and in humans. Inhibition of release of antidiuretic hormone (ADH) (115), antagonism of the renal tubular action of ADH (116), and increase in the glomerular filtration rate (117) have all been implicated in the mechanism. Release of atrial natriuretic factor has also been suggested to contribute to the diuretic mechanism of α_2 agonists (118, 119).

Hematologic System

Aggregation of platelets is induced by α_2 agonists at high concentrations (120). In the clinical setting, this effect is probably offset by a decrease in circulating catecholamines.

Use of α_2 Agonists in Anesthetic Practice

Preanesthetic Administration

A single dose of clonidine of 0.3 mg has the same pharmacokinetic and pharmacodynamic profile whether administered orally or sublingually (121). Therefore, the sublingual route can be predictably used in fasting patients, those having difficulty swallowing, or those who are unable to absorb drugs through the gastrointestinal tract. Rectal administration of 2.5 $\mu g \cdot kg^{-1}$ of clonidine in children, approximately 20 minutes before induction of anesthesia, achieves plasma concentrations within the range known to be clinically effective in adults (122).

Since sedation, anxiolysis, and antisialogogue action are attractive attributes in a premedication agent, administration of α_2 agonists is well-suited this purpose (58, 123-125). Devcic, Muzi, and Ebert (126) studied the influence of clonidine (approximately 3.5 $\mu g \cdot kg^{-1}$) on the sympathoexcitatory response to desflurane in volunteers. Clonidine significantly attenuated the rapid increases in blood pressure and heart rate during the transition between low and high doses of desflurane. In a comparative study, Weiskopf and colleagues (127) reported clonidine to be as efficacious as either esmolol or fentanyl in attenuating the sympathoexcitatory response to desflurane in volunteers. Similarly, the sympathoexcitatory response to intravenous ketamine, 1.0 $mg \cdot kg^{-1}$, was attenuated by oral clonidine, 5 $\mu g \cdot kg^{-1}$, as evidenced by the smaller increment in blood pressure (128). Clonidine premedication also blunted hypertension and tachycardia, as well as increments in plasma catecholamine concentrations during a stepwise increase in isoflurane concentration by mask anesthesia (129).

Another benefit of α_2 agonists as premedication is their ability to potentiate the anesthetic action of other agents and to reduce anesthetic requirements during surgery. This effect is universally observed regardless of the type of anesthetic, whether intravenous, volatile, or regional blockade. For example, premedication with oral clonidine, 5 $\mu g \cdot kg^{-1}$, reduced fentanyl requirements for induction and intubation by 45% in patients undergoing aortocoronary bypass surgery (130). In a similar patient population, clonidine was shown to reduce sufentanil requirement by 40% (131). Preoperative clonidine (5 $\mu g \cdot kg$) decreased the dose of droperidol to maintain hemodynamic stability in patients undergoing aortic surgery (132). Thiopental and propofol requirements for induction are also reported to be reduced by preanesthetic treatment with clonidine or dexmedetomidine, although the former interaction may be based on a pharmacokinetic mechanism (122, 133-135). The decreased requirement for induction and maintenance anesthetic agents may result in a quicker emergence from anesthesia, although this possibility has yet to be rigorously studied. Using auditory evoked potentials as a measure of recovery from the sedative effects of clonidine and diazepam, a cohort of elderly clonidine-treated patients exhibited faster recovery (136).

Ota and colleagues (137) systematically studied the effect of increasing doses (75 to 300 μg) of oral clonidine on regression of sensory anesthesia following subarachnoid administration of hyperbaric tetracaine in patients undergoing gynecologic and urologic surgery. Earlier, these investigators had established that the optimal timing for oral premedication was 1 hour (138). The prolonging effect of oral clonidine increased in a dose-dependent manner and reached a maximal effect at 150 μg in which the duration of the block doubled. Four patients in the highest-dose group (300 μg) developed bradycardia. When compared with intrathecal fentanyl, oral clonidine (200 μg) shortened the onset time of tetracaine's sensory block and prolonged the duration of sensory and motor block (139). Although no significant interaction occurred between clonidine and fentanyl, clonidine premedication did increase the incidence of hypotension and bradycardia.

Premedication with oral clonidine (approximately 3 $\mu g \cdot kg^{-1}$) prolonged sensory and motor block from lidocaine spinal anesthesia (140). Although no subjects had hypotension or bradycardia, the incidence of sedation was greater when the volunteers were pretreated with clonidine. When clonidine (3 $\mu g \cdot kg^{-1}$) was combined with bupivacaine intrathecally, the duration of both the motor and sensory block increased (141). Although blood pressure and heart rate were lower in patients receiving clonidine, the need for analgesia postoperatively was also less. Klimscha and colleagues (142) compared the hemodynamic and analgesic effects of spinal versus epidural clonidine alone and in combination with bupivacaine. Intrathecal, but not epidural, clonidine decreased mean arterial pressure significantly compared with bupivacaine alone. Although the onset time required to surgical anesthesia was unaffected by clonidine, the duration of spinal and epidural anesthesia was increased more than twofold. The mechanism of action does not involve pharmacokinetic alterations of local anesthetic disposition (143). From the data included in these studies, it is now possible both qualitatively and quantitatively to enhance conduction blockade with α_2 agonists by various routes of administration. Unfortunately, we are still no closer to understanding the mechanism of these local anesthetic-enhancing qualities.

The successful application of α_2 agonists to patients at the extreme ages of life is now established (144, 145). The elderly patient population appears to be most likely to benefit from the sympatholytic effects of the drug because of the prevalence of coronary artery disease and hypertension in this group (56, 58). In patients between 4 and 12 years, the combination of 4 $\mu g \cdot kg^{-1}$ clonidine and 30 $\mu g \cdot kg^{-1}$ atropine orally, 105 minutes before coming to the operating room, was more effective than diazepam at promoting anxiolysis and sedation (145). The degree to which heart rate can be increased with atropine is attenuated in pediatric patients (146), although bradycardia is not more likely to occur when atropine is used prophylactically. As in adults, the dose of induction agents can be reduced in the pediatric population (147). The quality and duration of block produced by bupivacaine caudal-epidural anesthesia is enhanced when clonidine, rather than epinephrine, is added to the injectate (148).

An extension of the pharmacologic properties of α_2 agonists is the development of severe bradycardia and hypotension (122, 125, 149). Bradycardia can be preempted by the prophylactic use of an anticholinergic agent (atropine or glycopyrrolate), although the increment in heart rate is significantly less in both adults and children (150). Conversely, hypotension responds in an exaggerated fashion to treatment with ephedrine (151). The pressor response to phenylephrine has been reported in clonidine-treated (5 $\mu g \cdot kg^{-1}$ orally) awake or anesthetized (enflurane-nitrous oxide) patients (152). The magnitudes of maximal mean blood pressure increases in the clonidine group (26 $\pm$ 7%, [mean $\pm$ SD] for awake and 32 $\pm$ 15% for anesthetized subjects) were greater ($p < 0.05$) than in the control group (13 $\pm$ 7% for awake and 18 $\pm$ 7% for anesthetized subjects). These data suggest that α_1-adrenoceptor-mediated vasoconstriction is enhanced following oral clonidine and that restoration of blood pressure can be achieved effectively by either ephedrine or phenylephrine, in small doses, in clonidine-premedicated hypotensive patients.

Intraoperative Administration

To determine whether the addition of clonidine to a standardized general anesthetic regimen safely provides postoperative sympatholysis for patients with known or suspected coronary artery disease, Ellis and colleagues (153) randomly allocated patients undergoing elective major noncardiac surgery to receive either placebo or clonidine by a combination of oral and transdermal routes. Clonidine reduced enflurane requirements, intraoperative tachycardia, and myocardial ischemia. Although decrements in heart rate were maintained during the first 5 postoperative hours, the incidence of postoperative myocardial ischemia did not differ between the two groups.

Although α_2 agonists have been recognized to possess potent analgesic and sedative effects, these agents have not been used as sole anesthetic agents. Several reports have described intraoperative administration of α_2 agonists. Talke and associates (154) reported on the safety of the perioperative infusion of dexmedetomidine in patients undergoing vascular surgery. The combination of oral and transdermal clonidine (which maintained the plasma concentration of clonidine at therapeutic levels) provided lower anesthetic requirements, greater hemodynamic stability, more rapid recovery from anesthesia, and a decreased requirement for postoperative morphine for pain control in patients undergoing lower abdominal operations (155). In patients undergoing abdominal aortic grafting, perioperative infusion of clonidine (7 μg/kg over 120 minutes) after aortic declamping may reduce norepinephrine, epinephrine, and vasopressin concentrations during the recovery period (156). Although more hemodynamic stability is obtained, higher fluid volumes are required during the postoperative period. Moreover, intraoperative clonidine infusion (a loading dose of 4 μg/kg following 2 μg/kg/h until closure of the peritoneum) can enhance the quality of postoperative analgesia by morphine (157). A significant reduction in postoperative shivering episodes follows the intraoperative administration of clonidine.

Another route of administration of the α_2 agonists is into the intrathecal or epidural space to potentiate local anesthetic agents. Intrathecal clonidine (150 μg) prolonged bupivacaine spinal anesthesia in elderly patients undergoing hip surgery, and this technique was superior to the addition of epinephrine (200 μg) to bupivacaine (158). Concerning epidural anesthesia, addition of clonidine to epidural lidocaine was reported to augment its anesthetic potency. Another merit of epidural clonidine during the surgical period is to provide sedation and relative hemodynamic stability, compared with plain lidocaine or lidocaine with epinephrine (159). Epidural and intravenous clonidine have both been shown to decrease postoperative opiate narcotic requirements (160, 161). Intraoperative administration of clonidine (4 μg/kg in 20 minutes, followed by 2 μg/kg/h) reduced the analgesic demands, improved the pain visual analog scores, and provided greater patient satisfaction (162). Epidural clonidine reduced the intra- and postoperative analgesic requirements when compared with the same dose given by the intravenous route, although the plasma concentrations were less in the epidural group (163).

Gabriel and colleagues (164) showed that, in the presence of clonidine, the electroencephalographic spectral indices reflected a deeper anesthetic state even though the end-expiratory isoflurane concentration was reduced by 50%. Kulka and colleagues (165) systematically examined the dose-response effect of intravenous clonidine (2, 4, or 6 $\mu g \cdot kg^{-1}$) on the sympathoadrenal response to surgical stimulation in patients undergoing coronary artery bypass graft surgery. Although the two higher doses were equally effective at blocking the hemodynamic and catecholamine responses to stimulation, this was not apparent at the lower dose. Murga and associates examined the effect of epidural clonidine on fentanyl requirements in patients undergoing general anesthesia with a "nitrous-narcotic" technique for abdominal hysterectomy (166). Epidural clonidine decreased fentanyl requirements, improved cardiovascular stability, reduced pain intensity, and decreased the need for postoperative analgesia in the recovery room.

Data from these studies continue to stress the anesthetic-sparing qualities of the α_2 agonists in patients undergoing general anesthesia. Whether the use of lower concentrations of the other anesthetics will be associated with a better outcome is not addressed. However, with lower doses of "fixed agents," a faster emergence from general anesthesia may be anticipated, with a commensurate decrease in time in the postanesthesia care unit.

Postoperative Analgesia

Eisenach and colleagues examined the postoperative analgesic effect of epidural clonidine or fentanyl, alone or in combination, in patients after cesarean section (167). Although these investigators showed that the required dose of each analgesic could be reduced by about 50% when the drugs were used in combination, these data do not reveal a synergistic interaction. A possible reason for the lack of synergy, which has been repeatedly demonstrated in animal studies, was the large variability in the patients who received fentanyl alone. In another study involving patients who had undergone cesarean section, Capogna and associates (168) showed a dose-dependent increase in the duration of epidural morphine-local anesthetic analgesia when clonidine (75 or 150 μg) was included in the mixture. Moreover, the need for redosing was diminished in the patients who received clonidine. In a further study involving patients who had undergone cesarean section, the addition of either clonidine or epinephrine (which also activates α_2-adrenergic receptors) to epidural sufentanil decreased the number of administrations of sufentanil by patient-controlled analgesia (PCA) (169). Patients undergoing gastrectomy with a combined general and epidural anesthetic technique received epidural morphine with or without clonidine (3 $\mu g \cdot kg^{-1}$) for postoperative analgesia (170). The cumulative number of supplemental systemic morphine injections by PCA was less in those patients who received clonidine at each hour for 24 hours postoperatively ($p < 0.05$), whereas the Visual Analog Scale for pain was lower. In the clonidine-treated patients, the sedation score was higher, and mean blood pressure was lower. Conversely, patients undergoing hip replacement surgery did not have any reduction in PCA analgesic requirements (171) when a small dose of clonidine (75 μg) was added to intrathecal morphine.

Bernard's group (172) compared the analgesic efficacy, arterial blood gases, and pharmacokinetics of an intravenous infusion of fentanyl, 75 $\mu g \cdot h^{-1}$, and a mixture of fentanyl, 25 $\mu g \cdot h^{-1}$, plus clonidine, 0.3 $\mu g \cdot h^{-1}$, after surgery. Pain relief, sedation, and supplemental ketoprofen requirements were similar in both groups. The number of episodes of arterial desaturation (less than 90% for more than 20 seconds) was 106 in 4 of the patients in the fentanyl group (versus none in the clonidine-fentanyl group). Mean arterial blood pressure, plasma clearance, and the elimination rate constant of fentanyl were lower in the clonidine-fentanyl group than in the fentanyl alone group. In an interesting study, Rockemann and colleagues (173) compared the analgesic effects of epidural clonidine (8 $\mu g \cdot kg^{-1}$) alone, with a lower dose (4 $\mu g \cdot kg^{-1}$) in combination with morphine (2 mg), or morphine (50 $\mu g \cdot kg^{-1}$) alone in patients undergoing pancreatectomy. Patients who received epidural solutions containing clonidine had earlier onset and a longer duration of analgesia than when morphine alone was used. Hemodynamicaly, the clonidine-treated patients had a rate-dependent decrease in cardiac output.

To reduce the side effects without affecting the analgesic property, continuous epidural administration following bolus injection of clonidine (800 μg bolus followed by 20 $\mu g/h$) is advocated as an alternative method. With this continuous treatment, more than 6 hours of analgesia has been observed following cesarean section (174). In comparison with single-dose clonidine administration, several reports have described the effectiveness of combining epidural administration of clonidine with local anesthetics or opioids. Adding 150 μg of clonidine to epidural fentanyl, morphine, and bupivacaine resulted in longer duration of postoperative analgesia (175-177). This has now been extended to pediatric patients receving combinations of clonidine and bupivacaine by the caudal route (178). Substitution of bupivacaine with 2-chloroprocaine antagonizes the analgesic action of clonidine (179); a similar finding has been observed with opiate narcotics (180). The efficacy of intrathecal clonidine (150 μg) as a sole analgesic agent after cesarean section without remarkable side effects has focused attention on this use (181, 182).

Systemic administration of clonidine for postoperative analgesia has also been reported. Bonnet and associates compared the analgesic effect (visual analog scale) of intramuscular clonidine (2 $\mu g \cdot kg^{-1}$) with the same dose of epidural clonidine after minor operations (orthopedic or perineal surgery) (183). Both onset and duration of analgesia after intramuscular clonidine were comparable with epidural clonidine. In addition, although the peak plasma concentration of clonidine was higher in the intramuscular group, side effects, including hypotension, bradycardia, and drowsiness, were similar. Another possible route of systemic administration of α_2 agonists for postoperative analgesia is intravenous. Intravenous clonidine, 150 μg, produced analgesic effects similar to those of morphine, 5 mg, in patients after orthopedic surgery (184). In one case report, oral clonidine was used as an analgesic agent in a patient who had undergone pheochromocytoma resection, after insufficient analgesic effects with epidural local anesthetics and opioids (185).

Perioperative as well as postoperative administration of clonidine can decrease oxygen consumption and episodes of shivering during recovery from anesthesia (186-188). The antishivering effect can be demonstrated with a small dose (189). This feature provides further justification for using this agent in patients with coronary artery disease. α_2 Agonists improve pain control in postoperative patients in several settings, although whether these compounds exert a potent enough analgesic effect to be used as the sole analgesic agent except in specialized settings (e.g, postpartum) is still unclear. The use of α_2 agonists alone for postsurgical analgesia does not seem to be effective unless these agents are given in extremely high doses or in parturient patients. In other settings, the combination of α_2 agonists with opiate narcotics appears to provide durable analgesia with fewer side effects than when either type of agent is used alone.

Use in Disease States

Two groups of surgical patients in whom the beneficial effects of α_2 agonists have already been demonstrated are those suffering from hypertension and those with glaucoma. In both groups, the beneficial effects relate to the pharmacologic action of this class of drug in interrupting the pathogenic process. Currently, investigators are studying the potential myocardial ischemia and infarction-reducing effect of α_2 agonists including dexmedetomidine and mivazerol. The data with clonidine, although encouraging, are inconclusive (190). Another group of patients likely to benefit from α_2 agonists are those undergoing neurosurgical procedures because of the putative neuroprotective, intracranial pressure-reducing, induced hypotensive, and sympatholytic actions of these drugs. Again, preliminary data are encouraging (191), but more rigorous studies are needed.

Miscellaneous Uses

Because of a potent analgesic property, α_2 agonists may be useful in the relief of pain other than in the postoperative period. Epidural clonidine produces effective analgesia in a dose-dependent fashion (100 to 900 μg) with few side effects in patients with neuropathic pain (192). Epidural clonidine is also a useful therapeutic adjunct in the management of patients with refractory reflex sympathetic dystrophy (RSD) (193). Transdermal application of clonidine also relieves hyperalgesia in patients with RSD (194). This effect, confined to the skin region beneath the patch, suggests a peripheral mechanism. Transdermal clonidine is useful in the relief of painful diabetic neuropathy (195).

Anecdotal reports demonstrate that intrathecal clonidine in combination with morphine or hydromorphone can attenuate the pain of cancer, and the combination is an excellent alternative approach to control of the pain of terminal cancer (196-197). One case report suggested that intrathecal clonidine is effective in pain relief, even after tolerance to intrathecal morphine has developed (198). This phenomenon indicates the possibility that temporary pain control can be provided by clonidine to allow the morphine-tolerant patient to recapture sensitivity to morphine.

In conclusion, the use of α_2 agonists, either alone or in combination, is becoming widespread in anesthesia. The original enthusiasm for this class of compound for its plethora of beneficial effects appears to have been justified, based on the more recent clinical studies. This chapter provides the practitioner with a working knowledge of the mechanism of action, physiology, and pharmacology of this novel class of anesthetic agent.

The initial promise of this class of agent is now being fulfilled with the development of more highly selective compounds. In the next decade, the field will continue to evolve with the clinical introduction of the second generation of α_2 agonists, notably dexmedetomidine, a more selective, specific, and efficacious compound than the prototype, clonidine. Furthermore, formulations allowing several different routes of administration, ranging from transdermal to neuraxial, will further extend clinical utility of these drugs. These novel compounds will help to define, more precisely, the clinical utility of this interesting class of compounds in intravenous anesthesia.

REFERENCES

1. Lands AM, Arnold A, McAuliff JP. A study of the adrenotropic receptors. Am J Physiol 1948;153:586–600.
2. Bylund DB, U'Pritchard DC. Characterization of alpha-1 and alpha-2 adrenergic receptors. Int Rev Neurobiol 1983;24:343–431.
3. Bylund DB. Subtypes of α_2-adrenoceptors: pharmacological and molecular biological evidence converge. Trends Pharmacol Sci 1988;9:356–361.
4. Kyte J, Doolittle RFA. A simple method for displaying the hydropathic character of a protein. J Mol Biol 1982;157:105–132.
5. Henderson R, Baldwin JM, Ceska TA, et al. Model for the structure of bacteriorhodopsin based on high-resolution electron microscopy. J Mol Biol 1990;213:899–929.
6. Raymond JR, Hnatowich M, Caron MG, Lefkowitz RJ. Stucture-function relationships of G-protein-coupled receptors, ADP-ribosylating toxins and G proteins. In Moss J, Vaughn ASM, eds. Washington, DC: 1990.
7. Toon S, Hopkins KJ, Aarons L, et al. Rate and extent of absorption of clonidine from a transdermal therapeutic system. J Pharm Pharmacol 1989;41:17–21.
8. Lonnqvist PA, Bergendahl HTG, Eksborg S. Pharmacokinetics of clonidine after rectal administration in children. Anesthesiology 1994;81:1097–1101.
9. Scheinin H, Virtanen R, McDonald E. Medetomidine, a novel α_2-adrenoceptor agonist: a review of its pharmacodynamic effects. Prog Neuropsychopharmacol Biol Psychiatry 1989; 13:635–651.
10. Ernsberger P, Meeley MP, Mann JJ, Reis DJ. Clonidine binds to imidazole binding sites as well as α_2-adrenoceptors in the ventrolateral medulla. Eur J Pharmacol 1987;134:1–13.
11. Zonnenechein R, Dement S, Atlas D. Imidazoline receptors in rat liver cells: a novel receptor or a subtype of alpha 2-adrenoceptors? Eur J Pharmacol 1990;190:203–215.
12. Tibirica E, Feldman J, Mernet D, et al. A midazoline-specific mechanism for the hypotensive effect of clonidine: a study with yohimbine and idazoxan. J Pharmacol Exp Ther 1991;256:606–613.
13. Salonen M, Reid K, Maze M. Synergistic interaction between α_2-adrenergic agonists and benzodiazepines in rats. Anesthesiology 1992;76:1004–1011.
14. Correa-Sales C, Rabin B C, Maze M. A hypnotic response to dexmedetomidine, an α_2 agonist, is mediated in the locus coeruleus in rats. Anesthesiology 1992;76:948–952.
15. deSarro GB, Ascioti C, Froio F, et al. Evidence that locus coeruleus is the site where clonidine and drugs acting at $alpha_1$ and $alpha_2$ adrenoceptors affect sleep and arousal mechanisms. Br J Pharmacol 1987;90:675–685.
16. Doze VA, Chen BX, Maze M. Dexmedetomidine produces a hypnotic-anesthetic action in rats via activation of central α_2 adrenoceptors. Anesthesiology 1989;71:75–79.
17. Correa-Sales C, Reid K, Maze M. Pertussis toxin mediated ribosylation of G proteins blocks the hypnotic response to an alpha 2 agonist in the rat. Pharmacol Biochem Behav 1992; 43:723–727.
18. Correa-Sales C, Nacif-Coelho C, Reid K, Maze M. Inhibition of adenylate cyclase in the locus coeruleus mediates the hypnotic response to an alpha 2 agonist in the rat. J Pharmacol Exp Ther 1992;263:1046–1049.
19. Nacif-Coelho C, Correa-Sales C, Chang LL, Maze M. Perturbation of ion channel conductance alters the hypnotic response to the alpha 2 adrenergic agonist dexmedetomidine in the locus coeruleus of the rat. Anesthesiology 1994;81:1527–1534.
20. Carabine UA, Milligan KR, Moore JA. Adrenergic modulation of preoperative anxiety: a comparison of temazepam, clonidine and timolol. Anesth Analg 1991;73:633–637.
21. Ferrari F, Tartoni PL, Margiafico V. B-HT 920 antagonizes rat neophobia in the X-maze test. Arch Int Pharmacodyn Ther 1989;298:71–74.
22. Wright RMC, Carabine UA, Orr DA, et al. Preanesthetic medication with clonidine. Br J Anaesth 1990;65:628–635.
23. Uhde TW, Stein MB, Vittone BJ, et al. Behavioral and physiologic effects of short-term and long-term administration of clonidine in panic disorder. Arch Gen Psychiatry 1989;46:170–177.
24. Puzantian T, Hart LL. Clonidine in panic disorder. Ann Pharmacother 1993;27:1351–1353.
25. Soderpalm B, Engel JA. Biphasic effects of clonidine on conflict behavior: involvement of different alpha-adrenoceptors. Pharmacol Biochem Behav 1988;30:471–477.
26. Pertovaara A, Kauppila T, Jyasjarvi E, Kalso E. Involvement of suptraspinal and spinal segmental alpha-2-adrenergic mechanisms in the medetomidine-induced antinociception. Neuroscience 1991;44:705–714.
27. Wang YC, Su DR, Lin MT. The site and mode of analgesic actions exerted by clonidine in monkeys. Environ Neurol 1985; 90:479–488.
28. Yaksh TL, Reddy SVR. Studies in primates on the analgesic effeects associated with intrathecal actions of opiates, $alpha_2$ adrenergic agonists, and baclofen. Anesthesiology 1981;54:451–467.
29. Fielding S, Wilder J, Hynes M, et al. A comparison of clonidine with morphine for antinociceptive and anti-withdrawal actions. J Pharmacol Exp Ther 1978;207:899–905.
30. Omote k, Kitahata L, Collins JG, et al. Interaction between opi-

ate subtype and $alpha_2$ adrenergic agonists in suppression of noxiously evoded activity of WDR neurons in the spinal dorsal horn. Anesthesiology 1991;74:737–743.
31. Ossipov MH, Harris S, Lloyd P, et al. Antinociceptive interaction between opioids and medetomidine: systemic additivity and spinal synergy. Anesthesiology 1990;73:1227–1235.
32. Meert TF, DeKock M. Potentiation of the analgesic properties of fentanyl-like opioids with α_2-adrenoceptor agonists in rats. Anesthesiology 1994;81:677–688.
33. Spaulding TC, Fielding S, Venafro JJ, Lal H. Antinociceptive activity of clonidine and its potentiation of morpnine analgesia. Eur J Pharmacol 1979;58:19–25.
34. Wilcox GL, Carlsson KH, Jochim A, Jurna I. Mutual potentiation of antinociceptive effects of morphine and clonidine on motor and sensory response in rat spinal cord. Brain Res 1987; 405:84–93.
35. Ossipov MH, Harris S, Lloyd P, Messineo E. An isobolographic analysis of the antinociceptive effect of systemically and intrathecally administered combination of clonidine and opiates J Pharmacol Exp Ther 1990;255:1107–1116.
36. Eisenach JC, DeAngelo R, Taylor C, Hood DD. An isobolographic study of epidural clonidine and fentanyl after cesarean section. Anesth Analg 1994;79:285–290.
37. Jaakola ML, Salonen M, Lehinen R, Scheinin H. The analgesic action of dexmedetomidine, a novel $alpha_2$-adrenoceptor agonist, in healthy volunteers. Pain 1991;46:281–285.
38. Pauppila T, Kemppainen P, Tanila H, Pertovaara A. Effect of systemic medetomidine, an $alpha_2$ adrenoceptor agonist, on experimental pain in humans. Anesthesiology 1991;74:3–8.
39. Brown DA. G-proteins and potassium currents in neurons. Annu Rev Physiol 1990;52:215–242.
40. Sullivan AF, Kalso EA, McQuay HJ, Dickenson AH. The antinociception actions of dexmedetomidine on dorsal horn neuronal responses in the anaesthetized rat. Eur J Pharmacol 1992; 215:127–133.
41. Stevens SW, Monasky MS, Yaksh TL. Spinal infusion of opiate and $alpha_2$ agonists in rats: tolerance and cross-tolerance studies. J Pharmacol Exp Ther 1988;244:63–70.
42. Gold MS, Redmond DE, Kleber HD. Clonidine blocks acute opiate withdrawal symptoms. Lancet 1978;2:599–602.
43. Gerra G, Marcato A, Caccavari R, et al. Clonidine and opiate receptor antagonists in the treatment of heroin addiction. J Subst Abuse Treat 1995;12:35–41.
44. Ashton H. Benzodiazepine withdrawal: outcome in 50 patients. Lancet 1987;82:665–671.
45. Cushman P Jr, Sowers J. Alcohol withdrawal syndrome: clinical and hormonal responses to α_2 adrenergic treatment. Alcoholism 1989;13:361–364.
46. Yam PC, Forbes A, Knox WJ. Clonidine in the treatment of alcohol withdrawal in the intensive care unit. Br J Anaesth 1992; 68:106–108.
47. Gourlay S, Forbes A, Marriner T, et al. A placebo-controlled study of three clonidine doses for smoking cessation. Clin Pharmacol Ther 1994;55:64–69.
48. Detweiler DJ, Eisenach JC, Tong C, Jackson C. A cholinergic interaction in $alpha_2$ adrenoceptor-mediated antinociception in sheep. J Pharmacol Exp Ther 1993;265:536–542.
49. Naguib M, Yaksh TL. Antinociceptive effects of spinal cholinesterase inhibition and isobolographic analysis of the interaction with μ and α_2 receptor systems. Anesthesiology 1994; 80:1338–1348.
50. Hood DD, Eisenach JC, Tong C, et al. Cardiorespiratory and spinal cord blood flow effects of intrathecal neostigmine methylsylfate, clonidine, and their combination in sheep. Anesthesiology 1995;82:428–435.
51. Kaukinen S, Pyykko K. The potentiation of halothane anesthesia by clonidine. Acta Anaesthesiol Scand 1979;23:107–111.
52. Bloor BC, Flack WE. Reduction in halothane anesthetic requirement by clonidine, an α_2 adrenergic agonist. Anesth Analg 1982;61:741–745.
53. Maze M, Vickery RG, Merlone SC, Gaba DM. Anesthetic and hemodynamic effects of the $alpha_2$ adrenergic agonists, azepexole, in isoflurane-anesthetized dogs. Anesthesiology 1988; 68:689–694.
54. Segal IS, Vickery RG, Walton JK, et al. Dexmedetomidine diminishes halothane anesthetic requirements in rats through a postsynaptic $alpha_2$ adrenergic receptors. Anesthesiology 1988; 69:818–823.
55. Vickery RG, Sheridan BS, Segal IS, Maze M. Anesthetic and hemodynamic effects of the stereoisomers of medetomidine, an $alpha_2$-adrenergic agonist, in halothane-anesthetized dogs. Anesth Analg 1988;67:611–615.
56. Ghignone M, Calvillo O, Quintin L. Anesthesia for ophthalmic surgery in the elderly: the effects of clonidine on intraocular pressure, perioperative hemodynamics, and anesthesia requirement. Anesthesiology 1988;68:707–716.
57. Jaakola ML, Ali-Melkkila T, Kanto J, et al. Dexmedetomidine reduces intraocular pressure, intubation responses and anaesthetic requirements in patients undergoing ophthalmic surgery. Br J Anaesth 1992;68:570–575.
58. Kumar A, Bose S, Phattacharya A, et al. Oral clonidine premedication for elderly patients undergoing intraocular surgery. Acta Anaesthesiol Scand 1992;36:159–164.
59. Hoffman WE, Cheng MA, Thomas C, et al. Clonidine decreases plasma catecholamines and improves outcome from incomplete ischemia in the rat. Anesth Analg 1991;73:460–464.
60. Hoffman WE, Kochs E, Werner C, et al. Dexmedetomidine improves neurologic outcome from incomplete ischemia in the rat. Anesthesiology 1991;75:328–332.
61. Maier C, Steinberg GK, Sun GH, et al. Neuroprotection by the $alpha_2$ adrenoceptor agonist, dexmedetomidine, in a focal model of cerebral ischemia. Anesthesiology 1993;79:306–312.
62. Maiese K, Pek L, Berger SB, Reis DJ. Reduction in focal cerebral ischemia by agents acting at imadazole receptors. J Cereb Blood Flow Metab 1992;12:53–63.
63. Zornow NH, Fleischer JE, Scheller MS, et al. Dexmedetomidine, an $alpha_2$-adrenergic agonist, decreases cerebral blood flow in the isoflurane-anesthetized dog. Anesth Analg 1990;70:624–630.
64. Morrison SF, Ge YZ. Adrenergic modulation of a spinal sympathetic reflex in the rat. J Pharmacol Exp Ther 1995;273:380–385.
65. Jonge A De, Timmerman PBMWM, Zweiten PA Van. Participation of cardiac presynaptic α_2 adrenoceptors in the bradycardic effects of clonidine and analogues. Naunyn Schmiedebergs Arch Pharmacol 1981;317:8–12.
66. Dukes ID, Williams EMV. Effects of selective α_1-, α_2-, β_1- and β_2-adrenoceptor stimulation on potentials and contractions in the rabbit heart. J Physiol 1984;355:523–546.
67. Housemans PR. Effects of dexmedetomidine on contractility, relaxation and intracelluar calcium transients of isolated ventricular myocardium. Anesthesiology 1990;73:919–922.
68. Ruffolo RR. Distribution and function of peripheral alpha-adrenoceptors on the cardiovascular system. Pharmacol Biochem Behav 1985;22:827–833.
69. Chillian WN. Functional distribution of α_1 and α_2 adrenergic receptors in coronary microcirculation. Circulation 1991; 84:2108–2122.
70. Miyamoto MI, Rockman HA, Guth BD, et al. Effect of alpha-adrenergic stimulation on regional contractile function and myocardial blood flow with and without ischemia. Circulation 1991;84:1715–1724.
71. Heusch G, Schipke J, Thamer V. Clonidine prevents sympathetic initiation and aggravation of poststenotic myocardial ischemia. J Cardiovasc Pharmacol 1985;7:1176–1182.
72. Cocks TM, Angus JA. Endothelium-dependent relaxation of

coronary arteries by noradrenaline and serotonin. Nature 1983; 305:627–630.
73. Hori M, Kitakaze M, Tamai J, et al. Alpha$_2$-adrenoceptor stimulation can augment coronary vasodilation maximally induced by adenosine in dogs. Am J Physiol 1989;257:H132–H140.
74. Schmeling WT, Kampine JP, Roerig DL, Warltier DC. The effects of the stereoisomers of the alpha$_2$ adrenergic agonist medetomidine on systemic and coronary hemodynamics in conscious dogs. Anesthesiology 1991;75:499–511.
75. Frisk-Holmberg M, Paalzow L, Wibell L. Relationship between the cardiovascular effects and steady-state kinetics of clonidine in hypertension: demonstration of a therapeutic window in man. Eur J Clin Pharmacol 1984;26:309–313.
76. Kubo T, Misu Y. Pharmacological characterization on the α-adrenoceptor responsible for a decrease of blood pressure in the nucleus tractus solitari of the rat. Naunyn Schmiedebergs Arch Pharmacol 1981;317:120–125.
77. Svensson TH, Bunney BS, Aghajanian GK. Inhibition of both noradrenergic and serotonergic neurons in brain by the alpha-adrenergic agonist clonidine. Brain Res 1975;92:291–306.
78. Ross CA, Ruggiero DA, Reis DJ. Projections from the nucleus tractus solitarii to the rostal ventrolateral medulla. J Comp Neurol 1985;242:511–534.
79. Unnerstall J, Kopajtic TA, Kuhar MJ. Distribution of alpha$_2$ agonists binding sites in the rat and human central nervous system: analysis of some functional, autonomic correlates of the pharmacology effects of clonidine and related adrenergic agents. Brain Res Rev 1984;7:69–101.
80. Ernsberger P, Guiliano R, Willette N, Reis D. Role of imidazole receptors in the vasodepressor response to clonidine analogs in the rostral ventrolateral medulla. J Pharmacol Exp Ther 1990; 253:408–418.
81. Tibirica E, Feldman J, Mermet C, et al. Selectivity of rilmenidine for the nucleus reticularis lateralis, a ventrolateral medullary structure containing imidazoline-preferring receptors. Eur J Pharmacol 1991;209:213–221.
82. Aantaa R, Scheinin M. Alpha$_2$-adrenergic agents in anaesthesia. Acta Anaesthesiol Scand 1993;37:433–448.
83. Bousquet P, Feldman J, Schwartz J. Central cardiovascular effects on a adrenergic drugs: differences between catecholamines and imidazolines. J Pharmacol Exp Ther 1984;230:232–236.
84. Bousquet P, Feldman J, Tibirica E, et al. New concepts on the central regulation of blood pressure. Am J Med 1989;87:10s–13s.
85. Hayashi Y, Sumikawa K, Maze M, et al. Dexmedetomidine prevents epinephrine-induced arrhythmias through stimulation of central alpha$_2$ adrenoceptors in halothane-anesthetized dogs. Anesthesiology 1991;75:113–117.
86. Kamibayashi T, Hayashi Y, Sumikawa K, et al. A role of vagus nerve in antiarrhythmic effects of doxazosin and dexmedetomidine on halothane-epinephrine arrhythmias. Anesthesiology 1995;83:992–999.
87. Zornow MH, Maze M, Dyck JB, Shafer SL. Dexmedetomidine decreases cerebral blood flow velocity in humans. J Cereb Blood Flow Metab 1993;13:350–353.
88. Fale A, Kirsch JR, McPherson RW. Alpha$_2$-adrenergic agonist effects on normocapnic and hypercapnic cerebral blood flow in the dog are anesthetic dependent. Anesth Analg 1994;79:892–898.
89. McPherson RW, Traystman RJ. Effect of dexmedetomidine on cerebrovascular response to hypoxia during isoflurane anesthesia. Anesthesiology 1991;75:A174.
90. Anderson RJ, Hart GR, Crumpler CP, Lerman MJ. Clonidine overdoses: report of six cases and review of the literature. Ann Emerg Med 1989;10:107–112.
91. Olsson JM, Pruitt AW. Management of clonidine ingestion in children. J Pediatr 1983;103:646–650.
92. Eisenach JC. Intravenous clonidine produces hypoxia by a peripheral α_2 adrenergic mechanism. J Pharmacol Exp Ther 1988; 244:247–252.
93. Nguyen D, Abdul-Rasool I, Ward D, et al. Ventilatory effects of dexmedetomidine, atipamezole, and isoflurane in dogs. Anesthesiology 1992;76:573–579.
94. Garty M, Ben-Zvi Z, Harwity A. Interaction of clonidine and morphine with lidocaine in mice and rats. Toxicol Appl Pharmacol 1989;101:255–260.
95. Penon C, Ecoffey C, Cohen SE. Ventilatory response to carbon dioxide after epidural clonidine injection. Anesth Analg 1991; 72:761–764.
96. Bailey PL, Sperry RJ, Johnson GK, et al. Respiratory effects of clonidine alone and combined with morphine in humans. Anesthesiology 1991;74:43–48.
97. Javis DA, Duncan SR, Segal IS, Maze M. Ventilatory effects of clonidine alone and in the presence of alfentanil, in human volunteers. Anesthesiology 1992;76:899–905.
98. Lindgren BR, Ekstrom T, Anderson RG. The effect of inhaled clonidine in patients with asthma. Am Rev Respir Dis 1986; 134:266–269.
99. Issa FG. Effect of clonidine in obstructive sleep apnea. Am Rev Respir Dis 1992;145:435–439.
100. Grossman A, Weerasuriya K, Al-Damluji S, et al. Alpha$_2$ adrenoceptor agonists stimulate growth hormone secretion but have no acute effects on plasma cortisol under basal conditions. Horm Res 1987;25:65–71.
101. Deveasa J, Arce V, Lois N, et al. α_2 Adrenergic agonism enhances the growth hormone (GH) response to GH-releasing hormone through an inhibition of hypothalmic somatostatin release in normal man. J Clin Endocrinol Metab 1990;71:1581–1588.
102. Deveasa J, Diaz MJ, Tresquerres AI, et al. Evidence that α_2 adrenergic pathways play a major role in growth hormine (GH) neuroregulation: α_2 adrenergic agonism counteracts the inhibitory effects of muscarinic cholinergic receptor blockade on the GH response to GH-releasing hormone, while α_2 adrenergic blockade diminishes the potentiating effect of increased cholinergic tone on such stimulation in normal men. J Clin Endocrinol Metab 1991;73:251–256.
103. Maze M, Virtanen R, Daunt D, et al. Effects of dexmedetomidine, a novel imidazole sedative-anesthetic agent, on adrenal stereogenesis: in vivo and in vitro studies. Anesth Analg 1991; 73:204–208.
104. Lange SV. Presynaptic regulation of catecholamine release. Biochem Pharmacol 1974;23:1793–1800.
105. Gutman Y, Boonyaviroj P. Suppression by noradrenaline of catecholamine secretion from adrenal medulla. Eur J Pharmacol 1974;28:384–86.
106. Wada A, Sakurai S, Kobayashi H, et al. Alpha$_2$-adrenergic receptors inhibit catecholamine secretion from bovine adrenal medulla. Brain Res 1982;252:189–191.
107. Powis DA, Baker PF. Alpha$_2$-adrenoceptors do not regulate catecholamine secretion by bovine adrenal medullary cells: a study with clonidine. Mol Pharmacol 1986;29:134–141.
108. Regunathan S, Evinger MJ, Meeley M, Reis D. Effects of clonidine and other imidazole-receptor binding agents on second messenger systems and calcium influx in bovine adrenal chromaffin cells. Biochem Pharmacol 1991;42:2011–2018.
109. Angel I, Langer SZ. Adrenergic-induced hyperglycemia in anaesthetized rats: involvement of peripheral α_2 adrenoceptors. Eur J Pharmacol 1988;154:191–196.
110. Massara F, Limone P, Cagliero E, et al. Effects of naloxone on the insulin and growth hormone responses to alpha-adrenergic stimulation with clonidine. Acta Endocrinol 1983;103:371–375.
111. Karhuvaara S, Kallio AM, Salonen M, et al. Rapid reversal of alpha$_2$-adrenoceptor agonist effects by atipamezole in human volunteers. Br J Clin Pharmacol 1991;31:160–165.
112. Blandiaai C, Bernardini MC, Vizi ES, Tacca M Del. Modulation of gastric acid secretion by peripheral presynaptic α_2 adreno-

ceptors at both sympathetic and parasympathetic pathways. J Auton Pharmacol 1990;10:305–312.

113. Orko R, Pouttu J, Ghignone M, et al. Effect of clonidine on hemodynamic responses to endotracheal intubation and gastric acidity. Acta Anaesthesiol Scand 1987;31:325–329.
114. McArthur KE, Anderson DS, Durbin TE, et al. Clonidine and lidamidine to inhibit watery diarrhea in a patient with lung cancer. Ann Intern Med 1982;96:323–325.
115. Peskind ER, Raskind MA, Leake RD, et al. Clonidine decreases plasma and cerebrospinal fluid arginine vasopressin but not oxytocin in humans. Neuroendocrinology 1987;46:395–400.
116. Stanton B, Puglisi E, Gellai M. Localization of alpha$_2$-adrenoceptor-mediated increase in renal Na^+, K^+, and water excretion. Am J Physiol 1987;252:F1016–F1021.
117. Strandhoy JW. Role of alpha$_2$ receptors in the regulation of renal function. J Cardiovasc Pharmacol 1985;7 (suppl 8):S28–S33.
118. Chen M, Lee J, Huang BS, et al. Clonidine and morphine increase atrial natriuretic peptide secretion in anesthetized rats. Proc Soc Exp Biol Med 1989;191:299–303.
119. Hamaya Y, Nishikawa T, Dohi S. Diuretic effect of clinidine during isoflurane, nitrous oxide, and oxygen anesthesia. Anesthesiology 1994;81:811–819.
120. Ruffolo RR, Nichols AJ, Hieble JP. Functions mediated by alpha$_2$ adrenergic receptors In: Limbird LE, ed. The alpha$_2$ adrenergic receptors. Clifton, NJ: Humana Press, 1988:187–280.
121. Cunningham FE, Baughman VL, Peters J, Laurito CE. Comparative pharmacokinetics of oral versus sublingual clonidine. J Clin Anesth 1994;6:430–433.
122. Lonnqvist PA, Bergendahl HT, Eksborg S. Pharmacokinetics of clonidine after rectal administration in children. Anesthesiology 1994;81:1097–1101.
123. Aho M, Lehtinen AM, Erkola O, et al. The effects of intravenous administered dexmedetomidine on perioperative hemodynamics and isoflurane requirements in patients undergoing abdominal hysterectomy. Anesthesiology 1991;74:112–118.
124. Aho M, Erkola OA, Scheinen H, et al. Effect of intravenous administered dexmedetomidine on pain after laparoscopic tubal ligation. Anesth Analg 1991;73:112–118.
125. Carabine UA, Wright PMC, Moore J. Preanaesthetic medication with clonidine: a dose-response study. Br J Anaesth 1991;67: 79–83.
126. Devcic A, Muzi M, Ebert TJ. The effects of clonidine on desflurane-mediated sympathoexcitation in humans. Anesth Analg 1995;80:773–779.
127. Weiskopf RB, Eger EI II, Noorani M, Daniel M. Fentanyl, esmolol, and clonidine blunt the transient cardiovascular stimulation induced by desflurane in humans. Anesthesiology 1994; 81:1350–1355.
128. Tanaka M, Nishikawa T. Oral clonidine premedication attenuates the hypertensive response to ketamine. Br J Anaesth 1994; 73:758–762.
129. Tanaka S, Tsuchida H, Namba H, Namiki A. Clonidine and lidocaine inhibition of isoflurane-induced tachycardia in humans. Anesthesiology 1994;81:1341–1349.
130. Ghignone M, Quintin L, Duke PC, et al. Effects of clonidine on narcotic requirements and hemodynamic response during induction of fentanyl anesthesia and endotracheal induction. Anesthesiology 1986;64:36–42.
131. Flack JW, Bloor BC, Flack WE, et al. Reduced narcotic requirement by clonidine with improved hemodynamic and adrenergic stability in patients undergoing coronary surgery. Anesthesiology 1987;67:11–19.
132. Engelman E, Lipszyc M, Gilbart E, et al. Effects of clonidine on anesthetic requirements and hemodynamic response during aortic surgery. Anesthesiology 1989;71:178–187.
133. Buhrer M, Mappes A, Lauber R, et al. Dexmedetomidine decreases thiopental dose requirement and alters distribution pharmacokinetics. Anesthesiology 1994;80:1216–1227.
134. Aantaa RE, Kanto JH, Scheinen M, et al. Dexmedetomidine, an α_2 adrenergic agonist, reduces anesthetic requirements for patients undergoing minor gynecological surgery. Anesthesiology 1990;73:230–235.
135. Richard MJ, Skues MA, Jarvis AP, Prys-Roberts C. Total i.v. anaesthesia with propofol and alfentanin: dose requirements for propranolol and the effect of premedication with clonidine. Br J Anaesth 1990;65:157–163.
136. Kumar A, Tandon OP, Bhattacharya A, et al. Recovery from pre-operative sedation with clonidine-brain stem auditory evoked response. Anaesthesia 1994;49:533–537.
137. Ota K, Namiki A, Iwasaki H, Takahashi I. Dose-related prolongation of tetracaine spinal anesthesia by oral clonidine in humans. Anesth Analg 1994;79:1121–1125.
138. Ota K, Namiki A, Iwasaki H, Takahashi I. Dosing interval for prolongation of tetracaine spinal anesthesia by oral clonidine in humans. Anesth Analg 1994;79:1117–1120.
139. Singh H, Liu J, Gaines GY, White PF. Effect of oral clonidine and intrathecal fentanyl on tetracaine spinal block. Anesth Analg 1994;79:1113–1116.
140. Liu S, Chiu AA, Neal JM, et al. Oral clonidine prolongs lidocaine spinal anesthesia in human volunteers. Anesthesiology 1995;82:1353–1359.
141. Niemi L. Effects of intrathecal clonidine on duration of bupivacaine spinal anaesthesia, haemodynamics, and postoperative analgesia in patients undergoing knee arthroscopy. Acta Anaesthesiol Scand 1994;38:724–728.
142. Klimscha W, Chiari A, Krafft P, et al. Hemodynamic and analgesic effects of clonidine added repetitively to continuous epidural and spinal blocks. Anesth Analg 1995;80:322–327.
143. Boico O, Bonnet F, Mazoit JX. Effects of epinephrine and clonidine on plasma concentrations of spinal bupivacaine. Acta Anaesthesiol Scand 1992;36:684–688.
144. Filos KS, Patroni O, Goudas LC, et al. A dose-response study of orally administered clonidine as premedication in the elderly: evaluating hemodynamic safety. Anesth Analg 1993; 77:1185–1192.
145. Mikawa K, Maekawa N, Nishina K, et al. Efficacy of oral clonidine premedication in children. Anesthesiology 1993;79:926–931.
146. Nishina K, Mikawa K, Maekeawa N, et al. Oral clonidine premedication blunts the heart rate response to intravenous atropine in awake children. Anesthesiology 1995;82:1126–1130.
147. Nishina K, Mikawa K, Maekawa N, et al. Clonidine decreases the dose of thiamylal required to induce anesthesia in children. Anesth Analg 1994;79:766–768.
148. Jamali S, Monin S, Begon C, et al. Clonidine in pediatric caudal anesthesia. Anesth Analg 1994;78:663–666.
149. Aantaa RE, Kanto J, Scheinen H. Intramuscular dexmedetomidine, a novel α_2 adrenoceptor agonist, as premedication for minor gynaecological surgery. Acta Anaesthesiol Scand 1991; 35:283–288.
150. Nishikawa T, Dohi S. Oral clonidine blunts the heart rate response to intravenous atropine in humans. Anesthesiology 1991;75:217–222.
151. Nishikawa T, Kimura T, Taguchi N, Dohi S. Oral clonidine preanesthetic medication augments the pressor responses to intravenous ephedrine in awake or anesthetized patients. Anesthesiology 1991;74:705–710.
152. Inomata S, Nishikawa T, Kihara S, Akiyoshi Y. Enhancement of pressor response to intravenous phenylephrine following oral clonidine medication in awake and anaesthetized patients. Can J Anaesth 1995;42:119–125.
153. Ellis JE, Drijvers G, Pedlow S, et al. Premedication with oral and transdermal clonidine provides safe and efficacious postoperative sympatholysis. Anesth Analg 1994;79:1133–1140.
154. Talke P, Jain U, Leung J, et al. Effects of perioperative dexmedetomidine infusion in patients undergoing vascular surgery. Anesthesiology 1995;82:620–633.
155. Segal IS, Javis DJ, Duncan SR, et al. Clinical efficacy of oral-

transdermal clonidine combinations during the perioperative period. Anesthesiology 1991;74:220–225.
156. Quintin L, Roudot F, Roux C, et al. Effect of clonidine on the circulation and vasoactive hormones after aortic surgery. Br J Anaesth 1991;66:108–115.
157. DeKock M, Pichon G, Scholtes JL. Intraoperative clonidine enhances postoperative morphine patient-controlled analgesia. Can J Anaesth 1992;39:537–544.
158. Racle JP, Benkhadra A, Poy JY, Gleizal B. Prolongation of isobaric bupivacaine spinal anesthesia with epinephrine and clonidine for hip surgery in the elderly. Anesth Analg 1987;66:442–446.
159. Nishikawa T, Dohi S. Clinical evaluation of clonidine added to lidocaine solution for epidural anesthesia. Anesthesiology 1990; 73:853–859.
160. Motsh J, Graber E, Ludwig K. Addition of clonidine enhances postoperative analgesia from epidural morphine: a double blind study. Anesthesiology 1990;73:1066–1073.
161. Bernard JM, Hommeril JL, Passuti N, Pinaud M. Postoperative analgesia by intravenous clonidine. Anesthesiology 1991; 75:577–582.
162. DeKock M, Lavandhomme P, Scholtes JL. Intraoperative and postoperative analgesia using intravenous opioid, clonidine and lignocaine. Anaesth Intensive Care 1994;22:15–21.
163. DeKock M, Crochet B, Morimont C, Scholtes JL. Intravenous or epidural clonidine for intra- and postoperative analgesia. Anesthesiology 1993;79:525–531.
164. Gabriel AH, Faryniak B, Sojka G, et al. Clonidine: an adjunct in isoflurane N_2O/O_2 relaxant anaesthesia. Effects on EEG power spectra, somatosensory and auditory evoked potentials. Anaesthesia 1995;50:290–296.
165. Kulka PJ, Tryba M, Zenz M. Dose-response effects of intravenous clonidine on stress response during induction of anesthesia in coronary artery bypass graft patients. Anesth Analg 1995; 80:263–268.
166. Murga G, Samso E, Valles J, et al. The effect of clonidine on intra-operative requirements of fentanyl during combined epidural/general anaesthesia. Anaesthesia 1994;49:999–1002.
167. Eisenach JC, D'Angelo R, Taylor C, Hood DD. An isobolographic study of epidural clonidine and fentanyl after cesarean section. Anesth Analg 1994;79:285–290.
168. Capogna G, Celleno D, Zangrillo A, et al. Addition of clonidine to epidural morphine enhances postoperative analgesia after cesarean delivery. Reg Anesth 1995;20:57–61.
169. Vercauteren MP, Vandeput DM, Meert TF, Adriaensen HA. Patient-controlled epidural analgesia with sufentanil following caesarean section: the effect of adrenaline and clonidine admixture. Anaesthesia 1994;49:767–771.
170. Anzai Y, Nishikawa T. Thoracic epidural clonidine and morphine for postoperative pain relief. Can J Anaesth 1995;42:292–297.
171. Grace D, Bunting H, Milligan KR, Fee JP. Postoperative analgesia after co-administration of clonidine and morphine by the intrathecal route in patients undergoing hip replacement. Anesth Analg 1995;80:86–91.
172. Bernard JM, Lagarde D, Souron R. Balanced postoperative analgesia: effect of intravenous clonidine on blood gases and pharmacokinetics of intravenous fentanyl. Anesth Analg 1994; 79:1126–1132.
173. Rockemann MG, Seeling W, Brinkmann A, et al. Analgesic and hemodynamic effects of epidural clonidine, clonidine/morphine, and morphine after pancreatic surgery: a double-blind study. Anesth Analg 1995;80:869–874.
174. Mendez R, Eisenach JC, Kashtan K. Epidural clonidine analgesia after cesarean section. Anesthesiology 1990;73:848–852.
175. Carabine UA, Milligan KR, Moore J. Extradural clonidine and bupivacaine for postoperative analgesia. Br J Anaesth 1992; 68:132–135.
176. Carabine UA, Milligan KR, Mulholland D, Moore J. Extradual clonidine infusions for analgesia after total hip replacement. Br J Anaesth 1992;68:338–343.
177. Rostaing S, Bonnet F, Levron JC, et al. Effects of epidural clonidine on analgesia and pharmacokinetics of epidural fentanyl in postoperative patients. Anesthesiology 1991;75:420–425.
178. Lee JJ, Rubin AP. Comparison of a bupivacaine-clonidine mixture with plain bupivacaine for caudal analgesia in children. Br J Anaesth 1994;72:258–262.
179. Huntoon M, Eisenach JC, Boese P. Epidural clonidine after cesarean section. Anesthesiology 1992;76:187–193.
180. Camann WR, Hartigan PM, Gilbertson LI, et al. Chloroprocaine antagonism of epidural opioid analgesia: a receptor-specific phenomenon. Anesthesiology 1990;73:860–863.
181. Filos KS, Goudas LC, Patroni O, Polyzou V. Hemodynamic and analgesic profile after intrathecal clonidine in humans: a dose-response study. Anesthesiology 1994;81:591–601.
182. Filos KS, Goudas LC, Patroni O, Polyzou V. Intrathecal clonidine as a sole analgesic for pain relief after cesarean section. Anesthesiology 1992;77:174–267.
183. Bonnet F, Boico O, Rostaining S, et al. Clonidine-induced analgesia in postoperative patients: epidural versus intramuscular administration. Anesthesiology 1990;72:423–427.
184. Tryba M, Zenz M, Strumpf M. Clonidine i.v. is equally effective as morphine i.v. for postoperative analgesia: a double blind study. Anesthesiology 1991;75:A1085.
185. Okuyama A, Sugimoto H, Takahisa M, et al. Oral clonidine relieved postoperative pain after pheochromocytoma resection. J Anesth 1995;9:289–291.
186. Delaunay L, Bonnet F, Duvaldestin P. Clonidine decreases postoperative oxygen consumption in patients recovering from general anaesthesia. Br J Anaesth 1991;67:397–401.
187. Quintin L, Viale JP, Annat G, et al. Oxygen uptake after major abdominal surgery: effect of clonidine. Anesthesiology 1991; 74:236–241.
188. Joris J, Banache M, Bonnet F, et al. Clonidine and ketanserin both are effective treatment for postanesthetic shivering. Anesthesiology 1993;79:532–539.
189. Capogna G, Celleno D. IV clonidine for post-extradural shivering in parturients: a preliminary study. Br J Anaesth 1993; 71:294–295.
190. Dorman BH, Zucker JR, Verrier ED, et al. Clonidine improves perioperative myocardial ischemia, reduces anesthetic requirement, and alters hemodynamic parameters in patients undergoing coronary artery bypass surgery. J Cardiothorac Vasc Anesth 1993;7:386–395.
191. Traill R, Gillies R. Clonidine premedication for craniotomy: effects on blood pressure and thiopentone dosage. J Neurosurg Anesthesiol 1993;5:171–177.
192. Eisenach JC, Rauck RL, Buzzanel C, Lysak S. Epidural clonidine analgesia for intractable cancer pain: phase 1. Anesthesiology 1989;71:647–652.
193. Rauck RL, Eisenach JC, Jackson K, et al. Epidural clonidine treatment for refractory reflex sympathetic dystrophy. Anesthesiology 1993;79:1163–1169.
194. Davis KD, Treede RD, Raja SN, et al. Topical application of clonidine releives hyperalgesia in patients with sympathetically maintained pain. Pain 1991;47:309–317.
195. Zeigler D, Lynch SA, Muir J, et al. Transdermal clonidine versus placebo in painful diabetic neuropathy. Pain 1992;48:403–408.
196. Coombs D, Saunder RL, Fratkin JD, et al. Continous intrathecal hydromorphine and clonidine for intractable cancer pain. J Neurosurg 1986;64:890–894.
197. vanEssen EJ, Bovill JG, Ploeger EJ, Beerman H. Intrathecal morphine and clonidine for control of intractable cancer pain: a case report. Acta Anaesthesiol Belg 1988;39:109–112.
198. Coombs D, Saunders RI, Lachance D, et al. Intrathecal morphine tolerance: use of intrathecal clonidine, DADLE, and intraventricular morphine. Anesthesiology 1985;62:358–363.

21 Intravenous Drug Interactions

H. Ronald Vinik

Many current theories of anesthesia assume that a single, common molecular mechanism produces anesthesia. However, clinicians understand that general anesthesia has several components including analgesia, anxiolysis, amnesia, unconsciousness, and suppression of somatic (motor), cardiovascular, and hormonal responses to surgery. The actions of intravenous agents are more easily recognized because they often have a predominant, if not a specific, reaction to influencing particular receptors. For example, opiates have a predominant analgesic action but also produce a sedative hypnotic component at higher doses. Often, this "pure" opioid reaction is incomplete, and patients have been described as pain free, immobile, and yet still aware. However, the addition of a subhypnotic dose of a benzodiazepine with the opiate combines to produce a state of general anesthesia.

In an editorial, Kissin indicates that a wide spectrum of pharmacologic actions of different drugs can be used to create the state of general anesthesia by targeting the components of anesthesia including hypnosis, analgesia, amnesia, and suppression of reflexes (1). The spectrum of effects that constitutes the state of general anesthesia should not be considered to result from a single anesthetic action even if it is produced by one drug, that is, an inhalation agent. These effects are produced by separate pharmacologic actions that are not easily recognized because of insufficient specificity of the actions of inhalational agents. Intravenous agents, however, are generally considered to produce more specific actions.

SPECIFICITY OF ACTION

Several groups of drugs administered intravenously can provide anesthesia similar to that provided by inhalational agents by acting on specific receptors within the central nervous system (CNS). Receptor-mediated action is defined by a specific response that is dose dependent and may be reversible with a specific antagonist. Intravenous anesthetic agents used include barbiturates, benzodiazepines, etomidate, ketamine, propofol, and steroid anesthetics. All have specific, or at least well-defined, binding sites.

Classic theories of anesthesia are based on unitary, nonspecific mechanisms of anesthetic action in which one anesthetic may be freely replaced by another. Such hypotheses predict that combinations of anesthetic agents should have an additive effect. This has been confirmed for several inhalational agents (2, 3). Because intravenous agents have different and specific mechanisms of action, one can expect drug interactions. These interactions may be additive, synergistic, or even antagonistic.

INTERACTIONS OF INTRAVENOUS ANESTHETICS DRUGS

In intravenous anesthesia, the following different interactions can occur:

1. Physicochemical, in which the two different drugs may be incompatible when mixed because of, for example, large pH differences, which cause precipitation.
2. Pharmacokinetic, when one drug (a) changes or competes for protein binding sites and consequently alters the availability of active unbound drug at the receptor site or (b) alters the distribution or metabolism of the second drug.
3. Pharmacodynamic, which can occur at the receptor site when drug A modulates the receptor sensitivity to drug B, that is, with barbiturates and benzodiazepines, at their common gammamino receptor complex. A potent interaction occurs between benzodiazepines and opiates, however, at separate sites that are probably mediated by other liberated neurotransmitters.

4. Physiologic, in which drugs acting at different receptors do not interact as such, but may produce the same physiologic effect; for example, a cholinergic drug and a β blocker both produce bradycardia but mediated by different mechanisms.

Consequences of Drug Interactions

The commonly described interactions in anesthesia usually relate to the potential for toxicity. A well-recognized example is the use of meperidine in patients taking monoamine oxidase inhibitors, with potentially fatal results. Drug interactions need not be detrimental. Interactions may be beneficial if they are quantifiable, predictable, consistent, and controllable.

Quantification of Intravenous Anesthetic Action

To measure the effect of combining two agents, dose-response curves are determined for the individual agents separately and then for the combination using a probit procedure. These curves are then compared with isobolographic analysis.

Use of Isobolographic Analysis

A more precise means of measuring drug interactions is the use of isobolographic analysis. This is the most commonly used analytic technique of this type of interaction (4). On an isobole diagram, points on the x and y axes represent the potency expressed as the 50% effective dose (ED_{50}) for a particular effect of each of the two agents alone (5). A straight line defines the fractional combinations of two agents that would be expected to have the same potency if the interaction between them were additive only. If the reference point for the effect of a combination of two agents falls significantly to the left of the additive line, synergism is inferred.

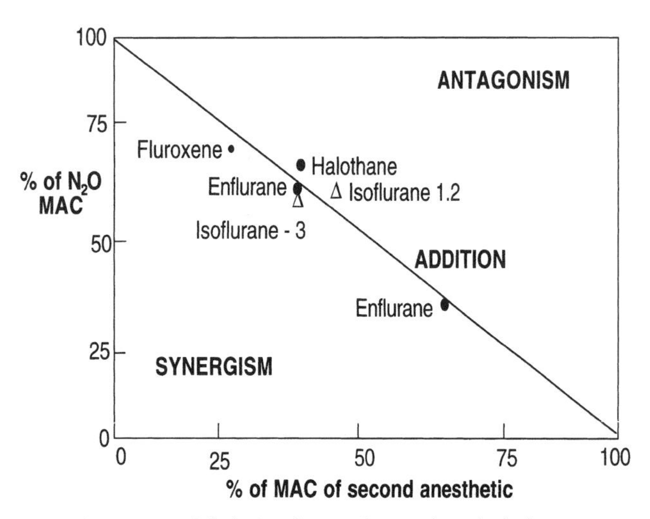

FIGURE 21-1. Inhalational agent interactions: isobologram.

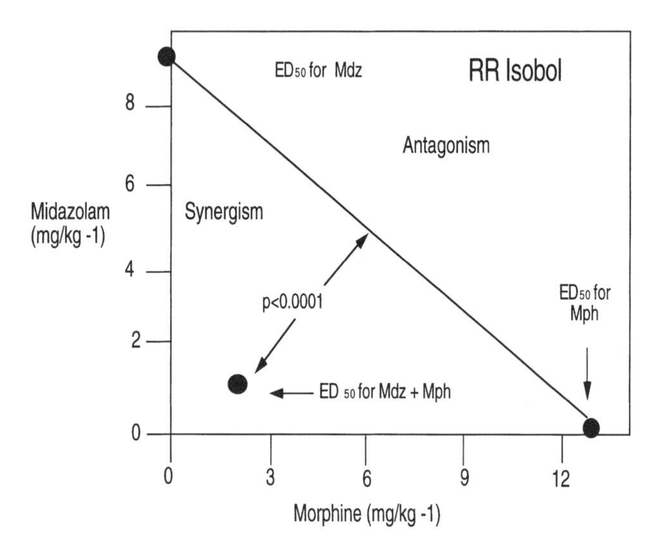

FIGURE 21-2. Sedative and hypnotic midazolam-morphine interactions in rats. (From Kissin I, Brown PT, Bradley EL Jr. Sedative and hypnotic midazolam-morphine interactions in rats. Anesth Analg 1990;71:137–143.)

In Figure 21-1, combinations of various volatile agents are used with the minimum alveolar concentration (MAC) (that which prevents movement to a painful stimulus in 50% of patients) as an end point. The combinations fall near the additive (diagonal) line, confirming that the effects of combining these drugs are only additive. In contrast, an intravenous combination of benzodiazepine and an opiate (6) is clearly synergistic (Fig. 21-2).

Midazolam-Thiopental Synergism

Midazolam-thiopental-pentobarbital anesthetic synergism has been reported in animal experiments and in surgical patients (7, 8). Barbiturates allosterically enhance benzodiazepine binding to the benzodiazepine receptor (9). Therefore, the potentiating effect of thiopental sodium can be explained by the ability of barbiturates to modulate the benzodiazepine receptor. A study in rats (6) indicated that benzodiazepine-barbiturate anesthetic synergism is not one sided, and small doses of midazolam potentiate the hypnotic effect of pentobarbital to the same extent that pentobarbital potentiates thiopental sodium-induced unconsciousness in humans (10). To prove that this effect occurs with a low subhypnotic dose of midazolam, we used this drug in an intravenous dose of 0.02 mg/kg, less than one-tenth the ED_{50} value for midazolam-induced unconsciousness (11).

Fifty healthy unpremedicated adult patients who

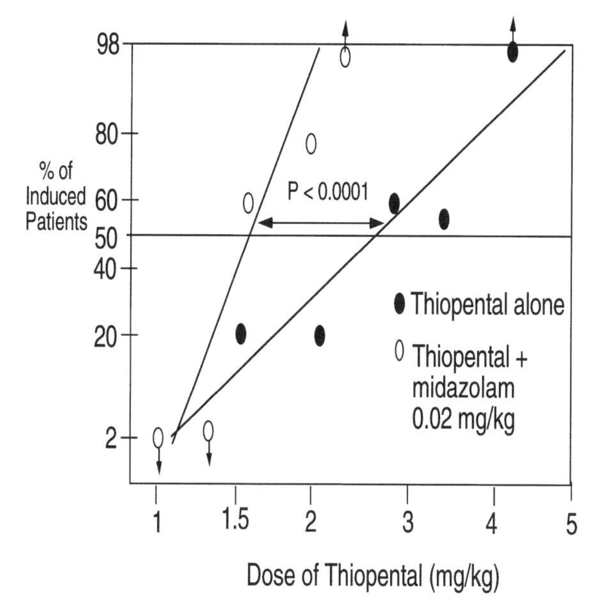

FIGURE 21-3. Thiopental-midazolam interaction: dose-response curve. (From Vinik HR, Kissin I. Midazolam for coinduction of thiopental anesthesia in patients [Abstract]. Anesthesiology 1990;73 [suppl 3]:A1216.)

were scheduled for elective surgery were assigned to one of the two groups in which a thiopental dose-response curve for unconsciousness (and loss of the eyelash reflex) was determined with and without the addition of midazolam. With a fixed dose of midazolam, thiopental was administered at five dose levels, varying from 1 to 4 mg, with five patients in each dose group. Midazolam or saline was injected intravenously first, followed 1 minute later by thiopental. The dose-response curves were determined with probit analysis (12). The study groups did not differ in age, weight, or sex.

The thiopental sodium dose-response curve for the induction of anesthesia is shown in Figure 21-3. A 96% increase in hypnotic potency was obtained with the combination of thiopental and midazolam compared with thiopental alone. The addition of midazolam changed the position of the curves so the ED_{50} point was shifted to the left along the dose axis and the slope of the curve became steeper. The degree of synergism resulted in a 49% reduction in the ED_{90} of thiopental, from 3.87 to 1.97 mg/kg. The effect of midazolam was more pronounced at the upper end of the curve, as shown more clearly in Table 21-1. At a time when midazolam reduced the thiopental sodium ED_{99} value from 5.75 to 2.37 mg/kg ($p < 0.02$), the ED_{50} value was decreased only from 2.38 to 1.57 mg/kg ($p < 0.001$) and the ED_{01} value did not change at all. Thus, the least sensitive patients showed the maximum synergism.

TABLE 21-1. Changes in Thiopental Sodium Anesthetic Potency Induced by Midazolam 0.02 mg/kg

Level of Response	Thiopental Sodium (mg/kg) Saline	Midazolam	Change in Thiopental Sodium Potency (%)	p-value
ED_{01}	0.98	1.40	—	NS
ED_{10}	1.46	1.25	+17	NS
ED_{30}	1.95	1.42	+37	$p < 0.05$
ED_{50}	2.38	1.57	+52	$p < 0.001$
ED_{70}	2.90	1.72	+69	$p < 0.001$
ED_{90}	3.87	1.97	+96	$p < 0.005$
ED_{99}	5.75	2.37	+143	$p < 0.02$

NS, not significant.

Opioid-Benzodiazepine Hypnotic Interaction

A marked degree of mutual hypnotic synergism has been demonstrated in similarly designed studies with opiates and benzodiazepines. Figure 21-4 shows that the ED_{50} for induction with alfentanil is 0.13 mg/kg, which can be reduced to 0.027 mg/kg by adding a small dose of midazolam 0.02 mg/kg, 1 minute before the alfentanil. Figure 21-5 demonstrates that the synergism is not one sided and is also potent. A subanalgesic dose of alfentanil 0.003 mg/kg significantly potentiates the hypnotic effect of midazolam, reducing the ED_{50} of midazolam from 0.27 to 0.14 mg/kg. The dose of alfentanil, 0.003 mg/kg, had been demonstrated to be subanalgesic in a previous study (15). The threshold for analgesia was determined to be statistically significant at 0.015 mg/kg. This indicates that the drug alfentanil, primarily an analgesic, can have potent hypnotic effects when combined with a benzodiazepine. A dose of 20 μg/kg alfentanil reduced the

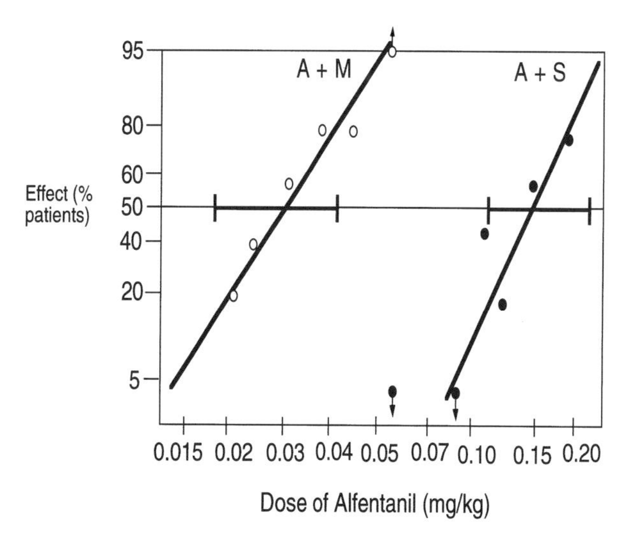

FIGURE 21-4. Alfentanil (A)-midazolam (M)-hypnotic (S)-interaction. (From Vinik HR, Bradley EL Jr, Kissin I. Midazolam-alfentanil synergism for anesthetic induction in patients. Anesth Analg 1989;69:213–217.)

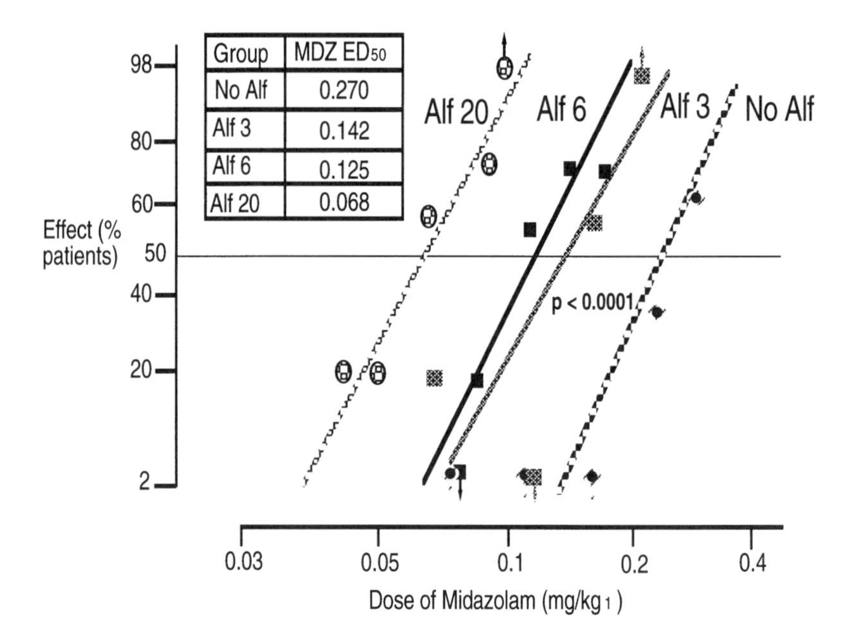

FIGURE 21-5. Midazolam (MDZ)-alfentanil (Alf)-hypnotic interaction. (From Vinik HR, Bradley EL Jr, Kissin I. Midazolam-alfentanil synergism for anesthetic induction in patients. Anesth Analg 1989; 69:213–217.)

ED_{50} of midazolam to 0.07 mg/kg, a premedication dose if used alone.

In a similarly designed study, Tverskoy and colleagues (13) demonstrated that a small dose of thiopental, 0.7 mg/kg, when added to a range of midazolam doses, produced marked synergism for hypnotic effect and resulted in a reduction of the hypnotic ED_{50} of midazolam, and these investigators concluded that the midazolam-thiopental interaction resulted in mutual potentiation. These interactions represent an approximately 74% reduction in the individual components. The interaction between alfentanil (0.02 mg/kg) and propofol is only additive, not synergistic, for hypnosis (Fig. 21-6) (17). The ED_{90} for propofol alone was 1.62 mg/kg, which was reduced to 1.24 mg/kg by the addition of alfentanil at 0.020 mg/kg. The difference between propofol alone and the combination of propofol and alfentanil was not significant at the ED_{50} level. The midazolam-propofol interaction, however, is synergistic (Fig. 21-7) (18) and is similar to the midazolam-thiopental interaction. Figure 21-7 shows that, for propofol alone, one study showed that the ED_{90} was 1.88 mg/kg, but this was reduced to 1.03 mg/kg with the addition of midazolam 0.02 mg/kg ($p < 0.02$). This result is probably a reflection of the propofol mechanism, which also activates γ-aminobutyric receptors.

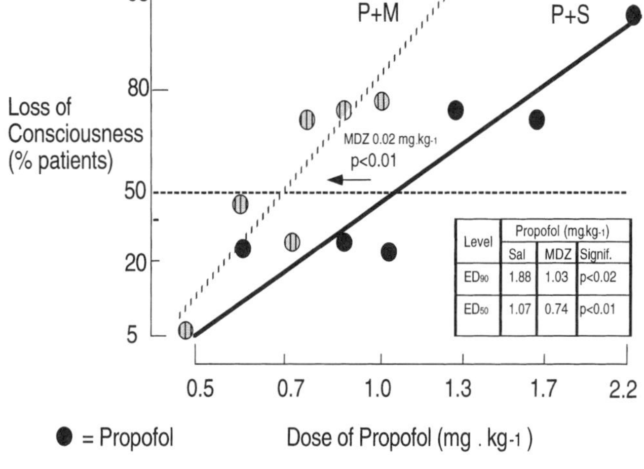

Level	Propofol (mg.kg-1)		
	Sal	MDZ	Signif.
ED_{90}	1.88	1.03	p<0.02
ED_{50}	1.07	0.74	p<0.01

FIGURE 21-7. Propofol (P)-midazolam (MDZ)-hypnotic interaction. S and Sal, Salbutamol.

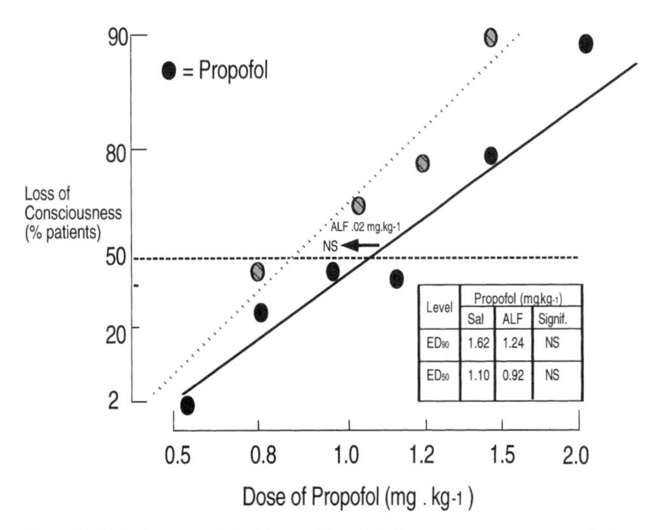

Level	Propofol (mg.kg-1)		
	Sal	ALF	Signif.
ED_{90}	1.62	1.24	NS
ED_{50}	1.10	0.92	NS

FIGURE 21-6. Propofol-alfentanil (ALF)-hypnotic interaction. Sal, Salbutamol. (From Vinik HR. Propofol-alfentanil hypnotic interaction [Abstract]. Anesth Analg 1991;7 [suppl 2]:S308.)

ADDITIVE INTERACTIONS

Anesthesiologists are familiar with the additive interaction between inhalational agents and do not expect an enhanced (or synergistic) result when combining two volatile agents. Similarly, interactions with intravenous agents may be only additive, implying no pharmacodynamic interaction between the two agents. Examples of additive reactions are ketamine-thiopental (19) and ketamine-midazolam (20) interactions, which are additive for hypnotic, as well as antinociceptive, actions. This lack of synergism can be explained by the different mechanism of action of ketamine. Ketamine inhibits excitatory transmission by decreasing depolarization of cell membranes through blockade of N-methyl-D-aspartate receptors. This mechanism differs from the allosteric stimulation of receptors of γ-aminobutyric acid receptor-chloride channel complex, and it is therefore not surprising that synergism is absent.

ANTAGONIST INTERACTIONS

An example of antagonistic interactions among intravenous anesthetics is related to the antinociceptive components of anesthesia. Diazepam-opiate combinations have been shown to be synergistic for hypnotic interaction (21). Morphine and fentanyl anesthetic interactions with diazepam demonstrate relative antagonism in rats (22). The antagonism observed was relative in that no increased need for one drug was noted when another one was added. This interaction may more accurately be referred to as infra-additive rather than antagonistic. Another mechanism for diminishing an effect of one drug by adding a second drug can be demonstrated with morphine antinociception. Morphine has both a spinal and a supraspinal antinociceptive action. Adjunctive anesthetic agents can diminish the supraspinal morphine component by inhibiting the activation of descending inhibitory pathways. The morphine-halothane interaction, which leads to suppression of heart rate increase to a noxious stimulus, is an example of this type of antagonism (23).

TRIPLE SYNERGISM

The hypnotic effects of propofol, midazolam, and alfentanil have been studied in equipotent combinations. Binary and triple combinations were compared in a similar population of healthy, unpremedicated patients (24). The results (Fig. 21-8 and Table 21-1) showed that the triple combination was synergistic for the hypnotic effect and demonstrated significant reductions of the ED_{50} doses for combinations of drugs compared with the individual drugs alone ($p < 0.0001$). In this experiment, the triple combination reduced the induction dose of propofol by 86%. The effects of the triple combination were not statistically different from those of the binary combination of midazolam and alfentanil.

PHARMACOKINETIC MECHANISMS OF INTERACTION

The pharmacokinetic component of drug interactions occurs when one drug alters the ability of another drug to be available at the site of its action. An example is the effect on cardiac output, particularly when a bolus dose of a drug such as thiopental is given. The hemodynamic depressive effect is to slow redistribution and, consequently, the plasma effect site ratio of concurrently administered drugs. This effect was well il-

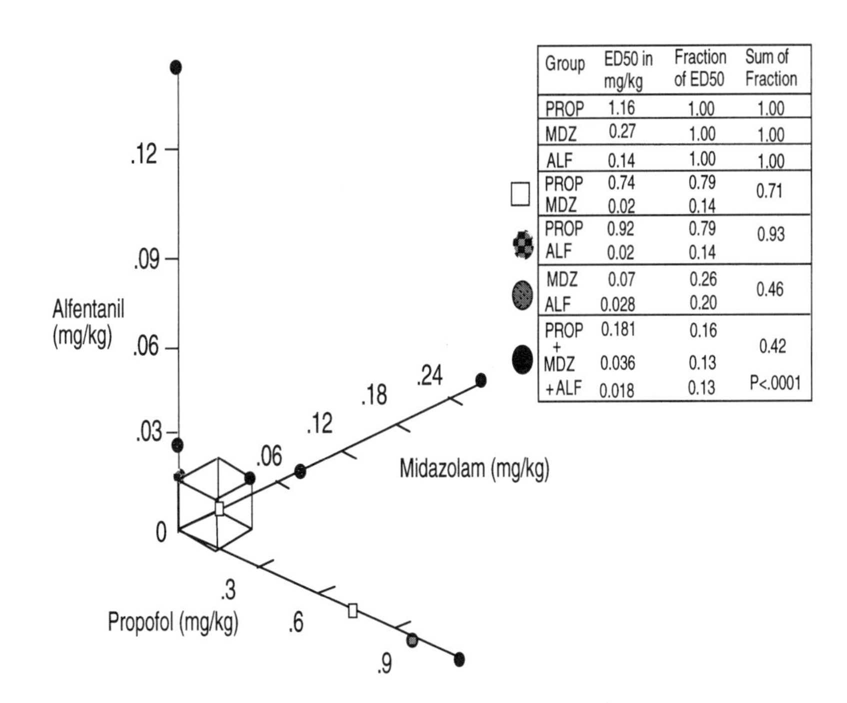

Group	ED50 in mg/kg	Fraction of ED50	Sum of Fraction
PROP	1.16	1.00	1.00
MDZ	0.27	1.00	1.00
ALF	0.14	1.00	1.00
PROP MDZ	0.74 0.02	0.79 0.14	0.71
PROP ALF	0.92 0.02	0.79 0.14	0.93
MDZ ALF	0.07 0.028	0.26 0.20	0.46
PROP + MDZ +ALF	0.181 0.036 0.018	0.16 0.13 0.13	0.42 P<.0001

FIGURE 21-8. Propofol (PROP)-midazolam (MDZ)-alfentanil (ALF) combinations: demonstrate the effect of so-called triple synergism.

lustrated by Crankshaw (25), who showed that two equal doses of thiopental administered intravenously 80 seconds apart produced a much higher plasma concentration after the second dose (see Fig. 21-8). Protein binding affects the amount of free active drug at the CNS effect site. When a highly protein bound drug is rapidly administered intravenously, the binding capacity of plasma proteins may be temporarily exceeded, resulting in a high concentration of unbound active drug, which produces a more intense reaction at the receptor site. Consequently, competitive displacement by one drug from plasma protein binding sites magnifies the effect of the other drug, which is freed to react at the effector site.

The α_2-adrenergic agonists (e.g., clonidine and dexmedetomidine) can be used to reduce the dose requirement of intravenous and volatile anesthetics (36, 37). Dexmedetomidine (38) reduces the MAC of volatile agents by a pharmacodynamic interaction. The mechanism of interaction between dexmedetomidine and thiopental appears to be related to pharmacokinetics (38). A combination of thiopental and dexmedetomidine resulted in a 30% decrease in the dose of thiopental for equal suppression of the electroencephalogram (EEG). The calculated plasma concentration at the effect site was the same in both groups, indicating that the interaction was not pharmacodynamic; that is, dexmedetomidine did not change CNS sensitivity to thiopental. Rather, the effect was pharmacokinetic in that blood pressure, heart rate, and cardiac output are decreased by α_2 agonists, and consequently, volume of distribution and intercompartmental shifts are changed by these hemodynamic effects. The results are similar to those seen with concurrent β-blocker drugs, which also decrease circulating catecholamines.

A reduction in MAC by α_2 agonists is evidence of a pharmacodynamic interaction and is not explained by any pharmacokinetic alteration of volatile agents by dexmedetomidine. These observations may indicate that EEG burst suppression is unrelated to movements as defined by MAC values. Alternatively, dexmedetomidine has a different mechanism of interaction for barbiturates than for volatile anesthetics.

DETERMINATION OF PHARMACOKINETIC COMPONENT OF DRUG INTERACTION

Because drug concentrations at the site of action in the brain cannot be measured, they have to be estimated. These estimates are based on steady-state concentrations achieved over time and, therefore, are presumed to allow equilibration between plasma and effect site. Equilibration can be achieved by using pharmacokinetic model-driven infusions with the use of computers administered for rapid equilibration of the plasma and the effect site.

PHARMACODYNAMIC MECHANISMS FOR ANESTHETIC DRUG INTERACTIONS

One can determine an interaction with a dose-related or brain concentration (by using steady-state blood concentrations) analysis. If both analyses show the same degree of synergism, then the interaction is determined by pharmacodynamic mechanisms. If the synergism is manifested only by the dose-related analysis, then the mechanism is pharmacokinetic. This principle is demonstrated in the study by Kissin and associates (21) who examined interactions using intravenous doses and also brain concentrations of the drugs used. The hypnotic synergism between morphine and diazepam was shown to be similar when the concentrations used were expressed as fractions of the brain concentration when used alone did not differ from the dose-related analysis. The authors concluded that the diazepam-morphine interaction is pharmacodynamic. Further evidence for the pharmacodynamic nature of the interaction is seen when the results of the interaction differ for different components of anesthesia. In a rat study (26, 27) assessing the interaction for a combination of morphine and thiopental (6), investigators found a synergistic interaction for the righting reflex (hypnotic effect), whereas they found an antagonistic response to the ability of the combination to block the motor response to a noxious stimulus. This outcome difference is obviously not related to a pharmacokinetic mechanism.

When combinations of intravenous anesthetic agents are given, the degree of sedation and hypnosis cannot be predicted from the doses of the individual drugs, unless the effect of a possible interaction is known and measured. The combination of propofol and ketamine has been used for total intravenous anesthesia. Hui (39) has shown that no interaction occurs between propofol and ketamine when these agents are used for induction of anesthesia for either hypnotic effect or anesthetic effect, as determined by response to a transcutaneous 5-second, 50-Hz tetanic stimulus. Additionally, they found that the apnea threshold of propofol was not altered by the addition of ketamine. The clinical effect of this additive interaction was complimentary for hemodyamic effects. The usual increase in heart rate and blood pressure induced by sympathetic stimulation with ketamine was canceled by the opposing effect of propofol, which decreases hemodynamic response by decreasing systemic vascular resistance and myocardial contractility with resulting improved cardiovascular stability.

The literature indicates a discrepancy in the reports of mechanism of interaction between propofol and opiates. Administration of propofol and alfentanil in bolus doses for induction of anesthesia indicates additivism or (17) a borderline synergism (28, 29). Propofol-fentanyl combinations are only additive (30). However, when using steady-state plasma concentrations, reports indicate that propofol blood concentrations required for loss of consciousness are reduced from 3.30 to 1.18 μg/ml when concomitant alfentanil concentrations are 400 μg/ml (31). A similar effect was described for fentanyl (32). When different methods of analysis are used, results can be difficult to compare; however, the pharmacodynamic propofol-opioid interaction when determined using blood concentration analysis is clearly more synergistic than when using dose-related analysis. A possible explanation for this discrepancy may be related to pharmacokinetic effects of drugs given in bolus doses on cardiac output, altered volume of distribution, or overwhelming the protein-binding capacity of highly bound drugs. These effects enhance the effect of the concomitantly administered drug because of a pharmacokinetic interaction rather than a pharmacodynamic interaction.

CLINICAL ADVANTAGES OF SYNERGISTIC DRUG INTERACTIONS

Drug interactions significantly enhance the hypnotic effects of certain combinations when these agents are given concurrently for peak effect. As McKay (33) indicated, the nature and degree of side effects provoked by the interactions between intravenous anesthetics determine whether the findings of hypnotic synergism are of any clinical value.

It may be possible to use smaller, less toxic doses if the synergism has a greater effect on hypnosis than on undesired end points such as cardiovascular depression. The view (34) that a combination of intravenous anesthetics should be regarded as a new "drug" with individual properties, rather than merely reflecting the known properties of the individual agents, deserves serious consideration. Synergistic drugs significantly reduce the component doses required for a hypnotic effect. In the thiopental-midazolam study, my colleagues and I also demonstrated a differential reduction in the dose for the primary induction agent. The patients who were least sensitive to the drug showed the greatest degree of synergism, so those who originally required 5 mg/kg of thiopental needed only 2 mg/kg when 0.02 mg/kg midazolam was given concurrently. This has the effect of reducing interpatient variability and makes the patient's hypnotic response more predictable and consistent.

Utility of Drug Interactions

Interactions among biologically active agents are important for several reasons. Combinations of agents are used clinically for the therapeutic advantage they may provide over single agents. The best evidence of these advantages comes from the treatment of malignant disease and of infections in which oncologists and infectious disease specialists have clearly demonstrated enhanced survival by using combination therapy.

These smaller doses of cytotoxic drugs should produce less toxic side effects. However, not all interactions among these drugs are beneficial, and some may cause toxicity. Interactions are generally described as synergistic, additive, or antagonistic. Synergism implies an enhanced or potentiated effect. An additive effect is only a summation of individual drug agents; that is, no interaction occurs. Antagonism is one drug's diminishing the effect of another. In Figure 21-3, which shows the midazolam-thiopental interaction, and in Figure 21-7, which shows the midazolam-propofol interaction, the slope of dose-response curve steepens when midazolam is added, indicating clear differences when the single induction agents thiopental or propofol are used alone or when used concurrently with a small dose of midazolam 0.02 mg/kg (one-tenth of the ED_{50} of midazolam alone). First, the dose of thiopental of propofol is reduced by approximately 50%. Second, the change in slope shows that the synergism for hypnosis is greatest in the patients who are least sensitive to the drug. The clinical correlation of this effect is that not only is the dose reduced, but also it is disproportionately reduced for the patients who are least sensitive. This, in effect, decreases interpatient variability, consequently making induction doses of thiopental or propofol more predictable and consistent when used with small coinduction doses of midazolam.

Utility of Triple Synergism

Benzodiazepine-opioid hypnotic interactions are synergistic. Figure 21-9 indicates that the combination of midazolam and alfentanil reduced each component by 74% for the hypnotic end point of loss of consciousness in patients (28). The addition of propofol, however, did not significantly increase the degree of synergism. The clinical combination of midazolam, alfentanil, and propofol, when given in reduced doses rapidly, has clinical applications because of the following pharmacologic effects:

1. The dose of propofol is markedly reduced.
2. Onset is accelerated compared with the individual drugs. Induction is consistently achieved in 45 seconds or less with individually subhypnotic doses.

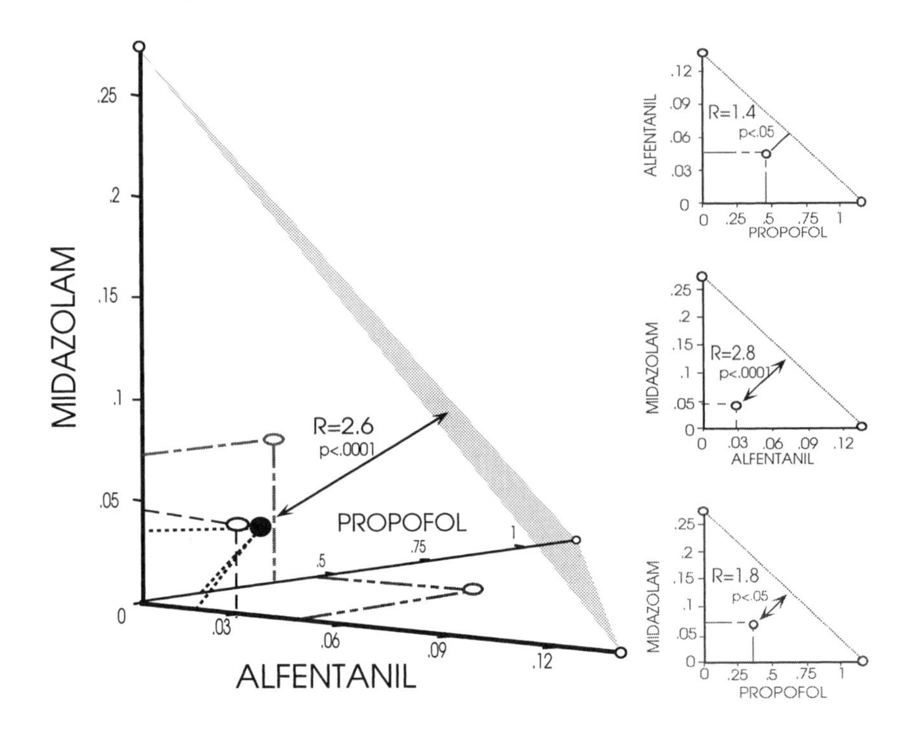

FIGURE 21-9. Binary *versus* triple synergism: isobolographic comparisons.

3. Hemodynamic response to intubation is markedly blunted even when intubation occurs 60 seconds after induction.
4. Intraocular pressure is controlled below baseline after succinylcholine administration (35).

The reduction of the dose of propofol for induction of anesthesia is significantly reduced (49%) by the addition of midazolam (28). In one study, the addition of alfentanil alone to propofol had an additive effect and reduced the ED_{90} from 1.62 to 1.24 mg/kg (Fig. 21-10). However, the triple combination resulted in an 86% reduction of propofol. These results are shown graphically by a progressively steepening of the dose response curve of propofol. The steep slope of the midazolam, alfentanil, and propofol curve confirms the reduction of the dose of propofol. This dose-response curve clearly demonstrates that the combination is more predictable for hypnotic effect. The steep dose-response effect decreases the dose range and, more important, the interpatient variability, by having greater synergism in the insensitive patient. The patients at the upper end of the curve who require higher doses have been made more predictable. This reduction in inter-

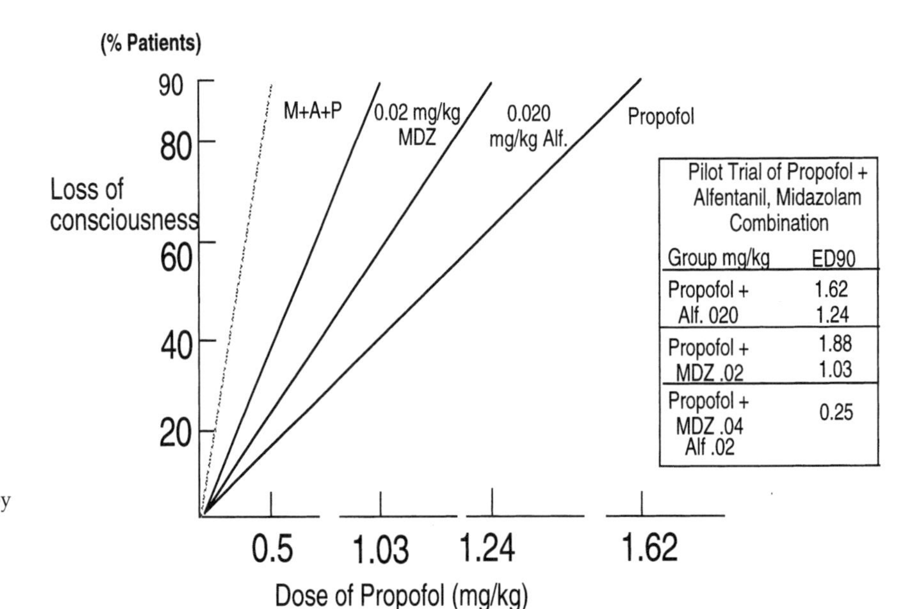

FIGURE 21-10. This composite of three different studies shows the progressive reduction of the induction dose of propofol by the addition of alfentanil and midazolam singly and then the combination of alfentanil (Alf) plus midazolam (MDZ) to propofol (M+A+P; broken line).

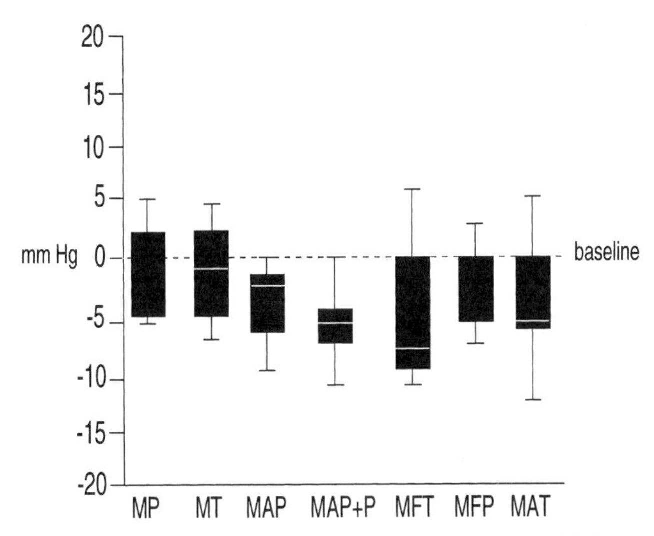

FIGURE 21-11. Intraocular pressure changes after succinylcholine. A, Alfentanil; F, fentanyl; M, midazolam; P, propofol; T, thiopental. n = 94. The minimum and maximum pressure are indicated by the ticks above and below each box.

patient variability by use of the triple combination has implications for the cost of anesthetic drugs. Because 30% of propofol's cost is attributed to waste because of the need to discard the excess drug after a single use, by using a predictable dose regimen (because of reduced interpatient variability), waste can be reduced. Moreover, more economical packaging, such as 10-ml prefilled syringes, would eliminate most waste and would also reduce incidence of infection as a further benefit.

In an example of the clinical benefit of using appropriate combinations (35), intraocular pressure (IOP) was measured after succinylcholine using different combinations of induction agents. Only the midazolam, alfentanil, and propofol combinations maintained intraocular pressure below baseline (Fig. 21-11). However, after intubation even this group of agents did not control IOP unless 50% more propofol was given before intubation (Fig. 21-12).

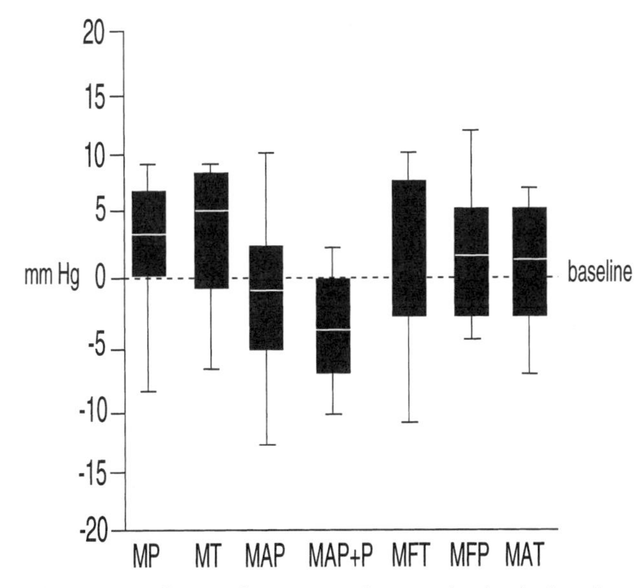

FIGURE 21-12. Intraocular pressure changes after intubation. A, Alfentanil; F, fentanyl; M, midazolam; P, propofol; T, thiopental.

IMPORTANCE OF PHARMACODYNAMIC INTERACTION

A clear understanding of pharmacodynamic principles in drug interaction enables the clinician to maximize the efficacy and to minimize the toxicity of drug combination therapy. Many examples of appropriate combinations are evident when treating severe hypertension, cancer, major bacterial infections, and the prevention of transplant rejection. The underlying rationale for using drugs with different mechanisms of action includes promotion of synergistic beneficial pharmacologic effects and avoidance of additive side effects by dose reductions and decreasing tolerance, such as in large infusion or sedation in the intensive care unit.

EFFECT OF DRUG INTERACTIONS ON THE COST OF INTRAVENOUS ANESTHETIC TECHNIQUES

Burgeoning health care costs have precipitated the revolution in the health care industry. Managed care and capitation programs have directed attention to cost containment (Table 21-2). Anesthesia personnel have been told to reduce the cost of drugs used in the operating room. To a large extent, this recommendation has been driven by hospital pharmacies which are trying to reduce drug budgets in the face of new and expensive additions to the formulary. Hospital formula additions are usually determined by the lowest bidder if the new drugs are declared to be therapeutic equivalents. Consequently, more expensive drugs are only added if they have a clear therapeutic advantage. For example, pharmacists question the advantage of propofol over thiopental when an induction dose costs five times more (based on average wholesale price and corrected for relative potency). Cost of maintenance of anesthesia with nitrous oxide 65% and a generic inhalational agent at a 2-L flow rate can be reduced to less than $3 a MAC hour. Compare an average propofol infusion at $25 per hour (based on 100 to 150 μg/kg/min in a 70-kg patient). The responsibility of the anesthesiologist is to justify the use of the more expensive drug by choosing the agent with a clear clinical advantage and preferably a superior outcome. The increased cost of a new drug can also be justified if it

TABLE 21-2. Costs of Intravenous Anesthetic Agents*

Generic Name	Strength	Average Wholesale Price (Red Book) ($)	US $ Cost/mg	Cost of Standard Induction US Dosage (70-kg/$)
Thiopental	500 mg	8.44	0.017	4.76 (4 mg/kg)
	2% 5 g	34.75	0.007	1.96
Etomidate	2 mg/ml 20 ml	27.41	0.68	14.28 (0.3 mg/kg)
Propofol	20 ml	12.85	0.06	8.40 (2 mg/kg)
	50 ml	32.25	0.06	8.40 (2 mg/kg)
Methohexital	500 mg/50 ml	11.49	0.023	2.41 (1.5 mg/kg)
Ketamine	200 mg/20 ml	9.70	0.048	5.04 (1.5 mg/kg)
Midazolam	2 mg/2 ml	4.25	2.12	4.25 (2 mg) (small sedative dose)
	5 mg/5 ml	9.35	1.87	9.35 (5 mg) (medium sedative dose)
	10 mg/2 ml	21.00	2.10	21.00 (10 mg) (large sedative dose)
Lorazepam	2 mg	9.78	2.45	9.78
	4 mg	11.49	2.87	11.49
Diazepam	5 mg	2.44	.49	2.44
	10 mg/kg	2.81	.28	2.81
Fentanyl	0.100 mg	2.06	—	2.06 (0.1 mg)
	1 mg/20 ml	13.98	13.98	13.98 (0.1 mg)
Alfentanil	1 gm	7.50		7.50 (1 mg)
	2.5 mg	13.44	5.37	13.44
Sufentanil	0.050/1 ml	13.57		2.71 (0.01 mg)
	0.1 mg/2 ml	24.06		2.40 (0.01 mg)

Anatomy of Anesthetic Drug Costs

This table compares average wholesale prices published in the red book. However, these prices may be irrelevant to a particular pharmacy because of special purchasing arrangements.

Acquisition Costs

A hospital pharmacy rarely pays the average wholesale price because:
- It belongs to a purchasing group that negotiates a special price for members.
- The pharmacy is managed by another party.
- A contract price has been negotiated with the supplier.
- A special deal is contingent on other purchases.

Price to Patient or Insuror

For hospitals to balance their budgets, administration fees are added to acquisition costs of drugs. These administration costs vary from region to region and hospital to hospital and often bear no relation to the original acquisition cost. This occurs, for example when operating room costs are packaged and not itemized and results in apparently unrelated charges that are often bizarre (e.g., thiopental, $85 for a $4 item). The amount the patient pays is often totally unrelated to the original acquisition cost of the drug.

Wastage

Drug benefits can be reduced without sacrificing the advantages of newer drugs by:
- Avoiding waste; often drugs are unnecessarily drawn up for quick availability and then discarded at the end of the case.
- To comply with single usage protocol, ampules of propofol, for example, can be fractionated into separated syringes from a larger ampule and used on several patients.
- Drug interaction studies have shown that concurrent use of interacting drugs not only decreases the dose but reduces interpatient variability response; this enables the clinician to give precise premeasured doses because the required dose of the combination is predictable.

Even though anesthetic drugs represent less than 5% of the cost of operating room services, anesthesia personnel must be aware of relative costs to use therapeutically equivalent drugs at lower cost.

It would be reprehensible to deprive patients of the potential benefit of appropriate medication if it costs slightly more.

**This table lists the average wholesale price (red book, November 1995) of frequently used intravenous anesthetic agents, sedative hypnotics, and analgesics. Only the available lowest quoted prices are shown. These often vary with different generic manufacturers. Drugs available in prefilled syringes are more expensive. The last column gives prices of accepted induction doses in a typical 70-kg patient for the five induction agents. Costs of three different benzodiazepines are shown for various sedative doses. The analgesics cost is shown in the last column (for equivalent potency). Fentanyl has one-tenth the potency of sufentanil and is 10 times more potent than alfentanil.*

results in savings in other areas, for example, if the new drug enables quicker recovery or fewer side effects that result in earlier discharge and decreased nursing costs. Pharmacists and hospital administrators should understand that the costs of anesthetic drugs are minor compared with overall operating costs. The cost of an operating room is at least $600 an hour, and the overall costs of anesthesia drugs are less than 5% of the operating room costs (40). Anesthesiologists have unique expertise which should allow them to assess cost-to-benefit ratios of particular drugs and the logical reasons for drug preferences. They should encourage administrators not to define costs too narrowly because this could be counterproductive for good patient care.

In conclusion, anesthesia providers have lagged behind in the elucidation and application of synergistic drug interactions to achieve improved patient outcomes. Oncologists have used synergistic combinations of chemotherapeutic drugs with great success. Combinations of antibiotics have major therapeutic advantages in cases of resistant microorganisms. The mechanisms of the interactions include pharmacodynamic and kinetic components. Our analyses of single doses differ from those of investigators who have used steady-state infusions and extrapolated effect site concentrations. These interactions need to be better understood by practicing anesthesiologists so they can shed the image of "alchemist in the operating room." The application of rigorous defined pharmacologic principles to intravenous anesthesia should enhance patients' well-being.

REFERENCES

1. Kissin I. General anesthetic action: an obsolete notion? [Editorial]. Anesth Analg 1993;76:215–218.
2. Eger EI II. Anesthetic uptake and action. Baltimore: Williams & Wilkins, 1974:17.
3. Torri G, Damia G, Fabiani ML. Effect of nitrous oxide on the anaesthetic requirement of enflurane. Br J Anaesth 1974;46:468–472.
4. Berenbaum MC. What is synergy? Pharmacol Rev 1989;41:93–141.
5. Quasha AL, Eger EI II, Tinker JT. Determination and application of MAC. Anesthesiology 1980;53:315–334.
6. Kissin I, Brown PT, Bradley EL Jr. Sedative and hypnotic midazolam-morphine interactions in rats. Anesth Analg 1990; 71:137–143.
7. Kissin I, Mason JO III, Bradley EL Jr. Pentobarbital and thiopental anesthetic interactions with midazolam. Anesthesiology 1987;67:26–31.
8. Tverskoy M, Fleyshman G, Bradley EL Jr, Kissin I. Midazolam-thiopental anesthetic interaction in patients. Anesth Analg 1988;67:342–345.
9. Leeb-Lundberg F, Snowman A, Olsen RW. Barbiturate receptors are coupled to benzodiazepine receptors. Proc Natl Acad Sci U S A 1980;77:7468–7474.
10. Vinik HR, Kissin I. Midazolam for coinduction of thiopental anesthesia inpatients [Abstract]. Anesthesiology 1990;73(suppl 3):A1216.
11. Kissin I, Vinik HR. Midazolam potentiates thiopental sodium anesthetic induction in patients. J Clin Anesth 1991;3:367–370.
12. Finney DJ. Probit analysis. 3rd ed. London: Cambridge University Press, 1971.
13. Tverskoy M, Fleyshman G, Bradley EL Jr, Kissin I. Midazolam-thiopental anesthetic interaction in patients. Anesth Analg 1988;67:342–345.
14. Vinik HR, Bradley EL Jr, Kissin I. Midazolam-alfentanil synergism for anesthetic induction in patients. Anesth Analg 1989; 69:213–217.
15. Castillo R, Battito F, Bradley EL Jr. Does midazolam antagonize the analgesic effect of alfentanil in patients? Anesthesiology 1989; 71 (suppl 3A):A116.
16. Kissin I, Vinik HR, Castillo R, Bradley EL Jr. Alfentanil potentiates midazolam-induced unconsciousness in subanalgesic doses. Anesth Analg 1990;71:65–69.
17. Vinik HR, propofol-alfentanil hypnotic interaction [Abstract]. Anesth Analg 1991;7(suppl 2):S308.
18. Short TG, Chui PT. Propofol and midazolam act synergistically in combination. Br J Anaesth 1991;67:539–545.
19. Royblat L, Katz J, Rozentsveig V, et al. Anaesthetic interaction between thiopentone and ketamine. Eur J Anaesthesiol 1992; 9:307–312.
20. Hong W, Short TG, Hui WC. Hypnotic and anesthetic interactions between ketamine and midazolam in female patients. Anesthesiology 1993;79:1227–1232.
21. Kissin I, Brown PT, Bradley EL Jr, et al. Diazepam-morphine hypnotic synergism in rats. Anesthesiology 1989;70:689–694.
22. Kissin I, Brown PT, Bradley EL Jr. Morphine and fentanyl anesthetic interacts with diazepam: relative antagonism in rats. Anesth Analg 1990;71:236–241.
23. Kissin I, Kerr CR, Smith R. Morphine-halothane interaction in rats. Anesthesiology 1984;60:553–561.
24. Vinik HR, Kissin I. Propofol-midazolam-alfentanil combination: is hypnotic synergism present? [Abstract] Anesth Analg 1993;76(suppl 2):S450.
25. Crankshaw D. Hypnotics in infusion anaesthesia: with particular reference to thiopentone. Anaesth Intensive Care 1987; 15:90–96.
26. Kissin I, Mason JO III, Bradley EL Jr. Morphine and fentanyl hypnotic interactions with thiopental. Anesthesiology 1987; 67:331–335.
27. Kissin I, Mason JO III, Bradley EL Jr. Morphine and fentanyl interactions with thiopental in relation to movement response to noxious stimulation. Anesth Analg 1986;65:1149–1154.
28. Vinik HR, Bradley EL Jr, Kissin I. Triple anesthetic combination: propofol-midazolam-alfentanil. Anesth Analg 1994;78:354–358.
29. Short TG, Plummer JL, Chui PT. Hypnotic and anaesthetic interactions between midazolam, propofol and alfentanil. Br J Anaesth 1992;69:162–167.
30. Ben-Shlomo I, Finger J, Bar-Av E, et al. Propofol and fentanyl act additively for induction of anaesthesia. Anaesthesia 1993; 48;111–113.
31. Vuyk J, Griever GER, Engbers FHM, et al. The interaction between propofol and alfentanil during induction of anesthesia. Anesthesiology 1994;81:A400.
32. Smith C, McEwan AI, Jhaveri R, et al. The interaction of fentanyl on the Cp_{50} of propofol for loss of consciousness and skin incision. Anesthesiology 1994;81:820–828.
33. McKay AC. Synergism among i.v. anaesthetics. Br J Anaesth 1991;67:1–3.
34. Short TG, Plummer JL, Chui PT. Hypnotic and anaesthetic interactions between midazolam, propoful and alfentanil. Br J Anaesth 1992;69:162–167.
35. Vinik HR. Intraocular pressure (IOP) changes during rapid se-

quence induction with succinylcholine or rocuronium. Anesth Analg 1995;80:S530.

36. Ghignone M, Quintin L, Duke PC, et al. Effects of clonidine on narcotic requirements and hemodynamic response during induction of fentanyl anesthesia and endotracheal intubation. Anesthesiolgoy 1986;64:36–42.
37. Ghignone M, Noe C, Calvillo O, Quintin L. Anesthesia for opthalmic surgery in the elderly: the effects of clonidine of intraocular pressure, perioperative hemodynamics, and anesthetic requirement. Anesthesiology 1988;68:707–716.
38. Buhrer M, Mappes A, Lauber R, et al. Dexmedetomidine decreases thiopental dose requirement and alters distribution pharmacokinetics. Anesthesiology 1994;80:1216–1227.
39. Hui TW. Additive interactions between propofol and ketamine when used for anesthesia induction in femal patients. Anesthesiology 1995;82:641–648.
40. Lubarsky DA, Smith LR, Glass PSA. Comparison of maintenance drug costs of isoflurane, desflurane, sevoflurane and propofol with OR and PACU labor costs during a 60 minute outpatient procedure. Anesthesiology 1995;30(suppl 3A):A1035.

VI SPECIAL PATIENT POPULATIONS

22 Intravenous Anesthesia for Pediatric Patients

Mehernoor F. Watcha

Children fear injections, and their struggles during the placement of intravenous cannulae have led many anesthesiologists in the United States to induce anesthesia with inhalation agents before attempting venous cannulation. Although the availability of EMLA (eutectic mixture of local anesthetics) cream has permitted painless venipuncture, children still fear the approach of adults bearing needles. In contrast to practices in the United States, the induction of anesthesia with intravenous agents is more common in Europe. However, regardless of the induction technique, traditionally anesthesia was maintained with inhalation agents because of the experience of prolonged awakening when barbiturates and ketamine were used for total intravenous anesthesia (TIVA) (1, 2). The availability of new intravenous agents with higher systemic clearances and more rapid metabolism has rekindled interest in TIVA. This technique avoids the problems associated with the use of more conventional inhalation agents (i.e., renal and hepatic toxicity, mutagenicity, and teratogenicity). In addition, the safe and reliable administration of inhalation agents requires specialized and expensive equipment to vaporize the agent and a method to scavenge and evacuate waste gases, to reduce exposure of medical personnel to residual concentrations of agents. These drugs may also have an adverse effect on the ozone layer. In contrast, intravenous agents can be administered without special devices, and scavenging of waste gases is not necessary during TIVA.

The ideal anesthetic for TIVA should be water-soluble, nonirritating, and stable in aqueous solutions, have a long shelf life, possess analgesic and amnestic properties, and produce a rapid, smooth onset of hypnosis without cardiorespiratory depression.* Finally, this agent should be able to be rapidly redistributed or undergo fast biotransformation to inactive, nontoxic metabolites so recovery of consciousness would be fast when the administration of the drug is terminated. No such agent is currently available, but various drugs have been used for this purpose, including propofol, short-acting opioids (fentanyl, alfentanil, sufentanil, and remifentanil), ketamine, etomidate, and midazolam. This chapter reviews the use of TIVA in children.

PROPOFOL

Propofol was introduced in clinical practice in the United States in 1989. Initial reports concentrated on its use for induction of anesthesia, but the realization that propofol's pharmacokinetics results in a rapid, clear emergence from anesthesia and lack of cumulative effects even after prolonged administration encouraged its use as a maintenance anesthetic drug (3). Data are available on the experiences with propofol for induction and maintenance of anesthesia in children, along with information about its recovery characteristics (3).

Induction Characteristics

The fast onset and smooth transition from the awake to the anesthetized state in unpremedicated children, along with a short, predictable duration of action, has made propofol a highly satisfactory induction agent, comparable to thiopental. Early reports suggested that a propofol dose of 2.8 mg/kg was required for loss of eyelash reflex in unpremedicated children, whereas 2.0 mg/kg was sufficient in children premedicated with trimeperazine (4). Aun and associates determined the dose-response relationship of propofol in 300 unpremedicated healthy Chinese children, by using the loss of eyelash reflex and acceptance of a face mask as the

*White PF, Way WL, Trevor AJ: Ketamine-Its pharmacology and therapeutic uses. Anesthesiology 1982;56:119–36

end point (1). An age-related reduction in the dose requirements was noted, and these authors recommended a dose between 2.5 and 3.5 mg/kg, similar to the recommendations of Hannallah and colleagues and Patel and associates, who studied children in the United States and the United Kingdom, respectively (2, 4). Manschot and colleagues concluded that 2.5 mg/kg is an appropriate induction dose for children aged 3 to 15 years if it is preceded by alfentanil, 5 μg/kg, but a sleep response to a lower dose of 1.5 mg/kg was noted more often in older children (5). Westrin determined that the median effective dose (ED_{50}) for induction of anesthesia with propofol was 3.0 ± 0.2 mg/kg in infants aged 1 to 6 months and 2.4 ± 0.1 mg/kg in children aged 10 to 16 years (6). An intravenous dose of 3 mg/kg appears to induce anesthesia satisfactorily in most children.

Pain on injection of propofol is noted in 28 to 60% of patients and remains a significant drawback to its use for induction of anesthesia (1, 7-9). This pain may be ameliorated by the use of large antecubital veins and by the administration of small doses of lidocaine or opioid analgesics before injecting propofol (2). Cameron and associates have determined that lidocaine, 0.2 mg/kg, is the minimum effective dose required to prevent pain when propofol is injected into a vein on the dorsum of the hand in children (10). Hiller and Saarnivaara have demonstrated that pretreatment with alfentanil, 15 or 20 (but not 10) μg/kg, is as effective in preventing pain on induction as adding 10 mg lidocaine to the syringe with the induction dose of propofol (7).

The cardiovascular effects of an induction dose of propofol were studied by these authors and others (8, 11, 12). Induction of anesthesia was associated with a reduction in heart rate and blood pressure (13). Heart rate reductions of 10 to 20% were noted, with a prolongation of the corrected QT interval and a higher incidence of bradycardia and junctional rhythms than following induction with thiopental (14). The reduction of blood pressure after the administration of propofol was less in children than in adults, and cardiovascular measurements usually remain in the clinically acceptable range (12, 15, 16). Possible mechanisms for the hypotension may relate to the following: 1) its action on peripheral vasculature (vasodilatation); 2) decreased myocardial contractility; 3) resetting of the baroreflex activity; and 4) inhibition of the sympathetic nervous system outflow. Aun and colleagues noted that blood pressure decreases after induction with propofol were greater than after thiopental (16). However, reductions in cardiac index, as measured by two-dimensional echocardiography and pulsed Doppler measurements, did not differ significantly following induction of anesthesia with propofol or thiopental. The decrease in systemic vascular resistance was similar in toddlers who received either of the two intravenous induction agents, but in older children, the decrease was markedly greater following propofol (16). The concomitant use of propofol, alfentanil, and succinylcholine warrants careful monitoring for severe bradycardia and hypotension (7, 17). Bradycardia in this patient population may be an even greater problem if clonidine (or dexmedetomidine) is used as a preanesthetic sedative. Similarly, the incidence of vagally mediated bradycardia during surgical stimulation (e.g., oculocardiac reflex during strabismus surgery) is higher when propofol is used compared with inhalation agents (17, 18). However, Martin and associates noted that blood pressure measurements tended to be higher in children receiving propofol anesthesia compared with those receiving volatile inhalation agents (8).

Because propofol appears to suppress airway reflexes more effectively than thiopental, conditions for insertion of a laryngeal mask airway (LMA) are better when propofol has been used for induction (19). In a study of 60 children aged 4 to 9 years, Allsop and associates showed that an LMA was inserted successfully in 35%, 70%, and 90% of children who received intravenous propofol, 2.5, 3.0, or 3.5 mg/kg, respectively (20). Propofol has also been used to facilitate tracheal intubation without the use of muscle relaxants. When used alone, propofol, 3.5 mg/kg, provided poor intubating conditions (21). However, the addition of alfentanil, 40 μg/kg, resulted in more acceptable conditions compared with the use of lower doses of alfentanil (20 μg/kg), with or without lidocaine (22). Hiller and Saarnivaara noted that pretreatment with alfentanil also diminished the hemodynamic responses to tracheal intubation (7, 22).

The incidence of apnea after induction of anesthesia with propofol and thiopental is similar in unpremedicated children, but the addition of benzodiazepines and opioids for premedication increases apnea in the propofol group (2, 6, 9, 22). Although hiccups have not been reported as frequently with propofol as with thiopental, induction of anesthesia with propofol is associated with a higher incidence (21 to 28%) of spontaneous choreiform movements, dystonic flexion, twisting, or extension movements suggestive of a subcortical origin (23). These movements can be reduced by administering higher doses of propofol or by the concomitant use of opioids or droperidol (24).

Despite the increased frequency of apnea with a propofol induction, the incidence of airway obstruction has been lower than in children receiving potent inhalation agents for induction (2, 8). Data also indicate that propofol, unlike halothane, does not inhibit hypoxic pulmonary vasoconstriction or affect pulmonary gas exchange. In patients undergoing neurosurgical procedures, Mendoza and colleagues demonstrated that halothane, but not propofol, increased intrapulmonary shunt and alveolar-arterial oxygen tension differences (25). Few data are available regarding the effect of propofol on pulmonary gas exchange in children. In animal studies, the pulmonary uptake of propofol was affected by the timing of the concomitant administration of fentanyl. When given 30 seconds before propofol, fentanyl reduced pulmonary uptake, but no significant effects were noted when fentanyl was given 3 to 10 minutes before propofol (26).

Maintenance and Recovery Characteristics

Although propofol has been used for both induction (single dose) and maintenance (continuous infusion) of anesthesia in children, few data are available on the use of propofol for TIVA in children (8, 18, 25, 27). Although TIVA avoids the use of both nitrous oxide (N_2O) and volatile agents, it is a more common practice to administer N_2O with a propofol infusion. The infusion rate that provides satisfactory conditions varies with the surgical stimulus (28). Hannallah and associates have stated that the average maintenance propofol dose required to prevent movement during surgery was 267 ± 83 μg/kg/min (15). However, much lower doses are required for sedation for noninvasive radiologic procedures. A loading dose of 2 mg/kg, followed by an infusion at 100 μg/kg/min, provided satisfactory conditions for computed tomography (CT) scans (29). For painful procedures such as bone marrow aspirates or lumbar puncture, infusion rates between 100 and 300 μg/kg/min may be required (30).

The popularity of propofol in adult outpatient anesthesia is based on the rapidity of recovery and the decreased incidence of postoperative emesis. Blood concentrations decrease rapidly following the termination of propofol infusions because of the large volume of distribution and fast metabolism of the drug. In several studies, standard recovery end points (eye opening, response to commands, ambulation, oral intake, and discharge readiness) occurred earlier in children receiving propofol versus halothane (25, 31). In ambulatory surgery, rapid recovery and the absence of emesis are desired goals and have contributed to the popularity of propofol in this field. Because more than 70% of pediatric procedures requiring anesthesia are performed on an outpatient basis in the United States, maintenance of anesthesia with propofol following N_2O sedation or mask inductions has been advocated in this patient population (8). Small children who awaken earlier may appear to have an increased need for sedation and analgesia in the postanesthetic care unit (PACU), leading to delays in discharge (11, 17). Other factors that may delay awakening after propofol include excemine premedication, the concomitant use of long-acting opioids, and the use of fixed infusion rates rather than adjustments in infusion rates as clinically warranted. In a study of 156 children undergoing outpatient surgery while receiving propofol or halothane anesthesia, Martin and colleagues failed to demonstrate a difference in recovery times. However, both groups of patients received an oral narcotic-based premedicant along with morphine during surgery (8).

With the introduction of inhaled agents that have low blood gas partition coefficients (e.g., sevoflurane and desflurane), clinically important differences in awakening after propofol anesthesia compared with inhalation agents are no longer evident, although statistically significant differences have been reported. A meta-analysis of studies of propofol and desflurane anesthesia in adults noted no statistically significant differences in the time to following commands after discontinuation of desflurane versus propofol (32). Yet, patients who received propofol were discharged to home a mean of 17 minutes (range 4 to 30 minutes) more quickly than patients who received desflurane (32). Similarly, earlier awakening with sevoflurane has not been translated into earlier discharge after ambulatory surgery. Institutional protocols that insist on a minimum stay in phase I and II recovery areas may limit any benefits derived from earlier recovery with propofol.

The newer inhalation agents are not associated with a decrease in the incidence of postoperative nausea and vomiting, and the reduced emesis rate continues to be a major advantage for the use of propofol in outpatient procedures (7, 8, 17, 18, 33). For example, up to 60 to 80% of children undergoing strabismus surgery with halothane anesthesia vomit in the postoperative period compared with 16 to 20% with propofol (17, 18, 34, 35). Similarly, Martin and associates noted a significant decrease in emesis (18% versus 34%) in children receiving propofol rather than a volatile agent during various outpatient surgical procedures (8). Propofol may even have an antiemetic effect in children undergoing chemotherapy (36) and in adults with nausea in the PACU (37). However, this effect in the PACU is short-lived. Other investigators have also suggested that the effect of intraoperative use of propofol on the incidence of postoperative emesis is limited to the immediate postoperative period, and postdischarge emesis rates do not differ between children who received propofol or an inhalation agent during strabismus surgery (35). Emesis rates may be more affected by the use of adjuvants such as N_2O and opioids than by specific anesthetic agents in this patient population (18, 38).

Investigators have suggested that the use of propofol regimens for outpatient anesthesia is cost-effective because it results in more rapid recovery, decreased postoperative nausea and vomiting, and a shorter time to being judged "fit for discharge" (39). Sung and colleagues reported that patients receiving propofol spent 15 minutes less in the more labor-intensive phase I recovery area compared with patients receiving a standard thiopental-isoflurane regimen (40). However, these authors did not include the costs of wasted propofol, infusion equipment and supplies, and the potential decrease in costs of the inhalation regimen with the use of low fresh gas flows (41). Marais and associates used a computer simulation of the flow of patients through a recovery room area and claimed that the preferential use of propofol over a thiopental-isoflurane regimen would be associated with a 25% reduction in nursing costs (42). These comparisons were based on theoretic savings of nursing costs and not actual savings (i.e., decreased overtime or decreased hiring of operating room and PACU personnel).

A definitive study is still required to confirm that propofol usage is associated with real cost savings in busy institutions with long surgical waiting lists (43). This type of study must go beyond merely demonstrating earlier recovery in the operating room and PACU with propofol, to show that its use is associated with decreased times to actual discharge, reduced hiring of nurses and support personnel, or the completion of at least one additional case in the same operating room session. In a study that limited the perspective to that of the chief financial officer of a health maintenance organization, the use of propofol for induction and maintenance of anesthesia reduced the total cost of surgery by $202.71, compared with the costs of using thiopental-isoflurane anesthesia in intra-abdominal surgical procedures with a duration of less than 4 hours (39). Pharmacoeconomic studies should also be performed from the perspective of the patient and from society as a whole. The measurement of the effect of anesthetics on the time to return to normal activities is most important, but it has not been included in clinical trials. In pharmacoeconomic studies of the choice of anesthetic drugs in pediatric patients, data should be obtained on the time a child's caretaker can return to their regular work inside or outside the house. Patient satisfaction will become an important measure of the quality of care, and some validated measurement tool of these intangible costs will have to be established (43).

Pharmacokinetics

The blood concentration curves of propofol are best fitted to a three-compartment model, with an initial short half-life (1.5 to 4.2 minutes) when redistribution occurs, followed by a second phase (9.3 to 56 minutes) associated with a high metabolic clearance in the liver and at other sites and a large volume of distribution, and a final third phase (209 to 475 minutes) that reflects the slow elimination from poorly perfused tissues (9, 44-46). The volume of distribution of the central compartment is larger for propofol in children than in adults (343 versus 228 ml/kg). The pharmacokinetics of propofol is not appreciably altered in children or adults with morbid obesity, renal failure, or cirrhosis (47-51). The clearance of propofol has been reported to be 32 to 57 ml/kg/min in children compared with 27 mg/kg/min for adults (52). Therefore, higher doses are required to achieve and maintain the same blood levels in children compared with adults. In addition, the theoretic target concentration required to maintain an adequate depth of anesthesia may be higher in children than in adults (52). A target propofol blood concentration of 5 mg/ml would successfully induce anesthesia in the majority of adult patients premedicated with temazepam without major hemodynamic or respiratory side effects (53). In children who have not received any opioids, mean blood propofol levels of 6.6 mg/ml have been stated to be necessary to prevent movement with surgical stimuli (54). These blood levels may be achieved by a dose of 1.5 to 2.0 mg/kg in adults, but higher doses (3 to 3.5 mg/kg) have been recommended for satisfactory induction of anesthesia and the prevention of movement with skin incision in children (54).

A major problem with pharmacokinetic studies in children is the need to draw frequent and relatively large volumes of blood at multiple points in time. When only a few samples are drawn, an increased potential exists that measurement errors will result in large errors in the estimate of pharmacokinetic parameters. Newer approaches have been made to provide reasonable estimates of these parameters in a population using a small number of samples from individual patients. These include the "naive pooled data," sparse sampling and the "mixed-effects modeling" approaches (55). In the pooled data approach, all data are analyzed allowing for differences in fixed effects, but not in random variation among individuals. The mixed effects model also permits random variation among individuals and requires software such as the NONMEM program. Kataria and colleagues have shown no appreciable differences among the traditional two-stage, pooled-data, and the mixed-effects approaches (45).

The clinical usefulness of pharmacokinetic data in the daily practice of clinical anesthesia has been questioned. Computer-assisted controlled infusion (CACI) devices that constantly adjust the infusion rate with the stated aim of achieving and maintaining a desired blood level of a drug have been tested in human patients (28). Although the pumps may achieve a desired blood level if they are programmed with appropriate data, adjustments still need to be made in the infusion rates during an operation, because these desired blood levels change with the degree of surgical stimulation. Coetzee and associates have shown that the choice of a pharmacokinetic model did not make much clinical difference in the quality of anesthesia (56). Marsh and colleagues have demonstrated that these devices need to be programmed with data from children and not adults to avoid a systematic overprediction of actual blood propofol concentrations (52). However, the limited availability of such data in children, along with ethnic and interpatient variability in pharmacokinetics, may reduce the clinical usefulness of such devices (9, 57, 58). In one study, there were no differences in recovery from anesthesia after induction and maintenance with a computerized, target-controlled infusion of propofol or with a propofol-halothane technique (59). In another similar study, recovery after minor surgical procedures was much slower when propofol was administered by a pharmacokinetic model-controlled syringe pump compared with techniques that used propofol-halothane, thiopental-halothane, or halothane alone (60). This group claimed that the mean blood concentration required for satisfactory anesthesia was 6.6 (range 3 to 11) mg/ml, and the mean blood concentration at the time of waking, which occurred 40 minutes after switching off the infusion, was 0.86 (range 0.40 to 1.45) mg/ml (54).

Browne and colleagues examined the dose requirements of propofol in children to prevent patient movement with skin incision (27). These authors administered alfentanil as a loading dose of 65 or 85 μg/kg, followed by an infusion of 50 or 65 μg/kg/h, respectively, and propofol given by a three-stage manual infusion scheme designed to achieve and maintain a steady-state blood concentration (27). The mean effective whole blood concentration of propofol associated with a suppression of movement response in 95% of subjects was 3.87 and 4.26 mg/ml, when the high and low doses of alfentanil were administered. This study suggested a loading dose of 1.3 to 1.5 mg/kg of propofol, followed by an initial infusion of 13 to 15 mg/kg/h for the first 10 minutes, 10 to 12 mg/kg/h for the next 10 minutes, and a final infusion rate of 8 to 10 mg/kg/h would prevent patient movement in 95% of cases (27). As expected, the higher doses were required when less alfentanil was used.

The doses suggested by the manual infusion scheme of Browne and associates are useful starting guidelines for clinical practice in which further adjustments in the infusion rates are based on signs of light anesthesia (e.g., tearing, hypertension, tachycardia) in an individual patient. The concomitant administration of opioids, N_2O, regional block, or other anesthetic agent reduces the requirements of propofol. Similar adjustments are necessary when a computer-controlled infusion device is used, even though fentanyl pretreatment or concomitant administration of epidural bupivacaine does not significantly affect propofol's pharmacokinetics (20, 61).

Specific Situations Where Propofol May Be Advantageous

Propofol is safe to use in patients predisposed to malignant hyperthermia (MH) because in vivo and in vitro tests have failed to demonstrate an MH response (62). Hence, propofol has been widely used in patients at high risk of this complication. The rapid onset and offset of action of propofol and its low incidence of emesis have made it an attractive choice in ambulatory surgery, particularly in operations associated with a high incidence of emesis (e.g., strabismus correction, middle ear surgery) (3, 18, 34, 38, 47). Propofol has also been used to good effect when quick emergence from anesthesia is required following brief, but intensely stimulating procedures (e.g., following microlaryngeal surgery, when the patient needs to be wide awake to protect the airway). In some of these microlaryngeal procedures, the anesthesiologist may not be able to provide inhalation agents by a tracheal tube, and yet it is essential to keep the child still (63). TIVA with propofol has been shown to be highly effective in this situation (64). Although tracheal intubation without neuromuscular blockade is possible if large doses of propofol are used, the drug does not have an effect at the neuromuscular junction, and it has been used in patients with myasthenia gravis (21, 65, 66). In fact, severe muscle spasms during electrical stimulation of nerve rootlets has made propofol unacceptable as the primary anesthetic during selective dorsal rhizotomy procedures (67). However, propofol has been recommended for use in other neurosurgical procedures, particularly when N_2O is avoided because of concerns of air embolism and when brain swelling precludes the use of potent inhalation agents (68-70). Because propofol can induce electroencephalograhic silence without affecting somatosensory evoked potential monitoring, it has a role in aneurysmal and sterotactic surgery (19, 70-72).

With the advent of small, portable microprocessor-controlled infusion devices, the advantages of TIVA with propofol have been appreciated in situations where space for anesthesia machines is limited (e.g., during radiologic imaging) and during transport. Martin and colleagues have described their experiences using propofol for a patient who needed to be kept anesthetized while being moved between separate locations for myelography, CT, and spinal biopsy (73). Subanesthetic doses of propofol have been used for sedation for radiologic or diagnostic procedures such as cardiac catheterization, transesophageal echocardiography, and repetitive cranial radiation. Lebovic and associates used propofol for sedation during cardiac catheterization and noted significantly shorter recovery times compared with children receiving ketamine (74). Marcus and associates have described the successful use of propofol for diagnostic, outpatient transesophageal echocardiography in children with complex, congenital heart conditions (75).

Propofol is particularly advantageous in the magnetic resonance imaging (MRI) suite where a simple, safe technique of rapid induction and fast recovery is necessary, but the dynamic magnetic field limits the use of ferrous materials (76, 77). The patient must not move during the scanning procedure, but placement in the long, enclosed MRI tube and loud noises of the MRI scanner have made this a terrifying experience for both adults and children. Sedation is often necessary, but limited access to the airway, the need for special pulse oximeters and other monitoring equipment, and pressures from hospital administrators for efficient use of the time a patient spends in the MRI suite have made this area a particularly challenging environment for safe and effective sedation. Frankville and colleagues determined that a loading dose of 2 mg/kg propofol followed by an infusion at 100 μg/kg/min provides adequate sedation without patient movement during MRI scans (29). Kain and associates made a partial analysis of the costs associated with the use of barbiturates and propofol sedation for radiologic imaging procedures and suggested that increased efficiency in the flow of patients through the radiologic suite compensates for the higher costs of propofol (78). However, these authors did not consider the costs of providing an anesthesiologist for sedation when propofol is used. The use of propofol by nonanesthesiologists is controversial, and many institutions limit its use to anesthesiologists. Reports of respiratory depression with all the drugs used for TIVA, including propofol, have been published (30, 79-81). Patients receiving sedatives and anesthetics outside the operating room need the same careful attention and close monitoring as those in operating suites (82). Personnel skilled in airway management must be available when these drugs are used (82).

Many disorders that traditionally required major, open surgical procedures in operating rooms are now managed with minimally invasive procedures using fiberoptic scopes and specialized catheters. Compared with the older, open surgical procedures, performance of the newer operations often requires more time and expensive instruments. Claims of cost-effectiveness of the newer surgical techniques are based on the more rapid recovery of patients, shorter hospital stays, and the ability to perform these procedures in adults receiving sedation and local anesthesia. In children, usually deeper levels of sedation and general anesthesia are often required (83). Propofol is useful in these procedures because it can provide the full continuum from mild conscious sedation to general anesthesia in a dose-dependent fashion.

Propofol's greatest attributes are its pharmacokinetic properties and recovery profile, which result in a rapid, clear emergence and lack of cumulative effects even after prolonged administration. Compared with other intravenous anesthetics, the induction dose of propofol is associated with a relatively higher incidence of respiratory depression, short-lived apnea, and blood pressure reduction that may occasionally be marked. Many interventional radiologic procedures have been performed in children with cardiac conditions. Early fears of increased hypotension and cardiac depression with the use of propofol have been allayed with greater experience. This drug has been used successfully in radiofrequency ablation of aberrant cardiac conduction tracts (84), transcatheter closure of ventricular septal defects (85), and noncardiac surgery in children with heart defects (86). Cost considerations of longer stays in the intensive care unit (ICU) after large doses of opioids during open heart surgery have lead to the introduction of the "fast-track" method of using lower doses of opioids along with propofol infusions during cardiopulmonary bypass. Early extubation of the trachea is the goal of this technique (87). Whether overall mortality and morbidity are reduced with this technique in pediatric patients remains to be seen. Evidence suggests lower mortality in children who receive continuous infusions of opioids during the postoperative period compared with those who receive inhalation agents during surgery and intermittent opioids for analgesia after the operation (88).

Although propofol has been used for long-term sedation in adult patients undergoing ventilation in the ICU (89), reports of neurologic dysfunction following the termination of the infusion in children have raised some questions about its use in this patient population (90, 91). In addition, five cases of metabolic acidosis and fatal myocardial failure have been reported in children with respiratory infections who received prolonged, high-dose infusions of propofol for sedation during mechanical ventilation. Autopsies on three of these five children showed fatty infiltration of the liver (92). Microembolism from the lipid vehicle of propofol may be responsible for circulatory obstruction in critically ill children (93). Although no data suggest that adding propofol to the therapeutic regimens of pediatric ICU patients is associated with increased morbidity, propofol should probably not be used in this population until more data on its safety are available (94). Clusters of sepsis have been reported in surgical patients who received propofol, and careful attention to aseptic technique is required during the filling of syringes with propofol (95).

OPIOIDS

Alfentanil

The pharmacokinetics of alfentanil makes it attractive for use in short surgical procedures. It is rapid in onset, with a large margin of safety and stable hemodynamic properties. Its small volume of distribution and short elimination half-life have led to its use as a total opioid anesthetic and as a supplement to propofol during TIVA (7, 23, 27). It has also been used with N_2O as part of a so-called "balanced technique." Mulroy and colleagues have demonstrated that alfentanil, 12.5 to 50

μg/kg, is safe in children when combined with N_2O alone or with N_2O and halothane. This loading dose does not blunt the response to surgical incision, and a larger initial dose or continuous infusion is necessary (96). van Beem and associates have demonstrated that continuous infusions of alfentanil and vecuronium during N_2O anesthesia are useful in patients undergoing vertebral column surgery, because this regimen permits monitoring by both evoked cortical somatosensory potentials and an intraoperative wake-up tests (97). Markovitz and associates have demonstrated that alfentanil does not increase intracranial pressure in children with hydrocephalus during N_2O-isoflurane anesthesia (98).

Alfentanil has also been used as an adjuvant to decrease fasciculations caused by succinylcholine and for sedation of neonates undergoing painful procedures while being mechanically ventilated (99). However, alfentanil can induce muscle rigidity that can interfere with mechanical ventilation, and gas exchange after alfentanil is administered may occur only after muscle relaxants are given (100). Alfentanil has been useful for sedation during cardiac catheterization in children aged 1 to 17 months (101). In this study, the induction and maintenance dose requirements were less in cyanotic compared with noncyanotic infants (induction 21 $\pm$ 6 versus 28 $\pm$ 8 μg/kg; maintenance rate 29 $\pm$ 10 versus 34 $\pm$ 3 μg/kg/h). The mean plasma concentration of alfentanil during maintenance of sedation was 79 $\pm$ 23 ng/ml (101).

Alfentanil is also useful as an opioid anesthetic in children undergoing surgical repair of congenital heart disease. The pharmacokinetics of alfentanil before and after cardiopulmonary bypass has been studied by Hollander and associates (102). They noted an increase in the volume of distribution and a decrease in the normalized area under the concentration-time curve after bypass. These changes may not necessarily be accompanied by changes in clinical effect because the latter are related to the free fraction of alfentanil. Postoperative emesis and other side effects noted with alfentanil anesthesia do not seem to be greater than with other fentanyl derivatives such as sufentanil.

Sufentanil

Sufentanil has also been used for TIVA in pediatric cardiac anesthesia. In a landmark study by Anand and Hickey, markers of the physiologic stress response and perioperative outcome were compared in infants randomized to receive deep intraoperative anesthesia with high-dose sufentanil followed by postoperative infusions of opioids or light anesthesia with halothane and morphine, followed by intermittent morphine and diazepam postoperatively (88). In this important study, the group receiving light anesthesia had more severe hyperglycemia and lactic acidemia during surgery, higher blood levels of lactate and acetoacetate after surgery, and an increased incidence of sepsis, metabolic acidosis, disseminated intravascular coagulation, and death (88). This study has suggested that postoperative analgesia attenuates the stress response and may reduce the vulnerability of these neonates to postoperative complications. The current financial pressures to reduce the stay of patients in the ICU needs to be balanced against the findings of this study. Although the "fast track" early extubation technique may be effective for the less complicated congenital heart disorders such as atrial septal defects and ventricular septal defects without pulmonary hypertension, whether this approach is appropriate for children with the more complex cyanotic heart defects is unclear. Caution is essential before applying data from adult studies to the pediatric cardiac population.

Barankay and colleagues followed up the Anand-Hickey study with a study comparing sufentanil alone with sufentanil with flunitrazepam in children undergoing primary correction of tetralogy of Fallot (103). The sufentanil-flunitrazepam technique was associated with greater hemodynamic stability and prevented elevations of plasma epinephrine and norepinephrine during surgical stimulation. Guay and associates studied the pharmacokinetics of sufentanil in healthy children (104). The volume of distribution when expressed as a function of body weight was 1.5 times greater than values reported in adults. However, when the volume of distribution was expressed as a function of body surface area, no differences were noted. The clearance of sufentanil in the children studied by Guay and colleagues was twice as rapid as that previously reported by other investigators in adults. This finding suggests that children require a higher maintenance dose of sufentanil than adults and may explain the results of the study by Baranky and associates (103).

Remifentanil

Remifentanil is the latest derivative of fentanyl and has recently been approved for widespread clinical use in the United States and Europe (105). This drug is a pure μ-opioid receptor agonist with little binding at the other opioid receptor sites. The chemical structure of this 4-anilidopiperidine derivative of fentanyl possesses an ester side chain that is susceptible to tissue esterase hydrolysis and rapid elimination (106-108). The major metabolite of remifentanil, GI90291, is eliminated more slowly but is also much less potent and unlikely to make a significant contribution to the overall effect of remifentanil. Studies in adults suggest that remifentanil is a potent analgesic with sedative actions, and has a significant effect in reducing the minimum alveolar concentration of inhalation agents. Although synergy with intravenous hypnotics is modest for loss of consciousness, synergy in reducing movement and hemodynamic responses to surgical or other noxious stimuli is profound. As with other fentanyl derivatives, its use is associated with hemodynamic stability, attenuated stress responses, ventilatory depression, muscle rigidity, nausea, itching, and high-amplitude, low frequency electroencephalographic activity (105, 109, 110). The respiratory depressant activity may be antagonized by naloxone (111). At present, few, if any, published data are available on the use of remifentanil in children.

KETAMINE

The body of knowledge and experience with ketamine in children is vast. This agent is particularly useful in handling the uncontrollable child when all other methods have failed because it is effective by the intramuscular route (112). Ketamine is useful when the availability of vaporizers and other anesthetic equipment is limited, such as in the field of war or in some developing countries (113). Newer uses and routes of administration are being found for this old drug. It has been given orally and intranasally for sedation of children before surgery (114-118). Ketamine has also been administered in the caudal epidural space with or without bupivacaine and is effective in controlling postoperative pain (119). Ketamine is useful in burn patients undergoing multiple procedures and in military medicine when a ready supply of compressed gases may not be available (79, 120).

The analgesic qualities of ketamine have lead to its use in the postoperative period in children undergoing positive pressure ventilation and in children undergoing painful procedures such as bone marrow biopsies, suture of lacerations, and dental procedures (121-125). Although ketamine was formerly considered to preserve respiratory function and to be used with spontaneous ventilation, more recent studies have shown that oxygen desaturation may occur (79, 80, 126). The increased use of ketamine outside the operating rooms by persons without skills in airway management should be viewed with caution (80, 121, 124, 127). Respiratory arrest has been reported with intramuscular ketamine (78). In previously premature babies undergoing surgical procedures during regional anesthesia, the addition of ketamine for sedation increased the incidence of postoperative apnea (128, 129). In another study of 76 adults and 64 children scheduled for peripheral surgery, patients were randomly allocated to spontaneously breathe room air or 40% oxygen during TIVA with ketamine (130). Continuous pulse oximetry monitoring revealed oxygen desaturation ($SpO_2 < 92\%$) immediately after induction of anesthesia in 20 adults and 9 children breathing room air and in only 3 adults breathing oxygen ($p < 0.05$). Respiratory abnormalities were sufficiently severe to warrant tracheal intubation in 2 patients. The large decrease in oxygen saturation sometimes observed requires that trained personnel be present and that equipment for tracheal intubation be available whenever ketamine is used.

Ketamine was historically used in cardiac catheterization laboratories because it was believed to have little effect on the cardiovascular system and spontaneous ventilation could be maintained. Audenaert and colleagues studied the cardiorespiratory effects of preanesthetic sedative medications including nasal ketamine (5 mg/kg) with midazolam (0.2 mg/kg), oral meperidine (3 mg/kg) with pentobarbital (4 mg/kg), and rectal methohexital (30 mg/kg) (131). Although the ketamine-midazolam combination produced no significant cardiovascular or respiratory effects, the meperidine-barbiturate combination decreased heart rate, mean arterial pressure, cardiac index, respiratory rate, and oxygen saturation without altering stroke volume. Rectal methohexital increased heart rate with a coincident decrease in stroke volume, but it had no other positive or negative cardiac or respiratory effect (131).

Wolfe and colleagues studied the hemodynamic effects of ketamine, hypoxia, and hyperoxia in 14 children with surgically treated congenital heart disease who lived in areas at or higher than 1200 m above sea level (132). These authors made simultaneous measurements of pulmonary artery and aortic pressures, thermodilution cardiac outputs, and blood gases in room air (16% oxygen) and with ketamine infusion (132). Reaction to hypoxia identified 3 groups: normal, intermediate, and hyperresponsive. The normal responders had normal resistance ratios (0.11) in room air and had little resistance ratio response to hypoxia (+0.02), hyperoxia (−0.03), or ketamine (+0.01). The intermediate responders had a slightly higher but normal resistance ratio (0.20) in room air and a moderate reaction to hypoxia (+0.13), hyperoxia (−0.08), and ketamine (+0.11). The hyperresponders had an elevated resistance ratio (0.42) in room air and a striking reaction to hypoxia (+0.65), hyperoxia (−0.17), and ketamine (+0.49). Hypoxia and ketamine had a greater effect on resistance ratio than hypoxia alone in patients with reactive pulmonary vascular beds. These authors concluded that ketamine should not be used in children undergoing diagnostic procedures to establish operability based on pulmonary vascular resistance or pulmonary vascular reactivity (132).

Hickey and colleagues described their experience in 122 children undergoing transcatheter closure of an atrial septal defect (133). They used a loading dose of intravenous ketamine, 0.25 to 0.5 mg/kg, along with midazolam, 0.1 to 0.2 mg/kg, and followed it with a continuous intravenous infusion of ketamine at 1 to 1.5 mg/kg/h, along with midazolam at 0.1 mg/kg/h. Supplemental boluses of ketamine and midazolam were administered as required. Although most of their patients were breathing spontaneously during the procedure, these investigators elected to intubate the trachea and control ventilation in 29 patients to provide better conditions. However, 2 of their spontaneously breathing patients developed apnea or airway obstruction and required tracheal intubation on a semiurgent basis. This finding indicates the need for careful monitoring of the respiratory status by a designated team member who has no other duties assigned during the procedure (133).

Ketamine was also used as part of a TIVA technique by Kubota and associates in Japan when propofol and sufentanil were not available (134). These authors used droperidol, ketamine, and fentanyl. A loading dose of 1 to 1.5 mg/kg^{-1} ketamine was administered intravenously, along with fentanyl, 1 to 2 μg/kg. This was followed by a continuous infusion of ketamine at 1 to 1.5 mg/kg/h accompanied by bolus doses of fentanyl up to a total of 5 to 10 μg/kg. Satisfactory conditions were reported in a series of 56 children, including some with cerebral palsy (134).

These data indicate that ketamine has a place in pediatric anesthesia, but it must be used with caution because unexpected respiratory complications may occur. Careful monitoring of pediatric patients during sedation is essential regardless of the drug chosen for sedation (81).

MIDAZOLAM AND FLUMAZENIL

Midazolam is a water-soluble benzodiazepine with a relatively short duration of action. These properties have made it popular for sedation during various procedures including preanesthetic sedation. Oral doses of 0.5 to 0.75 mg/kg have been shown to be highly effective and do not delay recovery from surgery (114, 136-141). The lack of an effect of midazolam on cardiac electrophysiology has made this agent useful for sedation when the cardiologist attempts to induce reentrant arrhythmia during electrophysiologic studies (135). Midazolam has also been used to induce anesthesia. However, because children have a variable response to a given dose of midazolam, the drug must be titrated to effect, and other agents such as propofol, ketamine, or opioids may be needed to complete induction (133). Jones and colleagues studied the cardiovascular and recovery effects of intravenous induction with thiopental, 4 mg/kg, propofol, 2.5 mg/kg, or midazolam, 0.5 mg/kg, in children (12). The midazolam-treated group took longer to identify themselves compared with both the propofol-treated ($p = 0.005$) and the thiopental-treated groups ($p = 0.02$), but no difference was reported in the groups in time to eye opening. Psychomotor performance on awakening was significantly worse in the midazolam group compared with the propofol ($p < 0.03$) and thiopental groups ($p < 0.02$). Drug blood levels correlated weakly with both methods of psychomotor assessment ($r \geq 0.6$). Within 1 hour, patients in all groups were equally awake, cooperative, and coordinated (12).

The pharmacokinetics of midazolam after oral, rectal, nasal, and intravenous administration is known for the pediatric population (136-138). In neonates, the clearance of midazolam is slower than in older children (139). These data have been used to develop CACI devices. Kern and associates anesthetized 17 pediatric patients undergoing cardiac surgery with CACI using age-appropriate pharmacokinetic models for administering sufentanil and midazolam (140). Predicted CACI plasma concentrations were correlated with assayed plasma drug concentrations at eight predefined intervals, and the authors noted that plasma levels predicted by CACI provided a reasonable approximation of measured plasma concentrations for both drugs. They concluded that the CACI system was an acceptable and easy-to-use alternative to inhalation anesthesia using calibrated vaporizers (140).

Midazolam has been widely used in the ICU for sedation of children undergoing positive pressure ventilation and has been shown to be effective compared with placebo in neonates (141). In adult studies, propofol was noted to be a better sedative for this purpose (89). However, as described earlier, the possibility of cardiac failure in children receiving propofol for sedation in the ICU has led to a return to midazolam and fentanyl infusions (142). In burn patients, midazolam infusions have been used for an average of 16.5 days (range 4 to 56 days) to reduce narcotic requirements, decrease anxiety, and improve the tolerance of dressing changes (143). However, tolerance does develop, and a wide range of infusion rates have been used, with an initial average rate of 0.045 mg/kg/h (range 0.01 to 0.09 mg/kg/h), and a maximum mean rate of 0.11 mg/kg/h (range 0.04 to 0.35 mg/kg/h). Although no hypotension or problems weaning from mechanical ventilation were seen, two (8.3%) children experienced reversible neurologic abnormalities attributed to midazolam infusion but made full neurologic recoveries (143). Tolerance and neurologic abnormalities following long-term midazolam infusions have been reported by others (144, 145). The development of tolerance and the expense of midazolam infusions in these patients have led some ICUs to use longer-lasting drugs such as lorazepam and diezepam.

Withdrawal symptoms have been reported when midazolam infusions have been discontinued (146). Hughes and associates noted that 49 out of 53 critically ill infants and children who had received midazolam for sedation in a regional ICU were fully alert within 4 hours of midazolam's discontinuance, but 4 patients took 6 hours to 1 week to become fully alert (147). These 4 children demonstrated abnormal behavior starting within 12 hours of discontinuation of midazolam and lasting for 3 hours to 1 week (147). The overall incidence of adverse effects of midazolam in the patients studied was 17%. Because many of these patients were also receiving opioid infusions, medications to decrease these side effects should include longer-acting opioids. Oral medications (methadone, lorazepam) have been used to decrease these withdrawal-related side effects (148).

The availability of a specific benzodiazepine antagonist, flumazenil, has renewed interest in the use of midazolam (31). However, flumazenil has a shorter half-life than midazolam, and hence patients must be carefully watched to prevent resedation (31, 149). Flumazenil is useful to reverse the effects of benzodiazepine for an intraoperative wake-up test in children undergoing spinal fusion with midazolam infusions (150). In a placebo-controlled study, the effects of flumazenil on awakening were examined in 40 healthy children who received 0.5 mg/kg midazolam orally for sedation and 0.5 mg/kg intravenously for induction of anesthesia (151). Psychomotor performance was tested by the time to complete a post-box toy. Flumazenil rapidly antagonized midazolam-induced hypnosis in children and was associated with minimal change in cardiorespiratory variables. Children receiving flumazenil awoke approximately four times faster and identified themselves nearly three times sooner. In the flumazenil-treated group, 65% could complete the post-box toy at 10 minutes, compared with none of the placebo group. No cases of resedation were reported, but 1 child did not awaken for 30 minutes after intravenous administration of flumazenil, 1.0 mg. The mean total dose of flumazenil administered in this study was 0.024 ± 0.019 mg/kg (151). Other investigators have administered flumazenil rectally in the ICU to reverse the effects of midazolam (152).

In conclusion, TIVA has the advantages of not requiring special equipment and of not having environmental side effects. The advent of propofol has raised interest in this technique. This intravenous anesthetic agent is characterized by a rapid onset and offset of action, pain on injection, and a low incidence of emesis. It has a role in pediatric anesthesia for ambulatory surgery and for procedures performed outside the operating suite such as MRI, interventional radiology, and CT scans. Older agents such as ketamine and short-acting opioids (e.g., alfentanil and remifentanil) are also useful for TIVA. Finally, the use of flumazenil may hasten emergence from anesthesia when larger doses of midazolam have been administered.

REFERENCES

1. Aun CST, Short SM, Leung DHY, Oh TE. Induction dose-response of propofol in unpremedicated children. Br J Anaesth 1992;68:64–67.
2. Hannallah RS, Baker SB, Casey W, et al. Propofol: effective dose and induction characteristics in unpremedicated children. Anesthesiology 1991;74:217–219.
3. Smith I, White PF, Nathanson M, Gouldson R. Propofol: an update on its clinical use. Anesthesiology 1994;81:1005–1043.
4. Patel DK, Keeling PA, Newman GB, Redford P. Induction dose of propofol in children. Anaesthesia 1988;43:949–952.
5. Manschot HJ, Meursing AE, Axt P, et al. Propofol requirements for induction of anesthesia in children of different age groups. Anesth Analg 1992;75:876–879.
6. Westrin P. The induction dose of propofol in infants 1–6 months of age and in children 10–16 years of age. Anesthesiology 1991;74:455–458.
7. Hiller A, Saarnivaara L. Injection pain, cardiovascular changes and recovery following induction of anaesthesia with propofol in combination with alfentanil or lignocaine in children. Acta Anaesthesiol Scand 1992;36:564–568.
8. Martin TM, Nicolson SC, Bargas MS. Propofol anesthesia reduces emesis and airway obstruction in pediatric outpatients. Anesth Analg 1993;76:144–148.
9. Valtonen M, Lisalo E, Kanto J, Rosenberg P. Propofol as an induction agent in children: pain on injection and pharmacokinetics. Acta Anaesthesiol Scand 1989;33:152–155.
10. Cameron E, Johnston G, Crofts S, Morton NS. The minimum effective dose of lignocaine to prevent injection pain due to propofol in children. Anaesthesia 1992;47:604–606.
11. Hiller A. Comparison of cardiovascular changes during anaesthesia and recovery from propofol-alfentanil-nitrous oxide and thiopental-halothane-nitrous oxide anaesthesia in children undergoing otolaryngological surgery. Acta Anaesthesiol Scand 1993;37:737–741.
12. Jones RD, Visram AR, Chan MM, et al. A comparison of three induction agents in paediatric anaesthesia: cardiovascular effects and recovery. Anaesth Intens Care 1994;22:545–555.
13. Short SM, Aun CS. Haemodynamic effects of propofol in children. Anaesthesia 1991;46:783–785.
14. Saarnivaara L, Hiller A, Oikkonen M. QT interval, heart rate and arterial pressures using propofol, thiopentone or methohexitone for induction of anaesthesia in children. Acta Anaesthesiol Scand 1993;37:419–423.
15. Hannallah RS, Britton JT, Schafer PG, et al. Propofol anaesthesia in paediatric ambulatory patients: a comparison with thiopentone and halothane. Can J Anaesth 1994;41:12–18.
16. Aun CS, Sung RY, O'Meara ME, et al. Cardiovascular effects of i.v. induction in children: comparison between propofol and thiopentone. Br J Anaesth 1993;70:647–653.
17. Larsson S, Asgeirsson B, Magnusson J. Propofol-fentanyl anesthesia compared to thiopental-halothane with special reference to recovery and vomiting after pediatric strabismus surgery. Acta Anaesthesiol Scand 1992;36:182–186.
18. Watcha MF, Simeon RM, White PF, Stevens JL. Effect of propofol on the incidence of postoperative emesis after strabismus surgery in children. Anesthesiology 1991;75:204–209.
19. Traast HS, Kalkman CJ. Electroencephalographic characteristics of emergence from propofol/sufentanil total intravenous anesthesia. Anesth Analg 1995;81:366–371.
20. Allsop E, Innes P, Jackson M, Cunliffe M. Dose of propofol required to insert the laryngeal mask in children. Paediatr Anaesth 1995;5:47–51.
21. Wessen A, Persson PM, Nilsson A, Hartvig P. Concentration-effect relationships of propofol after total intravenous anesthesia. Anesth Analg 1993;77:1000–1007.
22. Hiller A, Klemola UM, Saarnivaara L. Tracheal intubation after induction of anaesthesia with propofol, alfentanil and lidocaine without neuromuscular blocking drugs in children. Acta Anaesthesiol Scand 1993;37:725–729.
23. Borgeat A, Dessibourg C, Popvic V, et al. Propofol and spon-

taneous movements: an EEG study. Anesthesiology 1991;74: 24–27.
24. Borgeat A, Fuchs T, Wilder-Smith O, Tassonyi E. The effect of nalbuphine and droperidol on spontaneous movements during induction of anesthesia with propofol in children. J Clin Anesth 1993;5:12–15.
25. Mendoza CU, Suarez M, Castaneda R, et al. Comparative study between the effects of total intravenous anesthesia with propofol and balanced anesthesia with halothane on the alveolar-arterial oxygen tension difference and on the pulmonary shunt. Arch Med Res 1992;23:139–142.
26. Matot I, Neely CF, Katz RY, Marshall BE. Fentanyl and propofol uptake by the lung: effect of time between injections. Acta Anaesthesiol Scand 1994;38:711–715.
27. Browne BL, Prys-Roberts C, Wolf AR. Propofol and alfentanil in children: infusion technique and dose requirement for total i.v. anaesthesia. Br J Anaesth 1992;69:570–576.
28. Shafer SL. Advances in propofol pharmacokinetics and pharmacodynamics. J Clin Anesth 1993;5 (suppl 1):14S–21S.
29. Frankville DD, Spear RM, Dyck JB. The dose of propofol required to prevent children from moving during magnetic resonance imaging. Anesthesiology 1993;79:953–958.
30. McDowall RH, Scher CS, Barst SM. Total intravenous anesthesia for children undergoing brief diagnostic or therapeutic procedures. Acta Anaesthesiol Belg 1995;7:273–280.
31. Jensen AG, Moller JT, Lybecker H, Hansen PA. A random trial comparing recovery after midazolam-alfentanil anesthesia with and without reversal with flumazenil, and standardized neurolept anesthesia for major gynecologic surgery. J Clin Anesth 1995;7:63–70.
32. Dexter F, Tinker JH. Comparisons between desflurane and isoflurane or propofol on time to following commands and time to discharge: a metaanalysis. Anesthesiology 1995;83:77–82.
33. Borgeat A, Popovic V, Meier D, Schwander D. Comparison of propofol and thiopental/halothane for short duration ENT surgical procedures in children. Anesth Analg 1990;71:511–515.
34. Snellen FT, Vanacker B, Van Aken H. Propofol-nitrous oxide versus thiopental sodium-isoflurane-nitrous oxide for strabismus surgery in children. J Clin Anesth 1993;5:37–41.
35. Reimer EJ, Montgomery CJ, Bevan JC, et al. Propofol anaesthesia reduces early postoperative emesis after paediatric strabismus surgery. Can J Anaesth 1993;40:927–933.
36. Scher CS, Amar D, McDowall RH, Barst SM. Use of propofol for the prevention of chemotherapy-induced nausea and emesis in oncology patients. Can J Anaesth 1992;39:170–172.
37. Borgeat A, Wilder-Smith OH, Suter PM. The nonhypnotic therapeutic applications of propofol. Anesthesiology 1994;80:642–656.
38. Weir PM, Munro HM, Reynolds PI, et al. Propofol infusion and the incidence of emesis in pediatric outpatient strabismus surgery. Anesth Analg 1993;76:760–764.
39. Suver J, Arikian SR, Doyle JJ, et al. Use of anesthesia selection In controlling surgery costs in an HMO hospital. Clin Ther 1995; 17:561–571.
40. Sung YF, Reiss N, Tilette T. The differential cost of anesthesia and recovery with propofol-nitrous oxide anesthesia versus thiopental sodium-isoflurane-nitrous oxide anesthesia. J Clin Anesth 1991;3:391–394.
41. Philip BK, Mushlin PS, Manzi D, et al. Isoflurane versus propofol for maintenance of anesthesia for ambulatory surgery [Abstract]. Anesthesiology 1992;77 (suppl):44A.
42. Marais ML, Maher MW, Wetchler BV, et al. Reduced demands on recovery room resources with propofol (Diprivan). Anesthesiol Rev 1989;16:29–40.
43. Fulton BF, Goa KL. Propofol: a pharmacoeconomic appraisal of its use in day case surgery. Pharmacoeconomics 1996;2:168–178.
44. Jones RD, Chan K, Andrew LJ. Pharmacokinetics of propofol in children. Br J Anaesth 1990;65:661–667.
45. Kataria BK, Ved SA, Nicodemus HF, et al. The pharmacokinetics of propofol in children using three different data analysis approaches. Anesthesiology 1994;80:104–122.
46. Saint-Maurice C, Cockshott ID, White M, Kenny GNC. Pharmacokinetics of propofol in young children after a single dose. Br J Anaesth 1989;63:667–670.
47. Bryson HM, Fulton BR, Faulds D. Propofol: an update of its use in anaesthesia and conscious sedation. Drugs 1995;50:513–559.
48. Kirvela M, Olkkola KT, Rosenberg PH, et al. Pharmacokinetics of propofol and haemodynamic changes during induction of anaesthesia in uraemic patients. Br J Anaesth 1992;68:178–182.
49. Raoof AA, van Obbergh LJ, Verbeeck RK. Propofol pharmacokinetics in children with biliary atresia. Br J Anaesth 1995; 74:46–49.
50. Nathan N, Debord J, Narcisse F, et al. Pharmacokinetics of propofol and its conjugates after continuous infusion in normal and in renal failure patients: a preliminary study. Acta Anaesthesiol Belg 1993;44:77–85.
51. Servin F, Farinotti R, Haberer JP, Desmonts JM. Propofol infusion for maintenance of anesthesia in morbidly obese patients receiving nitrous oxide: a clinical and pharmacokinetic study. Anesthesiology 1993;78:657–665.
52. Marsh B, White M, Morton N, Kenny GN. Pharmacokinetic model driven infusion of propofol in children. Br J Anaesth 1991;67:41–48.
53. Chaudhri S, White M, Kenny GNC. Induction of anesthesia using a target controlled infusion system. Anaesthesia 1992; 47:551–553.
54. Short TG, Aun CS, Tan P, et al. A prospective evaluation of pharmacokinetic model controlled infusion of propofol in paediatric patients. Br J Anaesth 1994;72:302–306.
55. Fisher DM. Propofol in pediatrics: lessons in pharmacokinetic modeling [Editorial comment]. Anesthesiology 1994;80:2–5.
56. Coetzee JF, Glen JB, Wium CA, Boshoff L. Pharmacokinetic model selection for target controlled infusions of propofol: assessment of three parameter sets. Anesthesiology 1995;82:1328–1345.
57. Jones RD, Chan K, Andrew LJ, et al. Comparative pharmacokinetics of propofol in Chinese adults and children. Methods Find Exp Clin Pharmacol 1992;14:41–47.
58. Vandermeersch E, Van Hemelrijck J, Byttebier G, Van Aken H. Pharmacokinetics of propofol during continuous infusion for pediatric anesthesia. Acta Anaesthesiol Belg 1989;40:161–165.
59. Doyle E, McFadzean W, Morton NS. IV anaesthesia with propofol using a target-controlled infusion system: comparison with inhalation anaesthesia for general surgical procedures in children. Br J Anaesth 1993;70:542–545.
60. Aun CS, Short TG, O'Meara ME, et al. Recovery after propofol infusion anaesthesia in children: comparison with propofol, thiopentone or halothane induction followed by halothane maintenance. Br J Anaesth 1994;72:554–558.
61. De Gasperi A, Cristalli A, Noe L, et al. Fentanyl pre-treatment does not affect the pharmacokinetic profile of an induction dose of propofol in adults. Eur J Anaesth 1994;11:89–93.
62. McKenzie AJ, Couchman KG, Pollock N. Propofol is a "safe" anaesthetic agent in malignant hyperthermia susceptible patients. Anaesth Intens Care 1992;20:165–168.
63. Shikowitz MJ, Abramson AL, Liberatore L. Endolaryngeal jet ventilation: a 10-year review. Laryngoscope 1991;101:455–461.
64. Perrin G, Colt HG, Martin C, et al. Safety of interventional rigid bronchoscopy using intravenous anesthesia and spontaneous assisted ventilation: a prospective study. Chest 1992;102:1526–1530.
65. McConaghy P, Bunting HE. Assessment of intubating conditions in children after induction with propofol and varying doses of alfentanil. Br J Anaesth 1994;73:596–599.

66. Rowe R, Andropoulos D, Heard M, et al. Anesthetic management of pediatric patients undergoing thoracoscopy. J Cardiothorac Vasc Anesth 1994;8:563–566.
67. Riegle EV, Gunter JB, Lagueruela RG, et al. Anesthesia for selective dorsal rhizotomy in children. J Neurosurg Anesthesiol 1992;4:182–187.
68. Bone ME, Bristow A. Total intravenous anaesthesia in stereotactic surgery: one year's clinical experience. Eur J Anaesth 1991;8:47–54.
69. Weglinski MR, Perkins WJ. Inhalational versus total intravenous anesthesia for neurosurgery: theory guides, outcome decides. J Neurosurg Anesthesiol 1994;6:290–293.
70. Taniguchi M, Nadstawek J, Pechstein U, Schramm J. Total intravenous anesthesia for improvement of intraoperative monitoring of somatosensory evoked potentials during aneurysm surgery. Neurosurgery 1992;31:891–897.
71. Ravussin P, de Tribolet N. Total intravenous anesthesia with propofol for burst suppression in cerebral aneurysm surgery: preliminary report of 42 patients. Neurosurgery 1993;32:236–240.
72. Ravussin P, de Tribolet N, Wilder-Smith OH. Total intravenous anesthesia is best for neurological surgery. J Neurosurg Anesthesiol 1994;6:285–289.
73. Martin LD, Pasternak LR, Pudimat MA, et al. Total intravenous anesthesia with propofol in pediatric patients outside the operating room. Anesth Analg 1992;74:609–612.
74. Lebovic S, Reich DL, Steinberg LG, et al. Comparison of propofol versus ketamine for anesthesia in pediatric patients undergoing cardiac catheterization. Anesth Analg 1992;74:490–494.
75. Marcus B, Steward DJ, Khan NR, et al. Outpatient transesophageal echocardiography with intravenous propofol anesthesia in children and adolescents. J Am Soc Echocardiogr 1993;6:205–209.
76. Vangerven M, Van Hemelrijck J, Wouters P, et al. Light anaesthesia with propofol for paediatric MRI. Anaesthesia 1992; 47:706–707.
77. Tobin JR, Spurrier EA, Wetzel RC. Anaesthesia for critically ill children during magnetic resonance imaging. Br J Anaesth 1992;69:482–486.
78. Kain ZN, Gaal DJ, Kain TS, et al. A first-pass cost analysis of propofol versus barbiturates for children undergoing magnetic resonance imaging. Anesth Analg 1994;79:1102–1106.
79. Smith JA, Santer LJ. Respiratory arrest following intramuscular ketamine injection in a 4-year-old child. Ann Emerg Med 1993; 22:613–615.
80. Pesonen P. Pulse oximetry during ketamine anaesthesia in war conditions. Can J Anaesth 1991;38:592–594.
81. Greene CA, Gillette PC, Fyfe DA. Frequency of respiratory compromise after ketamine sedation for cardiac catheterization in patients less than 21 years of age. Am J Cardiol 1991;68:1116–1117.
82. Statement of the American Academy of Pediatrics, Committee on Drugs: Guidelines for the monitoring and management of pediatric patients during and after sedation for diagnostic and therapeutic procedures. Pediatrics 1992;88:1286–1287.
83. Javorski JJ, Hansen DD, Laussen PC, et al. Paediatric cardiac catheterization: innovations. Can J Anaesth 1995;42:310–329.
84. Lavoie J, Walsh EP, Burrows FA, et al. Effects of propofol or isoflurane anesthesia on cardiac conduction in children undergoing radiofrequency catheter ablation for tachydysrhythmias. Anesthesiology 1995;82:884–887.
85. Laussen PC, Hansen DD, Perry SB, et al. Transcatheter closure of ventricular septal defects: hemodynamic instability and anesthetic management. Anesth Analg 1995;80:1076–1082.
86. Burrows FA. Anaesthetic management of the child with congenital heart disease for non-cardiac surgery. Can J Anaesth 1992;39:R60–R70.
87. Burrows FA, Taylor RH, Hillier SC. Early extubation of the trachea after repair of secundum-type atrial septal defects in children. Can J Anaesth 1992;39:1041–1044.
88. Anand KJ, Hickey PR. Halothane-morphine compared with high-dose sufentanil for anesthesia and postoperative analgesia in neonatal cardiac surgery. N Engl J Med 1992;326:1–9.
89. Aitkenhead AR, Pepperman ML, Willatts SM, et al. Comparison of propofol andmidazolam for sedation in critically ill patients. Lancet 1989;2:704–709.
90. Trotter C, Serpell MG. Neurological sequelae in children after prolonged propofol infusion. Anaesthesia 1992;47:340–342.
91. Reynolds LM, Koh JL. Prolonged spontaneous movement following emergence from propofol/nitrous oxide anesthesia. Anesth Analg 1993;76:192–193.
92. Parke TJ, Stevens JE, Rice ASC, et al. Metabolic acidosis and fatal myocardial failure after propofol infusion in children: five case reports. Br Med J 1992;305:613–616.
93. Gempeler F, Elston AC, Thompson SP, Park GR. Propofol and intralipid cause creaming of the serum from critically ill patients. Anaesthesia 1994;49:17–20.
94. Meakin G. Role of propofol in paediatric anaesthetic practice. Paediatr Anaesth 1995;5:147–149.
95. Bennett SN, McNeil MM, Bland LA, et al. Postoperative infections traced to contamination of an intravenous anesthetic, propofol. N Engl J Med 1995;333:147–154.
96. Mulroy JJ, Davis PJ, Rymer DB, et al. Safety and efficacy of alfentanil and halothane in pediatric surgical patients. Can J Anaesth 1991;38:445–449.
97. van Beem H, Koopman-van Gemert A, Kruls H, Notermans SL. Spinal monitoring during vertebral column surgery under continuous alfentanil infusion. Eur J Anaesthesiol 1992;9:287–291.
98. Markowitz BP, Duhaime AC, Sutton L, et al. Effects of alfentanil on intracranial pressure in children undergoing ventriculoperitoneal shunt revision. Anesthesiology 1992;76:71–76.
99. Yli-Hanakla A, Randell T, Varpula T, Lindgren L. Alfentanil inhibits muscle fasciculations caused by suxamethonium in children and young adults. Acta Anaesthesiol Scand 1992; 36:588–591.
100. Pokela ML, Ryhanen PT, Koivisto ME, et al. Alfentanil-induced rigidity in newborn infants. Anesth Analg 1992;75:252–257.
101. Rautiainen P. Alfentanil infusion for sedation in infants and small children during cardiac catheterization. Can J Anaesth 1991;38:980–984.
102. den Hollander JM, Hennis PJ, Burm AG, et al. Pharmacokinetics of alfentanil before and after cardiopulmonary bypass in pediatric patients undergoing cardiac surgery: part 1. J Cardiothorac Vasc Anesth 1992;6:308–312.
103. Barankay A, Richter JA, Henze R, et al. Total intravenous anesthesia for infants and children undergoing correction of tetralogy of Fallot: sufentanil versus sufentanil-flunitrazepam technique. J Cardiothorac Vasc Anesth 1992;6:185–189.
104. Guay J, Gaudreault P, Tang A, et al. Pharmacokinetics of sufentanil in normal children. Can J Anaesth 1992;39:14–20.
105. Dershwitz M, Randel GI, Rosow CE, et al. Initial clinical experience with remifentanil, a new opioid metabolized by esterases. Anesth Analg 1995;81:619–623.
106. Egan TD, Lemmens HJ, Fiset P, et al. The pharmacokinetics of the new short-acting opioid remifentanil (GI87084B) in healthy adult male volunteers [See comments]. Anesthesiology 1993; 79:881–892.
107. Glass PS, Hardman D, Kamiyama Y, et al. Preliminary pharmacokinetics and pharmacodynamics of an ultra-short-acting opioid: remifentanil (GI87084B). Anesth Analg 1993;77:1031–1040.
108. Westmoreland CL, Hoke JF, Sebel PS, et al. Pharmacokinetics of remifentanil (GI87084B) and its major metabolite (GI90291) in patients undergoing elective inpatient surgery. Anesthesiology 1993;79:893–903.
109. Hoffman WE, Cunningham F, James MK, et al. Effects of remifentanil, a new short-acting opioid, on cerebral blood flow,

brain electrical activity, and intracranial pressure in dogs anesthetized with isoflurane and nitrous oxide. Anesthesiology 1993;79:107–113.
110. Sebel PS, Hoke JF, Westmoreland C, et al. Histamine concentrations and hemodynamic responses after remifentanil. Anesth Analg 1995;80:990–993.
111. Amin HM, Sopchak AM, Esposito BF, et al. Naloxone-induced and spontaneous reversal of depressed ventilatory responses to hypoxia during and after continuous infusion of remifentanil or alfentanil. J Pharmacol Exp Ther 1995;274:34–39.
112. Scott K, Eltringham RJ. Anesthetic dilemmas. Br J Hosp Med 1992;47:357.
113. Leppaniemi AK. Where there is no anaesthetist. . . . Br J Surg 1991;78:245–246.
114. Alderson PJ, Lerman J. Oral premedication for paediatric ambulatory anaesthesia: a comparison of midazolam and ketamine. Can J Anaesth 1994;41:221–226.
115. Tobias JD, Phipps S, Smith B, Mulhern RK. Oral ketamine premedication to alleviate the distress of invasive procedures in pediatric oncology patients. Pediatrics 1992;90:537–541.
116. Kentrup H, Skopnik H, Menke D, et al. Midazolam and ketamine as premedication in colonoscopies: a pharmacodynamic study. Int J Clin Pharmacol Ther Toxicol 1994;32:82–87.
117. Louon A, Reddy VG. Nasal midazolam and ketamine for paediatric sedation during computerised tomography. Acta Anaesthesiol Scand 1994;38:259–261.
118. Weksler N, Ovadia L, Muati G, Stav A. Nasal ketamine for paediatric premedication. Can J Anaesth 1993;40:119–121.
119. Naguib M, Sharif AM, Seraj M, et al. Ketamine for caudal analgesia in children: comparison with caudal bupivacaine. Br J Anaesth 1991;67:559–564.
120. Zhang WX. Combined ketamine, diazepam and procaine intravenous anesthesia in operations on burn patients: a report of 893 cases. Chung Hua Cheng Hsing Shao Shang Wai Ko Tsa Chih 1991;7:184–185.
121. Qureshi FA, Mellis PT, McFadden MA. Efficacy of oral ketamine for providing sedation and analgesia to children requiring laceration repair. Pediatr Emerg Care 1995;11:93–97.
122. Pruitt JW, Goldwasser MS, Sabol SR, Prstojevich SJ. Intramuscular ketamine, midazolam, and glycopyrrolate for pediatric sedation in the emergency department. J Oral Maxillofac Surg 1995;53:13–17; discussion 18.
123. Hartvig P, Larsson E, Joachimsson PO. Postoperative analgesia and sedation following pediatric cardiac surgery using a constant infusion of ketamine. J Cardiothorac Vasc Anesth 1993; 7:148–153.
124. Barr EB, Wynn RL. IV sedation in pediatric dentistry: an alternative to general anesthesia. Pediatr Dent 1992;14:251–255.
125. Abrams R, Morrison JE, Villasenor A, et al. Safety and effectiveness of intranasal administration of sedative medications (ketamine, midazolam, or sufentanil) for urgent brief pediatric dental procedures. Anesth Prog 1993;40:63–66.
126. Pederson L, Benumof J. Incidence and magnitude of hypoxaemia with ketamine in a rural African hospital. Anaesthesia 1993;48:67–69.
127. Green SM. The safety of ketamine for emergency department pediatric sedation [Letter]. J Oral Maxillofac Surg 1995;53:1232–1233.
128. Tashiro C, Matsui Y, Nakano S, et al. Respiratory outcome in extremely premature infants following ketamine anaesthesia. Can J Anaesth 1991;38:287–291.
129. Webster AC, McKishnie JD, Kenyon CF, Marshall DG. Spinal anaesthesia for inguinal hernia repair in high-risk neonates. Can J Anaesth 1991;38:281–286.
130. Joly LM, Benhamou D. Ventilation during total intravenous anaesthesia with ketamine. Can J Anaesth 1994;41:227–231.
131. Audenaert SM, Wagner Y, Montgomery CL, et al. Cardiorespiratory effects of premedication for children. Anesth Analg 1995; 80:506–510.
132. Wolfe RR, Loehr JP, Schaffer MS, Wiggins JW Jr. Hemodynamic effects of ketamine, hypoxia and hyperoxia in children with surgically treated congenital heart disease residing greater than or equal to 1,200 meters above sea level. Am J Cardiol 1991; 67:84–87.
133. Hickey PR, Wessel DL, Streitz SL, et al. Transcatheter closure of atrial septal defects: hemodynamic complications and anesthetic management. Anesth Analg 1992;74:44–50.
134. Kubota T, Takagi Y, Hasimoto H, Ishiara H. Clinical study of total intravenous anesthesia with droperidol, fentanyl and ketamine: application for pediatric patients. Masui 1991;40:1843–1851.
135. Yip AS, McGuire MA, Davis L, et al. Lack of effect of midazolam on inductibility of arrhythmias at electrophysiological study. Am J Cardiol 1992;70:593–597.
136. Malinovsky JM, Populaire C, Cozian A, et al. Premedication with midazolam in children: effect of intranasal, rectal and oral routes on plasma midazolam concentrations. Anaesthesia 1995; 50:351–354.
137. Feld L, Negus JB, White PF. Oral midazolam preanesthetic medication in pediatric outpatients. Anesthesiology 1990; 73:831–834.
138. Malinovsky JM, Lejus C, Servin F, et al. Plasma concentrations of midazolam after i.v., nasal or rectal administration in children. Br J Anaesth 1993;70:617–620.
139. Jacqz-Aigrain E, Daoud P, Burtin P, et al. Pharmacokinetics of midazolam during continuous infusion in critically ill neonates. Eur J Clin Pharmacol 1992;42:329–332.
140. Kern FH, Ungerleider RM, Jacobs JR, et al. Computerized continuous infusion of intravenous anesthetic drugs during pediatric cardiac surgery. Anesth Analg 1991;72:487–492.
141. Jacqz-Aigrain E, Daoud P, Burtin P, et al. Placebo-controlled trial of midazolam sedation in mechanically ventilated newborn babies. Lancet 1994;344:646–650.
142. Rosen DA, Rosen KR. Midazolam for sedation in the paediatric intensive care unit. Intensive Care Med 1991;17 (suppl 1):S15–S19.
143. Sheridan RL, McEttrick M, Bacha G, et al. Midazolam infusion in pediatric patients with burns who are undergoing mechanical ventilation. J Burn Care Rehabil 1994;15:515–518.
144. Shelly MP, Sultan MA, Bodenham A, Park GR. Midazolam infusions in critically ill patients. Eur J Anaesthesiol 1991;8:21–27.
145. Bergman I, Steeves M, Burckart G, Thompson A. Reversible neurologic abnormalities associated with prolonged intravenous midazolam and fentanyl administration. J Pediatr 1991; 119:644–649.
146. van Engelen BG, Gimbrere JS, Booy LH. Benzodiazepine withdrawal reaction in two children following discontinuation of sedation with midazolam. Ann Pharmacother 1993;27:579–581.
147. Hughes J, Gill A, Leach HJ, et al. A prospective study of the adverse effects of midazolam on withdrawal in critically ill children. Acta Paediatr 1994;83:1194–1199.
148. Tobias JD, Deshpande JK, Gregory DF. Outpatient therapy of iatrogenic drug dependency following prolonged sedation in the pediatric intensive care unit. Intensive Care Med 1994; 20:504–507.
149. Collins S, Carter JA. Resedation after bolus administration of midazolam to an infant and its reversal by flumazenil. Anaesthesia 1991;46:471–472.
150. Eldar I, Lieberman N, Shiber R, et al. Use of flumazenil for intraoperative arousal during spine fusion. Anesth Analg 1992; 75:580–583.
151. Jones RD, Lawson AD, Andrew LJ, et al. Antagonism of the hypnotic effect of midazolam in children: a randomized, double-blind study of placebo and flumazenil administered after midazolam-induced anaesthesia. Br J Anaesth 1991;66:660–666.
152. Lopez-Herce J, Lopez de Sa E, Garcia de Frias E. Reversal of midazolam sedation with rectal flumazenil in children. Crit Care Med 1994;22:1204.

23 Use of Intravenous Techniques in the Elderly

Alice L. Landrum

The appropriate use of intravenous anesthetic agents in the elderly patient is a subject of increasing importance for all anesthesiologists. Western industrialized nations are now experiencing an aging of their populations as a result of a demographic change from high to low mortality (1). The United Nations organization projects that from 1980 until 2000 the elderly population (> 65 years of age) will increase by 66% (2). In the United States, the population of the so-called elderly elderly (i.e., aged 85 years and older) increased by 33% during the 1980s, compared with an increase of only 10% in the overall population (3). Currently, the elderly population accounts for about one-third of annual health care expenditures in the United States (4).

As the elderly continue to make more demands on the health care system, anesthesiologists must be prepared to provide safe and efficient anesthetics for this rapidly growing segment of the population. It is important to understand how the elderly patient's physiology affects the pharmacologic response to intravenous agents and how these drugs affect the elderly patient's physiologic response.

PHARMACOLOGIC ISSUES

The elderly are more sensitive to the central nervous system (CNS) effects of intravenous anesthetics and risk developing adverse drug reactions (5, 6). The causes of decreased dose requirements in the elderly are multifactorial, including age-related physiologic changes, pathologic conditions, and environmental and genetic factors (7) (Table 23-1). Physiologic changes in the elderly affecting the pharmacokinetics or the pharmacodynamics of each intravenous agent probably play a significant role, but attempts to determine which factors are the most important have been inconclusive. Physiologic changes in the elderly may not parallel chronologic aging. In addition, specific physiologic processes may age at different rates within one individual (8). The lack of uniformity in physiologic changes, coupled with the influence of acquired diseases and environmental factors, leads to a high incidence of interindividual variability in dose requirements. The pharmacokinetics of intravenous agents involves distribution, redistribution, metabolism, and excretion events. Age-related physiologic changes that can affect distribution include changes in protein binding, body composition, and tissue perfusion. Plasma albumin levels fall by only about 12.5% in healthy elderly patients (9). However, even greater decreases occur in the presence of cirrhosis, renal failure, malnutrition, and rheumatoid arthritis (10). The effects of decreased albumin levels vary according to the extent that the drug is bound and depends on metabolism by the liver for elimination (10). α_1-acid glycoprotein (AAG) does not change in the healthy elderly subject (10). AAG is an acute-phase reactant that rises after trauma, surgery, stroke, and myocardial infarction and in infection, cancer, heart failure, and chronic airway disease (11). Plasma globulin levels rise with increasing age (12), a possible factor in drug resistance. However, the significance of plasma protein binding changes in the elderly patient is small when compared with the greater changes produced by disease states (13). For individual drugs, the clinical significance of protein binding depends on the degree of binding.

Changes in body composition include a decrease in total body water as a result of diminished lean body mass (14, 15) and an increase in body fat content (16). These changes in body composition can decrease the volume of distribution of water-soluble drugs (i.e., ethanol) and can increase the volume of distribution of fat-soluble drugs (i.e., thiopental). The volume of dis-

TABLE 23-1. Physiologic Changes in Aging that May Affect Pharmacokinetics of Intravenous Drugs

Change	Process Affected
Body water ↓	Distribution
Lean body mass ↓	
Body fat ↑	
Plasma albumin ↓	
Plasma globulin ↑	
α_1-Acid glycoprotein with disease	
Tissue perfusion changes ↑	
Liver mass ↓	Metabolism
Liver blood flow ↓	
Glomerular filtration ↓	Excretion
Renal plasma flow ↓	
Renal tubular function ↓	

tribution for water-soluble or hydrophilic drugs correlates well with lean body mass, making lean body mass a more accurate predictor of the required loading dose than actual (measured) weight. Because the volume of distribution is smaller, plasma concentration per unit dose is higher in the elderly (5). The volume of distribution for lipophilic drugs such as thiopental and diazepam correlates better with total body weight (17). When the volume of distribution is larger, the plasma concentration per unit dose is lower. If the clearance is unchanged, then the half-life and duration of action will be longer (5). Increasing evidence suggests that lean body mass is a better predictor of determining initial dosages for both hydrophilic and lipophilic drugs (17). The decrease in lean body mass in the elderly could help explain, in part, the decrease in dose requirements to obtain the desired response.

Changes in tissue perfusion may occur as a result of changing cardiac function. A decline in early diastolic left ventricular filling is a hallmark of the normal aging process. As the left atrial size increases, there is a compensatory augmentation of the atrial contribution to left ventricular filling. These changes in cardiac function predispose the elderly to elevated left atrial pressures and symptoms of pulmonary congestion when combined with conditions such as hypertension or coronary artery disease. Even older male athletes with a long history of endurance training exhibit this impairment in early diastolic left ventricular filling (18). As a result of changes in perfusion, both hepatic blood flow and renal blood flow decrease, whereas cerebral circulation, coronary circulation, and skeletal muscle circulation increase (19). In general, drugs with high hepatic extraction ratios have lower clearance rates and higher plasma concentrations in the elderly. Lower tissue perfusion may lengthen the time required to transport drugs to tissues and may delay the time to peak effect (20). For example, lower induction doses for thiopental reflect slower redistribution in the aged patient (21, 22).

Age-related physiologic changes affecting metabolism include reduced liver mass and reduced liver blood flow (23-25). Liver mass may decline by 25 to 35% with age (24), whereas liver blood flow may fall as much as 40% between the ages of 20 and 90 years (23). Changes in liver enzyme activity are probably due to environmental or disease-related factors rather than to the aging process itself. Direct measurement of both the activity and amount of human liver microsomal monooxygenases (enzymes responsible for hepatic phase I drug metabolism) has demonstrated the absence of significant age-dependent differences (26, 27). Similarly, current data indicate that the activities of glucuronyl transferases and sulfotransferases (enzymes responsible for phase II conjugation reactions) do not change significantly in aging humans (28). Reduced hepatic drug clearance is primarily due to reduced liver volume and decreased liver blood flow (26). Drugs with high hepatic extraction ratios (>0. 7), such as opioid analgesics, have lowered clearance in the elderly as a result of their dependence on liver blood flow (5).

Age-related changes affecting excretion are primarily related to changes in renal function. One of the most predictable pharmacokinetic alterations associated with aging is the reduction in renal clearance of drugs. In 1950, Davies and Shock (29) demonstrated with cross-sectional analysis that glomerular filtration and renal blood flow decline with age. Other investigative groups subsequently showed declines in measures of renal tubular function (30, 31). As part of the Baltimore Longitudinal Study of Aging, Rowe and associates (31), using both cross-sectional analysis and longitudinal data covering a 10-year period, reported a decline in creatinine clearance with increasing age. However, more recent longitudinal studies over a 23-year period using the same population employed by Rowe and associates reported that one-third of all subjects had no decrease in renal function, and a small group actually showed an increase in the creatinine clearance rate (32). These longitudinal studies of renal function have demonstrated that great variability exists among individuals and have cast doubt on the concept of a predictable "age-related decline" in renal function. Nevertheless, the majority of elderly patients do exhibit declines in creatinine clearance, which is the basis for the common clinical practice of giving smaller doses of renally excreted drugs to elderly patients. This documented variability in renal function reinforces the importance of titration of drug dosages according to individual patients' needs (5). For over 30 years, we have unequivocally accepted the idea that declining renal function is a natural result of aging. The foregoing findings from the Baltimore Longitudinal Study on renal function highlight the difficulties of interpreting data from most age-related studies regarding the influence of physiologic changes on the pharmacokinetics of intravenous anesthetic drugs.

Limitations of many of the physiologic studies involving elderly patients include inadequate sample size, cross-sectional analysis rather than longitudinal analysis, and frequent use of subjects who are institutionalized or who have complicating preexisting diseases (26). The environmental influences of cigarettes, caffeine, and alcohol may not have been considered, as well as gender-related issues such as differences in body composition between men and women. As a result of the many confounding influences on physiologic changes, no satisfactory definition of normal aging exists. Interindividual variability is a common feature of most of the physiologic functions influenced by the aging process. Therefore, intravenous anesthetics must be carefully titrated to meet the needs of the individual patient (5).

Few clinical studies have examined the effects of age on the pharmacodynamics of intravenous agents. The pharmacodynamics of intravenous anesthetic agents is difficult to study in the elderly for several reasons. Pharmacodynamic studies have to be designed to examine specific populations of drug receptors. This accomplishment is difficult in humans, and the validity of extrapolating results from animal models has been questioned (8). In vivo studies are also complicated by changes in pharmacokinetics and by compensatory mechanisms such as baroreceptor reflexes (8). Changes in drug sensitivity (pharmacodynamics) cannot be validated without accounting for alterations in a drug's pharmacokinetics (or plasma concentrations) (33). The rapid changes in plasma concentration that result from a drug's redistribution make it difficult to correlate drug concentrations and effect. Methodologic problems include the effects of gender, associated diseases, and the type of pharmacodynamic measure used to assess drug effect. Currently, no standard objective measure of CNS response exists (33, 34). Dynamic responses studied include response to vocal stimulus, movement to painful stimuli, saccadic eye movement velocity, tremor, postural sway, and specific changes in the electroencephalogram (e.g., EEG spectral edge or bispectral index) (33).

Age-related physiologic changes that can affect pharmacodynamics involve alterations in the quantity and activity of receptors in the CNS. With increasing age, brain size decreases (35) as a result of a loss of neurons. CNS receptors appear to have a reduced affinity for neurotransmitter molecules (36). Within the peripheral nervous system, one sees attrition of afferent conduction pathways and deterioration of electrical conductance along motor pathways (37). Neuromuscular junctions develop thickening of the postjunctional membrane and spread beyond the motor end plate (38). In addition is an age-related decrease in the number and density of motor end plate units. Decreased muscular activity leads to "downregulation" of skeletal muscle acetylcholine receptors (39). Although neurons in the sympathoadrenal pathways undergo attrition and fibrosis, plasma levels of epinephrine and norepinephrine are increased (40, 41). In spite of higher plasma levels of catecholamines, autonomic end-organ responsiveness is reduced (42).

Most of the clinical studies investigating the effects of age on pharmacodynamics have examined the peripheral adrenergic receptors. With aging, a well-documented decline occurs in the responsiveness of cardiac β_1 receptors to an infusion of isoproterenol (43). Vascular relaxation mediated by β_2 receptors also decreases with age (42). As previously mentioned, in vivo studies are complicated by changes in pharmacokinetics and by compensatory mechanisms such as baroreceptor reflexes (8).

In vitro studies using isolated tissue (e.g., vascular smooth muscle rings, papillary muscle strips, gastrointestinal smooth muscle, or blood components) avoid these complications. Numerous radioligand studies examining the numbers and affinities of autonomic receptors on isolated human cells give conflicting results. Studies on the effect of aging on the numbers of α_2 adrenoceptors on platelets have reported an increase (44), a decrease (45), or no change (46) in receptor numbers with increasing age. There does not seem to be any change in the number of β adrenoceptors on lymphocytes from elderly subjects (47), but some data suggest that β receptors' affinity for agonists may be reduced (48). However, the relevance of receptors on platelets or lymphocytes to those on innervated tissue is unclear (8).

The study of β adrenoreceptors on isolated lymphocytes has several limitations (49). Lymphocytes contain only β_2 receptors, whereas the heart has mostly β_1 receptors (50) such that changes in β_2 receptors on lymphocytes may not reflect in vivo changes in β_1 receptor properties. The stimulus to adrenergic receptors on lymphocytes may be underestimated because the exposure of lymphocytes to catecholamines is limited by the concentration in the blood. Innervated solid organs have their receptors exposed to additional "local" concentrations of norepinephrine, which is released at nerve endings in close proximity to the receptors (49). The circulating levels of norepinephrine are even higher in elderly subjects (40, 41), perhaps as a result of "spill-over" from sympathetic nerve endings (51). The cellular response of the elderly patient to β-adrenergic agonists is clearly diminished, but the mechanisms responsible for these changes at the receptor level are still unclear. The most likely explanations include a decrease in the number of high-affinity receptors, a decrease in the affinity of the receptors, an impairment in the activity of adenyl cyclase, or a decrease in cyclic adenosine monophosphate (cAMP)-dependent protein kinase activity (52, 53).

COMMONLY USED INTRAVENOUS ANESTHETIC DRUGS (TABLE 23-2)

Hypnotics

Ultrashort-acting Barbiturates

The dose of thiopental required for induction and maintenance of anesthesia may vary significantly among individuals even within comparable groups (54). The elderly patient usually requires a lower dose of thiopental (on the basis of kilograms of body weight) for induction of anesthesia when compared with younger adults (54-57). However, enough variation in response exists within the elderly population that determining the optimal dose is an uncertain exercise (57, 58). Pharmacokinetic studies have yielded conflicting results regarding age-related changes in the early disposition of thiopental. Earlier investigations using three-compartment models reported that elderly patients had a larger volume of distribution and a prolongation of their elimination half-life (58-60), as well as a higher "free" fraction of thiopental in the plasma (58). More recent studies using population-based models suggest that changes in rapid intercompartmental clearance and lean body mass play a more important role in determining the induction dose requirements of elderly patients (62, 64).

Many closely correlated factors influence the pharmacokinetic profile of thiopental. For example, the influence of body weight is difficult to isolate from the influence of age because body weight tends to change with age (61). Investigators have developed various models to describe populations of subjects. Stanski and Maitre (62) used the NONMEM model (nonlinear mixed effects model) (63) to reexamine thiopental pharmacokinetics and pharmacodynamics on the CNS using the EEG. With this type of population analysis, they reported that the V_1 and metabolic clearance rate were proportional to body weight, and rapid intercompartmental clearance ($V_1 \times K_{12}$) decreased with increasing age. However, a variability of 30 to 70% in thiopental distribution kinetic parameters was noted. Because thiopental distribution depends on cardiovascular function, these authors postulated that variability in cardiac function (and cardiac output) may explain the high degree of variability in pharmacokinetic parameters.

Avram and associates (64) used a concurrent indocyanine green (ICG) model to investigate the pharmacokinetic basis for increased sensitivity of the elderly to thiopental. Using early arterial sampling and

TABLE 23-2. Use of Intravenous Agents in the Elderly

Intravenous Agent	Special Considerations in the Elderly
Hypnotics	
Ultrashort-acting barbiturates	↓ Onset time, so titrate slowly ↑ Elimination half-life No change in sensitivity Large or repeated boluses does not ablate movement but could ↑ recovery
Benzodiazepenes	↑ Sensitivity Duration of sedative effects does not correlate with duration of plasma elimination half-lives
Ketamine	Hypertension and tachycardia Hallucinations Minimal respiratory effects
Etomidate	↓ Dose required to reach EEG end point −Ionotropic effect on aged heart Preserves sympathetic responses Inhibits adrenocortical function
Propofol	↓ Induction dose requirement Hypotension Impairs baroreceptor regulatory mechanism Greater risk for respiratory depression
Opioids	
Morphine	↑ Sensitivity ↓ Clearance Changes in ventilatory control
Meperidine	Postoperative delirium, which may be result of potent metabolite (normeperidine)
Fentanyl	↑ Sensitivity More disturbed ventilatory pattern
Sufentanil	High hepatic extraction ratio means that decreases in liver blood flow will ↑ activity
Alfentanil	Variations in protein binding influence dose required for clinical effect
Remifentanil	Rapid emergence associated with ↑ in mean arterial pressure and heart rate
Neuromuscular blockers	
Succinylcholine	Elderly men have ↓ levels of plasma cholinesterase
Pancuronium	↑ Effect due to ↓ renal clearance
Vecuronium	↑ Effect due to ↓ hepatic blood flow
Pipercuronium	↑ Onset time but no change in rate of recovery
Rocuronium	↑ Effect due to ↓ hepatic blood flow
D-Tubocurarine	↑ Effect due to ↓ renal clearance and hepatic blood flow
Atracurium	Slightly ↑ initial dose required as result of ↑ volume of distribution. Slight ↑ in steady state dose requirement may be due to ↓ in muscle activity and downregulation of acetylcholine receptors
Doxacurium	↑ Onset time and ↑ effect
Mivacurium	↑ Effect (up to 30% longer)
Cisatracurium	↑ Onset time but no change in recovery profile
Neuromuscular antagonists	
Neostigmine	↑ Duration of action
Pyridostigmine	↑ Duration
Edrophonium	Brief maximal duration of action
Neostigmine + Atropine	Significant dysrhythmias
Neostigmine + Glycopyrrolate	Fewer dysrhythmias
Edrophonium + Atropine	Minimal change in heart rate but similar incidence of atrial and junctional dysrhythmias

simultaneous modeling of thiopental disposition with that of ICG, they attempted to describe the early distribution of thiopental. With this model, intercompartmental clearance (Cl21) from V_1 to the rapidly equilibrating peripheral volume, V_2, decreased 35% between the ages of 20 and 80 years. However, these investigators also noted considerable interindividual variation that did not correlate with increasing age. From their analysis, Avram and associates concluded that dose adjustments should not be made on the basis of age alone. Lean body mass may be the best predictor of optimal thiopental dosing because cardiac output appears to correlate with change in intercompartmental clearance. Lean body mass is more closely related to cardiac output than either total body mass or body surface area. Doses should be based on physiologic or pathophysiologic factors rather than on age alone.

When elderly patients receive the same induction dose (4 mg/kg) as younger patients, their recovery is longer (65). Because thiopental has a low hepatic extraction ratio (0.15) (66), metabolism is less important than redistribution in terminating its initial effect after a single bolus dose. With repeated boluses (or continuous infusion), elimination becomes dependent on intrinsic hepatic enzyme activity and the degree of plasma protein binding. In this situation, metabolism becomes more relevant, and recovery from thiopental can be significantly prolonged (66).

Clinical studies have not demonstrated age-related changes in the CNS pharmacodynamics of thiopental. Homer and Stanski in 1985 (67) obtained pharmacodynamic data from a group of patients aged 19 to 88 years by observing the power spectral analysis of the EEG when infusion of thiopental was administered until the EEG produced a burst-suppression pattern with isoelectric periods. The total dose required to achieve early burst suppression decreased linearly with age, but arterial sampling demonstrated no relationship between age and the steady-state thiopental serum concentration producing half the maximal EEG slowing (Fig. 23-1). These data suggest that brain sensitivity does not change with age. Stanski and Maitre in 1990 (62) also examined thiopental's pharmacodynamics in the elderly with the NONMEM model. No age-related change in brain responsiveness was noted when they analyzed the EEG spectral edge versus time data. In studying the relationship of the thiopental concentration, clinical anesthetic depth, and the EEG, Hung and associates (68) concluded that the thiopental concentration required to ablate the movement response to intubation was so high (> than 80 μg/ml) that conventional induction doses of thiopental (4 to 5 mg/kg) could not achieve the plasma concentrations necessary to prevent movement in response to noxious stimuli. The clinical implication of this finding for elderly patients is that large or repeated boluses may not completely ablate movement during induction or maintenance of anesthesia, but they significantly prolong recovery. Although methohexital has early distribution kinetics similar to that of thiopental, the clearance and elimination half-time of the two drugs differ significantly. Methohexital's clearance is greater, and its resultant elimination half-time is significantly shorter. The high hepatic extraction ratio of methohexital (0.5) implies that the clearance of methohexital largely depends on hepatic blood flow (69). Because liver volume and liver blood flow decline with age (23, 24), the systemic clearance of methohexital may fall. However, age-related changes in hepatic drug elimination are multifactorial (70).

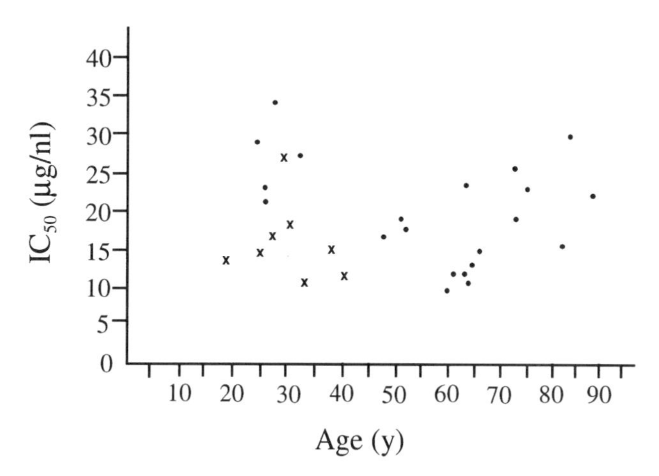

FIGURE 23-1. Brain sensitivity (IC_{50}) versus age. IC_{50} is the serum concentration of thiopental needed to cause one-half of the maximum electroencephalographic slowing and is a measure of brain sensitivity to the drug. The circles represent surgical patients who underwent arterial blood sampling, whereas the crosses represent volunteer subjects who underwent venous blood sampling. (From Homer TD, Stanski DR. The effect of increasing age on thiopental disposition and anesthetic requirement. Anesthesiology 1985;62:714–724.)

Benzodiazepines

Benzodiazepines provide effective anxiolysis, sedation, and amnesia even at low doses. At higher intravenous doses, these compounds can be used for anesthetic induction and maintenance. A widespread clinical impression exists that the elderly are more sensitive to the central depressant effects of benzodiazepines (33). Reports of adverse reactions associated with the use of benzodiazepines support this clinical impression (71); however, biologic mechanisms are still unclear (33). Aging can alter the distribution, clearance, and elimination of intravenous benzodiazepines. Clearance appears to be the pharmacokinetic parameter most affected by the aging process.

The benzodiazepines utilized most commonly in the operating room as intravenous sedatives and induction agents are diazepam, lorazepam, and midazolam. Differences in their metabolism influence the manner in which aging affects their clearance. All three benzodiazepines undergo metabolism in the liver, but diazepam and midazolam undergo oxidative metabolism by hydroxylation, whereas lorazepam undergoes conjugation by nonoxidative glucuronidation (72). The process of conjugation is less susceptible to outside influences such as enzyme induction or changes in hepatic perfusion, a finding that helps to explain why the clearance of lorazepam is unchanged by age (73). Both diazepam (74) and midazolam have reduced clearance in the elderly population; however, clearance of midazolam in the healthy elderly decreases to a lesser extent than that of diazepam. In addition, metabolism of midazolam appears to be affected by gender in that it is reduced in elderly men but not in elderly women (75, 76). Of the three drugs, midazolam plasma levels decrease most rapidly in the elderly such that it has the shortest plasma elimination half-life of the currently available parenteral benzodiazepines. Midazolam's higher hepatic extraction ratio allows for greater hepatic clearance and, therefore, greater overall clearance. Conditions that decrease hepatic perfusion decrease the clearance of midazolam. For example, liver disease causes a greater delay in the psychomotor recovery rate from midazolam sedation compared with diazepam (77).

Elderly patients require smaller doses of intravenous diazepam and midazolam to achieve a given anxiolytic or hypnotic effect (78, 79). Reidenberg and associates (78) studied elderly patients undergoing elective cardioversion and reported a negative correlation of age with measured plasma concentration and dose of diazepam required to obtain a specific sedative end point. Cook and associates (79) had similar findings when studying patients who received intravenous diazepam for dental procedures or endoscopy. Jacobs and associates (80) used intravenous midazolam for induction before elective coronary artery bypass grafting and reported that the plasma concentration associated with loss of responsiveness to verbal commands decreased with increasing age. Altered (or enhanced) sensitivity in the elderly is probably explained by changes in benzodiazepine receptor occupancy and cellular function (80); however, no age-related differences have been documented in benzodiazepine receptor number or affinity (81).

The importance of benzodiazepine receptors is highlighted by the observation that the different plasma elimination half-life values of the benzodiazepines do not correlate with the duration of their pharmacodynamic (sedative) effects. In one review of the literature comparing intravenous midazolam with diazepam, most of the studies showed similar sedative recovery rates (82). Differences in the observed sedative effects of benzodiazepines probably depend more on receptor affinity (83, 84). Benzodiazepines with a high reception affinity have prolonged elimination from the CNS, which correlates with a prolongation in the duration of their clinical effects and with lower therapeutic dosages (i.e., increased potency). For example, lorazepam has a more rapid elimination from plasma than diazepam, but it has a longer duration of pharmacologic activity on the CNS and is more potent.

Of the three commonly used benzodiazepines, lorazepam is the most potent and possesses the greatest affinity for benzodiazepine receptors (84, 85). Lorazepam's elimination half-life from cerebrospinal fluid is significantly longer than from plasma. Diazepam, the least potent, has lower receptor affinity such that its elimination half-life values from cerebrospinal fluid and plasma are similar. Although lorazepam does not have an active metabolite, diazepam has an active metabolite (desmethyldiazepam), which has a greater affinity for the benzodiazepine receptor (86). Midazolam has 1- and 4-hydroxy metabolites that have less CNS activity than the parent compound (87). The presence of a more potent active metabolite explains why long-term use of diazepam in the elderly can prolong its clinical effects. With short-term use, however, diazepam's clinical activity is shorter than that of lorazepam and is similar to that of midazolam.

Ketamine

The effects of ketamine on the cardiovascular system coupled with minimal effects on respiratory drive have made ketamine a useful drug for anesthetizing elderly critically ill patients. However, concern exists regarding ketamine's effects in patients with ischemic heart disease. Elderly patients anesthetized with ketamine have a consistent increase in heart rate and blood pressure. There appears to be an enhanced cardiostimulatory response to ketamine in patients with chronic hypertension. Elderly hypovolemic patients can become hypotensive after a dose of ketamine because of its direct negative inotropic effects. Ketamine can produce vivid dreams during induction and disorientation during emergence (88). When elderly patients anesthetized with ketamine and nitrous oxide were compared with a middle-aged population undergoing major intra-abdominal and intrathoracic procedures, the only significant difference between the two age groups was a higher systolic pressure in the recovery room for the elderly group (89).

Waxman and associates (90) investigated the cardiovascular effects of an induction dose of ketamine in critically ill adults with pulmonary artery catheters. A single induction dose varying from 24 to 144 mg produced significant decreases in cardiac performance and in peripheral oxygen transport. Subsequently, Pederson and associates (91) compared a low-dose infusion of ketamine with a thiopental bolus as an induction agent for 12 high-risk patients (5 of whom were older than 65 years). Using thoracic impedance cardiography, these investigators reported that ketamine infusion produced less depression of the cardiovascular system than thiopental, but both induction agents provoked ischemia in elderly patients with coronary artery disease. The initial increases in cardiac output, systemic blood pressure, and heart rate that occur after induction with ketamine tend to plateau after 3 to 5 minutes and return to baseline values after 10 to 20 minutes (92). Successful techniques for blunting the cardiovascular stimulation as well as the postanesthetic (psychomimetic) emergence reactions include the use of benzodiazepines (93, 94), thiopental, an investigational α_2 agonist, and an investigational α agonist, dexmedetomidine (95).

Information regarding the pharmacokinetics of ketamine in the elderly suggest that onset is rapid following intravenous administration, and emergence occurs within 15 minutes (87, 96); however, in one report, an elderly patient slept for 18 hours after a 50-minute hip-pinning procedure (97). Because ketamine is metabolized extensively by hepatic microsomal enzymes and has a high hepatic extraction ratio, changes in liver blood flow can affect its clearance. The reduced liver blood flow reported in the elderly decreases the clearance of ketamine and prolongs its duration of action. Unfortunately, no studies have specifically addressed age-related changes in the pharmacodynamics of ketamine. Because ketamine can exert a negative inotropic effect on ischemic myocardium (88, 90, 91), it is prudent to lower the induction dose for an elderly critically ill patient. However, for the healthy elderly patient, no data support the need to reduce the usual induction dose.

Etomidate

Etomidate has a different chemical structure than thiopental; however, aging appears to alter the dose-response relationship in a similar manner (98). The dose of etomidate required to reach a specific EEG end point decreases with increasing age. An 80-year-old patient requires less than half the dose of etomidate to reach the same stage EEG end point as a 22-year-old subject. This decrease in dose requirement appears to be the result of age-related changes in pharmacokinetics rather than pharmacodynamics because the relationship between the etomidate blood levels and maximal median frequency slowing of the EEG is similar. The elderly patient also requires half as long as the younger patient to reach a similar blood concentration of etomidate (98). The initial distribution volume in the elderly is decreased because of age-related physiologic changes (e.g., declining cardiac output, renal blood flow, hepatic perfusion).

The major advantage of etomidate as an induction agent is its hemodynamic stability. However, in elderly patients with compromised cardiovascular function, etomidate may have significant negative inotropic effects (99). Using invasive monitors, etomidate has decreased systolic, diastolic, and mean arterial pressure, as well as the heart rate and cardiac index. In addition, myocardial blood flow and oxygen consumption are decreased. Coronary perfusion pressure and cardiac output can be decreased following an induction dose of etomidate; however, perfusion is adequate because of a decrease in myocardial oxygen demand. Etomidate appears to have a negative iontropic effect on the aged heart (99). Because etomidate can impair cardiovascular performance, it should be used with caution in elderly patients with severe coronary or cerebral atherosclerosis.

Etomidate preserves both sympathetic outflow and autonomic reflexes (100). This preservation of sympathetic responses explains why etomidate can maintain hemodynamic stability. Nevertheless, the induction dose of etomidate should be decreased in patients with significant atherosclerotic disease. A major concern with the use of etomidate in critically ill patients is related to the direct inhibitory effect on adrenocortical function, resulting in suppression of cortisol production (101). The adrenosuppressive effects of etomidate last for 5 to 10 hours after a single induction dose (102). Continuous administration of etomidate for sedation of critically ill patients may result in significantly increased mortality (103). However, no evidence indicates increased mortality after the use of a single bolus dose of etomidate for induction of anesthesia.

Propofol

Propofol's rapid emergence and increased metabolic clearance rate compared with thiopentol (104) make it especially desirable in the elderly. In a multi-institutional study looking at more than 25,000 patients receiving propofol for induction or maintenance of anesthesia, an age older than 65 years was associated with prolonged time to awakening ($>$ 15 minutes after cessation of all anesthesia) (105). The pharmacokinetics of propofol is altered by aging as a result of decreases in cardiac function and hepatic blood flow. Propofol plasma concentrations are higher immediately after injection in the elderly as the result of a lower distribution volume (106). In addition, the total body clearance of propofol is lower in the elderly.

The pharmacodynamics of propofol also appears to be changed as a result of the aging process. Older patients require less propofol for induction of anesthesia (107, 108), and doses in excess of 1.75 mg/kg can cause significant hypotension and prolonged apnea in the elderly (107). Increasing age is also reported to decrease the propofol concentration required for loss of consciousness (107). When bolus doses of propofol are used for induction of anesthesia, systemic blood pressure is reduced, and the magnitude of decrease is greater in the elderly (99, 106, 107). As a result, the incidence of hypotension is significantly higher (30%) in patients over the age of 65 years (109). Causes of the decrease in systemic blood pressure include direct relaxant effects on vascular smooth muscle (110), as well as negative inotropic effects on the myocardium (111). Another important factor contributing to hypotension is inhibition of the sympathetic nervous system and further impairment of baroreflex regulatory mechanisms (112). For elderly patients with coexisting pulmonary disease, propofol can produce bronchodilation (113), thereby increasing dynamic compliance and decreasing peak inspiratory pressures (114, 115). However, the elderly patient who is receiving propofol for sedation during local or regional anesthesia may be at greater risk for central respiratory depression because propofol significantly depresses the hypoxic ventilatory response (116).

Opioids

Morphine

Elderly patients are more sensitive to opioid analgesics than young adults. Bellville and associates (117) suggested that age was an important determinant of the initial intramuscular dose of morphine. Kaiko recommended that age be used as a guide for the dosing interval rather than for the size of the initial bolus dose (118). Kaiko and his colleagues reported that the duration of relief with intramuscular morphine was significantly longer in the elderly. In 1982, Kaiko and associates (119) summarized the results of five studies examining the pharmacokinetics of intravenous morphine and concluded that plasma clearance of morphine is decreased by 50% in older subjects. Owen and colleagues (120) confirmed this observation using a single 10-mg intravenous dose of morphine. The older group had lower plasma clearance rates, and the morphine concentration in the peripheral compartment was higher in the older age group. Increased morphine concentration at analgesic receptors in the peripheral compartment may explain the increased drug effect in older patients. Increased sensitivity of the elderly to morphine probably has both a pharmacokinetic and a pharmacodynamic basis. The effects of morphine on minute volume of ventilation and end-tidal carbon dioxide tension are both similar in older and younger patients. However, after an intravenous dose of morphine (10 mg/70 kg), elderly patients have more frequent periods of apnea or periodic breathing (121). At a comparable pharmacodynamic end point (i.e., decrease in minute ventilation or increase in arterial carbon dioxide), the elderly appear to experience greater decreases in ventilation in the presence of morphine and are at greater risk for hypoxia (122).

Meperidine

As with morphine, the pharmacokinetics of meperidine is also influenced by aging. The free fraction of meperidine correlates with the patient's age (123). The decreased protein binding of meperidine in the elderly can increase the volume of distribution and decrease the rate at which meperidine is metabolized by the liver. Herman and associates (124) studied the pharmacokinetics of meperidine in seven elderly and six younger males and found a greater volume of distribution in the elderly, resulting in lower initial plasma concentrations. No age-related differences were seen in clearance rates or terminal elimination half-life values. The use of meperidine for analgesia may be a contributing factor to postoperative delirium in elderly patients (125), possibly related to the accumulation of its primary metabolite, normeperidine, in the presence of renal insufficiency.

Fentanyl

Studies of the pharmacokinetics of fentanyl in the elderly have yielded conflicting results. Based on a small sample size and short sampling interval, Bentley and colleagues (126) concluded that older patients had increased fentanyl concentrations, prolonged terminal elimination half-life values, and decreased clearance rates. Subsequent studies (122, 127-129) involving more prolonged sampling failed to confirm the finding of a decreased clearance rate and prolonged elimination half-life of fentanyl in elderly. However, Singleton and associates (122) did report higher initial plasma concentrations in elderly patients because of a smaller volume of distribution at steady state. Furthermore, Scott and Stanski (129) reported that the fast intercompartmental clearance rate decreased with age.

A pharmacodynamic explanation may play a more important role in the decreased fentanyl requirement in elderly patients. The dose of fentanyl required to induce EEG slowing decreases significantly with increasing age (a 50% decrease was noted from age 20 to 89 years) (129). Fentanyl-induced ventilatory depression (130) is directly related to the plasma fentanyl concentrations (127). If patients are hyperventilated, fentanyl-induced ventilatory depression may persist for more than 5 hours (127). Elderly patients may have greater impairment of ventilatory function after opioid-based anesthesia (131-133). Another adverse effect of fentanyl is impaired memory and behavioral performance (134). Elderly patients have a high incidence of mental status changes (135) after balanced anesthesia. Anesthetic drugs that impair memory and behavior may cause elderly patients to have a more significant decrement in CNS function. The problems related to disturbed ventilation and changes in mental status along with the decreased opioid dose requirements suggest that pharmacodynamic changes in the elderly play a significant role in their enhanced sensitivity to fentanyl.

Sufentanil

Sufentanil is highly bound to plasma proteins (92.5%), in particular AAG. This plasma protein level is not affected by aging but is affected by coexisting disease processes. Therefore, changes in protein binding could influence the onset of action of sufentanil.

Sufentanil's metabolism is primarily hepatic, with a 71% hepatic extraction ratio. Decreases in liver blood flow either as the result of aging or in response to inhalational agents or abdominal retraction influence the kinetics of sufentanil. Studies of sufentanil in the elderly have yielded conflicting results. Hudson and associates (136) reported a positive correlation of elimination half-life and volume of distribution at steady state with age. However, the small sample size and the type of surgical procedure, abdominal aortic surgery, may have had a significant effect on the disposition of sufentanil. Lechmann and associates (137) examined patients ranging in age from 24 to 77 years and did not find a significant correlation with age. A subgroup of patients receiving isoflurane had a positive correlation between the volume of distribution and the elimination half-life with age. Helmers and associates in 1994 (138) compared 12 elderly (65 to 87 years) with 12 younger patients (17 to 43 years) who were undergoing orthopedic surgery and found no difference in the values for sufentanil's elimination half-life, clearance, or volume of distribution.

Alfentanil

Analogous to sufentanil, alfentanil is highly protein bound (91%) to glycoproteins, especially AAG (139). Unlike the other opioid analgesics, alfentanil has a low pKa value of 6.5 such that at a pH of 7.40 the diffusible fraction (8%) is greater than that of fentanyl or sufentanil (140). As a result of its relatively large diffusible fraction and lipid solubility, an intravenous dose of alfentanil can rapidly reach the brain (140). The pKa and protein-binding characteristics of alfentanil may play a role in the wide variation among individuals in their responses to standard doses of the opioid analgesic. In elderly patients, the most consistent pharmacokinetic findings are a decrease in the alfentanil clearance rate and an increase in the terminal elimination half-life with age (129, 141, 142), suggesting that the maintenance infusion rate should be decreased in these patients.

With respect to pharmacodynamic changes with aging, Scott and Stanski (129) reported that the dose of alfentanil required to produce EEG slowing decreased by 50% from age 20 to 89 years. Lemmens and associates (143) examined the pharmacodynamics of alfentanil administered as part of a balanced anesthetic technique in premedicated patients undergoing surgery for breast cancer. The pharmacodynamic end points included changes in systolic blood pressure and heart rate and the onset of sweating, flushing, skeletal movement, swallowing, and grimacing (or eye) movement. Comparing the older and younger groups, these investigators failed to find a significant difference in the plasma concentration effect relation at intubation or skin incision. However, a higher incidence of muscle rigidity occurred in the older patients, and the alfentanil dose requirement was decreased in the older group. In a second study, Lemmens and associates (144) found a high incidence of muscle rigidity, bradycardia, hypotension, and postoperative ventilatory depression in elderly patients (aged 65 to 86 years).

In 1992, Lemmens and associates (145) examined the relationship of protein binding with the pharmacodynamic effects of alfentanil. In patients aged 21 to 85 years, a significant correlation existed between the plasma concentration effect relationship and the free fraction of alfentanil. However, these investigators failed to find a correlation between plasma concentration effect and age. Of importance, 45% of the observed variability in the response to alfentanil was related to protein binding. Variations in protein binding can result in different total plasma alfentanil concentrations to achieve the same effect.

Remifentanil

This newest opioid analgesic is an analog of fentanyl with a unique ester structure that may offer distinct advantages in elderly outpatients because of its rapid onset and short duration of action. Because it is rapidly metabolized by nonspecific tissue esterases, remifentanil's duration of action and elimination are independent of liver or renal function. Pharmacokinetic data suggest that clearance is not affected by aging (146). However, few data are available regarding remifentanil's kinetics in patients over 65 years of age. One study examined the hemodynamic effects of remifentanil in subjects over 70 years of age. In 3 of the 18 subjects, the remifentanil infusion had to be discontinued because of significant hypotension. Within 10 minutes after terminating the infusion, all the volunteers experienced rapid awakening, with sudden increases in blood pressure and heart rate. In 3 patients, treatment with labetolol was required because of pain-induced cardiovascular stimulation (147).

Neuromuscular Blocking Drugs and Their Antagonists

The pharmacokinetics of muscle relaxants appears to be altered in elderly patients. Changes in the distribution and elimination of muscle relaxants develop as a result of changes in body composition and decreases in organ function. Distribution may be affected by a decrease in total body fluid, lean body mass, cardiac output, and protein binding. Elimination can be prolonged by decreases in cardiac output, renal blood flow, glomerular filtration rate, and splanchnic blood flow (148). The concentration effect relationship at the neuromuscular junction does not appear to be changed by age; however, controversy exists regarding the pharmacodynamics of atracurium in the elderly.

Succinylcholine

Elderly men have decreased levels of plasma cholinesterase, resulting in a lower rate of succinylcholine hydrolysis (149). Although this change should prolong succinylcholine's duration of action, this has not been a problem in the healthy elderly patient.

Nondepolarizing Neuromuscular Blockers

AMINOSTEROIDS

PANCURONIUM. Pancuronium has a prolonged effect in elderly patients because of decreased plasma clearance secondary to delayed urinary excretion. The elimination half-life of pancuronium may be twice as long in elderly patients, contributing to a prolonged recovery rate (150).

VECURONIUM. Vecuronium is structurally related to pancuronium; however, its primary mode of elimination is by the hepatic rather than the renal route of administration. Because the aging process results in a decline of hepatic blood flow, the elderly population has reduced plasma clearance of vecuronium and a prolonged duration of action (151, 152). The sensitivity of the neuromuscular junction to vecuronium appears to be the same in the young and the elderly (151).

PIPERCURONIUM. This long-acting nondepolarizing relaxant is structurally related to pancuronium and is primarily eliminated by the renal route. Onset of action is prolonged in the elderly, but spontaneous recovery and sensitivity at the neuromuscular junction are similar in the young and elderly (148). The duration of action and elimination of pipercuronium do not appear to be affected by age.

ROCURONIUM. Rocuronium's onset of action may be prolonged in the elderly (153, 154). The onset time depends primarily on cardiac output, which may be diminished in the elderly. The volume of distribution and plasma clearance of rocuronium are decreased (153), and its duration of action is significantly prolonged in the elderly (153, 154). These pharmacokinetic changes can be explained by a decrease in total body water and liver mass, as well as the decrease in hepatic blood flow that accompanies the aging process. However, the potency is similar in the elderly and the young (154, 153).

BENZYLISOQUINOLONES

D-TUBOCURARINE. The initial and apparent volumes of distribution of d-tubocurarine (d-TC) are diminished in the elderly, reflecting the age-related changes in the volume of extracellular fluid. The clearance of d-TC is also impaired such that the elimination half-life value and duration of action are prolonged (155).

ATRACURIUM. The elimination of atracurium at physiologic pH and temperature depends on spontaneous degradation through Hofmann elimination and ester hydrolysis (156). Thus, age-related changes in liver and kidney function do not affect atracurium's activity (157). The elimination of atracurium can be prolonged as a result of an increase in the volume of distribution in the elderly, even though the total clearance rate is similar in elderly and young adults (158). The larger volume of distribution also contributes to an increase in the initial loading dose in the elderly. However, the increase in the elimination half-life may prolong recovery (158).

The pharmacodynamics of atracurium can be altered in elderly patients. Beemer and Bjorksten (159) found that patients over 70 years old had a slight increase in the steady-state plasma concentration of atracurium required to achieve 90% paralysis. Other investigators have also suggested that steady-state dose requirements for atracurium are slightly increased in the elderly (157, 160). This change may result from a decrease in muscular activity rather than an effect of age per se because most elderly patients are less active than younger patients. Muscle acetylcholine receptors are upregulated and downregulated in response to muscular activity. Exercise increases sensitivity to neuromuscular blocking drugs, and decreased muscular activity reduces sensitivity (39, 161). Therefore, elderly patients may require higher plasma concentrations of atracurium to achieve the same effect as in younger patients (159).

DOXACURIUM. This long-acting muscle relaxant is eliminated by renal and hepatobiliary pathways, as well as by slow hydrolysis by plasma cholinesterase. The volume of distribution of doxacurium is significantly larger in the elderly; however, the elimination half-life and clearance values are not significantly prolonged (162). Yet recovery times from doxacurium in the elderly tend to be prolonged and are more variable (162, 163). The onset of blockade is longer in the elderly, but the intensity of the block at equivalent dosages is similar in the young and elderly (163). The delay in onset is the result of age-related decline in cardiac function and muscle perfusion. These observations suggest that elderly patients respond in a manner similar to that of young patients to a standard dose of doxacurium. The elderly have a longer duration of surgical relaxation, and maintenance doses can be administered at less frequent intervals.

MIVACURIUM. For the elderly, the duration of action of mivacurium may be up to 30% longer, but the duration of action of mivacurium is still shorter for the elderly than that of any of the other available nondepolarizing muscle relaxants because of its unique plasma cholinesterase metabolism. The onset of action of mivacurium is similar to that of atracurium and vecuronium. If mivacurium is administered slowly (or individual doses), histamine release is minimized such that changes in heart rate and arterial pressure are similar for both the young and the elderly (164).

CISATRACURIUM. Cisatracurium is one of the more potent stereoisomers of atracurium. The onset of action to 90% paralysis is delayed by approximately 1 minute in the elderly, but the recovery profile is not changed by aging. The volume of distribution of cisatracurium is larger but the clearance is the same in the elderly, and the elimination half-life value is minimally prolonged. Changes in pharmacokinetics with aging appear to be minor and are not associated with significant prolongation of recovery time (165).

Antagonists of Neuromuscular Blockade

The duration of action of most of the intermediate- and long-acting muscle relaxants is prolonged in the elderly. Consequently, one must be aware of the actions of the neuromuscular antagonists. The duration of action of neostigmine and of pyridostigmine is prolonged in the aged patient (166). In contrast, the maximum duration of edrophonium's action is brief in the elderly, even though the plasma clearance is decreased and the elimination half-life is prolonged. The elderly also require a higher concentration of edrophonium to achieve the same reversal effect as in the young (167). As a result of edrophonium's brief maximum duration of action in the elderly, neostigmine or pyridostigmine would be a better choice for antagonizing long-acting muscle relaxants in elderly patients.

The antagonism of muscle relaxation is associated with changes in heart rate and rhythm as a result of effects of the anticholinergic and anticholinesterase drugs on the autonomic nervous system. These effects may prove clinically significant in the elderly patient with cardiac disease (168). Although the mixture of anticholinesterases and anticholinergics used for antagonism of residual blockade normally produces no significant problems, dysrhythmias and severe conduction disturbances can occur (169). The incidence of dysrhythmias in the postoperative period is greater in elderly patients who have received the combination of neostigmine and atropine compared with a neostigmine-glycopyrrolate combination. Therefore, the latter combination appears to be more appropriate for the elderly (169, 170). Edrophonium and atropine are both shorter-acting agents than neostigmine and glycopyrrolate, and therefore, they may be associated with fewer dysrhythmias. Cronnelly and associates (171) reported that the combination of edrophonium and atropine produced minimal changes in heart rate and an incidence of atrial and junctional dysrhythmias similar to that associated with neostigmine and atropine. Currently, no controlled studies have demonstrated a significant advantage of edrophonium atropine over neostigmine glycopyrrolate in the elderly population (172).

REFERENCES

1. Martin LG. Population aging policies in East Asia and the United States. Science 1991;251:527–531.
2. Warnes AM. The demography of aging. In: Davenport HT, ed. Anaesthesia and the Aged Patient. London: Blackwell Scientific Publications, 1988:9–26.
3. Goldsmith MF, ed. Demographers ponder the aging of the aged and await unprecedented looming elder boom. JAMA 1993; 269:2331–2332.
4. Burner ST, Waldo DR, Mukusick DR. National health expenditure projections through 203D. Health Care Financing Rev 1992;14:1–2.
5. Woodhouse KW. Pharmacokinetics of drugs in the elderly. J R Soc Med 1994;87 (suppl):2–4.
6. Castleden CM, Pickles H. Suspected adverse drug reactions in elderly patients reported to the Committee on Safety of Medicines. Br J Clin Pharmacol 1988;26:347–353.
7. Montamat SC, Cusack BJ, Vestal RE. Management of drug therapy in the elderly. N Engl J Med 1989;321:303–309.
8. Leslie C, Scott P, Caird F. Principal alterations to drug kinetics and dynamics in the elderly. Med Lab Sci 1992;49:319–325.
9. Greenblatt DJ. Reduced serum albumin concentration in the elderly: a report from the Boston Collaborative Drug Surveillance Program. J Am Geriatr Soc 1979;27:20–2.
10. Veering B, Burm A, Souverijn J, et al. The effect of age on serum concentrations of albumin and a_1-acid glycoprotein. Br J Clin Pharmacol 1990;29:201–206.
11. Piafsky KM. Disease-induced changes in the plasma binding of basic drugs. Clin Pharmacokinet 1980;5:246–262.
12. Cammarata RJ, Rodnan GP, Fennell RH. Serum anti-a-globulin and antinuclear factors in the aged. JAMA 1967;199:115–118.
13. Wood M. Plasma drug binding: implications for anesthesiologists. Anesth Analg 1986;65:786–804.
14. Fulop T Jr, Worum I, Scongor J, et al. Body composition in elderly people. Gerontology 1985;31:6–14.
15. Cohn SH, Vartsky D, Yasumura S, et al. Compartmental body composition based on total-body nitrogen, potassium, and calcium. Am J Physiol 1980;239:E524-E530.
16. Novak LP. Aging, total body potassium, fat-free mass, and cell mass in males and females between ages 18 and 85 years. J Gerontol 1972;4:438–443.
17. Morgan DJ, Bray KM. Lean body mass as a predictor of drug dosage: implications for drug therapy. Clin Pharmacokinet 1994;26:292–307.
18. Fleg JL, Shapiro EP, O'Connor F, et al. Left ventricular diastolic filling performance in older male athletes. JAMA 95;273:1371–1375.
19. Bender AD. The effect of increasing age on the distribution of peripheral blood flow in man. J Am Geriatr Soc 1965;13:192–198.
20. Dawling S, Crom P. Clinical pharmacokinetic considerations in the elderly: an update. Clin Pharmacokinet 1989;17:236–263.
21. Christensen JH, Andreasen F, Jansen JA. Pharmacokinetics and pharmacodynamics of thiopentone: a comparison between young and elderly patients. Anaesthesia 1982;37:398–404.
22. Stanski DR, Maitre PD. Population pharmacokinetics and pharmacodynamics of thiopental: the effect of age revisited. Anesthesiology 1990;72:412–422.
23. Wynne HA, Cope LH, Mutch E, et al. The effect of age upon liver volume and apparent liver blood flow in healthy man. Hepatology 1989;9:297–301.
24. Marchesini G, Bua V, Brunori A, et al. Galactose elimination capacity and liver volume in aging man. Hepatology 1988; 8:1079–1083.
25. Swift CG, Homeida M, Halliwell M, Roberts CJC. Antipyrine disposition and liver size in the elderly. Eur J Clin Pharmacol 1978;14:149–152.

26. Schumucker DL, Woodhouse KW, Wang RK, et al. Effects of age and gender on in vitro properties of human liver microsomal monooxygenase. Clin Pharmacol Ther 1990;48:365–374.
27. Brodie MJ, Boobis AR, Bulpitt CJ, Davies DS. Influence of liver disease and environmental factors on hepatic monooxygenase activity in vitro. Eur J Clin Pharmacol 1981;20:39–46.
28. Herd B, Wynne H, Wright P, et al. The effect of age on glucuronidation and sulphation of paracetamol by human liver fractions. Br J Clin Pharmacol 1991;32:768–770.
29. Davies DF, Shock NW. Age changes in glomerular filtration rate, effective renal plasma flow, and tubular excretory capacity in adult males. J Clin Invest 1950;29:496–507.
30. Miller JH, McDonald RK, Shock NW. Age changes in the maximal rate of renal tubular reabsorption of glucose. J Gerontol 1952;7:196–200.
31. Rowe JW, Andres R, Tobin JD, et al. The effect of age on creatine clearance in men: a cross-sectional and longitudinal study. J Gerontol 1976;31:155–163.
32. Lindeman RD, Tobin J, Shock NW. Longitudinal studies on the rate of decline in renal function with age. J Am Geriatr Soc 1995; 33:278–285.
33. Greenblatt DJ, Shader RI, Harmatz JS. Implications of altered drug disposition in the elderly: studies of benzodiazepines. J Clin Pharmacol 1989;29:866–872.
34. Prys-Roberts C. Anaesthesia: a practical or impractical construct? Br J Anaesth 1987;59:1341–1345.
35. Schwartz M, Creasey H, Grady CL, et al. Computed tomographic analysis of brain morphometrics in 30 healthy men aged 21 to 81 years. Ann Neurol 1985;17:146–157.
36. Dax EM. Receptors and associated membrane events in aging. Rev Biol Res Aging 1958;2:315–336.
37. Dorfman LJ, Bosley TM. Age-regulated changes in peripheral and central nerve conduction in man. Neurology 1979;29:38–44.
38. Tomonaga M. Histochemical and ultra-structural changes in senile human skeletal muscle. J Am Geriatr Soc 1977;25:125–131.
39. Martyn JA, White DA, Gronert GA, et al. Up and down regulation of skeletal muscle acetylcholine receptors. Anesthesiology 1992;76:822–843.
40. Ziegler MG, Lake CR, Kopin IJ. Plasma noradrenaline increases with age. Nature 1976;261:333–335.
41. Prinz PN, Vitiello MV, Smallwood RG, et al. Plasma norepinephrine in normal young and aged men: relationship with steep. J Gerontol 1984;39:561–567.
42. Pan HY, Hoffman BB, Pershe RA, Blaschke TF. Decline in beta adrenergic receptor-mediated vascular relaxation with aging in man. J Pharmacol Exp Ther 1986;239:802–807.
43. Vestal RE, Wood AJ, Shank DG. Reduced beta-adrenoceptor sensitivity in the elderly. Clin Pharmacol Ther 1979;26:181–186.
44. Yokoyama M, Kusui A, Sakamoto S, Fukuzaki H. Age-associated increments in human platelet alpha-adrenoceptor capacity: possible mechanism for platelet hyperactivity to epinephrine in aging man. Thromb Res 1984;34:287–295.
45. Brodde D-E, Anlauf M, Graben N, Bock KD. Age-dependent decrease of α_2-adrenergic receptor number in human platelets. Eur J Pharmacol 1982;81:345–347.
46. Davis PB, Silski C. Aging and the α_2-adrenergic system of the platelet. Clin Sci 1987;73:507–513.
47. Abrass IB, Scarpace PJ. Human lymphocyte beta-adrenergic receptors are unaltered with age. J Gerontol 1981;36:298–301.
48. Fuldman RD, Limbird LE, Nadcau J, et al. Alterations in leukocyte β-receptor affinity with aging. N Engl J Med 1984; 310:815–819.
49. Smiley RM, Pantuck CB, Chadburn A, Knowles DM. Downregulation and desensitization of the β-adrenergic receptor system of human lymphocytes after cardiac surgery. Anesth Analg 1993;77:653–661.
50. Brodde D-E. β_1 and β_2-adrenoceptors in the human heart: properties, function and alterations in chronic heart failure. Pharmacol Rev 1991;43:203–242.
51. Rubin PC, Scott PJW, McLean K, Reid JL. Noradrenaline release and clearance in relation to age and blood pressure in man. Eur J Clin Invest 1982;12:121–125.
52. Montamat SC, Davies AD. Physiological response to isoproterenol and coupling of beta-adrenergic receptors in young and elderly human subjects. J Gerontol 1989;44:M100-M105.
53. Scarpace PJ. Decreased β-adrenergic responsiveness during senesence. Fed Proc 1986;45:51–54.
54. Christensen JH, Adreansen F. Individual variation in response to thiopental. Acta Anaesthesiol Scand 1978;22:303–313.
55. Dundee JW. The influence of body weight, sex and age on the dosage of thiopentone. Br J Anaesth 1954;26:164–173.
56. Dundee JW, Hassard TH, McGowan WA, Henshaw J. The induction dose of thiopentone. Anaesthesia 1982;37:1176–1184.
57. Muravchick S. Effect of age and premedication on thiopental sleep dose. Anesthesiology 1984;61:333–336.
58. Jung D, Mayersohn M, Perrier D, et al. Thiopental disposition as a function of age in female patients undergoing surgery. Anesthesiology 1982;56:263–268.
59. Christensen JH, Andreasen F, Jansen JA. Influence of age and sex on the pharmacokinetics of thiopentone. Br J Anaesth 1981; 53:1189–1195.
60. Christensen JH, Andreasen F, Jansen JA. Thiopentone sensitivity in young and elderly women. Br J Anaesth 1983;5:33–40.
61. Hull CJU. Pharmacokinetics for anaesthesia. Oxford: Butterworth-Heinemann, 1991:263.
62. Stanski DR, Maitre PO. Population pharmacokinetics and pharmacodynamics of thiopental: the effect of age revisited. Anesthesiology 1990;72:412–422.
63. Verotta D, Sheiner LB. Simultaneous modeling of pharmacokinetics and pharmacodynamics: an improved algorithm. Comp Appl Biosci 1987;3:345–349.
64. Avram JM, Krejcic TC, Henthorn TK. The relationship of age to the pharmacokinetics of early drug distribution: the concurrent disposition of thiopental and indocyanine green. Anesthesiology 1990;72:403–411.
65. Sear JW, Cooper GM, Kumar V. The effect of age on recovery: a comparison of the kinetics of thiopente and althesin. Anaesthesia 1983;38:1158–1161.
66. Burch PG, Stanski DR. The role of metabolism and protein binding in thiopental anesthesia. Anesthesiology 1983;58:146–152.
67. Homer TD, Stanski DR. The effect of increasing age on thiopental disposition and anesthetic requirement. Anesthesiology 1985;62:714–724.
68. Hung OR, Varvel JR, Shafer SL, Stanski DR. Thiopental pharmacodynamics. II. Quantification of clinical and electroencephalographic depth of anesthesia. Anesthesiology 1992;77:237–244.
69. Hudson RJ, Stanski DR, Burch PG. Pharmacokinetics of methohexital and thiopental in surgical patients. Anesthesiology 1983;59:215–219.
70. Vestal RE. Aging and determinants of hepatic drug clearance. Hepatology 1989;9:331–334.
71. Ray W, Griffin M, Schaffner W, et al. Psychotropic drug use and the risk of hip fracture. N Engl J Med 1987;316:363–369.
72. Castledon CM, Swift CG. Hypnotics, sedatives and anticonvulsants. In: Swift CG, ed. Clinical pharmacology in the elderly. New York: Marcel Dekker, 1987:281–341.
73. Kraus JW, Desmond PV, Marshall JP, et al. Effects of aging and liver disease on disposition of lorazepam. Clin Pharmacol Ther 1978;24:411–419.
74. MacKlon AF, Barton M, James D. Rawlings MD. The effect of age on the pharmacokinetics of diazepam. Clin Sci 980;49:479–483.

75. Greenblatt DJ, Abernathy DR, Locniskar A, et al. Effect of age, gender and obesity on midazolam kinetics. Anesthesiology 1984;61:27–35.
76. Holazo AA, Winkler MB, Patel IH. Effects of age, gender and oral contraceptives on intramuscular midazolam pharmacokinetics. J Clin Pharmacol 1988;28:1040–1045.
77. Hamdy N, Kennedy H, Nicholl J, Triger D. Sedation for gastroscopy: a comparative study of midazolam and diazemuls in patients with and without cirrhosis. Br J Clin Pharmacol 1986; 22:643–647.
78. Reidenberg MM, Levy M, Warner H, et al. Relationship between diazepam dose, plasma level, age and central nervous system depression. Clin Pharmacol Ther 1978;23:371–374.
79. Cook PJ, Flanagan R, James IM. Diazepam tolerance: effect of age, regular sedation, and alcohol. Br Med J 1984 ;289:351–353.
80. Jacobs JR, Reves JG, Marty J, et al. Aging increases pharmacodynamic sensitivity to the hypnotic effect of midazolam. Anesth Analg 1994;80:143–148.
81. Sunhara T, Inoue O, Kobayashi K, et al. No age-related changes in human benzodiazepine receptor binding measured by PET with [110]Ro 15–4513. Neurosci Lett 1993;159:207–210.
82. Ariano RE, Kassun DA, Aronson KJ. Comparison of sedative recovery time after midazolam versus diazepam administration. Crit Care Med 1994;22:1492–1496.
83. Cheng EY. Sedative recovery rate with midazolam is no faster than with diazepam. ACP J Club 1995;March-April:40.
84. Colburn WA, Jack ML. Relationships between CSF drug concentrations, receptor binding characteristics and pharmacokinetic and pharmacodynamic properties of selected 1,4-substantiated benzodiazepines. Clin Pharmacol 1987;13:179–190.
85. Ochs HR, Busse J, Greenblatt DJ, Allen MD. Entry of lorazepam into cerebrospinal fluid. Br J Clin Pharmacol 1980;10:405–406.
86. Arendt RM, Greenblatt DJH, Liebisch DC, et al. Determinants of benzodiazepam brain uptake: lipophilicity versus binding affinity. Psychopharmacology 1987;93:72–76.
87. Zeigler WH, Schalch E, Leishman B, Eckert M. Comparison of the effects of intravenously administered midazolam, triazolam and their hydroxy metabolites. Br J Clin Pharmacol 1983; 16:635–695.
88. Lorhan PH, Lippman M. A clinical appraisal of the use of ketamine hydrochloride in the aged. Anesth Analg 1971;50:448–451.
89. Vaughan RW, Stephen CR. Abdominal and thoracic surgery in adults with ketamine, nitrous oxide, and d-tubocurarine. Anesth Analg 1974;53:271–280.
90. Waxman K, Shoemaker WC, Lippman M. Cardiovascular effects of anesthetic induction with ketamine. Anesth Analg 1980; 58:355–358.
91. Pederson T, Engbek J, Klausen NO, et al. Effects of low-dose ketamine and thiopentone on cardiac performance and myocardial oxygen balance in high-risk patients. Acta Anaesthesiol Scand 1982;26:235–239.
92. Tweed WA, Minuck M, Mymin D. Circulatory response to ketamine anesthesia. Anesthesiology 1972;37:613–619.
93. White PF. Comparative evaluation of intravenous agents for rapid sequence induction-thiopental, ketamine, and midazolam. Anesthesiology 1982;57:279–284.
94. Marlow R, Reich DL, Neustein S, Silvay G. Haemodynamic response to induction of anaesthesia with ketamine/midazolam. Can J Anaesth 1991;38:844–848.
95. Levanen J, Makela M-L, Scheinin H. Dexmedetomidine premedication attenuates ketamine-induced cardiostimulatory effects and post anesthetic delirium. Anesthesiology 1995; 82:1117–1125.
96. Idvall J, Ahlgren I, Aronsen KF, Stenberg P. Ketamine infusions: pharmacokinetics and clinical effects. Br J Anaesth 1979; 51:1167–1173.
97. Sussman DR. A comparative evaluation of ketamine anesthesia in children and adults. Anesthesiology 1974;40:459–464.
98. Arden JR, Holley FO, Stanski DR. Increased sensitivity to etomidate in the elderly: initial distribution versus altered brain response. Anesthesiology 1986;65:19–27.
99. Larsen R, Rathgeber J, Bagdahn A, et al. Effects of propotolon cardiovascular dynamics and coronary blood flow in geriatric patients. Anaesthesia 1988;43 (suppl):25–31.
100. Ebert TJ, Muzi M, Berens R, et al. Sympathetic responses to induction of anesthesia in humans with propofol or etomidate. Anesthesiology 1992;76:725–733.
101. Wagner RL, White PE. Etomidate inhibits adrenocortical function in surgical patients. Anesthesiology 1984;61:647–651.
102. Fragen RJ, Shanks CA, Molten A, Avram M. Effects of etomidate on hormonal responses to surgical stress. Anesthesiology 1984;61:652–656.
103. Ledingham IM, Watt I. Influence of sedation on mortality in critically ill multiple trauma patients. Lancet 1983;2:127D.
104. Shafer SL. Advances in propofol pharmacokinetics and pharmacodynamics. J Clin Anesth 1993;5 (suppl 1):145–215.
105. Apfelbaum JL, Trasela TH, Hug CC, et al. The initial clinical experience of 1819 physicians in maintaining anesthesia with propofol: characteristics associated with prolonged time to awakening. Anesth Analg 1993;77:S10-S14.
106. Kirkpatrick T, Cockshott D, Douglas EJ, Nimmo WS. Pharmacokinetics of propofol (Diprivan) in elderly patients. Br J Anaesth 1988;60:146–150.
107. Dundee JW, Robinson FP, McCollum J, Patterson CC. Sensitivity to propofol in the elderly. Anaesthesia 1986;41:482–485.
108. Smith C, McGwan AL, Jhaveri R, et al. The interaction of fentanyl on the CP_{50} of propofol for loss of consciousness and skin incision. Anesthesiology 1994;81:820–828.
109. Hug CC, McLeskey CH, Nahrwold ML, et al. Hemodynamic effects of propofol: data from over 25, 000 patients. Anesth Analg 1993;77:821–829.
110. Muzi M, Berens RA, Kampine JP, Ebert TJ. Venodilation contributes to propofol-mediated hypotension in humans. Anesth Analg 1992;74:877–883.
111. Mulier JP, Wouters PF, Van Aken H, et al. Cardiodynamic effects of propofol in comparison with thiopental: assessment with a transesophageal echocardiographic approach. Anesth Analg 1991;72:28–35.
112. Ebert TJ, Muzi M, Berens R, et al. Sympathetic responses to induction of anesthesia in humans with propofol or etomidate. Anesthesiology 1992;76:725–733.
113. Pizov R, Brown RH, Weiss YS, et al. Wheezing during induction of general anesthesia in patients with and without asthma. Anesthesiology 1995;82:1111–1116.
114. Conti G, Dell'Utri D, Vilardi V, et al. Propofol induces bronchodilation in mechanically ventilated chronic obstructive pulmonary disease (COPD) patients. Acta Anaesthesiol Scan 1993; 37:105–109.
115. DeSouza G, Delisser E, Turry P, Gold M. Comparison of propofol with isoflurane for maintenance of anesthesia in patients with chronic obstructive pulmonary disease: use of pulmonary mechanics, peak flow rates and blood gases. J Cardiothorac Vasc Anesth 1994;9:24–28.
116. Blouin RT, Seifert HA, Babenco H, et al. Propofol depresses the hypoxic ventilatory response during conscious sedation and isohypercapnia. Anesthesiology 1993;79:1177–1182.
117. Bellville JW, Forrest WH Jr, Miller E, Brown BW. Influence of age on pain relief from analgesics. JAMA 1971;217:1835–1841.
118. Kaiko RF. Age and morphine analgesia in cancer patients with postoperative pain. Clin Pharmacol Ther 1980;28:823–826.
119. Kaiko RF, Wallenstein SL, Rogers AG, et al. Narcotics in the elderly. Med Clin North Am 1982;66:1079–1089.
120. Owen JA, Sitar DS, Berger L, et al. Age-related morphine kinetics. Clin Pharmacol Ther 1983;34:364–368.

121. Arunasalam K, Davenport HT, Painter S, Jones JG. Ventilatory response to morphine in young and old subjects. Anaesthesia 1983;38:529–533.
122. Singleton MA, Rosen JL, Fisher DM. Pharmacokinetics of fentanyl in the elderly. Br J Anaesth 1988;60:619–622.
123. Mather LE, Tucker GT, Pflug AE, et al. Meperidine kinetics in man: intravenous injection in surgical patients and volunteers. Clin Pharmacol Ther 1975;17:21–30.
124. Herman RJ, McAllister CB, Branch RA, Wilkinson GR. Effects of age on meperidine disposition. Clin Pharmacol Ther 1985; 37:19–24.
125. Marcantonio ER, Juarez G, Goldman L, et al. The relationship of postoperative delirium with psychoactive medications. JAMA 1994;272:1518–1522.
126. Bentley JB, Borel JD, Nenad RE, Gillespie TJ. Age and fentanyl pharmacokinetics. Anesth Analg 1982;61:968–971.
127. Cartwright P, Prys-Roberts C, Gill K, et al. Ventilatory depression related to plasma fentanyl concentrations during and after anesthesia in humans. Anesth Analg 1983;62:966–974.
128. Hudson RJ, Thomson IR, Cannon JE, et al. Pharmacokinetics of fentanyl in patients undergoing abdominal aortic surgery. Anesthesiology 1986;64:334–338.
129. Scott JC, Stanski DR. Decreased fentanyl and alfentanil dose requirements with age: a simultaneous pharmacokinetic and pharmacodynamic evaluation. J Pharmacol Exp Ther 1987; 240:159–166.
130. Scamman FL, Ghoncim MM, Korttilak K. Ventilatory and mental effects of alfentanil and fentanyl. Acta Anaesthesiol Scand 1984;28:63–67.
131. Kronenberg RS, Drage CW. Attenuation of the ventilatory and heart rate responses to hypoxia and hypercapnia with aging in normal man. J Clin Invest 1973;52:1812–1819.
132. Martinez D, Zamel N, Bradley D, Phillipson EA. Effects of aging on the peripheral chemoreflex during sleep in healthy men. Am Rev Respir Dis 1984;129:244A–250A.
133. Shore ET, Millman RP, Silage DA, et al. Ventilatory and arousal patterns during sleep in normal young and elderly subjects. J Appl Physiol 1985;59:1607–1615.
134. Veselis RA, Reinsel RA, Feshchenko VA, et al. Impaired memory and behavioral performance with fentanyl at low plasma concentrations. Anesth Analg 1994;79:952–960.
135. Jorm AF, Korten AE, Henderson AS. The prevalence of dementia: A quantitative integration of the literature. Acta Psychiatr Scand 1987;76:465–479.
136. Hudson RJ, Bergstrom RG, Thomson IR, et al. Pharmacokinetics of sufentanil in patients undergoing abdominal aortic surgery. Anesthesiology 1989;70:426–431.
137. Lechmann KA, Sipakis K, Gasparini R, VanPeer A. Pharmacokinetics of sufentanil in general surgical patients under different conditions of anaesthesia. Acta Anaesthesiol Scand 1993; 37:176–180.
138. Helmers J, Van Leenwen L, Zuurmond W. Sufentanil pharmacokinetics in young adult and elderly surgical patients. Eur Anaesthesiol 1994;11:181–185.
139. Belpaire FM, Bogaert MG. Binding of alfentanil to human a_1-acid glycoprotein, albumin and serum. Int J Clin Pharmacol 1991;29:96–102.
140. Hullo CJ. Pharmacokinetics fo anaesthesia. Oxford: Butterworth-Heinemann, 1991:310.
141. Helmers H, Van Peer A, Woestenborghs R, et al. Alfentanil kinetics in the elderly. Clin Pharmacol Ther 1984;36:239–243.
142. Hudson RJ, Thomson IR, Burgess PM, Rosenbloom M. Alfentanil pharmacokinetics in patients undergoing abdominal aortic surgery. Can J Anaesth 1991;38:61–67.
143. Lemmens H, Bovill JG, Hennis PJ, Burm A. Age has no effect on the pharmacodynamics of alfentanil. Anesth Analg 1988; 67:956–960.
144. Lemmens H, Bovill JG, Burm A, Hennis PJ. Alfentanil infusion in the elderly. Anaesthesia 1988;43:850–856.
145. Lemmens H, Burm A, Bovill JG, et al. Pharmacodynamics of alfentanil: the role of plasma protein binding. Anesthesiology 1992;76:65–70.
146. Westmoreland CL, Hoke JF, Sebel PS, et al. Pharmacokinetics of remifentanil (G187084B) and its major metabolite (G190291) in patients undergoing elective inpatient surgery. Anesthesiology 1993;79:893–903.
147. Minto CF, Schnider TW, Cohane CA, et al. The hemodynamic effects of remifentanil in volunteers over 70 years. Anesthesiology 1994;81:A11.
148. Ornstein E, Matteo RS, Schwartz AE, et al. Pharmacokinetics and pharmacodyanics of pipecuronium bromide (Arduan) in elderly surgical patients. Anesth Analg 1992;74:841–844.
149. Shanor SP, Vantlees GR, Baart N, et al. The influence of age and sex on human plasma and red cell cholinesterase. Am J Med Sci 1961;242:357–361.
150. Duvaldestin P, Saada J, Berger JL, et al. Pharmacokinetics, pharmacodynamics, and dose-response relationships of pancuronium in control and elderly subjects. Anesthesiology 1982; 56:36–40.
151. Rupp SM, Castagnoli KP, Fisher DM, Miller RD. Pancuronium and recuronium pharmacokinetics and pharmacodynamics in younger and elderly adults. Anesthesiology 1987;67:45–49.
152. Lein CA, Matteo RS, Ornstein E, et al. Distribution, elimination, and action of vecuronium in the elderly. Anesth Analg 1991; 73:39–42.
153. Matteo RS, Ornstein E, Schwartz AE, et al. Pharmacokinetics and pharmacodynamics of rocuronium (Org 9426) in elderly surgical patients. Anesth Analg 1993;77:1193–1197.
154. Bevan DR, Fiset P, Balendran P, et al. Pharmacodynamic behavior of rocuronium in the elderly. Can J Anaesth 1993;40:127–132.
155. Matteo RS, Backus WW, McDaniel DD, et al. Pharmacokinetics and pharmacodynamics of d-Tubocurarine and metocurine in the elderly. Anesth Analg 1985;64:23–29.
156. Hughes R, Chapple OJ. The pharmacology of a tracurium: a noncompetitive neuromuscular blocking agent. Br J Anaesth 1981;53:31–44.
157. D'Hollander AA, Luyckx C, Barvbais L, DeVille A. Clinical evaluation of atracurium besylate requirement for a stable muscle relaxation during surgery: lack of age-related effects. Anesthesiology 1983;59:237–240.
158. Kitts JB, Fisher DM, Canfell PC, et al. Pharmacokinetics and pharmacodynamics of atracurium in the elderly. Anesthesiology 1990;72:272–275.
159. Beemer GH, Bjorksten AR. Pharmacodynamics of atracurium in clinical practice: effect of plasma potassium, patient demographics and concurrent medication. Anesth Analg 1993; 76:1288–1295.
160. Brandon BW, Cook DR, Woelfel SK, et al. Atracurium infusion requirements in children during halothane, isoflurane and narcotic anesthesia. Anesth Analg 1985;64:471–476.
161. Gronert GA, White DA, Shafer SL, Mattco RS. Exercise produces sensitivity to metocurine. Anesthesiology 1989;70:973–977.
162. Dresner DL, Basta SJ, Ali HH, et al. Pharmacokinetics and pharmacodynamics of doxacurium in young and elderly patients during isoflurane anesthesia. Anesth Analg 1990;71:498–502.
163. Koscielniak-Neilsen ZJ, Law-Min JC, Donati F, et al. Dose-response relations of doxacurium and its reversal with neostigmine in young adults and healthy elderly patients. Anesth Analg 1992;74:845–850.
164. Maddineni VR, McCoy EP, Mirakhur RK, et al. Mivacurium in the elderly: comparison of neuromuscular and hemodynamic effects with adults. Anesthesiology 1993;79:A964.

165. Ornstein E, Lein CA, Matteo RS, et al. Pharmacodynamics and pharmacokinetics of cisatracurium in geriatric surgical patients. Anesthesiology 1996;86:520–525.
166. Young WL, Mattco RS, Ornsterin E. Duration of Action of neostigmine and pyridostigmine in the elderly. Anesth Analg 1988; 67:775–778.
167. Matteo RS, Young WL, Ornstein E, et al. Pharmacokinetics and pharmacodynamics of edrophonium in elderly surgical patients. Anesth Analg 1990;71:334–339.
168. Owens WD, Waldbaum LS, Stephen CR. Cardiac dysrhythmias following reversal of neuromuscular blocking agents in geriatric patients. Anesth Analg 1978;57:186–190.
169. Urguhart ML, Ramsey FM, Royster RL, et al. Heart rate and rhythm following an edrophonium/atropine mixture for antagonism of neuromuscular blockade during fentanyl/N_2O/O_2 or isoflurane/N_2O/O_2 anesthesia. Anesthesiology 1987;67:561–565.
170. Muravchick S, Owens WD, Felts JA. Glycopyrrolate and cardiac dysrhythmias in geriatric patients after reversal of neuromuscular blockade. Can Anaesth Soc J 1979;26:22–25.
171. Cronnelly R, Morris RB, Miller RD. Edrophonium: duration of action and atropine requirement in humans during halothane anesthesia. Anesthesiology 1982;57:261–266.
172. Landrum AL, Krechel SK. Trends in geriatric anesthesia. In: Lake C, ed. Advances in anesthesia. vol 12. St. Louis: Mosby-Year Book, 1995:226–271.

24 Use of Intravenous Techniques in Ambulatory Patients

Ian Smith and Dori Ann McCulloch

Ambulatory anesthesia is a rapidly expanding subspecialty. In the United States, well over half of all elective operations are now performed on an ambulatory basis. In other parts of the world, considerable growth is occurring in outpatient surgery, stimulated by the desire for greater value for money spent on the health care system. Depending on the nature of the operative procedure and the preferences of the patient, ambulatory surgery may be performed with the patient under general anesthesia, regional anesthesia, or local (infiltration) anesthesia. In addition, sedative techniques may be utilized, either alone or to supplement local anesthesia.

Whatever technique is chosen, the ideal ambulatory anesthetic should combine a smooth and pleasant induction of anesthesia with optimum intraoperative conditions, a rapid return of protective reflexes and recovery of cognitive function, adequate postoperative analgesia, and a low incidence of side effects. Intravenous anesthetic agents are routinely used for the induction of general anesthesia, and these drugs may also be administered for maintenance of anesthesia, either by intermittent bolus injection or by continuous infusion. Furthermore, by infusing lower doses of these same agents, anesthesiologists can provide controllable levels of sedation to supplement local and regional anesthetic techniques.

This chapter reviews the pharmacology of intravenous anesthetic agents commonly used for general anesthesia and intraoperative sedation of ambulatory patients.

INTRAVENOUS INDUCTION AGENTS

The use of intravenous drugs for induction of anesthesia has become universally accepted in all but a few special circumstances. Intravenous anesthetics produce a rapid, smooth loss of consciousness that is associated with a higher degree of patient acceptance than inhalation of anesthetic vapors. Over the years, many compounds have been developed for intravenous induction of anesthesia. Although some of these early compounds are still in use (e.g., thiopental), others have fallen out of use or have not progressed beyond the experimental stage (e.g., propanidid, Althesin). Meanwhile, the search continues for compounds that more closely approach the theoretical "ideal" induction agent (1). For use in ambulatory anesthesia, such an agent must be associated with rapid and complete recovery, as well as with a low incidence of side effects, especially postoperative nausea and vomiting.

Barbiturates

Since its introduction by Lundy and Waters in 1935, thiopental has remained the induction agent against which all others are judged. Associated with rapid induction and minimal side effects, thiopental remains an inexpensive and dependable induction agent for procedures lasting more than 60 minutes (2). Although initial awakening after thiopental may be reasonably rapid, complete recovery from its sedative effects may be delayed by accumulation and a long elimination half-life. This delayed recovery is an important limitation to the use of thiopental for outpatient procedures.

Methohexital is also a barbiturate compound that, like thiopental, produces a rapid induction of anesthesia. It was extremely popular for ambulatory procedures before the availability of propofol because awakening and recovery occur more rapidly than with thiopental (3, 4). For example, following induction of anesthesia for outpatient dental extraction with methohexital, 50% of patients in one study returned to preoperative values using the Maddox wing test within 12.5 minutes of the end of anesthesia (3). In contrast, 70% of patients receiving thiopental for induction of anesthesia still had significant ocular divergence 30 minutes after discontinuation of the maintenance halothane-nitrous oxide (N_2O) anesthetic (3). Similarly, following outpatient urologic surgery in which anesthesia was maintained with enflurane, choice reaction time (a standard test of psychomotor function) returned to preoperative values within an hour of the end of surgery when methohexital was used as the induction agent, whereas it was still impaired 2 hours following thiopental administration (5). Furthermore, choice reaction time was within 80 milliseconds of baseline values 30 minutes after anesthesia induced by methohexital, but was prolonged by almost 300 milliseconds at 30 minutes the same time after thiopental (5). Although clinical recovery was significantly faster after methohexital compared with thiopental when these agents were administered as a single dose to healthy volunteers, simulated driving skills were significantly impaired 6 to 8 hours after either induction agent (6). Although methohexital represents an improvement over thiopental in terms of early recovery characteristics, it clearly is not ideal in this respect. Furthermore, methohexital is associated with more undesirable side effects than thiopental during the induction period, including pain on injection, myoclonic movements, and hiccups (7).

Etomidate

The pharmacokinetic properties of the imidazole derivative, etomidate, suggest that it should be a suitable induction agent for ambulatory anesthesia. Induction is similarly rapid to that with the available barbiturates, but it is associated with greater cardiovascular stability (8). Emergence is slightly faster than with thiopental (9), whereas emergence and early recovery appear comparable with those associated with methohexital (8, 10). More widespread use of etomidate is primarily limited by an unacceptably high incidence of side effects. Pain on injection is common, although this can be reduced by the addition of lidocaine. Venous irritation and phlebitis may also occur with etomidate; one series reported an incidence as high as 42% (11). Thrombophlebitis may persist for up to 10 days and represents significant morbidity in an ambulatory patient. The pain and venous sequelae are almost certainly due to the hyperosmolality of etomidate caused by the use of propylene glycol as a solvent. Reformulation of etomidate in a starch-derived solvent appears to reduce the incidence of pain and thrombophlebitis significantly (11).

Myoclonic movements are also frequently observed with etomidate, although these movements are not associated with epileptic activity on the electroencephalogram. Prior administration of fentanyl (or other opioids) can reduce these involuntary movements (12). The primary factor limiting the use of etomidate in ambulatory patients, however, is the high incidence of postoperative nausea and vomiting (9, 13). Both myoclonus and postoperative nausea appear to be consequences of etomidate itself, rather than the solvent, and are not prevented by reformulation.

Ketamine

Ketamine has unique properties among the intravenous anesthetic agents. In addition to its sedative-hypnotic properties, which result in a light, dissociative sleep, it is also a potent analgesic, permitting it to be used as the sole anesthetic agent without the requirement for pain-relieving adjuvants. Delusions, vivid dreams, and other hallucinogenic-like emergence phenomena complicate the use of ketamine in the ambulatory setting (14). These psychomimetic emergence reactions can be minimized by benzodiazepine pretreatment (15, 16), or by coadministration of ketamine with other sedative-hypnotic medications (17, 18). Even when ketamine is "tamed" (19), however, it still has a slower and less predictable onset of action, as well as a longer recovery time than other available agents, and is therefore rarely used for induction or maintenance of ambulatory anesthesia.

Steroid Anesthetics

Certain naturally occurring and synthetic steroids have anesthetic properties (20). Most steroid anesthetics have proved difficult to solubilize, however. In the early 1970s, a mixture of alphaxalone and alphadalone in a Cremophor solution was investigated under the trade name of Althesin. Initial results indicated the apparent advantages of a rapid onset of action, excellent cardiovascular stability, and a short duration of action. Althesin was marketed for several years in the United Kingdom and in other parts of Europe and gained widespread acceptance for ambulatory anesthesia. It was withdrawn from clinical practice, however, after several reports of severe anaphylactic reactions, which were probably related to the Cremophor EL solvent (12). Nevertheless, this drug served as a good example of the favorable properties of steroid anesthesia. Some interest remains in alphaxalone (the more active compound of the two components in Althesin), although attempts to prepare a stable lipid emulsion have proved unsuccessful to date (12).

Pregnenolone (3α-hydroxy–5β-pregnane–20-one) is a naturally occurring metabolite of progesterone. It has been known to possess anesthetic properties, but as with other steroid anesthetics, its development has been delayed by the problem of finding a suitable solvent. A preparation of pregnenolone emulsified in soybean oil (eltanolone) has been developed and is undergoing worldwide clinical investigations. In common with other steroid anesthetics, eltanolone appears to be associated with excellent hemodynamic stability (21, 22). The therapeutic index of eltanolone is 6 to 8 times greater than that of the established intravenous anesthetics (23), and it even exceeds that of other anesthetic steroids (20, 23). Induction of anesthesia with eltanolone is generally smooth (22–25), but it appears to be slower compared with other intravenous agents (23). Compared with propofol, pain on injection and apnea are not commonly observed during induction of anesthesia with eltanolone (24–27). Eltanolone satisfactorily induces anesthesia in 50% of unpremedicated patients when the agent is administered in a dose of 0.44 mg•kg^{-1} (25), whereas 0.5 mg•kg^{-1} is effective in 90% (24). Direct comparative studies suggest that eltanolone is three to four times more potent than propofol and seven times more potent than thiopental when it is used for induction of anesthesia (26).

Initial emergence from a single dose of pregnenolone emulsion is somewhat slower than that from Althesin or propofol and is comparable to emergence from thiopental (23). Complete recovery of motor coordination occurs rapidly after initial awakening from pregnenolone (and propofol), however, but it is considerably delayed following thiopental administration (23). The longer duration of action with a single dose of eltanolone is confirmed in human patients by the finding that only 29% of patients in whom anesthesia was induced with eltanolone, 0.8 mg•kg^{-1}, required an incremental dose to maintain anesthesia lasting an average of 8 minutes, compared with 70% of a similar group of patients in whom anesthesia was induced with propofol, 2 mg•kg^{-1} (27). Emergence from eltanolone anesthesia was significantly slower compared with propofol (12 [4 to 23] minutes versus 4 [1 to 9] minutes, $p < 0.001$), and later clinical milestones (e.g., ability to tolerate oral fluids, to ambulate, and to void) were also delayed (Fig. 24-1). Psychomotor recovery and hospital discharge were also significantly delayed following brief anesthesia with eltanolone compared with propofol (27). The elimination half-life of eltanolone is short (0.9 to 1.4 hours), however, and its total body clearance is rapid (1.8 to 3.1 L•kg^{-1}•h^{-1}), suggesting a low potential for accumulation (22). Recovery times following successive doses of pregnenolone emulsion have been remarkably constant compared with other anesthetic agents (23), and recovery from anesthesia in human patients may possibly be more comparable to recovery from propofol after surgical procedures of slightly longer duration. Clearly, further investigation of eltanolone is required before recommendations can be made regarding its use in the ambulatory setting. Unfortunately, further commercial development of pregnenolone seems unlikely at the present time.

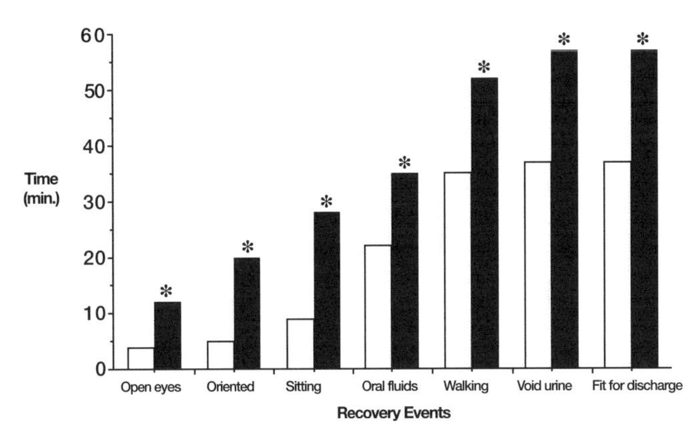

FIGURE 24-1. Median times required to reach the indicated emergence and recovery milestones following brief outpatient anesthesia with either propofol (open bars) or eltanolone (solid bars). *$p < 0.01$, from propofol group. (Data from Kallela H, Haasio J, Korttila K. Comparison of eltanolone and propofol in anesthesia for termination of pregnancy. Anesth Analg 1994; 79:512–516.)

Propofol

Propofol offers many advantages over the other available intravenous induction agents. It has become the induction agent of choice for ambulatory surgery because of its smooth and rapid onset of action, rapid recovery, and minimal postoperative side effects (28). The duration of clinical action of propofol is short, and recovery from its effects is rapid because of early redistribution and a high metabolic clearance rate (29). As a result of the rapid clearance of propofol, minimal accumulation of drug occurs, such that clinical recovery is still rapid after prolonged administration (30).

Propofol has been compared with a variety of other drugs as an outpatient anesthetic induction agent (Table 24-1). Compared with thiopental, propofol has generally been shown to result in a faster emergence or improved performance in psychomotor testing during the early recovery period in both adults and children (5, 31–36). Use of propofol in place of thiopental as the induction agent may even result in earlier discharge of outpatients from the ambulatory surgical facility when anesthesia is maintained with enflurane or isoflurane (33, 36). Obviously, recovery events are also influenced by the choice of maintenance anesthetic, and no differences were observed between propofol and thiopental when anesthesia lasting approximately 30 minutes or longer was maintained with halothane (37) or enflurane (34).

In comparison with other induction agents, the use of propofol results in less remarkable improvements in recovery (31, 38-40). For example, although propofol was associated with greater alertness, improved per-

TABLE 24-1. Comparison of Propofol with Alternative Induction Agents for Outpatient Anesthesia

Reference	Population	Adjuvants	Comparator	Maintenance	Principal Findings*
DeGrood et al, 1987 (31)†	30 laparoscopies	fentanyl	thiopental	isoflurane	Faster emergence and improved test results
Gupta et al, 1992 (32)	30 arthroscopies	alfentanil	thiopental	isoflurane	Improved test results for first 90 min of recovery
Chittleborough et al, 1992 (33)	40 dental	fentanyl	thiopental	enflurane	Faster emergence and discharge
Ding et al, 1993 (34)†	40 laparoscopies	fentanyl	thiopental	enflurane	Faster emergence, recovery times similar
Mackenzie & Grant, 1985 (5)†	40 urology		thiopental	enflurane	Greatly improved psychomotor performance
Rolly & Versichelen, 1985 (35)	30 females	fentanyl	thiopental	halothane-isoflurane	Faster emergence, later events not reported
Runcie et al, 1993 (36)	102 children		thiopental	halothane-isoflurane	Faster emergence, earlier discharge in older children only
Sanders et al, 1989 (37)	40 dental		thiopental	halothane	Similar emergence and recovery
O'Toole et al, 1987 (38)	50 females		methohexital	isoflurane	Faster emergence, improved test results at 20 min
Mackenzie & Grant, 1985 (5)†	40 urology		methohexital	enflurane	Improved psychomotor performance
Valanne & Korttila, 1985 (39)	73 oral surgery		methohexital	enflurane	Similar times to orientation and ambulation
DeGrood et al, 1987 (31)†	30 laparoscopies	fentanyl	etomidate	isoflurane	Nonsignificantly faster recovery
Norton & Dundas, 1990 (40)†	40 vasectomy		midazolam-flumazenil	isoflurane	Improved psychomotor performance

**Findings are expressed with respect to the propofol group.*

†This study was a multiple-group comparison but has been subdivided for ease of interpretation.

(Modified from Smith I, White PF, Nathanson M, Gouldson R. Propofol: an update on its clinical use. Anesthesiology 1994;81:1005–1043.)

formance on reaction time testing, and a shorter period of postoperative ataxia compared with methohexital in one study (38), differences in alertness and reaction times were no longer apparent 40 minutes after the end of anesthesia. Ataxia took almost an hour to resolve after methohexital administration, however (38). Compared with etomidate, propofol resulted in nonsignificantly faster eye opening and similar performance on simple pencil and paper tests 1 and 3 hours after anesthesia (31). Nevertheless, the use of propofol for induction of anesthesia resulted in a reduced incidence of postoperative side effects compared with methohexital and etomidate (5, 31, 38).

Following ambulatory surgery, postoperative nausea and vomiting are particularly undesirable not only because of the unpleasantness of these symptoms for the patient, but also because they can significantly delay discharge and may even necessitate an unanticipated admission to hospital. Several investigators have reported a reduced incidence of these complications when propofol is used for induction of anesthesia (31, 33), and increasing evidence indicates that propofol possesses direct antiemetic properties (41–45).

Unfortunately, propofol is not completely devoid of unwanted side effects. It can produce more profound hypotension than other induction agents (46), primarily as a result of peripheral vasodilatating effects (47). Slow administration (30 to 60 seconds) and adequate hydration significantly reduce the magnitude of its hypotensive action, however. Propofol also causes pain on injection, which may be minimized by the use of large (anticubital) veins or prophylactic administration of lidocaine (48). Unlike etomidate, propofol is not associated with phlebitis. Propofol may also improve the mood of patients in the postoperative period (49), producing a euphoric state, which appears to be well received by patients.

INTRAVENOUS MAINTENANCE AGENTS

Maintenance of anesthesia using intravenous drugs may be preferable to the use of inhalational agents for many ambulatory procedures. Intravenous administration delivers the anesthetic directly into the circulation, without the need to traverse the airways and lungs. Volatile agents are often pungent and irritating to the airway, and this property can limit the rate at which the delivered concentration can be changed and hence can impede rapid deepening of anesthesia. Leaks in the breathing circuit may reduce the delivered anesthetic concentration while polluting the operating room environment and potentially risking inadequate anesthesia and awareness. Yet, intravenous techniques have primarily gained popularity for ambulatory patients because they may possibly improve the recovery profile or reduce the incidence of side effects (e.g., postoperative nausea and vomiting) compared with inhalation anesthesia.

All the agents used for intravenous induction of anesthesia can, in theory, be used to maintain anesthesia. If recovery is to be rapid after administration of these drugs for 30 to 90 minutes, however, careful consideration must be given to the pharmacokinetic properties of the induction agents. Following bolus administration, these intravenous drugs rapidly reach well-perfused tissues (including the brain) and induce anesthesia. If the drug rapidly redistributes into less well-perfused tissues (e.g., muscle), recovery from a single dose occurs rapidly. If the volume into which the drug redistributes is small, however, with repeated or continuous administration a state of equilibrium quickly occurs, the concentration in the central (e.g., central nervous system) circulation remains elevated, and recovery is delayed. Recovery times continue to be short after prolonged administration only if the drug is rapidly metabolized to an inactive form, or if the compartment to which it is redistributed is extremely large (e.g., fat). The concept of context-sensitive half-time has been introduced to describe recovery from anesthetic administration of varying duration (30). The "half-time" refers to the time taken for the plasma concentration to decrease by 50% following cessation of drug delivery, whereas the "context" relates to the preceding duration of drug administration. Of the intravenous anesthetic agents currently available, propofol appears the most suitable for use as a maintenance agent because it has a relatively short half-time, which is only slightly prolonged with increasing duration of administration. For example, the half-time of propofol is less than 25 minutes after infusions of 3 hours and only 50 minutes after 8 hours or more (30). In contrast, thiopental has a half-time of almost 2 hours after infusions lasting only 3 hours (30).

The theoretical advantage of propofol appears to be supported by clinical evidence from comparisons with other intravenous agents for maintenance of anesthesia (Table 24-2).(5, 17, 31, 50–65) Emergence is generally reported to occur earlier with propofol compared with other intravenous maintenance anesthetics. For extremely short procedures, later recovery events do not differ significantly between propofol and methohexital (51, 56), although the improved recovery following propofol becomes more apparent when anesthesia is of longer duration (53, 54). Compared with thiopental administration, the use of propofol can permit earlier hospital discharge (17), and differences in recovery have still been evident at 24 hours, demonstrating the prolonged activity of this barbiturate even after brief administration (59, 65).

In addition to decreasing emergence and recovery times when using propofol in place of alternative intravenous maintenance agents, several investigators have reported better quality of anesthesia with propofol. Compared with etomidate, intravenous anesthesia with propofol was more stable and easier to administer (31), whereas propofol produces better muscle relaxation and less hiccuping than either thiopental or methohexital, resulting in improved surgical conditions (53, 56). A reduced incidence of postoperative nausea and vomiting has also been reported after the use of propofol for induction and maintenance of anesthesia compared with etomidate (31), methohexital (51, 53), and thiamylal (57).

Several investigators have attempted to compare intravenous maintenance regimens with inhalational techniques in patients undergoing ambulatory surgery. This type of comparison is always controversial because of the difficulties in ensuring similar depths of anesthesia with both techniques. The end-expired concentration of volatile anesthetics can be measured on a breath-by-breath basis and correlated with minimum alveolar concentration values in an attempt to establish a consistent anesthetic depth. With intravenous anesthetics, one cannot measure the plasma drug concentration in real time. In any case, the correlation between plasma levels and clinical effect with intravenous anesthetics is often poor (66). Until an objective, anesthetic agent-independent monitor of depth of anesthesia is developed, the practitioner must rely on the use of clinical signs (67, 68). With volatile agents, changes in heart rate and blood pressure appear to reflect the depth of anesthesia. Indeed, monitoring the end-tidal anesthetic concentration does not appear to improve the ability to regulate anesthetic depth compared with the use of clinical signs alone (69, 70). With intravenous agents, however, these autonomic signs are less reliable, and patients may exhibit motor activity without any prior changes in hemodynamic variables. Motor responses and changes in the respiratory pattern appear to be the most reliable clinical indicators of anesthetic depth (66), but this information is lost when muscle relaxants and controlled ventilation are employed.

Comparisons between intravenous and volatile anesthetic maintenance techniques are also impaired by differences in the choice of the associated induction agent. For example, several authors have shown that induction and maintenance of anesthesia with propofol result in faster emergence and recovery than induction with thiopental and maintenance with halothane (71), enflurane (72, 73), or isoflurane (74–79). The slower recovery time seen with the inhaled techniques may possibly be due, in part, to the use of thiopental (versus propofol) for induction and may not be directly related to the use of volatile agents, however. Several investigators have compared intravenous and volatile maintenance techniques following induction of anesthesia with propofol. Although isoflurane has often been associated with slower awakening compared with propofol, few differences have been observed in

TABLE 24-2. Comparison of Propofol with Alternative Intravenous Techniques for Outpatient Anesthesia

Reference	Population	Adjuvants	Administration	Comparator	Principal Findings*
DeGrood et al, 1987 (31)†	31 laparoscopies	fentanyl	FRI	etomidate	Faster and more predictable recovery
Heath et al, 1988 (50)†	40 TOPs	alfentanil	IB	etomidate	Faster emergence, smoother induction
Cade et al, 1991 (51)	70 females	fentanyl	IB	methohexital	Faster recovery to ambulation
Cundy & Arunasalam, 1985 (52)	60 TOPs	fentanyl	IB	methohexital	Improved "quality" of anesthesia, less drowsiness
Doze et al, 1986 (53)	60 females	meperidine	VRI	methohexital	Earlier orientation and ambulation
Heath et al, 1988 (50)†	40 TOPs	alfentanil	IB	methohexital	Similar recovery times
Jakobsson et al, 1993 (17)†	100 TOPs	fentanyl	IB	methohexital	Similar discharge times, earlier recovery not reported
Kay & Healy, 1985 (54)†	60 cystoscopies	alfentanil	IB	methohexital	Faster emergence and psychomotor recovery
Mackenzie & Grant, 1985 (5)	40 orthopedic	papavaretum	VRI	methohexital	Faster emergence, smoother anesthetic
Noble & Ogg, 1985 (55)	50 TOPs	alfentanil	IB	methohexital	Similar emergence and recovery times
Ræder & Misvær, 1988 (56)†	50 D & Cs	alfentanil	IB	methohexital	Faster emergence, recovery times similar
Sampson et al, 1988 (57)	40 TOPs	—	IB	thiamylal	Faster emergence, later events not reported
Edelist, 1987 (58)	90 TOPs	—	IB	thiopental	Faster emergence and orientation
Heath et al, 1988 (50)†	40 TOPs	alfentanil	IB	thiopental	Faster emergence, recovery times similar
Heath et al, 1990 (59)	60 D & Cs	alfentanil	IB	thiopental	Reduced tiredness 24 h postoperatively
Henriksson et al, 1987 (60)	120 D & Cs	—	IB	thiopental	Faster emergence, later events not reported
Jakobsson et al, 1993 (17)†	100 TOPs	fentanyl	IB	thiopental	Faster discharge
Johnston et al, 1987 (61)	93 D & Cs	—	IB	thiopental	Faster emergence, later events not reported
Korttila et al, 1992 (62)	12 volunteers	—	2 boluses	thiopental	Faster emergence and psychomotor recovery
Nielsen et al, 1991 (63)	57 females	diazepam	FRI	thiopental	Similar emergence and recovery times
Ræder & Misvær, 1988 (56)†	50 D & Cs	alfentanil	IB	thiopental	Faster emergence and psychomotor recovery
Ryom et al, 1992 (64)	76 females	meperidine	IB	thiopental	Similar performance in postoperative testing
Sanders et al, 1991 (65)	36 females	—	IB	thiopental	Faster emergence, improved performance at 24 h

**Findings are expressed with respect to the propofol group.*

†This study was a multiple-group comparison but has been subdivided for ease of interpretation.

TOP, Termination of pregnancy; D & C, dilatation and curettage; VRI, variable-rate infusion; FRI, fixed-rate infusion; IB, intermittent bolus doses.

(Modified from Smith I, White PF, Nathanson M, Gouldson R. Propofol: an update on its clinical use. Anesthesiology 1994;81:1005–1043.)

later recovery events or the time of hospital discharge (80-87). Similarly, following induction of anesthesia with propofol, the continued use of propofol for maintenance has not hastened recovery or discharge compared with enflurane (34, 87), desflurane (88, 89), or sevoflurane (90).

Although the use of "standardized" infusion regimens (80-82, 85) or fixed volatile anesthetic concentrations (80, 82, 83, 85) may have prevented comparisons from being made at equivalent depths of anesthesia, the use of intravenous adjuvants such as fentanyl and midazolam may possibly have masked small differences between techniques. Differences in recovery from propofol or from volatile anesthesia appear to be of little clinical significance. The substitution of propofol for a volatile anesthetic agent appears to produce a further decrease in the incidence of postoperative nausea and vomiting, however, even when propofol is used as an induction agent before the inhalation technique (34, 82, 88, 89, 91, 92). The use of propofol as a maintenance anesthetic may be advantageous for more prolonged outpatient procedures, because emergence, recovery, and discharge times have been significantly longer after isoflurane anesthesia lasting approxi-

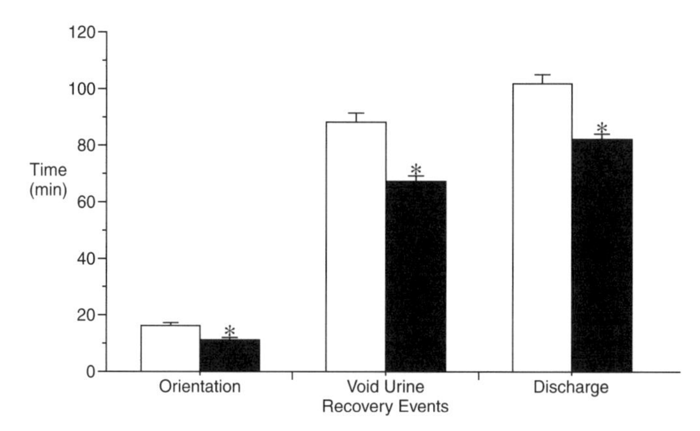

FIGURE 24-2. Emergence and recovery times following prolonged outpatient anesthesia (mean duration 3 hours) induced with propofol and maintained with either isoflurane (open bars) or propofol (solid bars). Values are mean ± standard error of mean. *$p < 0.01$, from isoflurane group. (Data from Valanne J. Recovery and discharge of patients after long propofol infusion vs isoflurane anaesthesia for ambulatory surgery. Acta Anaesthesiol Scand 1992; 36:530–533.)

mately 3 hours compared with a propofol-based technique (Fig.24-2) (91). Although infusions of propofol are frequently administered with N_2O, controversy exists as whether N_2O significantly reduces the propofol requirement (93, 94). Early recovery (e.g., emergence) appears to be faster in patients who receive propofol in combination with N_2O. Although omission of N_2O does not appear to reduce postoperative nausea and vomiting in adults (93), the incidence of this symptom is already low in outpatients undergoing many ambulatory procedures (94).

INTRAVENOUS ADJUVANT DRUGS

In contrast to the volatile agents, which possess hypnotic, analgesic, and muscle relaxant properties, the available intravenous anesthetics (with the exception of ketamine) tend to be almost pure sedative-hypnotics. Therefore, when intravenous agents are used to maintain anesthesia, patients have a greater requirement for adjuvant drugs. This requirement may have advantages, because balanced techniques allow independent titration of analgesic, amnestic, hypnotic, and muscle relaxant components to meet the needs of the individual patient. Furthermore, the simultaneous use of small doses of multiple drugs may offer advantages over the use of higher doses of a single drug. As patients are exposed to more compounds, however, the risks of unwanted drug interactions and side effects may also increase.

Supplementation of intravenous anesthetic techniques almost always involves the use of an opioid analgesic. Because opioid analgesics can also produce sedation and depression of mental function, rapid and short-acting analgesics such as fentanyl and alfentanil are the most widely used in outpatient anesthesia. For example, in one study, the use of fentanyl or alfentanil to supplement anesthesia maintained with methohexital improved the quality of anesthesia without delaying recovery (95). In another study, compared with fentanyl, an infusion of alfentanil resulted in improved intraoperative conditions by reducing unwanted patient movement when the drug was used to supplement a continuous methohexital infusion (96). In combination with propofol, an alfentanil infusion reduced the requirement for supplemental propofol boluses to treat clinical signs of inadequate anesthesia in one study (97). Despite the lower total propofol dose administered to patients receiving alfentanil, initial awakening was delayed, although later recovery events (including hospital discharge) were not affected (97). Use of alfentanil also reduced postoperative analgesic requirements and did not significantly increase the incidence of side effects, including postoperative nausea and vomiting (97). The use of agonist-antagonist or partial agonist drugs (e.g., dezocine) appears to offer no advantage over the pure μ-opioid receptor agonists (98). In the future, the availability of an ultrashort-acting opioid analgesic, remifentanil, may permit improved suppression of noxious stimuli when this agent is administered as an adjuvant during outpatient anesthesia. One hopes that the extremely short half-time of this novel opioid will facilitate rapid recovery and limit the severity and duration of adverse postoperative side effects such as nausea, vomiting, and ventilatory depression. The provision of effective analgesia in the postoperative period may be problematic, however, and may require prior treatment with local anesthetics or nonsteroidal anti-inflammatory drugs.

Many investigators have used short-acting opioid analgesics with N_2O for maintenance of ambulatory anesthesia. Although alfentanil-N_2O has been shown to permit faster awakening than halothane (99-101), enflurane (101, 102), or isoflurane (103), later recovery events have generally not been affected by the substitution of this short-acting opioid analgesic for volatile anesthetics. Similar results have been obtained with fentanyl (104, 105) and sufentanil (106). Furthermore, the use of opioid analgesics for anesthetic maintenance has been associated with an unacceptably high incidence of intraoperative apnea (99, 100), as well as postoperative nausea, vomiting, and retching (66). The incidence of these side effects severely limits the applicability of so-called nitrous-narcotic techniques in the ambulatory setting. It remains to be seen whether remifentanil will overcome some of these disadvantages of opioid-based anesthetic techniques for brief outpatient procedures.

Ketamine has been used as an analgesic adjuvant during intravenous anesthesia as an alternative to the opioids. A loading dose of 0.5 to 1 $mg \cdot kg^{-1}$ followed by 1 to 2 $mg \cdot kg^{-1} \cdot h^{-1}$ has provided comparable intraoperative conditions with slightly improved hemodynamic stability compared with fentanyl, 3.5 $\mu g \cdot kg^{-1}$ and 1.5 $\mu g \cdot kg^{-1} \cdot h^{-1}$, when used to supplement a variable-rate propofol infusion (18). Although emergence times were similar with both techniques in this study, later recovery events were significantly delayed in those patients who had received ketamine. Postoperative dizziness and confusion were more likely to be reported by patients who had received ketamine, although these symptoms apparently did not affect their overall satisfaction with the technique. No patient experienced dreaming or hallucinations (18). In contrast, when ketamine, 20 mg, was used to supplement propofol anesthesia for brief gynecologic surgery, dreaming was reported by 58% of patients, compared with 22% when fentanyl, 100 μg, was used as the primary analgesic (17). The use of ketamine in this investigation was not associated with any other adverse side effects and did not delay hospital discharge (17). Despite the analgesic properties of ketamine, a higher proportion of patients receiving intraoperative ketamine reported pain at the time of hospital discharge compared with those receiving fentanyl (48% versus 8%) (17). Thus, ketamine does not appear to be a particularly useful adjuvant during outpatient intravenous anesthesia.

The α_2-agonist drugs have analgesic-sparing effects and can significantly reduce the requirements for sedative, anesthetic, and opioid-analgesic agents. Both clonidine and dexmedetomidine have been used as adjuvants to existing intravenous anesthetics. For example, premedication with dexmedetomidine, 0.5 $\mu g \cdot kg^{-1}$ (which is the most highly selective α_2 agent), permitted a 30% reduction in the dose of thiopental required to induce and to maintain anesthesia for brief gynecologic surgical procedures (107). In addition, dexmedetomidine pretreatment appeared to reduce the stress response associated with surgery and also facilitated early recovery (107). Following laparoscopic sterilization, a slightly lower dose of dexmedetomidine (0.4 $\mu g \cdot kg^{-1}$) provided effective pain relief and significantly reduced requirements for supplemental opioid analgesia (108). Unfortunately, the use of the α_2-agonist drugs has been associated with an unacceptably high incidence of side effects, including bradycardia and excessive sedation, which can delay discharge following ambulatory surgery. The future role of these agents in the outpatient setting is yet to be defined.

INTRAVENOUS AGENTS FOR SEDATION

Ambulatory surgery does not always require general anesthesia. Many procedures can be performed safely utilizing simple infiltration with local anesthesia, whereas regional anesthesia, intravenous analgesia, and peripheral nerve blocks can be used for more extensive operations. The operating room can be a frightening environment, however, and many patients dislike being "awake" during their operation. Furthermore, injection of local anesthetics is often painful, as is the pressure resulting from traction on deep tissue planes, as well as the need to remain immobile for long periods on an uncomfortable operating table. The addition of sedative-hypnotic, anxiolytic, and analgesic drugs can make local anesthetic-based techniques more acceptable to most ambulatory patients.

Benzodiazepines are highly effective anxiolytic drugs that also provide variable degrees of sedation and amnesia. The majority of these compounds have extremely long durations of effect and contribute to delayed recovery after ambulatory procedures. Midazolam, however, has a short duration of action after a single dose and is commonly used in ambulatory patients. Additional advantages of midazolam over other available benzodiazepines include its water solubility and lack of venous irritation. Although midazolam is relatively short acting, accumulation can occur after multiple doses or prolonged administration, producing residual sedation and amnesia that can delay recovery after ambulatory surgery. In addition, the sedative effects of midazolam are also more prolonged in elderly patients.

Investigators have attempted to find alternative sedative agents that would permit rapid recovery after more prolonged surgical procedures. Attention has naturally focused on the use of subanesthetic doses of intravenous anesthetic agents. When variable-rate infusions of etomidate, methohexital, and midazolam were titrated to achieve a clinically acceptable sedation level for operations performed with the patient under regional anesthesia, outpatients receiving midazolam were significantly more sedated during the early recovery period and demonstrated slower recovery of cognitive function compared with either of the other two groups (109). However, midazolam provided superior amnesia for intraoperative events. In addition, methohexital required more frequent dose adjustments to produce the desirable sedation level, whereas etomidate was associated with a high incidence of postoperative headache and a tendency to more postoperative nausea (109).

The properties that make propofol desirable for ambulatory anesthesia are also beneficial when the drug is administered at lower doses for intraoperative sedation (28). During orthopedic surgery with the patient under regional anesthesia, a mean infusion rate of 3.8 $mg \cdot kg^{-1} \cdot h^{-1}$ resulted in patients who were asleep, but arousable to command (110). This relatively deep level of sedation was easily maintained by adjusting the infusion rate, and patients were awake within 4 minutes of discontinuing the propofol infusion (110).

Constant infusions of propofol, 0.5 to 4 mg•kg^{-1}•h^{-1}, produced dose-dependent increases in the level of sedation during urologic surgery with the patient under regional anesthesia and were all associated with rapid recovery (111). Optimal sedation in this elderly male population appeared to be achieved with a propofol infusion of approximately 2 mg•kg^{-1}•h^{-1} of propofol, although variations in patient response make it essential to vary the infusion rate to the desired effect.

Several investigators have compared propofol with midazolam for use as sedatives during local and regional anesthesia. Titration of the sedative infusion was reported to be easier with propofol compared with midazolam, resulting in a lower incidence of oversedation (112). In addition, propofol resulted in significantly less postoperative sedation, drowsiness, confusion, clumsiness, and amnesia compared with midazolam (112). Other workers achieved comparable levels of sedation during spinal anesthesia with propofol, 3.7 mg•kg^{-1}•h^{-1}, and midazolam, 0.27 mg•kg^{-1}•h^{-1}, but awakening was significantly faster following discontinuation of propofol (2 minutes versus 9 minutes, respectively) (113). Furthermore, psychomotor function was impaired for up to 2 hours after discontinuing midazolam, whereas propofol produced no clinically demonstrable effect 30 minutes after the end of the operation (113). In another investigation, patients receiving midazolam, 0.04 mg•kg^{-1}•h^{-1}, required up to 2 hours for full recovery, compared with 15 minutes following propofol, 2.65 mg•kg^{-1}•h^{-1} (114).

With the availability of the specific benzodiazepine antagonist, flumazenil, investigators proposed that the delayed recovery following midazolam could be overcome by "reversing" residual sedation. Indeed, after operations lasting approximately 1 hour and requiring an average of 10 mg of midazolam, the use of flumazenil, 1 mg, permitted discharge of patients up to 20 minutes earlier compared with "natural" recovery from the sedative effects of midazolam (115). However, recovery from the midazolam-flumazenil technique was no more rapid than when a propofol infusion was used to provide intraoperative sedation (115). Furthermore, once patients had recovered from propofol, they remained clearheaded for the remainder of their postoperative course. In contrast, the antagonist activity of flumazenil diminished before the residual sedative effects of midazolam had resolved, resulting in a recurrence of sedation in approximately one-third of the patients after they had been discharged home (115). The recurrence of sedation away from the hospital environment could be problematic for some patients who have undergone ambulatory surgery.

Sedative drugs may also be used alone, without local anesthetics, to facilitate diagnostic and investigational procedures. For example, midazolam is frequently administered as the sole sedative agent for endoscopy and bronchoscopy. Propofol has also been used to provide sedation for both upper and lower gastrointestinal endoscopy. In one study, satisfactory conditions and complete amnesia for the diagnostic procedure were obtained with an average propofol infusion rate of 4.3 mg•kg^{-1}•h^{-1} (116). In a comparison with midazolam, recovery was more rapid with fewer "hangover effects" following propofol sedation (117). Because of the ease with which the transition to general anesthesia can be made, however, propofol is an unsuitable agent for procedures in which sedation is provided by nonanesthesiologists.

Amnesia for intraoperative events appears to be less profound with propofol compared with midazolam (111–113, 118) and is not reliably produced by subhypnotic doses of propofol (111). Amnesia following propofol rarely persists into the postoperative period, with the advantage that patients are more likely to remember important postoperative information and instructions. When intraoperative amnesia is desirable, it can be achieved reliably by administering a small dose of midazolam (e.g., 1 to 2 mg) in addition to propofol (119). As well as improving intraoperative amnesia, the combination of midazolam and propofol also results in improved anxiolysis and greater sedation, without significantly prolonging recovery. Nevertheless, care should be exercised when using the drug combination because synergistic interactions may occur, with respect to both desirable and adverse effects. For example, the combination of fentanyl, 2 μg•kg^{-1}, with midazolam, 50 μg•kg^{-1}, resulted in apnea in half of a group of volunteers (120), whereas neither drug produced apnea when it was administered alone.

SUMMARY

In summary, intravenous anesthesia permits independent regulation of all the components necessary for successful anesthesia or sedation. An intravenous technique also permits the avoidance of hazards associated directly with inhaled agents and does not impede the delivery of adequate inspired concentrations of oxygen. Intravenous anesthesia allows recovery that is at least as rapid and complete as that following maintenance by inhalational agents, and it may reduce the incidence and severity of postoperative side effects. Some of the more recently introduced intravenous anesthetic drugs (e.g., propofol) have clinical properties that are particularly well suited to the field of ambulatory surgery. The combination of smooth, effective anesthesia with a rapid recovery and favorable side effect profile ensures that these agents will be of value in ambulatory anesthesia for some time to come. Newer drugs continue to be developed that may offer further advantages in the future. The steroid anesthetics represent a group of compounds with considerable potential that is yet to be fulfilled. Improvements in intravenous drug delivery and monitoring systems, combined with the optimal use of adjuvants, will ensure a bright future for intravenous sedative and anesthetic techniques in the ambulatory setting.

REFERENCES

1. White PF. Comparative evaluation of intravenous agents for rapid sequence induction: thiopental, ketamine and midazolam. Anesthesiology 1982;57:279–284.
2. White PF. Clinical pharmacology of intravenous induction drugs. Int Anesthesiol Clin 1988;26:98–104.
3. Hannington-Kiff JG. Measurement of recovery from outpatient general anaesthesia with a simple ocular test. Br Med J 1970; 3:132–135.
4. Cooper GM. Recovery from anaesthesia. Clin Anaesth 1984; 2:145–162.
5. Mackenzie N, Grant IS. Comparison of the new emulsion formulation of propofol with methohexitone and thiopentone for induction of anaesthesia in day cases. Br J Anaesth 1985;57:725–731.
6. Korttila K, Linnoila M, Ertama P, Häkkinen S. Recovery and simulated driving after intravenous anesthesia with thiopental, methohexital, propanidid, or alphadione. Anesthesiology 1975; 43:291–299.
7. Whitwam JG, Manners JM. Clinical comparison of thiopentone and methohexitone. Br Med J 1962;I:1663–1665.
8. Miller BM, Hendry JGB, Lees NW. Etomidate and methohexitone: a comparative clinical study in out-patient anaesthesia. Anaesthesia 1978;33:450–453.
9. Horrigan RW, Moyers JR, Johnson BH, et al. Etomidate vs thiopental with and without fentanyl: a comparative study of awakening in man. Anesthesiology 1980;52:362–364.
10. Craig J, Cooper GM, Sear JW. Recovery from day-case anaesthesia: comparison between methohexitone, Althesin and etomidate. Br J Anaesth 1982;54:447–451.
11. Doenicke A, Roizen MF, Nebauer AE, et al. A comparison of two formulations for etomidate, 2-hydroxypropyl-β-cyclodextrin (HPCD) and propylene glycol. Anesth Analg 1994;79:933–939.
12. Dundee JW. After thiopentone: a review of recent history. Baillieres Clin Anaesthesiol 1991;5:272–281.
13. Watcha MF, White PF. Postoperative nausea and vomiting: its etiology, treatment, and prevention. Anesthesiology 1992; 77:162–184.
14. Figallo EM, McKenzie R, Tantisira B, et al. Anaesthesia for dilatation, evacuation and curettage in outpatients: comparison of subanaesthetic doses of ketamine and sodium methohexitone-nitrous oxide anaesthesia. Can Anaesth Soc J 1977;24:110–117.
15. Lilburn JK, Dundee JW, Nair SG, et al. Ketamine sequelae: evaluation of the ability of various premedicants to attenuate its psychic actions. Anaesthesia 1978;33:307–311.
16. White PF, Way WL, Trevor AJ. Ketamine: its pharmacology and therapeutic uses. Anesthesiology 1982;56:119–136.
17. Jakobsson J, Oddby E, Rane K. Patient evaluation of four different combinations of intravenous anaesthetics for short outpatient procedures. Anaesthesia 1993;48:1005–1007.
18. Guit JBM, Koning HM, Coster ML, et al. Ketamine as analgesic for total intravenous anaesthesia with propofol. Anaesthesia 1991;46:24–27.
19. Coppel DL, Bovill JG, Dundee JW. The taming of ketamine. Anaesthesia 1973;28:293–296.
20. Clarke RSJ. Steroid anaesthesia [Editorial]. Anaesthesia 1992; 47:285–286.
21. Høgskilde S, Carl P, Sjøntoft E, et al. Cardiovascular alterations following iv infusion of pregnanolone emulsion and its vehicle [Abstract]. Acta Anaesthesiol Scand 1991;35:89.
22. Carl P, Høgskilde S, Nielsen JW, et al. Pregnanolone emulsion: a preliminary pharmacokinetic and pharmacodynamic study of a new intravenous anaesthetic agent. Anaesthesia 1990;45:189–197.
23. Eriksson H, Haasio J, Kortilla K. Comparison of eltanolone and thiopental in anaesthesia for termination of pregnancy. Acta Anaesth Scand 1995;39:479–484.
24. Rajah A, Powell H, Morgan M. Eltanolone for induction of anaesthesia and to supplement nitrous oxide for minor gynaecological surgery. Anaesthesia 1993;48:951–954.
25. Powell H, Morgan M, Sear JW. Pregnanolone: a new steroid intravenous anaesthetic. Anaesthesia 1992;47:287–290.
26. Van Hemelrijck J, Muller P, Van Aken H, White PF. Relative potency of eltanolone, propofol, and thiopental for induction of anesthesia. Anesthesiology 1994;80:36–41.
27. Kallela H, Haasio J, Korttila K. Comparison of eltanolone and propofol in anesthesia for termination of pregnancy. Anesth Analg 1994;79:512–516.
28. Smith I, White PF, Nathanson M, Gouldson R. Propofol: an update on its clinical use. Anesthesiology 1994; 81:1005–1043.
29. Shafer SL, Stanski DR. Improving the clinical utility of anesthetic drug pharmacokinetics [Editorial]. Anesthesiology 1992; 76:327–330.
30. Hughes MA, Glass PSA, Jacobs JR. Context-sensitive half-time in multicompartment pharmacokinetic models for intravenous anesthetic drugs. Anesthesiology 1992;76:334–341.
31. DeGrood PMRM, Harbers JBM, Van Egmond J, Crul JF. Anaesthesia for laparoscopy: a comparison of five techniques including propofol, etomidate, thiopentone and isoflurane. Anaesthesia 1987;42:815–823.
32. Gupta A, Larsen LE, Sjöberg F, et al. Thiopentone or propofol for induction of isoflurane-based anaesthesia for ambulatory surgery? Acta Anaesthesiol Scand 1992;36:670–674.
33. Chittleborough MC, Osborne GA, Rudkin GE, et al. Double-blind comparison of patient recovery after induction with propofol or thiopentone for day-case general anaesthesia. Anaesth Intensive Care 1992;20:169–173.
34. Ding Y, Fredman B, White PF. Recovery following outpatient anesthesia: use of enflurane versus propofol. J Clin Anesth 1993;5:447–450.
35. Rolly G, Versichelen L. Comparison of propofol and thiopentone for induction of anaesthesia in premedicated patients. Anaesthesia 1985;40:945–948.
36. Runcie CJ, Mackenzie SJ, Arthur DS, Morton NS. Comparison of recovery from anaesthesia induced in children with either propofol or thiopentone. Br J Anaesth 1993;70:192–195.
37. Sanders LD, Isaac PA, Yeomans WA, et al. Propofol-induced anaesthesia: double-blind comparison of recovery after anaesthesia induced by propofol or thiopentone. Anaesthesia 1989; 44:200–204.
38. O'Toole DP, Milligan KR, Howe JP, et al. A comparison of propofol and methohexitone as induction agents for day case isoflurane anaesthesia. Anaesthesia 1987;42:373–376.
39. Valanne J, Korttila K. Comparison of methohexitone and propofol ("Diprivan") for induction of enflurane anaesthesia in outpatients. Postgrad Med J 1985;61 (suppl 3):138–143.
40. Norton AC, Dundas CR. Induction agents for day-case anaesthesia: a double-blind comparison of propofol and midazolam antagonised by flumazenil. Anaesthesia 1990;45:198–203.
41. McCollum JSC, Milligan KR, Dundee JW. The antiemetic action of propofol. Anaesthesia 1988;43:239–240.
42. Scher CS, Amar D, McDowall RH, Barst SM. Use of propofol for the prevention of chemotherapy-induced nausea and emesis in oncology patients. Can J Anaesth 1992;39:170–172.
43. Borgeat A, Wilder-Smith OHG, Saiah M, Rifat K. Subhypnotic doses of propofol possess direct antiemetic properties. Anesth Analg 1992;74:539–541.

44. Borgeat A, Wilder-Smith OHG, Suter PM. The nonhypnotic therapeutic applications of propofol. Anesthesiology 1994; 80:642–656.
45. Schulman SR, Rockett CB, Canada AT, Glass PSA. Long-term propofol infusion for refractory postoperative nausea: a case report with quantitative propofol analysis. Anesth Analg 1995; 80:636–637.
46. Grounds RM, Twigley AJ, Carli F, et al. The haemodynamic effects of intravenous induction: comparison of the effects of thiopentone and propofol. Anaesthesia 1985;40:735–740.
47. Monk CR, Coates DP, Prys-Roberts C, et al. Haemodynamic effects of a prolonged infusion of propofol as a supplement to nitrous oxide anaesthesia. Br J Anaesth 1987;59:954–960.
48. Johnson RA, Harper NJN, Chadwick S, Vohra A. Pain on injection of propofol: methods of alleviation. Anaesthesia 1990; 45:439–442.
49. Zacny JP, Lichtor JL, Coalson DW, et al. Subjective and psychomotor effects of subanesthetic doses of propofol in healthy volunteers. Anesthesiology 1992;76:696–702.
50. Heath PJ, Kennedy DJ, Ogg TW, et al. Which intravenous induction agent for day surgery? A comparison of propofol, thiopentone, methohexitone and etomidate. Anaesthesia 1988; 43:365–368.
51. Cade L, Morley PT, Ross AW. Is propofol cost-effective for day-surgery patients? Anaesth Intensive Care 1991;19:201–204.
52. Cundy JM, Arunasalam K. Use of an emulsion formulation of propofol ("Diprivan") in intravenous anaesthesia for termination of pregnancy: a comparison with methohexitone. Postgrad Med J 1985;61 (suppl 3):129–131.
53. Doze VA, Westphal LM, White PF. Comparison of propofol with methohexital for outpatient anesthesia. Anesth Analg 1986;65:1189–1195.
54. Kay B, Healy TEJ. Propofol ("Diprivan") for outpatient cystoscopy: efficacy and recovery compared with Althesin and methohexitone. Postgrad Med J 1985;61 (suppl 3):108–114.
55. Noble J, Ogg TW. The effect of propofol ("Diprivan") and methohexitone on memory after day case anaesthesia [Abstract]. Postgrad Med J 1985;61 (suppl 3):103–104.
56. Ræder JC, Misvær G. Comparison of propofol induction with thiopentone or methohexitone in short outpatient general anaesthesia. Acta Anaesthesiol Scand 1988;32:607–613.
57. Sampson IH, Plosker H, Cohen M, Kaplan JA. Comparison of propofol and thiamylal for induction and maintenance of anaesthesia for outpatient surgery. Br J Anaesth 1988;61:707–711.
58. Edelist G. A comparison of propofol and thiopentone as induction agents in outpatient surgery. Can J Anaesth 1987;34:110–116.
59. Heath PJ, Ogg TW, Gilks WR. Recovery after day-case anaesthesia: a 24-hour comparison of recovery after thiopentone or propofol anaesthesia. Anaesthesia 1990;45:911–915.
60. Henriksson B-À, Carlsson P, Hallén B, et al. Propofol vs thiopentone as anaesthetic agents for short operative procedures. Acta Anaesthesiol Scand 1987;31:63–66.
61. Johnston R, Noseworthy T, Anderson B, et al. Propofol vs thiopental for outpatient anesthesia. Anesthesiology 1987;67:431–433.
62. Korttila K, Nuotto EJ, Lichtor JL, et al. Clinical recovery and psychomotor function after brief anesthesia with propofol or thiopental. Anesthesiology 1992;76:676–681.
63. Nielsen J, Jenstrup M, Gerdes NU, et al. Awakening and recovery of simple cognitive and psychomotor functions 2 h after anaesthesia for day-case surgery: total intravenous anaesthesia with propofol-alfentanil versus thiopentone-alfentanil. Eur J Anaesthesiol 1991;8:219–227.
64. Ryom C, Flarup M, Suadicani P, et al. Recovery following thiopentone or propofol anaesthesia assessed by computerized coordination measurements. Acta Anaesthesiol Scand 1992; 36:540–545.
65. Sanders LD, Clyburn PA, Rosen M, Robinson JO. Propofol in short gynaecological procedures: comparison of recovery over 2 days after anaesthesia with propofol or thiopentone as sole anaesthetic agents. Anaesthesia 1991;46:451–455.
66. White PF, Coe V, Shafer A, Sung M-L. Comparison of alfentanil with fentanyl for outpatient anesthesia. Anesthesiology 1986; 64:99–106.
67. White PF. Clinical uses of intravenous anesthetic and analgesic infusions. Anesth Analg 1989;68:161–171.
68. Stanski DR. Monitoring depth of anesthesia. In: Miller RD, ed. Anesthesia. New York: Churchill Livingstone, 1990:1001–1029.
69. Wang J, Liu J, Klein KW, White PF. Effects of end-tidal gas monitoring and flow rates on hemodynamic stability and the recovery profile. Anesth Analg 1994;79:538–544.
70. Liu J, Klein KW, Griffin JD, White PF. Does monitoring end-tidal isoflurane concentration improve titration during general anesthesia? J Clin Anesth 1995.
71. Puttick N, Rosen M. Propofol induction and maintenance with nitrous oxide in paediatric outpatient dental anaesthesia. Anaesthesia 1988;43:646–649.
72. Millar JM, Jewkes CF. Recovery and morbidity after daycase anaesthesia: a comparison of propofol with thiopentone-enflurane with and without alfentanil. Anaesthesia 1988;43:738–743.
73. Price ML, Walmsley A, Swaine C, Ponte J. Comparison of a total intravenous anaesthetic technique using a propofol infusion, with an inhalational technique using enflurane for day case surgery. Anaesthesia 1988;43 (suppl):84–87.
74. Doze VA, Shafer A, White PF. Propofol-nitrous oxide versus thiopental-isoflurane-nitrous oxide for general anesthesia. Anesthesiology 1988;69:63–71.
75. Gold MI, Sacks DJ, Grosnoff DB, Herrington CA. Comparison of propofol with thiopental and isoflurane for induction and maintenance of general anesthesia. J Clin Anesth 1989;1:272–276.
76. Sung YF, Reiss N, Tillette T. The differential cost of anesthesia and recovery with propofol-nitrous oxide anesthesia versus thiopental sodium-nitrous oxide anesthesia. J Clin Anesth 1991; 3:391–394.
77. Korttila K, Östman P, Faure E, et al. Randomized comparison of recovery after propofol-nitrous oxide versus thiopentone-isoflurane-nitrous oxide anaesthesia in patients undergoing ambulatory surgery. Acta Anaesthesiol Scand 1990;34:400–403.
78. Marais ML, Maher MW, Wetchler BV, et al. Reduced demands on recovery room resources with propofol (Diprivan) compared to thiopental-isoflurane. Anesth Rev 1989;16:29–40.
79. Lim BL, Low TC. Total intravenous anaesthesia versus inhalational anaesthesia for dental day surgery. Anaesth Intensive Care 1992;20:475–478.
80. Herregods L, Capiau P, Rolly G, et al. Propofol for arthroscopy in outpatients. Comparison of three anaesthetic techniques. Br J Anaesth 1988;60:565–569.
81. Larsen LE, Gupta A, Ledin T, et al. Psychomotor recovery following propofol or isoflurane anaesthesia for day-care surgery. Acta Anaesthesiol Scand 1992;36:276–282.
82. Marshall CA, Jones RM, Bajorek PK, Cashman JN. Recovery characteristics using isoflurane or propofol for maintenance of anaesthesia: a double-blind controlled trial. Anaesthesia 1992; 47:461–466.
83. Milligan KR, O'Toole DP, Howe JP, et al. Recovery from outpatient anaesthesia: a comparison of incremental propofol and propofol-isoflurane. Br J Anaesth 1987;59:1111–1114.
84. Nightingale JJ, Lewis IH. Recovery from day-case anaesthesia: comparison of total i.v. anaesthesia using propofol with an inhalation technique. Br J Anaesth 1992;68:356–359.
85. Zuurmond WWA, Van Leeuwen L, Helmers JHJH. Recovery from propofol infusion as the main agent for outpatient arthros-

copy: a comparison with isoflurane. Anaesthesia 1987;42:356–359.
86. Oikkonen M. Propofol vs isoflurane for gynaecological laparoscopy. Acta Anaesthesiol Scand 1994;38:110–114.
87. Pollard BJ, Bryan A, Bennett D, et al. Recovery after oral surgery with halothane, enflurane, isoflurane or propofol anaesthesia. Br J Anaesth 1994;72:559–566.
88. Van Hemelrijck J, Smith I, White PF. Use of desflurane for outpatient anesthesia: a comparison with propofol and nitrous oxide. Anesthesiology 1991;75:197–203.
89. Rapp SE, Conahan TJ, Pavlin DJ, et al. Comparison of desflurane with propofol in outpatients undergoing peripheral orthopedic surgery. Anesth Analg 1992;75:572–579.
90. Fredman B, Nathanson MH, Smith I, et al. Sevoflurane for outpatient anesthesia: a comparison with propofol. Anesth Analg 1995;81:823–828.
91. Valanne J. Recovery and discharge of patients after long propofol infusion vs isoflurane anaesthesia for ambulatory surgery. Acta Anaesthesiol Scand 1992;36:530–533.
92. Green G, Jonsson L. Nausea: the most important factor determining length of stay after ambulatory anaesthesia. A comparative study of isoflurane and/or propofol techniques. Acta Anaesthesiol Scand 1993;37:742–746.
93. Sukhani R, Jurie J, Jabamoni R. Propofol for ambulatory gynecologic laparoscopy: does omission of nitrous oxide alter postoperative emetic sequelae and recovery? Anesth Analg 1994; 78:831–835.
94. Lindekær AL, Skielboe M, Guldager H, Jensen EW. The influence of nitrous oxide on propofol dosage and recovery after total intravenous anaesthesia for day-case surgery. Anaesthesia 1995;50:397–399.
95. Cooper GM, O'Connor M, Mark J, Harvey J. Effect of alfentanil and fentanyl on recovery from brief anaesthesia. Br J Anaesth 1983;55:179S–182S.
96. Dachowski MT, Kalayjian R, Angelillo JC, Dolan EA. Continuous infusion of methohexital and alfentanil hydrochloride for general anesthesia in outpatient third molar surgery. J Oral Maxillofac Surg 1989;47:233–237.
97. Smith I, Van Hemelrijck J, White PF. Efficacy of esmolol versus alfentanil as a supplement to propofol-N_2O anesthesia. Anesth Analg 1991;73:540–546.
98. Ding Y, White PF. Comparative effects of ketorolac, dezocine, and fentanyl as adjuvants during outpatient anesthesia. Anesth Analg 1992;75:566–571.
99. Cartwright DP. Recovery after anaesthesia with alfentanil or halothane. Can Anaesth Soc J 1985;32:479–483.
100. Moss E, Hindmarch I, Pain AJ, Edmondson RS. Comparison of recovery after halothane or alfentanil anaesthesia for minor surgery. Br J Anaesth 1987;59:970–977.
101. Biswas TK, Hatch PD. A comparison of alfentanil, halothane and enflurane as supplements for outpatient urological surgery. Anaesth Intensive Care 1989;17:275–279.
102. Howie MB, Hoffer LJ, Kryc J, et al. A comparison of enflurane with alfentanil anaesthesia for gynaecological surgery. Eur J Anaesthesiol 1989;6:281–294.
103. Short SM, Rutherfoord CF, Sebel PS. A comparison between isoflurane and alfentanil supplemented anaesthesia for short procedures. Anaesthesia 1985;40:1160–1164.
104. Azar I, Karambelkar DJ, Lear E. Neurologic state and psychomotor function following anesthesia for ambulatory surgery. Anesthesiology 1984;60:347–349.
105. Rising S, Dodgson MS, Steen PA. Isoflurane vs fentanyl for outpatient laparoscopy. Acta Anaesthesiol Scand 1985; 29:251–255.
106. Zuurmond WWA, Van Leeuwen L. Recovery from sufentanil anaesthesia for outpatient arthroscopy: a comparison with isoflurane. Acta Anaesthesiol Scand 1987;31:154–156.
107. Aantaa R, Kanto J, Scheinin M, et al. Dexmedetomidine an α_2-adrenoceptor agonist, reduces anesthetic requirements for patients undergoing minor gynecologic surgery. Anesthesiology 1990;73:230–235.
108. Aho MS, Erkola OA, Scheinin H, et al. Effect of intravenously administered dexmedetomidine on pain after laparoscopic tubal ligation. Anesth Analg 1991;73:112–118.
109. Urquhart ML, White PF. Comparison of sedative infusions during regional anesthesia: methohexital, etomidate and midazolam. Anesth Analg 1989;68:249–254.
110. Mackenzie N, Grant IS. Propofol for intravenous sedation. Anaesthesia 1987;42:3–6.
111. Smith I, Monk TG, White PF, Ding Y. Propofol infusion during regional anesthesia: sedative, amnestic and anxiolytic properties. Anesth Analg 1994;79:313–319.
112. White PF, Negus JB. Sedative infusions during local and regional anesthesia: a comparison of midazolam and propofol. J Clin Anesth 1991;3:32–39.
113. Wilson E, Mackenzie N, Grant IS. A comparison of propofol and midazolam by infusion to provide sedation in patients who receive spinal anaesthesia. Anaesthesia 1988;43 (suppl):91–94.
114. Fanard L, Van Steenberge A, Demeire X, van der Puyl F. Comparison between propofol and midazolam as sedative agents for surgery under regional anaesthesia. Anaesthesia 1988;43 (suppl):87–89.
115. Ghouri AF, Ramirez Ruiz MA, White PF. Effect of flumazenil on recovery after midazolam and propofol sedation. Anesthesiology 1994;81:333–339.
116. Dubois A, Balatoni E, Peeters JP, Baudoux M. Use of propofol for sedation during gastrointestinal endoscopies. Anaesthesia 1988;43:75–80.
117. Patterson KW, Casey PB, Murray JP, et al. Propofol sedation for outpatient upper gastrointestinal endoscopy: comparison with midazolam. Br J Anaesth 1991;67:108–111.
118. Pratila MG, Fischer ME, Alagesan R, et al. Propofol versus midazolam for monitored sedation: a comparison of intraoperative and recovery parameters. J Clin Anesth 1993;5:268–274.
119. Taylor E, Ghouri AF, White PF. Midazolam in combination with propofol for sedation during local anesthesia. J Clin Anesth 1992;4:213–216.
120. Bailey PL, Pace NL, Ashburn MA, et al. Frequent hypoxemia and apnea after sedation with midazolam and fentanyl. Anesthesiology 1990;73:826–830.

25 Use of Intravenous Techniques in Critically Ill Patients

Michael B. Howie

Patients who are critically ill present challenges for practitioners of anesthesiology because these patients undergo many different pathophysiologic changes, resulting in alterations in tissue blood flow, fluid compartment volumes, plasma protein levels, and end-organ metabolic and excretory function. All these changes may alter the pharmacokinetic profile of intravenous anesthetic drugs. Cardiac output falls in hypovolemia, with resulting changes in drug kinetics. Dynamic changes in distribution and elimination of intravenous anesthetic occur as a result of continuous variation in cardiac output and tissue blood flow (1). Drugs used in the treatment of the critically ill (e.g., inotropes or vasodilators) further affect the pharmacokinetics of anesthetic drugs.

Ischemia and reduced tissue perfusion lead to cellular damage and impaired organ function. Compensatory mechanisms include autoregulation of tissue blood flow, increased sympathetic nervous system activity, alterations in body fluid distribution, and increased synthesis of plasma proteins. In circulatory failure, oxygen delivery and consumption are lower than metabolic demands, leading to increased anerobic metabolism and acidosis. As a result, acidic drugs are less ionized and basic drugs are more ionized, thereby affecting their passage across membranes. As the degree of ionization is increased, movement is reduced, leading to lower drug levels at the effector site or trapping of the drug once it has arrived at the site of action. An inverse relationship has been described between hydrogen ion concentration and the degree of plasma protein binding of basic drugs. Thus, acidosis leads to a greater free fraction of drug in the plasma and more drug available in an active form for diffusion into tissues (2, 3).

During respiratory acidosis, central nervous system (CNS) levels of morphine are 20% higher in the first few minutes after bolus injection than in a normal physiologic state. This finding is presumably due to reduced protein binding and increased cerebral blood flow. CNS levels decline at a slower rate, possibly because of trapping of the basic drugs such as morphine within the brain secondary to increased ionization from the reduced pH (4). In liver impairment, drug elimination depends on whether the drug has a high extraction ratio, in which case it is efficiently removed from the blood by the liver, or a low extraction ratio, with metabolism dependent on hepatic enzyme activity, so-called flow- or capacity-limited metabolism, respectively (5). The level of plasma proteins and the degree of drug binding vary. The effects of these alterations in free drug concentration produce consequent changes in the drug's volume because only the free fraction of the drug is available for diffusion into the tissues. All acid glycoprotein levels increase in response to stress. In contrast, thiopental binds to albumin, and many basic drugs also bind to this plasma protein.

INTRAVENOUS ANESTHETICS

For all intravenous induction of anesthesia, the rate of induction depends on the rate of delivery of free drug to its site of action in the CNS. Reductions in cardiac output slow induction times. This effect results from the need to preserve cerebral blood flow and the reduction in initial volume caused by underperfusion of other tissues. In shock states, these factors may hasten induction and may also significantly reduce dosage requirements.

Thiopental

In addition to the effects noted previously, impairment of renal and hepatic function and changes in plasma protein binding alter the pharmacokinetics of thiopental in shock. In renal impairment, binding of thiopental is reduced even in the absence of hypoalbuminemia (6). Ghoneim and colleagues reported decreased protein binding in patients with impaired renal function (7). Because the decreased binding was greater than could be explained by the degree of uremia and hypoalbuminemia, these investigators suggested that accumulated nitrogenous compounds possibly played a role. Reduced protein binding in hepatic impairment is accounted for by hypoalbuminemia (7). However, bilirubin also competes with some acidic drugs for binding sites.

Propofol

A prolonged elimination half-life may contribute to a slowed awakening after prolonged infusions of propofol in critically ill patients. Propofol is associated with flow-dependent liver metabolism. In a study by Servin and associates, four of five patients with hepatic dysfunction showed a delayed recovery and reduced clearance from a propofol infusion given during surgery for portocaval shunt. Such shunting reduces liver blood flow and, therefore, reduces metabolism of drugs such as propofol with flow-dependent kinetics (8).

Midazolam

In critically ill patients, midazolam has prolonged sedation as a result of altered hepatic blood flow and has impaired metabolic capacity (9). Marked pharmacokinetic variability has been reported in critically ill patients receiving midazolam infusions for sedation in the intensive care unit (ICU) (10).

Neuromuscular Blocking Drugs

The reduction in muscle blood flow in critically ill patients slows the onset of neuromuscular blockade. However, recovery depends on drug receptor disassociation and is therefore unaffected. Dose requirements of nondepolarizing agents are increased following thermal injury, with the dose requirement of pancuronium increased 2.5-fold in burned children (11). Pancuronium is only 10% protein bound, and therefore, increases in protein binding following thermal injury are unlikely to explain this effect. Investigators have speculated that increases in the number of acetylcholine receptors may be responsible for the decreased responsiveness, a mechanism believed to cause the hyperkalemic response to succinylcholine following thermal injury.

In shock states, the potential exists for renal and hepatic impairment. Before the introduction of atracurium and vecuronium, all non-depolarizing neuromuscular blockers were heavily dependent on the kidney for their elimination (12). As a result, atracurium and vecuronium have become the agents of choice in critically ill patients. Fahey and colleagues investigated the pharmacokinetics of atracurium in patients with and without renal failure and found no difference in the pharmacokinetic variables (13). Ward and colleagues found no pharmacokinetic changes when atracurium was administered to patients with fulminant hepatic failure (14). The independence of atracurium pharmacokinetics from renal and hepatic function is due in part to its elimination by Hoffman degradation and ester hydrolysis, even though Fischer and associates suggested that only half the plasma clearance of atracurium could not be accounted for in this way (15).

Lynam and associates found that the duration of action of vecuronium was significantly prolonged in renal failure (16), as a result of decreased clearance of vecuronium from the plasma. In healthy patients, 15 to 20% of an injected dose depends on the kidney for its elimination. The pharmacokinetics of vecuronium in renal impairment appears to be more variable than that of atracurium. Because 40 to 50% of vecuronium is excreted in the bile, its elimination half-life would be expected to be prolonged in the presence of liver disease. Cholestatic jaundice is associated with a 50% reduction in the clearance of vecuronium (17). Therefore, vecuronium should be used with caution in patients with impaired liver function, particularly if marked cholestasis exists.

HYPOVOLEMIA

In hypovolemic patients, several important conclusions emerge from a review of the medical literature (18). First, wide interpatient and interstudy variations exist. Second, with the exception of ketamine, which stimulates the cardiovascular system, all intravenous anesthetics decrease blood pressure by removing sympathetic tone, depressing the myocardium, increasing venous pooling, reducing venous return, producing bradycardia, and decreasing systemic vascular resistance. Third, depending on the anesthetic agent and the dose selected, hemodynamic depression may be caused by more than one of these mechanisms. Thiopental for example, reduces arterial blood pressure by three different mechanisms (i.e., venous dilatation and peripheral pooling of blood, decreased sympathetic tone leading to reduction of system vascular resistance, and myocardial depression both by a direct effect of the drug and indirectly by inhibition of sympathetic output) (19-22). Fourth, the severity of hemodynamic depressant effects differs among intravenous anesthetics. For equivalent hypnotic doses, etomidate is the least depressant, diazepam, midazolam, and thiopental are intermediate, and propofol is the most depressant.

Hypovolemia is characterized by compensatory hemodynamic responses that include central catecholamine output and stimulation of the neuroregulatory mechanisms. Tachycardia and vasoconstriction are useful in maintaining the systemic blood pressure within normal limits of depletion as long as the intravascular volume is less that 10 to 15% of the total blood volume. In addition to direct cardiovascular depression, intravenous anesthetics inhibit central catecholamine output and blunt the baroreflex response, resulting in peripheral vasodilation and decreases in heart rate, all of which can cause hypotension in a previously compensated patient. Anesthetics vary in the direction and extent of their effects on each of these mechanisms. For example, ketamine stimulates central catecholamine secretion, whereas other intravenous agents decrease CNS sympathetic outflow. Furthermore, none of the intravenous anesthetics depress the baroreflex response to the degree observed with the inhalation anesthetics (23). The effects of intravenous anesthetics on baroreflex sensitivity are mild and shorter lasting than those of inhalation anesthetics and appear to correlate with the plasma drug concentrations (24).

The degree of intravascular volume depletion is the primary determinant of intravenous anesthetic use in hypovolemic patients. In the presence of profound hypotension (i.e., severe uncompensated hypovolemia), these agents almost invariably further decrease systemic blood pressure. There is no substitute for restoring the intravascular volume before induction of anesthesia. When this cannot be accomplished before emergency induction, selection of the anesthetic with the least cardiovascular depressant effect appears logical. Because of its stimulatory effects on the cardiovascular system, ketamine has been a popular choice in hypovolemic patients. In a prospective study by Lippman and colleagues (25) ketamine increased heart rate, blood pressure, and cardiac output in critically ill patients. However, these authors noted that wide variation in the response to ketamine can produce both positive and negative ionotropic effects (25). The decrease in systemic blood pressure produced by ketamine in some critically ill patients may be explained by the inability of the sympathomimetic effects of ketamine to counterbalance its direct negative ionotropic or vasodilator effect (26). This can result from inadequate release of catecholamines as a result of depleted catecholamine stores, excessive myocardial depression, or both. It is probably more important to administer smaller quantities of any of the intravenous anesthetics than given under normovolemic conditions. For emergency induction of anesthesia in normovolemic patients, ketamine, alone or in combination with midazolam (or thiopental), is associated with excellent hemodynamic stability (27).

CEREBRAL FUNCTION

Adequate cerebral perfusion pressure must be maintained during induction of anesthesia by avoiding decreases in systemic blood pressure without producing a rise in intracranial pressure. Ravussin and colleagues have suggested that total intravenous anesthesia (TIVA) is preferred for neurosurgery because of its cerebral vasoconstrictor and metabolic depressant properties (28). Volatile anesthetics are cerebral vasodilators, thus increasing cerebral blood flow, blood volume, and intracranial pressure. Volatile anesthetics also impair cerebral autoregulation and blood flow-metabolism coupling. In neurosurgical patients anesthetized with propofol, oxygen supply to the brain was improved compared with patients anesthetized with thiopental (29).

Assuming that intravascular volume is adequate and systemic blood pressure is normal, cerebral perfusion pressure depends on the intracranial pressure, which is determined by the four intracranial compartments: cerebrospinal fluid, blood, brain substance, and the presence of a lesion. An intravenous anesthetic technique that reduces, or at least does not increase, the volume of these components should be selected. Ketamine may increase intracranial bleeding by increasing the systemic pressure. Barbiturates reduce brain edema after head injury because they scavenge free radicals (30). With the exception of ketamine, which increases intracranial pressure by producing hypertension, all intravenous anesthetics cause a comparable degree of cerebrovascular constriction and reduction in the cerebral metabolic rate of oxygen (31).

The major drawback to the use of these agents is their cardiovascular depressant effect, which can reduce cerebral perfusion pressure. If the patient is hypotensive, a greater proportion of the induction technique should consist of opioid analgesics, thereby permitting a reduction of the hypnotic component. The hypertension and the intracranial pressure increases that normally accompany laryngoscopy and intubation can be effectively attenuated. Propofol has been used successfully to treat patients with head injuries both intraoperatively and for sedation in the ICU (32). This drug's short duration of effect, combined with its favorable effects on intracranial and cerebral perfusion pressures, makes it a useful drug for head-injured patients (33, 34).

MYOCARDIAL COMPROMISE

The effects of intravenous anesthetics including barbiturates, etomidate, propofol, and ketamine on systemic hemodynamics and left ventricular function have been extensively studied. Barbiturates (including both thiopental and methohexital) decrease indirect indices of myocardial contractility. Failure to maintain adequate perfusion is the result of cardiovascular system decompensation. Clinical signs vary, particularly among the elderly or when the result is insidious rather than massive. In some patients, relative hypotension may be the only evidence of a clinically significant problem. The ability to distinguish a patient at risk is improved by hemodynamic and biochemical measurements. Thus, a critically ill patient should have full hemodynamic monitoring before induction of anesthesia (35-38).

Thiopental decreases ventricular dP/dt_{max} in a dose-related manner in the isolated heart and depresses the tension development and the force-velocity relationship of atrial and ventricular muscle in vitro (39). These direct negative ionotropic actions combine with barbiturate-induced increases in venous capacitance, and transient decreases in central sympathetic nervous system tone produce the characteristic reductions in mean arterial pressure and cardiac output observed clinically during induction of anesthesia (40).

Barbiturate-induced alterations in intracellular calcium (Ca^{++}) homeostasis may have an impact on diastolic performance, as well as on systolic function. The hallmark of induction of anesthesia with etomidate is remarkable stability of systemic and pulmonary hemodynamics. Investigations in healthy patients (41) and in those with cardiovascular disease (42) have repeatedly demonstrated that etomidate produces minimal changes in hemodynamics. Modest decreases in mean arterial pressure, presumably resulting from declines in central sympathetic nervous system tone, venous return, and peripheral metabolism have been reported with higher doses of etomidate in patients with cardiac disease. Etomidate has been shown to have little effect on myocardial contractility of isolated normal and cardiomyopathic papillary muscle tissue, presumably because of its ability to maintain intracellular Ca^{++} for contractile activation (43).

Induction and maintenance of anesthesia with propofol are associated with significant decreases in systemic arterial pressure. Propofol-induced hypotension results from a combination of venous and arterial vasodilation and direct negative ionotropic effects. Propofol produces more direct myocardial depression than equivalent doses of thiopental and methohexital. Propofol does not alter the functional integrity of the sarcoplasmic reticulum, with the exception of a modest increase in Ca^{++} uptake.

The observation that ketamine can lead to acute hemodynamic decompensation in a subset of critically ill patients with impaired function of the sympathetic nervous system has stimulated exploration of the direct effects of this intravenous anesthetic agent on cardiovascular function. In most patients, ketamine can produce significant increases in heart rate and arterial pressure that can be attributed to the central and peripheral sympathomimetic actions of this drug (44). Ketamine blocks the reuptake of monamines, including norepinephrine, into adrenergic nerves, a mechanism of action similar to that of cocaine. Depletion of catecholamines may unmask the direct vasodilator and myocardial depressant actions of ketamine in patients at risk (45). The use of opioids as the major component of anesthesia in the management of patients with a compromised cardiovascular status is an accepted practice to minimize the risk of untoward (and unexpected) cardiovascular depression.

With the development of sedative-hypnotics, analgesics, and adjuncts with short and predictable durations of action, the practical application of TIVA has become a reality. The lessons learned in relatively healthy patients must be considered before applying these techniques to critically ill patients. Specific topics related to TIVA have generated much research over the past 5 years and include dose requirements for adequate anesthesia, computerized infusion delivery systems, and pharmacokinetic interactions between propofol and opioid analgesics.

Of paramount concern is the problem of intraoperative awareness. With TIVA, awareness of the patient under anesthesia is one of the major concerns. At present, anesthesiologists have no adequate monitors to ensure that patients are unconscious. We must rely on our clinical acumen and knowledge of the dose-effect relationships to prevent this awareness. Fortunately, the brain concentration required to ensure lack of recall in an individual patient appears to be lower than that required to suppress the somatic motor and autonomic responses (46).

The difficulty in assessing intraoperative awareness, especially in critically ill patients with minimal anesthesia, is a result of the patient's paralysis by muscle relaxants. The most reliable sign of inadequate anesthesia, namely, somatic (motor) movement, is no longer available. The minimum anesthetic concentration is a value that relates to the presence of movement in 50% of patients; however, all patients must be adequately anesthetized (47). In a study by van Leeuwen and associates, three infusion rates of propofol with a two-step infusion of alfentanil were compared. Each patient was given propofol, 2 mg/kg, and alfentanil, 600 μg/kg/h, for 10 minutes, followed by an infusion of alfentanil at 10 μg/kg/h. Propofol was infused at 2, 3, or 4 mg/kg/h for the duration of the surgery, and movements were treated with alfentanil (1 mg) and propofol (20 mg) as needed. All three infusion systems gave satisfactory anesthetic conditions. However, patients in the 2 mg/kg/h required more frequent supplemental injections of propofol. In addition, it is uncertain if these propofol infusion rates could have been used in critically ill patients (48).

When fixed doses of intravenous agents are used, their pharmacokinetic and pharmacodynamic effects vary according to the patient's existing physiology. A given dose of an anesthetic affects a patient with hemorrhagic shock differently from a hemodynamically stable patient. The hemodynamic state varies greatly during any surgical procedure, especially operations associated with large fluid shifts. Unlike a volatile anesthetic, once an intravenous drug is given, it cannot be retrieved. No real-time measures of intravenous drug-blood concentrations exist. Should the practitioner underestimate the blood loss or the degree of myocardial dysfunction, profound circulatory depression will result. Thus, minimal dosages of intravenous anesthetics should be administered to critically ill patients. Anesthesiologists should search for a combination of intravenous drugs that produces an adequate anesthetic state with minimal cardiovascular depression.

TOTAL INTRAVENOUS ANESTHESIA

Propofol has been shown to be an essential component of TIVA in healthy patients and can be used safely in critically ill patients. Induction or maintenance of anesthesia with propofol frequently is associated with significant decreases in systemic arterial blood pressure. The circulatory depression observed with propofol can be attributed to both venodilation and arterial vasodilation with subsequent decreases in left ventricular preload. In contrast, other studies have implied that propofol may produce direct myocardial depression, contributing to the significant decrease in arterial blood pressure observed during propofol anesthesia (49).

Pagel and Warltier have suggested that many cardiovascular studies assess myocardial contractility indirectly, implying that changes in inotropic state depend on ventricular loading conditions. End-systolic pressure dimension relations may manifest less linearity and are relatively insensitive to decreases in contractile states at lower ranges of systemic pressure. These workers investigated the direct effects of propofol on regional myocardial contractility in chronically instrumented dogs. Using the preload recruitable stroke work relationship to assess contractility, this technique is a linear extension of the traditional Frank-Starling concept and has been shown to be independent of heart rate and load. By integrating data from the entire cycle, this technique has been shown to reflect global ventricular performance closely and suggests that propofol produces a dose-dependent depression of myocardial contractility. The preload recruitable stroke work decreases approximately 23%, 32%, 39%, and 48%. The magnitude of the negative inotropic action observed with even a moderate dose of propofol is comparable to that produced by 1.0 MAC of isoflurane (49), a finding suggesting that the significant decreases in systemic arterial blood pressure observed with a continuous propofol anesthetic can be attributed to a combination of the direct negative inotropic actions of the drug, as well as its effects on peripheral arterial and venous vascular tone.

Park and Lynch (50) compared the actions of propofol and thiopental on myocardial contractility using the isometric tension of isolated ventricular papillary muscle preparation. Propofol applied in intralipid emulsion caused dose-dependent depression of contractions at all stimulation rates, whereas intralipid alone had no effect. The myocardial depression may not rapidly reverse with a decline in the propofol serum concentrations. The highly hydrophobic nature of propofol may decrease its washout from the myocardium. At least a threefold higher concentration of propofol was required to obtain the same degree of depression observed with thiopental (46).

When opioids are given in combination with propofol to decrease intubation-associated hypertension, the drug combination can increase the hypotensive effect during the subsequent postintubation period. Billard and associates (51) reported that the mean decrease in systolic blood pressure after propofol was 28 mm Hg when no fentanyl was administered, 53 mm Hg after 2 μg/kg of fentanyl, and 50 mm Hg after 4 μg/kg. Hemodynamic response to intubation was decreased by the administration of fentanyl proportional to the preinduction dose of fentanyl (51).

The dilemma in treating critically ill patients relates to the need to attenuate the hemodynamic response to intubation and other noxious stimuli, without overdosing a patient for subsequent events. Propofol may induce a greater degree of hypotension before intubation relative to other hypnotic agents, yet this dose may not suppress the postintubation hypertensive response. The relationship between the plasma and the biophase (k_{e0}) must be considered such that the maximal effects of both the opioid and hypnotic are used to advantage. The k_{e0} for propofol is only 2.9 minutes, compared with 6.4 minutes for fentanyl. The time interval between fentanyl and subsequent propofol administration must be sufficient to achieve the peak predicted biophase concentration of both drugs. Intubation must be performed at the time of optimal maximal muscle relaxation. The blood pressure increase after intubation with propofol does not seem to be modified by increasing the fentanyl dose above 2 μg/kg, which only destabilizes the circulatory system.

The depth of anesthesia provided by propofol is not the main factor in determining the hemodynamic response to intubation. The level of analgesia provided by the opioid analgesic appears to be the major factor. The hemodynamic response to intubation can be suppressed with a fentanyl dose of 8 μg/kg, given in combination with propofol 1.5 mg/kg to premedicated patients (52). The addition of fentanyl, 2 or 4 μg/kg, to an induction dose of propofol increases the amplitude of prestimulation hypotension, but the hypertensive response to intubation is decreased.

Use of a moderate dose of opioid supplemented by a hypnotic agent appears to be the best course for a critically ill patient, but the sequence of administration must be carefully planned. Propofol produces significant hypotension in critically ill patients; however, an infusion of propofol to maintain hypnosis during the maintenance period may be associated with less hemodynamic instability (53, 54). Hall and colleagues utilized propofol as a means to decrease the amount of opioid and to shorten extubation time such that patients could be moved to intermediate care facilities, thereby utilizing scarce ICU resources more efficiently. This study was carried out in patients with reduced ventricular function using anesthetic techniques that provided stable intraoperative hemodynamics with minimal myocardial depression while permitting early tracheal extubation. Cardiac patients were assigned randomly to receive two propofol anesthetic regimens consisting of: (1) propofol, 1 to 2 mg/kg, and sufentanil 0.03 μg/kg/min (fixed rate), plus propofol, 50 to 200 μg/kg/min as a variable-rate infusion for maintenance of anesthesia; or (2) sufentanil, 5 μg/kg for induction, and propofol, 50 to 200 μg/kg/min variable-rate infusion for maintenance of anesthesia. A third group received sufentanil, 5 μg/kg, for induction of anesthesia and were maintained with enflurane. No group differences were noted in hemodynamics or inotropic requirements to separate from cardiopulmonary bypass. A lower incidence of myocardial lactate production (an indicator of ischemia) was noted in patients receiving sufentanil and a variable-rate propofol infusion for maintenance of anesthesia. This was in a population of patients whose myocardial function was definitely impaired. Compared with a previous study by Hall and associates (55), the patients in this study had a higher incidence of ischemia. However, if compared with a population having reduced ejection fractions, these techniques may have been associated with a lower incidence of ischemia (55). Patients with impaired ventricular function have an element of compensated heart failure and tend to have increased cardiac filling pressures that may benefit from the vasodilation produced by propofol. The favorable recovery profile is one of the primary reasons for using propofol. Any technique that must satisfy the criteria for early extubation should include propofol. However, it may not be possible to produce the best technique in terms of intraoperative hemodynamic stability with sufentanil and propofol and yet have early recovery times in patients with compromised cardiac function. Countering the early noxious stimuli with effective doses of an opioid analgesic at the onset of anesthesia does seem to be part of a good technique, however.

The careful dosing of propofol for induction of anesthesia is important in critically ill patients. Induction is often associated with marked decreases in systemic arterial pressure, which has at least three components to its production: 1) after load reduction; 2) preload decrease; and 3) negative ionotropic effect. Mulier and colleagues obtained data in humans using the end-systolic pressure volume relation as an index of myocardial contractility (56). This parameter was decreased significantly during low- and high-dose propofol anesthesia. End-diastolic volume as an index of preload remained stable, as did the cardiac output. Although thiopental maintained a stable cardiac output, a compensatory increase in heart rate occurred. The reflex tachycardia during thiopental anesthesia does not occur with propofol in the presence of similar reductions in arterial pressure (56). These findings indicate a more pronounced baroreflex inhibition during propofol anesthesia. Thus, lower doses of propofol combined with an opioid can produce smaller decreases in blood pressure, benefiting the hydraulic pressure relationship of the coronary circulation. Manara and colleagues found that alfentanil, 50 μg/kg, and propofol, 0.5 mg/kg, followed by infusions of alfentanil and propofol, produced good protection against hemodynamic responses to intubation, skin incision, and sternotomy (57). Alterations in the infusion rates in anticipation of painful surgical stimuli plus the use of adjunct agents (e.g., nitroglycerin) were believed to improve hemodynamic stability. These authors further stated that propofol and alfentanil infusions allow for separate control of the hypnotic and analgesic components without the hemodynamic consequences of adding volatile agents, or large doses of opioid analgesics, which may result in prolonged ventilatory support in the ICU after surgery (57).

The effect of propofol differs between young and elderly patients. Older patients have a more pronounced tendency toward arterial hypotension after equal dosages of propofol. These differing physiologic effects of propofol may be related to the higher incidence of concurrent disease in the elderly, a smaller volume of distribution, and an increase in the free plasma fraction of drug (58). A comparison of intravenous anesthetics requires the use of equianesthetic doses. Rolly and Versichelen found the relative potency of propofol compared with thiopental to be 1:2.6 in humans. Thus, 1.5 mg/kg of propofol corresponds to 4 mg/kg of thiopental, and 2.5 mg/kg of propofol corresponds to 6.5 mg/kg thiopental (59). Because the hemodynamic effects of propofol are varied and complex, care should be taken to administer a reduced dose to critically ill and elderly patients (60). In many elderly patients, induction of anesthesia is adequate with a dose of 1.5 mg/kg, and these patients do not suffer the hemodynamic consequences associated with the usual dose in healthier younger patients. The decrease in peripheral vascular resistance produced by propofol can be extremely deleterious in elderly patients who may not have the ability to respond by an increase in heart rate caused by concurrent cardiac medications (e.g., β blockers or calcium antagonists). Because the direct effects of propofol on vascular smooth muscle are proportional to the blood concentration, the practitioner should avoid administering a normal dose of propofol to the elderly patient with preexisting diseases.

Rouby and colleagues studied patients who had artificial heart implants and found that, 5 minutes after injection of propofol, the mean arterial pressure was decreased by 39% (compared with only 21% after thiopental). Similarly, right atrial pressure was decreased by 50% after propofol (versus only 20% with thiopental). Given that cardiac output was maintained constant throughout the study, these results suggest that propofol (2.5 mg/kg) is a more potent dilator of venous and arterial beds than thiopental (5 mg/kg) (61). It seems that any bolus form of propofol above 1.5 mg/kg can be deleterious to a critically ill patient. Carefully administered, almost insignificant, doses of propofol should be initiated in this type of patient, and if propofol is used, preload must be enhanced (i.e., fluid bolus) to conserve cardiac output.

Propofol also produces vasodilation independent of endothelial function. Evidence suggests that propofol relaxes aortic smooth muscle by blocking voltage-gated Ca^{++} channels that regulate extracellular reflux of Ca^{++} (62). Propofol can produce relaxation of arterial rings, which are devoid of neuronal and hormonal influence. The endothelium does not play a major role in propofol-induced vasodilation. The circulatory changes associated with any intravenous anesthetic also depend on the conditions of vascular tone before administration of the agent. Thus, critically ill patients may have high sympathetic and vascular tone before surgery, and the induction of anesthesia produces its hemodynamic effects, in part, by removing this awake tone. Critically ill patients may be well compensated by using vasodilators that can decrease the sympathetic tone. Thus, careful assessment of the patient's awake tone and the effect of concurrent medications should be performed before induction of anesthesia.

Studies on the action of anesthetics on diastolic function are important because many of these agents alter the rate and extent of ventricular filling, factors that play a critical role in the mechanical efficiency of the heart. Even so-called stimulatory drugs such as ketamine can lead to acute cardiovascular decompensation in critically ill patients with impaired sympathetic nervous system function. Pagel and colleagues found that ketamine profoundly depresses both active (ventricular relaxation) and passive (regional myocardial stiffness) phases of diastole in the presence of autonomic nervous system blockade. However, no alteration of diastolic function, as measured by isovolumetric relaxation or passive diastolic compliance, was observed with propofol. Thus, use of ketamine (versus propofol) may produce more acute cardiac decompensation in catecholamine-depleted, critically ill patients (63).

OPIOIDS AS A COMPONENT OF INTRAVENOUS ANESTHESIA

Opioid analgesics are an important component of general anesthesia in critically ill patients because they effectively block somatic and autonomic responses to painful stimuli during surgery, while producing minimal effects on cardiovascular stability. Opioids do not reliably produce unconsciousness and should be combined with hypnotic and amnestic agents. In surgical patients, opioids are characterized by large interindividual variability in their pharmacodynamics and pharmacokinetics. During surgery, different plasma opioid concentrations are required to suppress acute hemodynamic responses to different surgical stimuli. Consequently, the opioid dosage needs to be tailored to the individual patient and adjusted during surgery to result in adequate anesthesia and rapid recovery. Opioids are occasionally used as sole anesthetics in critically ill patients because of the concern of myocardial depression.

During intravenous anesthesia, opioids are commonly combined with other agents to produce unconsciousness. Ideally, combinations that reduce the dose requirements of the individual components decrease side effects and increase the recovery profile (64). To achieve a stable anesthetic course and rapid recovery, the rate of anesthetic infusions should be varied according to a patient's needs and intraoperative responses. The anesthetics should be given with the knowledge that each component lessens the need for the other, and minimal amounts of each drug should be used during surgery.

Sufentanil is the most potent opioid clinically available. The steady-state plasma concentration that causes half the maximal electroencephalographic slowing (IC_{50}) is one twelfth (0.68 ng/ml) that of fentanyl (8.1 ng/ml). The IC_{50} of alfentanil and remifentanil are 520 and 14.7 ng/ml, respectively (65). However, drug potency (based on steady-state drug concentrations) cannot be applied to the clinical situation in which bolus injections are administered, infusion rates are changed, and steady-state plasma concentrations simply do not exist. Although fentanyl is alleged to be 60 times more potent than alfentanil, the clinical (bolus) dose ratio between alfentanil and fentanyl is the order of 10:1. The explanation for this discrepancy is that the central volume of distribution is four to six times larger for fentanyl than for alfentanil, and initially more fentanyl is needed to fill the central compartment.

Whereas fentanyl, sufentanil, alfentanil, and remifentanil are phenylpiperidine analgesics, remifentanil has an ester linkage that is hydrolyzed by nonspecific tissue esterases. Fentanyl and its newer analogs are moderately to highly lipid soluble, enabling them rapidly to diffuse through lipid membranes, including the blood-brain barrier. The pKa of the weak bases alfentanil and remifentanil is lower than the plasma pH, which means they will be un-ionized at physiologic pH. A high diffusable fraction results in a large concentration gradient and a fast diffusion to the effect site, contributing to a rapid onset of analgesic effect. Alfentanil and remifentanil have the highest diffusable fraction and the fastest onset of drug action. However, this effect may not be beneficial in a critically ill patient who may need a more gentle onset of the drug's action. Intermittently changing the plasma concentration of alfentanil or remifentanil according to the anticipated surgical stimuli and the needs of the individual patient results in greater hemodynamic stability and more rapid recovery.

Basic lipophilic drugs such as the opioids, bind to α_1-acid glycoproteins. Since α_1-acid glycoprotein is an acute-phase reactant protein, it increases in illness as a result of inflammation, malignancy, and trauma. Differences in protein concentration and, consequently, differences in tissue binding may be of clinical importance. The opioid drug dosage should be reduced in the elderly patient, because both pharmacodynamic changes are common in this patient population. The combination of opioids with other intravenous anesthetics can profoundly alter the plasma concentration-effect relationship. Vuyk and colleagues have demonstrated that alfentanil requirements are significantly higher when the drug is administered as a supplement to 66% nitrous oxide compared with supplementation of a hypnotic concentration of propofol (4 μg/ml) (66).

For a fentanyl and midazolam combination, an additive effect with respect to hypnosis has been demonstrated. During induction of anesthesia, an opioid analgesic is often used to suppress the hypertensive response to intubation. However, the addition of an opioid may aggravate hypotension in the time between induction and intubation and the post-intubation period, when preparing and draping of the patient takes place. Of the opioids currently available, sufentanil's higher potency and more rapid elimination may make it the opioid of choice in the critically ill. Crozier and associates used a staging program to induce anesthesia in patients who were undergoing abdominal surgery with either sufentanil-midazolam or fentanyl-midazolam as part of a TIVA technique. The induction dose of opioid was 1.5 μg/kg of sufentanil or 10 μg/kg of fentanyl administered in two injections. The midazolam infusion was started as soon as the opioid effect was noted. Midazolam was infused in two stages (1.1 mg/kg^{-1} for 10 minutes, then 0.3 mg/kg^{-1}/h^{-1}) aiming at a steady-state plasma concentration of approximately 500 to 600 ng/ml^{-1}, at which time unconsciousness was ensured. Two to three minutes after starting the midazolam infusion, the remainder of the initial opioid dose was given. Thirty minutes after induction, an opioid infusion was started at 1.5 μg/kg^{-1}/h^{-1} for sufentanil or 10 μg/kg^{-1}/h^{-1} for fentanyl. Additional injections of sufentanil or fentanyl were given whenever patients had clinical signs of insufficient anesthesia (67). This technique approaches the variable-rate process of induction that should take place with critically ill patients. Divided doses of all induction drugs should be used, and careful infusion should be administered as a maintenance technique. The midazolam dosages should be decreased in elderly and critically ill patients.

When high-dose opioid techniques are used, bradycardia is a risk during induction and may require treatment with atropine. Bradycardia is always a concern with critically ill patients who are taking β blockers or calcium antagonists. If the baseline heart rate is less than 50 beats per minute, pancuronium can be used as the muscle relaxant, allowing its vagolytic properties to counter the vagal effect of the opioid analgesic. Another concern related to high-dose opioid techniques is chest wall rigidity. Muscle relaxation should be given early in the sequence of induction when opioids are used to avoid this complication. When large doses of midazolam are administered, reversal with flumazenil may be required at the end of surgery. However, reversal drugs should be avoided in critically ill patients, and the anesthetic regimen should be planned so the residual effects can benefit the patient in the postoperative recovery period (67).

TIVA technique with sufentanil and midazolam can provide a hemodynamically stable perioperative course and can prevent acute hemodynamic stress responses during major abdominal surgery. The initial decrease in blood pressure can be avoided by administering a lower dose of midazolam during the initial (loading) phase. Sedation and amnesia at induction can be achieved with small doses of midazolam 2–5 mgiv before administering the opioid analgesic. Continued hypnosis can be ensured by using a propofol infusion during the maintenance phase of anesthesia

(68). Propofol is associated with excellent cardiovascular stability when it is infused for maintenance of cardiac anesthesia (54). Use of propofol is associated with faster recovery characteristics than midazolam and can be continued into the postoperative period until the patient is ready for extubation. Sedation and residual analgesia are necessary to prevent abrupt wakening and agitation following major surgery.

If a patient is so hemodynamically unstable that any anesthetic technique will compromise the circulatory system, minimal (if any) intravenous anesthesia should be used. A pure opioid anesthetic supplemented with small doses of the benzodiazepine lorazepam, 0.5 to 2 mg, can produce an unconscious amnestic state in the unstable critically ill patient. For maintenance of anesthesia, additional lorazepam can be administered in combination with a constant infusion of sufentanil, 0.03μg/kg/min, which can be reduced by 0.005- to 0.01-μg/kg^{-1}/min^{-1} increments at hourly intervals. If the condition of the patient improves, midazolam or propofol can be added as a constant infusion (e.g., midazolam, 0.5 to 1 μg/kg/min infusion, or propofol 25 to 75 μg/kg^{-1}/min^{-1}). The interaction of benzodiazepine and opioids is synergistic with respect to their hypnotic effect, and lorazepam and sufentanil appear to be superadditive. The combinations may be even more synergistic when using three drugs (e.g., midazolam, sufentanil, and propofol).

A TIVA technique provides for rapid recovery but is unlikely to be successful if administration of the opioid is not carefully tailored to provide for an early extubation. As with other anesthetic agents, infusion of opioids for progressively long periods can lead to slow recovery and prolonged time to extubation (54, 69). Remifentanil represents an exciting development in the pharmacology of intravenous opioids. Like alfentanil, it produces a rapid onset of intense analgesia, with typical opioid effects such as respiratory depression, bradycardia, and moderate hypotension when administered in high doses. The novel aspect of the drug relates to its mechanisms of metabolism, consisting of hydrolysis of an ester link by nonspecific esterases. The drug has pharmacokinetic properties that produce a recovery profile independent of its duration of infusion (70). The potential exists to provide intense intraoperative analgesia, without postoperative respiratory depression. Thus, the effects of a high-dose opioid technique can be achieved using remifentanil without the postoperative consequences. The subsequent absence of postoperative analgesia may be a problem and may require a continued low-dose infusion or administration of traditional opioid analgesics. The rapid offset of remifentanil enhances its value in critically ill patients with marked pharmacokinetic and dynamic variability as a result of their unstable physiologic state during the perioperative period.

In summary, the introduction of an intravenous drug is a commonly used method for inducing anesthesia in a critically ill patient. As a result of the rapid transfer of the drug into the effect compartment, cardiovascular collapse may ensue. This untoward situation can be avoided by injecting a lower dose of intravenous anesthetics and analgesics to achieve a target concentration that can be manipulated either upward or downward with the same ease associated with the use of a vaporizer delivering volatile anesthetics. A target-controlled delivery system can facilitate titration of intravenous anesthetics according to the surgical conditions and the individual patient's anesthetic and analgesic requirements.

With the introduction of rapid and short-acting intravenous drugs, TIVA has become an attractive alternative for critically ill patients. Of the intravenous anesthetics, propofol has the most satisfactory pharmacokinetic profile for maintenance of anesthesia, with a rapid recovery after prolonged infusions. When used as an induction agent in critically ill patients, propofol can induce hypotension in the presence of impaired cardiac function, hypovolemia, and advanced age. In these cases, small doses of a benzodiazepine and an opioid analgesic are probably the safest technique for induction of anesthesia.

Critically ill patients need to be carefully protected against the pressor responses to noxious stimuli, and opioids are the safest and most effective form of protection. However, prolonged infusion of opioids can lead to a slow recovery and delayed extubation after major surgery in the criticaly ill population. Remifentanil produces rapid onset of intense analgesia and can be used for maintenance of anesthesia while ensuring a rapid recovery profile unaffected by the duration of the infusion. Because general anesthesia cannot be optimally achieved with any single intravenous agent, the rational use of combinations of sedative and analgesic drugs with synergistic interactions can provide ideal perioperative conditions for anesthetizing the critically ill patient without the complication of intraoperative awareness or a prolonged recovery period.

REFERENCES

1. Swinekoe CV, Reilley CS. Pharmacokinetics of the shocked state. Anesth Pharmacol Rev 1994;2:92–102.
2. Waller ES. Pharmacokinetic principles of lidocaine dosing in relation to disease state. J Clin Pharmacol 1981;21:181–194.
3. Woosley RL. Pharmacokinetics and pharmacodynamics and antiarrhythmic agents in patients with congestive heart failure. Am Heart J 1987;114:1280–1291.
4. Finck AD, Berkowitz BA, Hempstead J, Ngai SH. Pharmacokinetics of morphine: effect of hypercarbia on serum and brain concentrations in the dog. Anesthesiology 1977;47:407–410.
5. Blaschke TF. Protein binding and kinetics of drugs in liver disease. Clin Pharmacokinet 1977;2:32–44.
6. Ghoneim MM, Pandya HB, Kelley SE, et al. Binding of thio-

pental to plasma proteins: effects on distributions in the brain and heart. Anesthesiology 1976;45:635–639.
7. Ghoneim MM, Pandya HB. Plasma protein binding of thiopental in patients with impaired renal or hepatic function. Anesthesiology 1975;42:545–549.
8. Servin F, Cockshott ID, Farinotti R, et al. Pharmacokinetics of propofol infusion in patients with cirrhosis. Br J Anaesth 1990; 65:177–183.
9. Byatt CM, Lewis LD, Dawling S, Cochrane GM. Accumulation of midazolam after repeated dosage in patients receiving mechanical ventilation in an intensive care unit. Br Med J 1984; 289:799–800.
10. Shafer A, Doze VA, White PF. Pharmacokinetic variability of midazolam infusions in critically ill patients. Crit Care Med 1990;18:1039–1041.
11. Martyn JA, Liu LM, Szyfelbein SK, et al. The neuromuscular effects of pancuronium in burned children. Anesthesiology 1983;59:561–564.
12. Miller RD. Pharmacokinetics of atracurium and other non-depolarizing neuromuscular blocking agents in normal patients and those with renal or hepatic dysfunction. Br J Anaesth 1986; 58 (suppl 1):11S–13S.
13. Fahey MR, Rupp SM, Fischer DM, et al. The pharmacokinetics and pharmacodynamics of atracurium in patients with and without renal failure. Anesthesiology 1984;61:699–702.
14. Ward S, Neill EA. Pharmacokinetics of atracurium in acute hepatic failure (with acute renal failure). Br J Anaesth 1983; 55:1169–1172.
15. Fischer DM, Canfell PC, Fahey MR, et al. Elimination of atracurium in humans: contribution of Hoffman elimination and ester hydrolysis vs. organ-based elimination. Anesthesiology 1986;665:6–12.
16. Lynam DP, Cronnelly R, Castagnoli KP, et al. The pharmacodynamics and pharmacokinetics of vecuronium in patients anesthetized with isoflurane with normal renal function or with renal failure. Anesthesiology 1988;69:227–231.
17. Arden JR, Lynam DP, Castagnoli KP. Vecuronium in alcoholic liver disease: a pharmacokinetic and pharmacodynamic analysis. Anesthesiology 1988;68:771–776.
18. Capan, Levon. Intravenous agents. In: Grande C, ed. Textbook of trauma anesthesia and critical care. St. Louis: Mosby, 1993:468–478.
19. Eckstein JW, Hamilton WK, McCammand JM. The effect of thiopental on peripheral venous tone. Anesthesiology 1961; 22:525.
20. Wabon WE, Seely E, Smith AC. The action of thiopentone on vascular distensibility of the hand. Br J Anaesth 1962;34:19.
21. Joyce JT, Roizen MF, Eger E II. Effect of thiopental induction on sympathetic activity. Anesthesiology 1983;59:19–22.
22. Conway CM, Ellis DB. The hemodynamic effects of short acting barbiturates: a review. Br J Anaesth 1969;41:534.
23. Marty J, Gauzit R, Lefevre P, et al. Effects of diazepam and midazolam on baroreflex control of heart rate and on sympathetic activity in humans. Anes Analg 1986;65:113–119.
24. Ebert TJ, Kotrly KJ, Madsen KE, et al. Fentanyl-diazepam anesthesia with or without N_2O does not attenuate cardiopulmonary baroreflex-mediated vasoconstrictor responses to controlled hypovolemia in humans. Anesth Analg 1988;67: 548–554.
25. Lippman M, Appel PL, Mok MS, Shoemaker WC. Sequential cardiorespiratory patterns of anesthesia induction with ketamine in critically ill patients. Crit Care Med 1983;11:730–734.
26. White PF, Ham J, Way WL, Trevor AJ. Pharmacology of ketamine isomers in surgical patients. Anesthesiology 1981;52:231–78.
27. White PF, Ham J, Way WL, Trevor AJ. Pharmacology of ketamine isomers in surgical patients. Anesthesiology 1981;52:231–278.
28. Ravussin P, de Tribolet N, Wilder-Smith OHG. Total intravenous anesthesia is best for neurologic surgery. J Neurosurg Anesth 1994;6:285–289.
29. Hoper J, Gaab MR, Batz M, Feyerherd F. Local oxygen supply to the cerebral cortex during thiopental and propofol anesthesia. Anaesthetist 1994;43:534–548.
30. Artru AA. Dose related changes in the rate of cerebrospinal fluid formation and resistance to reabsorption of cerebro-spinal fluid following administration of thiopental, midazolam and etomidate in dogs. Anesthesiology 1988;69:541–546.
31. Shaprio HM, Wyte SR, Harris AB. Ketamine anaesthesia in patients with intracranial pathology. Br J Anaesth 1972;44:1200–1204.
32. Smith I, White PF, Nathanson M, Gouldson R. Propofol: an update on its clinical uses. Anesthesiology 1994;81:1005–1043.
33. Vandesteene A, Trempont V, Engelman E, et al. Effect of propofol on cerebral blood flow and metabolism in man. Anaesthesia, 1988;43 (suppl):42–43.
34. Wright PJ, Murray RJ. Penetrating craniocerebral airgun injury: anaesthetic management with propofol infusion and review of recent reports. Anaesthesia 1989;44:219–221.
35. Seltzer JL, Gerson JI, Allen FB. Comparison of the cardiovascular effects of bolus vs. incremental administration of thiopentone. Br J Anaesth 1980;52:527–530.
36. Sonntag H, Hellberg K, Schenk HD, et al. Effects of thiopental (Trapanal) on coronary blood flow and myocardial metabolism in man. Acta Anaesthesiol Scand 1975;19:69–78.
37. Reiz S, Balfors E, Friedman A, et al. Effects of thiopentone on cardiac performance, coronary hemodynamics and myocardial oxygen consumption in chronic ischemic heart disease. Acta Anaesthesiol Scand 1981;25:103–110.
38. Fischler M, Dubois C, Brodaty D, et al. Circulatory responses to thiopentone and tracheal intubation in patients with coronary artery disease: effects of pretreatment with labetalol Br J Anaesth 1985;57:493–496.
39. Stowe DF, Bosnjak ZJ, Kampine JP. Comparison of etomidate, ketamine, midazolam, propofol and thiopental on function and metabolism of isolated hearts. Anesth Analg 1992;74:547–558.
40. Pagel P, Warltier D. Anesthetics and left ventricular function. In: Warltier D, ed. Ventricular function. Baltimore: Williams & Wilkins, 1995:213–252.
41. Criado A, Maseda J, Navarro E, et al. Induction of anaesthesia with etomidate: hemodynamic study of 36 patients. Br J Anaesth 1980;52:803–806.
42. Gooding JM, Weng JT, Smith RA, et al. Cardiovascular and pulmonary responses following etomidate induction of anesthesia in patients with demonstrated cardiac disease. Anesth Analg 1979;58:40–41.
43. Prakash O, Dhasmana KM, Verdouw R, Saxena PR. Cardiovascular effects of etomidate with emphasis on regional myocardial blood flow and performance. Br J Anaesth 1981;53:591–599.
44. Lundy PM, Gverzdys S, Frew R. Ketamine: evidence of tissue specific inhibition of neuronal and extraneuronal catecholamine uptake processes. Can J Physiol Pharmacol 1985;63:298–303.
45. Pagel PS, Kampine JP, Schmeling WT, Warltier DC. Ketamine depresses myocardial contractility as evaluated by the preload recruitable stroke work relationship in chronically instrumented dogs with autonomic nervous system blockade. Anesthesiology 1992;76:564–572.
46. Prys-Roberts C. Total intravenous anesthesia: assessment of adequacy. ASA Review Course. 53–56.
47. Raftery S. Total intravenous anaesthesia. Curr Opin Anaesthesiol 1991;4:522–529.
48. van Leeuwen L, Zuurmond WW, Deen L, Helmers HJ. Total intravenous anaesthesia with propofol, alfentanil, and oxygen-air: three different dosage schemes. Can J Anaesth 1990;37:282–286.

49. Pagel PS, Warltier DC. Negative inotropic effects of propofol as evaluated by the regional preload recruitable stroke work relationship in chronically instrumented dogs. Anesthesiology 1993;78:100–108.
50. Park WK, Lynch C III. Propofol and thiopental depression of myocardial contracility: a comparative study of mechanical and electrophysiologic effects in isolated guinea pig ventricular muscle. Anesth Analg 1992;74:395–405.
51. Billard V, Moulla F, Bourgain JL, et al. Hemodynamic response to induction and intubation: propofol/fentanyl interaction. Anesthesiology 1994;81:1384–1393.
52. Vermeyen KM, Erpels FA, Janssen LA, et al. Propofol-fentanyl anaesthesia for coronary bypass surgery in patients with good left ventricular function. Br J Anaesth 1987;59:1115–1120.
53. Massey NJ, Sherry KM, Oldroyd S, Peacock JE. Pharmacokinetics of an infusion of propofol during cardiac surgery. Br J Anaesth 1990;65:475–479.
54. Mora CT, Duke C, Torjman MC, White PF. Effect of anesthetic technique on the hemodynamic response and recovery profile after coronary revascularization. Anesth Analg 1995;81:900–910.
55. Hall RI, Murphy JT, Landymore R, et al. Myocardial metabolic and hemodynamic changes during propofol anesthesia for cardiac surgery in patients with reduced ventricular function. Anesth Analg 1993;77:680–689.
56. Mulier JP, Wouters PF, Van Aken H, et al. Cardiodynamic effects of propofol in comparison with thiopental: assessment with a transesophageal echocardiographic approach. Anesth Analg 1991;72:28–35.
57. Manara AR, Monk CR, Bolsin SN, Prys-Roberts C. Total i.v. anaesthesia with propofol and alfentanil for coronary artery bypass grafting. Br J Anaesth 1991;66:716–718.
58. Scheepstra GL, Booij LH, Rutten CL, Coenen LG. Propofol for induction and maintenance of anaesthesia: comparision between younger and older patients. Br J Anaesth 1989;62:54–60.
59. Rolly G, Versichelen L. Comparison of propofol and thiopentone for induction of anaesthesia in premedicated patients. Anaesthesia 1985;40:945–948.
60. Azari DM, Cork RC. Comparative myocardial depressive effects of propofol and thiopental. Anesth Analg 1993;77:324–329.
61. Rouby JJ, Andreev A, Leger P, et al. Peripheral vascular effects of thiopental and propofol in humans with artificial hearts. Anesthesiology 1991;75:32–42.
62. Jenstrup M, Nielsen J, Fruergard K, et al. Total i.v. anaesthesia with propofol-alfentanil or propofol-fentanyl. Br J Anaesth 1990;64:717–722.
63. Pagel PS, Schmeling WT, Kampine JP, Warltier DC. Alteration of canine left ventricular diastolic function by intravenous anesthetics in vivo. Anesthesiology 1992;76:419–425.
64. Lemmens JHM. Opioids in intravenous anesthesia. Anesth Pharmacol Rev 1995;3:67–73.
65. Scott JC, Cooke JE, Stanski DR. Electroencephalographic quantitation of opioid effect: comparative pharmacodynamics of fentanyl and sufentanil. Anesthesiology 1991;74:34–42.
66. Vuyk J, Lim T, Engbers FH, et al. Pharmacodynamics of alfentanil as a supplement to propofol or nitrous oxide for lower abdominal surgery in female patients. Anesthesiology 1993;78:1035–1045.
67. Crozier TA, Langenbeck M, Muller J, et al. Total intravenous anesthesia with sufentanil-midazolam for major abdominal surgery. Eur J Anaesth 1994;11:449–459.
68. Taylor E, Ghouri AF, White PF. Midazolam in combination with propofol for sedation during local anesthesia. J Clin Anesth 1992;4:213–216.
69. White M. Why total intravenous anesthesia. Anesth Pharmacol Rev 1995;3:6–13.
70. Egan TD, Lemmens HJ, Fiset P, et al. The pharmacokinetics of the new short acting opioid remifentanil (GI87084B) in healthy adult male volunteers. Anesthesiology 1993;79:881–892.

VII CONTROVERSIES IN INTRAVENOUS ANESTHESIA

26A Intravenous Drug Delivery Devices and Computer Control*

Talmage D. Egan

Anesthesiologists routinely utilize various sophisticated devices for the delivery of intravenous drugs. The gravity-driven infusion systems in widespread use just a few years ago are primitive compared with the convenience, accuracy, and precision provided by today's infusion pumps. However, although modern infusion systems are remarkably advanced, they still fall short of the convenience and theoretical appeal associated with the delivery of inhaled anesthetics by an agent-specific vaporizer. Emulation of the clinical convenience and pharmacokinetic-dynamic exactness provided by vaporizers is perhaps the ultimate goal in the development of infusion devices for intravenous anesthetics. The effort to achieve that goal has led to the integration of computerized infusion pump technology with modern pharmacokinetic-pharmacodynamic concepts.

The aims of this chapter are to summarize briefly the history of intravenous drug delivery devices, to contrast intravenous *versus* inhaled anesthetic delivery systems, to develop the concept of the computer-controlled infusion pump (CCIP) as an "intravenous vaporizer," to survey the current status of computer-controlled drug delivery, and to forecast areas of future advancement.

HISTORICAL BACKGROUND

The development of intravenous drug delivery devices has been a slow process punctuated by major advances spanning over four centuries, as summarized in Figure 26A-1 (1). Gaining direct access to the circulation for the administration of drugs was first accomplished shortly after Harvey's description of the circulatory system when Christopher Wren injected opium into a human vein by means of a feather quill attached to an animal bladder in 1657. More than two centuries later, convenient access to the circulation was made possible with the development of the hollow hypodermic needle by Frances Rynd.

With access to the circulation achieved, the development of intravenous drug delivery systems then focused primarily on the accurate administration of fluid. Beginning with the syringe and simple gravity-driven devices, which were the mainstay delivery method until recently, this development effort culminated in the production of highly accurate, convenient, "calculator" pumps, complete with sophisticated options.

More recent research efforts have attempted to achieve greater pharmacokinetic exactness by combining existing computerized pump technology with modern clinical pharmacology. High-resolution pharmacokinetic modeling has made it possible to program pumps to control the infusion rate according to a drug's pharmacokinetic parameters. Rather than setting an infusion rate, as with calculator pumps, the user of these devices identifies a desired plasma or effect site concentration (i.e., "open-loop" control). The pharmacokinetic model-driven pump then calculates and sets the appropriate infusion rates over time to achieve the targeted concentration.

In a similar fashion, "closed-loop" control infusion devices extend this marriage of infusion pump technology and modern pharmacology to achieve pharmacodynamic exactness. Making use of complete pharmacokinetic-dynamic models, such devices alter the infusion rate according to a real-time measure of drug effect, thus "closing the loop" between pharma-

*This chapter has been adapted and expanded with permission from Egan TD. Intravenous drug delivery systems: toward an intravenous vaporizer. J Clin Anesth 1996;8:8S-14S, a summary of a presentation delivered at the fourth annual meeting of the Society for Intravenous Anesthesia, Atlanta, Georgia October 20, 1995.

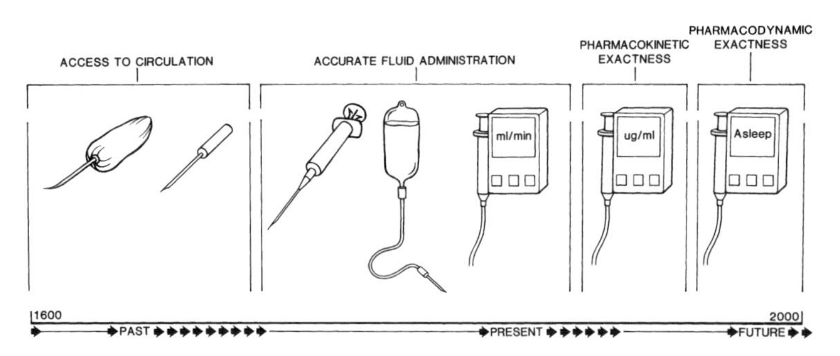

FIGURE 26A-1. A summary of important advances in the development of intravenous drug delivery devices. Convenient access to the circulation and accurate fluid administration were the initial challenges to be addressed, whereas increased pharmacokinetic-pharmacodynamic exactness using computers is now the focus of research activity. (From Egan TD. Intravenous drug delivery systems: toward an intravenous vaporizer. J Clin Anesth 1996;8:8S–14S.)

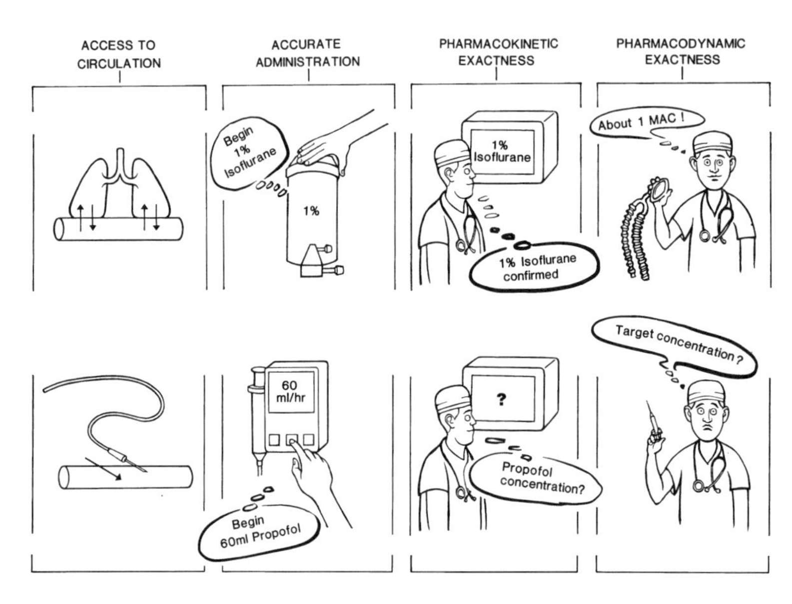

FIGURE 26A-2. A cartoon contrasting volatile versus intravenous delivery systems. Gaining access to the circulation indirectly by the lungs affords a fundamental advantage over direct intravenous access because the equilibration of gas across the alveoli to the pulmonary capillaries prevents perpetual drug uptake. (From Egan TD. Intravenous drug delivery systems: toward an intravenous vaporizer. J Clin Anesth 1996;8:8S–14S.)

cokinetics and pharmacodynamics. The anesthesiologist's specified degree of drug effect is achieved by providing feedback to the combined pharmacokinetic-dynamic model.

INTRAVENOUS *VERSUS* VOLATILE DELIVERY SYSTEMS

Administering volatile anesthetic through the lung by a calibrated vaporizer has several fundamental advantages. These advantages are a function of gaining access to the circulation indirectly through the lung and are summarized in the upper panel of Figure 26A-2. Because uptake of inhaled anesthetic progressively diminishes as equilibrium between the alveolar and pulmonary capillary partial pressures is approached, the setting on the vaporizer is a proportional reflection of the concentration in the blood and at the site of drug action in the central nervous system (CNS). In other words, because of this equilibration process, the partial pressure in the blood cannot rise beyond the partial pressure of the inhaled gas. This enables relatively accurate administration. Moreover, the expired concentration can be measured and confirmed with modern respiratory gas monitoring, ensuring pharmacokinetic exactness. Finally, the clinical meaning of the measured concentration is well described and is standardized in terms of minimum alveolar concentration (MAC), providing pharmacodynamic exactness.

In contrast, when access to the circulation is gained directly, there is nothing to prevent the indefinite uptake of drug, as depicted in the lower panel of Figure 26A-2. Thus, without the aid of a computer model, the infusion rate of an intravenous anesthetic agent does not reveal much about the resulting concentration in the blood, preventing entirely accurate administration. Furthermore, as yet no capability exists to measure the concentration of intravenous anesthetics in real time, preventing equivalent pharmacokinetic exactness. Finally, even if concentrations of intravenous agents were measurable in the clinical setting, the meaning of a given concentration is not yet well understood; that is, a thoroughly researched and widely appreciated analog of MAC for the intravenous agents is not available, so pharmacodynamic exactness equivalent to the volatile anesthetics is not yet possible.

Because practitioners have not had an intravenous anesthetic delivery device capable of targeted administration, they are not accustomed to thinking in terms of the appropriate plasma concentration for a given intravenous anesthetic technique and specific type of surgical stimulation as when using inhaled drugs. When delivering inhaled anesthetics with an agent-specific vaporizer, practitioners think in terms of the appropriate expired concentration. In contrast, when delivering intravenous drugs with a syringe pump, anesthetists think in terms of infusion rates, not concentrations. Thus, today's calculator pumps, although accurate and sophisticated, fall short of the theoretical appeal and practical convenience associated with the delivery of volatile anesthetic through the lung.

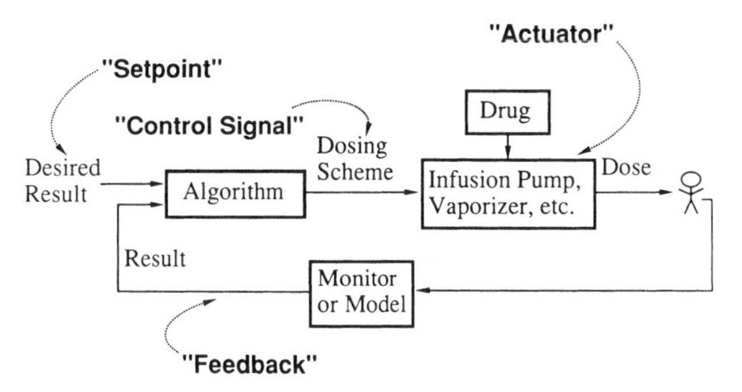

FIGURE 26A-3. A schematic diagram of computer-controlled drug delivery. Note that the primary difference between open and closed loop control is the origin of the feedback signal (see text for complete explanation). (From Reves JG, Jacobs JR, Glass P. Intravenous anesthetic drug delivery in anesthesia. International Anesthesia Research Society Review Course Lectures, 1992:29–34.)

COMPUTER-CONTROLLED DRUG DELIVERY AS AN INTRAVENOUS VAPORIZER

CCIPs have made progress towards the concept of a "vaporizer" for intravenous drugs because they address the fundamental limitation associated with delivering drugs directly into the circulation. Constant rate infusions result in continuous drug uptake. CCIPs, in contrast, gradually decrease the rate of infusion based on the drug's pharmacokinetics. Known in its general form as the BET (i.e., bolus, elimination, and transfer) method (2), the dosing scheme determined by a CCIP accounts for the initial concentration after a bolus dose and the subsequent drug distribution and clearance while an infusion is ongoing.

Using some variation of this BET method, CCIPs compute a prediction of the drug concentration at frequent intervals based on the drug's pharmacokinetic parameters and the drug dosage previously administered. The computer's prediction of the current drug concentration serves as the feedback to the system in formulating future dosage rates. The CCIP changes the infusion rates at frequent intervals, sometimes as often as every 10 seconds, to "hone in" on the targeted concentration.

Delivery of drug by a CCIP therefore requires a different knowledge base on the part of the physician. Rather than setting an infusion rate based on clinical experience and recommendations from the anesthesia literature, the anesthesiologist using a CCIP designates a target concentration, and the CCIP calculates the infusion rates necessary to achieve and maintain the concentration over time. Successful use of a CCIP thus requires knowledge of the therapeutic concentrations appropriate for the specific anesthetic technique and the prevailing surgical stimulus.

Drug delivery by a CCIP according to a pharmacokinetic model has been described by various names in the anesthesia literature. Computer-assisted continuous infusion (CACI), target-controlled infusion (TCI), and model-based drug delivery are all methods of computerized delivery using "open-loop" systems in that no feedback from the patient is considered by the pump infusion control mechanism. The computer prediction of the current drug concentration is the only control signal evaluated by the pump. The anesthesiologist must assess the adequacy of the patient response and must change the target concentration as necessary.

"Closed-loop" computer-controlled drug delivery is fundamentally different in that the computer control mechanisms evaluate a real-time measure of drug effect, such as muscle relaxation, heart rate, or blood pressure, and adjust drug delivery based on that measure. Figure 26A-3 schematically summarizes the difference between open-loop and closed-loop control.

As noted in Figure 26A-3, the origin of the feedback signal is the primary difference between open-loop and closed-loop drug delivery. With both types of delivery, the anesthesiologist determines the "setpoint" or desired result. For open-loop delivery, the setpoint is a plasma or effect site concentration; the setpoint for closed-loop delivery is a desired level of drug effect. During closed-loop control, the feedback signal is provided by a monitor such as a peripheral nerve stimulator or an electroencephalogram (EEG). The open-loop feedback signal, in contrast, is provided by a mathematic model that predicts the current drug concentration. For both types of delivery, the computer's control algorithm considers differences between the setpoint and the feedback signal and generates a "control signal." This control signal alters the pump (or "actuator") behavior to achieve the desired setpoint.

REMAINING CHALLENGES IN THE DEVELOPMENT OF COMPUTER-CONTROLLED INFUSION PUMPS

Although open-loop CCIPs have made progress toward the concept of a vaporizer for intravenous drugs, significant challenges remain. Not surprisingly, these challenges are the same as those faced historically by the developers of intravenous delivery systems: accurate fluid administration, pharmacokinetic precision, and pharmacodynamic exactness.

Whether the goal is open-loop or closed-loop control, the computerized pump must be capable of delivering the desired volume of fluid accurately. Because potent intravenous anesthetics are dissolved or suspended in small volumes of fluid, this issue is not trivial. Today's pumps have by and large successfully met this challenge in that they are accurate to about ±5 to 10% even when the infusion rates are altered by computer as often as every 10 seconds (3, 4). However, unsolved problems exist relating to pump performance. For example, pump mechanisms are often not smooth enough to deliver a truly continuous infusion; that is, there are instantaneous flow rate errors that accumulate over time for which the pump does not ever fully compensate (5).

From a bioengineering perspective, other challenges center around the perplexities of optimal system control. When applied to computerized drug delivery, system control refers to the fine tuning of the pump's drug administration algorithm to reach and maintain the targeted drug concentration or desired level of drug effect within an acceptable time frame and with an acceptable margin of error. As portrayed in Figure 26A-3, a control system attempts to manage some output (the controlled variable, such as the drug concentration in the blood) based on information provided by an input signal (the feedback, such as the prediction of current drug concentration).

The fine tuning of the control system can be surprisingly complex because the system must attempt to achieve a multitude of goals, some of which are diametrically opposed. As illustrated in Figure 26A-4, for example, the control system must provide acceptable performance with regard to the time to induction (time to reaching the target), the degree of overshoot, the time to stability, the extent of oscillation at steady state, and the maximum deviation from the target. In addition, the system must be capable of responding appropriately to perturbation (such as a period when the syringe pump is off because the syringe must be changed or when there is artifactual disturbance of the feedback signal).

The control mechanisms of these computerized pumps must also account for the problem of plasma-effect site dysequilibrium. This issue is important in that the effect site or "biophase" concentrations, not the plasma concentrations, best correlate with drug effect (6). Although plasma has arbitrarily been the target site for many CCIP applications, the effect site is the more logical target (7). When targeting the plasma, a significant delay occurs in the achievement of a stable level of drug effect for many drugs; targeting the effect site results in a faster attainment of therapeutic concentrations in the biophase (8).

Figure 26A-5 illustrates the difference between targeting the plasma and targeting the effect site. The smooth, unvarying time course of the setpoint when targeting the plasma creates an illusion of precise control when, in fact, the effect site concentrations (and therefore the degree of drug effect) are lagging behind the plasma, resulting in a less than smooth time course of drug effect. When targeting the effect site, one sees a more rapid rise in effect site concentrations with a time course of drug effect that more accurately parallels the time course of surgical stimulation.

Having adequately addressed most of these engineering challenges, many of the remaining knowledge gaps are now in the area of clinical pharmacology. Current pharmacokinetic-dynamic models cannot adequately account for the significant variability observed in human drug disposition and response (9, 10). More-

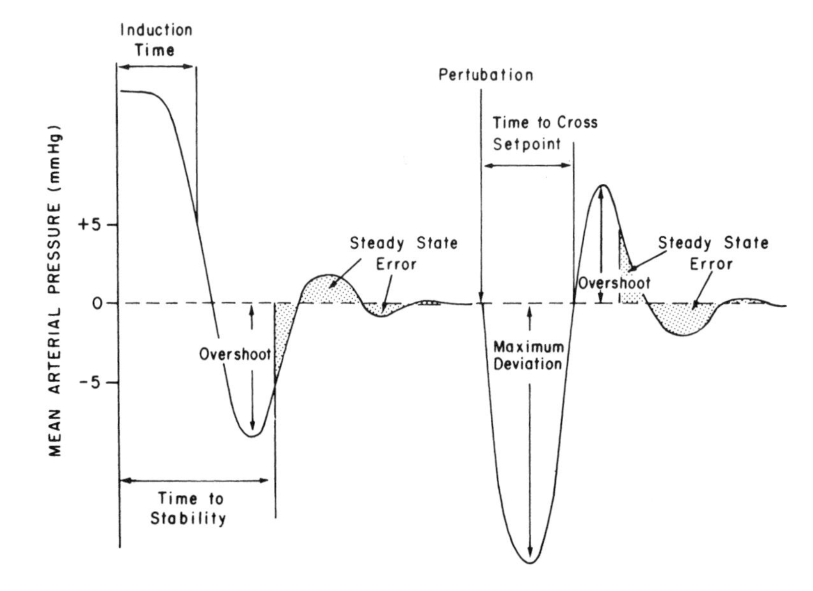

FIGURE 26A-4. An example of a closed-loop delivery system using nitroprusside to control arterial blood pressure. The drug infusion control mechanisms must address a host of issues, including time to induction, degree of overshoot, and magnitude of steady-state error. (From Westenskow DR, Meline L, Pace NL. Controlled hypotension with sodium nitroprusside: anesthesiologist versus computer. J Clin Monit 1987; 3:80–86.)

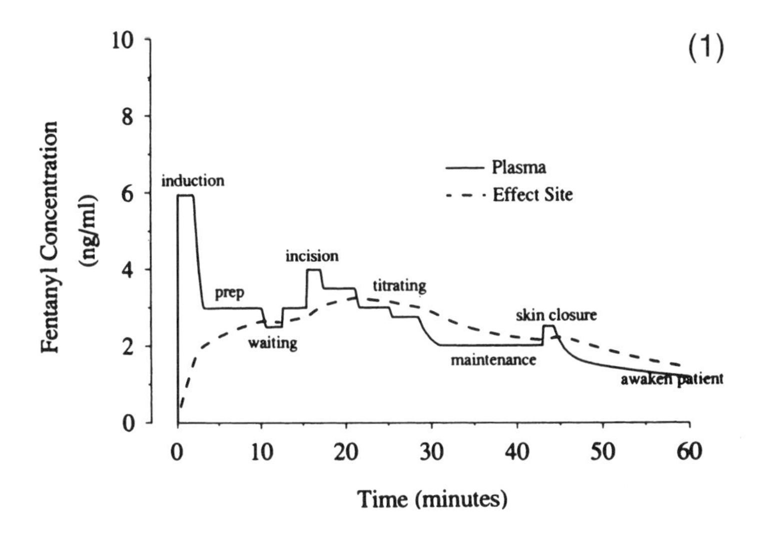

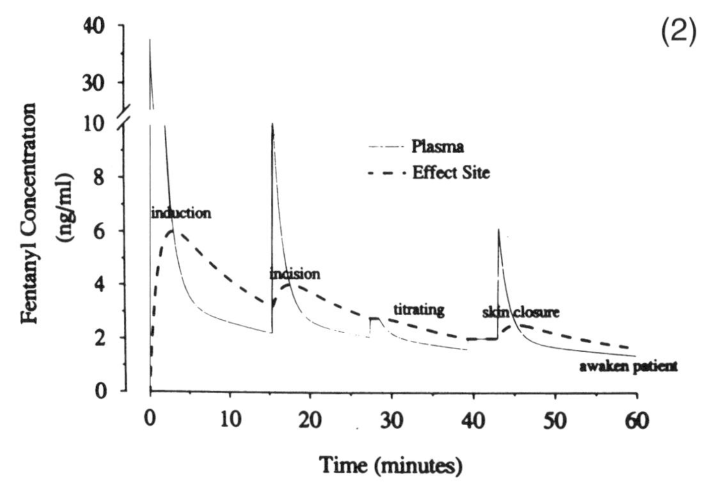

FIGURE 26A-5. Two simulations of computerized fentanyl delivery illustrating the difference between targeting the plasma and targeting the effect site. The upper panel targets the plasma; the lower panel targets the effect site. When targeting the effect site, there is a more rapid rise in effect site concentrations with a time course of drug effect that more accurately parallels the time course of surgical stimulation. (From Shafer SL, Gregg KM. Algorithms to rapidly achieve and maintain stable drug concentrations at the site of drug effect with a computer controlled infusion pump. J Pharmacokinet Biopharm 1992;20:147–169.)

over, the therapeutic windows for intravenous anesthetics when used as part of diverse anesthetic techniques for a broad array of surgical stimuli are not well defined. In particular, the interactions of different classes of intravenous agents when used as part of a total intravenous anesthetic have not yet been precisely quantified. What initial sufentanil target concentration would be reasonable, for example, when anesthetizing a 78-year-old man who is undergoing thoracotomy using a propofol infusion after midazolam premedication? What propofol target concentration would be appropriate for conscious sedation during a hernia repair under spinal anesthesia in a 30-year-old man? Highly sophisticated pharmacokinetic-dynamic modeling techniques are making significant strides in addressing these knowledge gaps (11-14).

A related and critical obstacle preventing the implementation of completely automated, closed-loop delivery of anesthesia by a computer is the lack of an adequate means of monitoring the depth of anesthesia. Because the anesthetic state is such a complex function of unconsciousness, amnesia, analgesia, motionlessness, and autonomic depression, the search for an adequate depth of anesthesia monitor remains an elusive "Holy Grail" of anesthesia research activity (15). Closed-loop administration of anesthetics requires meaningful pharmacodynamic feedback. Although such feedback is available for some components of the anesthetic state (e.g., muscle relaxation, hemodynamics), it is not yet possible to quantify the complete anesthetic state when using numerous drugs. New EEG signal-processing techniques are showing promise in terms of measuring hypnosis (16), but the technology necessary to measure other components of the anesthetic state such as analgesia remains elusive.

CURRENT STATE OF THE ART

The best current computer-controlled drug delivery systems reflect tremendous progress in technology and clinical pharmacology over the last decade. Various pumps that are programmed according to pharmacokinetic or pharmacodynamic models are in use throughout the world. These machines are at differing stages of development, ranging from experimental prototypes to marketed products. They have been used in association with many different intravenous anesthetic agents, including the opioids, sedative-hypnotics, and muscle relaxants. Applied in both clinical and research settings, these advanced gadgets are yielding promising results.

The Stanpump program is one example of a widely utilized open-loop CCIP. Developed by Shafer and colleagues at Stanford University, as the name suggests, Stanpump is versatile in that it can deliver any anesthetic for which a suitable pharmacokinetic model is available. As with most other experimental CCIPs, the performance of the device is typically good, with a median absolute performance error of approximately 20 to 30%, as shown in Figure 24A-6 (17). Stanpump has also been applied in small animal research with comparable performance (18).

A similar CACI system has been developed at Duke University by Jacobs and colleagues for applications in anesthesiology. Although it can be used clinically with excellent results (19), this system has been especially useful in human clinical pharmacology experiments in which a steady-state level of drug effect at a specified concentration is absolutely essential. Performing drug interaction experiments such as volatile anesthetic MAC reduction by opioids is just one example of how this technology can be exploited (13).

Perhaps the open-loop infusion system closest to becoming a commercially available device in the United States is the TCI system for propofol developed by Kenny and colleagues in the United Kingdom (20). This device has been specifically packaged for commercial use and thus is complete with a user-friendly interface. After extensive clinical application around the world, this device is yielding promising results in a variety of settings (21, 22). Known as the Diprifusor™, the device is now approved for patient use in Europe and elsewhere.

Some computer-controlled delivery devices do not utilize standard compartmental models. One such device is the "computer-assisted intravenous anaesthesia system" developed by Crankshaw and colleagues in Australia (23). This CCIP is unique in that it is based on the plasma drug efflux method, a nonparametric, error-correcting method for determining the optimal infusion rate-time profile for producing a constant plasma concentration. The performance associated with this method is typically better than CCIPs that utilize compartmental models, but the versatility of the device is limited in that the user must be satisfied with a single, preset plasma concentration because the infusion rate-time profiles are devised for one concentration target only (e.g., 100 μg/L for alfentanil) (24).

Although numerous closed-loop infusion devices have been developed for the administration of neuromuscular blockers and anithypertensive agents such as nitroprusside (25, 26), development of closed-loop devices for the administration of complete anesthesia has been hampered by the lack of an adequate monitor of "depth of anesthesia." Schuttler and colleagues have developed closed-loop infusion systems that utilize the EEG median frequency as the feedback signal. Having first developed a system using methohexital, they now

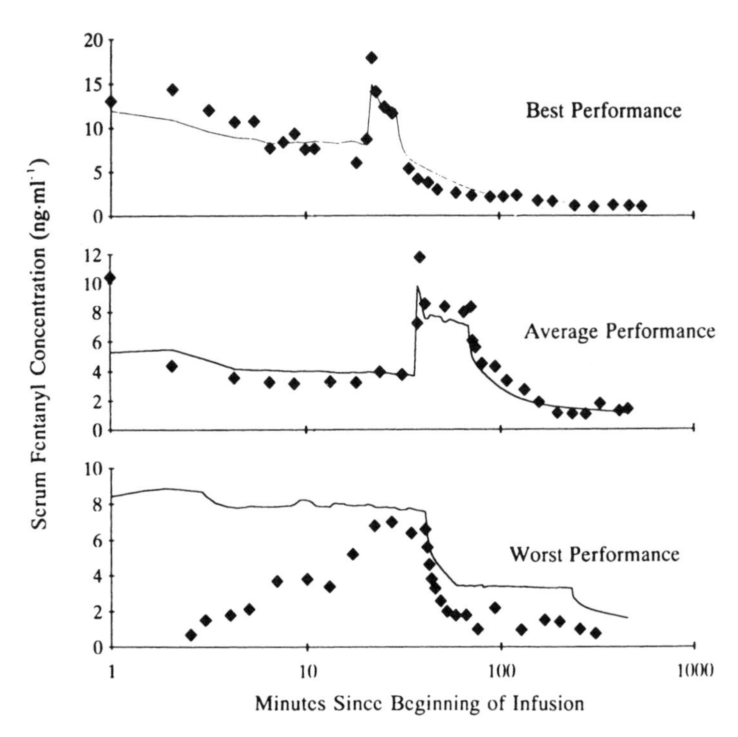

FIGURE 26A-6. The best, median, and worst performance of Stanpump when used to administer fentanyl to 21 patients. The line represents the predicted concentration, and the diamonds represent the measured concentrations. (From Shafer SL, Varvel JR, Aziz N, Scott JC. Pharmacokinetics of fentanyl administered by computer controlled infusion pump. Anesthesiology 1990;73:1091–1102.)

have a device that infuses alfentanil by open-loop control and propofol by closed-loop control (27, 28). Both the earlier device using methohexital and the more recent device using the combination of drugs have yielded clinically satisfying results. Kenny and colleagues have developed a similar closed-loop device that utilizes auditory evoked potentials as the feedback signal (29).

At the University of Utah, Kern and colleagues have developed a closed-loop system for the administration of neuromuscular blockers that is unique because it utilizes minibolus drug administration instead of a continuous infusion (5). The theoretical advantage of this method is that bolus administration avoids the instantaneous flow rate errors associated with the pump "start-up" time.

FUTURE DIRECTIONS

The future will no doubt bring exciting advances in computer-controlled drug delivery. Because adequate pump technology is largely in place, improvements in computerized delivery will come as a result of advances in clinical pharmacology.

For example, some pharmacokinetic parameter sets for a given drug clearly perform better than others for drug delivery by computer. Why parameter sets estimated from one study would perform better than those from another is unclear. Some evidence suggests that pharmacokinetic parameters estimated from computerized delivery perform better than those estimated from noncomputerized delivery (17). Which compartmental model pharmacokinetic parameters sets perform best and why is an area of intense investigation (30, 31).

CCIPs may eventually move beyond the utilization of simple compartmental models. It is conceivable that CCIPs could utilize hybrid models that incorporate elements of physiology (32). These hybrid models may improve pump performance by taking into account physiologic processes such as drug recirculation or patient variables such as cardiac output and renal function. Similarly, closed-loop CCIP control mechanisms may eventually include advanced "fuzzy logic" techniques, the rules of which are intended to emulate the actual control actions of a clinical expert (33).

Another area of research focus relates to CCIP performance. How does one define good performance? Measures of performance such as the median absolute performance error, median performance error, divergence, and wobble have been proposed as a means of standardizing the assessment of performance (34). Recognized standards of performance are necessary to make comparisons among devices and parameter sets.

A related area requiring investigation is the comparison of CCIP drug delivery versus traditional methods of delivery in terms of outcome. Can specific indicators of perioperative outcome such as cost be improved through the use of CCIPs? There is some suggestion that CCIP-delivered anesthetics can improve various surrogate outcome measures such as hemodynamic stability (35), but this area remains largely unexplored.

The application of computer-controlled drug delivery will likely expand outside the operating room environment. Sedation of mechanically ventilated patients in the intensive care unit and analgesia of postoperative patients in surgical wards are just two examples of possible application for target-controlled drug delivery outside the operating room (36, 37). Figure 26A-7 is an example of the integration of patient-controlled analgesia technology with the concept of target-controlled drug delivery.

Even if computer-controlled drug delivery never gains truly widespread acceptance in clinical medicine, its role in clinical pharmacology research is already solidified. It is impossible to make meaningful pharmacodynamic observations without controlling the pharmacokinetic aspects of an experiment. Computer-controlled drug delivery enables an investigator to establish a steady-state drug level near a target concentration. Using CCIPs for pharmacokinetic control of a pharmacodynamic experiment has become a frequently applied method in clinical pharmacology research in anesthesia (11, 12, 38).

Another firmly entrenched research application of CCIPs is the use of simulation. Through simulation of

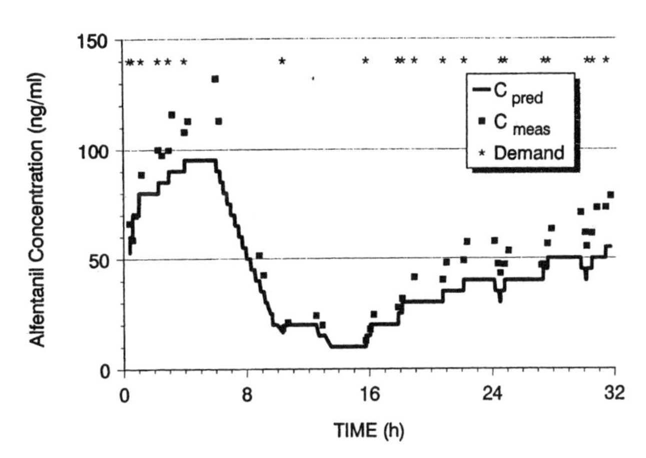

FIGURE 26A-7. Patient-controlled analgesia using an open-loop computer-controlled infusion of alfentanil, an example of target-controlled drug delivery outside the operating room. The line represents the targeted concentration; the squares represent the actual measured concentrations. The asterisks indicate a patient demand for increased analgesia. (From van den Nieuwenhuyzen MCO, Engbers FHM, Burm AGL, et al. Computer controlled infusion of alfentanil versus patient controlled administration of morphine for postoperative analgesia: a double blind randomized trail. Anesth Analg 1995;81:671–679.)

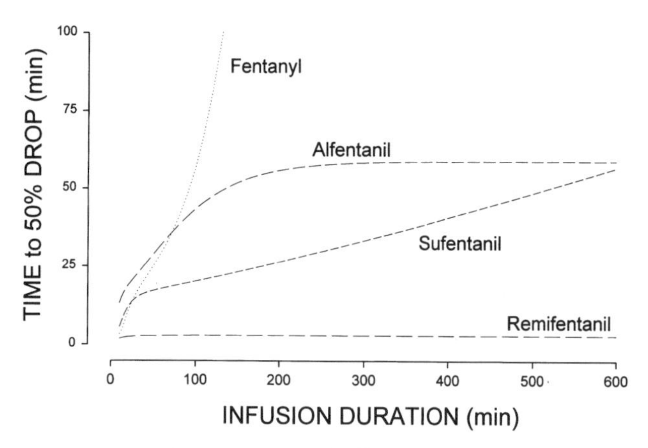

FIGURE 26A-8. Context-sensitive half-time simulations for remifentanil and the currently marketed fentanyl congeners. Context-sensitive half-times are a common application of computer-controlled infusion pump simulation. (From Egan TD, Lemmens HJM, Fiset P, et al. The pharmacokinetics of the new short-acting opioid remifentanil (GI87084B) in healthy adult male volunteers. Anesthesiology 1993; 79:881–892.)

computer-controlled drug delivery, investigators can make comparisons about the clinical pharmacology of two drugs that are not possible in any other way. The context-sensitive half-time is just one example of CCIP simulation (39, 40). Defined as the time required to achieve a 50% decrease in the plasma drug concentration after termination of a continuous infusion targeted to maintain a constant concentration, context-sensitive half-times have been utilized to compare the pharmacokinetics of the newer opioid remifentanil with the currently available opioids as in Figure 26A-8 (41). Through CCIP simulation, one can also compare the decay in effect site concentrations that occur after administration of an "equipotent" infusion (i.e., an infusion targeted to a concentration that produces 50% of maximal effect) (42).

In the future, in addition to cost, perhaps the biggest hurdle that may impede the widespread application of CCIPs will be physician familiarity. Switching from empirically based dosage regimens to target control will require a new mindset of clinicians. A sound understanding of fundamental pharmacokinetic-dynamic modeling principles will be necessary to implement with confidence computer-controlled drug delivery in the clinical setting. This switch will represent a revolution akin to the high-technology monitoring techniques embraced by anesthesiologists over the last 20 years.

ACKNOWLEDGMENTS

The expert assistance of Mr. John Kilbourn in providing the drawings for this manuscript is gratefully acknowledged.

REFERENCES

1. Vandam LD. Intravenous anesthesia: history, currency, prospects. Mt Sinai J Med 1983;50:316–322.
2. Schwilden H. A general method for calculating the dosage scheme in linear pharmacokinetics. Eur J Clin Pharmacol 1981; 20:379–386.
3. Currie J, Owen H, Ilsley AH. Rate controlled analgesia: a laboratory evaluation of a new infusion device. Anaesth Intensive Care 1990;18:555–559.
4. Conner SB, Quill TJ, Jacobs JR. Accuracy of drug infusion pumps under computer control. IEEE Trans Biomed Eng 1992; 39:980–982.
5. Kern SE, Westenskow DR. Biophase based mini-bolus delivery as an alternative to continuous infusion for drugs that exhibit a biophase lag. J Pharmacokinet Biopharm (in press).
6. Jacobs JR, Reves JG. Effect site equilibration time is a determinant of induction dose requirement. Anesth Analg 1993;76:1–6.
7. Shafer SL, Gregg KM. Algorithms to rapidly achieve and maintain stable drug concentrations at the site of drug effect with a computer controlled unfusion pump. J Pharmacokinet Biopharm 1992;20:147–169.
8. Jacobs JR, Williams EA. Algorithm to control effect compartment drug concentrations in pharmacokinetic model-driven drug delivery. IEEE Trans Biomed Eng 1993;40:993–999.
9. Crankshaw DP. Variability and anesthetic agents. Anaesth Pharmacol Rev 1994;2:271–279.
10. Hull CJ. How far can we go with compartmental models? Anesthesiology 1990;72:399–402.
11. Ausems ME, Hug CC, Stanski DR, Burm AGL. Plasma concentrations of alfentanil required to supplement nitrous oxide anesthesia for general surgery. Anesthesiology 1986;65:362–373.
12. Vuyk J, Lim T, Engbers FHM, et al. The pharmacodynamic interaction of propofol and alfentanil during lower abdominal surgery in women. Anesthesiology 1995;83:8–22.
13. McEwan AI, Smith C, Dyar O, et al. Isoflurane minimum alveolar concentration reduction by fentanyl. Anesthesiology 1993;78:864–869.
14. Stanski DR, Maitre PO. Population pharmacokinetics and pharmacodynamics of thiopental: the effect of age revisited. Anesthesiology 1990;72:412–422.
15. Prys-Roberts C. Anaesthesia: a practical or impossible construct? Br J Anaesth 1987;59:1341.
16. Sigl JC, Chamoun NG. An introduction to bispectral analysis for the electroencephalogram. J Clin Monit 1994;10:392–404.
17. Shafer SL, Varvel JR, Aziz N, Scott JC. Pharmacokinetics of fentanyl administered by computer controlled infusion pump. Anesthesiology 1990;73:1091–1102.
18. Gustafsson LL, Ebling WF, Osaki E, et al. Plasma concentration clamping in the rat using a computer controlled infusion pump. Pharm Res 1992;9:800–807.
19. Glass PSA, Jacobs JR, Smith LR, et al. Pharmacokinetic model driven infusion of fentanyl: assessment of accuracy. Anesthesiology 1990;73:1082–1090.
20. White M, Kenny GNC. Intravenous propofol anaesthesia using a computerised infusion system. Anaesthesia 1990;45:204–209.
21. Church JA, Stanton PD, Kenny GNC, Anderson JR. Propofol for sedation during endoscopy: assessment of a computer controlled infusion system. Gastrointest Endosc 1991;37:175–179.
22. Skipsey IG, Colvin JR, Mackenzie N, Kenny GNC. Sedation with propofol during surgery under local blockade: assessment of a target controlled infusion system. Anaesthesia 1993;48:210–213.
23. Crankshaw DP, Morgan DJ, Beemer GH, Karasawa F. Preprogrammed infusion of alfentanil to constant arterial plasma concentration. Anesth Analg 1993;76:556–561.

24. Shafer SL. Constant versus optimal plasma concentrations. Anesth Analg 1993;76:467–469.
25. Jaklitsch RR, Westenskow DR, Pace NL, et al. A comparison of computer-controlled versus manual administration of vecuronium in humans. J Clin Monit 1987;3:269–276.
26. Westenskow DR, Meline L, Pace NL. Controlled hypotension with sodium nitroprusside: anesthesiologist versus computer. J Clin Monit 1987;3:80–86.
27. Schwilden H, Schuttler J, Stoeckel H. Closed loop feedback control of methohexital anesthesia by quanitative EEG analysis in humans. Anesthesiology 1987;67:341–347.
28. Schuttler J, Kloos S, Ihmsen H, Schwilden H. Clinical evaluation of a closed-loop dosing device for total intravenous anesthesia based on EEG depth of anesthesia monitoring. Anesthesiology 1992;77:A501.
29. Kenny GNC, McFadzean W, Mantzaridis H, Fisher AC. Closed loop control of anesthesia. Anesthesiology 1992;77:A328.
30. Coetzee JF, Glen JB, Wium CA, Boshoff L. Pharmacokinetic model selection for target controlled infusions of propofol: assessment of three parameter sets. Anesthesiology 1995;82:1328–1345.
31. Vuyk J, Engbers FHM, Burm AGL, et al. Performance of computer-controlled infusion of propofol: an evaluation of five pharmacokinetic parameter sets. Anesth Analg 1995;81:1275–1282.
32. Wada DR, Ward DS. The hybrid model: a new pharmacokinetic model for computer controlled infusion pumps. IEEE Trans Biomed Eng 1994;41:134–142.
33. Mason DG, Edwards ND, Linkens DA, Reilly CS. Performance assessment of a fuzzy controller for atracurium-induced neuromuscular block. Br J Anaesth 1996;76:396–400.
34. Varvel JR, Donoho DL, Shafer SL. Measuring the predictive performance of computer-controlled infusion pumps. J Pharmacokinet Biopharm 1992;20:63–94.
35. Ausems ME, Vuyk J, Hug CC, Stanski DR. Comparison of a computer-assisted infusion versus intermittent bolus administration of alfentanil as a supplement to nitrous oxide for lower abdominal surgery. Anesthesiology 1988;68:851–861.
36. Barr J, Egan TD, Feeley TW, Shafer SL. The pharmacokinetics and pharmacodynamics of computer controlled propofol infusions in ICU patients. Clin Pharmacol Ther 1993;53:185.
37. van den Nieuwenhuyzen MCO, Engbers FHM, Burm AGL, et al. Computer controlled infusion of alfentanil versus patient controlled administration of morphine for postoperative analgesia: a double blind randomized trail. Anesth Analg 1995; 81:671–679.
38. Fiset P, Lemmens HJM, Egan TD, et al. Pharmacodynamic modeling of the electroencephalographic effects of flumazenil in healthy volunteers sedated with midazolam. Clin Pharmacol Ther 1995;58:567–582.
39. Shafer SL, Varvel JR. Pharmacokinetics, pharmacodynamics and rational opioid selection. Anesthesiology 1991;74:53–63.
40. Hughes MA, Glass PSA, Jacobs JR. Context-sensitive half-times in multicompartment pharmacokinetic models for intravenous anesthetic drugs. Anesthesiology 1991;76:334–341.
41. Egan TD, Lemmens HJM, Fiset P, et al. The pharmacokinetics of the new short-acting opioid remifentanil (GI87084B) in healthy adult male volunteers. Anesthesiology 1993;79:881–892.
42. Egan TD, Minto CF, Hermann DJ, et al. Remifentanil versus alfentanil: comparative pharmacokinetics and pharmacodynamics in healthy adult male volunteers. Anesthesiology 1996; 4:821–833.

26B European Perspective

Gavin N. C. Kenny and Nick Sutcliffe

Europeans have been active in the field of intravenous anesthesia from the earliest days. In 1656, Sir Christopher Wren of England first used the intravenous administration to induce anesthesia in dogs and humans. In 1845, Francis Rynd of Scotland developed the hollow hypodermic needle. The Frenchman Pierre Cyprien Ore pioneered the use of intravenous chloral hydrate in 1874. Finally, August Bier of Germany described the intravenous regional technique of local anesthesia in the early 1900s.

In more recent years, the conservative nature of the United States Food and Drug Administration has meant that European physicians have had access to new anesthetic drugs earlier than their American colleagues. This has been a double-edged sword in that agents such as Althesin and propanidid were withdrawn before being released in the United States because of the high incidence of adverse reactions. Likewise, prolonged intravenous infusions of etomidate interfere with steroid synthesis and are associated with an increased mortality in critically ill patients (1, 2). These rapidly metabolized drugs are more suited to total intravenous anesthesia (TIVA) compared with barbiturate compounds. Experienced gained in Europe with TIVA using these agents has been valuable, particularly regarding propofol, which was first introduced into the United Kingdom in 1984. This drug is particularly suited to continuous infusion techniques because of its rapid metabolism, high clearance, and low propensity for accumulation, even in patients with hepatic disease (3, 4).

One major difference between Europe and the United States has been the higher incidence of anesthesia with spontaneous ventilation administered by European anesthesiologists. Anesthesiologists rely more on regional anesthesia, particularly in the Scandinavian countries. These differences in clinical practice have several implications for TIVA. First, the maintenance of spontaneous respiration gives valuable clues to the depth of anesthesia; however, a narrow "therapeutic window" exists within which the blood concentration must be maintained to provide adequate surgical anesthesia without excessive respiratory depression. Second, the use of local and regional techniques allows a "lighter" plane of general anesthesia (or deep sedation) to be maintained with an intravenous hypnotic infusion.

DELIVERY SYSTEMS: EQUIPMENT

The infusion devices commonly used in nursing care are generally unsuitable for the specialized tasks of induction and maintenance of intravenous anesthesia. These devices lack essential performance characteristics and safety features.

Any device used to deliver TIVA should meet the following criteria:

1. The device should be capable of a wide range of infusion rates to facilitate both induction (e.g., 1000 ml/h) and maintenance of anesthesia (e.g., 0 to 300 ml/h).
2. The device should incorporate a rechargeable battery source to provide continuous electrical power and automatic switchover in the event of disconnection from the main electrical supply. Interruption of power should not alter any aspect of performance or lead to any loss of stored data. Battery life should be adequate to provide anesthesia for prolonged periods, and the device should indicate battery charge status.
3. The device should be simple to operate, each aspect of its function should require confirmatory action, and abort facilities should be readily available. The internal software should contain appropriate "error traps" to prevent data input errors resulting in dangerously high infusion rates.
4. The device should be physically and electrically

robust, water resistant, and capable of surviving at least modest abuse. The device's internal control and communication systems should not be sensitive to electromagnetic fields and must comply with current standards of electrical and mechanical safety.

5. The device must deliver accurate infusion rates over the entire operating range. Most devices tend to be inaccurate at extremely low infusion rates, so it may be preferable to dilute a drug to avoid the need for low infusion rates.
6. Modern standards of safety in anesthesia require the provision of comprehensive alarm facilities relating to incorrect size or make or malposition of the syringe, a syringe that is almost empty or completely empty, occlusion situations, low battery, and malfunction of the pump's internal mechanism.
7. The device should provide information relating to all modes of function (e.g., the drug infused, the current infusion rate, and total administered dose), as well as various alarm messages.
8. The system should ideally have the ability to log infusion data and be controllable by a remote computer.

PHARMACOKINETICS OF DRUG DELIVERY

The administration of a single dose of drug results in a peak blood concentration, which then decreases rapidly with time. Large bolus doses can result in an excessive blood concentration at the time of peak effect, with possible toxic side effects. Repeated single doses can be administered to maintain the drug effect, but this technique results in alternating "peak and trough" drug concentrations in the blood, with the potential for both toxic and subtherapeutic effects (Fig. 26B-1). This range may be acceptable for drugs with a wide therapeutic window, but it is inappropriate for the currently available rapid, short-acting intravenous anesthetic analgesic and muscle relaxant drugs. When drugs are administered by infusion at a constant rate, a considerable period (e.g., 4 to 5 times the distribution half-life) is required to achieve a true steady-state concentration (Fig. 26B-2), so induction time can be unacceptably long.

Pharmacokinetics describes the relationship between the dose of drug administered and the time course of the drug's concentration in the blood and tissues (5). When a drug is administered to a patient, the drug is simultaneously subjected to dilution, elimination, and distribution; the relationship between the quantity and time course of drug delivery and the resultant time course of drug concentration in the blood can be determined by performing complex mathematical calculations (see Chapter 2). Pharmacokinetic calculations can be used as a guide to the administration of intravenous drugs.

The pharmacokinetic behavior of many drugs can be described by a multicompartment model (Fig. 26B-3). This consists of a hypothetic central compartment into which the drug is infused and from which the drug is eliminated, together with one or more peripheral compartments into which the drug is distributed. The rate constants for the influx and efflux of drug from each compartment can be calculated from measuring drug concentrations in blood samples taken at intervals from patients after a drug bolus (6) or infusion (7). The mathematical model can then be used to generate an infusion regimen designed to maintain a particular blood concentration of anesthetic drug. These compartments are mathematical concepts and do not refer to any anatomic sites, although the drug concentration in the blood is considered to represent the concentration within the central compartment.

Using pharmacokinetic principles, the clinician can design an infusion regimen based on a bolus dose followed by a manually adjusted stepped infusion with

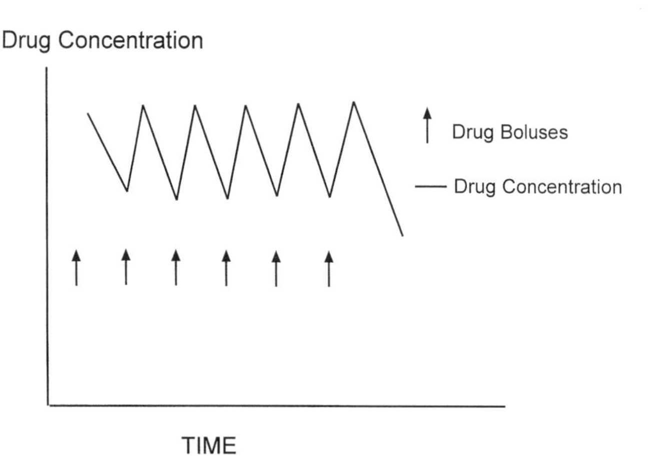

FIGURE 26B-1. Changes in drug concentration with time within the blood during repeated bolus dosing of drug.

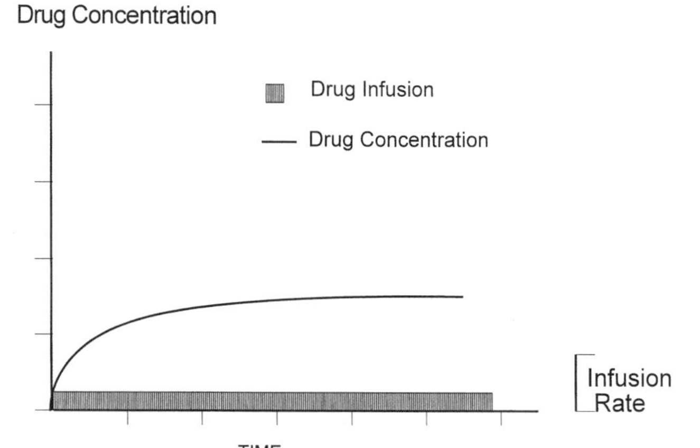

FIGURE 26B-2. Changes in drug concentration with time within the blood during a zero order infusion of drug.

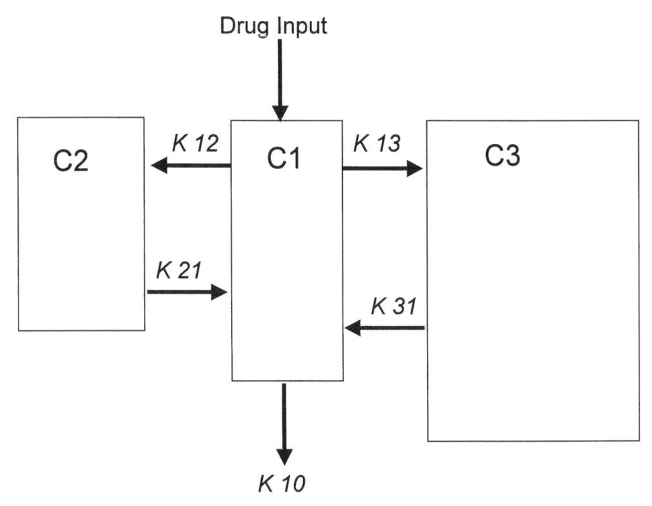

FIGURE 26B-3. Three-compartment pharmacokinetic model describing the distribution and elimination of an intravenous drug.

one or more rate changes over time. This method is designed to achieve a fixed blood concentration of anesthetic drug and has been proposed for the delivery of TIVA (8). Such an approach lacks flexibility, however, because it does not allow for a change in the drug concentration within the blood and therefore cannot accommodate variations in the level of surgical stimulation. Likewise, variations in patient susceptibility to a given concentration of anesthetic drug (pharmacodynamic variability) cannot be addressed with "fixed" infusion regimens. No single blood concentration of drug produces satisfactory anesthesia at all levels of surgical stimulation in all patients. Glass and his colleagues demonstrated marked variations in measured blood propofol concentrations required for different levels of surgical stimulation (9). Other researchers have shown that differences in protein binding may be responsible for much of the variability in the pharmacodynamics of alfentanil (10). Therefore, factors other than simple pharmacokinetics may alter the availability of anesthetic drugs at the site of action. Indeed, the pharmacodynamic variation may be greater than the observed pharmacokinetic variability (11). Thus, when using TIVA the clinician must be able to titrate the infusion regimen to a particular individual. It is essential to be able to change the blood concentration of anesthetic drug and the depth of anesthesia in response to variations in the level of surgical stress.

EFFECT SITE CONCENTRATION

Although anesthesiologists using TIVA tend to think in terms of blood concentrations of anesthetic drugs, the drug concentration at the site of action (effect site or biophase concentration) determines the effect of an anesthetic drug. Obviously, because the primary site of anesthetic action is somewhere within the brain, current technology does not permit us to measure the effect site concentration. Because the blood concentration and effect site concentration equilibrate over time, however, we can estimate the effect site concentration given a measure of drug effect. Figure 26B-4 shows a theoretic plot of effect site concentration *versus* blood concentration during a rapid intravenous infusion of an anesthetic drug and following cessation of the infusion. Disequilibrium exists between blood concentration and effect site concentration of drug, the degree of which is related to the speed of drug transfer between blood and effect site, and the rapidity of the intravenous infusion. With a slow infusion rate, disequilibrium is less pronounced, and the peak blood and effect site concentrations occur almost simultaneously (Fig. 26B-5). Although measuring effect site concentration is not feasible, we can measure the drug

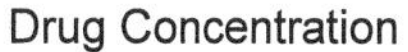

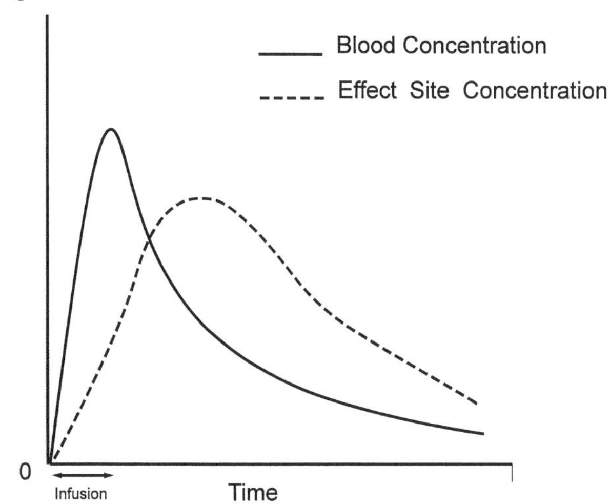

FIGURE 26B-4. Schematic representation of drug concentration within the blood and at the effect site, during a rapid infusion.

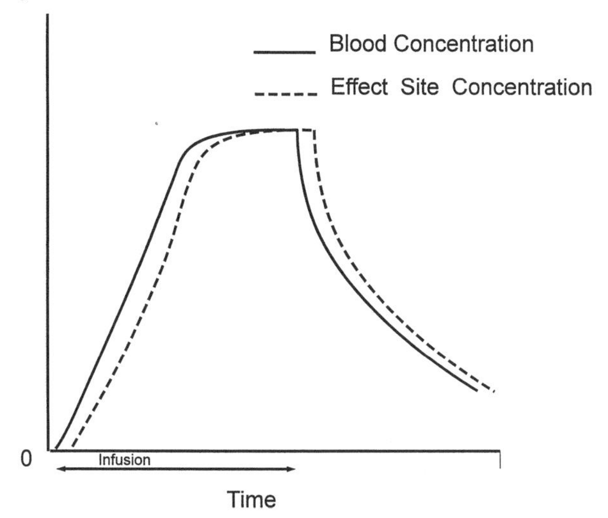

FIGURE 26B-5. Schematic representation of drug concentration within the blood and at the effect site, during a slow infusion.

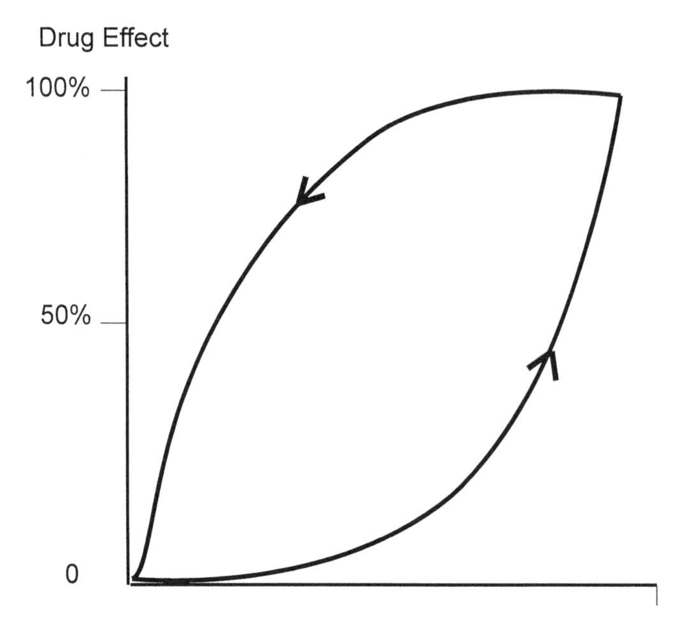

FIGURE 26B-6. Schematic representation of drug effect plotted against blood concentration of anesthetic drug.

effect within the central nervous system using the processed electroencephalographic (EEG) signal or an evoked response from the brain stem. This method allows construction of a blood concentration *versus* drug effect plot, which displays a degree of hysteresis related to the disequilibrium between blood concentration and effect site concentration of drug (Fig. 26B-6). Mathematical modeling can then be used to estimate the rate constant for the movement of drug between the blood and effect site (12, 13). Given this information, the effect site concentration can be estimated at any point in time during administration of the drug.

MANUAL SYSTEMS

Manually controlled infusion regimens designed to maintain a particular blood concentration of anesthetic drug can be derived from a pharmacokinetic model. An advantage of this technique is that no specialized infusion system is required. The anesthesiologist gives the required bolus dose, followed by a stepped infusion regimen that is manually adjusted at set time intervals. This method also has the advantage of avoiding regulatory issues raised when using specialized infusion equipment designed to change infusion rates "automatically" over time. Prys Roberts and colleagues have proposed a manually adjusted regimen for the delivery of propofol anesthesia (8). This regimen consists of a bolus of 1 mg/kg, followed by an infusion of 10 mg/kg/h for 10 minutes, reducing to 8 mg/kg/h for a further 10 minutes, followed by an infusion of 6 mg/kg/min for the duration of surgery. This regimen is designed to achieve a blood propofol concentration of 3 μg/ml. This type of infusion regimen lacks flexibility and often requires supplementation with other agents. Using this regimen with 70% nitrous oxide in oxygen and an opiate premedication, Tackley and colleagues found that they had to supplement TIVA with isoflurane in 25% of spontaneously breathing patients who were undergoing body surface surgery (14). Manually adjusted infusion regimens also require that the anesthesiologist alter the rate at set time intervals, a technique that requires careful attention in the early stages of anesthesia, with the potential for distraction from patient monitoring.

TARGET-CONTROLLED INFUSION SYSTEMS

The pharmacokinetic parameters describing the distribution and elimination of anesthetic and analgesic agents can be incorporated into computerized infusion systems designed to achieve and to maintain any desired target blood concentration of drug appropriate for an individual patient and level of surgical stimulation. Target-controlled infusion (TCI) systems designed to deliver propofol for anesthesia and sedation have been described by several groups (9, 15–17). In addition, TCI systems delivering alfentanil have also been described, for supplementation of propofol anesthesia (16) and for the provision of postoperative analgesia (18).

Description

TCI systems deliver variable infusion schemes based on a complex mathematical solution to the pharmacokinetic model. Patient factors such as weight and age are entered into the system together with a "target" blood propofol concentration. The control software then calculates and delivers a rapid infusion designed to achieve this target concentration, followed by a computer-controlled constantly adjusting infusion regimen calculated to maintain the target concentration. A new target concentration can be selected at any stage. If a higher target concentration is chosen, the system will deliver a further rapid infusion. If a lower concentration is chosen, the control software will stop the infusion until it has calculated that the new target concentration has been achieved, after which the system will control the infusion rate to maintain the new target concentration. This method is analogous to the use of a calibrated vaporizer in that anesthesiologists select a target concentration of intravenous agent just as they would an inspired concentration of volatile agent. The target concentration can than be adjusted according to the patient's response to surgery. Figure 26B-7 shows target blood propofol concentrations, in an individual patient receiving a TCI of propofol, together with the infusion rate profile delivered by the system to achieve these theoretical concentrations. TCI of propofol has been shown superior to manually adjusted regimens with respect to cardiovascular stability during anesthesia and ease of use (19). By selecting a lower target concentration of propofol, these systems can be used to provide sedation for endoscopy (20) and for surgery under local or regional blockade (21), as well as in patients in intensive care units. In fact, TCI is particularly suitable for operative procedures requiring postoperative sedation in the intensive care unit, because, at the end of surgery, a target concentration suitable for sedation can be selected to provide seamless drug delivery into the postoperative period. Two prototype TCI systems capable of delivering TCI of propofol are shown in Figure 26B-8, and these systems will be commerically available from 1996.

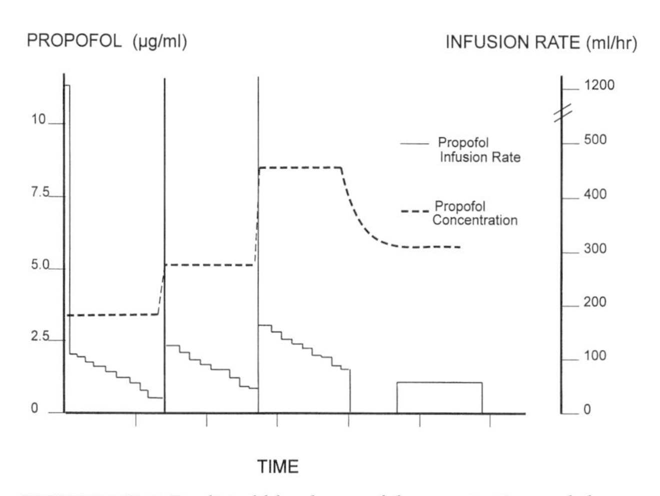

FIGURE 26B-7. Predicted blood propofol concentration and the concurrent infusion regimen during a target controlled infusion of propofol.

TCI systems can be evaluated in one of two ways: first, by comparison of measured and predicted blood concentrations of drug; and second, by clinical assessment of the quality of anesthesia delivered by the system.

Comparison of Measured and Predicted Drug Concentrations

During an evaluation study, anesthetic drug concentrations are measured in blood samples both during and after anesthesia and compared with the anesthetic concentrations predicted when using the delivery system. Pharmacokinetic performance is assessed by first calculating prediction error (PE) for each blood sample as follows:

$$\text{Prediction error } (\%) = \frac{\text{C(measured)} - \text{C(predicted)}}{\text{C(predicted)}}$$

where C is the anesthetic concentration.

The bias is defined as the mean prediction error and is a measure of the tendency of the delivery system to over- or underestimate the measured blood concentration in a given patient. Thus, if bias has a positive value, then the measured value is on average greater than the prediction and vice versa. Precision is defined as the mean value of the individual values of absolute

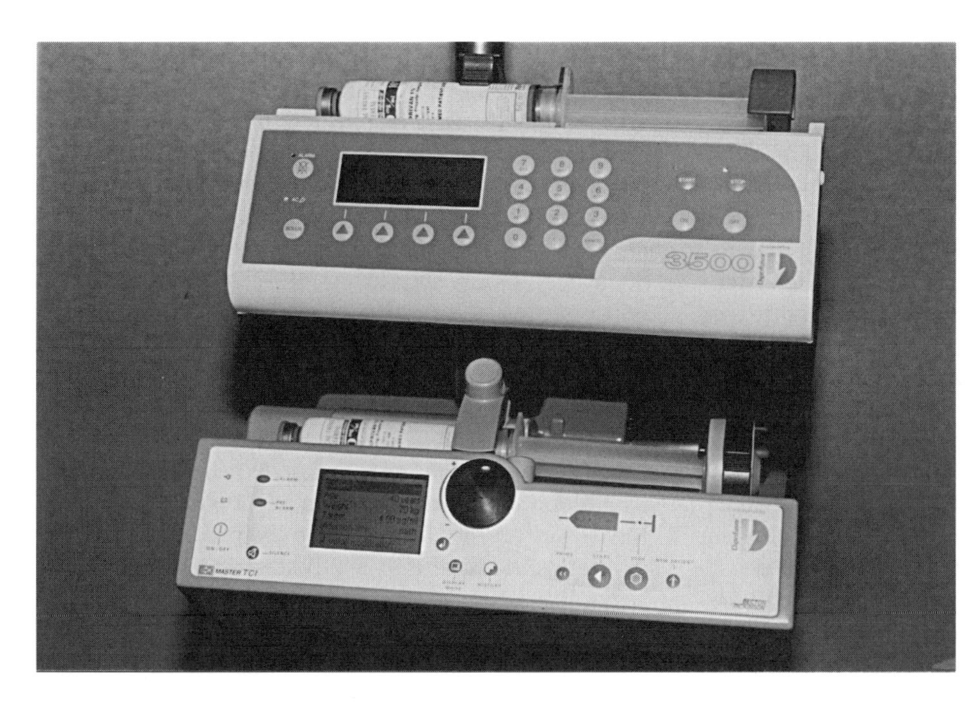

FIGURE 26B-8. Computer-controlled target-controlled infusion systems manufactured by Graseby Medical Ltd. (Colonial Way, Watford, Herts., UK) and Becton Dickinson and Co. (B.P. 3, 38590 Brézins, France).

prediction errors and is taken to be a measure of the degree of scatter of blood concentration values about the line of perfect prediction. Ideally, the delivery system should have a bias as close as possible to zero consistent with the smallest possible value for precision. Numerous factors affect pharmacokinetic performance.

The control software and hardware system must be capable of accurately implementing infusion regimens generated by the computer model, expressed by continuous mathematical functions. Currently available infusion devices are not capable of implementing such regimens precisely, however, and can only approximate them by delivering short stepped sequential zero order infusions. The degree of deviation of the delivered regimen from the theoretically ideal regimen described by the computer model depends on the update times employed and the resolution of the pump. The combination of computer and infusion pump must be validated together to detect any inconsistency between the volume that should be delivered and that which is actually administered by the infusion system (22).

Sources of Error

Technical errors in the administration of the infused drug lead to a discrepancy between the amount of drug prescribed and the amount delivered. Examples include extravasation of drug, stopcocks (taps) not opened, and incorrect concentration of drug in the syringe.

The sampling site is relevant because blood samples obtained simultaneously from different sites within the vascular system can give widely different values (23). Similarly, the time of sampling can affect the result because blood samples withdrawn during infusion at high flow rates when adequate mixing of the drug may not have occurred can produce abnormally high measurements of drug concentration (24–26). This phenomenon illustrates that the pharmacokinetic models with which the delivery devices are programmed are oversimplifications and do not reflect with complete accuracy the physiologic and pharmacokinetic processes that operate in the body.

The individual values of prediction error for each blood sample may vary considerably throughout the course of drug administration because of short-term changes in physiology that occur on exposure to different blood concentration of the anesthetic drug (e.g., dose-dependent pharmacokinetics) (27). Concurrent administration of adjuvant drugs may produce changes in the pharmacokinetics of the drug infused.

Pharmacokinetic mismatching between the delivery system and the study (patient) population is the most common source of high bias values. Usually, the pharmacokinetic model and its associated parameters are derived from a formal pharmacokinetic study of a small patient population in which a bolus dose of the drug is administered to each patient and pharmacokinetic modeling is performed on the basis of the subsequent decay of drug concentration in the individual patient's blood. This initial decay phase may be poorly characterized because of the effects of inadequate mixing and the necessity for rapid sampling. As a consequence, some of the derived parameters are inaccurate. The other major problem in this respect is that of inherent pharmacokinetic variability among surgical patients receiving similar drugs for the same type of operation.

Alternatively, data derived during and after drug infusions may be subjected to computer-based remodeling procedures to obtain the best patient model in terms of bias or precision in a retrospective fashion. For example, compared with adults, young children have an increased requirement for propofol (on a milligrams-per-kilogram basis) during anesthesia. This increased requirement is partly related to altered pharmacokinetic variables in the pediatric population (28). When the delivery system described by White and Kenny (15) was reprogrammed with revised pharmacokinetic parameters that more accurately described the elimination and distribution of propofol in children, better agreement was achieved between the measured and predicted blood concentrations in a subsequent prospective study (28).

During delivery of anesthesia using systems based on population pharmacokinetics, a degree of mismatch between the computer-based model and an individual patient's pharmacokinetic profile is inevitable. Much research is directed toward minimizing and describing this deviation. This problem will probably not be eliminated, unless it were possible to measure the true blood concentrations of an anesthetic drug online and feedback in real time the measurements directly to the TCI system. This method would allow correction of the pharmacokinetic model for each individual patient and would decrease or remove the variation between measured and predicted blood concentrations of the drug. In clinical situations, however, the delivery device does not have to be completely accurate in terms of achieving the selected target drug concentration. Such acquisition should certainly be optimized, but will not always be perfect. A bias of between 10 and 20% and an associated precision of less than 30% seem to be adequate for clinical practice (16). New sensors under development may be able to measure concentrations of anesthetic agents within the blood in real time (29), but questions whether a knowledge of actual true blood concentration of an anesthetic drug will allow the effect that it achieves to be predicted more accurately still remain. Probably, the pharmacodynamic variability of anesthetic drugs among and within patients is even more variable than the pharmacokinetics. This inherent variability is further increased by the influence of other relevant factors such as concurrent drug administration and intensity of surgical stimulus. Kenny and his colleagues have described the marked variations in measured blood propofol concentrations required for different levels of surgical stimulation (11). Similarly, Shafer has described the relationship among the propofol infusion rate, blood concentrations, anesthetic technique, and surgical stress (12).

In practice, however, the clinician titrates drug delivery to a particular effect using the TCI infusion device to achieve proportional changes based on pharmacokinetic principles. The variability of measured drug concentration in relation to that which is predicted is not confined to intravenous anesthesia. For inhalational anesthetics, investigators have demonstrated considerable variability of blood partial vapor pressures in relation to end-tidal partial pressure values, especially during periods of rapid change in inspired vapor concentrations (30–32).

Clinical Evaluation

Clinically, systems can be assessed by the way in which they affect patients in terms of drug side effects (or toxicity) and, subjectively, by the quality of anesthesia. Equally important are the ease of use and "user satisfaction" with respect to the anesthesiologist.

Quality of Anesthesia

Cardiovascular and respiratory depression occur frequently after a bolus dose of propofol, typical reductions in systolic blood pressure being in the order of 25%, with a frequency of apnea of 50% or more (33, 34). Decreasing the peak concentration achieved by inducing anesthesia with a continuous infusion may reduce the frequency of adverse effects (35). A similar improvement in the incidence of adverse cardiorespiratory effects was demonstrated by Chaudhri and colleagues, who studied 60 patients premedicated with temazepam (19). Patients were allocated randomly to receive an infusion of propofol designed to achieve and to maintain a target propofol concentration of 3, 4, or 5 μg/ml. Induction time was measured from the start of the infusion to loss of verbal contact. The success rate of inducing anesthesia within 3 minutes of achieving the target concentration was 40%, 75%, and 90% when the predicted target concentration was 3, 4, and 5 μg/ml, respectively. Significant reductions in arterial pressure occurred 3 minutes after achieving the target concentrations, but these reductions were about 15% of the baseline values compared with typical reductions of 25% reported following induction with bolus doses. The frequency of apnea and pain on injection was also low in all groups. Selecting a target propofol concentration of 5 μg/ml would successfully induce anesthesia in the majority of patients premedicated with temazepam without clinically significant hemodynamic or respiratory side effects.

Published reports from anesthesiologists who used TCI suggest that its ability to provide smooth control of induction in difficult anesthetic situations is a major clinical advantage (36–38). Alvis and colleagues reported fewer interventions and improved hemodynamic stability when they employed a TCI delivery device compared with a manual technique to infuse fentanyl during cardiac anesthesia (17). Similar benefits were reported using a TCI system for alfentanil to supplement nitrous oxide during lower abdominal surgery (39). Satisfactory cardiorespiratory stability with rapid recovery has also been reported using TCI with propofol to provide sedation in patients undergoing endoscopic procedures (20) and surgery under local anesthesia (40).

Ease of Use

One study has assessed the ease of use of TCI by anesthesiologists not previously exposed to the technique (41). Thirty anesthesiologists were instructed in the use of the TCI system and were then given a system for their own use. Their attitudes to administering TIVA with TCI propofol were assessed by questionnaire after a 12-week experience with the TCI system. The results showed that 27 of the 30 anesthesiologists had increased their use of propofol for maintenance of anesthesia, largely because of improved control and greater confidence regarding the predictability of the anesthetic effect. All the anesthesiologists in this study found it acceptable to titrate the target blood concentration of the anesthetic drug (rather than the infusion rate) against the patient's response to surgical stimulation.

Effective Blood Concentration (MAC Equivalence)

Although many reports have compared the relative effects of volatile and intravenous agents, designing comparative studies based on equipotent doses of the different anesthetics has been difficult. Anesthesiologists tend to consider the potency of volatile agents in terms of the minimum alveolar concentration (MAC) of the anesthetic required to prevent purposeful movement in 50% of patients in response to a noxious stimulus. Similarly, the effective blood concentration (EC_{50}) of propofol required to prevent response to surgical incision in 50% of patients can be determined. A study designed to express the potency of propofol in equivalent terms to MAC for volatile agents determined the EC_{50} and EC_{95} in female patients breathing either 100% oxygen or 67% nitrous oxide in oxygen (26). Propofol was administered by a TCI system programmed to maintain the blood propofol concentration at a predetermined target value, and the response to the initial skin incision was observed. The EC_{50} for patients who received propofol and nitrous oxide was 4.5 μg/ml and the EC_{95} was 4.7 μg/ml. For those who received only propofol, the EC_{50} and EC_{95} were 6.0 and 6.2 μg/ml, respectively. Such an approach allows the anesthesiologist to select with greater confidence a target blood concentration that produces adequate anesthesia and thereby minimizes the risk of awareness in patients who concurrently receive neuromuscular blocking agents. In addition, this method should enable more accurate comparisons to be made between the relative anesthetic and adverse effects of intravenous and inhalational agents by providing a better appreciation of equipotent doses.

Closed-loop Systems

In spite of the sophistication of TCI drug delivery, the anesthesiologist still has to rely on clinical judgment to assess drug effect and to alter the target concentration as appropriate. The whole process could be automated by a feedback loop if a reliable measurement of drug effect existed (i.e., brain monitor).

Patient-Controlled Analgesia

The efficacy of analgesia can only be assessed adequately by the individual patient receiving the analgesic medication. Therefore, the control signal in a closed-loop analgesia system must come from the patient's own degree of satisfaction with their pain control. Various systems offer patient-controlled analgesia (PCA). This is usually provided in the form of an intravenous bolus of an opioid analgesic in response to a button press by the patient. Such systems have been shown to be superior to intermittent intramuscular morphine with respect to the quality of analgesia (42, 43) and nursing satisfaction (44). Problems with this approach, however, are that patients require an initial bolus to achieve a therapeutic effect, and the system cannot keep the patient pain-free because the patient only initiates a bolus in response to pain. One way to overcome these deficiencies is to program into the system an initial bolus dose and a background continuous infusion. With drugs such as morphine, however, this method can lead to accumulation and respiratory depression. An alternative approach was adopted by Davies and colleagues (18). They described a TCI of alfentanil, which rapidly achieved the required level of analgesia because of the rapid onset of alfentanil's action. The target level was then altered by the nursing staff in response to the patient's request. This nurse-controlled system has been modified so the target concentration of alfentanil is increased in response to button presses by the patient (45). The control software also slowly reduces the target concentration over a period of time if no button presses are detected. An added safety feature is that the system can be linked to a pulse oximeter, so if the oxygen saturation falls below a predefined limit, the infusion will be rapidly be reduced by the computer until the saturation level rises above this preset limit.

Patient-Controlled Sedation

Studies have described the use of standard PCA infusion devices for the delivery of patient-controlled sedation with propofol, alfentanil, or midazolam. Hopkins and colleagues described patient-controlled neuroleptanalgesia in 22 patients who used a PCA pump to deliver a droperidol-alfentanil mixture during minor gynecologic surgery (46). The majority of patients remained detached, sedated, and pain-free during the procedure. Ghouri and co-workers assessed propofol, alfentanil, or midazolam self-administered using a PCA pump, to provide sedation during outpatient surgery performed with the patient under local analgesia (47). After intravenous premedication with midazolam 1 mg and fentanyl 50 μg, 90 patients were randomized to receive propofol, alfentanil, or midazolam when self-administered by a PCA pump. Patients were allowed to self-administer 2-ml bolus doses of alfentanil (250 μg/ml), midazolam (0.4 mg/ml), or propofol (10 mg/ml), with a lockout time of 3 minutes to supplement a basal infusion of the same drug at 5 ml/h. The authors noted that although all three regimens proved acceptable to the patients, the alfentanil regimen was associated with more episodes of desaturation ($SpO_2 < 90\%$) and an increased incidence of postoperative nausea and vomiting. Similarly, Zelcer and colleagues described patient-controlled administration of alfentanil by PCA pump in 80 patients having vaginal ovum-retrieval procedures. These investigators compared this technique with physician-controlled alfentanil administration and found the two regimens equally effective despite a lockout time of 3 minutes in the group administering their own sedation (48).

An alternative approach is to use a TCI with the control software increasing the target concentration in response to button presses by the patient. This system still requires a lockout period to allow the effect site concentration to equilibrate with that in the blood. A further enhancement to this system would be to program the control software to estimate the effect site drug concentration and only allow further increases in target concentration when blood and effect site drug concentration have equilibrated. This type of system for administering propofol is currently under investigation for providing patient-controlled sedation during radiologic and other procedures (Kenny, personal communication).

Closed-loop Anesthesia

To deliver closed-loop anesthesia, a measurement of depth of anesthesia is required. Considerable efforts have been made over the years to develop a reliable index of anesthetic depth. Most attempts have been based on some form of processed EEG. The compressed spectral array (CSA) analyzes time segments of the raw EEG and provides a measure of the distribution of the power contained within the signal. Separate epochs of EEG activity are recorded, and the power contained within different frequencies is calculated and displayed, usually as a series of troughs and peaks. Under anesthesia, power shifts to the lower frequencies and provides a guide to the extent of global cerebral suppression. The spectral edge is the frequency below which is contained 95% of the total power in the CSA and provides a measure of the upper edge of the power spectrum. This EEG parameter has been shown to decrease with increasing concentrations of anesthetic, but a poor correlation exists between the spectral edge frequency and the anesthetic concentration during the transition from deep to light anesthesia (49).

The median frequency represents the midpoint of the power distribution in the CSA and is the frequency below and above which lies 50% of the total power in the EEG. The median frequency has been suggested to be an accurate indicator of depth of anesthesia in that it appears to have a close relationship with drug concentrations in both the uptake and elimination phases (49). Moreover, a satisfactory level of anesthesia is reported to occur at a median frequency of 2 to 3 Hz (50). Different types of anesthetic agent appear to produce varying patterns of CSA in anesthetized patients, however. The recording of discrete time epochs of EEG can also lead to difficulties in analysis during periods of burst suppression activity in the EEG. Bispectral analysis of the EEG is an additional technique that has been suggested to correlate best with the level of anesthesia (51, 52) and sedation (53) (Figure 26B-9).

Changes in RR interval of the electrocardiogram, so-called heart rate variability (54) and changes in lower esophageal contraction (55, 56) have also been proposed as an index of anesthetic depth. None of these techniques have proved reliable enough for routine clinical use for closed-loop anesthesia. The combination of heart rate variability and the processed EEG signal may prove more useful in judging depth of anesthesia and sedation during commonly used balanced anesthetic techniques.

The auditory evoked potential (AEP) has been investigated as an alternative measure of the depth of anesthesia. It is obtained by delivering auditory stimuli in the form of clicks to earphones at a frequency of 6 to 12 Hz. The EEG activity is recorded after each click from three electrodes placed on the scalp, and several hundred EEG sweeps are filtered and averaged to produce the AEP. Thornton and colleagues have reported that the AEP provides a reproducible guide to the level of anesthesia obtained with many different anesthetic agents and responds appropriately to different levels of surgical stimulation (57). A single parameter derived from the AEP has been used to control the deliv-

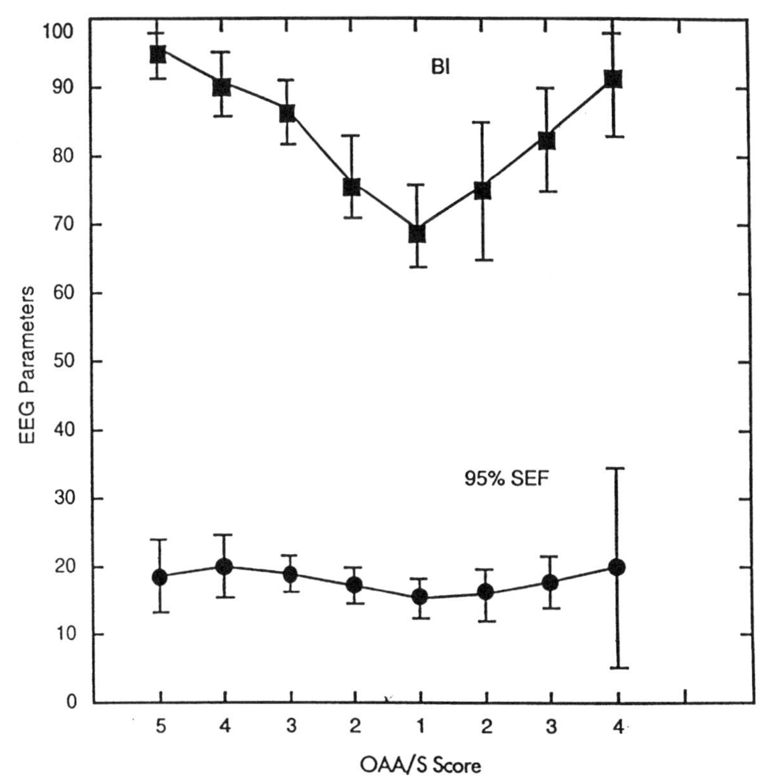

FIGURE 26B-9. EEG-bispectral index (BI) and 95% spectral edge frequency (95% SEF) as a function of the level of midazolam-induced sedation during the onset and recovery phases. The EEG parameters are mean ± S.E. (*Adapted from* Liu J, Singh H, White PF. EEG bispectral analysis predicts the depth of midazolam-induced sedation. An esthesiology 1996;84:64–69.

ery of propofol in patients breathing spontaneously during surgery (58). No patient was aware during the surgical procedures. Although the patients recalled hearing the clicks as their last memory before loss of consciousness, none of the patients were concerned by the clicks, and all were prepared to have the same anesthetic in the future. Closed-loop control of anesthesia will probably not become a routine part of anesthetic practice in the near future, but it offers the possibility of providing a valuable and unbiased assessment technique to examine the effects of supplementary drugs and to compare equipotent doses of different intravenous and volatile agents.

In summary, European physicians have been involved in the evolution of intravenous anesthesia and analgesia from an early stage. The concurrent use of regional anesthesia and of a spontaneous respiration technique for general anesthesia is widespread in Europe, and TIVA is particularly suitable for this approach. Newer intravenous anesthetic and analgesic agents such as propofol and remifentanil possess pharmacokinetic profiles well-suited to TIVA, and these agents have been available in Europe for longer than in the United States. Therefore, European anesthesiologists have more experience with sophisticated intravenous delivery systems. In the past, the potential advantages of TIVA over inhalation techniques were offset by the greater ease of use of calibrated vaporizers, compared with manually adjusted infusion regimens. The development of TCI systems has taken much of the "guess work" out of the use of TIVA, however, and allows flexible control of the depth of anesthesia and sedation in a manner analogous to the use of the calibrated vaporizer for delivering inhaled agents. The development of equipment capable of measuring parameters related to the depth of anesthesia (e.g., EEG bispectral and AEP), have allowed closed-loop TIVA to become a useful research tool. Perhaps this technique will be available for routine clinical use in the near future.

REFERENCES

1. Ledingham IM, Watt I. Influence of sedation on mortality in critically ill multiple trauma patients [Letter]. Lancet 1983; 1:1270.
2. Fellows IW, Bastow MD, Byrne AJ, Allison SP. Adrenocortical suppression in multiply injured patients: a complication of etomidate treatment. Br Med J Clin Res Ed 1983;287:1835–1837.
3. Servin F, Cockshott ID, Farinotti R, et al. Pharmacokinetics of propofol infusions in patients with cirrhosis. Br J Anaesth 1990; 65:177–183.
4. Gray PA, Park GR, Cockshott ID, et al. Propofol metabolism in man during the anhepatic and reperfusion phases of liver transplantation. Xenobiotica 1992;22:105–114.
5. Hull CJ. Pharmacokinetics and pharmacodynamics. Br J Anaesth 1979;51:579–594.
6. Cook DR, Freeman JA, Lai AA, et al. Pharmacokinetics of mivacurium in normal patients and in those with hepatic or renal failure. Br J Anaesth 1992;69:580–585.
7. Gepts E, Jonckheer K, Maes V, et al. Disposition kinetics of propofol during alfentanil anaesthesia. Anaesthesia 1988;43 (suppl):8–13.
8. Prys-Roberts FL, Dixon J, Lewis GT, et al. Induction and maintenance of propofol anaesthesia: a manual infusion scheme. Anaesthesia 1988;43 (suppl):14–17.
9. Glass PS, Markham K, Ginsberg B, Hawkins ED. Propofol concentrations required for surgery. Anesthesiology 1989;71:A273.
10. Lemmens HJ, Burm AG, Bovill JG, et al. Pharmacodynamics of alfentanil: the role of plasma protein binding. Anesthesiology 1992;76:65–70.
11. Kenny GN, McFadzean WA, Mantzaridis H. Propofol requirements during closed-loop anesthesia. Anesthesiology 1993; 79:A329.
12. Shafer SL. Advances in propofol pharmacokinetics and pharmacodynamics. J Clin Anesth 1993;5:14S–21S.
13. Buhrer M, Maitre PO, Crevoisier C, Stanski DR. Electroencephalographic effects of benzodiazepines. II. Pharmacodynamic modeling of the electroencephalographic effects of midazolam and diazepam. Clin Pharmacol Ther 1990;48:555–567.
14. Tackley RM, Lewis GT, Prys Roberts C, et al. Computer controlled infusion of propofol. Br J Anaesth 1989;62:46–53.
15. White M, Kenny GN. Intravenous propofol anaesthesia using a computerised infusion system. Anaesthesia 1990;45:204–209.
16. Schüttler J, Kloos S, Schwilden H, Stoeckel H. Total intravenous anaesthesia with propofol and alfentanil by computer-assisted infusion. Anaesthesia 1988;43 (suppl):2–7.
17. Alvis JM, Reves JG, Govier AV, et al. Computer-assisted continuous infusions of fentanyl during cardiac anesthesia: comparison with a manual method. Anesthesiology 1985;63:41–49.
18. Davies FW, White M, Kenny GN. Postoperative analgesia using a computerised infusion of alfentanil following aortic bifurcation graft surgery. Int J Clin Monit Comput 1992;9:207–212.
19. Chaudhri S, White M, Kenny GN. Induction of anaesthesia with propofol using a target-controlled infusion system. Anaesthesia 1992;47:551–553.
20. Church JA, Stanton PD, Kenny GN, Anderson JR. Propofol for sedation during endoscopy: assessment of a computer-controlled infusion system. Gastrointest Endosc 1991;37:175–179.
21. Skipsey IG, Colvin JR, Mackenzie N, Kenny GN. Sedation with propofol during surgery under local blockade: assessment of a target-controlled infusion system. Anaesthesia 1993;48:210–213.
22. Kenny GN, White M. A portable target controlled propofol infusion system. Int J Clin Monit Comput 1992;9:179–182.
23. Major E, Aun C, Yate PM, et al. Influence of sample site on blood concentrations of ICI 35868. Br J Anaesth 1983;55:371–375.
24. Chiou WL. Potential pitfalls in conventional pharmocokinetic studies: effects of the initial mixing of drug in blood and the pulmonary first-pass elimination. J Pharmacokinet Biopharm 1979;7:527–536.
25. White M, Kenny GN. Evaluation of a computerised propofol infusion system. Anesthesiology 1989;71:A278.
26. Davidson JA, McLeod AD, Howie JC, et al. The effective concentration$_{50}$ for propofol with and without 67% nitrous oxide. Acta Anaesthesiol Scand 1993;37:458–464.
27. Sear JW, Diedericks J, Foex P. Continuous infusions of propofol administered to dogs: effects on ICG and propofol disposition. Br J Anaesth 1994;72:451–455.
28. Marsh BJ, White M, Morton N, Kenny GN. Pharmacokinetic model driven infusion of propofol in children. Br J Anaesth 1991;67:41–48.
29. Merlo S, Yager P, Burgess LW. Development of fiber optic sensor for detection of general anesthetics and other small molecules. In: D'Argenio DZ, ed. Advanced methods of pharmocokinetic and pharmacodynamic systems analysis. New York: Plenum, 1991:155–170.

30. Carpenter RL, Eger EI. Alveolar-to-arterial-to-venous anesthetic partial pressure differences in humans. Anesthesiology 1989;70:630–635.
31. Dwyer RC, Fee JP, Howard PJ, Clarke RS. Arterial washing of halothane and isoflurane in young and elderly adult patients. Br J Anaesth 1991;66:572–579.
32. Frei FJ, Zbinden AM, Thomson DA, Rieder HU. Is the end-tidal partial pressure of isoflurane a good predictor of its arterial partial pressure? Br J Anaesth 1991;66:331–339.
33. Price ML, Walmsley A, Swaine C, Ponte J. Comparison of a total intravenous anaesthetic technique using a propofol infusion, with an inhalational technique using enflurane for day case surgery. Anaesthesia 1988;43 (suppl):84–87.
34. Goodman NW, Black AMS, Carter JA. Some ventilatory effects of propofol as a sole anaesthetic agent. Br J Anaesth 1980; 59:1497–1503.
35. Peacock JE, Lewis RP, Reilly CS, Nimmo WS. Effect of different rates of infusion of propofol for induction of anaesthesia in elderly patients. Br J Anaesth 1990;65:346–352.
36. Crofts SL, Hutchison GL. General anaesthesia and undrained pneumothorax: the use of a computer-controlled propofol infusion. Anaesthesia 1991;46:192–194.
37. Donnelly JA, Webster RE. Computer-controlled anaesthesia in the management of bronchopleural fistula. Anaesthesia 1991; 46:383–384.
38. MacKenzie RE, McFadzean WA. A difficult airway managed by computer? Anaesthesia 1992;47:633–634.
39. Ausems ME, Vuyk J, Hug CC Jr, Stanski DR. Comparison of a computer-assisted infusion versus intermittent bolus administration of alfentanil as a supplement to nitrous oxide for lower abdominal surgery. Anesthesiology 1988;68:851–861.
40. Skipsey IG, Colvin JR, Kenny GN. Sedation with propofol during surgery under regional blockade. Br J Anaesth 1991;67:218–219P.
41. Taylor I, White M, Kenny GN. Assessment of the value and pattern of use of a target controlled propofol infusion system. Int J Clin Monit Comput 1993;10:175–180.
42. Wasylak TJ, Abbott FV, English MJM, Jeans MJ. Reduction of post-operative morbidity following patient-controlled morphine. Can J Anaesth 1990;37:726–731.
43. Kenady DE, Wilson JF, Schwartz RW, et al. A randomized comparison of patient-controlled versus standard analgesic requirements in patients undergoing cholecystectomy. Surg Gynecol Obstet 1992;174:216–220.
44. Aitken HA, Kenny GN. Use of patient-controlled analgesia in postoperative cardiac surgical patients: a survey of ward staff attitudes. Intensive Care Nursing 1990;6:74–78.
45. Irwin MG, Jones RD, Visram AR, Kornberg JP. A patient's experience of a new postoperative patient-controlled analgesic technique. Eur J Anaesth 1994;11:413–415.
46. Hopkins D, Shipton EA, Tissandie JP. Extending patient-controlled analgesia to patient-controlled neuroleptanalgesia. S Afr J Surg 1992;30:168–170.
47. Ghouri AF, Taylor E, White PF. Patient-controlled drug administration during local anesthesia: a comparison of midazolam, propofol, and alfentanil. J Clin Anesth 1992;4:476–479.
48. Zelcer J, White PF, Chester S, et al. Intraoperative patient-controlled analgesia: an alternative to physician administration during outpatient monitored anesthesia care. Anesth Analg 1992;75:41–44.
49. Arden JR, Holley FO, Stanski DR. Increased sensitivity to etomidate in the elderly: initial distribution versus altered brain response. Anesthesiology 1986;65:19–27.
50. Schwilden H, Stoeckel H. Effective therapeutic infusions produced by closed-loop feedback control of methohexital administration during total intravenous anesthesia with fentanyl. Anesthesiology 1990;73:225–229.
51. Kearse LA Jr, Manberg P, DeBros F, et al. Bispectral analysis of the electroencephalogram during induction of anesthesia may predict hemodynamic responses to laryngoscopy and intubation. Electroencephalogr Clin Neurophysiol 1994;90:194–200.
52. Kearse LA Jr, Manberg P, Chamoun N, et al. Bispectral analysis of the electroencephalogram correlates with patient movement to skin incision during propofol/nitrous oxide anesthesia. Anesthesiology 1994;81:1365–1370.
53. Liu J, Singh H, White PF. EEG bispectral analysis predicts the depth of midazolam-induced sedation. Anesthesiology 1996; 84:64–69.
54. Pomfrett CJ, Sneyd JR, Barrie JR, Healy TE. Respiratory sinus arrhythmia: comparison with EEG indices during isoflurane anaesthesia at 0.65 and 1.2 MAC. Br J Anaesth 1994;72:397–402.
55. Evans JM, Davies WL. Monitoring Anesthesia. In: Sear JW, ed. Clinics in anesthesiology. Philadelphia: WB Saunders, 1984:242–262.
56. Sessler DI, Stoen R, Olofsson CI, Chow F. Lower esophageal contractility predicts movement during skin incision in patients anesthetised with halothane but not with nitrous oxide and alfentanil. Anesthesiology 1989;70:42–46.
57. Thornton C, Konieczko K, Jones JG, et al. Effect of surgical stimulation on the auditory evoked response. Br J Anaesth 1988; 60:372–378.
58. Kenny GN, McFadzean WA, Mantzaridis H, Fisher AC. Closed-loop control of anesthesia. Anesthesiology 1992;77:A328.

26C Australian Perspective

David P. Crankshaw

The modern anesthesiologist desires fixed-rate infusions, as well as sophisticated variable-rate infusions, based on drug pharmacokinetics and pharmacodynamics. Neither electronic nor mechanical technology is a limiting factor in the development of complex drug-infusion delivery systems. A confirmation of this concept is apparent in many of the routinely used critical care devices (e.g., ventilators and defibrillators) that perform calculations including feedback on physiologic signals. Clearly, technology is not the limiting step. The general lack of development of infusion technology is in stark contrast to the numerous peer-reviewed journal articles, reviews, and textbooks that describe the value of pharmacokinetic prediction in achieving clinical goals. Although it is technically simple to compute a mathematic function in real time and to use this to set a delivery rate, infusion pumps capable of performing this task have not reached the commercial marketplace.

Specific tables detailing stepped infusion rates required to achieve and maintain a specified target drug concentration in surgical patients have been described for various anesthetic drugs (1). Pharmacokinetic models, designed to predict therapeutic concentrations when the target concentration is altered, have also been described (2). These systems usually incorporate the names of drugs, as well as data that specify infusion rates, reflecting the pharmacokinetic properties of each drug. The question is why, if the technology is available and the theory is well-known, do no commercial devices exist?

REGULATION OF THERAPEUTIC PRODUCTS

Therapeutic goods include both chemical substances and medical devices. These goods are regulated separately in Australia by the Drug Safety and Evaluation Branch and the Therapeutic Devices Branch of the Commonwealth Department of Health and Social Services. These branches operate under separate sets of regulations and perform different functions. For drugs, a therapeutic claim is based on demonstrated safety and efficacy in achieving some clinical goal in a defined patient population. Safety must be demonstrated by evaluating animal data where larger or prolonged exposure has been undertaken. Efficacy is established by clinical trials in representative patient populations. This involves evaluation of the ability of the formulation to achieve therapeutic levels, evaluation of the ability of the drug to achieve therapeutic end points against stated claims for the drug, and a determination of the incidence of any short- or long-term side effects resulting from its administration. All this evaluation must be conducted over a range of therapeutic situations corresponding to the situations in which the drug is likely to be used. This stipulation generally requires multicenter trials and is a time-consuming and expensive process involving a large bureaucracy and considerable expenditure both for the conduct of the trials and for the preparation of the documentation.

In contrast, most devices perform a clearly defined function and do not usually require clinical studies to determine whether they are capable of achieving this function. A constant-rate infusion device, for example, requires evaluation of quality in the design and manufacturing process to ensure reliability, compliance with relevant safety and performance standards according to the specifications of the device, and finally certification that labeling is appropriate and accurate. This straightforward process does not involve clinical trials and hence has a relatively small cost.

TARGET-CONTROLLED INFUSION DEVICE

If one analyzes a preprogrammed target-controlled infusion (TCI) device, it is clear that therapeutic claims are made for the device and the device consists of two distinct parts. The first part is a predictive control system that provides a control signal specifying the rate at which the drug must be delivered. This system contains the name of one or more drugs, some data, and mathematic capability relating to each drug that is used to generate the control signal. The second part is the underlying infusion system, controlled by a microprocessor. It is the same as a device designed for fixed-rate delivery of drugs, except the rate is varied from time to time according to a control message from the controller (first part), in contrast to its being altered by the operator.

Provided an infusion system accurately translates the control signal into the drug delivery rate specified by the control system, the therapeutic claims must be for the control system and not for the delivery system itself. The high cost of validating therapeutic claims clearly makes approval of an integrated TCI system extremely expensive. This additional cost for development and evaluation adds markedly to the unit cost, and furthermore, such evaluation must be repeated each time the control system is added to or altered in any way.

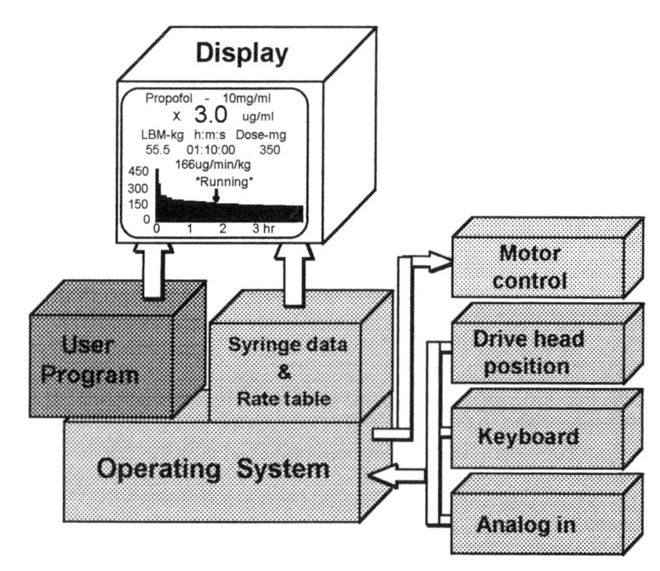

FIGURE 26C-1. Block diagram of the functional components of a proposed target-controlled infusion (TCI) device. The pale shaded area is the basic device implementing target-controlled step programs entered by the operator. The User Program, shown in darker shading, is loaded to perform a specific function for which separate regulatory approval is required. The pattern of all infusion patterns is continuously displayed.

USE OF THE PHYSICIAN'S KNOWLEDGE

An alternative to an integrated TCI system is a purpose-built device suitable for being programmed by the user. In this way, one or more tables of infusion information and the name of the table may be entered. The infusion rate can then be scaled according to the size of the patient and further scaled according to an assessment of the clinical requirement. Simple infusion rate profiles are contained in the product information for intravenous anesthetic drugs. For example, a bolus of propofol, 2.0 to 2.5 mg/kg, followed by a profile consisting of 10 mg/kg/h for 10 minutes, 8 mg/kg/h for 10 minutes, then 6 mg/kg/h thereafter is recommended by Zeneca/ICI Pharmaceuticals (3). This regimen reflects, among others, the clinical studies of Prys-Roberts and colleagues (4). If a suitable infusion device is programmed with such a profile, the physician decides on the method of infusion for the particular drug and clinical situation. This avoids the regulatory process in favor of the preferable process of medical education. It is, after all, the physician who chooses the drug, fills the syringe, and sets the target concentration. The addition of a variable-rate infusion pattern that the physician can vary at any time would seem more appropriate than government regulation of this aspect of patient care. An infusion pump with basic features to permit variable-rate delivery according to simple tabulated patterns would be a great improvement over existing technology.

Knowledge of physicians can be enhanced by utilizing published tables of delivery rates as a function of patient body weight and of delivery rates to achieve various clinical end points from the medical literature and to avoid mandatory adherence to commercial programs. Interested commercial parties can, of course, make recommendations by way of product information that most physicians would find useful (5). By allowing the physician to be responsible for the drug delivery program, the overall magnitude of the delivery rate pattern can be established according to the weight of the patient and modified as necessary according to the clinical assessment. Simple scaling of the overall magnitude of a variable-rate infusion pattern, determined by the physician and not by the supplier of the infusion device, permits practical administration of intravenous anesthetic drugs without the need for complex computation and prediction capability in the device and hence avoids the need for an evaluation of the device in terms of its therapeutic efficacy. This process is already well understood by anesthetists in their day-to-day use of volatile anesthetic agents.

The ability to set an infusion pump to deliver a variable-rate pattern already exists in the Versitaper function of the IMED Gemini Series of infusion pumps. An extension of this design is to permit a basic pattern to be scaled according to the size of the patient, such as based on total body weight (TBW). This type of function is seen in the Baxter Autosyringe syringe pumps. The combination of these two design features would be major advances in the implementation of intravenous anesthesia.

A further refinement, still within the confines of existing infusion pump technology, is to provide a "scaling factor" for use by the operator. For example, by programming an infusion profile for a target concentration of propofol of 1 μg/ml, this scaling factor becomes numerically equal to the expected arterial blood or target propofol concentration in the central nervous system (CNS). A table of infusion rates as a function of time using infusion pattern from previous studies to achieve a therapeutic propofol concentration of 1 μg/ml in the arterial blood is programmed into the pump and, with scaling by a factor of 10, would be expected to result in a concentration range up to 10 μg/ml. A similar pattern has been published for the opioid analgesic alfentanil (6). Hence, a simple but effective TCI device can be produced for anesthesiologists without involvement of the regulatory agencies. The responsibility for creating a device containing infusion patterns and appropriate scaling factors is entirely that of the physician-programmer. This type of device would rely on published data and the knowledge that the pattern must be appropriate to the needs of a particular patient. This approach places the responsibility on the education process and avoids the risk that predictions made by evaluators of therapeutic goods (e.g., regulatory agencies) at one or more sites are not referable to all sites or patients.

OTHER SUPPLIERS CAN OBTAIN APPROVAL FOR INFUSION REGIMENS

The process of physician programming of infusion devices can be facilitated if pharmaceutical companies are prepared to provide recommendations for drug-specific information and to provide the complex mathematic algorithms needed to compute delivery rates and support clinical trials to establish the efficacy of a particular delivery method. This information could then be incorporated in a separate module suitable for loading into an already approved syringe pump. Incorporation of this information could occur by uploading a control program to reside in the infusion pump or by attachment of a physically discrete *programming module*. Specific programming modules would perhaps achieve better results than an individual physician programming an operator-designed infusion scheme, and would permit the manufacturer of a new drug (e.g., remifentanil) to recommend a delivery pattern based on the results of clinical trials and to protect the control program from inappropriate modification. This type of module would, of course, become a *therapeutic device* separate from the infusion pump, and the data supporting its efficacy would become the responsibility of the supplier of the module. Any module that takes over the decision-making process from the individual physician would require approval as an additional therapeutic modality.

FEATURES OF CURRENT INFUSION DEVICES

In considering the design of any new syringe pump, it is important to specify which features already exist in clinical practice because this simplifies the regulatory process. Certain features improve the functionality of basic fixed-rate infusion devices. These features are in no way predictive, but already perform scaling procedures on values entered by the physician. The typical features include the following:

1. An ability to alter characteristics of the device using a *setup mode* so that rate limits, drug units displayed on the screen, alarm signals, pressure limits, syringes to be used, dose rates to be used, and communication settings may be altered. These programming features can only be entered using a sequence of button presses not normally implemented by the user (e.g., IVAC Model 770). This permits incorporation of protocols, by agreement between the biomedical engineering department and physicians, that are "locked in" until protocols are revised and thus avoids inadvertent alteration.
2. An ability to view the features and programs that have been inserted and locked in before and during operation by the individual practitioner (e.g., IVAC Model 770).
3. An ability of a device to learn settings from another device (e.g., IVAC Model 770).
4. An ability to program a sequence of delivery rates indirectly by entering a series of set volumes of drug solution and the times over which that volume must be given, thereby allowing the pump to calculate the actual delivery rate (e.g., IMED Gemini PC-1 or PC-2).
5. An ability to enter an infusion rate, the patient's body weight, and the concentration of the drug and then to display the rate of delivery in a standardized form for easy interpretation (e.g., Graseby 3400).
6. An ability to scale bolus and infusion rate to the patient's body weight (e.g., Baxter Autosyringe Model AS20GH-2).

Each of these examples illustrates features that extend the capability of a simple syringe pump. These features alter the way the device functions or displays information by performing simple *calculations* without having to predict what will occur in the patient.

DESIGNING A NEW DEVICE

The device must have an liquid crystal diode (LCD) display that can present entered data in graphic form so the pattern prescribed by the physician can be observed and transcription errors identified before use of the device. When the device is delivered from the manufacturer, it should contain software functions that permit the practitioner to perform the following functions:

1. To enter one or more sets of delivery rates and the time intervals during which each rate will operate.
2. To name each of the sets of infusion rates so a particular set may be chosen and the name of the set displayed during the operation.
3. To indicate whether this rate is to be scaled to individual weight, body surface area, or some other measure of patient size.
4. To enter a scaling factor or multiplication factor that will increase or decrease the overall size of the delivery rate pattern.
5. To suggest a starting value for this multiplication factor and also the range of values for the multiplication factor that practitioners deem suitable for the anesthetic drug.
6. To enter symbols (or characters) that identify the multiplication (or scaling) factor on the screen of the device.

During the operation, multiplication factors may be altered from the keyboard. The purpose of the multiplication factor is to permit the operator to adjust the overall magnitude of the preset pattern of infusion rates while maintaining its overall pattern.

EXTENSIONS TO BASIC TABLE FUNCTIONS

An enhancement to the basic ability to download tables and to scale them to clinical need is an ability to upload programs that perform more sophisticated functions. A standardized environment that permits uploading of software from an external data module or communications port would meet this need. This uploaded software can be a combination of data and control software.

The specification for this interface must include the provision of a control signal to the infusion device for interpretation of keyboard signals as well as control of the display. Before the start of the operation, a display containing a tabulated infusion scheme would appear and would indicate the pattern that would be followed using the initial settings of the program. With a standardized computer interface, a range of medical applications could be implemented by independent suppliers. These programs would then work in devices from various manufacturers, provided each adhered to the standard interface.

UPLOADABLE COMPUTERIZED INFUSION SCHEMES

Alarm System Based on Physiologic Signals

This additional program permits sampling and analysis of an analog signal based on a physiologic function, and it generates an alarm and infusion "shut off" if preset limits are exceeded.

Patient-controlled Drug Administration

This system permits the physician to enter a set of parameters for infusing a sedative-hypnotic (e.g., midazolam, methohexitol, or propofol) or an opioid analgesic (e.g., morphine, meperidine, hydromorphone, or fentanyl) by the intravenous route of administration or local anesthetics by the epidural route. Delivery using this mode typically involves a series of pulses of drug administration (i.e., bolus doses) in which the rate and duration of the pulse are defined. In addition, a background (basal) infusion rate may be selected. Pulses of drug are usually triggered by the patient's pressing a "momentary closure" push button switch connected to a digital input. The program permits the operator to set the number of bolus doses that can be delivered in a set period. The software can store the usage pattern and can display it as text or graphics.

Delivery Based on Feedback from a Biologic Signal

This type of program implements a control algorithm to maintain a physiologic variable within limits according to an electrical signal indicating the magnitude of a given physiologic variable. A widely used example is the control of arterial blood pressure by infusion of cardiovascular drugs that can increase or decrease the resistance of the circulatory system or can alter the function of the heart. Delivery of an anesthetic agent can also be adjusted according to a signal derived from the spontaneous electrocardiogram, pulse oximeter, or capnograph or from the CNS using an EEG or evoked response.

Predictive Models of Patient Drug Concentration

Plasma Drug Efflux

An extension of the rate-time table of the physician program mode is implementation of the plasma drug efflux (PDE) function. With this system, drug infusion rates are generated according to predictions of the rates required to maintain a constant arterial blood concentration of an infused drug in the arterial blood. Infusion rate data are entered in the form of tables of values of infusion rate against the time period that the rate is to run. A table may contain a single set of infusion rates or multiple infusion rate profiles, in which each is associated with a range-specified target arterial blood concentration. The first column of each table specifies a series of time intervals during which each corresponding delivery rate is to run before switching to the next delivery rate. Subsequent columns contain sets of infusion rates, normalized to 1.0 μg/ml of target propofol concentration and 1.0 kg of lean body mass (LBM), corresponding to each time period. Each column is headed by a specific target concentration (C_T, μg/ml) to identify the infusion-rate profile contained in that column. Subsidiary tables may store a factor known to alter the overall relationship between the infusion rate and time (e.g., the addition of nitrous oxide) or a specific patient population (e.g., children, geriatric patients). During the operation in the PDE mode, similar calculations are performed to the standard mode. However, in this case, the multiplication factor is actually the predicted arterial target concentration, which is expressed in units of micrograms of drug per milliliter of arterial blood, and the tabulated values are expressed in terms of units of PDE (i.e., milliliters of blood cleared of drug per minute per kilogram of subject TBW or LBM) (1). The major feature of the PDE function is the ability to modify the infusion rate according to predicted changes in the PDE according to the target concentration.

Compartmental Pharmacokinetic Model

Another form of prediction is the compartmental pharmacokinetic model (CPM), certain examples of which use microconstants for a one-, two-, or three-compartment pharmacokinetic model, to predict an infusion rate pattern suitable for establishing and maintaining the target concentration as it is varied by the operator. Microconstants describing the particular model are identified by a name usually referring to the relevant drug. For example, V_1 (ml/kg LBM) and k_{10} (per minute) for a one-compartment model, V_1, k_{10}, k_{12}, and k_{21} for a two-compartment model or V_1, k_{10}, k_{12}, k_{21}, k_{13}, and k_{31} for a three-compartment model. If the site of action of the drug is remote from the arterial circulation, a further rate constant may be necessary (k_{e0}) to predict the transfer of drug to the effect site. This model requires an appropriate mathematic model to generate the delivery rate control signal and the predicted arterial (or effect site) concentration during the operation.

Complex Predictive Model

The PDE approach is valid for establishing and maintaining a range of arterial blood concentrations provided rate-time tables are available to cover the values of target concentration used. In contrast to the Kenny TCI model, the method used to derive PDE does not incorporate methods for predicting infusion requirements to make step changes from one target concentration value to another once the infusion is under way. The complex predictive model (CPM) is widely used to predict dosing requirements for making step changes in target concentration. Because the CPM is derived from drug elimination profiles, it does not allow for concentration-dependent changes in the model that are known to occur with intravenous anesthetics (e.g., propofol). The CPM is also unlikely to model sudden changes in target concentration accurately because of the abstraction of the mamillary compartmental model from the system of tubes and variably perfused tissues that constitute the body. New approaches to modeling, using deconvolution or neural networks to derive more sophisticated simulations, are likely to emerge in the future. A system permitting uploading data and software into a device with a standardized interface permits progress in research in the development of these computer-driven models. An adequate operator interface, as well as computational capability, will permit prompt implementation of these methods as they become available in the future.

In conclusion, by analysis of the nature of a TCI device, one can separate the predictive component from the basic features controlled by the operator. The implementation of a range of features found in existing infusion devices into one device would permit the anesthesiologist to use relatively sophisticated infusion patterns and to adapt these to body size and to the patient's clinical need. With sophisticated predictive models, practical intravenous anesthesia could be achieved with a level of sophistication surpassing that characteristic of inhalation anesthesia.

REFERENCES

1. Crankshaw DP. Variability and anaesthetic agents. Anaesth Pharmacol Rev 1994;2:271–279.
2. Glass PSA, Jacobs JR, Reeves JG. Intravenous anesthetic delivery. In: Miller RD, ed. Anesthesia. New York: Churchill Livingstone, 1990:85–104.
3. Introduction to infusion anaesthesia with Diprivan. Hawthorn VIC, Australia: Oxford Clinical Communications, 1995.
4. Prys-Roberts FL, Dixon J, Lewis GTR, et al. Induction and maintenance of propofol anaesthesia. Anaesthesia 1988;43 (suppl): 14–17.
5. Target controlled infusion (TCI) in anaesthesia. Cheshire, England: Zeneca Pharmaceuticals, 1995.
6. Crankshaw DP, Morgan DJ, Beemer GH, Karasawa F. Preprogrammed infusion of alfentanil to constant arterial plasma concentration. Anesth Analg 1993;76:556–561.

27 Monitoring the Adequacy of Intravenous Anesthesia

Ron Flaishon, Eric Lang and Peter S. Sebel

Surgery induces both physiologic and psychologic disturbances. During an operation, respiratory, hemodynamic, endocrine, and other perturbations may result from the surgical trauma, anesthesia, or concurrent disease. Although anesthesiologists have the ability to monitor many physiologic parameters, we lack a universally accepted method of monitoring the adequacy of anesthesia. This chapter reviews the concept of anesthesia, approaches to monitoring the adequacy of anesthesia, and current technologies that may lead to a useful monitor of anesthetic adequacy.

Dioscorides, the Greek philosopher, was the first to use the term "anesthesia" to describe the narcotic effect of the plant *Mandragora* (1). One of the first definitions of anesthesia in modern history appeared in the 1751 edition of Bailey's English dictionary, in which the term anesthesia was defined as "defect in sensation." Years later, Oliver Wendell Holmes used the term "anesthesia" to describe the state that made surgical procedures possible. Modern anesthesia combines analgesia, amnesia, hypnosis, suppression of somatic, motor, cardiovascular, and hormonal response, and muscular relaxation. These aspects of anesthesia can be optimally achieved by using one or more drugs with different pharmacologic effects. Following the introduction of neuromuscular blocking agents (NMBAs), the problem of patients' being aware during their operation but unable to communicate their plight became more prominent. The classic clinical signs of inadequate anesthesia such as movement, eyeball movement, respiratory rhythm and rate, and tidal volume are lost when NMBAs are used. Hemodynamic and other signs of light anesthesia may not detect insufficient anesthesia because of the pharmacologic effects of anesthetic agents or other drugs used during surgery. For example, opioids may block the sympathetic response (2), and α- and β-receptor blocking agents may attenuate the hypertensive or tachycardic response (3).

The methods used to define anesthetic adequacy are extremely varied, ranging from anecdotal descriptions of light, moderate, or deep anesthesia (4) to concepts such as minimal alveolar concentration (MAC) of volatile anesthetics that allow us to compare anesthetic potency (5, 6), to electrophysiologic methods (7). Heart rate and blood pressure are clinically measurable components, and sweat and lacrimation may be observed, but analgesia and unconsciousness (involving both hypnosis and amnesia) are virtually impossible to define and to evaluate. No universal end point or monitor serves as the basis for the rational administration of drugs to achieve unconsciousness. To date, absence of recall is the only criterion for hypnosis and amnesia, but it is neither objective nor reliable.

ADEQUACY OF THE ANESTHETIC STATE

Over the years, many definitions of the term "anesthetic state" have been proposed, and many ways to describe anesthetic adequacy have been suggested. After the introduction of ether in the nineteenth century, the first modern definitions of anesthetic state and depth of anesthesia began to appear. Wendell Holmes defined anesthesia as the state in which the patient is insensible to the trauma of surgery. In a letter to the *Lancet* in 1847, Plomley described the depth of ether anesthesia in three stages: intoxication, excitement, and narcosis (8).

Guedel, in 1937 (9), used clinical signs such as muscular tone and respiratory, hemodynamic, and ocular signs to describe four stages of ether anesthesia. The first stage is characterized by analgesia, amnesia, sedation, preservation of eyelid reflex, and regular breathing with both diaphragm and intercostal muscles. The second stage (delirium) is an excitatory phase manifested by unconscious excitement and uninhibited activity, irregular and unpredictable ventilation, mydriasis, and preserved eyelid reflex. The third phase is surgical anesthesia, which is subdivided into four planes. The first plane is characterized by slight somatic relaxation, regular respiration, and active ocular muscles. In the second plane, inspiration is shorter than exhalation with an inspiratory pause, and the eyes are immobile. Plane three brings about relaxation of the abdominal muscles and loss of eyelid reflex. In plane four, paradoxic rib cage movement occurs, and the pupils are dilated. Guedel's fourth stage is respiratory paralysis, flaccid muscles, and the occurrence of respiratory arrest, as well as cardiovascular collapse. At that time, this stage probably culminated with the death of the patient, but today, with the availability of mechanical ventilation and cardiovascular support, many of our patients would survive this phase. Artusio in 1954 (10) further divided the first stage into three planes. In the first plane, the patient does not experience amnesia or analgesia. During the second plane, the patient is completely amnestic but experiences only partial analgesia. Only in the third plane does the patient have complete amnesia and analgesia. Although these clinical signs and stages were relevant and could be effectively utilized during the administration of ether, cyclopropane, and chloroform anesthesia, their effectiveness is questionable with the use of other volatile agents and of intravenous anesthetics and combination of opioids and other drugs in modern anesthetic practice and with current monitoring techniques. For example, Spackman and associates (11) showed that isoflurane alone did not attenuate the hemodynamic response to laryngoscopy, even at concentrations that caused burst suppression of the electroencephalogram (EEG), a finding suggesting that anesthesia and analgesia were mediated by different mechanisms.

Detecting and monitoring depth of anesthesia, as described by Guedel and Artusio, became even more difficult with the introduction of d-tubocurarine. The use of NMBAs eliminated many of the clinical signs of anesthetic depth: the rate, rhythm, and volume of respiration and the degree of muscle relaxation induced by the anesthetic (12), as well as eyeball movement. Seven of the nine components of Guedel's classification involved skeletal muscle activity. The two remaining, pupil size and lacrimation, are clinically inadequate to judge anesthetic adequacy, especially when opioid analgesics are used. Woodbridge, in 1957 (13), described anesthesia using the four-component concept: sensory block, reflex block, motor block, and "mental" block. Some 30 years, later Pinsker (14) proposed another concept, suggesting that paralysis, unconsciousness, and attenuation of stress are the necessary components of anesthesia. Pinsker also described anesthesia as a "sickness," like shock, being complex and involving many different components. These two theories do not necessarily differ. Pinsker set the end point of anesthetic state, whereas Woodbridge described the way to achieve it.

In 1987, Prys-Roberts redefined the elements that he considered relevant to the concept of anesthetic depth (15). In his editorial, Prys-Roberts suggested that if pain is considered a "conscious perception of noxious stimulus," then "a state of anesthesia" can be defined as drug-induced unconsciousness in which the patient neither perceives nor recalls pain. Prys-Roberts considers loss of consciousness as an all-or-none quantal phenomenon. Thus, no degrees or variable depths of anesthesia exist. According to this theory, surgery causes noxious stimuli resulting in a series of somatic (i.e., pain and movement), autonomic, and hemodynamic responses that may be modified by different drugs. He has defined anesthesia in terms of the drugs producing unconsciousness and modification of noxious stimuli, and he has classified drugs by their pharmacologic properties rather than by their ability to produce components of the state of anesthesia. Autonomic responses are divided into three categories: 1) the pseudomotor response, consisting of sweating; 2) the hemodynamic response, consisting of increased sympathetic activity resulting in increase in arterial blood pressure and heart rate; and 3) the release of stress hormone, which is impossible to measure in real time and is extremely difficult to eliminate completely. Figure 27-1 illustrates a scheme of responses to noxious stimuli and the order in which they are suppressed. Prys-Roberts considers analgesia, neuromuscular blockade, and suppression of autonomic activity as discrete pharmacologic events that are not components of anesthesia but are supplementary to it. The inclusion of neuromuscular blockade in the definition of the

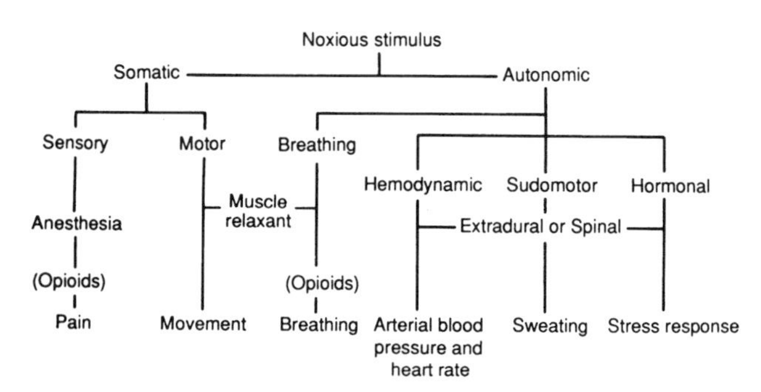

FIGURE 27-1. The clinically relevant responses to the noxious stimulus of operation, the severity, and the order by which they are eliminated (from left to right). (From Prys-Roberts C. Anaesthesia: a practical or impractical construct? Br J Anaesth 1987;11:1341–1345.)

anesthetic state is both illogical and confusing, because neuromuscular blockade is not a component of anesthesia, nor is it a substitute for inadequate anesthesia. The only features common to all anesthetics are the suppression of sensory perception and the production of unconsciousness.

Kissin (16) defined anesthesia as prevention of psychologic and somatic adverse effects of surgery using different pharmacologic agents. He further noted that a wide spectrum of pharmacologic actions including analgesia, anxiolysis, amnesia, unconsciousness, suppression of somatic motor response, and hemodynamic and hormonal responses to the surgical stimuli can be used to create an anesthetic state. Kissin and Gelman (17) suggested that attenuation of the stress response involves not only sensory block and analgesia, but also synergistic interaction between drugs (18). Like Prys-Roberts, Kissin views general anesthesia as a spectrum of separate pharmacologic actions produced by one or more drugs. The combination of these effects is anesthesia; however, goals may vary according to the needs of the individual patient and the surgeon.

Considering Kissin's (16) and Prys-Robert's (15) theories, the term "depth of anesthesia" may be inappropriate. According to their theories, anesthesia is composed of distinct effects that may be achieved by one or more drugs. One drug may induce several effects by different pharmacologic mechanisms. For example, opioids may act by two mechanisms, one receptor specific and the other related to lipid solubility. Weston and Roth (19) suggested that volatile anesthetics act through multiple site and mechanisms. Depending on the dose, inhaled anesthetics may abolish perception of pain, stop movement (MAC) (20), attenuate autonomic response (MAC-BAR, described later in this chapter) (21), and provide some skeletal muscle relaxation. Opioids are analgesic at low doses, but they may be used as induction agents at high doses (e.g., fentanyl, 50 to 150 μg/kg) (22, 23); however, at the same time, they may cause muscle rigidity (23). Combinations of drugs may complicate the monitoring of anesthetic adequacy. For example, Kissin and associates (2) demonstrated that the combination of opioids and barbiturates was synergistic in blocking the righting reflex, but antagonistic in blocking the response to tail clamp. These investigators concluded that the anesthetic effect of an agent could have several components with different mechanisms. A common practice in anesthesia is to administer several different drugs to achieve amnesia, sedation, analgesia, and paralysis, whereas the stress response is usually attenuated using opioids or specific central or peripheral sympathetic blocking drugs. Significant interpatient variability in the requirement for sedatives and analgesics exists (24). Some patients require only mild sedation for a minor surgical procedure, whereas others need to be heavily sedated or even anesthetized. Anesthetic techniques used for minor surgical procedures are different from those used for major cardiothoracic and neurosurgery procedures. Anesthetic requirements also differ according to the surgical procedure and the relative degrees of stimulation. Ausems and associates (24) found that the Cp_{50}) (the plasma concentration of a drug causing 50% chance of suppressing a response to stimulus) of alfentanil was lower for breast surgery than for lower abdominal surgery, with still higher doses required for upper abdominal surgery (Fig. 27-2).

The term "depth of anesthesia" and the definition of stages are irrelevant in the modern practice of anesthesia. Anesthesia is neither deep nor light, and it may or may not be adequate. The practitioner should tailor anesthesia to a specific patient undergoing specific surgery and monitor the adequacy of anesthesia. For the purposes of this chapter, anesthesia is defined

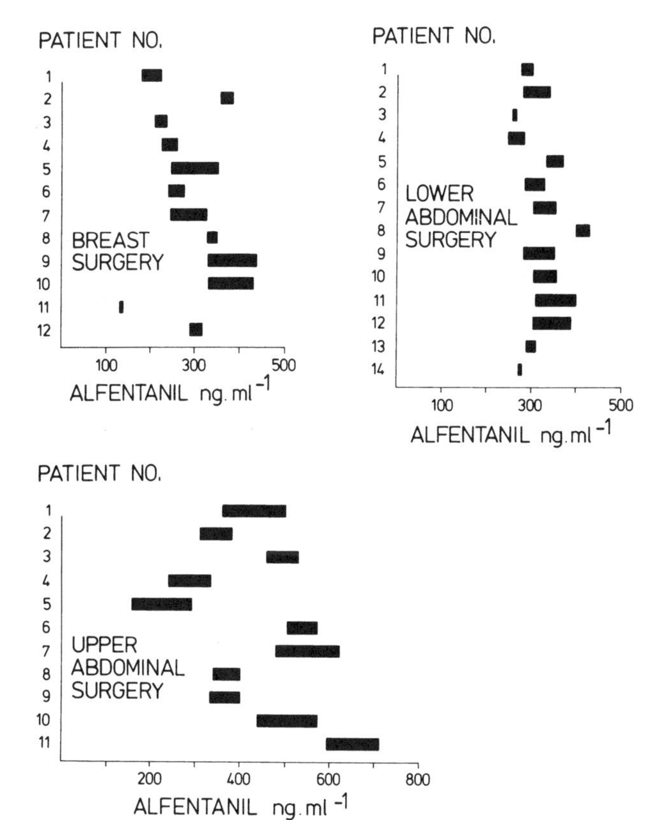

FIGURE 27-2. The relationship of alfentanil plasma concentration to responsiveness of patients during breast surgery and lower and upper abdominal surgery. Each bar represents the highest concentration associated with a response and the lowest concentration associated with no response, for each patient. Note the high variability in the upper abdominal surgery group. (From Ausems ME, Hug CC, Stanski DR, Burm AG. Plasma concentrations of alfentanil required to supplement nitrous oxide anesthesia for general surgery. Anesthesiology 1986;65:362–373.)

as a transient state of unconsciousness with analgesia and amnesia.

AWARENESS, MEMORY, AND RECALL DURING ANESTHESIA

Patients' awareness of surgical procedures still occurs in the clinical practice of anesthesia. The occurrence of awareness and recall increased after the introduction of NMBAs, and it is one of the major causes of patients' complaints and legal claims (25).

Awareness is a state of being aware (i.e., being conscious, watchful, vigilant, informed, and able to respond to command) (7). Memory is the ability to receive, modify, store, and retrieve informational stimuli (26). In the 1970s, psychologists divided memory into explicit and implicit states. Explicit memory involves the conscious recollection of previous input with reference to a specific event or stimuli. Implicit memory refers to any effect on experience, thoughts, feeling, or action without any direct recollection of a past event that may have contributed to it (27). Recall may be considered synonymous with explicit memory (7). The terms awareness, recall, and memory should be distinguished. A patient may be aware during surgery and may obey commands, but may have no recall of any intraoperative event. Russell (28) studied 25 patients who were anesthetized with nitrous oxide (N_2O), using the isolated forearm technique (IFT). Eleven patients responded to command (wakeful), and 9 opened their eyes during surgery, but only 1 patient had an actual recall of an intraoperative event. In another study of 36 women undergoing cesarean section using the IFT under general anesthesia, 12 women followed commands, but only 3 had any recall (29). Patients may not be aware during surgery or have any recall postoperatively, but they may still have implicit memory (30, 31). For example, patients can demonstrate implicit memory for a story played during general anesthesia (32). Subconscious learning may also occur during anesthesia. For example, patients who were played positive suggestions during anesthesia required less analgesia (33) and had a better postoperative course than those who did not receive suggestions (31). Implicit memory may be manifested by acute or chronic psychosis or by nightmares years after surgery (34). One retrospective study (35) reported a 30% incidence of postoperative sleep disturbances and an 18% incidence of nightmares following anesthesia without any relationship with recall or awareness.

The occurrence of recall varies with the anesthetic technique and the operation. Up to 0.5% of patients paralyzed during surgery may recall events related to their operation (36). Other studies report an incidence of 0.2 to 2% (37–39), but it may be as high as 4% (7). The incidence of awareness and recall is greater in high-risk and hemodynamically unstable patients and in those undergoing emergency surgery (probably because of the use of lower doses of anesthetic and analgesic drugs) (40). In a study of patients who underwent surgery for trauma (41), 43% of the hemodynamically unstable patients had intraoperative recall, compared with 11% of the more stable patients who received higher doses of anesthetics. Some patients described recall and awareness as their worst hospital experience. Inadequate anesthesia and awareness can lead to postoperative or post-traumatic psychologic disorders (34, 35). The detection and diagnosis of awareness and recall and prompt commencement of appropriate therapy may help to prevent the development of chronic disorders.

Currently, reliable and predictable methods to detect intraoperative awareness in real time are not available. The only method to detect awareness and recall in the paralyzed patient is the postoperative interview. More important, the patient may deny any recall unless queries are properly phrased. In addition, recall of some events may be elicited only by hypnosis (42, 43).

MOVEMENT AS A MEASURE OF ANESTHETIC ADEQUACY

Movement in response to skin incision is a useful sign for monitoring anesthetic adequacy and comparing anesthetic potency. In 1963, Merkel and Eger first introduced the concept of MAC as the minimum alveolar concentration of halothane needed to prevent gross purposeful movement in response to supramaximal noxious stimulus in 50% of subjects (20). This concept was first described for halothane in dogs, but it was later extended to humans and to other volatile anesthetics (44). In human patients, the initial skin incision represents a reproducible stimulus. The concentration of volatile anesthetics required to eliminate the motor response to skin incision (MAC) is higher than that required for loss of consciousness (MAC awake) (45) but lower than the concentration needed to block adrenergic response to painful stimuli (MAC-BAR) (21). Movement in response to surgical stimulation cannot be used as a measure of anesthetic adequacy in the presence of complete neuromuscular blockade. To avoid neuromuscular blockade when not surgically indicated is prudent, however, because preservation of some neuromuscular function enables the anesthetized patient to alert the anesthesiologist to inadequate anesthesia.

Does movement represent the effect of anesthetics on the central nervous system (CNS)? Several studies have demonstrated that the neuroanatomic structures of the forebrain are not required to mediate somatic responsiveness in reaction to surgical stimulation. Rampil and associates reported that precollicular decerebration did not alter the ability of general anesthetics to block somatic response (46). These investigators demonstrated that the MAC of isoflurane in decerebrate animals was 1.26%, not different from the 1.3% found in the control group. These investigators also reported (47) that MAC of isoflurane did not change after hypothermic spinal cord transaction. They concluded that somatic motor responsiveness and its sensitivity to isoflurane appeared to be unaltered despite acute loss of descending cortical and bulbar controls, a finding suggesting that the site of anesthetic inhibition of motor response may be in the spinal cord. Confirming evidence was forthcoming from Antognini and Schwartz (48), who preferentially anesthetized the brain with isoflurane using two bypass circuits. Oxygen and isoflurane were delivered to the brain by a bubble oxygenator. When isoflurane was delivered only to the brain, the concentration required to block movement was 2.9%, compared with 1.2% before bypass, suggesting that brain structures are a relatively important means of depressing somatic responsiveness. Borges and Antognini (49) studied MAC in animals in which the brain was isolated from the rest of the body. While isoflurane concentration in the brain was maintained at 0.2 to 0.3%, isoflurane was also delivered to the lungs and MAC was determined. These investigators showed that isoflurane MAC for the body after bypass was 0.8%, as compared with 1.4% before bypass. Confirming evidence also comes from a study that found that ischemic forebrain injury does not alter the MAC of halothane, a finding again indicating that anatomic foci for motor responses elicited during MAC determination are localized at levels caudal to the forebrain (50). King and Rampil (51) found that isoflurane depresses spinal motor neuron excitability, suggesting that this effect may play an important role in the provision of surgical immobility. These studies raise the possibility that, although the brain is a major site of action of the inhaled anesthetics, the movement response may be at least partly mediated by spinal structures.

Jacoby and associates (52) studied patients' response to tetanic nerve stimulation, trapezius muscle squeeze, and laryngoscopy and correlated the response to the thiopental plasma concentration using a computer-controlled infusion. EEG became isoelectric at thiopental plasma concentration while the Cp_{50} for intubation was 78.8 μg/ml, without any alteration in the EEGs of 50 μg/ml, with movement. From this study, one can conclude that movement is a more sensitive sign than the EEG in monitoring adequacy of anesthesia, assuming that providing adequate anesthesia involves prevention of movement in response to a pain stimulus and that prevention of movement in response to surgical stimulus involves both analgesia and hypnosis. The electromyograph (EMG) can also be used to monitor muscle activity (53). The EMG has little predictive value, however, and has not been useful in the presence of NMBAs.

IFT is a method whereby the patient's forearm is isolated from neuromuscular blockade through the use of a tourniquet before administration of the NMBA drug. In this manner, the patient can move the forearm in response to inadequate anesthesia or in response to command, although the rest of the body is paralyzed. IFT has been employed as a monitor of anesthetic adequacy and a monitor of awareness in the presence of NMBAs (54–57). To increase the specificity of the IFT, this method was modified by Wang and associates (58) to include written communication with the isolated forearm. When used clinically, the IFT can interfere with surgery (59), and it can be difficult to implement in the operating room (39, 56, 60, 61). Excessive arm movement can be avoided with the use of a restraining band (56). The technique should not be maintained for over 20 minutes because of the risk of ischemia (39) and petechial hemorrhages (57). IFT can be difficult to interpret, because movement may range from spinal reflex activity to substantive evidence of wakefulness (60). Some investigators have not been able to correlate signs of light anesthesia or postoperative recall to the isolated arm movement response, suggesting that the occurrence of purposeful movement in an isolated extremity is not a good predictor of intraoperative recall (57, 59, 62). As mentioned before, awareness may occur without recall (28).

CLINICAL SIGNS OF ADEQUATE ANESTHESIA

Adequacy or depth of anesthesia is routinely estimated by observing blood pressure, heart rate, respiratory rate, rhythm, and depth, muscle tonus, ocular signs, lacrimation, and diaphoresis. Evans and associates (63) used a scoring system based on blood pressure (P), heart rate (R), and sweat (S) and tear (T) formation (i.e., PRST score). Each index is assigned a score of 1 or 2, resulting in nine levels from 0 to 8. For most applications, an anesthetized patient is allocated scores from 0 to 4, with any score above 2 considered an unacceptable response.

The heart rate and electrocardiogram can be used to monitor anesthetic adequacy. For example, an increase in the degree of respiratory sinus arrhythmia accompanies decreases in the depth of propofol anesthesia (64). Although these signs are most extensively used to monitor anesthesia, they are indirect and nonspecific, they are modified by disease, drugs, and surgical technique, and the degree of interpatient variability is high. These clinical signs are not always helpful in detecting awareness under anesthesia. For example, patients may be completely awake with no change in the foregoing signs (22, 23). Moerman and associates (65) reported 26 cases of awareness and recall, of which 12 patients' records were available for review. Of these 12 patients, only 5 experienced hypertension during surgery, and tachycardia was observed in 3 patients. Cullen and colleagues (66) studied hemodynamic, respiratory, and ocular signs to estimate the depth of anesthesia using inhaled anesthetics. Hypotension was the only clinical sign that correlated with an increase in the concentration of halothane and isoflurane. The addition of N_2O to halothane anesthesia caused an increase in the mean blood pressure. In patients anesthetized with halothane, heart rate, tidal volume, and pupillary diameter increased 1 minute after the surgical stimulus was applied, with no change in blood pressure or respiratory rate, and all clinical signs returned to preincision values 12 minutes later. The clinical response to stimulation was different when isoflurane was used, and it persisted for 1 hour. From this study, we can conclude that no single clinical sign is sufficiently specific and sensitive unless we also consider the patient, the anesthetic technique, the stimulus, and the length of anesthesia.

Ausems and associates (24) studied the response of 37 patients undergoing abdominal surgery under alfentanil-N_2O anesthesia. These investigators used an increase in systolic blood pressure and heart rate, movement, swallowing, coughing, grimacing, eye opening, lacrimation, flushing, and diaphoresis as clinical criteria to categorize the response. In this study, no single sign was conclusively consistent and sufficient to represent satisfactory anesthesia. Glass and associates (67) studied 18 patients during fentanyl-N_2O anesthesia. In their study, 7 patients moved in response to skin incision, but only 2 of them manifested an acute hemodynamic response. One of the conclusions from this study was that movement is a more sensitive indicator of inadequate anesthesia than an acute heart rate and blood pressure response. Dutton and associates (68) reported that heart rate and blood pressure changes did not predict movement to skin incision when isoflurane-N_2O was used, but it did have a predictive value when fentanyl was added. EEG was a better predictor of movement than hemodynamic response in this study.

The traditional approach to hemodynamic signs may lead to misinterpretation. Increasing the dose of the anesthetic does not necessarily cause bradycardia or hypotension. Hudson and associates (69) found that, with increasing thiopental dose, a progressive slowing of the EEG and a decrease in blood pressure were noted, whereas heart rate increased. A rapid increase in the inspired concentration of desflurane may induce an increase in both heart rate and blood pressure as a result of sympathoadrenal activation (70, 71). The hemodynamic response may vary, depending on the drugs used. For example, an anesthetic dose of propofol may result in a decrease in blood pressure, in contrast to the minimal hypotensive response seen after etomidate, probably because of differing effects of these drugs on the sympathetic nervous system (72).

As mentioned earlier, other clinical signs (e.g., diaphoresis and lacrimation) have been utilized to estimate anesthetic adequacy, but they too are neither sensitive nor specific (28). In a study of 30 parturient women undergoing nonemergency cesarean section (73), the occurrence of awareness and hemodynamic and motor response was high, but signs such as eye centering, pupil size, and sweat were inconclusive. Hilgenberg reported a case of awareness during mitral valve replacement in which the patient had no hemodynamic changes, diaphoresis, lacrimation, or movement to indicate that anesthesia was inadequate (22). Diaphoresis loses its diagnostic value in the presence of temperature changes. During a lengthy surgical procedure that involves massive blood transfusion, hypothermia can also attenuate this response. In the periods before and after cardiac bypass, the patient's temperature is actively changed from deep hypothermia to relative hyperthermia, thereby modifying the "sweat" response. Moreover, in certain periods, large shifts in fluid balance result in changes in the pharmacokinetics of the anesthetic drugs. Recall of surgery and postoperative sleep disturbances are higher in these patients (7). Mydriasis as a sign of inadequate anesthesia, and sympathetic activation loses its specificity and sensitivity after ocular operation, or when ophthalmologic drugs, opioids, or atropine are used.

Hemodynamic response to noxious stimulus does not necessarily imply awareness, light anesthesia, or even the perception of pain. During organ harvesting from brain-dead cadavers, hemodynamic changes have been observed in response to the skin incision (74, 75). Hemodynamic and somatic responses to noxious stimuli may not only involve the CNS, but may also be mediated by spinothalamic tracts and adrenal medullary stimulation by reflex spinal arc (76). Dissection and manipulation of the aorta in cardiac surgery may cause tachycardia and hypertension that is not always manageable with analgesic and anesthetic drugs, but may require the use of vasoactive drugs (6, 43). Monk and associates (77) evaluated intraoperative hemodynamic and stress hormone responses when either isoflurane, alfentanil, or trimethaphan was used to treat hypertension in patients anesthetized with alfentanil and N_2O. Despite differing patterns of hormonal responses, the investigators failed to a demonstrate clinical advantage of any of the drugs. The hemodynamic profile was much the same for the three groups. The conclusion from this study is that the hemodynamic and hormonal stress response may be managed by anesthetic, analgesic, or sympathetic blocking drugs.

Thus, blood pressure, heart rate, ocular signs, lacrimation, and sweat are not useful in predicting responses to noxious stimuli. During anesthesia without any stimulus, these parameters do not correlate with the anesthetic dose or concentration, nor can they help to detect intraoperative awareness and recall.

INDIRECT MEASURES OF ANESTHETIC ADEQUACY

Facial electromyography (FACE) records summed facial electromyographic voltages over the frontalis, corrugator, zygomatic, and orbicularis oculi muscles with surface electrodes. The facial muscles are relatively resistant to NMBAs. The pattern of muscular tension (i.e., a grimace or a smile) may be useful in monitoring anesthetic adequacy (78). To date, insufficient research has been performed, and further studies will be required to determine the utility of FACE as a monitor of adequate anesthesia.

The measurement of lower esophageal contractility (LEC) was proposed as a noninvasive method to monitor anesthetic adequacy (63, 79). Increasing concentrations of inhaled anesthetics were found to decrease LEC. Thornton and associates (80) found no correlation between plasma concentrations of propofol and LEC. Sessler and associates (81) conducted a controlled study and found that LEC could predict movement in response to skin incision in patients anesthetized with of halothane; however, no correlation was found between LEC and movement in response to skin incision in patients anesthetized with alfentanil and N_2O. LEC may also relate to the nature and intensity of surgery. Thomas and Aitkenhead (82) found that both spontaneous LEC and provoked LEC after skin incision were greater in women undergoing hysterectomy than in those undergoing varicose vein surgery. Glycopyrrolate and other anticholinergic agents reduce the incidence of spontaneous esophageal contractility. Other investigators have suggested that LEC is inappropriate for assessing adequacy of anesthesia (83–85). As a result of these findings, LEC has not gained popularity as a monitor of anesthetic adequacy.

ELECTROPHYSIOLOGIC APPROACHES TO MONITORING ANESTHETIC ADEQUACY

Various electrophysiologic approaches to monitoring anesthetic adequacy have been used with varying degrees of success. These include spontaneous EEG, various processed EEG transformations, such as median frequency (MF), spectral edge frequency (SEF), and bispectral (BIS) index. Brain stem evoked responses represent another method of attempting to monitor anesthetic adequacy using auditory evoked responses (AER).

Electroencephalographic Measures

Because the brain is the primary site of action of general anesthetics, it is reasonable to assume that the EEG, which represents the electrical activity of the brain, contains useful data for assessing adequacy of anesthesia. The EEG is a noninvasive monitor of cerebral activity in the unconscious patient and is related to cerebral blood flow and metabolism (15). The spontaneous EEG represents cortical electrical activity derived from summated excitatory and inhibitory postsynaptic activity. This electrical activity has direct physiologic correlates relevant to anesthesia and has been employed in pharmacodynamic and pharmacokinetic studies involving many anesthetic drugs (86–89). All anesthetics and analgesic drugs change the raw EEG signal (90) and may alter the EEG in a different fashion. For example, although isoflurane and enflurane are two isomers with the same chemical structure, they have different effects on the EEG. Isoflurane causes EEG depression and at 2 MAC produces burst suppression and an isoelectric EEG (91), whereas the equivalent concentration of enflurane produces generalized spike and wave activity. Thiopental causes transient EEG activation and burst suppression (92), in contrast to opioids, which produce progressive, predictable slowing of the EEG without burst suppression (87) (Fig. 27-3). Despite possessing

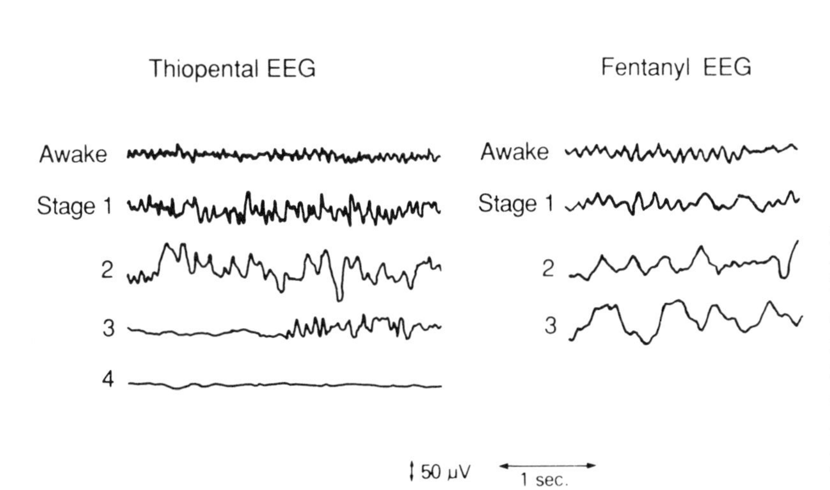

FIGURE 27-3. The electroencephalographic (EEG) pattern of increasing plasma concentration of thiopental (left) and fentanyl (right). Low plasma concentration of thiopental produces increase in frequency and amplitude. As the concentration increases, both amplitude and frequency decrease. In stage 3, thiopental produces burst suppression and finally an isoelectric EEG. Fentanyl has its maximal effect in stage 3, that is, large and slow waves without burst suppression. (From Reference 92.)

unique drug specific changes, it is still possible to characterize the anesthetic response (e.g., consciousness) using EEG measures such as the BIS index (Fig. 27-4).

Previous attempts have been made to use the EEG as a monitor of anesthetic adequacy. The raw EEG has limited use as an anesthesia monitor because of the complexity of the signals and the difficulties in online analysis and interpretation; thus, several processed and computerized EEG techniques have been proposed. The use of a mathematical technique known as Fourier analysis allows the raw EEG signal to be digitized and separated into sine waves. The power spectrum is then calculated from the individual components (93) (Fig. 27-5). The data may then be presented as a linear display, compressed spectral array (CSA), in which individual time fragments (epochs) are plotted above one another, creating a "hill and valley" pattern. The gray scale display also known as density modulated spectral array (DSA) is shown in Figure 27-6. Each epoch is displayed as a line of varying density, or a series of dots of various size. The SEF reduces the power spectrum to a single number that represents the frequency below which 95% of the total power is present (94) (see Fig. 27-7). It has long been thought to correlate with anesthetic adequacy (95, 96). SEF correlates well with plasma concentrations of opioids (86) and thiopental (69, 92) and may be useful in predicting the hemodynamic response to laryngoscopy and intubation (95). It may also be used to guide opioid administration to reduce drug dose and the magnitude of hemodynamic responses (96). Other workers have been unable to correlate SEF with hemodynamic responses (97). Dutton and colleagues found it a good predictor of movement to trocar insertion with a variety of anesthetic techniques (68). In another study, however, SEF was not useful in predicting movement at skin incision during 1 MAC isoflurane anesthesia (98).

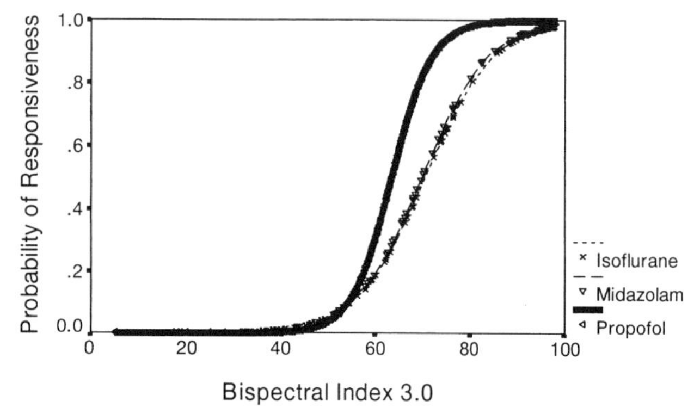

FIGURE 27-4. The relationship between the EEG-BIS (bispectral) index and the probability of a response to verbal command (consciousness) in volunteers receiving increasing concentrations of either isoflurane, midazolam or propofol. (Data from Kearse L, Rosow C, Sebel P, Bloom M, Glass P, Howell S. Greenwald S. "The Bispectral Index Correlates With Sedation/Hypnosis and Recall: Comparison Using Multiple Agents." Anesthesiology 83(3A):A507, 1995.)

The MF of the EEG power spectrum (the frequency above and below which 50% of the EEG power resides) (99) has also been studied during anesthesia. An MF of less than 5 Hz is associated with unconsciousness during etomidate (100) or methohexital (101) anesthesia. The MF has also been used in an adaptive feedback control algorithm for the closed-loop control of propofol (102) anesthesia and other anesthetic techniques using etomidate and methohexital (101, 103, 104) and alfentanil-N_2O anesthesia (105).

Drummond and associates investigated five processed EEG parameters and assessed their value as predictors of imminent arousal (spontaneous movement, coughing, or eye opening) from isoflurane-N_2O anesthesia (106). Although some of the EEG parameters, thresholds, including MF, SEF 90%, and total power of the EEG, predicted arousal with sensitivity of 90% and specificity of 82 to 90%, no measure was reliable enough to serve as the sole predictor of imminent arousal. Another study using isoflurane anesthesia found that awakening was always preceded by an abrupt decrease in EEG power; however, on emergence from fentanyl-N_2O anesthesia, no change in the EEG power spectrum was noted (99). These EEG parameters appear to provide potentially useful trend information regarding changing levels of anesthesia, but none is sufficiently reliable to be used as the sole indicator of anesthetic depth.

The conventional EEG analysis does not use all the information provided by the EEG. Power spectral analysis assumes a Gaussian, stationary, and first-order (linear) model of the frequencies within the EEG (i.e., the amplitudes of the EEG are normally distributed, the statistical properties do not change over time, and the frequency constituents are uncorrelated). Under this assumption, the EEG is considered to be made up by a linear superimposition of statistically independent sinusoidal wave components. Only frequency and power estimates are considered, whereas phase information is generally ignored. In reality, however, biologic systems exhibit significant nonlinear complexities that do not conform to the assumptions of conventional power spectral analysis. To overcome this limitation, the EEG-BIS provides a means by which quadratic (second-order) interactions can be quantified (107, 108). It does so by quantifying the phase coupling between any two frequencies and a third frequency (harmonic) at their sum (or difference). The extent of the coupling between two frequencies (bicoherence)

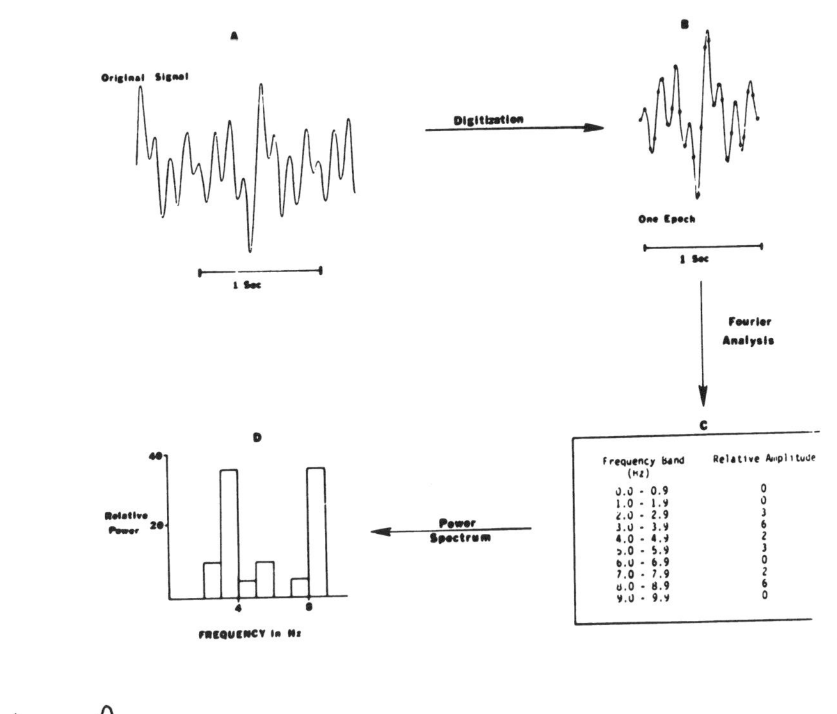

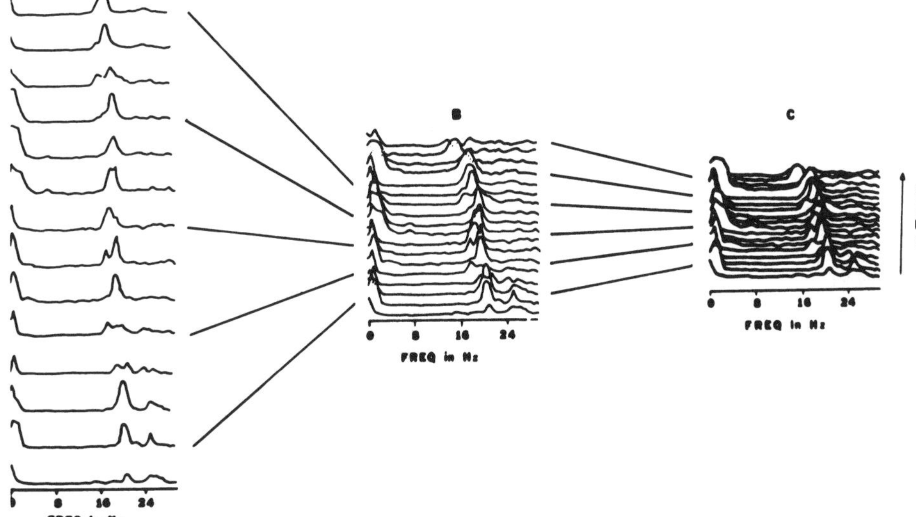

FIGURE 27-5. A schematic representation of the power spectrum analysis. The top panel is the original signal before and after digitalization. In the middle panel, one epoch is transformed using Fourier analysis to its component from which the power spectrum is calculated. The bottom panel shows a series of epochs plotted closely above one another creating a "hill and valley" pattern of compressed spectral array. (From Levy WJ, Shapiro HM, Maruchak G, Meathe E. Automated EEG processing for intraoperative monitoring: A comparison of techniques. Anesthesiology 1980;53:223–236.)

can vary from 0% (if no harmonic is generated) to 100% (if a harmonic is generated for the duration of the period analyzed) (Fig. 27-8). BIS provides a more comprehensive description of the information available from Fourier analysis than the power spectrum, thus allowing the construction of a better profile of changes that take place in the EEG under a variety of clinical conditions.

As mentioned earlier, movement is an unequivocal sign of inadequate anesthesia (52, 54) and a measure of anesthetic potency (20). The value of BIS to predict movement in response to skin incision has been studied retrospectively (109, 110). It has been shown to predict patient movement in response to skin incision during isoflurane-oxygen anesthesia, a finding that may be valuable in the paralyzed patient. This study was limited in that only responses to volatile anesthetic agents were assessed. Subsequently, BIS was demonstrated to predict movement in response to surgical skin incision with either propofol-alfentanil or isoflurane-alfentanil (111, 112) anesthesia. BIS was found to be a more accurate predictor of patient movement during propofol-N_2O anesthesia than the power spectrum or the plasma propofol concentration (112). The EEG-BIS was superior to MAC concentration in predicting hemodynamic response to skin incision (113). However, BIS was not independent of anesthetic technique. BIS values were not significantly different between patients who moved at skin incision during propofol-alfentanil anesthesia and those who did not move during

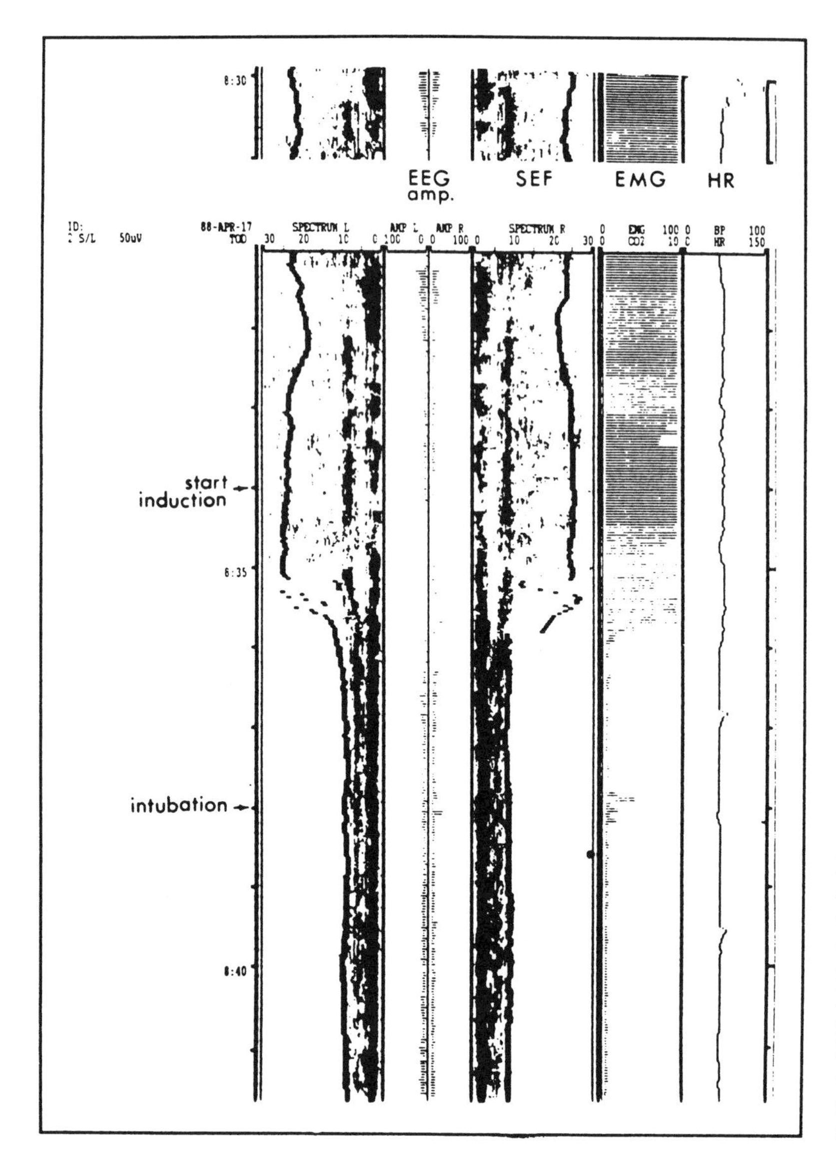

FIGURE 27-6. The density modulation configuration of the power spectrum in an awake patient and during induction of anesthesia for cardiac surgery, using fentanyl and midazolam. Spectral edge frequency (SEF) 95% is represented by the bold line. EEG, Electroencephalography; EMG, electromyography; HR, heart rate. (From Sidi A, Halimi P, Cotev S. Estimating anesthetic depth by electroencephalography during anesthetic induction and intubation in patients undergoing cardiac surgery. J Clin Anesth 1990;2:101–107.)

A Signal made up of 3 Independent Sine Waves: 2 Hz, 3 Hz. and 5 Hz.

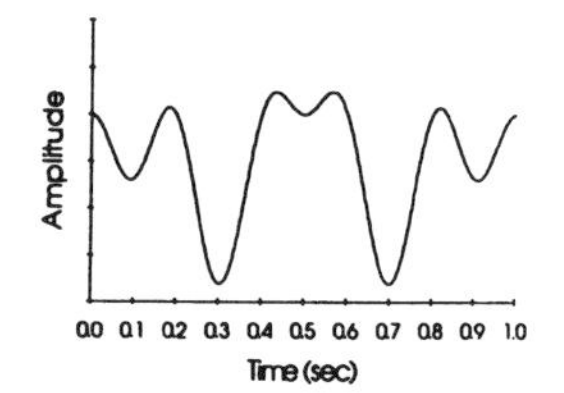

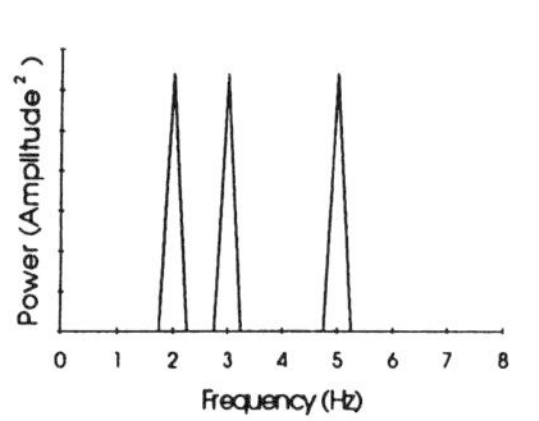

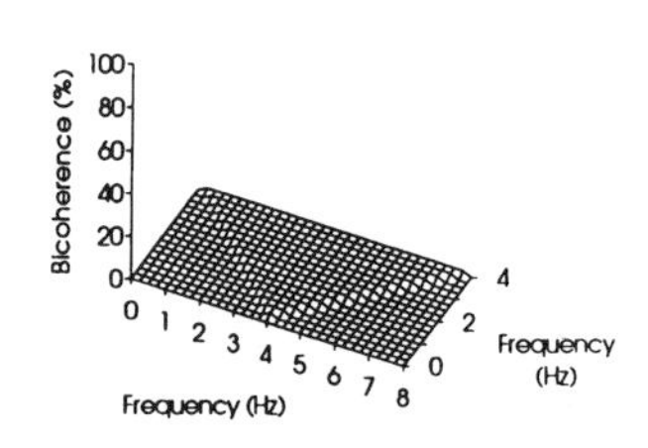

A Signal made up of the sum of 2 Independent Sine Waves (2 Hz and 3 Hz) and their Harmonic at 5 Hz.

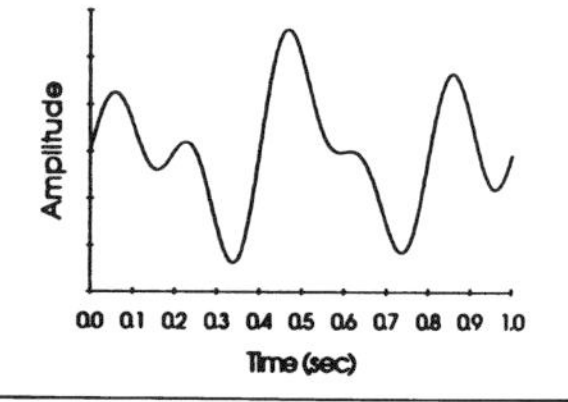

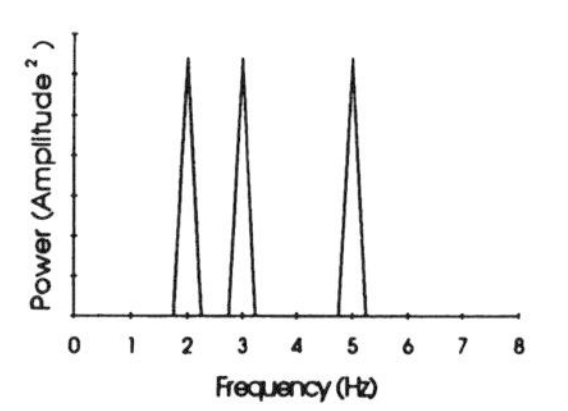

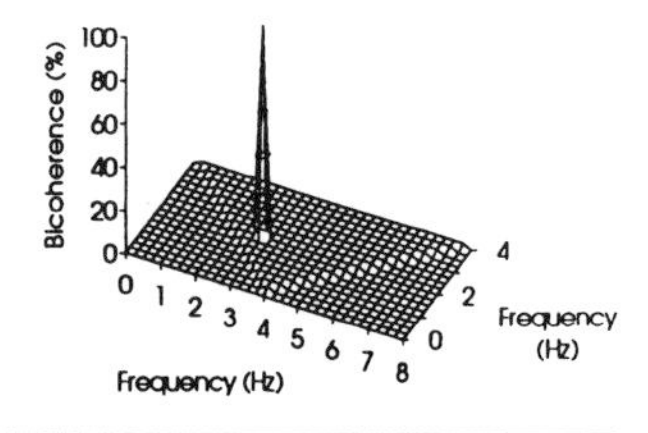

FIGURE 27-7. Comparison of electroencephalographic (EEG) analysis using power spectrum and bispectrum. The upper and lower left panels are simulated EEG tracing containing 2-, 3-, and 5-Hz components. The middle panels are the power spectra of the EEG, and the right panels represent the bispectral analysis of the EEG. In the upper panel, the EEG component has no phase relationship, whereas in the lower panel the 5-Hz component is a harmonic of the 2- and 3-Hz signal. Although the raw EEG looks different, the power spectra are identical, but the peak is clearly seen at the lower right panel. (Data from Sebel PS, Bowles SM, Saini V, Chamoun N. EEG bispectrum predicts movement during thiopental/isoflurane anesthesia. J Clin Monit 1995;11:83–91.)

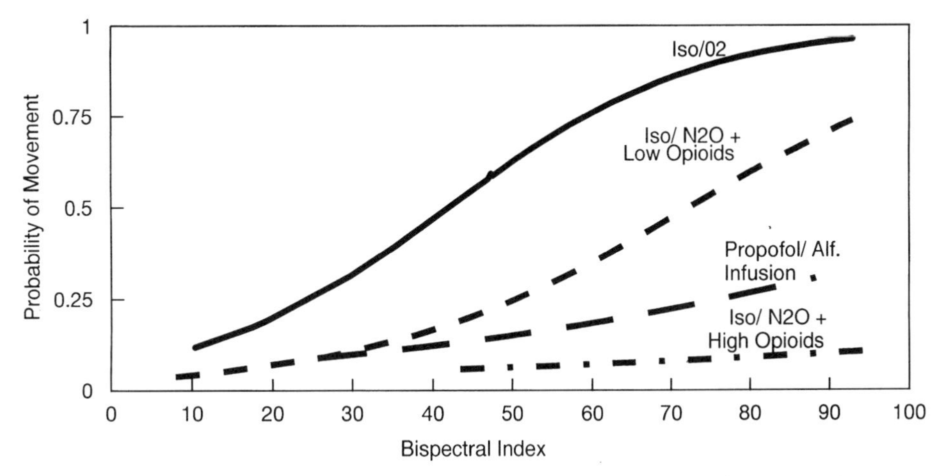

FIGURE 27-8. The relationship between the BIS and the probability of movement in response to skin incision in patient receiving different anesthetic regimens. Note that when increasing amounts of opioids are used, the probability of response to incision is reduced dramatically at all BIS levels. From Sebel PS, Rampil I, Cork R, White PF, Smith NT, Glass P, Jopling M, Chamoun N. Bispectral analysis (BIS) for monitoring anesthesia: comparison of anesthetic techniques. Anesthesiology Sep 1994 81(34):A1488.

isoflurane-alfentanil anesthesia (111, 112). A relationship between BIS and anesthetic depth using an opioid-based anesthetic has also been demonstrated (114). In a large multicenter study, using a variety of anesthetic techniques, patient movement in response to surgical skin incision was investigated (115). The relationship between the EEG-BIS and the probability of patient movement in response to skin incision was dependent on the anesthetic technique (Fig. 27-8). Specifically, patients with apparently "light" EEG profiles with high doses of opioids did not move at incision, thus supporting a distinction between the analgesic and hypnotic effects of the agents used (115). When hypnotic drugs such as propofol or isoflurane were used as the primary anesthetic agent, a good correlation was noted between BIS and the probability of response to incision. Movement in response to a surgical incision reflects both a reaction to a stimulus (which can be reduced below a sensitivity threshold by opioid analgesics) and the "responsiveness" of the brain that is modified primarily by hypnotic agents.

Evoked Responses

Many studies suggest that auditory stimuli can be perceived intraoperatively and that AER may be useful in monitoring adequacy of anesthesia (32). The AER is a series of waves representing the electrical activity that occurs in response to a sound stimulus and is induced in various regions of the auditory pathway from the cochlea to the cortex, as shown in Figure 27-9. A repeated auditory stimulus is applied, and the resultant EEG is averaged during the interval immediately after the stimulus. Thus, the nonstimulus-related portion of the background EEG is eliminated, and the specific evoked potential remains. Once this is achieved, the responses are reproducible and appear similar in different subjects. The AER may be divided to several segments according to the anatomic area of origin and the elapsed time following the auditory stimulus. The brainstem AER (BAER) is the early component of the AER that occurs in the first 8 milliseconds following the stimulus and originates in the brainstem. The middle latency auditory evoked response (MLAER) comprises potentials occurring between 8 and 100 milliseconds after stimulation and related to neural activity within the thalamus and primary auditory cortex (32, 116). The late cortical response occurs between 50 and 1000 milliseconds and reflects activation of the frontal cortex (116). Because the late cortical component is affected by attention, sleep, and sedation (117, 118), it is of limited utility in assessing anesthetic effects. Various investigations have reported conflicting results of the effect of propofol on BAER (80, 119). Most anesthetic and analgesic drugs such as volatile anesthetics (120,121), diazepam (122), ketamine (123), and fentanyl (in doses up to 50 μg/kg) (124) do not affect BAER (Figs. 27-10 to 27-12). Extremely high doses of thiopental (up to 77.5 mg/kg) prolong the latency of the BAER, with no significant alterations in amplitude (125). The BAER was not affected by the combination of isoflurane-fentanyl or of propofol-fentanyl (126). As opposed to BAER, studies using AER have demonstrated graded linear dose-related prolongations of waves latency and decrease of amplitude with most anesthetics. A dose-related effect on the early cortical components of the AER has also been demonstrated (127–129). Propofol produces dose-related increases in latency and decreases in amplitude of the early cortical response similar to the changes observed with volatile anesthetics, etomidate, and Althesin (80) (see Fig. 27-10).

Thornton and colleagues found that etomidate and Althesin produce dose-related prolongations in the amplitude and latency of the waves in the cortical com-

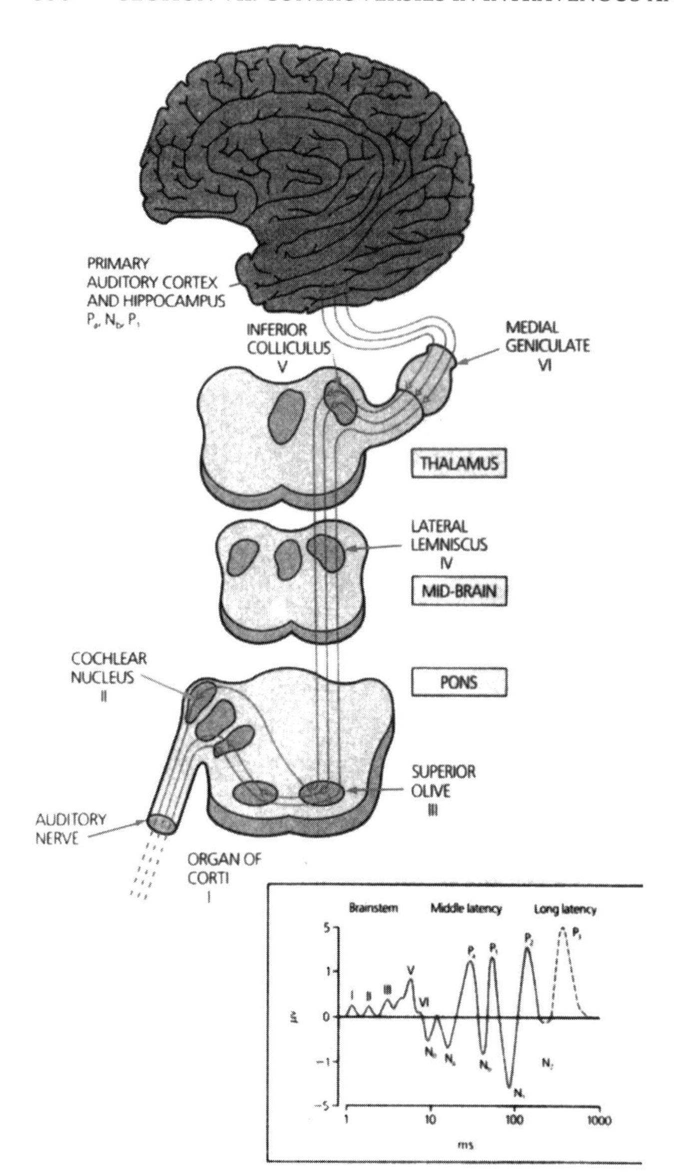

FIGURE 27-9. The brain pathway of the auditory signal. Waves I to VI are originated in the brain stem in the marked sites. The middle latency waves arise from the primary auditory cortex, and the long latency waves arise in other cortical associated areas. (From Ghoneim MM, Block RI. Learning and consciousness during general anesthesia. Anesthesiology 1992;76:279–305.)

ponent of the AER, in contrast to the BAER, in which no effect of the drugs was seen (130, 131). These investigators suggested that the intravenous anesthetics have little effect on neural function below the level of the superior colliculus and that the similarity between anesthetic effects on the middle latency component of the AER may be useful in assessing adequacy of anesthesia. Based on several of their studies, Thornton and associates (132) concluded that early cortical waves show graded changes depending on the surgical stimulus with at least six anesthetic drugs. Confirmatory evidence has come from the work of Schwender and associates (126), who found that BAER did not change from the awake pattern in patients anesthetized with isoflurane-fentanyl or propofol-fentanyl, in contrast to the MLAER, which showed a marked decrease in amplitude and increase in latency. These changes were not significant when fentanyl was used as the sole anesthetic. Opioids, even after large "induction" doses, did not affect the MLAER (133). In the bottom panel of Figure 27-11 is an example of a patient anesthetized with high-dose fentanyl. The authors of this study (133) suggested that opioids, even in large doses, do not provide reliable suppression of the auditory stimulus processing during general anesthesia, an observation that can explain the high occurrence of awareness and recall during high-dose opioid "anesthesia." These authors also concluded that inadequate suppression of the auditory stimulus processing may be associated with cardiovascular changes during sternotomy.

The amplitude and latencies of the BAER did not change during induction of anesthesia with ketamine (123), as shown in the top panel of Figure 27-11, suggesting that ketamine did not adequately suppress the perception and processing of sensory stimuli, a finding

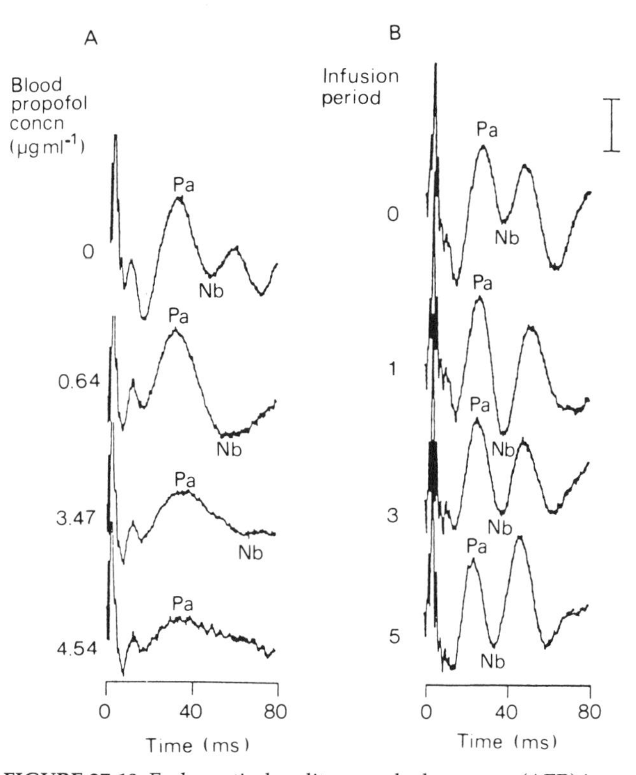

FIGURE 27-10. Early cortical auditory evoked response (AER) in a patient given propofol (A) and a patient given saline (B). Note the decrease in amplitude and increase in latency, and the lack of change in the brain stem AER (BAER) in A. (From Thornton C, Konieczko KM, Knight AB, et al. Effect of propofol on the auditory evoked response and oesophageal contractility. Br J Anaesth 1989; 63:411–417.)

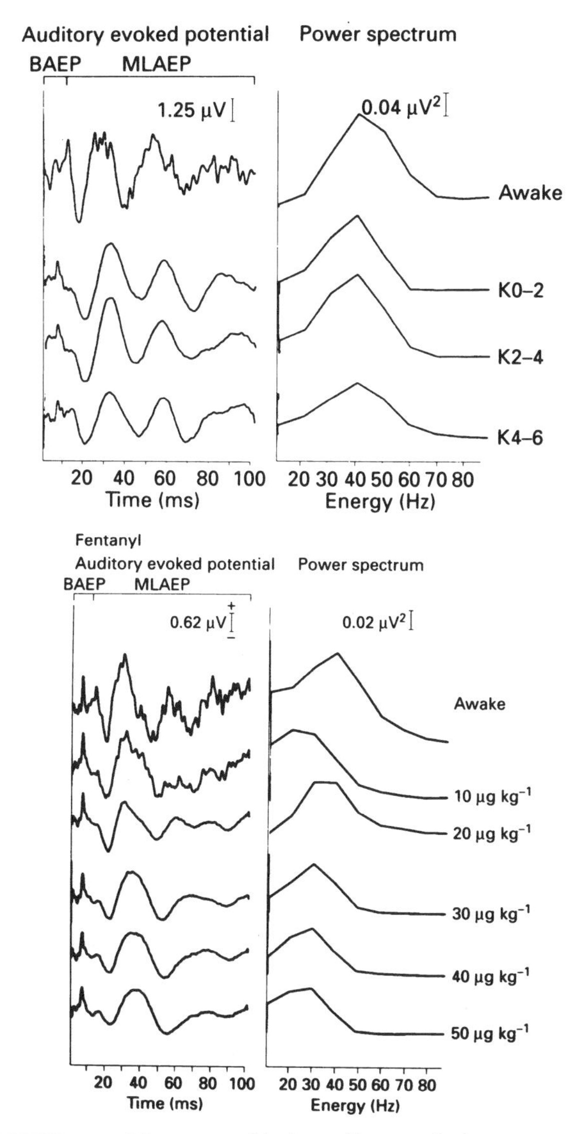

FIGURE 27-11. The top panel is the auditory evoked response (AER) tracing of a patient anesthetized with ketamine. Data are shown from the awake patient and at 0 to 2, 2 to 4, and 4 to 6 minutes. The BAER is easily identified unchanged. The middle latency AER (MLAER) shows large amplitude and characteristic periodic waveform that are unchanged from the awake pattern. The bottom panel shows the effect on the AER tracing of different doses of fentanyl. (From Schwender D, Klasing S, Madler C, et al. Mid-latency auditory evoked potentials during ketamine anaesthesia in humans. Br J Anaesth 1993;71:629–632.)

that may partially explain the high incidence of dreams and hallucinations associated with ketamine. In patients undergoing cardiac surgery, high-amplitude and periodic AER waveforms were found to correlate with implicit memory (32) (see Fig. 27-12). Thornton and colleagues (134), using the IFT in patients anesthetized with enflurane and N_2O, concluded that characteristic patterns in the AER indicate potential awareness. Although these findings indicate that the AER (particularly the middle latency component) may be a promising method of anesthetic adequacy monitoring, further research will be required before one can determine the clinical utility of AER monitoring.

Anesthetic adequacy can also be monitored by the 40-Hz auditory steady-state response (ASSR). The ASSR is a sinusoidal electrical response of the brain to repeated auditory stimuli and appears when the rate of stimulus delivery is sufficiently rapid to produce overlapping of the responses to individual stimuli. This response is most prominent for stimulus rates near 40 Hz, and the amplitude is reduced by 50% during sleep (135). Several features of the ASSR make it a potential candidate for monitoring the level of consciousness during anesthesia. The ASSR is a steady-state equivalent of the transient middle latency response that shows graded, dose-related amplitude reduction with general anesthetics (135). Plourde and

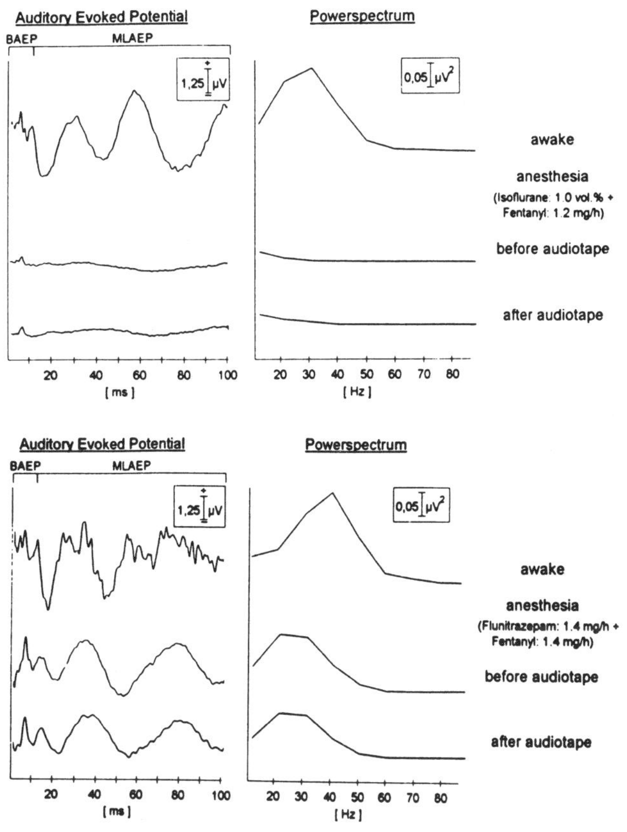

FIGURE 27-12. The tracing of auditory evoked response (AER) (left panel) and power spectrum (right panel) of two patients undergoing cardiac surgery. The top panel is the AER tracing of a patient without implicit memory; brain stem AER (BAER) can be identified easily as in the awake state, whereas middle latency AER (MLAER) is severely attenuated. The lower panel is the electroencephalogram of a patient with implicit memory. The MLAER continue to show high amplitude and periodic waveform. (From Schwender D, Kaiser A, Peter K, Poppel E. Midlatency auditory evoked potentials and explicit and implicit memory in patients undergoing cardiac surgery. Anesthesiology 1994;80:493–501.)

associates evaluated ASSR during balanced anesthesia with thiopental, fentanyl, and isoflurane (with and without N_2O) (135). The ASSR was reduced significantly at the end of the induction period and decreased below noise levels during surgical anesthesia. It increased significantly during emergence and recovery, although the amplitude during recovery remained significantly lower than the preinduction values. A subsequent study evaluated the ASSR in patients undergoing cardiac surgery anesthetized with high-dose sufentanil (136). The ASSR was present before induction, was greatly attenuated or abolished with loss of consciousness, and reappeared at low amplitude 5 to 10 minutes later and remained attenuated until the end of surgery. The amplitude increased with early signs of awakening in the intensive care unit. Thus, the ASSR appears to be a potential tool for monitoring adequacy of anesthesia.

PHARMACOLOGIC APPROACHES TO MEASURING ANESTHETIC ADEQUACY

Depth of anesthesia has been most commonly characterized by the drug effect, like the concept of MAC defined by Eger and associates (5). Eger et al considered the plasma concentration of the inhaled agent to be constant throughout surgery and a good approximation to the alveolar concentration at equilibrium. Drug uptake from the lungs depended on the cardiac output, ventilation-perfusion ratio, mode of mechanical ventilation, hemodynamic state, and atelectasis, all of which can change during operation (137). Although no method of measuring actual plasma concentrations in real time is available, MAC is unaffected by the type of stimulation, provided a maximal stimulus is applied (20). Noxious stimuli are not always maximal, however, and response differences may be noted when the skin is incised in different parts of the body (24). Using MAC as a guide to the delivery of adequate anesthesia ensures us that only 50% of patients will not move in response to noxious stimulus, meaning that they are not adequately anesthetized. Using the 95% effective dose (ED_{95}) of anesthetics instead of the median effective dose (ED_{50}) (MAC) ensures us that our patients have only a 5% chance of moving at surgical stimulus, but this does not represent adequate anesthesia for all patients. To identify patients who move is impossible when NMBAs are used. A 1-MAC concentration of the volatile anesthetic does not necessarily blunt the stress response of surgery because it takes higher concentration to block this response (i.e., MAC-BAR) (21). Thus, MAC may not be used to monitor the adequacy of anesthesia; however, it is a useful method for comparing potencies of different anesthetics.

Pharmacokinetic and pharmacodynamic concepts govern the relationship between drug dose and response. The body's interactions with the drug through distribution, metabolism, and elimination govern the concentration of the drug that is ultimately available at the site of action (or biophase). The ideal site for measurement of an anesthetic drug concentration is in the biologic fluids immediately surrounding the effect site where the anesthetic agent exerts its pharmacologic action. Although this is not possible in clinical practice, slow administration allows time for equilibrium with the effect site such that direct measurement of plasma drug concentrations can be related to the drug concentrations at the effect site. Rapid intravenous administration of anesthetic drugs causes a disequilibrium between plasma drug concentration and effect site drug concentration. The disposition of drug in the effect site can be mathematically modeled and is known as the k_{e0} (138). This rate constant can then be used to estimate the half-time of equilibration between plasma drug concentration and effect site concentration, as well as the concentration of drug at the effect site (139). Context-sensitive half-time refers to the time required for the effect site drug concentration to decrease by 50% (140). The context-sensitive half-time was found to be a much better predictor of the intravenous anesthetic duration of action than its elimination half-time (140, 141).

Drug effect can be modeled as a function of drug concentration. Ideally, drug effect has a stable baseline with minimal variability, an effect that measurably increases as the drug concentration is increased, and a maximal plateau after which an increase in drug concentration has no effect. The midpoint between baseline and maximal effect is known as the Cp_{50}, or the plasma concentration of drug that results in 50% of the maximal effect. This parameter is used to compare drug potency and individual sensitivity to a drug. The use of the foregoing pharmacokinetic and pharmacodynamic parameters can be helpful in delivering anesthesia that is adequate to the patient and the procedure, but these parameters cannot be used to assess and monitor the adequacy of anesthesia.

Pharmacodynamic modeling has been used to relate clinical signs of inadequate opioid anesthesia to plasma concentrations of the drug (24). These investigators were able to describe the alfentanil concentration versus response relationship for different perioperative stimuli. Intubation required significantly higher plasma concentrations of alfentanil than did skin incision. Skin closure required significantly lower plasma concentrations than did skin incision. The rapid blood-brain equilibration of alfentanil means that a given plasma concentration has a close relationship with the effect site concentration (86). Glass and associates have applied a similar concept to administering fentanyl using a computer-assisted continuous infusion device to provide constant plasma fentanyl concentrations (67). Because of the longer k_{e0}, a significant amount of time was allowed between establishing the constant plasma concentration of fentanyl and applying the noxious stimuli. The approaches provide important insight into the correlation between plasma opioid concentration and clinical assessment of anesthetic adequacy (141).

Given the difficulty of measuring drug concentration in real time, the minimum infusion rate (MIR) has been proposed to compare requirements for intravenous anesthetic agents (142). The MIR is the minimum infusion rate necessary to prevent somatic response to skin incision in 50% of patients, from which the ED_{50} and ED_{95} can be estimated using pharmacokinetic formulations. This concept confronts some of the limitations of studies investigating the relationship between bolus doses of intravenous anesthetics and specific responses. The method makes use of the movement response, which is analogous to the MAC concept for inhaled anesthetic agents. Unfortunately, MIR is not helpful because it depends on the drug's pharmacokinetics and the CNS responsiveness. MIR ignores accumulation of drugs; thus, it is a time-dependent measure. Maintaining steady-state effect site concentrations is difficult using the MIR concept.

The relationship between plasma concentrations of thiopental and clinical measures of anesthetic adequacy have also been investigated (143). Hung and associates (144) used a computer-controlled infusion to maintain varying plasma concentrations of thiopental. At each thiopental site effect concentration, response to verbal command, 50-Hz electrical tetanus, laryngoscopy, intubation, and finally skin incision was assessed. Cp_{50} values (the probability of no movement in response to each stimulus) were calculated using logistic regression. Intubation required significantly higher thiopental concentrations than did laryngoscopy, trapezius muscle squeeze, electrical tetanus, and verbal responsiveness.

Combinations of intravenous anesthetic agents and opioids have also been investigated (145). A constant plasma concentration of propofol was maintained while alfentanil was titrated to clinical response. Propofol had a significant interaction with alfentanil by decreasing the dose and concentration of alfentanil needed for adequate anesthesia. The combination of opioids and inhaled anesthetics has also been studied by determining the MAC-reducting effects of opioid analgesics (6, 146, 147). Such studies are important in that opioid analgesics and intravenous anesthetics are commonly used concurrently and are rarely employed alone as single anesthetic agents. Quantification of these relationships is important in monitoring adequacy of anesthesia.

CLOSED-LOOP FEEDBACK-CONTROLLED ADMINISTRATION OF ANESTHETICS

The use of target-controlled infusion (TCI) systems, like the computer-assisted continuous infusion (CACI) device described previously, with appropriate measures of anesthetic adequacy, has allowed the development of closed-loop control systems. Several studies have been published, most utilizing the EEG. Schwilden and colleagues (105) used the MF of the EEG power spectrum as the feedback signal for the administration of alfentanil. The same group also studied the administration of propofol (102) and methohexital (103) using this system (102). They concluded that this system uses a relevant therapeutic end point and has the potential to be useful in assessing and defining analgesic and anesthetic dose requirements. Other investigators successfully employed the same feedback signal to administer total intravenous anesthesia (TIVA) using propofol and alfentanil (148).

Robb and associates administered enflurane (149) and isoflurane (150) with the aid of a closed-loop feedback system. They used a vaporizer that was modified to allow it to be driven by a computer controller. Systolic blood pressure was used as the feedback signal. These investigators achieved satisfactory blood pressure control, and the anesthetic state was clinically acceptable to an independent observer. The foregoing systems have several limitations, however. All those presented so far use only one parameter as a feedback signal (e.g., blood pressure or EEG). As discussed earlier, no one sign or monitor can be used alone to monitor adequacy of anesthesia. These systems control the administration of only one drug, a technique that is rarely used. These systems do not take into consideration the type of surgery, specific surgical stimuli (e.g., manipulation of the adrenal gland or the aorta), or concurrently administered drugs. The available feedback systems are not sufficiently flexible (150) and do not have reliable fail-safe devices.

Greenhow and associates (151) describe a real-time expert system for advice and control (RESAC) of anesthesia. This system has been developed to advise on the concentration of volatile anesthetics by merging clinical information with online measurements. RESAC was programmed to receive information from monitors connected to the computer or directly from the keyboard. The information RESAC required was patient data, blood pressure, heart rate, pupil movement and size, diaphoretic, respiratory signs, and dose of opioid administered, as well as information on the desired physiologic ranges. RESAC then produced a text commentary on the adequacy of anesthesia, couched in advisory terms. Although not a closed-loop feedback system, the method of using an online expert system has exciting potential. A future approach to the problem will involve a neural network method, investigating a multitude of clinical signs to determine the degree of adequacy of anesthetic drugs.

IDEAL MONITOR OF DEPTH OF ANESTHESIA

Although the "ideal" anesthetic effect monitor does not exist, it may never exist because we are dealing a complex biologic system with an indefinite number of normal and abnormal variables and variants. Variable responses to different stimuli, drugs, and drug combinations also occur. The characteristics of the ideal hypothetic index monitor would include the following: 1) it should be noninvasive; 2) have a graded response; 3) the information presented by the monitor should provide an estimation of the adequacy of anesthesia independent of anesthetic technique or agent used; 4) be independent of the length and time of the operation; 5) predictive of events (e.g., movement); 6) effective during the recovery phase; 7) it should correlate with the anesthetic concentrations; 8) possess physiologic borders; 9) incorporated in a closed-loop feedback system with fail-safe features; 10) output should be simple and easy to interpret by the anesthesiologist; 11) the signal should be robust; 12) the output should include advisory information on analgesia and sedation, as well as awareness; and 13) it should detect decreasing adequacy of anesthesia in the presence of equipment failure and malfunction.

The most reliable monitor of patient responses to date has been the anesthesiologist, with his or her senses, experience, and knowledge. The current definitions of "anesthesia" and "anesthetic adequacy" are controversial. All anesthetics display some relationship among administered dose, plasma concentration, and clinical effect. However, the details of these relationships are not clearly understood. To date, no single clinical method and no single monitor can consistently monitor anesthetic adequacy. In the future, an integrated physiologic monitor may provide more useful information on the depth of intravenous anesthesia.

REFERENCES

1. White DC. Anaesthesia: a privation of the senses: an historical introduction and some definitions. In: Rosen M, Lunn JN, eds. Consciousness, awareness, and pain in general anesthesia. London: Butterworth, 1987:1.
2. Kissin I, Mason JO, Bradley EL. Morphine and fentanyl hypnotic interaction with thiopental. Anesthesiology 1987;67:331–335.
3. Kelly JS, Roy RC. Intraoperative awareness with propofol-oxygen total intravenous anesthesia for microlaryngeal surgery. Anesthesiology 1992;77:207–209.
4. Cullen SC, Larson CP. Evaluation of anesthetic depth. In: Essentials of anesthetic practice. Chicago: Year Book, 1974:77.
5. Eger EI, Saidman LJ, Brandstater B. Minimum alveolar anesthetic concentration: a standard of anesthetic potency. Anesthesiology 1965;26:756–763.
6. Westmoreland CL, Sebel PS, Gropper A. Fentanyl or alfentanil decreases the minimum alveolar anesthetic concentration of isoflurane in surgical patients. Anesth Analg 1994;78:23–28.
7. Ghoneim MM, Block RI. Learning and consciousness during general anesthesia. Anesthesiology 1992;76:279–305.
8. Plomley F. Operation upon the eye. Lancet 1847;1:134.
9. Guedel AE. Inhalational anesthesia: a fundamental guide. New York: Macmillan, 1937.
10. Artusio JF. Di-ethyl ether analgesia: a detailed description of the first stage of ether analgesia in man. J Pharmacol Exp Ther 1954;111:343–348.
11. Spackman TN, Messick JM, Sharbrough FW. Isoflurane anesthesia at depths producing a burst suppression EEG pattern does not attenuate the hemodynamic response to intubation [Abstract]. Anesthesiology 1991;75:A355.
12. Robson JG. Measurement of depth of anaesthesia. Br J Anaesth 1969;41:785–788.
13. Woodbridge P. Changing concept concerning depth of anesthesia. Anesthesiology 1957;18:536–550.
14. Pinsker MC. Anesthesia: a pragmatic construct. Anesth Analg 1986;65:819–827.
15. Prys-Roberts C. Anaesthesia: a practical or impractical construct? Br J Anaesth 1987;11:1341–1345.
16. Kissin I. General anesthetic action: an obsolete notion? Anesth Analg 1993;76:215–218.
17. Kissin I, Gelman S. Three components of anesthesia: one more reason to accept the concept. Anesth Analg 1987;66:98.
18. Kissin I, Brown PT. Reserpine-induced changes in anesthetic action of fentanyl. Anesthesiology 1985;62:597–600.
19. Weston GA, Roth SH. Differential actions of volatile anaesthetic agents on a single isolated neurone. Br J Anaesth 1986;58:1390–1396.
20. Merkel G, Eger EI. A comparative study of halothane and halopropane anesthesia. Anesthesiology 1963;24:346–357.
21. Roizen MF, Horrigan RW, Frazer BM. Anesthetic doses blocking adrenergic (stress) and cardiovascular responses to incision-MAC BAR. Anesthesiology 1981;54:390–398.
22. Hilgenberg JC. Intraoperative awareness during high-dose fentanyl-oxygen anesthesia. Anesthesiology 1981;54:341–343.
23. Hug CC, Moldenhauer CC. Does opioid "anesthesia" exist? Anesthesiology 1990;73:1–4.
24. Ausems ME, Hug CC, Stanski DR, Burm AG. Plasma concentrations of alfentanil required to supplement nitrous oxide anesthesia for general surgery. Anesthesiology 1986;65:362–373.
25. Aitkenhead AR. Risk management in anaesthesia. J Med Def Union 1991;4:86–90.
26. Stedman's medical dictionary. Baltimore: Williams & Wilkins, 1990.
27. Kihlstrom JF. Implicit memory function during anesthesia. In: Bonke B, Sebel PS, Winograd E, eds. Memory and awareness in anesthesia. Englewood Cliffs, NJ: Prentice Hall, 1993:10–30.
28. Russell IF. Comparison of wakefulness with two anaesthetic regimens. Br J Anaesth 1986;58:965–968.
29. Russell IF. Balanced anesthesia: does it anesthetize? Anesth Analg 1985;64:941–942.
30. Jones JG, Konieczko K. Hearing and memory in anaesthetised patients. Br Med J 1986;292:1291–1293.
31. Jelicic M, Bonke B, Appelboom DK. Indirect memory for words presented during anaesthesia. Lancet 1990;336:249.
32. Schwender D, Kaiser A, Peter K, Poppel E. Midlatency auditory evoked potentials and explicit and implicit memory in patients undergoing cardiac surgery. Anesthesiology 1994;80:493–501.
33. Caseley-Rondi G, Merikle PM, Bowers KS. Unconscious cog-

nition in the context of general anesthesia. Consciousness Cogn 1994;3:166–195.
34. Suresh D. Nightmares and recovery from anesthesia. Anesth Analg 1991;72:404–405.
35. Brimacombe J, Macfie AG. Peri-operative nightmares in surgical patients. Anaesthesia 1993;48:527–529.
36. Aitkenhead AR. Awareness during anaesthesia: what should the patient be told? Anaesthesia 1990;45:351–352.
37. Mainzer J Jr. Awareness, muscle relaxants and balanced anesthesia. Can Anaesth Soc J 1979;26:386–393.
38. Sandin R, Nordstrom O. Awareness during total I.V. anesthesia. Br J Anaesth 1993;71:782–787.
39. Breckenridge JL, Aitkenhead AR. Awareness during anaesthesia: a review. Ann R Coll Surg Engl 1983;65:94–95.
40. Robinson RJS, Boright WA, Ligier B, et al. The incidence of awareness and amnesia for perioperative events, after cardiac surgery with lorazepam and fentanyl anesthesia. J Cardiothorac Vasc Anesth 1987;1:524.
41. Bogetz MS, Katz JA. Recall of surgery for major trauma. Anesthesiology 1984;61:6–9.
42. Levinson BW. States of awareness during general anaesthesia. Br J Anaesth 1965;37:544–546.
43. Blacher RS. Awareness during surgery. Anesthesiology 1984; 61:1–2.
44. Stevens WC, Dolan WM, Gibbons RT, et al. Minimum alveolar concentrations (MAC) of isoflurane with and without nitrous oxide in patients of various ages. Anesthesiology 1975;42:197–200.
45. Newton DEF, Thornton C, Konieczko K, et al. Levels of consciousness in volunteers breathing sub-MAC concentrations of isoflurane. Br J Anaesth 1990;65:609–615.
46. Rampil IJ, Mason P, Singh H. Anesthetic potency (MAC) is independent of forebrain structures in the rat. Anesthesiology 1993;78:707–712.
47. Rampil IJ. Anesthetic potency is not altered after hypothermic spinal cord transection in rats. Anesthesiology 1994;80:606–610.
48. Antognini JF, Schwartz K. Exaggerated anesthetic requirements in the preferentially anesthetized brain. Anesthesiology 1993; 79:1244–1249.
49. Borges M, Antognini JF. Does the brain influence somatic responses to noxious stimuli during isoflurane anesthesia? Anesthesiology 1994;81:1511–1515.
50. McFarlane C, Warner DS, Dexter F, Ludwig PA. Minimum alveolar concentration for halothane in the rat is resistant to effects of forebrain ischemia and reperfusion. Anesthesiology 1994;81:1206–1211.
51. King BS, Rampil IJ. Anesthetic depression of spinal motor neurons may contribute to lack of movement in response to noxious stimuli. Anesthesiology 1994;81:1484–1492.
52. Jacoby LL, Allan LG, Collins JC, Larwill LK. Memory influences subjective experience: noise judgments. J Exp Psychol Learn Mem Cogn 1988;14:240–247.
53. Chang T-L, Dworsky WA, White PF. Use of continuous electromyography for monitoring depth of anesthesia. Anesth Analg 1988;67:521–25.
54. Jessop J, Jones JG. Conscious awareness during general anesthesia-what are we attempting to monitor? Br J Anaesth 1991; 66:635–637.
55. Tunstall ME. Detecting wakefullness during general anesthesia for caesarean section. Br Med J 1977;1:1321.
56. Russell IF. Concious awareness during general anesthesia: depth of anesthesia. In: Jones JG, ed. Bailliere's clinical anesthesiology. London: Bailliere Tindall, 1989:511–532.
57. Bogod DG, Orton JK, Yau HM, Oh TE. Detecting awareness during general anesthetic caesarean section: an evaluation of two methods. Anaesthesia 1990;45:279–284.
58. Wang M, Russell IF, Charlton PF, Conlon J. An experimental simulation of anesthetic awareness and validation of the isolated forearm technique. In: Sebel PS, Bonke B, Winograd E, eds. Memory and awareness in anesthesia. Englewood Cliffs, NJ: Prentice Hall, 1993:434–446.
59. Breckenridge JL, Aitkenhead AR. Isolated forearm technique for detection of wakefulness during general anesthesia. Br J Anaesth 1981;53:665–666.
60. Millar K, Watkinson N. Recognition of words presented during general anesthesia. Ergonomics 1989;26:585–594.
61. Russell IF. Auditory perception under anesthesia. Anaesthesia 1979;34:211.
62. Russell IF. Midazolam-alfentanil: an anesthetic? An investigation using the isolated forearm technique. Br J Anaesth 1993; 70:42–46.
63. Evans JM, Bithell JF, Vlachonikolis IG. Relationship between lower oesophageal contractility, clinical signs, and halothane concentration during general anaesthesia and surgery in man. Br J Anaesth 1987;59:1346–1355.
64. Pomfrett CJD, Barrie JR, Healy TEJ. Respiratory sinus arrhythmia: an index of light anaesthesia. Br J Anaesth 1993;71:212–217.
65. Moerman N, Bonke B, Oosting J. Awareness and recall during general anesthesia. Anesthesiology 1993;79:454–464.
66. Cullen DJ, Eger EI II, Stevens WC, et al. Clinical signs of anesthesia. Anesthesiology 1972;36:21–36.
67. Glass PSA, Doherty M, Jacobs JR, et al. Plasma concentration of fentanyl, with 70% nitrous oxide, to prevent movement at skin incision. Anesthesiology 1993;78:842–847.
68. Dutton RC, Smith WD, Smith NT. Does the EEG predict anesthetic depth better than cardiovascular variables? [Abstract.] Anesthesiology 1990;73:A532.
69. Hudson RJ, Stanski DR, Saidman LJ, Meathe E. A model for studying depth of anesthesia and acute tolerance to thiopental. Anesthesiology 1983;59:301–308.
70. Weiskopf RB, Moore MA, Eger EI II, et al. Rapid increase in desflurane concentration is associated with greater transient cardiovascular stimulation than with rapid increase in isoflurane concentration in humans. Anesthesiology 1994;80:1035–1045.
71. Ebert TJ, Muzi M, Lopatka CW. Neurocirculatory responses to sevoflurane in humans: a comparison to desflurane. Anesthesiology 1995;83:88–95.
72. Ebert TJ, Muzi M, Berens R, et al. Sympathetic responses to induction of anesthesia in humans with propofol or etomidate. Anesthesiology 1992;76:725–733.
73. Schultetus RR, Hill CR, Dharamraj CM, et al. Wakefulness during cesarean section after anesthetic induction with ketamine, thiopental, or ketamine and thiopental combined. Anesth Analg 1986;65:723–728.
74. Larson MD. Surgically induced hypertension in brain dead patients. Anesth Analg 1985;64:1030.
75. Wetzel RC, Setzer N, Stiff JL, Rogers MC. Hemodynamic response in brain dead organ donor patients. Anesth Analg 1985; 64:125–128.
76. Guyton AC. The autonomic nervous system: the adrenal medulla. In: Textbook of medical physiology. Philadelphia: WB Saunders, 1991:667–678.
77. Monk TG, Mueller M, White PF. Treatment of stress response during balanced anesthesia: comparative effects of isoflurane, alfentanil, and trimethaphan. Anesthesiology 1992;76:39–45.
78. Lang E, Bennett HL, Sebel PS, Sigl J. Comparison of bispectral EEG (BIS), facial electromyography (FACE), and hemodynamic responses as predictors of loss and return of consciousness following propofol [Abstract]. Anesthesiology 1994;81:475.
79. Evans JM, Davies WL, Wise CC. Lower oesophageal contractility: a new monitor af anaesthesia. Lancet 1984;1:1151–1154.
80. Thornton C, Konieczko KM, Knight AB, et al. Effect of propofol

on the auditory evoked response and oesophageal contractility. Br J Anaesth 1989;63:411–417.
81. Sessler DI, Stoen R, Olofsson CI, Chow F. Lower esophageal contractility predicts movement during skin incision in patients anesthetized with halothane, but not with nitrous oxide and alfentanil. Anesthesiology 1989;70:42–46.
82. Thomas DI, Aitkenhead AR. Relationship between lower oesophageal contractility and type of surgical stimulation. Br J Anaesth 1990;64:306–310.
83. Raftery S, Enever G, Prys-Roberts C. Oesophageal contractility during total I.V. anaesthesia with and without glycopyrronium. Br J Anaesth 1991;66:566–571.
84. Watcha MF, White PF. Failure of LEC to predict patient movement during skin incision in anesthetized children. Anesthesiology 1989;71:664–668.
85. Ghouri AF, Monk TG, White PF. Electroencephalogram spectral edge frequency, lower esophageal contractility and autonomic responsiveness during general anesthesia. J Clin Monit 1993;9:176–185.
86. Scott JC, Ponganis KV, Stanski DR. EEG quantitation of narcotic effect: the comparative pharmacodynamics of fentanyl and alfentanil. Anesthesiology 1985;62:234–241.
87. Scott JC, Cooke JE, Stanski DR. Electroencephalographic quantitation of opioid effect: comparative pharmacodynamics of fentanyl and sufentanil. Anesthesiology 1991;74:34–42.
88. Homer TD, Stanski DR. The effect of increasing age on thiopental disposition and anesthetic requirement. Anesthesiology 1985;62:714–724.
89. Stanski DR, Maitre PO. Population pharmacokinetics and pharmacodynamics of thiopental: the effect of age revisited. Anesthesiology 1990;72:412–422.
90. Clark DL, Rosner BS. Neurophysiologic effects of general anesthetics. I. The electroencephalogram and sensory evoked responses in man. Anesthesiology 1973;38:564–582.
91. Neigh JL, Garman JK, Harp JR. The electroencephalogram pattern during anesthesia with Ethrane. Anesthesiology 1971; 35:482–487.
92. Bührer M, Maitre PO, Hung OR, et al. Thiopental pharmacodynamics. Defining the pseudo-steady-state serum concentration-EEG effect relationship. Anesthesiology 1992;77:226–236.
93. Levy WJ, Shapiro HM, Maruchak G, Meathe E. Automated EEG processing for intraoperative monitoring: a comparison of techniques. Anesthesiology 1980;53:223–236.
94. Rampil IJ, Holzer JA, Quest DE, et al. Prognostic value of computerized EEG analysis during carotid endarterectomy. Anesth Analg 1983;62:234–241.
95. Rampil IJ, Matteo RS. Changes in EEG spectral edge frequency correlate with the hemodynamic response to laryngoscopy and intubation. Anesthesiology 1987;67:139–142.
96. Sidi A, Halimi P, Cotev S. Estimating anesthetic depth by electroencephalography during anesthetic induction and intubation in patients undergoing cardiac surgery. J Clin Anesth 1990; 2:101–107.
97. White PF, Boyle WA. Relationship between hemodynamic and electroencephalographic changes during general anesthesia. Anesth Analg 1989;68:177–181.
98. Dwyer R, Rampil IJ, Eger EI, Bennett HL. The EEG does not predict movement in response to surgical incision at 1.0 MAC isoflurane [Abstract]. Anesthesiology 1991;75:A1025.
99. Long CW, Shah NK, Loughlin C, et al. A comparison of EEG determinants of near-awakening from isoflurane and fentanyl anesthesia: spectral edge, median power frequency, and delta ratio. Anesth Analg 1989;69:169–173.
100. Schwilden H, Schüttler J, Stoeckel H. Quantitation of the EEG and pharmacodynamic modelling of hypnotic drugs: etomidate as an example. Eur J Anaesth 1985;2:121–130.
101. Schwilden H, Schüttler J, Stoeckel H. Closed loop feedback control of methohexital anesthesia by quantitative EEG analysis in humans. Anesthesiology 1987;67:341–347.
102. Schwilden H, Stoeckel H, Schüttler J. Closed-loop feedback control of propofol anaesthesia by quantitative EEG analysis in humans. Br J Anaesth 1989;62:290–296.
103. Schwilden H, Stoeckel H. Effective therapeutic infusions produced by closed-loop feedback control of methohexital administration during total intravenous anesthesia with fentanyl. Anesthesiology 1990;73:225–229.
104. Schwilden H, Schuttler J, Stoeckel H. Quantitation of the EEG and pharmacodynamic modelling of hypnotic drugs: etomidate as an example. Eur J Anesthesiol 1985;2:121–131.
105. Schwilden H, Stoeckel H. Closed-loop feedback controlled administration of alfentanil during alfentanil-nitrous oxide anaesthesia. Br J Anaesth 1993;70:389–393.
106. Drummond JC, Brann CA, Perkins DE, Wolfe DE. A comparison of median frequency, spectral edge frequency, a frequency band power ratio, total power, and dominance shift in the determination of depth of anesthesia. Acta Anaesthesiol Scand 1991;35:693–699.
107. Huber PJ, Kleiner B, Gasser T, Dumermuth G. Statistical methods for investigating phase relations in stationary stochastic processes. IEEE Trans Audio Electroacoust 1971;19:78–86.
108. Sigl J, Chamoun N. An introduction to bispectral analysis for the electroecephlogram. J Clin Monit 1994;10:392–404.
109. Sebel PS, Bowles SM, Saini V, Chamoun N. Accuracy of EEG in predicting movement at incision during isoflurane anesthesia [Abstract]. Anesthesiology 1992;75:A446.
110. Sebel PS, Bowles SM, Saini V, Chamoun N. EEG bispectrum predicts movement during thiopental/isoflurane anesthesia. J Clin Monit 1995;11:83–91.
111. Vernon JM, Bowles SM, Sebel PS, Chamoun N. EEG bispectrum predicts movement at incision during isoflurane or propofol anesthesia [Abstract]. Anesthesiology 1992;55:A502.
112. Vernon JM, Lang E, Sebel PS, Manberg P. Prediction of movement using bispectral EEG during propofol/alfentanil or isoflurane/alfentanil anesthesia. Anesth Analg 1995;80:780–785.
113. Lien CA, Berman M, Saini V, et al. The accuracy of the EEG in predicting hemodynamic changes with incision during isoflurane anesthesia [Abstract]. Anesth Analg 1992;74:S187.
114. Kearse LA, Saini V, deBros F, Chamoun N. Bispectral analysis of EEG may predict anesthetic depth during narcotic induction [Abstract]. Anesthesiology 1991;75:A175.
115. Sebel PS, Rampil IJ, Cork RC, et al. Bispectral analysis (BIS) for monitoring anesthesia: comparison of anesthetic techniques [Abstract]. Anesthesiology 1994;81:1488.
116. Picton TW, Hillyard SA, Krausz HI, Galambos R. Human auditory evoked potentials. I. Evaluation of components. Electroencephalogr Clin Neurophysiol 1974;36:179–190.
117. Picton TW, Hillyard SA. Human auditory evoked potentials. II. Effects of attention. Electroencephalogr Clin Neurophysiol 1974;36:191–199.
118. Milligan KR, Lumsden J, Howard RC, et al. Use of auditory evoked responses as a measure of recovery from benzodiazepine sedation. J R Soc Med 1989;82:595–597.
119. Chassard D, Joubaud A, Colson A, et al. Auditory evoked potentials during propofol anaesthesia in man. Br J Anaesth 1989; 62:522–526.
120. Thornton C, Heneghan CPH, James MF, Jones JG. Effects of halothane or enflurane with controlled ventilation on auditory evoked potentials. Br J Anaesth 1984;56:315–322.
121. Newton DEF, Thornton C, Creagh-Barry P, Doré CJ. Early cortical auditory evoked response in anaesthesia: comparison of the effect of nitous oxide and isoflurane. Br J Anaesth 1989; 62:61–65.
122. Loughnan BL, Sebel PS, Thomas DI, et al. Evoked potentials following diazepam or fentanyl. Anaesthesia 1993.

123. Schwender D, Klasing S, Madler C, et al. Mid-latency auditory evoked potentials during ketamine anaesthesia in humans. Br J Anaesth 1993;71:629–632.
124. Samra SK, Lilly DJ, Rush NL, Kirsh MM. Fentanyl anesthesia and human brain-stem auditory evoked potentials. Anesthesiology 1984;61:261–265.
125. Drummond JC, Todd MM, U HS. The effect of high dose sodium thiopental on brain stem auditory and median nerve somatosensory evoked responses in humans. Anesthesiology 1985;63:249–254.
126. Schwender D, Haessler R, Klasing S, et al. Mid-latency auditory evoked potentials and circulatory response to loud sounds. Br J Anaesth 1994;72:307–314.
127. Thornton C, Catley DM, Jordan C, et al. Enflurane anaesthesia causes graded changes in the brainstem and early cortical auditory evoked response in man. Br J Anaesth 1983;55:479–485.
128. Sebel PS, Ingram DA, Flynn PJ, et al. Evoked potentials during isoflurane anaesthesia. Br J Anaesth 1986;58:580–585.
129. Schmidt JF, Chraemmer-Jorgensen B. Auditory evoked potentials during isoflurane anaesthesia. Acta Anaesthesiol Scand 1986;30:378–380.
130. Thornton C, Heneghan CPH, Navaratnarajah M, et al. Effect of etomidate on the auditory evoked response in man. Br J Anaesth 1985;57:554–561.
131. Thornton C, Heneghan CPH, Navaratnarajah M, Jones JG. Selective effect of althesin on the auditory evoked response in man. Br J Anaesth 1986;58:422–427.
132. Thornton C, Konieczko K, Jones JG, et al. Effect of surgical stimulation on the auditory evoked response. Br J Anaesth 1988; 60:372–378.
133. Schwender D, Rimkus T, Haessler R, et al. Effects of increasing doses of alfentanil, fentanyl and morphine on mid-latency auditory evoked potentials. Br J Anaesth 1993;71:622–628.
134. Thornton C, Barrowcliffe MP, Konieczko KM, et al. The auditory evoked response as an indicator of awareness. Br J Anaesth 1989;63:113–115.
135. Plourde G, Picton TW. Human auditory steady-state response during general anesthesia. Anesth Analg 1990;71:460–468.
136. Plourde G, Boylan JF. The auditory steady state response during sufentanil anaesthesia. Br J Anaesth 1991;66:683–691.
137. Eger EI II. Uptake and distribution. In: Miller RD, ed. Anesthesia. New York: Churchill Livingstone, 1994:101–121.
138. Hull CJ, Van Been HBH, Sibbald MA, Watson MJ. A pharmacodynamic model for pancuronium. Br J Anaesth 1978;50:1113–1121.
139. Shafer SL, Varvel JR. Pharmacokinetics, pharmacodynamics, and rational opioid selection. Anesthesiology 1991;74:53–63.
140. Hughes MA, Glass PSA, Jacobs JR. Context-sensitive half-time in multicompartment pharmacokinetic models for intravenous anesthetic drugs. Anesthesiology 1992;76:334–341.
141. Youngs EJ, Shafer SL. Pharmacokinetic parameters relevant to recovery from opioids. Anesthesiology 1994;81:833–842.
142. Sear JW, Phillips KC, Andrews CJH, Prys-Roberts C. Dose-response relationships for infusions of Althesin or methohexitone. Anaesthesia 1983;38:931–936.
143. Becker KE Jr. Plasma levels of thiopental necessary for anesthesia. Anesthesiology 1978;49:192–196.
144. Hung OR, Varvel JR, Shafer SL, Stanski DR. Thiopental pharmacodynamics. II. Quantitation of clinical and electroencephalographic depth of anesthesia. Anesthesiology 1992;77:237–244.
145. Hung OR, Varvel JR, Shafer SL, Stanski DR. Pharmacodynamics of alfentanil as a supplement to propofol or nitrous oxide for lower abdominal surgery in female patients. Anesthesiology 1993;78:1036.
146. Murphy MR, Hug CC. The anesthetic potency of fentanyl in terms of its reduction of enflurane MAC. Anesthesiology 1982; 57:485–488.
147. McEwan AI, Smith C, Dyar O, et al. Isoflurane minimum alveolar concentration reduction by fentanyl. Anesthesiology 1993;78:864–869.
148. Schüttler J, Kloos S, Ihmsen H, Schwilden H. Clinical evaluation of a closed-loop dosing device for total intravenous anesthesia based on EEG depth of anesthesia monitoring [Abstract]. Anesthesiology 1992;77:A501.
149. Robb HM, Asbury AJ, Gary WM, Linkens DA. Towards a standardized anaesthetic state using enflurane and morphine. Br J Anaesth 1991;66:358–364.
150. Robb HM, Asbury AJ, Gray WM, Linkens DA. Towards a standardized anaesthetic state using isoflurane and morphine. Br J Anaesth 1993;71:366–369.
151. Greenhow SG, Linkens DA, Asbury AJ. Pilot study of an expert system adviser for controlling general anaesthesia. Br J Anaesth 1993;71:359–365.

28 Controlling the Stress Response

Erik P. Vandermeulen

The surgical stress response is a complex array of endocrine, hemodynamic, metabolic, and inflammatory changes initiated by surgically-induced injury. The resulting hypermetabolic state causes a substrate flow from storage areas toward vital organs and the site of injury. Such a response may contribute to a higher incidence of perioperative cardiovascular, pulmonary, and gastrointestinal complications, thereby increasing morbidity and even mortality following major surgery (1, 2). Several studies have investigated the modification or abolishment of this stress reaction by inhalational, intravenous, or regional anesthetic techniques. However, except for studies involving regional anesthesia, few have evaluated the effects of such an intervention on clinical outcome. In fact, no conclusive data are available to evaluate the effects of limiting the stress response on postoperative mortality and morbidity (3).

EFFECT OF SURGERY ON THE STRESS RESPONSE

Surgical trauma and the resulting tissue damage initiate a nociceptive signal originating from the site of injury (Fig. 28-1) (4). This signal is transmitted to the central nervous system (CNS) by somatosensory and sympathetic afferents (5, 6), including small myelinated (Aδ), unmyelinated (C), and even some fast conducting fibers. In addition, tissue injury causes the release of electrolytes and chemical mediators (e.g., potassium (K^+), bradykinin, prostaglandins, substance P, histamine) (7, 8). The synergistic action of this complex mixture of mediators (also known as the inflammatory soup) sensitizes peripheral nociceptors and further stimulates the inflammatory response and the release of substance P from vesicles in the peripheral terminals of unmyelinated C fibers. The inflammatory response also includes activation of the complement, coagulation, and fibrinolytic cascades. Increasing evidence also suggests an important role for the immune system in the local and systemic responses to stress. Locally released cytokines such as interleukins and tumor necrosis factor are involved in the multitude of metabolic, immunologic, and hematopoietic changes of stress response (9-12).

The afferent impulses carried by both neural and humoral pathways stimulate the hypothalamopituitary axis causing the release of stress hormones (e.g., catecholamines, cortisol, glucagon, growth hormone, aldosterone, and antidiuretic hormone [ADH] or vasopressin). The magnitude of this response is proportional to the degree of surgical injury sustained by the patient (13). A first phase (the so-called ebb phase) is dominated by catecholamines and is characterized by increased gluconeogenesis, hyperglycemia, supranormal protein and fat mobilization, and sodium and water retention. The second phase (the so-called flow phase) is dominated by steroid and peptide hormones and is characterized by a sustained catabolic reaction. A progressive return toward baseline metabolic conditions occurs over a period of days to weeks following elective surgery (9, 14).

INFLUENCE OF ANESTHESIA ON THE STRESS RESPONSE

Traditionally, opioid analgesics have been the primary agents used during general anesthesia to blunt the neuroendocrine response to surgical stimulation. Although profound analgesia should inhibit the metabolic response to surgery, such a relationship has not always been shown (15). Furthermore, sedative-hypnotics, α_2-adrenergic agonists, and nonsteroidal anti-inflammatory drugs (NSAIDs) are capable of modulating the stress response to surgery by altering the level of consciousness or by a direct effect on the

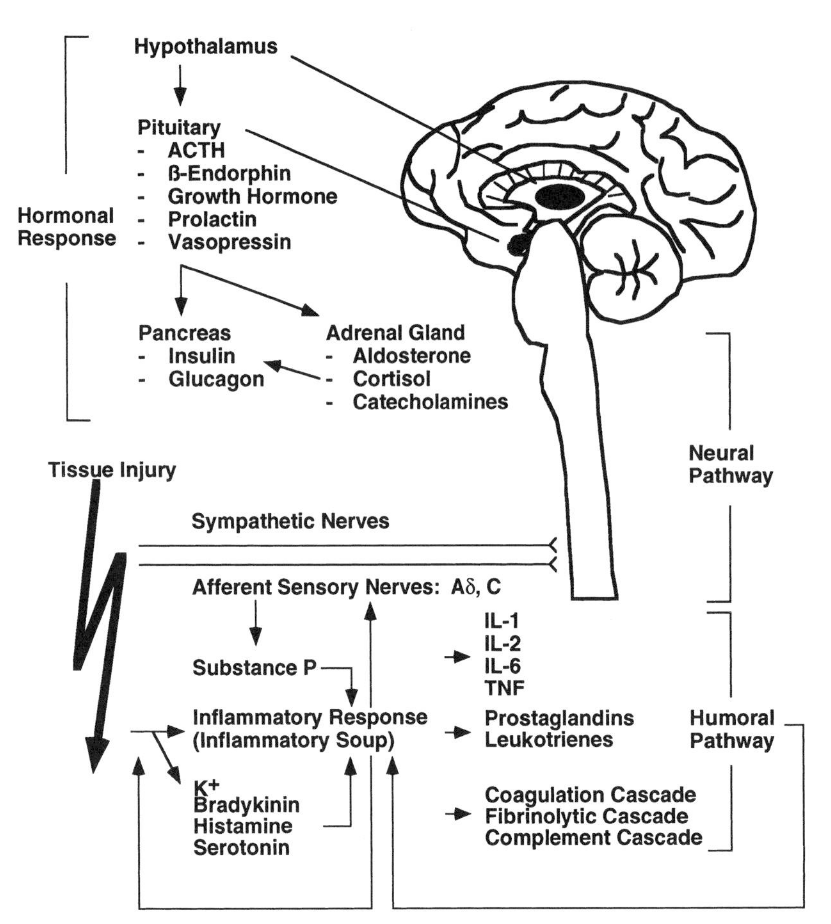

FIGURE 28–1. Different mechanisms in the stress response to tissue injury. Surgical tissue injury initiates a nociceptive signal that is transmitted to the central nervous system by somatosensory (Aδ, C) and sympathetic nerve fibers (the neural pathway), and causes the release of electrolytes and chemical mediators (the inflammatory soup). This inflammatory soup sensitizes the primary afferent nociceptors (Aδ, C) and further enhances the inflammatory reaction with the release of substance P, cytokines, and activation of the arachidonic acid (prostaglandins, leukotrienes), coagulation, complement, and fibrinolytic cascades (the humoral pathway). Both the neural and humoral input into the hypothalamopituitary axis cause the release of different stress hormones (the hormonal response). ACTH, Adrenocorticotropic hormone; IL, interleukin; TNF, tumor necrosis factor.

neuroendocrinologic response to surgically induced injury.

Inhalation Anesthetics

The volatile anesthetics are still widely used in general anesthesia. Although their exact mechanisms of action remain unclear, several hypotheses have been proposed (16). A widely accepted general principle of anesthetic pharmacology is that synaptic communication between neurons is essential for CNS function. Drug-induced, reversible impairment of this communication causes amnesia, analgesia, loss of consciousness, and even muscle relaxation. Earlier work suggested that deeper levels of inhalation anesthesia would cause a more pronounced attenuation of the stress response (17). However, in a subsequent study, higher doses of halothane did not result in a supplemental reduction of stress hormones in patients undergoing abdominal hysterectomy (18). Similarly, general anesthesia with enflurane (19), isoflurane (20), desflurane, or sevoflurane (21) does not completely prevent the perioperative rise in the plasma levels of different stress hormones. When the stress response to surgery during halothane anesthesia was compared to that during a balanced technique with morphine (22) or fentanyl (23, 24), significantly lower stress hormone levels were found in patients who had received the opioid-based regimens. In contrast, enflurane was more effective than neuroleptanesthesia in preventing the sympathoadrenal response to surgery (25, 26). Finally, total intravenous anesthesia (TIVA) with propofol-alfentanil proved superior to a conventional isoflurane anesthesia technique in suppressing the stress response to invasive stimuli (27).

The mechanism by which volatile anesthetics may have a limited blocking effect on the surgical stress response is believed to be twofold. First is the general anesthetic effect of these compounds. Second, halothane and enflurane have been shown to reduce the adrenal release of catecholamines (28, 29). In conclusion, volatile anesthetics have a small (if any) effect on the suppression hypothalamopituitary reaction to surgical stimulation.

Intravenous Anesthetics

Sedative-Hypnotics

BARBITURATES. Barbiturates have been one of the cornerstones of anesthesia practice since the 1960s. The postsynaptic γ-aminobutyric $acid_A$ ($GABA_A$) receptor complex appears to be the most likely site of action for barbiturate-mediated sedative-hypnotic effects (Table 28-1) (30). Activation of the $GABA_A$ receptor complex by hypnotic barbiturates increases the chloride permeability of neurons and thus membrane conductance, which reduces the excitability of the postsynaptic neurons. Moreover, the affinity of GABA binding to the $GABA_A$ receptor is potentiated by barbiturates, increasing the number of available GABA receptors and slowing the dissociation of GABA from its receptors.

Although it is widely accepted that barbiturates are hyperalgesic (or antianalgesic), recent information has shown barbiturate-mediated depression of spinal nociceptive neurotransmission. Because $GABA_A$ receptors are also found in spinal cord neurons, barbiturates may possibly exhibit antinociceptive effects at the spinal level (31-34). However, suppression of nociceptive neurotransmission is not effective until anesthetic drug concentrations are acheived. Furthermore, specific groups of barbiturates (or their derivatives) may have unique properties that reduce the descending inhibition from higher centers responsible for processing nociceptive stimuli at the level of the spinal cord. These hyperalgesic (or antianalgesic) properties may not be shared by other barbiturates or other widely used sedative-hypnotic agents.

Some evidence suggests that thiopental has limited metabolic and endocrine effects (see Table 28-1). Despite unchanged serum insulin levels, a slight increase in blood glucose levels can be detected (35). Plasma cortisol levels are decreased, but no influence on the adrenocortical response to surgery is noted (36, 37). Whether ADH secretion is increased remains controversial (38).

ETOMIDATE. Interaction of the imidazole derivative etomidate with specific subpopulations of the $GABA_A$ receptor causes an almost fourfold increase in GABA-ergic inhibition and thereby inhibits neuronal excitability (see Table 28-1) (30). Although initial reports suggested that etomidate was capable of profoundly blunting the normal hormonal response to surgery, subsequent reports suggested an increased mortality in critically ill patients subjected to long-term sedation with etomidate infusions (39, 40). Moreover, the drug inhibited the adrenocortical, but not the catecholamine, response to surgery (see Table 26-1) (36, 41). Etomidate was also shown to lack any analgesic activity, as evidenced by its inability to block the sympathetic response to laryngoscopy and intubation unless combined with an opioid analgesic (42, 43). The absence of adrenocortical response during and after etomidate anesthesia was a result not of suppression of nociception (44), but of adrenocortical enzyme

TABLE 28-1. Sedative-Hypnotic Drugs and the Stress Response to Surgery

Drugs	Mechanisms (References)	Hormonal Effects (References)
Barbiturates	$GABA_A$ receptor: CNS depression (30)	↓ ACTH (36)
		↑ ADH (38)
	Spinal $GABA_A$ receptor: inhibition of nociceptive neurotransmission (31, 32)	↑ Blood glucose (35)
		↓ Plasma cortisol (36)
	Hypothalamopituitary axis (36, 38)	
Etomidate	$GABA_A$ receptor: CNS depression (30)	↑ ACTH (36, 41, 44, 45)
		↓ Plasma cortisol (36, 41, 44, 45)
	Adrenocortical enzyme inhibition (41, 44, 45)	
Propofol	$GABA_A$ receptor: CNS depression (30)	↓ ADH (52)
		↓ ACTH (50)
	Spinal $GABA_A$ receptor: Inhibition of nociceptive neurotransmission (33, 34, 46, 47)	↑ Prolactin (50)
		↓ Plasma cortisol (50–52)
		↓ Plasma epinephrine (52)
	Hypothalamopituitary axis (central noradrenergic inhibition) (37, 48–53)	↓ Plasma norepinephrine (50–52)
Benzodiazepines	$GABA_A$ receptor: CNS depression (30)	↓ ACTH (58–60, 62)
		↓ β-Endorphin (58–60)
	Hypothalamopituitary Axis (56–62)	↓ Catecholamines (56, 57)
		↓ Plasma cortisol (58–60)
	Inflammatory response (cytokines) (63)	
Ketamine	Loss of consciousness	↑ ACTH (66, 77, 78)
	Thalamoneocortical projection system (depression) (64)	↑ ADH (78)
		↑ Plasma cortisol (66, 77, 78)
		↑ Plasma epinephrine (66, 78)
	Medullary reticular formation (depression) (64, 70–72)	↑ Plasma norepinephrine (66, 78)
		↑ Prolactin (77)
	Analgesia	
	Opiate receptors in central and peripheral nervous system (64, 71, 72)	
	NMDA-receptor antagonism (73–76)	
	Hypothalamopituitary axis (stimulation) (88)	
	Increased release and decreased reuptake of catecholamines (84–87)	

GABA, γ-Aminobutyric acid; ACTH, adrenocorticotropic hormone; ADH, antidiuretic hormone; NMDA, N-methyl-D-aspartate.

(mitochondrial 17α- and 11β-hydroxylase) inhibition, causing a decrease in cortisol, 17α-hydroxyprogesterone, and aldosterone production with a concomitant increase in adrenocorticotropic hormone (ACTH) and cortisol precursors (45).

PROPOFOL. Propofol is an alkyl phenol anesthetic agent (2,6-diisopropylphenol) that possesses a unique pharmacokinetic and dynamic profile, enabling rapid and smooth recovery and minimal postoperative confusion and nausea. The primary mechanism by which propofol exerts its anesthetic actions appears to be also mediated by the $GABA_A$ receptor-activated chloride channel (see Table 28-1) (30). Even though some studies suggest that propofol may have spinal antinociceptive effects, analgesic properties have not been demonstrated (34, 46, 47). Propofol has been shown to blunt the hemodynamic response to laryngoscopy and intubation more effectively than thiopental, but this differential effect may be related to its cardiovascular actions rather than to its analgesic activity, and the blunting of the hyperdynamic response is enhanced in the presence of opioid analgesics (see Table 28-1) (48, 49). The use of propofol as an anesthetic agent for electroconvulsive therapy showed a reduction in prolactin, ACTH, and cortisol levels in comparison with patients treated with thiopental (50). This decrease in prolactin may have been related to the reduction in seizure duration, whereas the reduction in ACTH and cortisol secretion was probably mediated through a reduction of central noradrenergic activity and the generalized cerebral depressant effect of propofol. Two studies have demonstrated that supplementary doses of propofol, in association with baseline analgesia provided by fentanyl or alfentanil, are effective in controlling acute hemodynamic and hormonal responses to surgical stimuli during TIVA. Glass and associates reported that supplemental doses of propofol were superior to supplemental boluses of fentanyl in the treatment of acute hemodynamic responses during surgery (51). In contrast, Monk and associates found no differences when supplemental doses of propofol were compared with boluses of alfentanil (52). Finally, the ACTH stimulation and adrenocortical response to surgery appear to be well maintained during propofol anesthesia (37, 53-55).

BENZODIAZEPINES. Benzodiazepine agonists have a wide spectrum of clinically relevant effects that are useful during intravenous anesthesia, including hypnosis, sedation, anxiolysis, and amnesia. In addition, benzodiazepines have anticonvulsant and centrally mediated muscle relaxant properties. The extent to which all of these properties are present differs among the benzodiazepines. The mechanism of action of benzodiazepines has been well described in the anesthesia literature. Benzodiazepines produce their clinical effects by activating the postsynaptic $GABA_A$-receptor complex, which also includes the benzodiazepine receptor (see Table 28-1) (30).

Benzodiazepines have been used for intravenous sedation and induction of general anesthesia in the operating room and for sedation in the operating room and intensive care unit. Because of its water solubility, as well as its rapid onset and short duration of action, midazolam has become the benzodiazepine of choice in anesthesia. When anesthesia was induced with a combination of midazolam and fentanyl, the hemodynamic response to laryngoscopy and endotracheal intubation was effectively attenuated, and levels of circulating catecholamines were decreased (see Table 28-1) (56). The administration of midazolam (or diazepam) before induction of general anesthesia caused a significant decrease in plasma norepinephrine and a transient depression of the baroreflex control function of the heart rate (57). Moreover, maintenance of anesthesia with a midazolam-based infusion in patients undergoing superficial orthopedic surgery reduced the secretion of cortisol, ACTH, and β-endorphin after surgery (58). These findings were consistent with those found in patients having abdominal surgery under midazolam-based anesthesia (59, 60). Midazolam was also found to reduce the physiologic and hormonal response to hypotensive episodes that occurred during the course of anesthesia and surgery (61).

Unlike etomidate, which directly suppresses cortisol production in the adrenal gland, benzodiazepines reduce the adrenal response to surgery by decreasing ACTH secretion, suggesting a direct influence of these drugs on the centrally mediated hypothalamopituitary axis (62). Furthermore, induction of anesthesia with intravenous midazolam induced a marked and delayed inhibition of the production of lipopolysaccharide-induced production of interleukin-1β, tumor necrosis factor, and interleukin-6 by monocytes (63). These cytokines have been closely linked to the surgical stress response (11, 12).

Benzodiazepines are effective in blunting the surgical stress response, not only by their sedative-hypnotic effect, but also by their direct influence on the hypothalamopituitary axis and the immunologic changes occurring during and after surgery.

KETAMINE. The phencyclidine derivative ketamine is different from most other anesthetic induction agents because it possesses a clinically significant analgesic effect and does not normally depress the cardiovascular and respiratory systems (64, 65). Commerically available ketamine is a racemic mixture of two isomers, S-(−)-ketamine and R-(−)-ketamine (66, 67). The anesthetic potency of the S-(+)-enantiomer was found to be three times higher that of the R-(−)-ketamine isomer. Ketamine's primary site of action is the thalamoneocortical projection system, where it selectively depresses neuronal function while stimulating parts of the limbic system (see Table 28-1) (68, 69). Neural transmission in the medullary reticular formation is also inhibited (70). A partial explanation for the analgesic properties of ketamine may be its occupation of opiate receptors in the brain and spinal cord (64, 71, 72). Finally, ketamine may also cause inhibition of dorsal horn wide dynamic range neurons, because of its interaction with the spinal N-methyl-D-aspartate (NMDA) receptor (73-76).

In patients, ketamine produces a dissociative state of anesthesia that resembles normal sleep and profound analgesia in which most (but not all) protective reflexes are maintained. When ketamine was used in combination with midazolam during trauma surgery, significant increases in ACTH, cortisol, and prolactin were detected (see Table 28-1) (77). Although midazolam was able adequately to block the intraoperative rise in catecholamine levels, these stress hormones increased during the postoperative period. In a study involving young, healthy volunteers, Adams and associates were able to demonstrate significant increases in the plasma levels of epinephrine, norepinephrine, ACTH, and cortisol following the intravenous injection of S-(−)-ketamine (66). The same authors reported significant increases in plasma catecholamines, ADH, ACTH, and cortisol in geriatric patients undergoing orthopedic surgery under TIVA with S-(−)- or R-(−)-ketamine (78). Therefore, these investigators recommended the use of a more potent hypnotic agent in combination with ketamine to provide adequate control of the hemodynamic and surgical stress parameters. No difference was noted in the endocrine or cardiovascular effects of the ketamine isomers (79, 80).

The limited efficacy of ketamine for controlling the surgical stress response may partly be explained by the direct effects of the drug on the endocrine and cardiovascular systems. The principal mechanism by which ketamine stimulates the circulatory system appears to be centrally mediated (81-83). The drug has been shown to stimulate the sympathoneural release of norepinephrine and to inhibit the intra- and extraneuronal uptake of catecholamines (84-87). Data from an experimental study also suggest a direct influence on the pituitary-adrenal axis, causing the release of ACTH and aldosterone (88). Although ketamine provides both sleep and analgesia, it produces insufficient control of the surgical stress response. The combination of ketamine and a sedative-hypnotic drug (e.g., thiopental, midazolam, diazepam, or propofol) overcomes this problem and provides excellent anesthetic conditions (77, 89-91).

Opioids

The preoperative administration of high doses of morphine (4 to 5 mg/kg), fentanyl (50 to 100 μg/kg), or one its newer analogs, alfentanil (1.2 mg/kg) or sufentanil (7 to 20 μg/kg), produces a marked reduction in the hormonal response to surgery (Table 28-2). The release of epinephrine, norepinephrine or dopamine (92-96), cortisol (92, 94-98), growth hormone (92, 97-100), aldosterone (24), β-endorphin (23), and vasopressin (24, 95, 100) is significantly suppressed during high-dose opioid anesthesia. A marked decrease in the surgical stress response was also described when more modest doses of fentanyl (101, 102), alfentanil (52, 103), or sufentanil (104) were supplemented with nitrous oxide or an inhalation anesthetic agent. Suppression of stress hormone secretion occurred throughout the operation and during the early postoperative period when major (noncardiac) surgery (92, 93, 101, 102) was performed. During cardiac surgery, inhibition of the neuroendocrine response was limited to the precardiopulmonary bypass period irrespective of the dose of opioid medication (94, 104-107). Philbin and associates demonstrated a ceiling effect with respect to the dose of fentanyl or sufentanil in patients undergoing elective coronary artery bypass surgery (108). The dose-related effects of opioids on stress response modulation are similar to their ceiling effects on the requirements of volatile anesthetic agents (109-112). Further increases in dosage of opioid analgesics do not result in additional inhibition of the stress response

TABLE 28-2. Opioids and the Stress Response to Surgery

Mechanisms (Reference)	Type of Surgery (Reference)	Hormonal Effects (References)
Analgesia:	Abdominal Surgery (92, 93, 99, 101, 102, 128, 130, 195)	↓ ACTH (97, 101, 102, 128)
Opiate receptors in the central and peripheral nervous system (118–120)	Cardiac Surgery* (23, 24, 94, 96, 97, 99)	↓ ADH (24, 52, 95, 100, 103)
		↓ Aldosterone (24, 100)
Peripheral opiate receptors (121–126)	Urologic Surgery (103)	↓ β-Endorphin (23, 101, 128, 131, 132)
		↑ Enkephalin (133–136)
Hypothalamopituitary axis (127–138)		↓ Catecholamines (92–95, 98, 104, 105, 140)
		↓ Cortisol (52, 92, 94, 95, 98, 99, 101–103, 105, 106, 128, 130)
		↓ Growth hormone (92, 98–100, 102, 130, 195)

**Effect on stress response limited to precardiopulmonary bypass period.*
ACTH, Adrenocorticotropic hormone; ADH, antidiuretic hormone.

(108, 113, 114). Moreover, high-dose opioid anesthesia may induce epileptiform activity in subcortical structures with extensive endogenous opioid pathways (e.g., the limbic system) (115). In contrast, some evidence indicates that the epidural use of opioids may produce a more complete blockade of the hormonal response to surgical stimuli (116, 117).

The mechanisms by which opioid analgesics are capable of producing these clinical effects are not clearly understood, but a dual mechanism appears to be involved (see Table 28-2). First is the central analgesic effect of opiates. By acting on specific opiate receptors in the CNS, opiates are capable of producing pain relief and reducing nociceptive input to higher brain centers. Interaction with receptors in the periaqueductal gray produces activation of a descending pain inhibiting system, thereby reducing afferent nociceptive impulses reaching the hypothalamus (118, 119). Opioids also produce a direct analgesic action on the nucleus reticularis of the brain and the substantia gelatinosa of the spinal cord (120). More recent evidence has suggested that opiates may produce analgesia by binding to peripheral primary nociceptive afferent nerve endings (121-126). Finally, opioid analgesics may be capable of directly influencing centrally mediated neuroendocrine responses. Several different hypothalamic receptors have been identified that can be stimulated by opioids and can thereby modify hormonal secretion (127-130). Exogenous opiates may possibly inhibit the secretion of endogenous opiates (e.g., β-endorphin) by a negative-feedback mechanism (131). Acting as both stress hormones and regulators of hypothalamic activity, β-endorphins lessen the release of corticotropin-releasing factor in response to incoming nociceptive neuronal impulses (131), thereby decreasing pituitary ACTH release (132). Experimental studies have reported the activation of proenkephalin gene in the hypothalamus in response to acute and chronic stress (133, 134). Investigators have also suggested that the administration of opioids before a stressor to stimulus may induce the proenkephalin gene in the hypothalamus (135). Thus, administering opioids preoperatively may alter the endogenous stress response in a manner that enhances autonomic stability and improves clinical outcome (136). Finally, increasing evidence suggests that both endogenous (e.g., endorphins, enkephalins, dynorphin) (133, 134, 137, 138) and exogenous (e.g., morphine) opioids (135, 139, 140) play important regulatory roles in the hypothalamopituitary reaction to surgery.

In summary, these data demonstrate that intravenous opioids are efficient in inhibiting the surgical stress response. Unfortunately, they seem to have a ceiling effect with respect to this inhibition, especially during the cardiopulmonary bypass period of cardiac surgery. In contrast, the epidural administration of opioids provides a more pronounced depression of the stress reaction than does intravenous administration. Increasing experimental (and clinical) evidence suggests a fundamental role for both endogenous and exogenous opioids in the modulation of the surgical stress response.

α_2-Adrenergic Agonists

The most commonly used α_2 agonist in clinical anesthetic practice is the antihypertensive drug clonidine. Newer and more selective α_2-adrenoceptor compounds (e.g., detomidine, dexmedetomidine) are currently undergoing clinical evaluation. The interaction of α_2 adrenoceptors and α_2-adrenergic agonists activates a complex effector system transduced by different guanine nucleotide binding proteins (G proteins) (Table 28-3) (141). The effector mechanisms involved include the following: 1) inhibition of adenylate cyclase; 2) acceleration of sodium-hydrogen ion (Na^+-H^+) exchange; 3) activation of K^+ channels; 4) inhibition of voltage-sensitive calcium (Ca^{++}) channels; and 5) an influence on phosphatidyl inositol turnover. These changes result in an altered transmembrane voltage (hyperpolarization) and neuronal hypoexcitability, effects that may explain the antinociceptive activity of α_2 agonists.

A potent inhibition of central sympaticoadrenal outflow can be demonstrated after the administration of clonidine (142). Whether this effect is caused by direct action on central sympathetic outflow or presynaptic

TABLE 28-3. α_2-Adrenoceptor Agonists and the Stress Response to Surgery

Mechanisms (References)	Type of Surgery (References)	Hormonal Effects (References)
α_2 Adrenoceptor in the central and peripheral nervous system (G-protein effector system); depressed neuronal excitability (141, 142, 158–161)	Abdominal surgery (152)	↓ ACTH (147)
Inhibition of central sympathetic outflow (presynaptic autoinhibitory α_2 adrenoceptors or direct effect) (142–145)	Cardiac surgery (153, 154)	↓ ADH (145)
Hypothalamopituitary axis (147, 148)	General surgery (150, 151)	↓ β-Endorphin (149)
Adrenal gland (only dexmedetomidine) (146)	Laparoscopic surgery (149)	↓ Catecholamines (149, 151, 153–157)
	Orthopedic surgery (143, 157)	↓ Cortisol (147)
	Vascular surgery (155, 156)	↓ Vasopressin (156)

ACTH, Adrenocorticotropic hormone; ADH, antidiuretic hormones.

autoinhibition of α_2 adrenoceptors is not clear (143, 144). Similar effects have been observed on ADH secretion (145). Although dexmedetomidine can inhibit adrenal steroidogenesis based on its imidazoline structure (146), this property is not shared by clonidine. However, clonidine has been shown to inhibit ACTH release directly, with a subsequent decrease in cortisol secretion in response to surgical stress (147, 148).

The hemodynamic response to intubation can be effectively attenuated by the preoperative intramuscular (149) or oral (150) administration of clonidine (see Table 28-3). Similar results were reported in hypertensive patients undergoing elective surgery (151), as well as in patients premedicated with intramuscular dexmedetomidine (152). Significant reductions in circulating catecholamines were found throughout coronary artery bypass operations when patients were treated perioperatively with clonidine (153, 154). Similarly, the adjunctive use of clonidine in aortic surgery reduced the need for supplemental analgesics and decreased norepinephrine levels throughout the procedure (155). In another study involving aortic surgery, the addition of a clonidine infusion after unclamping the aorta significantly reduced the circulating levels of epinephrine, norepinephrine, and ADH and limited the number of interventions required to maintain hemodynamic stability (156). A reduction in plasma epinephrine and norepinephrine was also reported after orally administered clonidine in patients having orthopedic surgery under spinal anesthesia (157). Finally, the β-endorphin response to laparoscopic surgery was effectively blunted by clonidine (149). The epidural (or intrathecal) use of α_2-adrenoceptor agonists was also found to inhibit the sympathoadrenal stress response to surgery effectively in both animals (158) and patients (142, 159). These effects can be explained by an α_2-agonist-mediated inhibition of the nociceptive neurotransmission at the level of the spinal cord (160, 161).

Overall, the adjunctive administration of α_2 agonists during the perioperative period improved hemodynamic stability, decreased the need for supplemental anesthetics and analgesics, and efficiently blocked the sympathoadrenal response to anesthesia and surgery (141, 162). Unfortunately, these drugs may also cause perioperative hypotension, bradycardia, and postoperative sedation. Most of these effects are revised by the selective α_2-adrenoceptor antagonist (e.g., atipamezole) (163). Therefore, α_2-adrenergic agonists may be extremely useful in the anesthetic management of patients at risk of developing major cardiovascular complications during anesthesia and surgery (152). However, in otherwise healthy persons, the hemodynamic and psychomotor side effects of these agents may outweigh any potential beneficial effects (152, 155, 164).

Nonsteroidal Anti-inflammatory Drugs

Increasing evidence indicates that intermediates in the arachidonic acid cascade may play an important role in the onset and maintenance of the inflammatory, immunologic, and metabolic responses to surgery (see Fig. 28-1) (7-9, 165). Furthermore, increases in plasma norepinephrine levels have been found to parallel the increase in core temperature values (166, 167), thus suggesting that hyperthermia has an influence on the activity of the hypothalamopituitary-adrenocortical axis. Investigators have also suggested that fever and infammatory substances (e.g., prostaglandin metabolites) may be important in the catabolic state associated with surgical stress (166-169). The febrile response has been mainly attributed to the release of interleukin-1 from macrophages. This cytokine enhances the synthesis of prostaglandin E_2, which then stimulates specific receptors in the hypothalamic thermoregulatory center (170). Moreover, catabolic hormones by themselves may contribute to postoperative hyperthermia (168). Whether these factors are also important during and after uncomplicated elective clean surgery still has to be established, although more and more evidence suggests that this indeed may be the case (171, 172).

NSAIDs significantly inhibit the peripheral production of prostanoids, thereby producing anti-inflammatory, antipyretic, and analgesic effects (Table 28-4). However, evidence suggests that the analgesia produced by NSAIDs may also be mediated by a central antinociceptive effect (173-177). As previously stated, prostanoids are thought to be involved in the metabolic response to surgery, a hypothesis implying that prostaglandin synthesis inhibitors can modulate the surgical stress response. Schulze and associates demonstrated a small but significant reduction in the hyperglycemic and cortisol responses in a study examining the effects of rectal and intravenous indomethacin in patients undergoing elective herniorraphy procedures under epidural anesthesia (172). In addition, the febrile response was completely abolished in indomethacin-treated patients. In contrast, Jensen and associates found an increase in blood sugar levels after inguinal herniorraphy in patients treated with a single dose of indomethacin (178). In a second and similar study, involving patients undergoing elective open cholecystectomy procedures under general anesthesia, Schulze and associates could not reproduce their previous findings even though excellent postoperative analgesia was provided by means of epidural opioids and intravenous indomethacin (179). Negative results were also reported in two other studies evaluating the effects of intravenous indomethacin or ketorolac on the surgical stress response after abdominal hysterectomy (180) or open cholecystectomy (181), respectively. A positive effect of rectal indomethacin on endocrine responses after a total gastrectomy under

TABLE 28-4. Nonsteroidal Anti-Inflammatory Drugs and the Stress Response to Surgery

Mechanisms (References)	Type of Surgery (References)	Hormonal Effects (References)
Irreversible inhibition of cyclooxygenase enzyme (7–9)	Abdominal surgery (178–181)	↓ Blood sugar (179)
Central antinociceptive effect (173–176)	General surgery (171, 172)	↑ Blood sugar (178, 180)
Modulating effect on catabolic response (166–170)		↓ Cortisol (171, 172, 181)
		↓ Urinary catecholamines (171)

TABLE 28-5. Local Anesthetics and the Stress Response to Surgery

Mechanisms (References)	Type of Surgery (References)	Hormonal Effects (References)
Central depressant (189, 190, 193)	Abdominal surgery (187, 191)	↓ Urinary catecholamines (191)
Depressant activity on afferent C-fibers (113)		
Antiinflammatory effects (191, 192)		

epidural anesthesia was reported by Asoh and associates (171). These investigators found a significantly lower incidence of postoperative fever, decreased urinary epinephrine and norepinephrine excretion, and lower plasma cortisol levels on the second and third postoperative days. This profile resulted in an improved nitrogen balance.

Taken together, these results demonstrate that the routine perioperative administration of NSAIDs does not appear useful in modulating the perioperative stress response. Although the intraoperative analgesic effects of these compounds are limited (182), a significant opioid-sparing effect has been shown during the postoperative period (183).

Local Anesthetics

Intravenous bolus injections of lidocaine can reduce the hypertensive and tachycardiac response to laryngoscopy and intubation (184) and can cause a 10 to 28% decrease in the minimum alveolar anesthetic concentration for nitrous oxide in humans and halothane in rats (Table 28-5) (185). Furthermore, a reduction in postoperative pain after single injections or short-term infusions of lidocaine has been reported (186-188).

The central depressant action of lidocaine is a possible explanation for its central analgesic properties (see Table 28-5) (189, 190). Moreover, amide local anesthetics have potent anti-inflammatory properties that may be related to their structural similarities to the steroids and antihistaminic compounds (191, 192). Local anesthetics may also influence the activation of afferent nerves and the inflammatory responses crucial in the generation of pain impulses after surgery and the associated sympathoadrenal stress response (193).

Wallin and associates found that the use of a perioperative lidocaine infusion in patients undergoing cholecystectomy suppressed tachycardia and hypertension and decreased the need for postoperative analgesics (191). Although no effect on perioperative plasma catecholamine or glucose levels was found, a significant reduction in the urinary catecholamine output was detected during the second postoperative day. Using a similar study design with comparable plasma levels of lidocaine, Birch and associates found no effects on perioperative hemodynamics, adrenocortical response to surgery, or postoperative analgesic requirements (194). Of significance, these authors only started the continuous lidocaine infusion after the first request for pain relief after surgery.

In conclusion, the available data regarding the influence of lidocaine on the sympathoadrenal stress response to surgery remain controversial. Even in studies showing a positive effect on the stress response, this effect was limited in magnitude and duration, and the benefits may not outweigh the risks associated with the intravenous administration of lidocaine.

Drug Combinations

The stresses imposed on the patient are continuously changing during surgery and anesthesia. The availability of more potent and fast-acting anesthetics and analgesics should enable a faster and more effective treatment of these reactions. However, clinical experience suggests that, even when analgesia is sufficient or the depth of anesthesia is adequate, an exaggerated stress response may occur during surgery. Although the consensus is that hyperdynamic stress reactions may respond to an increase in the depth of anesthesia, opinions differ on the best strategy to realize this goal. The most commonly used techniques include the administration of powerful, short-acting opioids or the use of supplementary sedative-hypnotic drugs. An alternative approach is the administration of drugs that block the external manifestations of the surgical stress reaction or some of its hormonal components.

Glass and associates found that supplemental doses of propofol in the presence of a constant infusion of fentanyl were more effective than propofol alone (or boluses of fentanyl with a propofol infusion) in blunting the hemodynamic response to surgery of the lower abdomen and lower limb (51). In a comparable study, Monk and associates found no significant difference in the treatment of acute hypertensive episodes during radical prostatectomy when they used a TIVA technique (52). The possible explanations for the differences between these two studies include the use of different opioids (fentanyl versus alfentanil) and dosage regimens (increase in infusion rate alone versus bolus dose plus an increase in infusion rate).

Monk and associates also studied the efficacy of alfentanil, isoflurane, or trimethaphan (a ganglionic blocker) in treating acute hemodynamic responses during retropubic dissection in patients undergoing radical prostatectomy procedures with a balanced anesthetic technique (103). Baseline analgesia was provided by a constant infusion of alfentanil. Although differing patterns of hormonal responses were found during the operation, the perioperative outcome was similar in all three treatment groups. However, even though trimethaphan-treated patients appeared to be adequately anesthetized, they continued to show a neuroendocrinologic response to surgery, with a sustained increase in plasma levels of both ADH and β-endorphin. In another study, Desborough and associates did not find an influence of trimethaphan-supplemented sufentanil anesthesia during cardiac surgery on perioperative catecholamine levels (195). Thus, sympatholytic drugs appear to produce a symptomatic rather than a causal remedy to the stress response. On the other hand, the elevated levels of β-endorphin represent an alternative form of analgesia (i.e., endogenous). Nevertheless, high levels of ADH can produce peripheral vasoconstriction, cardiac depression, and coronary artery vasoconstriction (196-198). Although sympatholytic techniques are associated with a rapid recovery from anesthesia, this approach may have a negative impact on end-organ function in patients with preexisting diseases. In contrast, premedication of patients undergoing abdominal hysterectomy with an angiotensin-converting enzyme inhibitor significantly reduced perioperative plasma and urinary norepinephrine levels while improving stroke volume and cardiac output (199). Finally, the addition of a specific hormonal blocking agent (e.g., somatostatin) to high-dose sufentanil anesthesia increased the suppression of the hormonal response to cardiac surgery (195).

Intravenous anesthetic agents that possess both hypnotic and analgesic properties may prove more effective in modulating the nociceptive input during intravenous anesthesia. This dualistic approach to the treatment of acute stress responses may, at least partially, explain the equivalence of propofol and alfentanil in blocking the stress responses during TIVA. The use of supplementary doses of a short-acting hypnotic with analgesic properties would offer distinct advantages over high doses of an opioid alone, because it would decrease the risk for postoperative opioid-related adverse events (e.g., sedation, nausea, vomiting, urinary retention, and respiratory depression). Two studies evaluated the use of different anesthetic techniques for elective craniotomy. Grundy and associates compared a thiopental-fentanyl infusion and a thiopental-sufentanil infusion with a balanced isoflurane-nitrous oxide technique (200). These authors did not find any significant differences among the three study groups, results also confirmed in a study by Todd and associates (201). A TIVA technique consisting of propofol and fentanyl induction, with maintenance with continuous infusions of propofol and fentanyl, was compared with a thiopental induction and maintenance with nitrous oxide-isoflurane with low-dose fentanyl, or a thiopental-fentanyl induction with a continuous fentanyl infusion and nitrous oxide-low-dose isoflurane for maintenance of anesthesia. Even though no hormone levels were measured, these authors found only modest differences in the hemodynamic, neurophysiologic, and recovery parameters among the three anesthetic treatment groups. More important, no difference was noted in either short-term or long-term outcome.

Preemptive Analgesia

During the last decade, basic scientific and clinical investigations have expanded our knowledge of the physiology of acute pain. Peripheral nociceptors (Aδ and C) are characterized by high thresholds and thus require intense stimuli to be activated. Peripheral tissue injury decreases pain threshold within the area of injury (primary hyperalgesia) and in the surrounding uninjured tissue (secondary hyperalgesia). The molecular mechanisms responsible for these phenomena are still being identified, but they are probably related to the local inflammatory response to tissue injury (i.e., peripheral sensitization) (8, 202). Investigators have also hypothesized that a similar process occurs in the dorsal horn of the spinal cord (203). An expansion of the receptive fields and a decrease in the threshold of the dorsal horn neurons disrupt the normal patterns of afferent stimulus processing in the CNS (i.e., central sensitization). Depending on the stimulus and the type of afferent impulses, a facilitated discharge of dorsal horn neurons ensues (the so-called windup phenomena). Moreover, the hyperexcitability of dorsal horn neurons also influences the activity in preganglionic sympathetic motoneurons, which, in turn, alter postganglionic sympathetic efferents and their interactions with primary sensory neurons (8). A positive feed-forward circuit is established in which sensory afferent input, central sensitization, and sympathetic outflow are acting in an additive (or even synergistic) fashion to modulate the pain response (4, 204). Investigators have suggested that further improvements in pain control will depend on the development of techniques 1) to prevent the occurrence of excitability changes in the CNS (i.e., CNS plasticity), 2) to depress or reverse these excitability changes, and 3) to prevent the disturbances that occur in the sympathetic nervous system (4).

Blocking peripheral sensory nerves with local anesthetics before the nociceptive stimulus is applied is one approach that can be used to prevent hyperexcitability changes within the CNS. Opioid analgesics may prove effective in preventing or even reversing the maladaptive plasticity of the CNS (4). However, except for a few studies involving the preemptive use of opioids (205-207) or lidocaine infiltration (208), data from clinical investigations assessing the existence of preemptive analgesia have consistently failed to demonstrate a preemptive analgesic effect. Whether the inability to demonstrate this phenomenon is related to flaws in the study design, misinterpretation of data, or the confounding effects of the analgesic drugs is not clear. In studies in which the investigators have reported preemptive analgesic effects, it is unclear whether such effects are related to a reduction in CNS hyperexcitability or improved timing of analgesic drug administration. Moreover, surgical trauma may differ significantly from the tissue injury caused under experimental conditions (209). Indeed, surgically induced trauma produces an intense and prolonged afferent nociceptive input to the CNS, consisting of a mixture of cutaneous, muscular, and visceral components. To complicate the situation further, a persistent inflammatory response is generated at the site of the tissue injury, extending the duration of central sensitization well into the postoperative period (210).

The possible influence of preemptive analgesia on the sympathoadrenal response to surgery has not yet been investigated. Because the nociceptive stimulus generated by surgical tissue injury initiates a whole cascade of inflammatory, metabolic, and cardiovascular events, effective preemptive analgesia may possibly have a supplemental effect on the sympathoadrenal response to surgery. However, further clinical investigations are necessary to elucidate this promising concept.

In conclusion, at present, no clear answer exists to the question regarding the best anesthetic regimen for preventing the stress response during surgery. Although data from clinical studies suggest that barbiturates, etomidate, propofol, benzodiazepines, opioids, and α_2-adrenergic agonists can decrease the hypothalamopituitary response to surgical stimuli, evidence is lacking to support the suggestion that this effect has a (beneficial) influence on clinical outcome. In fact, it must be concluded that until the catabolic hormonal) response to surgery can be totally prevented, attempts to establish a relationship among anesthetic technique, hormone secretion, and postoperative morbidity are premature (195, 211). Current data suggest that an experienced anesthetist sees no important differences between classic balanced anesthesia and a TIVA technique with respect to a patient's well-being during and after surgery.

REFERENCES

1. Kehlet H, Brand MR, Rem J. Role of neurogenic stimuli in mediating the endocrine-metabolic response to surgery. JPEN J Parenter Enteral Nutr 1980;4:152–156.
2. Kehlet H. Epidural analgesia and the endocrine-metabolic response to surgery: update and perspectives. Acta Anaesthesiol Scand 1984;28:125–127.
3. Scott NB, Kehlet H. Regional anaesthesia and surgical morbidity. Br J Surg 1988;75:299–304.
4. Woolf CJ. Recent advances in the pathophysiology of acute pain. Br J Anaesth 1989;63:139–146.
5. Raja SN, Meyer RA, Campbell JN. Peripheral mechanisms of somatic pain. Anesthesiology 1988;68:571–590.
6. Yaksh TL, Hammond DL. Peripheral and central substrates involved in the rostrad transmission of nociceptive information. Pain 1982;13:1–85.
7. Woolf CJ, Chong M-S. Preemptive analgesia: treating postoperative pain by preventing the establishment of central sensitization [Review]. Anesth Analg 1993;77:362–379.
8. Levine JD, Fields HL, Basbaum AI. Peptides and the primary afferent nociceptor. J Neurosci 1993;13:2273–2286.
9. Weissman C. The metabolic response to stress: an overview and update. Anesthesiology 1990;73:308–327.
10. Joris J, Cigarini I, Legrand M, et al. Metabolic and respiratory changes after cholecystectomy performed via laparotomy or laparoscopy. Br J Anaesth 1992;69:341–345.
11. Hall GM, Desborough JP. Interleukin-6 and the metabolic response to surgery. Br J Anaesth 1992;69:337–338.
12. Naito Y, Sunai T, Shingu K, et al. Responses of plasma adrenocorticotropic hormone, cortisol, and cytokines during and after upper abdominal surgery. Anesthesiology 1992;77:426–431.
13. Chernow B, Alexander R, Smallridge RC, et al. Hormonal responses to graded surgical stress. Arch Intern Med 1987; 147:1273–1287.
14. Weissman C, Hollinger I. Modifying systemic responses with anesthetic techniques. Anesth Clin North Am 1988;6:221–225.
15. Kehlet H. The stress response to surgery: release mechanisms and the modifying effect of pain relief. Acta Chir Scand Suppl 1988;550:22–28.
16. Koblin DD. Inhaled anesthetics: mechanisms of action. In: Miller RD, ed. Anesthesia. 4th ed. vol 1. New York: Churchill Livingstone, 1994:67–99.
17. Roizen MF, Horrigan RW, Frazer BM. Anesthetic doses blocking adrenergic (stress) and cardiovascular responses to incision: MAC BAR. Anesthesiology 1981;54:390–398.
18. Lacoumenta S, Paterson JL, Burrin J, et al. Effects of two differing halothane concentrations on the metabolic and endocrine responses to surgery. Br J Anaesth 1986;58:844–850.
19. Oyama T, Taniguchi K, Ishihara H, et al. Effects of enflurane anaesthesia and surgery on endocrine function in man. Br J Anaesth 1979;51:141–148.
20. Crozier TA, Morawietz A, Brobnik L, et al. The influence of isoflurane on peri-operative endocrine and metabolic stress responses. Eur J Anaesthesiol 1992;9:55–62.

21. Furuya K, Shimizu R, Hirabayashi Y, et al. Stress hormone responses to major intra-abdominal surgery during and immediately after sevoflurane-nitrous oxide anaesthesia in elderly patients. Can J Anaesth 1993;40:435–439.
22. Philbin DM, Coggins CH. Plasma antidiuretic hormone levels in cardiac surgical patients during morphine and halothane anesthesia. Anesthesiology 1978;49:95–98.
23. Cork RC, Hameroff SR, Weiss JL. Effects of halothane and fentanyl anesthesia on plasma β-endorphin immunoreactivity during cardiac surgery. Anesth Analg 1985;64:677–680.
24. Kono K, Philbin DM, Coggins CH, et al. Renal function and stress response during halothane or fentanyl anesthesia. Anesth Analg 1981;60:552–556.
25. Hamberger B, Järnberg P-O. Plasma catecholamines during surgical stress: differences between neurolept and enflurane anaesthesia. Acta Anaesthesiol Scand 1983;27:307–310.
26. Bickel U, Wiegand-Löhnert C, Fleischmann JW, et al. Different modulation of the perioperative stress hormone response under neurolept-anaesthesia or enflurane for cholecystectomy. Horm Metab Res 1991;23:178–184.
27. Holst D, Anger C, Bauch H-J. N_2O-supplemented intravenous anaesthesia versus inhalation anaesthesia: comparative study of sympatho-adrenergic reaction and postoperative vigilance. Anasthesiol Intensivmed Notfallmed Schmerzther 1993;28: 18–22.
28. Göthert M, Dreyer C. Inhibitory effect of halothane anesthesia on catecholamine release from the adrenal medulla. Naunyn Schmiedebergs Arch Pharmacol 1973;277:253–266.
29. Göthert M, Wendt J. Inhibition of adrenal medullary catecholamine secretion by enflurane. I. Investigations in vivo. Anesthesiology 1977;46:400–403.
30. Tanelian DL, Kosek P, Mody I, MacIver B. The role of the GABA$_A$ receptor/chloride channel complex in anesthesia. Anesthesiology 1993;78:757–776.
31. Kitahata LM, Ghazi-Saidi K, Yamashita M, et al. The depressant effect of halothane and sodium thiopental on the spontaneous and evoked activity of dorsal horn cells: lamina specificity, time course and dose dependence. J Pharmacol Exp Ther 1975; 195:515–521.
32. Kitahata LM, Saberski L. Are barbiturates hyperalgesic? [Editorial]. Anesthesiology 1992;77:1059–1061.
33. Jewett BA, Gibbs LM, Tarasiuk A, Kendig JJ. Propofol and barbiturate depression of spinal nociceptive neurotransmission. Anesthesiology 1992;77:1148–1154.
34. Anker-Møller E, Spangsberg N, Arendt-Nielsen L, et al. Subhypnotic doses of thiopentone and propofol cause analgesia to experimentally induced acute pain. Br J Anaesth 1991;66:185–188.
35. Kaniaris P, Katsilambros N, Castanas E. Relation between glucose tolerance and serum insuline levels in man before and after thiopental intravenous administration. Anesth Analg 1975; 54:718–721.
36. Fragen RJ, Shanks CA, Molteni A, Avram MJ. Effects of etomidate on hormonal responses to surgical stress. Anesthesiology 1984;61:652–656.
37. Fragen RJ, Weiss HW, Molteni A. The effect of propofol on adrenocortical steroidogenesis: a comparative study with etomidate and thiopental. Anesthesiology 1987;66:839–842.
38. Marsland AR, Bradley JP. Anaesthesia for renal transplantation: 5 years experience. Anaesth Intensive Care 1983;11:337–344.
39. Ledingham IM, Finlay WE, Watt I, McKee JI. Etomidate and adrenocortical function. Lancet 1983;1:1434.
40. Ledingham IM, Watt I. Influence of sedation on mortality in critically ill multiple trauma patients. Lancet 1983;1:1270.
41. Wagner RL, White PF. Etomidate inhibits adrenocortical function in surgical patients. Anesthesiology 1984;61:647–651.
42. Giese JL, Stockham RJ, Stanley TH, et al. Etomidate versus thiopental for induction of anesthesia. Anesth Analg 1985;64:871–876.
43. Nauta J, Stanley TH, de Lange S, et al. Anesthetic induction with alfentanil: comparison with thiopental, midazolam, and etomidate. Can Anaesth Soc J 1983;30:53–60.
44. Owen H, Spence AA. Etomidate [Editorial]. Br J Anaesth 1984; 56:555–557.
45. Wagner RL, White PF, Kan PB, et al. Inhibition of adrenal steroidogenesis by the anesthetic etomidate. N Engl J Med 1984; 310:1415–1421.
46. Briggs LP, Dundee JW, Bahar M, Clarke RSJ. Comparison of the effect of diisopropyl phenol (ICI 35 868) and thiopentone on response to somatic pain. Br J Anaesth 1982;54:307–311.
47. Wilder-Smith O, Borgeat A. Analgesia with subhypnotic doses of thiopentone and propofol. Br J Anaesth 1991;67:226–227.
48. Monk CR, Coates DP, Prys-Roberts C, et al. Haemodynamic effects of a prolonged infusion of propofol as a supplement to nitrous oxide anaesthesia. Br J Anaesth 1987;59:954–960.
49. Van Aken H, Meinhausen E, Prien T, et al. The influence of fentanyl and tracheal intubation on the hemodynamic effects of anesthesia induction with propofol/N_2O in humans. Anesthesiology 1988;68:157–163.
50. Mitchell P, Smythe G, Torda T. Effect of the anesthetic agent propofol on hormonal responses to ECT. Biol Psychol 1990; 28:315–324w.
51. Glass P, Dyar O, Jhavery R, et al. TIVA-Propofol and combinations of propofol with fentanyl. Anesthesiology 1991;75 (suppl):A44.
52. Monk TG, Ding Y, White PF. Total intravenous anesthesia: effects of opioid versus hypnotic supplementation on autonomic responses and recovery. Anesth Analg 1992;75:798–804.
53. Sebel PS, Lowdon JD. Propofol: a new intravenous anesthetic. Anesthesiology 1989;71:260–277.
54. Smith I, White PF, Nathanson M, Gouldson R. Propofol: an update on its clinical uses. Anesthesiology 1994;81:1005–1043.
55. Van Hemelrijck J, Weekers F, Van Aken H, et al. Propofol does not inhibit stimulation of cortisol synthesis. Anesth Analg 1995; 80:573–576.
56. Chræmmer-Jørgensen B, Hertel S, Strøm J, et al. Catecholamine response to laryngoscopy and intubation: the influence of three different drug combinations commonly used for induction of anaesthesia. Anaesthesia 1992;47:750–756.
57. Marty J, Gauzit R, Lefevre P, et al. Effects of diazepam and midazolam on baroreflex control of heart rate and on sympathetic activity in humans. Anesth Analg 1986;65:113–119.
58. Crozier TA, Beck D, Schlaeger M, et al. Endocrinological changes following etomidate, midazolam or methohexital for minor surgery. Anesthesiology 1987;66:628–635.
59. Desborough JP, Hall GM, Hart GR, Burrin JM. Midazolam modifies pancreatic and anterior pituitary hormone secretion during upper abdominal surgery. Br J Anaesth 1991;67:390–396.
60. Nilsson A, Persson MP, Hartvig P, Wide L. Effect of total intravenous anaesthesia with midazolam/alfentanil on the adrenocortical and hyperglycaemic response to abdominal surgery. Acta Anaesthesiol Scand 1988;32:379–382.
61. Glisson SN. Investigation of midazolam's influence on physiological and hormonal responses to hypotension. J Cardiovasc Pharmacol 1987;9:45–50.
62. Nilsson A. Autonomic and hormonal responses after the use of midazolam and flumazenil [Discussion 78]. Acta Anaesthesiol Scand Suppl 1990;92:51–54.
63. Taupin V, Jayais P, Descamps-Latscha B, et al. Benzodiazepine anesthesia in humans modulates the interleukin-1β, tumor necrosis factor-α and interleukin-6 responses of blood monocytes. J Neuroimmunol 1991;35:13–19.
64. White PF, Way WL, Trevor AJ. Ketamine: its pharmacology and therapeutic uses. Anesthesiology 1982;56:119–136.

65. White PF, Ham J, Way WL, Trevor AJ. Pharmacology of ketamine isomers in surgical patients. Anesthesiology 1981;52:231–278.
66. Adams H, Thiel A, Jung A, et al. Effects of S-(−)-ketamine on endocrine and cardiovascular parameters: recovery and psychomimetic reactions in volunteers [German]. Anaesthetist 1992;41:588–596.
67. Doenicke ARA, Mayer M, Adams HA, et al. The action of S-(−)-ketamine on serum catecholamine and cortisol: a comparison with ketamine racemate. Anaesthetist 1992;41:597–603.
68. Massopust LC, Wolin LR, Albin MS. Electrophysiologic and behavioral responses to ketamine hydrochloride in the rhesus monkey. Anesth Analg 1972;51:329–341.
69. Sparkes DL, Corssen G, Aizenman B, Black J. Further studies of the neural mechanisms of ketamine-induced anesthesia in the rhesus monkey. Anesth Analg 1975;54:189–195.
70. Ohtani M, Kikuchi H, Kitahata LM, et al. Effects of ketamine on nociceptive cells in the medial medullary reticular formation of the cat. Anesthesiology 1979;51:414–417.
71. Finck AD, Ngai SH. A possible mechanism of ketamine-induced analgesia. Anesthesiology 1979;51:S34.
72. Fratta W, Casu M, Belestrieri A, et al. Failure of ketamine to interact with opiate receptors. Eur J Pharmacol 1980;61:389–391.
73. Irifune M, Shimizu T, Nomoto M, Fukuda T. Ketamine-induced anesthesia involves the N-methyl-D-aspartate receptor-channel complex in mice. Brain Res 1992;596:1–9.
74. Klepstad P, Maurset A, Moberg ER, Øye I. Evidence of a role for NMDA receptors in pain perception. Eur J Pharmacol 1990;187:513–518.
75. Øye I, Paulsen O, Maurset A. Effects of ketamine on sensory perception: evidence for a role of N-methyl-D-aspartate receptors. J Pharmacol Exp Ther 1992;260:1209–1213.
76. Nagasaka H, Nagasaka I, Sato I, et al. The effects of ketamine on the excitation and inhibition of dorsal horn WDR neuronal activity induced by bradykinin injection into the femoral artery in cats after spinal cord transsection. Anesthesiology 1993;78:722–732.
77. Seitz W, Lübbe N, Hamkens A, Bornscheuer A. Combined midazolam-ketamine anesthesia in orthopedic surgery. Anaesthetist 1988;37:231–237.
78. Adams HA, Bauer R, Gebhart B, et al. Total i.v. anaesthesia with S-(−)-ketamine in geriatric orthopaedic surgery: endocrine stress response, cardiovascular reactions, and recovery. Anaesthetist 1994;43:92–100.
79. White PF, Schüttler J, Shafer A, et al. Comparative pharmacology of the ketamine isomers: studies in volunteers. Br J Anaesth 1985;57:197–203.
80. Schüttler J, Stanski DR, White PF, et al. Pharmacodynamic modeling of the EEG effects of ketamine and its enantiomers in man. J Pharmacokinet Biopharm 1987;15:241–253.
81. Chodoff P. Evidence for central adrenergic action of ketamine. Anesth Analg 1972;51:247–259.
82. White PF, Ham J, Way WL, Trevor AJ. Pharmacology of ketamine isomers in surgical patients. Anesthesiology 1981;52:231–278.
83. Wong DHW, Jenkins LC. An experimental study of the mechanism of action of ketamine on the central nervous system. Can J Anaesth 1974;21:57–67.
84. Hill GE, Wong KC, Shaw CL, et al. Interactions of ketamine with vasoactive amines at normothermia and hypothermia in the isolated rabbit heart. Anesthesiology 1978;48:315–319.
85. Nedergaard OA. Cocaine-like effect of ketamine on vascular adrenergic neurones. Eur J Pharmacol 1973;23:153–161.
86. Salt PJ, Barnes PK, Beswick FJ. Inhibition of neuronal and extraneuronal uptake of noradrenaline by ketamine in the isolated perfused rat heart. Br J Anaesth 1979;51:835–838.
87. Cook DJ, Housmans PR, Rorie DK. Effect of ketamine HCl on norepinephrine disposition in isolated ferret ventricular myocardium. J Pharmacol Exp Ther 1992;261:101–107.
88. Kudo M, Kudo T, Matsuki A, Ishihara H. Effects of ketamine on pituitary-adrenal axis in rats. Jpn J Anesthesiol 1993;42:552–556.
89. Zsigmond EK, Kothary SP, Kumar SM, Kelsch RC. Counteraction of circulatory side effects of ketamine by pretreatment with diazepam. Clin Ther 1980;3:28–32.
90. Hatano S, Keane DM, Boggs RE, et al. Diazepam-ketamine anaesthesia for open heart surgery: a micro-mini drip administration technique. Can Anaesth Soc J 1976;23:648–656.
91. Bidwai AV, Stanley TH, Graves CL, et al. The effects of ketamine on cardiovascular dynamics during halothane and enflurane anesthesia. Anesth Analg 1975;54:588–592.
92. Giesecke K, Hamberger B, Järnberg PO, et al. High- and low-dose fentanyl anaesthesia: hormonal and metabolic responses during cholecystectomy. Br J Anaesth 1988;61:575–582.
93. Kietzmann D, Larsen R, Rathgeber J, et al. Comparison of sufentanil-nitrous oxide anaesthesia with fentanyl-nitrous oxide anaesthesia in geriatric patients undergoing major abdominal surgery. Br J Anaesth 1991;67:269–276.
94. Stanley TH. Plasma catecholamines and cortisol responses to fentanyl-oxygen anesthesia for coronary-artery operations. Anesthesiology 1980;53:250–253.
95. Weiss BM, Schmid ER, Gattiker RI. Comparison of nalbuphine and fentanyl anesthesia for coronary artery bypass surgery. Anesth Analg 1991;73:521–529.
96. de Lange S, Stanley TH, Boscoe TM, et al. Catecholamine and cortisol responses to high dose sufentanil-O_2 and alfentanil-O_2 anesthesia during coronary surgery in man. Anesth Analg 1982;61:177–178.
97. Brandt MR, Korshin J, Prange Hansen A, et al. Influence of morphine anesthesia on the endocrine-metabolic response to open-heart surgery. Acta Anaesthesiol Scand 1978;22:400–412.
98. Sebel PS, Bovill JG, Schellekens APM, Hawker CD. Hormonal responses to high-dose fentanyl anaesthesia. Br J Anaesth 1981;53:941–947.
99. Reier CE, Georger JM, Kilman JW. Cortisol and growth hormone response to surgical stress. Anesth Analg 1973;52:1003–1010.
100. de Lange S, Boscoe MJ, Stanley TH, et al. Antidiuretic and growth hormone responses during coronary artery surgery with sufentanil-oxygen and alfentanil-oxygen anesthesia in man. Anesth Analg 1982;61:434–438.
101. Dubois M, Pickar D, Cohen M, et al. Effects of fentanyl on the response of plasma beta-endorphin immunoreactivity to surgery. Anesthesiology 1982;57:468–472.
102. Lacoumenta S, Yeo TH, Burrin JM, et al. Fentanyl and the β-endorphin, ACTH and glucoregulatory hormonal response to surgery. Br J Anaesth 1987;59:713–720.
103. Monk TG, Mueller M, White PF. Treatment of stress response during balanced anesthesia: comparative effects of isoflurane, alfentanil and trimethaphan. Anesthesiology 1992;76:39–45.
104. Vermeyen KM, Erpels FA, Beeckman CP, et al. Low-dose sufentanil-isoflurane anaesthesia for coronary artery surgery. Br J Anaesth 1989;63:44–50.
105. Bovill JG, Sebel PS, Fiolet JWT, et al. The influence of sufentanil on endocrine and metabolic responses to cardiac surgery. Anesth Analg 1983;62:391–397.
106. Walsh ES, Paterson JL, O'Riordan JBA, Hall GM. Effect of high-dose fentanyl anaesthesia on the metabolic and endocrine response to cardiac surgery. Br J Anaesth 1981;53:1155–1165.
107. Samuelson PN, Reves JG, Kirklin JK, et al. Comparison of sufentanil and enflurane-nitrous oxide anesthesia for myocardial revascularization. Anesth Analg 1986;65:217–226.
108. Philbin DM, Rosow CE, Schneider RC, et al. Fentanyl and sufentanil anesthesia revisited: how much is enough? Anesthesiology 1990;73:5–11.

109. Murphy MR, Hug CCJ. The anesthetic potency of fentanyl in terms of its reduction of enflurane MAC. Anesthesiology 1982; 57:485–488.
110. Lake CL, DiFazio CA, Moscicki JC, Engle JS. Reduction of halothane MAC: comparison of morphine and alfentanil. Anesth Analg 1985;64:807–810.
111. Hall RI, Murphy RI, Hug CCJ. The enflurane sparing effect of sufentanil in dogs. Anesthesiology 1987;67:518–525.
112. Hall RI, Szlam R, Hug CCJ. The enflurane sparing effect of alfentanil in dogs. Anesth Analg 1987;66:1287–1291.
113. Haley JE, Sullivan AF, Dickenson AH. Evidence for spinal N-methyl-D-aspartate receptor involvement in prolonged chemical nociception in the rat. Brain Res 1990;518:218–226.
114. Hug CC. Does opioid anesthesia exist? Anesthesiology 1990; 73:1–4.
115. Kearse LA, Koski G, Husain MV, et al. Epileptiform activity during opioid anesthesia. Electroencephalogr Clin Neurophysiol 1993;87:374–379.
116. Zwarts SJ, Hasenbos MAMW, Gielen MJM, Kho HG. The effect of continuous epidural analgesia with sufentanil and bupivacaine during and after thoracic surgery on the plasma cortisol concentration and pain relief. Reg Anesth 1989;14:183–188w.
117. Salomäki TE, Leppäluoto J, Laitinen JO, et al. Epidural versus intravenous fentanyl for reducing hormonal, metabolic, and physiologic responses after thoracotomy. Anesthesiology 1993; 79:672–679.
118. Mayer DJ, Wolfle TL, Akil H, et al. Analgesia from electrical stimulation in the brain stem of the rat. Science 1971;174:1351–1354.
119. Satoh M, Takagi H. Enhancement by morphine of the central descending inhibitory influence on spinal sensory transmission. Eur J Pharmacol 1971;14:60–65.
120. Yaksh TL, Rudy TA. Studies on the direct spinal action of narcotics in the production of analgesia in the rat. J Pharmacol Exp Ther 1977;202:411–416.
121. Joris JL, Dubner R, Hargreaves KM. Opioid analgesia at peripheral sites: a target for opioids released during stress and inflammation. Anesth Analg 1987;66:1277–1281.
122. Stein C, Millan MJ, Shippenberg TS, Herz A. Peripheral effects of fentanyl upon nociception in inflamed tissue of the rat. Neurosci Lett 1988;84:225–228.
123. Stein C, Comisel K, Haimeri E, et al. Analgesic effect of intraarticular morphine after arthroscopic knee surgery. N Engl J Med 1991;325:1123–1126.
124. Lawrence AJ, Joshi GP, Michalkiewicz A, et al. Evidence for analgesia mediated by peripheral opioid receptors in inflamed synovial tissue. Eur J Clin Pharmacol 1992;43:351–355.
125. Stein C. Peripheral mechanisms of opioid analgesia [Review]. Anesth Analg 1993;76:182–191.
126. Stein C. Peripheral and non-neuronal opioid effects. Curr Opin Anaesthesiol 1994;7:347–351.
127. Koenig JI, Mayfield MA, McCann SM, Krulich L. Differential role of the opioid μ and δ receptors in the activation of prolactin (PRL) and growth hormone (GH) secretion by morphine in the male rat. Life Sci 1984;34:1829–1837.
128. Grossman A, Besser GM. Opiates control ACTH through a noradrenergic mechanism. Clin Endocrinol 1982;17:287–290.
129. Desborough JP, Hall GM. Modification of the hormonal and metabolic response to surgery by narcotics and general anaesthesia. Clin Anaesthesiol 1989;3:317–334.
130. Hall GM, Lacoumenta S, Hart GR, Burrin JM. Site of action of fentanyl in inhibiting the pituitary-adrenal response to surgery in man. Br J Anaesth 1990;65:251–253.
131. Carr DB, Murphy MT. Operation, anesthesia and the endorphin system. Int Anesthesiol Clin 1988;26:199–205.
132. Plotsky PM. Opioid inhibition of immunoreactive corticotropin-releasing factor secretion into the hypophysial-portal circulation of rats. Regul Pept 1986;16:235–242.
133. Borsook D, Falkowski O, Burstein R, et al. Stress-induced regulation of a human proenkephalin-β-galaktosidase fusion gene in the hypothalamus of transgenic mice. Mol Endocrinol 1994; 8:116–125.
134. Lightman SL, Scott Young W III. Changes in hypothalamic preproenkephalin A mRNA following stress and opiate withdrawal. Nature 1987;328:643–645.
135. Borsook D, Falkowski O, Rosen H, et al. Opioids modulate stress-induced proenkephalin gene expression in the hypothalamus of transgenic mice: a model of endogenous opioid gene regulation by exogenous opioids. J Neurosci 1994;14:7261–7271.
136. Borsook D. Opioids and neurotrophic effects. Curr Opin Anaesthesiol 1994;7:352–357.
137. Harbuz MS, Rees RG, Lightman SL. HPA axis responses to acute stress and adrenalectomy during adjuvant-induced arthritis in the rat. Am J Physiol 1993;264:R179–R185.
138. McCubbin JA, Kaplan JR, Manuck SB, Adams MR. Opioidergic inhibition of circulatory and endocrine stress responses in cynomolgus monkeys: a preliminary study. Psychosom Med 1993;55:23–28.
139. Jiménez I, Fuentes JA. Subchronic treatment with morphine inhibits the hypertension induced by isolation stress in the rat. Neuropharmacology 1993;32:223–227.
140. Quinn MW, Wild J, Dean HG, et al. Randomised double-blind controlled trial of effect of morphine on catecholamine concentrations in ventilated pre-term babies. Lancet 1993;342:324–327.
141. Maze M. Alpha-2 adrenoceptor agonists: defining the role in clinical anesthesia. Anesthesiology 1991;74:581–605.
142. Kirnö K, Lundin S, Elam M. Epidural clonidine depresses sympathetic nerve activity in humans by a supraspinal mechanism. Anesthesiology 1993;78:1021–1027.
143. Hökfelt B, Hedeland H, Hansson B-G. The effect of clonidine and penbutolol, respectively on catecholamines in blood and urine, plasma renin activity and urinary aldosterone in hypertensive patients. Arch Int Pharmacodyn 1975;213:307–321.
144. Veith RC, Best JD, Halter JB. Dose-dependent suppression of norepinephrine appearance rate in plasma by clonidine in man. J Clin Endocrinol Metab 1984;59:151–155.
145. Peskind ER, Raskind MA, Leake RD, et al. Clonidine decreases plasma and cerebrospinal fluid arginine vasopressin but not oxytocin in humans. Neuroendocrinology 1987;46:395–400.
146. Maze M, Banks S, Daunt D, et al. Effect of dexmedetomidine, an imidazoline α_2-adrenergic agonist, on steroidogenesis: in vivo and in vitro studies. Eur J Pharmacol 1990;183:2343–2344.
147. Lanes A, Herrera A, Palacios A, Moncada G. Decreased secretion of cortisol and ACTH after clonidine administration in normal adults. Metabolism 1983;32:568–570.
148. Masala A, Satta G, Alagna S, et al. Effect of clonidine on stress-induced cortisol release in man during surgery. Pharmacol Res Commun 1985;17:293–298.
149. Aho M, Lehtinen A-M, Laaitikainen T, Korttila K. Effects of intramuscular clonidine on hemodynamic and plasma β-endorphin responses to gynaecologic laparoscopy. Anesthesiology 1990;72:797–802.
150. Laurito CE, Baughman VL, Becker GL, et al. The effectiveness of oral clonidine as a sedative/anxiolytic and as a drug to blunt the hemodynamic responses to laryngoscopy. J Clin Anesth 1991;3:186–193.
151. Ghignone M, Calvillo O, Quintin L. Anesthesia and hypertension: the effect of clonidine on perioperative hemodynamics and isoflurane requirements. Anesthesiology 1987;67:3–10.
152. Scheinin H, Jaakola M-L, Sjövall S, et al. Intramuscular dexmedetomidine as premedication for general anesthesia: a comparative multicenter study. Anesthesiology 1993;78:1065–1075.
153. Helbo-Hansen R, Fletcher R, Lundberg I, et al. Clonidine and the sympatico-adrenal response to coronary artery by-pass surgery. Acta Anaesthesiol Scand 1986;30:235–242.
154. Flacke JW, Bloor BC, Flacke WE, et al. Reduced narcotic requirement by clonidine with improved hemodynamic and adrener-

gic stability in patients undergoing coronary bypass surgery. Anesthesiology 1987;67:11–19.
155. Engelman E, Lipszyc M, Gilbart E, et al. Effects of clonidine on anesthetic drug requirements and hemodynamic response during aortic surgery. Anesthesiology 1989;71:178–187.
156. Quintin L, Roudot F, Roux C, et al. Effect of clonidine on the circulation and vasoactive hormones after aortic surgery. Br J Anaesth 1991;66:108–115.
157. Pouttu J, Tuominen M, Scheinin M, Rosenberg PH. Effects of oral clonidine premedication on concentrations of cortisol and monoamine neurotransmitters and their metabolites in cerebrospinal fluid and plasma. Acta Anaesthesiol Scand 1989;33:137–141.
158. Gaumann DM, Yaksh TL, Tyce GM. Effects of intrathecal morphine, clonidine, and midazolam on the somato-sympathoadrenal reflex response in halothane-anesthetized cats. Anesthesiology 1990;73:425–432.
159. Lund C, Qvitzau S, Greulich A, et al. Comparison of the effects of extradural clonidine with those of morphine on postoperative pain, stress responses, cardiopulmonary function and motor and sensory block. Br J Anaesth 1989;63:516–519.
160. Savola MKT, Woodley SJ, Maze M, Kendig JJ. Isoflurane and an a_2-adrenoceptor agonist suppress nociceptive neurotransmission in neonatal rat spinal cord. Anesthesiology 1991; 75:489–498.
161. Sullivan AF, Kalso EA, McQuay HJ, Dickenson AH. The antinociceptive actions of dexmedetomidine on dorsal horn neuronal responses in the anaesthetized rat. Eur J Pharmacol 1992; 215:127–133.
162. Longnecker DE. Alpine anesthesia: can pretreatment with clonidine decrease the peaks and valleys? Anesthesiology 1987; 67:1–2.
163. Aho M, Erkola O, Kallio A, et al. Comparison of dexmedetomidine and midazolam sedation and antagonism of dexmedetomidine with atipamezole. J Clin Anesth 1993;5:194–203.
164. Wright PMC, Carabine UA, McClune S, et al. Preanaesthetic medication with clonidin. Br J Anaesth 1990;65:628–632.
165. Lembeck F, Gamse R. Substance P in peripheral sensory processes. Ciba Found Symp 1982;91:35.
166. Kim YD, Lake CR, Lees DE, et al. Hemodynamic and plasma catecholamine responses to hyperthermic cancer therapy in humans. Am J Physiol 1979;237:H570–H574.
167. Weeke J, Gundersen HJG. The effect of heating and central cooling on serum TSH, GH, and norepinephrine in resting normal man. Acta Physiol Scand 1983;117:33–39.
168. Watters JM, Bessey PQ, Dinarello CA, et al. Both inflammatory and endocrine mediators stimulate host responses to sepsis. Arch Surg 1986;121:179–190.
169. Revhaug A, Michie HR, Manson McKJ, et al. Inhibition of cyclooxygenase attenuates the metabolic response to endotoxin in humans. Arch Surg 1988;123:162–170.
170. Dascombe MJ. The pharmacology of fever. Prog Neurobiol 1985;25:327–373.
171. Asoh T, Shirasaka C, Uchida I, Tsuji H. Effects of indomethacin on endocrine responses and nitrogen loss after surgery. Ann Surg 1987;206:770–776.
172. Schulze S, Schierbeck J, Hempel Spars B, et al. Influence of neural blockade and indomethacin on leukocyte, temperature, and acute phase protein response to surgery. Acta Chir Scand 1987; 153:255–259.
173. Malmberg AB, Yaksh TL. Antinociceptive actions of spinal nonsteroidal anti-inflammatory agents on the formalin test in the rat. J Pharmacol Exp Ther 1992;263:136–146.
174. Malmberg A, Yaksh T. Hyperalgesia mediated by spinal glutamate or substance P receptor blocked by spinal cyclooxygenase inhibition. Science 1992;257:1276–1279.
175. Malmberg AB. Pharmacology of the spinal action of ketorolac, morphine, ST-91, U50488H, and L-PIA on the formalin test and an isobolographic analysis of the NSAID interaction. Anesthesiology 1993;79:270–281.
176. Jurna K, Brune K. Central effect of the non-steroid anti-inflammatory agents, indomethacin, ibuprofen, and diclofenac, determined in C-fiber evoked activity in single neurones of the rat thalamus. Pain 1990;41:71–80.
177. Eisenach JC. Aspirin, the miracle drug: spinally, too? Anesthesiology 1993;79:211–213.
178. Jensen AG, Jensen VJ, Gregersen B, et al. Influence of a single dose of indomethacin on some biochemical changes and on postoperative intestinal paralysis following minor surgery: a prospective randomized double-blind study. Acta Anaesthesiol Scand 1990;34:624–627.
179. Schulze S, Roikjaer O, Hasselstrøm L, et al. Epidural bupivacaine and morphine plus systemic indomethacin eliminates pain but not systemic response and convalescence after cholecystectomy. Surgery 1988;103:321–327.
180. Engel C, Kristensen SS, Axel C, et al. Indomethacin and the stress response to hysterectomy. Acta Anaesthesiol Scand 1989; 33:540–544.
181. Varassi G, Panella L, Piroli A, et al. The effects of perioperative ketorolac infusion on postoperative pain and endocrine-metabolic response. Anesth Analg 1994;78:514–519.
182. Rich GF, Schacterle R, Moscicki JC, et al. Ketorolac does not decrease the MAC of halothane or depress ventilation in rats. Anesth Analg 1992;75:99–102.
183. Souter AJ, Fredman B, White PF. Controversies in the perioperative use of nonsteroidal antiinflammatory drugs. Anesth Analg 1994;79:1178–1190.
184. Abou-Madi MN, Keszler H, Jacoub JM. Cardiovascular reactions to laryngoscopy and tracheal intubation following small and large doses of intravenous lidocaine. Can Anaesth Soc J 1977;24:12–19.
185. Hines RSJ, DiFazio CA, Burney RG. Effects of lidocaine on the anesthetic requirements for nitrous oxide and halothane. Anesthesiology 1977;47:437–440.
186. Bartlett EE, Hutaserani O. Xylocaine for the relief of postoperative pain. Anesth Analg 1961;40:296–304.
187. Cassuto J, Wallin G, Högström S, et al. Inhibition of postoperative pain by continuous low-dose intravenous infusion of lidocaine. Anesth Analg 1985;64:971–974.
188. DeClive-Lowe SG, Desmond J, North J. Intravenous lignocaine anaesthesia. Anaesthesia 1958;13:138–146.
189. Foldes FF, Molloy R, McNall PG, Koukal LR. Comparison of toxicity of intravenously given local anesthetic agents in man. JAMA 1960;172:1493–1498.
190. Koppanyi T. The sedative central analgesic and anticonvulsant actions of local anesthetics. Am J Med Sci 1962;244:646–654.
191. Wallin G, Cassuto J, Högström S, et al. Effects of lidocaine infusion on the sympathetic response abdominal surgery. Anesth Analg 1987;66:1008–1013.
192. Ritchie JM, Greene NM. Local anesthetics. In: Goodman Gilman A, Rall T, et al, eds. Goodman and Gilman's The Pharmacological Basis of Therapeutics. 8th ed. New York: Pergamon Press, 1990:311–331.
193. Thøren P, Öberg B. Studies on the endoanesthetic effects of lidocaine and benzonatate on non-modulated nerve ending in the left ventricle. Acta Physiol Scand 1981;11:51–58.
194. Birch K, Jørgensen J, Chræmmer-Jørgensen B, Kehlet H. Effect of i.v. lignocaine on pain and the endocrine metabolic responses after surgery. Br J Anaesth 1987;59:721–724.
195. Desborough JP, Hall GM, Hart GR, et al. Hormonal responses to cardiac surgery: effects of sufentanil, somatostatin and ganglion block. Br J Anaesth 1990;64:688–695.
196. Boyle WA, Segel LD. Direct cardiac effects of vasopressin and their reversal by a vascular antagonist. Am J Physiol 1986; 251:734–741.

197. Ebert TJ, Cowley AW, Skelton M. Vasopressin reduces cardiac function and augments cardiopulmonary baroreflex resistance increases in man. J Clin Invest 1986;77:1136–1142.
198. Share L. Role of vasopressin in cardiovascular regulation. Physiol Rev 1988;68:1248–1284.
199. Böttcher M, Behrens JK, Møller EA, et al. ACE inhibitor premedication attenuates sympathetic responses during surgery. Br J Anaesth 1994;72:633–637.
200. Grundy BL, Pashayan AG, Mahla ME, Shah BD. Three balanced anesthetic techniques for neuroanesthesia: Infusion of thiopental sodium with sufentanil or fentanyl compared with inhalation of isoflurane. J Clin Anesth 1992;4:372–377.
201. Todd MM, Warner DS, Sokoll MD, et al. A prospective, comparative trial of three anesthetics for elective supratentorial craniotomy. Anesthesiology 1993;78:1005–1020.
202. Dray A, Perkins M. Bradykinin and inflammatory pain [Review]. Trends Neurosci 1993;16:99–104.
203. Coderre TJ, Katz J, Vaccarino AL, Melzac R. Contribution of central neuroplasticity to pathological pain: review of clinical and experimental evidence [Review]. Pain 1993;52:259–285.
204. Wall P. The prevention of postoperative pain. Pain 1988;33.
205. Katz J, Kavanagh B, Sandler A, et al. Preemptive analgesia: clinical evidence of neuroplasticity contributing to postoperative pain. Anesthesiology 1992;77:439–446.
206. Richmond CE, Bromley LM, Woolf CJ. Preoperative morphine pre-empts postoperative pain. Lancet 1993;342:73–75.
207. Amanor-Boadu SD, Jadad AR, Glynn CJ, et al. Influence of pre- and postoperative morphine administration on pain after body surface surgery: a double-blind randomized controlled study. In : Abstracts of the Seventh World Congress on Pain. Seattle: IASP Publications, 1993:538–539.
208. Ejlersen E, Andersen HB, Eliasen K, Mogensen T. A comparison between pre- and postincisional lidocaine infiltration on postoperative pain. Anesth Analg 1992;74:495–498.
209. McQuay HJ. Do preemptive treatments provide better pain control? In: Gebhart GF, Hammond DL, Jensen TS, eds. Proceedings of the Seventh World Congress on Pain, Progress in Pain Research and Management. Vol. 2. Seattle: IASP Press, 1994:709–723.
210. Dahl JB, Kehlet H. The value of pre-emptive analgesia in the treatment of postoperative pain. Br J Anaesth 1993;70:434–439.
211. Tuman KJ, McCarthy RJ, Spiess BD, et al. Does choice of anesthetic agent significantly affect outcome after coronary artery surgery? Anesthesiology 1989;70:189–198.

VIII CONCLUSIONS

29 Effect of Intravenous Anesthesia on Outcome

O.H.G. Wilder-Smith

Although the intravenous injection of anesthetic drugs is an "old" technique (the first intravenous injection of morphine was described in 1665 [1] by Sigmund), the exclusive use of intravenous drugs to produce anesthesia is a relatively new concept (2). The first attempt at intravenous anesthesia on a large scale was at Pearl Harbor in 1941 with thiopental, which was first introduced in the mid-1930s (3). The marked morbidity associated with its use by inexperienced anesthetists in the context of shocked patients led to the virtual abandonment of intravenous techniques by an entire generation of anesthetists. A decade later, the rehabilitation of intravenous anesthesia was pioneered by Laborit (4) and was elaborated as neuroleptanalgesia by DeCastro and Mundeleer (5). It was based on outcome factors because, for the first time, seriously ill patients could be anesthetized for long interventions with reliable safety. Considerations of outcome, fundamental to anesthesia since its inception (6), have to be rigorously applied to intravenous anesthetic techniques in the future.

In the last decade of the twentieth century, medicine faces escalating financial constraints and higher consumer expectations. As a primarily nontherapeutic medical activity that is perceived as technologically advanced and therefore costly, anesthesia is especially vulnerable to these trends, necessitating particular interest in cost-benefit relationships. Since the renaissance of total intravenous anesthesia (TIVA) following the introduction of propofol (7), discussion concerning the cost of new anesthetic drugs, whether justified or not, has become fashionable. Much more relevant than the direct cost of drugs, which forms only a small part of the health care budget, is the interest of society in financially efficient anesthesia, in which the balance of benefit (e.g., minimum consequence of illness) and cost (e.g., shortest possible hospitalization) is optimal. Patients have rightly become more demanding: they want to feel well after surgery and anesthesia, without pain, nausea, or other impairment. Our surgical colleagues have embraced increasingly less invasive procedures, and anesthesiologists must follow in offering increasingly less invasive anesthesia. Medical auditors want to know the long-term results of anesthesia-related procedures. Finally, anesthesiologists need to protect the roots of professionalism, by protecting the interests of patients to the highest ethical standards. All these trends and discussions must be faced with a heightened awareness and understanding of the interaction between outcome and anesthesia.

DEFINITIONS

Outcomes reflect the results of medical interventions. Clearly, the time at which the result of the intervention is assessed is of fundamental importance. Therefore, we must differentiate among immediate (up to 24 hours postoperatively), short (normally up to leaving the hospital), medium (the first year after surgery), and long-term outcomes. Practitioners must also distinguish between classes of outcomes, namely, between major end points with clear implications such as illness or death and intermediate or minor end points such as pain or prolonged time to awakening, whose relevance, particularly for long-term health or cost, is less clear.

The longer the period under consideration for outcome, the more effects enter into play for the result, making it increasingly difficult to assess the effect of a single intervention factor. Similarly, the rarer an outcome (e.g., death), the more difficult it is to prove the statistically significant effect of a given intervention factor. Both these considerations have resulted in the necessity of trials with increasingly rigid, standardized clinical protocols to reduce the number of confounding factors and large patient numbers to increase statistical power to prove the advantage of one medical intervention over another for rare long-term outcome (e.g., mortality), particularly in the context of ever-improving medical care. The importance of the last factor is demonstrated by the reduction in anesthesia-related mortality from 1:1000 in 1944 (8) to about 1:250,000 in 1986 (9).

Because large-scale, standardized trials are difficult, expensive, and time-consuming, the majority of outcome studies have understandably focused on shorter-term outcome and more frequently occurring or measurable end points. However, in the absence of studies relating short-term, and intermediate end points to long-term and major outcomes, the applicability of such investigations to discussions of overall cost-benefit equations for health care in modern society must be clearly reevaluated. Truly objective cost-benefit analysis of medical care therefore awaits more large long-term studies of major outcomes and detailed investigation of their relationship to short-term intermediate end points.

For practical purposes, however, we must at present make do with short-term intermediate end points for most of our choices in medical management. For anesthesia, both anesthetic and surgical outcomes must be studied in the context of the success of the anesthetic and of the way in which the anesthetic affected the result of surgery. In this chapter, the effect of intravenous anesthesia on intermediate outcome end points and their possible relationships to long-term and major outcomes are evaluated. The outcome differences between volatile and intravenous general anesthetic techniques are reviewed. However, the larger, better-documented, and better-known differences resulting from locoregional anesthetic techniques are outside the scope of this chapter. For purposes of this discussion, outcome includes only events outside the operating suite.

RECOVERY AFTER ANESTHESIA

Early awakening after anesthesia can be a desirable intermediate anesthetic outcome for two cost-related reasons: first, it may decrease recovery room or postanesthesia care unit (PACU) costs if it reduces the time spent there; second, it may reduce costs in the context of ambulatory (or day-case) surgery if it permits earlier discharge. However, cost reduction is not necessarily automatic because time spent in the PACU is often only charged in time steps much larger than the time gained by a more rapid recovery. In fact, higher throughput may actually require more staff without a concomitant increase in billable time, thus increasing cost. Apart from anecdotal evidence such as preventing accidents (10), early recovery from anesthesia has not been shown to affect surgical outcome.

Whether patients prefer to awaken more rapidly is unclear. It seems reasonable to assume that, once awake, patients appreciate a minimum of mental and motor impairment. This preference favors the use of intravenous hypnotics and muscle relaxants with a short duration of action and a short context-sensitive half-time (11). No study to date has been able to demonstrate convincing differences in mental or motor function end points between anesthetic regimens 24 to 48 hours after the operation. Much more important is postoperative analgesia, not only from the patient's point of view, but more particularly (as discussed later) from the standpoint of overall outcome. Although the use of short-acting opioids may be associated with faster recovery after anesthesia, this goal is not worth the price of increased postoperative pain. If ultrashort-acting opioids (e.g., remifentanil) are used for general anesthesia, adequate alternative provisions for analgesia must be made from awakening onward, such as locoregional block, nonsteroidal analgesic drugs, or other opioid analgesics.

Most studies of motor and mental recovery have compared volatile techniques (usually after intravenous induction) with propofol (with or without nitrous oxide [N_2O]) for ambulatory surgery (12-24) (Table 29-1). Comparisons with intravenous induction agents other than propofol or thiopental are rare. Studies comparing propofol TIVA with thiopental-isoflurane or halothane regimens demonstrate a consistently faster awakening with propofol, with a tendency to better early recovery (in the first 4 hours) (12, 14, 17). This advantage of propofol virtually disappears if isoflurane anesthesia is induced with propofol (12, 14-16, 18, 23, 24). Induction and maintenance of anesthesia with desflurane result in faster awakening than propofol, with no later difference in recovery (19, 22). In comparing propofol TIVA to sevoflurane with propofol or sevoflurane induction, no differences are apparent (24). In all these studies, volatile anesthesia without propofol was associated with a significantly higher incidence of postoperative nausea and vomiting (PONV), and the use of desflurane was associated with a higher influence of airway problems during anesthesia involving a face mask.

Few studies have carefully examined later recovery (e.g., return to work after surgery). Pollard and colleagues (23) demonstrated no differences after 12 hours between propofol TIVA and anesthesia maintained with volatile anesthetics in the context of outpatient oral surgery. In a study comparing short propofol and thiopental anesthesia in volunteers, Korttila and associates (25) were able to demonstrate better

TABLE 29-1. Recovery after Anesthesia: Propofol versus Volatile Anesthetics

Investigators (yr)	Reference	Comparison	Awakening	Early Recovery (1–4 h)	Later Recovery (4–48 h)	Tests
de Grood et al, 1987	12	PT vs T/iso	PT quicker	No difference at 1 and 3 h	NA	P-deletion
de Grood et al, 1987	12	PT vs P/iso	No difference	No difference	NA	P-deletion
Vinik et al, 1987	13	PT vs T/iso	PT faster	PT better at 1 h	NA	Trieger
Zuurmond et al, 1987	14	PT vs P/iso	No difference	No difference	NA	P-deletion MW
Milligan et al, 1987	15	PT vs P/iso	PT faster	No difference	NA	P-deletion CRT
Herregods et al, 1988	16	PT/N_2O vs P/iso	No difference	No difference	NA	Trieger, p-deletion
Puttick & Rosen, 1988	17	PT vs T/halo	PT faster	PT faster	NA	Clinical criteria
Nightingale and Lewis, 1990	18	PT-alfentanil vs P/iso	PT quicker	PT better at 1 h	NA	CRT, CFFT
Van Hemelrijk et al, 1991	19	PT/N_2O vs desflu	Desflu faster	No difference	NA	Clinical
Marshall et al, 1992	20	PT vs P/iso ± alfentanil	No difference	No difference	NA	MPMT
Ding et al, 1993	21	T/enflu vs P/enflu vs PT	PT faster vs thio/enflu	No difference	NA	Clinical
Lebenbom-Mansour et al, 1993	22	PT vs P/desflu vs desflu only	Trend desflu alone faster	No difference	NA	MPMT
Pollard et al, 1994	23	PT vs P/halo, P/enflu, P/iso	No difference	PT, P/enflu better 1–4 h	No difference; perform. improves up to 48 h	MPMT MW CRT
Fredman et al, 1995	24	PT vs P/sevo vs sevo only	No difference	No difference		Clinical criteria

NA, not applicable; P, propofol; T, thiopental; PT, propofol-TIVA; TT, thiopental-TIVA; iso, isoflurane; N_2O, nitrous oxide; enflu, enflurane; halo, halothane; desflu, desflurane; sevo, sevoflurane; MW, Maddox Wing test; CRT, choice reaction time; CFFT, critical flicker fusion test; MPMT, multiple psychomotor testing.

psychomotor function up to 5 hours after awakening from propofol anesthesia. In comparison, outpatients undergoing hernia repair with halothane anesthesia had impaired choice reaction time up to 48 hours postoperatively (26). However, bedrest alone can substantially impair psychomotor and cognitive function (27). Compared with patients receiving isoflurane-fentanyl anesthesia, patients undergoing major abdominal surgery under propofol-fentanyl TIVA (with or without N_2O) had better and faster late recovery in terms of vegetative symptoms, subjective control, and social orientation, with the differences being maximal 7 days after surgery (28). However, these differences were not reflected in shorter hospital stays (28).

With regard to other motor effects, Hiller and colleagues (29) were not able to demonstrate significant differences in postural stability either compared with baseline or between propofol-N_2O-alfentanil and thiopental-N_2O-halothane anesthesia in children 3 hours after minor otolaryngologic surgery. Bennett and associates (30), comparing anesthesia for minor surgery using either enflurane or propofol with N_2O, found no differences in gastric emptying using paracetamol absorption.

In summary, awakening after short anesthesia is faster after propofol than after thiopental or eltanolone induction (31, 32). If propofol is used as the induction agent, maintenance of anesthesia with propofol, isoflurane, desflurane, or sevoflurane has no clinically significant effect on early recovery. No significant differences resulting from a specific general anesthetic technique have been demonstrated 4 to 6 hours postoperatively, thus making effects on longer-term outcome by differences in recovery unlikely.

POSTOPERATIVE NAUSEA AND VOMITING (PONV)

The overall incidence of PONV has remained relatively constant at 20 to 30% since the introduction of halothane and concurrent demise of ether; intractable nausea and vomiting occur after about 1:1000 anesthetics (33). For ambulatory anesthesia, nausea has been shown to be the most important factor determining the length of stay in hospital (34). Comparing anesthetic maintenance with isoflurane only, propofol infusion for 25 minutes followed by isoflurane, and propofol infusion alone (34), the postoperative incidence of nausea requiring medical intervention was 44%, 13%, and 19% respectively. Mean hospital stay was 235 ± 90, 184 ± 56, and 197 ± 55 minutes, respectively, in the three groups, with nauseated patients staying an average of 267 ± 95 minutes compared with 185 ± 47 minutes for all non-nauseated patients. PONV causes extra cost not only because of longer hospital stays, but also because of the extra nursing (and perhaps physicians') efforts and additional materials (35). One American outpatient study has reported an extra direct cost of $15 per patient experiencing PONV (36). Thus, from a purely economic point of view, PONV is justifiably termed the "big little problem" (37).

Patients dislike PONV, particularly in the context of minor ambulatory surgery, and many consider it more debilitating than pain (38-40). The fear of PONV increases with a previous experience of PONV (39), and it may be even greater than the fear of pain. For example, in one study, 23% of patients expressed a fear of PONV compared with 14% who worried about postoperative pain (39). The occurrence of PONV is a strong reason for patients to rate their entire perioperative course poorly (41). Apart from patient dissatisfaction, vomiting can cause serious complications such as bronchial aspiration, rib fractures, gastric herniation, esophageal tears and rupture, muscular exhaustion, bleeding at the operation site, and increased suture tension (42). The latter two complications are particularly deleterious in the context of plastic, abdominal, intracranial, and intraocular surgery, particularly if associated with suture or wound dehiscence. Fluid and electrolyte imbalance can also follow protracted PONV. Although the short- and medium-term outcome implications of these emesis-associated complications can readily be imagined, definitive studies of their effects on long-term outcome are surprisingly lacking.

Many factors affect the incidence of PONV. The patient plays a role through gender (43), menstrual state (44), and previous history (45). Specific types of surgery (particularly strabismus surgery, orchidopexy, and adenotonsillectomy) and long operations are associated with higher rates of PONV (46). Mask ventilation and inexperienced anesthetists are also associated with higher incidences of PONV (47, 48). The drugs used during anesthesia can have a clear effect on the incidence of PONV. Extensive evidence indicates that the prophylactic administration of antiemetics reduces the incidence compared with placebo. Apart from the "classic" antiemetics droperidol and metoclopramide, the 5-hydroxytryptamine subgroup 3 (5-HT_3) receptor antagonists such as ondansetron, tropisetron, dolasetron, and granisetron effectively reduce PONV if these agents are given prophylactically (49). Droperidol and metoclopramide are less expensive than the 5-HT_3 antagonists, but they produce more side effects (49), such as dysphoria and sedation with droperidol and extrapyramidal phenomena with metoclopramide, all of which can be unpleasant for the patient. The 5-HT_3 antagonists seem free of major side effects (49), but whether they are better than conventional antiemetics for PONV prophylaxis is controversial, particularly for nausea (50) or opioid-associated nausea or vomiting (51). Regarding cost-effectiveness, one study found ondansetron to be more cost-effective than metoclopramide but less so than droperidol (52). Although the cost-effectiveness criteria used in this study have been criticized, a more recent prospective study has confirmed these findings (53).

The drugs used for anesthesia can influence the incidence of PONV (Table 29-2). As previously stated, the use of volatile agents as compared with propofol for the maintenance of anesthesia is clearly associated with more PONV (54), with little difference among the various volatile anesthetics (55). The effect of N_2O is variable and depends on the context of its use (56). Among the intravenous hypnotics, the introduction of propofol, with its direct antiemetic effect (57), has made a significant impact in reducing PONV, particularly if it is used during the maintenance period (58). Etomidate is associated with a high incidence of PONV (59), but the benzodiazepines seem to have little effect (60). The use of opioids, both intra- and postoperatively, markedly increases both nausea and vomiting

TABLE 29-2. Drugs Used During Anesthesia and Postoperative Nausea and Vomiting (PONV)

Drug Class	Specific Drugs	Effect on PONV	Comments	References
Volatiles/gases	Halothane, enflurane Isoflurane, desflurane	Higher vs propofol Maintenance	No clear differences among volatiles; depends on context	54, 55
	Nitrous oxide	Conflicting		56
IV hypnotics	Benzodiazepines	Little effect		60
	Etomidate	High incidence		59
	Propofol	Low incidence	Directly antiemetic	57, 58
Opioids	Morphine, fentanyl, meperidine	High incidence	Intra- & postop use, similar within group	61, 62
Myorelaxants	Vecuronium, atracurium, pancuronium, alcuronium	Panc > vec/atrac/alcuronium	Note reversal!	60
Anticholinesterases	Neostigmine	Increased incidence		64, 65
	Edrophonium	Decreased vs neostigmine	In children	65
Anticholinergics	Atropine	Decreased incidence vs glycopyrrolate		65, 66

(54, 61, 62). Such is also the case for patient-controlled analgesia (PCA), making the concurrent administration of antiemetics (e.g., droperidol or metoclopramide) with morphine PCA worthy of consideration (62). Replacing opioids with nonsteroidal anti-inflammatory agents such as ketorolac for postoperative analgesia reduces PONV (63). Finally, the avoidance of long-acting muscle relaxants such as pancuronium and of the need for subsequent antagonization is also effective in reducing PONV (60, 64-66).

In summary, the utilization of propofol for the maintenance of anesthesia seems to have a definite impact on PONV-associated postsurgical outcome when compared with volatile agents. The avoidance of opioids and long-acting myorelaxants provides another possible avenue to reduce PONV. However, decreases in PONV cannot be achieved if postoperative pain increases (67). The link between PONV reduction and possible improved long-term surgical outcome remains unproven.

GASTROINTESTINAL FUNCTION

Both anesthesia and surgery affect the gastrointestinal (GI) tract, mainly through changes in motility and perfusion. Anastomotic complications are a major risk factor after GI surgery, and as early as 1968, Whitaker (68) considered blood flow to be the single most important factor contributing to anastomotic healing. GI outcome is therefore likely to be influenced by changes in bowel perfusion, frequently resulting from hemorrhage and hypotension, but also because of flow redistribution secondary to anesthetic drugs. The mucosa is particularly vulnerable to consequently impaired blood supply, and this factor plays an important role in the healing of anastomoses and resistance to endotoxin and bacterial translocation.

The postoperative inhibition of GI motility is considered in large part to be due to a generalized increase in nervous, not but humoral, sympathetic activity (69-71). This is the result of both surgical and anesthetic influences. In general, motility after major non-GI surgery returns to normal within 4 to 5 days, with a shorter delay for more minor interventions (72). Gastric emptying is the most vulnerable to impairment (73), but it also recovers quickly, with the colon being slowest to return to normal motility (74). Although GI surgery causes more disturbance of motility than non-GI surgery, the degree of inhibition is not related to the amount of intraoperative handling of the gut (72). Pain and the associated increase in sympathetic tone inhibit gut motility, particularly gastric emptying (66).

Most investigators of GI function and outcome have focused on GI motility and perfusion, whereas little is known about direct effects of surgery and anesthesia on postoperative absorption or secretory activity of the GI tract. Impaired GI motility has clear outcome implications during all postoperative phases. In the immediate postoperative phase, impaired gastric emptying is associated with nausea and vomiting; if protective reflexes are depressed, pulmonary aspiration of gastric contents is a serious complication. In the short term, ileus is initially associated with electrolyte and water imbalance; if it persists, bacterial overgrowth and translocation of endotoxins with subsequent bacteremia, septic shock, and even multiple organ failure may occur (75-77). The problems of overgrowth and translocation are exacerbated in the presence of impaired mucosal perfusion (78). Ileus is associated with loss of fluid and electrolytes into the "third space"; apart from the immediate disturbances of electrolyte and water homeostasis, this causes tissue edema. The latter aggravates impaired tissue, particularly intestinal mucosal, perfusion and increases tension on suture lines. The bowel distention associated with ileus increases intra-abdominal pressure, resulting in diaphragmatic splinting, compounding the pulmonary complications of abdominal surgery (66).

Many anesthetic drugs have effects on GI function (Table 29-3). Volatile anesthetics generally decrease gastric emptying or colonic motility, but these effects wear off rapidly and normally have little clinical relevance (79-81). Intravenous hypnotics are considered to have only minor effects on GI motility, whereas the effects of N_2O remain controversial (82-86). In contrast, opioids are associated with major pertubations of GI function, with few differences described among the various opioid analgesics (87-92). Gastric emptying and large bowel motility are markedly depressed, whereas small intestinal contractility and pressure significantly increase. The latter increase is smaller with meperidine than with morphine (91, 92). Therefore, the use of meperidine for postoperative analgesia has been suggested to be associated with lower colonic anastomotic dehiscence rate than the use of morphine in small (or retrospective) studies (93, 94). The use of anticholinesterases such as neostigmine is followed by large increases in the frequency and intensity of large and small bowel contractions; these increases are not blocked by the concomitant use of anticholinergic agents (95-99). In addition, investigators have suggested that neostigmine reduces mesenteric blood flow, thus predisposing to bowel ischemia (100). Both factors together may explain the higher colonic anastomosis dehiscence rate when this reversal agent is used (101).

In summary, the evidence for an effect of the anesthetic technique on surgical outcome is stronger for postoperative GI function, particularly for anastomotic dehiscence, than for the other outcomes discussed so far. In this context, particular attention must be paid

TABLE 29-3. Gastrointestinal Function and Drugs Used in Anesthesia

Drug Class	Specific Drug	Gastric Effects	Small Intestine Effects	Large Intestine Effects	Comments	Reference
Volatiles/gases	Halothane	⇓ emptying	NA	⇓ colonic activity (rapid offset)	Colonic: CNR	79, 80
	Enflurane	⇓ emptying	NA	⇓ colonic activity (rapid offset)	Colonic: CNR	80, 81
	Nitrous oxide	NA	NA	⇔ (?⇓) activity (rapid offset)		82, 83
IV hypnotics	Thiopental	Minimal effects	NA	NA		84
	Propofol	Transiently ⇓ emptying	NA	NA		73
	Diazepam	⇑ pH, ⇓ vol. ⇑ emptying	NA	NA		85, 86
Opioids	Morphine	⇓⇓ emptying	⇑ contractility; ⇑ pressure	⇓⇓ motility; ⇑ pressure	Other opioids: similar	87-91
	Pethidine	⇓⇓ emptying	⇑ contractility; ⇑ pressure	⇓⇓ motility; ⇔ pressure	??⇓ anastomotic dehiscence?	87-90, 92-94
Anticholinergic	Atropine	⇓ emptying ++ in elderly	NA	NA		95, 96
	Glycopyrrolate	more than atropine	NA	NA		95
Anticholinesterases	Neostigmine	⇔ with atropine	⇑ freq./intensive/contractions	⇑ freq./intensive contractions	Not blocked by anticholinergics; ?⇑ anastomotic dehiscence	97-100

NA, not available; CNR, clinically not relevant; ⇑, increased; ⇓, decreased; ⇔, essentially unchanged.

to the use of opioids and the antagonism of muscle relaxants at the end of surgery.

CARDIOVASCULAR FUNCTION

Perioperative cardiovascular morbidity such as stroke or myocardial infarction is a major health problem. Of the 25 million patients who undergo noncardiac surgery in the United States per year, approximately 1 million are estimated to suffer significant cardiovascular morbidity postoperatively (102). The total hospital cost is estimated at $10 billion per year, with aftercare costing an additional $12 billion a year (102). Although the acute, intraoperative effects of different anesthetic regimens have been extensively investigated and discussed, little is known about their influence on immediate and short-term outcomes, and even less is known about medium- and long-term outcome. Studies demonstrating immediate and long-term influence on cardiovascular outcome have generally compared locoregional (mainly central neuraxial) techniques with balanced general anesthesia. Typical examples include the studies by Yeager and colleagues (103), by Tuman and associates (104), or by the Perioperative Ischemia Randomized Anesthesia Trial (PIRAT) study group (105, 106), which all demonstrated reduced postoperative complication rates or better surgical outcomes with regional anesthesia.

In comparing different anesthetic techniques, nonanesthetic factors generally demonstrate more prominent effects on outcome than the choice of the anesthetic agent. This finding was clearly demonstrated in a study by Tuman and colleagues involving patients who underwent coronary revascularization procedures. The study compared high-dose or moderate-dose fentanyl, sufentanil, ketamine-diazepam or halothane-based techniques and reported no differences regarding serious pulmonary, renal, or neurologic morbidity or in the duration of stay in the intensive care unit (107). Pedersen and colleagues came to similar conclusions regarding immediate and short-term cardiovascular morbidity in a study involving over 7000 patients receiving general anesthesia. These investigators reported an overall incidence of cardiovascular complications requiring intervention of 6.3% (108). Another study, involving over 17,000 patients, reported significant differences in intraoperative complications among halothane, enflurane, isoflurane, or fentanyl-based anesthetic techniques. However, these investigators were unable to demonstrate outcome differences in the first 7 postoperative days, particularly for major outcome end points (109). In the follow-up study (110), the major anesthetic drugs used were found (by multiple stepwise logistic regressions) to be significant predictors not only of severe cardiovascular outcomes, but also of any severe outcome including death.

Most of the studies mentioned (107-110) have compared the intraoperative use of intravenous or volatile agents without major differences in cardiovascular outcome. The absence or presence of long-duration postoperative ischemia as an immediate postoperative outcome may be the factor most significantly linked with long-term cardiac outcome (111, 112). In the context of intravenous anesthetic techniques, only the analgesic component has been demonstrated to influence cardiovascular outcome (113). Mangano and his Study of Perioperative Ischemia (SPI) group found that patients undergoing myocardial revascularization suffered fewer and less severe ischemic episodes (ST-segment change) in the intensive care unit when they were in a group receiving intense analgesia with sufentanil (1 μg/kg/h) for 18 hours from bypass onward than when they were in a group receiving intermittent bolus injections of morphine for analgesia during the same period (113). These differences did not extend beyond the period of intense analgesia, nor did they change short-term outcome for major end points such as fatal or nonfatal myocardial infarction (113). Medium- or long-term outcomes were not studied.

Although many articles have described the effects of different anesthetic and analgesic techniques on intraoperative cardiovascular function, much less is known about the effects of these techniques on postoperative cardiovascular morbidity. Effective antinociception appears to have some positive effect on postoperative myocardial ischemia, but the long-term implications of this improvement in short-term intermediate outcome remain unclear.

PULMONARY FUNCTION

Analogous to the findings for cardiovascular function, the effects of anesthesia on intermediate pulmonary outcome end points are considered to be most visible in the comparison of locoregional and general anesthetic techniques. Using historical controls, Watson and Allen (114) compared experiences of patients who underwent resections for esophageal cancer with or without epidural analgesia. These investigators reported an incidence of nonfatal and fatal respiratory complications in the general anesthesia group of 30% and 5%, compared with 13% and 0% in the epidural group. Short-term (30-day hospital) mortality was 9.8% in the general anesthesia group and 6.6% in the epidural group.

Outcome differences between volatile and intravenous techniques are generally immediate or short-term and usually involve the use of opioids. Opioids are well known for their respiratory depressant effects, a finding that explains a large part of their influence on short-term outcomes. Obviously, opioid analgesics with long durations of action are more frequently associated with postoperative respiratory depression than shorter-acting compounds. Preliminary evidence indicates that sufentanil may have a more favorable relationship between analgesia and respiratory depression than fentanyl (115). Respiratory complications may be aggravated by hangover of drugs that potentiate respiratory depression either directly or by depressing the patient's level of consciousness. Thus, respiratory complications in the immediate postoperative period are increased with the use of long-acting anesthetic drugs that potentiate respiratory depression (e.g., the long-acting benzodiazepines, diazepam, lorazepam, and flunitrazepam).

The respiratory depressant effects of opioid analgesics are evident in a multicenter study (110), comparing halothane, enflurane, isoflurane, and fentanyl anesthesia. The investigators reported that the major anesthetic drug used during surgery was a significant predictor of the number of severe perioperative respiratory complications. Another large study (108) found that the extent of pulmonary complications was significantly correlated with the use of muscle relaxants during maintenance of general anesthesia. The same study (108) also found that the avoidance of myorelaxant-associated complications depended much more on the choice of muscle relaxant (e.g., pancuronium) than on the manual evaluation of the response to train-of-four nerve stimulation (116). No peer-reviewed studies address the effects of general anesthetic agents on medium or long-term pulmonary outcomes. Similarly, the effect of different general anesthetic techniques on long-term pulmonary outcome remains unproven. In considering short-term and surrogate outcomes, most morbidity seems to stem from the use of opioid analgesics and longer-lasting myorelaxants. The advantage of locoregional techniques may be related to the reduction and even elimination of systemic opioid use after surgery.

NEUROLOGIC FUNCTION

Long-lasting disturbances of central nervous system (CNS) function (e.g., stroke, seizures, or disturbed consciousness) occur not only after intracranial surgery, but also after vascular (particularly carotid enarterectomy) and cardiac surgery. In the context of cardiac surgery, the rate of permanent neurologic deficit ranges between 1% and 5% (117, 118), with neurologic complications in the immediate to short-term postoperative period ranging from 7 to 11% (118). If one includes subtle alterations in cognitive function, the incidence rises to almost 80% (119, 120). Thus, any neuroprotective effect of a particular anesthetic technique could be expected to have outcome implications for these types of surgery, both in the short term as well as in the long term.

Many articles have been published in the anesthesia and neurology literature on the putative neuroprotective action of anesthetic drugs in animals. The intravenous anesthetics, especially the barbiturates, have been alleged to provide neuroprotection. The volatile agents (e.g., isoflurane) provide minimal if any neuroprotection. Barbiturates have demonstrated the most consistent neuroprotective effects in these models, not only because of the reliable cerebral metabolic depression they provide, but also because of their free radical scavenging effects, their anti-excitatory amino acid properties, and their ability to cause inverse vascular steal to ischemic brain areas (121, 122). Blockade of N-methyl-D-aspartate (NMDA)-receptors by the intravenous anesthetic ketamine or MK-801 (123, 124) has been shown to be neuroprotective in head injury or focal ischemia models, whereas AMPA-receptor blockers (e.g., NBQX) provide effective neuroprotection in generalized ischemia models, even when these agents are given well after the insult (125). In contrast, the use of N_2O generally worsens outcome in animal models of cerebral ischemia (121). However, evidence of improved clinical outcome effects has remained elusive for three reasons: first, the difficulty in translating from animal models to clinical situations; second, the differences between focal and generalized ischemia models; and third, the confounding effects of body temperature.

It is now generally accepted that mild hypothermia has significant neuroprotective effects (122) extending beyond those explicable solely by cerebral metabolic depression, and variations in body temperature may at least in part explain the positive results of different drugs as neuroprotectants (126). Unfortunately, the use of mild hypothermia in the context of neurosurgery has not so far proven successful (127) despite initial encouraging reports in head-injured patients (128). In considering focal versus generalized ischemia, one must realize that the maximum cerebral metabolic depression that can be produced by anesthetic drugs has only a minor impact in the context of generalized brain ischemia. Comparing cardiac arrest while the patient is awake versus during electroencephalographic (EEG) burst suppression, the extra energy available because of the preceding metabolic depression of EEG burst suppression translates into only about 15 seconds worth of extra preserved CNS membrane homeostasis (126), or a maximal shortening of the time to anoxic depolarization by 1 to 2 minutes (129). In focal or partial ischemic models, the magnitude of the improvement (e.g., in the ischemic penumbra), is much larger (129), explaining the enhanced success of neuroprotection in this context. Finally, animal brains sometimes react differently to ischemic stress than human brain tissue, and to extrapolate from the monoetiologic, closely controlled conditions imposed on animal ischemic models to the multietiologic problems of typical clinical brain ischemia is difficult.

Clinical neurosurgical studies comparing different anesthetic regimens have failed to demonstrate outcome differences beyond the immediate postoperative period (130, 131). More success has been achieved in the context of cardiac surgery, in which a single bolus of thiopental administered during cardiopulmonary bypass reduced postoperative neurologic deficit (132). In this successful study, ischemia was most likely focal, which is in keeping with animal studies. As predicted by animal studies, thiopental has little (if any) effect in comatose survivors of cardiac arrest (133).

Thus, although the question of neuroprotection by anesthesia remains unresolved and clinically unproven with respect to long-term outcomes, the evidence available tends to favor intravenous anesthesia with the barbiturates.

POSTOPERATIVE PAIN

The pain experienced by patients after surgery is unpleasant, and this alone is sufficient reason to avoid it in the postoperative period. The presence of pain postoperatively is associated with increased morbidity, thus providing another strong motivation for the effective use of pain-reducing anesthetic techniques and postoperative analgesia. Postoperative pain is associated with increased postoperative morbidity by reduced mobilization (e.g., venous or pulmonary thromboembolism or retention of pulmonary secretions and lung atelectasis). It also produces stress-induced sympathetic activation leading to increased oxygen demand and cardiac ischemia (or decompensation) or changes in the coagulation system and thromboembolic complications. Slower mobilization and the types of cardiovascular and pulmonary complications described previously increase the cost of care, both directly and by more prolonged hospitalization times.

Apart from immediate and short-term outcome considerations, increasing evidence suggests that pain, not only postoperatively but also intraoperatively, affects intermediate and possibly long-term outcomes. Longer-term effects of pain have been demonstrated for CNS sensory processing, for genetic expression, and for humoral immunity. Extensive animal evidence indicates that nociceptive stimuli (via Aδ, and even more effectively, C-fiber afferents) produce alterations in CNS somatosensory processing that are distinct from peripheral nociceptor sensitization (134-136). In animal models of nociceptive stimuli of limited intensity and duration, the effects of nociception on spinal CNS processing are primarily related to increased sensitization (134-136). Central sensitization consists of a reduction of sensory thresholds, an increased pain response to stimuli (e.g., allodynia), afterdischarging or even spontaneous dorsal spinal neuronal activity, and an extension of hypersensitive sensory fields beyond the damaged tissue area (i.e., secondary hyperalgesia). With longer-lasting C-fiber noxious stimulation, the dorsal horn neurons increasingly afterdischarge or discharge spontaneously, with these discharges in the absence of stimulation lasting for seconds up to minutes, a phenomenon termed "windup" (137).

Central sensitization plays an important role not only in postoperative pain, but also in the development of chronic pain syndromes (e.g., phantom pain after amputation) (134-136). The finding that analgesics are more potent in preventing central sensitization in animals if these agents are given before the noxious impulse than afterward led to the clinical concept of "preemptive analgesia" (138, 139). This concept postulates that analgesia instituted before nociception is more effective than that given afterward. Compared with analgesia after nociception, the pain and other consequences of the nociception are attenuated for significantly longer than the pharmacologic duration of action of the analgesic drug. Central sensitization is now known to result from the liberation of excitatory amino acids and neuropeptides by nociceptive afferents in the spinal dorsal horn (140). The activation of the NMDA receptor by the excitatory amino acid glutamate is necessary for the elicitation of central sensitization (141). Spinal NMDA-evoked sensitization in turn depends on the continuing presence of nitric oxide (NO) and subsequent soluble guanylate cyclase production, with NO playing the role of a retrograde neurotransmitter (142).

Ketamine, an NMDA-receptor antagonist, effectively blocks central sensitization after nociception in animal experiments (142). In experiments using the more clinically relevant formalin test in intact animals (Table 29-4), preemptive intrathecal morphine prevented central sensitization (143-145), whereas preemptive systemic opioids (morphine, alfentanil) combined with isoflurane were unable to do so (146). Postnociception intrathecal morphine was much less effective (145) for suppressing central sensitization. Preemptive volatile anesthetics alone produce a modest depression of spinal sensitization (143, 147). This effect is potentiated by the addition of opioids, particularly if they are administered intrathecally (143, 144). Even N_2O can produce dose-dependent preemptive analgesia, which can be antagonized by halothane (147, 148). The results of similar studies with the barbiturates and propofol are conflicting (147, 149).

The liberation of excitatory amino acids and neuropeptides in the area of the spinal dorsal horn not only changes sensory processing by a process of facilitation, but also leads to altered levels of second messengers (e.g., protein kinases) in the dorsal horn cells (136). The raised protein kinase levels have a positive feedback effect on the NMDA receptors and result in alterations of genetic expression by activating genes such as c-fos or jun-B (136, 150). These early intermediate genes are involved in the control of the production of regulatory substances such as the κ-agonist dynorphin and perhaps the δ-agonist enkephalin (136). Dynorphin is a complex modulator of hyperalgesia at the spinal level (151, 152). This nociception-induced alteration in genetic expression can be reduced by intrathecal morphine (150), which does not affect basal expression, in contrast to halothane or pentobarbital (153).

Page and Liebeskind et al have shown that, in rats undergoing tumor inoculation after abdominal surgery under volatile anesthesia, the rate of pulmonary metastasis is much higher 3 weeks later than in unoperated or anesthesia-only controls (154), and this effect is due to suppression of natural killer (NK) cell cytotoxic activity (155). The perioperative application of morphine to the rats reduces metastases to control

TABLE 29-4. Effect of Preemptive Anesthetic Agents on Postnociceptive Spinal Sensitization (PNSS) in the Rat Formalin Injection Model

Drug Class	Specific Drug	Route of Administration	Effect*	Comments	References
Volatiles/gases	Halothane	INH	0–41%	Contradictory despite similar doses and similar models	144, 147, 148
	Enflurane	INH	33%	—	147
	Isoflurane, Husoflurane	INH	33–51%	Dose-dependent	143, 147
	Desflurane	INH	58%	—	147
	Nitrous oxide	INH	29–49%	Dose-dependent, antagonized by naloxone or naltrexone	147, 148
Opioids	Morphine	IT	46–81%	Dose-dependent	143
IV hypnotics	Thiopental	IV	8%	—	147
	Phenobarbital	IV	29–79%	Dose-dependent	149
	Propofol	IV	7–41%	Contradictory despite similar doses and similar model	147, 149
Combinations	Nitrous oxide-halothane	INH	8%	—	147
	Morphine-halothane	IT/INH	82%	—	144
	Morphine-isoflurane	SC/INH	0%	—	146
	Alfentanil-isoflurane	SC/INH	16%	—	146

**Effect on percentage of reduction in number of phase II flinches compared with control.*

INH, Inhalation; IT, intrathecal; IV, intravenous; SC, subcutaneous.

levels and prevents NK cell activity suppression (154, 155). The effects of other anesthetics on this phenomenon have not been studied to date.

Can the postnociceptive spinal sensitization observed in animal models also be demonstrated after surgery in humans? An open study by Dahl and colleagues (156) of patients who underwent gynecologic surgery found evidence supportive of spinal sensitization using the spinal nociceptive flexion reflex (RIII-reflex) elicited by direct sural nerve stimulation. The same study also found decreased direct nerve stimulation pain thresholds in these patients. Using more physiologic dermatomal electric skin stimulation, the same group found increased sensory thresholds in dermatomes adjacent to hysterectomy incisions after surgery (157), suggesting the involvement of central inhibitory mechanisms. In a study measuring thresholds to dermatomal electric skin stimulation at multiple sites after spinal surgery, Wilder-Smith and associates (158) were able to demonstrate that generalized supraspinal inhibition or antinociception is the clinically predominant alteration to sensory processing after surgery (Fig. 29-1). Stress-induced analgesia is a well-known phenomenon (159) and has already been shown to be elicited by surgery in animals (160). By normalizing to a site distant to surgery (Fig. 29-2), this group was able to show the presence of postsurgical spinal sensitization, albeit dominated by supraspinal inhibition. Spinal sensitization was seen only in the patients anesthetized with isoflurane alone; this effect was suppressed by the addition of preemptive fentanyl. However, no difference was noted in clinical measures of pain (pain verbal rating scores, morphine consumption by PCA pump) between the two groups (158). Sensory changes had generally returned to baseline by 24 hours postoperatively, as in animal models (160).

Despite the success of the concept of preemptive analgesia in animal models and the demonstration of spinal sensitization after human surgery, the clinical exploitation of this idea in achieving reduced postoperative pain has proven difficult. In view of the predominance of supraspinal analgesia and the relatively short duration of sensory change after moderate surgical nociception, it is perhaps not surprising that those studies demonstrating differences in clinical pain parameters (e.g., pain rating scores or scales, morphine consumption using PCA devices) with preemptive analgesia have only been able to show modest advantages (139, 161). The most significant improvements resulting from preemptive analgesia have been demonstrated using locoregional anesthetic techniques (162, 163). Of the agents used for general anesthesia, the opioids (morphine) have been shown to produce modest but clinically detectable preemptive analgesia in some studies (164, 165). Another study looking not only at clinical pain but also at wound hyperalgesia has shown that ketamine supplementation of isoflur-

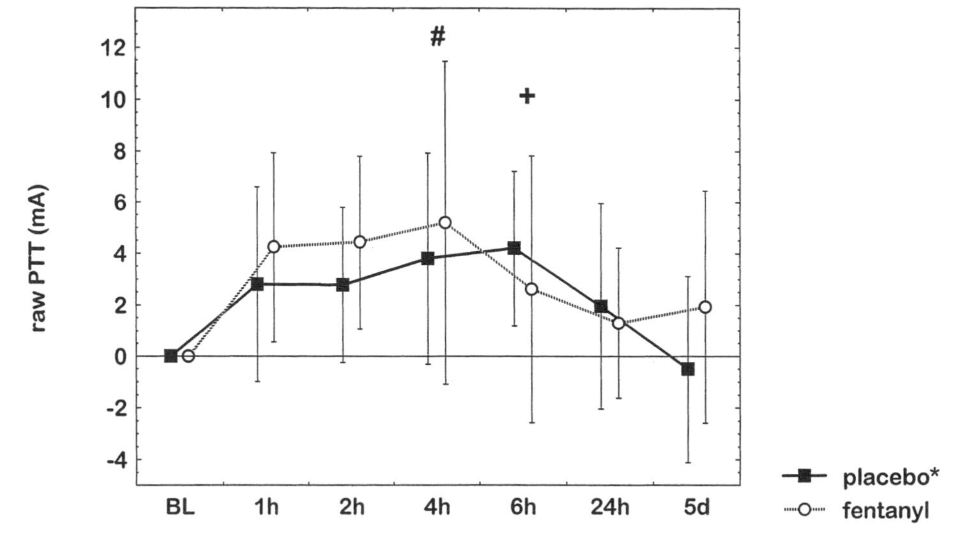

FIGURE 29-1. Change in raw pain tolerance thresholds (PTT) in milliamperes (mA) after herniated intervertebral disk surgery for patients receiving isoflurane-nitrous oxide-oxygen anesthesia supplemented with placebo (placebo group) or 3 μg/kg fentanyl just before induction. Thresholds are measured in the dermatome most affected by disk herniation using transcutaneous constant current electrical stimulation. Y-axis, Threshold change in milliamperes from baseline (BL) values; X-axis, time of measure after skin closure at the end of surgery. *Placebo group is different overall (ANOVA) from the fentanyl group over the entire time course. #Both groups are significantly different from BL. The minus sign indicates that only the placebo group is significantly different from BL. (Data from Wilder-Smith OHG, Tassonyi E, Senly C, et al. Surgical pain is followed not only by spinal sensitisation but also by supraspinal antinociception. Br J Anaesth 1996 (in press).)

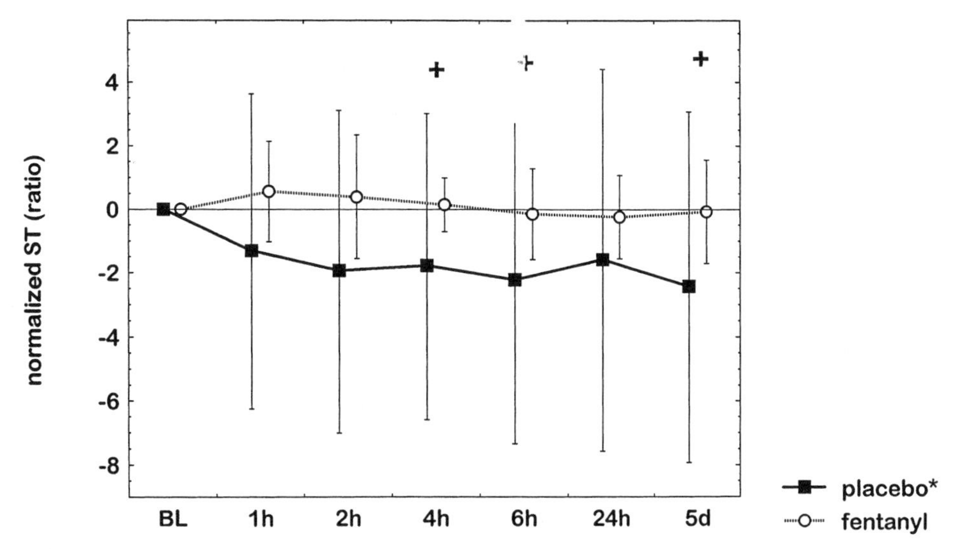

FIGURE 29-2. Change in normalized sensation thresholds (ST) in milliamperes (mA) after herniated intervertebral disk surgery for patients receiving isoflurane-nitrous oxide-oxygen anesthesia supplemented with placebo (placebo group) or 3 μg/kg fentanyl just before induction. Thresholds are measured in the dermatome most affected by disk herniation using transcutaneous constant current electrical stimulation. Threshold normalization is relative to the arm threshold by division; that is, the normalized threshold for the affected dermatome = (raw affected dermatome threshold)/(raw arm threshold). Y-axis, Change in normalized threshold (ratio) from baseline (BL) values; X-axis, time of measure after skin closure at the end of surgery. *Placebo group is different overall (ANOVA) from the fentanyl group over the entire time course. #Both groups are significantly different from BL. The minus sign indicates that only the placebo group is significantly different from BL. (Data from Wilder-Smith OHG, Tassonyi E, Senly C, et al. Surgical pain is followed not only by spinal sensitisation but also by supraspinal antinociception. Br J Anaesth 1996 (in press).)

ane anesthesia has preempting analgesic properties equivalent to those of fentanyl (166). No clinical data are available regarding preemptive analgesia and intravenous hypnotics (e.g., propofol or barbiturates), apart from a suggestion that children undergoing surgery with propofol-based (versus halothane-based) anesthesia may have less postoperative pain (167). As with all studies of preemptive analgesia with volatile agents and N_2O as the main anesthetic agents, the results are inconclusive.

The modulation of intra- and postoperative nociception seems promising for the improvement of intermediate outcomes. In addition to the opioid analgesics, the NMDA-blocker ketamine has also demonstrated promise in this direction. The link between ameliorated intermediate pain outcomes and major long-term outcomes remains unproven at present.

IMMUNOLOGIC FUNCTION

The length of anesthesia and surgery has long been known to correlate positively with the rate of postoperative infection (168), and the data of Liebeskind and associates (154, 155) incriminate the pain of surgery as another depressor of immune function. The direct effects of anesthetic agents on immune function have been extensively investigated (169). The depression of immune function by anesthesia and surgery affects both microbicidal and tumoricidal activity, thereby having the potential to affect outcomes not only in the immediate and short term, but particularly in the medium and long term by cancer surgery survival and recurrence rates.

Both anesthesia and surgery affect the systemic immune response, with some aspects activated and others depressed either during or after anesthesia and surgery (170). These alterations mainly depend on the extent of surgery, nutrition, and blood transfusion, with anesthesia playing a more minor role. The complement system is activated. Neutrophil migration and chemotaxis are generally decreased, whereas opsonization is slightly impaired and cytotoxic function remains intact. Monocyte and macrophage functions are also altered, with reduction of antigen processing and presenting capacity, increased phagocytosis after surgery, and modified monokine secretion. The humoral immune response is mildly depressed, and cell-mediated immunity is more inhibited postoperatively.

Locoregional anesthetic techniques have more positive effects on immune function than general anesthetic techniques. For example, spinal anesthesia is associated with clearly better neutrophilcidal activity (171), and epidural anesthesia minimizes changes in peripheral lymphocyte subpopulations after surgery (172). General anesthetic agents produce many effects on immune function (Table 29-5). The volatile anesthetics have greater effects on immune function than intravenous agents, in particular through depression of stimulated cytotoxic activity, which is a long-lasting effect (at least 11 days) (173-175). The volatile agents seem to have less influence on basal cytotoxic activity (173, 175). One study showed no alteration in the antibody response 2 weeks after antigen presentation (which occurred 1 week after volatile anesthesia) (176). Among the intravenous agents studied, pentobarbital seems to have the greatest effect in depressing the antibody response 3 weeks after anesthesia (176). This study found little difference between rats undergoing anesthesia only or anesthesia *and* surgery with regard to this antibody immune response (176). Other intravenous agents such as ketamine, methohexital, flunitrazepam, droperidol, fentanyl, and propofol seem to have only minor effects or effects apparent only at supraphysiologic concentrations (176-178). In the context of a minor surgical procedure, these agents seem to leave the white cell proliferative responses largely intact (178). Whether this applies to ill patients in the intensive care unit (179) needs further investigation.

The immunologic studies discussed have all used *in vitro* function of immune cells to assess their functional status. Although these tests are interesting surrogate markers of immune function that suggest that anesthetics have effects on microbicidal and tumoricidal activity after surgery, they do not necessarily predict how immune function in the intact human patient will respond. No published clinical outcome studies compare immunologic function using major outcomes such as tumor proliferation or infection rate with different general anesthetic regimens. In animal experiments, anesthesia has been shown to affect morbidity and mortality due to infection (180, 181) or malignancy (182, 183). Clinical evidence supporting the hypothesis that general anesthesia can contribute to the rapid

TABLE 29-5. Effects of Different General Anesthetic Agents on Various Immune Functions (IF)

Drug Class	Drugs	IF Affected	How IF affected	Comments	References
Volatiles/ gases	Halothane	Monocyte hydrogen peroxide production	Reduced	No effect on baseline phagocytosis	173
	Halothane	Neutrophil superoxide production	Reduced		174
	Halothane	Inhibition stimulation in naive NK cells, for at least 11 d	Inhibition stim in naive NK cells, for at least 11 d	Already stimulated NK cells: no effect on cyotoxicity	175
	Halothane	Antibody response (IgG) 3 wk postanesthesia; 2 wk postantigen	No effect	No difference between anesthesia-only and anesthesia-surgery	176
	Enflurane	Neutrophil superoxide production	Reduced		174
	Isoflurane	Neutrophil superoxide production	Reduced		174
	Isoflurane	Inhibition stim in naive NK cells, for at least 11 d	Inhibition stim in naive NK cells, for at least 11 d	As for halothane, somewhat more pronounced	175
IV hypnotics	Pentobarbital	Antibody response (IgG) 3 wk post-anesthesia; 2 wk postantigen	Clear reduction	No difference between anesthesia-only and anesthesia-surgery	176
	Ketamine-xylazine	Antibody response (IgG) 3 wk postanesthesia; 2 wk postantigen	Little effect	No difference between anesthesia-only and anesthesia-surgery	176
	Methohexital	PMNL function in vitro	⇓superoxide/peroxide production	Supraclinical concentrations	177
	Flunitrazepam	PMNL function in vitro	⇓superoxide anion production	Supraclinical concentrations	177
	Droperidol	PMNL function in vitro	No effect		177
	Propofol and fentanyl TIVA	Lymphocyte populations and functions	⇑T,B; ⇓memT; ⇑helpT; ⇓NK	Minor surgery; proliferative response: no effect	178
	Propofol	Lymphocyte proliferation response (ICU pats)	Reduced	Clinical concentrations	179
	Thiopental and fentanyl-nitrous oxide	Lymphocyte populations and functions	⇑T,B; ⇓memT; ⇓NK	Minor surgery; proliferative response: no effect	178

TIVA, Total intravenous anesthesia; NK, natural killer cells; PMNL, polymorphonuclear leukocyte; T,B, T or B lymphocytes; memT, memory T lymphocytes; helpT, T helper cells; ⇓, reduced; ⇑, increased.

spread of cancer after major surgery remains anecdotal (184, 185).

In summary, the influence of general anesthetic agents, in particular intravenous drugs, on intermediate or surrogate end points, which may be relevant to more major outcomes over longer periods, are discussed. On the whole, the connection between the surrogate end points and major outcomes remains poorly investigated and must be regarded as unproven at present. This lack of evidence is less marked for locoregional anesthetic techniques than for general anesthetic techniques. The alleged superiority of locoregional anesthesia is likely to be the result of better intra- and postoperative antinociception, and for the commonly used outcome measures discussed, the quality of modulation of nociception by general anesthesia may determine the clinical effects on outcome. In this respect, intravenous anesthetic and analgesic drugs are considered superior to volatile agents, a difference reflected in short-term and surrogate (or intermediate) end points, but not in longer-term and major outcome variables.

In conclusion, the lack of convincing effects on major and long-term surgical outcomes by general anesthetic techniques alone is a reflection of the multiple factors that influence outcome. The efforts of the anesthesiologist must always be seen in the context of the entire system of care for the surgical patient, including not only the anesthesia team in the operating suite, but also the operating surgeons, the recovery room nursing staff, and the intensive care team, as well as the nursing and medical staff caring for the patient in the postsurgical ward. Thus, although the choice of drug for anesthesia may have some effect on early and intermediate surgical outcome, the quality of the entire system providing medical care remains the major determinant of patient outcome after surgery (186).

REFERENCES

1. Atkinson RS, Rushman GB, Alfred Lee J. A synopsis of anaesthesia. Singapore: PG Publishing, 1984:243.
2. Weeser H, Scharpff W. Evipan, ein neues Einschlafmittel. Dtsch Med Wochenschr 1932;58:1205.
3. Lundy JS, Tovell RM. Thiopental, a new anesthetic agent. North West Med 1935;33:308.
4. Laborit H. Réflexions sur la potentialisation des anesthésiques généraux et les anesthésies combinées. Anesth Analg 1950; 7:289.
5. DeCastro J, Mundeleer P. Anesthésie sans barbituriques: la neuroleptanalgésie. Anesth Analg 1959;16:1022.
6. Snow J. On the inhalation of the vapour of ether in surgical operations. London: John Churchill, 1847.
7. Kay B, Rolly G. ICI 35868, a new intravenous induction agent. Acta Anaesthesiol Belg 1977;28:303–316.
8. Walters RM, Gillespie NA. Deaths in the operating room. Anesthesiology 1944;5:113–128.
9. Cohen MM, Duncan PG, Pope WDP, et al. A survey of 112,000 anaesthetics at one teaching hospital. Can Anaesth Soc J 1986; 33:22–31.
10. Warner MA, Shields SE, Chute CG. Major morbidity and mortality within 1 month of ambulatory surgery and anesthesia. JAMA 1993;270:1437–1441.
11. Hughes MA, Glass PSA, Jacobs JR. Context-sensitive half time in multicompartment pharmacokinetic models for intravenous anesthetic drugs. Anesthesiology 1991;76:334–341.
12. De Grood PM, Harbers JB, Van Egmond J, Crul JF. Anaesthesia for laparoscopy: a comparison of five techniques including propofol, etomidate, thiopentone and isoflurane. Anaesthesia 1987; 42:815–823.
13. Vinik HR, Shaw B, Mackrell T, Hughes G. A comparative evaluation of propofol for the induction and maintenance of anesthesia. Anesth Analg 1987;66:184S.
14. Zuurmond WWA, Van Leeuwen L, Helmers JHJH. Recovery from propofol infusion as the main agent for outpatient arthroscopy: a comparison with isoflurane. Anaesthesia 1987;42:356–359.
15. Milligan KR, O'Toole DP, Howe JP, et al. Recovery from outpatient anaesthesia: a comparison of incremental propofol and propofol-isoflurane. Br J Anaesth 1987;59:1111–1114.
16. Herregods L, Capiau P, Rolly G, et al. Propofol for arthroscopy in outpatients. Br J Anaesth 1988;60:565–569.
17. Puttick N, Rosen M. Propofol induction and maintenance with nitrous oxide in paediatric outpatient dental anaesthesia. Anaesthesia 1988;43:646–649.
18. Nightingale JJ, Lewis IH. Recovery from anaesthesia: a comparison of total intravenous anaesthesia with an inhalational technique. Br J Anaesth 1990;65:287–288.
19. Van Hemelrijk J, Smith I, White PF. Use of desflurane for outpatient anesthesia: a comparison with propofol and nitrous oxide. Anesthesiology 1991;75:197–203.
20. Marshall CA, Jones RM, Bajorek PK, Cashman JN. Recovery characteristics using isoflurane or propofol for maintenance of anaesthesia: a double-blind controlled trial. Anaesthesia 1992; 47:461–466.
21. Ding Y, Fredman B, White PF. Recovery following outpatient anesthesia: use of enflurane vs propofol. J Clin Anesth 1993; 5:447–450.
22. Lebenbom-Mansour MH, Pandit SK, Kothary SP, et al. Desflurane versus propofol anesthesia: a comparative analysis in outpatients. Anesth Analg 1993;76:936–941.
23. Pollard BJ, Bryan A, Bennett D, et al. Recovery after oral surgery with halothane, enflurane, isoflurane or propofol anaesthesia. Br J Anaesth 1994;72:559–566.
24. Fredman B, Nathanson MH, Smith I, et al. Sevoflurane for outpatient anesthesia: a comparison with propofol. Anesth Analg 1995;81:823–828.
25. Korttila K, Nuotto EJ, Lichtor JL, et al. Clinical recovery and psychomotor function after brief anesthesia with propofol or thiopental. Anesthesiology 1992;76:676–681.
26. Herbert M, Healey TEJ, Bourke JB, et al. Profile of recovery after general anaesthesia. Br J Anaesth 1983;286:1539–1542.
27. Edwards H, Rose EA, Schorow M, King TC. Post-operative deterioration in psychomotor function. JAMA 1981;245:1342–1343.
28. Kalman SH, Jensen AG, Ekberg K, Eintrei C. Early and late recovery after major abdominal surgery: comparison between propofol anaesthesia with and without nitrous oxide and isoflurane anaesthesia. Acta Anaesthesiol Scand 1993;37:730–736.
29. Hiller A, Pyykko I, Saarnivaara L. Evaluation of postural stability by computerised posturography following outpatient paediatric anaesthesia: comparison of propofol/alfentanil/ N_2O anaesthesia with thiopentone/halothane/N_2O anaesthesia. Acta Anaesthesiol Scand 1993;37:556–561.
30. Bennett MW, Bembridge JL, Shah MV. A comparison of the effect on gastric emptying of either enflurane or propofol given

during maintenance of anaesthesia for minor surgery. Anaesthesia 1994;49:675–677.
31. Kallela H, Haasio J, Korttila K. Comparison of eltanolone and propofol in anesthesia for termination of pregnancy. Anesth Analg 1994;79:512–516.
32. Eriksson H, Haasio J, Korttila K. Comparison of eltanolone and thiopental in anaesthesia for termination of pregnancy. Acta Anaesthesiol Scand 1995;39:479–484.
33. Watcha MF, White PF. Post-operative nausea and vomiting: do they matter? Eur J Anaesthesiol 1995;12 (suppl 10):18–23.
34. Green G, Jonsson L. Nausea: the most important factor determining length of stay after ambulatory anaesthesia. A comparative study of isoflurane and/or propofol techniques. Acta Scand Anaesthesiol 1993;37:742–746.
35. Norden JM, Hannallah RS, Patel RI, et al. Pharmaco-economics of vomiting: when is antiemetic prophylaxis cost effective in pediatric ambulatory surgery patients? Anesth Analg 1995; 80:S346.
36. Carroll NV, Miederhoff PA, Cox FM, et al. Costs incurred by outpatient surgical centers in managing postoperative nausea and vomiting. J Clin Anesth 1994;6:364–369.
37. Kapur PA. The big "little" problem [Editorial]. Anesth Analg 1991;73:751–755.
38. Lee PJ, Pandit SK, Green CR. Postanesthetic side effects in the outpatient: which are the most important? Anesth Analg 1995; 80:S271.
39. van Wijk MGF, Smalhout B. A postoperative analysis of the patient's view of anaesthesia in a Netherlands teaching hospital. Anaesthesia 1990;45:679–682.
40. Orkin FK. What do patients want? Preferences for immediate recovery. Anesth Analg 1992;74:S225.
41. Madej TH, Simpson KH. Comparison of the use of domperidone, droperidol and metoclopramide in the prevention of nausea and vomiting after gynaecological surgery. Br J Anaesth 1986;58:879–883.
42. Kenny GNC. Risk factors for postoperative nausea and vomiting. Anaesthesia 1994;49 (suppl):6–10.
43. Quinn AC, Brown JH, Wallace PG, Astbury AJ. Studies in postoperative sequelae: nausea and vomiting—still a problem. Anaesthesia 1994;49:62–65.
44. Beattie WS, Lindblad T, Buckley DM, Forrest JB. Menstruation increases the risk of nausea and vomiting after laparoscopy. Anesthesiology 1993;78:272–276.
45. Bredtmann RD, Herden HN,Teichmann W et al. Epidural anaesthesia in colonic surgery: results of a randomised prospective study. Br J Surg 1990;77:638–642.
46. Lerman J. Surgical and patient factors involved in postoperative nausea and vomiting. Br J Anaesth 1992;69 (suppl 1):24S–32S.
47. Havorka J, Korttila K, Erkola O. The experience of the person ventilating the lungs does influence postoperative nausea and vomiting. Acta Anaesthesiol Scand 1990;34:203–205.
48. Forrest JB, Cahalan MK, Rehder K, et al. Multicentre study of general anesthesia. II. Results. Anesthesiology 1990;72:262–268.
49. Watcha MF, White PF. Postoperative nausea and vomiting: its etiology, treatment and prevention. Anesthesiology 1992; 77:162–184.
50. Fisher DM. Surrogate end points: are they meaningful? Anesthesiology 1994;81:795–796.
51. Pitkanen MT, Niemi L, Tuominen MK, et al. Effect of tropisetron, a 5-HT_3 receptor antagonist, on analgesia and nausea after intrathecal morphine. Br J Anaesth 1993;71:681–684.
52. Watcha M, Smith I. Cost effectiveness analysis of antiemetic therapy for ambulatory surgery. J Clin Anesth 1994;41:291–294.
53. Tang J, Watcha MF, White PF. A comparison of costs and efficacy of ondansetron and droperidol as prophylactic antiemetic therapy for elective outpatient gynecologic procedures. Anesth Analg (in press).
54. Cohen MM, Duncan PG, DeBoer DP, Tweed WA. The postoperative interview: assessing risk factors for nausea and vomiting. Anesth Analg 1994;78:7–16.
55. Jones RM. Desflurane and sevoflurane: inhalational anaesthetics for the decade? Br J Anaesth 1990;65:526–536.
56. Rabey PG, Smith G. Anaesthetic factors contributing to postoperative nausea and vomiting. Br J Anaesth 1992;69 (suppl 1):40S–45S.
57. Borgeat A, Wilder-Smith OH, Saiah M, et al. Subhypnotic doses of propofol possess direct antiemetic properties. Anesth Analg 1992;74:539–541.
58. Raftery S, Sherry E. Total intravenous anaesthesia with propofol and alfentanil protects against nausea and vomiting. Can J Anaesth 1992;39:37–40.
59. Kestin IG, Dorje P. Anaesthesia for evacuation of retained products of conception: comparison between alfentanil plus etomidate with propofol plus thiopentone. Br J Anaesth 1987;59:364–368.
60. Haigh CG, Kaplan LA, Durham JM, et al. Nausea and vomiting after gynaecological surgery: a meta-analysis of factors affecting their incidence. Br J Anaesth 1993;71:517–522.
61. Weinstein MS, Nicolson SC, Schreiner MS. A single dose of morphine sulfate increases the incidence of vomiting after outpatient inguinal surgery in children. Anesthesiology 1994; 81:572–577.
62. Gan TJ, Alexander R, Fennelly M, Rubin AP. Comparison of different methods of administering droperidol in patient-controlled analgesia in the prevention of postoperative nausea and vomiting. Anesth Analg 1995;80:81–85.
63. Souter A, Freedman B, White PF. Controversies in the perioperative use of non-steroidal anti-inflammatory drugs. Anesth Analg 1994;79:1178–1190.
64. Ding Y, Fredman P, White PF. Use of mivacurium during laparoscopic surgery: effect of reversal drugs on postoperative recovery. Anesth Analg 1994;78:450–454.
65. Watcha MF, McCulloch DA, Tan TH, et al. Postoperative emesis in children is increased with the use of neostigmine-glycopyrrolate but not with edrophonium-atropine. Anesth Analg 1995;80:S543.
66. Ogilvy AJ, Smith G. The gastrointestinal tract after anaesthesia. Eur J Anaesthesiol 1995;12 (suppl 10):35–42.
67. Andersen R, Krogh K. Pain as a major cause of postoperative nausea. Can Anaesth Soc J 1976, 23:366–369.
68. Whitaker BL. Observations on the blood flow in the inferior mesenteric arterial system and the healing of colonic anastomoses. Ann R Coll Surg Engl 1968;43:89–95.
69. Glise H, Abrahamsson H. Reflex inhibition of gastric motility: pathophysiological aspects. Scand J Gastroenterol 1984;19 (suppl 89):77–82.
70. Douglas DM, Mann FC. The effects of some intra-abdominal procedures on intestinal activity. Gastroenterology 1943;1:513–517.
71. Dubois A, Henry DP, Kopin IJ. Plasma catecholamines and postoperative gastric emptying and small bowel propulsion in the rat. Gastroenterology 1975:68:466–469.
72. Graber JN, Schulte WJ, Condon RE, Cowles VE. Relationship of duration of postoperative ileus to extent and site of operative dissection. Surgery 1982;92:87–92.
73. Mushambi MC, Rowbotham DJ, Bailey SM. Gastric emptying after minor gynaecological surgery: the effect of anaesthetic technique. Anaesthesia 1992;47:297–299.
74. Dauchel J, Schang JC, Kachelhoffer J, et al. Gastrointestinal myoelectrical activity during the postoperative period in man. Digestion 1976;14:293–303.
75. Moss G, Regal ME, Lichtig LK. Reducing postoperative pain, narcotics and length of hospitalisation. Surgery 1986;90:206–210.
76. Runkel NSF, Moody FG, Smith GS, et al. Alterations in rat in-

testinal transit by morphine promotes bacterial translocation. Dig Dis Sci 1993;38:1530–1536.
77. Deitch EA. Simple intestinal obstruction causes bacterial translocation in man. Arch Surg 1989;124:699–701.
78. Deitch EA. The role of intestinal barrier failure and bacterial translocation in the development of systemic infection and multiple organ failure. Arch Surg 1990;125:403–404.
79. Schurizek BA, Willacy LHO, Kraglund K, et al. Effects of general anaesthesia with halothane on antroduodenal activity, pH and gastric emptying rate in man. Br J Anaesth 1989;62:129–137.
80. Condon RE, Cowles V, Ekborn GA, et al. Effects of halothane, enflurane and nitrous oxide on colonic motility. Surgery 1987; 101:81–85.
81. Schurizek BA, Willacy LHO, Kraglund K, et al. Effects of general anaesthesia with enflurane on antroduodenal activity, pH and gastric emptying rate in man. Eur J Anaesthesiol 1989; 6:265–279.
82. Pedersen FM, Wilken-Jensen C, Knudsen F, et al. The influence of nitrous oxide on recovery of bowel function after abdominal hysterectomy. Acta Anaesthesiol Scand 1993;37:692–696.
83. Krogh B, Jensen J, Henneburg SW, et al. Nitrous oxide does not influence operating conditions or postoperative course in colonic surgery. Br J Anaesth 1994;72:55–57.
84. Healy TEJ, Foster GE, Evans DF, Syed A. Effect of some iv anaesthetic agents on canine gastrointestinal activity. Br J Anaesth 1981;53:229–233.
85. Birnbaum D, Karmelli F, Tefera M. The effect of diazepam on human gastric secretion. Gut 1971;12:616–618.
86. Schurizek BA, Kraglund K, Andreasen F, et al. Gastrointestinal motility motility and gastric pH and emptying following ingestion of diazepam. Br J Anaesth 1988;61:712–719.
87. Nimmo WS, Heading RC, Wilson J, et al. Inhibition of gastric emptying and drug absorption by narcotic analgesics. Br J Clin Pharmacol 1975;2:509–513.
88. Ekborn G, Schulte WJ, Condon RE, et al. Effect of narcotic analgesics on bowel motility in subhuman primates. J Surg Res 1980;28:293–296.
89. Neely J. The effects of analgesic drugs on gastro-intestinal motility in man. Br J Surg 1969;56:925–929.
90. Yudioka H, Bogod DG, Rosen M. Recovery of bowel motility after surgery. Br J Anaesth 1987;59:581–584.
91. Painter NS, Truelove SC. The intraluminal pressure patterns in diverticulosis of the colon. Part II. The effect of morphine. Gut 1964;5:207–213.
92. Painter NS, Truelove SC. The intraluminal pressure patterns in diverticulosis of the colon. Part IV. The effect of pethidine and probanthine. Gut 1964;5:369–373.
93. Aitkenhead AR, Wishart HY, Peebles Brown DA. High spinal nerve block for large bowel anastamosis. Br J Anaesth 1978; 50:177–182.
94. Aitkenhead AR, Robinson S. Influence of morphine and pethidine on the incidence of anastamotic dehiscence after colonic surgery. Br J Anaesth 1990;64:230–231.
95. Clarke JM, Seager SJ. Gastric emptying following premedication with glycopyrrolate or atropine. Br J Anaesth 1983;55:1195–1199.
96. Rashid MU, Bateman DN. Effects of intravenous atropine on gastric emptying, paracetamol absorption, salivary flow and heart rate in young and elderly volunteers. Br J Clin Pharmacol 1990;30:25–34.
97. Schurizek BA. The effect of general anaesthesia on antroduodenal motility, gastric pH and gastric emptying in man. Dan Med Bull 1991;38:347–365.
98. Wilkins JL, Hardcastle JD, Mann CV, Kaufman L. Effects of neostigmine and atropine on motor activity of ileum, colon, and rectum of anaesthetised subjects. Br Med J 1970;1:793–794.
99. Child CS. Prevention of neostigmine-induced colonic activity: a comparison of atropine and glycopyrronium. Anaesthesia 1984;39:1083–1085.
100. Hunter AR. Colorectal surgery for cancer: the anaesthetist's contribution? Br J Anaesth 1986;58:825–826.
101. Aitkenthead AR. Anaesthesia and the gastro-intestinal system. Eur J Anaesthesiol 1988;5:73–112.
102. Mangano DT. Cardiac anesthesia risk management: multicenter outcome research. J Cardiothorac Vasc Anesth 1994;8 (suppl 1):10–12.
103. Yeager MP, Glass DD, Neff RK, Brinck-Johnson T. Epidural anesthesia and analgesia in high-risk surgical patients. Anesthesiology 1987;66:729–735.
104. Tuman KJ, McCarthy RJ, March RJ, et al. Effects of epidural anesthesia and analgesia on coagulation and outcome after major vascular surgery. Anesth Analg 1991;73;696–704.
105. Christopherson R, Beattie C, Frank S, et al. Perioperative morbidity in patients randomized to epidural or general anesthesia for lower extremity vascular surgery. Anesthesiology 1993; 79:422–434.
106. Rosenfeld BA, Beattie C, Christopherson R, et al. The effects of different anesthetic regimens on fibrinolysis and the development of postoperative arterial thrombosis. Anesthesiology 1993;79:435–443.
107. Tuman KJ, McCarthy RJ, Spiess BD, et al. Does choice of anesthetic agent significantly affect outcome after coronary artery surgery? Anesthesiology 1989;70:189–198.
108. Pedersen T, Eliasen K, Henriksen E. A prospective study of risk factors and cardiopulmonary complications associated with anaesthesia and surgery: risk indicators of cardiopulmonary morbidity. Acta Anaesthesiol Scand 1990;34:144–155.
109. Forrest JB, Cahalan MK, Rehder K, et al. Multicenter study of general anesthesia. II. Results. Anesthesiology 1990;72:262–268.
110. Forrest JB, Rehder K, Cahalan MK, Goldsmith CH. Multicenter study of general anesthesia. III. Predictors of severe perioperative adverse outcomes. Anesthesiology 1992;76:3–15.
111. Mangano DT, Browner WS, Hollenberg M, et al. Association of perioperative myocardial ischemia with cardiac morbidity and mortality in men undergoing non-cardiac surgery. N Engl J Med 1990;323:1781–1788.
112. Mangano DT. Perioperative cardiac morbidity. Anesthesiology 1990;72:153–184.
113. Mangano DT. Postoperative myocardial ischemia: therapeutic trials using intensive analgesia following surgery. Anesthesiology 1992;76:342–353.
114. Watson A, Allen PR. Influence of thoracic epidural analgesia on outcome after resection for esophageal cancer. Surgery 1994; 115:429–432.
115. Bailey PL, Streisand JB, East TD, et al. Differences in magnitude and duration of opioid-induced respiratory depression and analgesia with fentanyl and sufentanil. Anesth Analg 1990;70: 8–15.
116. Pedersen T. Complications and death following anaesthesia: a prospective study with special reference to the influence of patient-, anaesthesia-, and surgery-related risk factors. Dan Med Bull 1994;41:319–331.
117. Gardner TJ, Horneffer PJ, Manolio TA, et al. Stroke following coronary artery bypass grafting: a ten-year study. Ann Thorac Surg 1985;40:574–581.
118. Kuroda Y, Uchimoto R, Kaieda R, et al. Central nervous system complications after cardiac surgery: a comparison between coronary artery bypass grafting and valve surgery. Anesth Analg 1993;76:222–227.
119. Shaw PJ, Bates D, Cartlidge NEF, et al. Early intellectual dysfunction following coronary bypass surgery. Q J Med 1986; 225:59–68.
120. Ellis RJ, Wisniewski A, Potts R, et al. Reduction of flow rate and arterial pressure at moderate hypothermia does not result in

cerebral dysfunction. J Thorac Cardiovasc Surg 1980;71:173–180.
121. Ravussin P, de Tribolet N, Wilder-Smith OHG. Total intravenous anesthesia is best for neurological surgery. J Neurosurg Anesth 1994;6:285–289.
122. Todd MM, Warner DS. A comfortable hypothesis re-evaluated: cerebral metabolic depression and brain protection during ischemia. Anesthesiology 1992;76:161–164.
123. Shapira Y, Artru AA. Ketamine decreases cerebral infarct volume and improves neurological outcome following experimental head trauma in rats. J Neurosurg Anesth 1992;4:231–240.
124. Buchan AM, Slivka A, Xue D. The effect of the NMDA receptor antagonist MK-801 on cerebral blood flow and infarct volume in experimental focal stroke. Brain Res 1992;574:171–177.
125. Li H, Buchan AM. Treatment with an AMPA antagonist 12 h following severe normothermic forebrain ischemia prevents CA1 neuronal injury. J Cereb Blood Flow Metab 1993;13:933–939.
126. Drummond JC. Brain protection during anesthesia: a reader's guide. Anesthesiology 1993;79:877–880.
127. Baker KZ, Young WL, Stone JG, et al. Deliberate mild intraoperative hypothermia for craniotomy. Anesthesiology 1994; 81:361–367.
128. Shiozaki T, Sugimoto H, Taneda M, et al. Effect of mild hypothermia on uncontrollable intracranial hypertension after severe head injury. Neurosurgery 1993;79:363–368.
129. Siesjö BK. Pathophysiology and treatment of focal ischemia. Part II. mechanisms of damage and treatment. J Neurosurg 1992;77:337–354.
130. Todd MM, Warner DS, Sokoll MD, et al. A prospective comparative trial of three anesthetics for elective supratentorial craniotomy. Anesthesiology 1993;78:1005–1020.
131. Grundy BI, Pashayan AG, Mahla ME, Shah BD. Three balanced anesthetic techniques for neuroanesthesia: infusion of thiopental sodium with sufentanil or fentanyl compared with inhalation of isoflurane. J Clin Anesth 1992;4:372–377.
132. Nussmeier NA, Arlund C, Slogoff S. Neuropsychiatric complications after cardiopulmonary bypass: cerebral protection by a barbiturate. Anesthesiology 1986;64:165–170.
133. Brain resuscitation clinical trial I study group. Randomized clinical study of thiopental loading in comatose survivors of cardiac arrest. N Engl J Med 1986:314:397–403.
134. Woolf CJ. Evidence for a central component of post-injury pain hypersensitivity. Nature 1983;306:686–688.
135. Woolf CJ. Recent advances in the pathophysiology of acute pain. Br J Anaesth 1989;63:139–146.
136. Coderre TJ, Katz J, Vaccarino AL, Melzack R. Contribution of central neuroplasticity to pathological pain: review of clinical and experimental evidence. Pain 1993;52:259–285.
137. Mendell LM. Physiological properties of unmyelinated fiber projections to the spinal cord. Exp Neurol 1966;16:316–332.
138. Wall PD. The prevention of post-operative pain. Pain 1988; 33:289–290.
139. Woolf CJ, Chong MS. Preemptive analgesia: treating postoperative pain by preventing the establishment of central sensitization. Anesth Analg 1993;77:362–379.
140. Dubner R. Pain and hyperalgesia following tissue injury: new mechanisms and new treatments. Pain 1991;44:213–214.
141. Woolf CJ, Thompson SWN. The induction and maintenance of central sensitization is dependent on N-methyl-D-aspartic acid receptor activation: implications for post-injury pain hypersensitivity states. Pain 1991;44:293–299.
142. Meller ST, Gebhart GF, Nitric oxide (NO) and nociceptive processing in the spinal cord. Pain 1993;52:127–136.
143. Abram SE, Yaksh TL. Morphine, but not inhalation anesthesia, blocks post-injury facilitation. The role of preemptive suppression of afferent transmission. Anesthesiology 1993;78:713–721.
144. O'Connor TC, Abram SE. Halothane enhances suppression of spinal sensitization by intrathecal morphine in the rat formalin test. Anesthesiology 1994;81:1277–1283.
145. Chapman V, Haley JE, Dickenson AH. Electrophysiologic analysis of preemptive effects of spinal opioids on N-methyl-D-aspartate receptor-mediated events. Anesthesiology 1994;81: 1429–1435.
146. Abram SE, Olson EE. Systematic opioids do not suppress spinal sensitisation after subcutaneous formalin in rats. Anesthesiology 1994;80:1114–1119.
147. O'Connor TC, Abram SE. Inhibition of nociception-induced spinal sensitization by anesthetic agents. Anesthesiology 1995; 82:259–266.
148. Goto T, Marota JJ, Crosby G. Nitrous oxide induces preemptive analgesia in the rat that is antagonized by halothane. Anesthesiology 1994;80:409–416.
149. Goto T, Marota JJ, Crosby G. Pentobarbitone, but not propofol, produces pre-emptive analgesia in the rat formalin model. Br J Anaesth 1994;72:662–667.
150. Crosby G, Marota JJA, Goto T, Uhl GR. Subarachnoid morphine reduces stimulation-induced but not basal expression of preproenkephalin in the rat spinal cord. Anesthesiology 1994; 81:1270–1276.
151. Hylden JLK, Nahin RL, Traub RJ, Dubner R. Effects of spinal kappa-opioid receptor agonists on the responsiveness of nociceptive superficial dorsal horn neurons. Pain 1991;44:187–193.
152. Dubner R, Ruda MA. Activity-dependent neuronal plasticity following tissue injury and inflammation. Trends Neurosci 1992;15:96–103.
153. Marota JJ, Crosby G, Uhl GR. Selective effects of pentobarbital and halothane on c-fos and jun-B gene expression in rat brain. Anesthesiology 1992;77:365–371.
154. Page GG, Ben-Eliyahu S, Yirmiya R, Liebeskind JC. Morphine attenuates surgery-induced enhancement of metastatic colonisation in rats. Pain 1993;54:21–28.
155. Page GG, Ben-Eliyahu S, Liebeskind JC. The role of LGL/NK cells in surgery-induced promotion of metastasis and its attenuation by morphine. Brain Behav Immun 1994;8:241–250.
156. Dahl JB, Erichsen CJ, Fuglsang-Frederiksen A, Kehlet H. Pain sensation and nociceptive reflex excitability in volunteers and surgical patients. Br J Anaesth 1992;69:117–121.
157. Lund C, Hansen OB, Kehlet H. Effect of surgery on sensory threshold and somatosensory evoked potentials after skin stimulation. Br J Anaesth 1990;65:173–176.
158. Wilder-Smith OHG, Tassonyi E, Senly C, et al. Surgical pain is followed not only by spinal sensitisation but also by supraspinal antinociception. Br J Anaesth (in press).
159. Lewis JW, Cannon JT, Liebeskind JC. Opioid and non-opioid mechanisms of stress analgesia. Science 1980;208:623–625.
160. Jayaram A, Singh P, Carp HM. An enkephalinase inhibitor, SC 32615, augments analgesia induced by surgery in mice. Anesthesiology 1995;82:1283–1287.
161. Katz J. Pre-emptive analgesia: evidence, current status and future directions. Eur J Anaesthesiol 1995;12 (suppl 10):8–13.
162. Katz J, Kavanagh BP, Sandler AN, et al. Preemptive analgesia: clinical evidence of neuroplasticity of contributing to postoperative pain. Anesthesiology 1992;77:439–446.
163. Katz J, Clairoux M, Kavanagh BP, et al. Preemptive lumbar epidural anaesthesia reduces postoperative pain and patient-controlled morphine consumption after lower abdominal surgery. Pain 1994;59:395–403.
164. Richmond CE, Bromley LM, Woolf CJ. Preoperative morphine prevents postoperative pain. Lancet 1993;342:73–75.
165. Collis R, Brandner B, Bromley LM, Woolf CJ. Is there any advantage of increasing the pre-emptive dose of morphine or combining pre-incisional with postoperative morphine administration? Br J Anaesth 1995;74:396–399.

166. Tverskoy M, Oz Y, Isakson A, et al. Preemptive effect of fentanyl and ketamine on postoperative pain and wound hyperalgesia. Anesth Analg 1994;78:205–209.
167. Borgeat A, Popovic V, Meier D, Schwander D. Comparison of propofol and thiopenthal/halothane for short-duration ENT procedures in children. Anesth Analg 1990;71:536–540.
168. Cruse PJE, Foord R. A five-year prospective study of 23,649 surgical wounds. Arch Surg 1973;107:206–209.
169. Rubin G. The influence of alcohol, ether, and chloroform on natural immunity in its relation to leucocytosis and phagocytosis. J Inf Dis 1904;1:425–444.
170. Erskine R, Janicki P, Neil G, James MFM. Spinal anaesthesia but not general anaesthesia enhances neutrophil biocidal activity in hip arthroplasty patients. Can J Anaesth 1994;41:632–638.
171. Hashimoto T, Hashimoto S, Hori Y, et al. Epidural anaesthesia blocks changes in peripheral lymphocytes subpopulation during gastrectomy for stomach cancer. Acta Anaesthesiol Scand 1995;39:294–298.
172. Salo M. Effects of anaesthesia and surgery on the immune response. Acta Anaesthesiol Scand 1992;36:201–220.
173. Stevenson GW, Hall S, Rudnick J, et al. Halothane anesthesia decreases human monocyte hydrogen peroxide production: protection of monocytes by activation with gamma interferon. Immunopharmacol Immunotoxicol 1987;9:489–510.
174. Nakagawara M, Takeshige K, Takamatsu J, et al. Inhibition of superoxide production and Ca^{2+} mobilisation in human neutrophils by halothane, enflurane and isoflurane. Anesthesiology 1986;64:4–12.
175. Markovic SN, Knight PR, Murasko DM. Inhibition of interferon stimulation of natural killer cell activity in mice anesthetized with halothane or isoflurane. Anesthesiology 1993;78:700–706.
176. Lockwood LL, Silbert LH, Laudenslager ML, et al. Anesthesia-induced modulation of in vivo antibody levels: a study of pentobarbital, chloral hydrate, methoxyflurane, halothane, and ketamine/xylazine. Anesth Analg 1993;77:769–774.
177. Krumholz W, Demel C, Jung S, et al. The influence of intravenous anesthetics on polymorphonuclear leukocyte function. Can J Anaesth 1993;40:770–774.
178. Pirttikangas CO, Perttilä J, Salo M, et al. Propofol infusion anaesthesia and immune response in minor surgery. Anaesthesia 1994;49:13–16.
179. Pirttikangas CO, Perttilä J, Salo M. Propofol emulsion reduces proliferative responses of lymphocytes from intensive care patients. Intensive Care Med 1993;19:299–302.
180. Hansbrough JF, Zapata-Sirvent RL, Bartle EJ, et al. Alterations in splenic lymphocyte subpopulations and increased mortality.
181. Tait AR, DuBoulay PM, Knight PR. Alterations in the course of an histopathologic response to influenza virus infections produced by enflurane, halothane and diethyl ether anesthesia in ferrets. Anesth Analog 988;67:671–676.
182. Lundy J, Lovett EJH III, Hamilton S, Conran P. Halothane, surgery, immunosuppression and artificial pulmonary metastases. Cancer 1978;41:827–830.
183. Eggermont AMM, Steller EP, Sugarbaker PH. Laparotomy enhances intraperitoneal tumor growth and abrogates the antitumor effects of interleukin-2 and lymphokine-activated killer cells. Surgery 1987;102:71–78.
184. Jewell WR, Romsdahl MM. Recurrent malignant disease in operative wounds not due to surgical implantation from the resected tumor. Surgery 1965;58:806–809.
185. Lange PH, Hekmat K, Bosl G, et al. Accelerated growth of testicular cancer after cytoreductive surgery. Cancer 1978;45:1498–1506.
186. Lagasse RS, Steinberg ES, Katz RI, Saubermann AJ. Defining quality of perioperative care by statistical process control of adverse outcomes. Anesthesiology 1995;82:1181–1188.

30 Future of Intravenous Anesthesia

Stephen P. Lordon and Theodore H. Stanley

Intravenous anesthesia has existed since the mid-1600s in spite of difficulties of access to the circulatory system. Over the last three centuries, accurate fluid administration has become possible. Currently, intravenous anesthesia is focused on obtaining accurate pharmacokinetic data on drugs through prospective studies and computer modeling. Interest in intravenous anesthesia is growing as a result of the development of new intravenous agents with pharmacokinetic and pharmacodynamic profiles that allow more optimal control of anesthesia and more favorable recovery. Programmable infusion pumps administer these drugs more easily and accurately. Established drugs are being discovered to have new uses, incorporating innovative methods of drug delivery. Intravenous anesthesia in the future, however, will probably abandon nonselective, generalized administration of drugs for more selective, organ-specific "drug focusing." Organ-specific pharmacodynamic action may be achieved by using computers, externally applied electrical fields, monoclonal antibodies, magnetically controlled microspheres, or heat-sensitive liposomes containing receptor-specific drugs. Other future methods of anesthesia may involve intravenous administration of peptides that induce a temporary state of hibernation. Of critical importance, these new technologies will have to include easily understood features to be assimilated into everyday clinical practice.

No one drug provides all characteristics needed for anesthesia, namely, hypnosis, amnesia, analgesia, blockade of sympathetic and parasympathetic reflexes, and muscle relaxation. Typically, a combination of opioids, sedative-hypnotics, and muscle relaxants is utilized. If an ideal drug were available (1), it would possess these desirable pharmacodynamic properties, as well as a pharmacokinetic profile that would lead to a rapid predictable onset as well as rapid predictable recovery, independent of organ function and without depressing the cardiopulmonary, renal, or hepatic systems. It would be water soluble, stable in solution with a long shelf life, nonreactive with plastics, glass, or other container materials, reversible with a specific antagonist, and available in a concentrated formulation to avoid excess fluid administration. It would be nonallergenic, nonirritating to tissues, and nontoxic. Such a drug would have no active metabolites to prolong the action of the drug, and it would have no interactions with other drugs.

No currently available intravenous or inhalation anesthetic technique can meet all the foregoing requirements. In addition, no one general anesthetic technique has been demonstrated to provide an improved quality of anesthesia or outcome. Potent intravenous opioids and sedative hypnotics are commonly administered in combination with inhalation agents and muscle relaxants to produce "balanced anesthesia." The rationale for adding opioids to inhalation agents is to decrease the requirements for the inhalation agent, thereby reducing the cardiopulmonary depression and providing faster emergence. Each technique has clear advantages and disadvantages. Intravenous anesthesia has become a rapid, safe, and effective method of anesthetizing both adult and pediatric patients. Intravenous anesthesia has the clear advantage of providing control for each component of the anesthetic state independently, whether it be analgesia, amnesia, hypnosis, blockade of autonomic reflexes, or muscle relaxation, depending on the surgical needs. Intravenous anesthetic techniques cause no operating room air pollution, and the lungs are not dependent on transporting the anesthetic to its effective site. Total intravenous anesthesia (TIVA) is a method that replaces inhalation agents with a combination of intravenous anesthetics, analgesics, and muscle relaxants. It is the preferred method for thoracic surgery because high inspired oxygen concentrations can be administered, and inhibition of hypoxic pulmonary vasoconstriction is less problematic. If intravenous anesthetics are properly titrated, patients receiving them have less need for postoperative ventilator support. Intravenous anesthesia is also the method of choice for specific otolaryngologic procedures requiring jet ventilation. It is also the preferred method for patients with malignant hyperthermia. Several studies have demonstrated decreased nausea and vomiting with propofol compared with inhaled anesthetics (2). Intraoperative increases in prolactin and cortisol levels have been found to be more effectively blunted with intravenous (versus inhaled) anesthetics (3), and this action may protect against the stress response of surgery. In one study, early phases of recovery and discharge criteria were met sooner in patients receiving propofol as an alternative to thiopental-isoflurane (4). Finally, intravenous anesthesia is often the method of choice in rural areas and in military conflicts where anesthesia machines may be limited.

A major limitation to the widespread use of intravenous anesthetic techniques is the primitive delivery systems which are currently used (5). Inhaled anesthetics are considered to be more controllable, with safe and convenient delivery systems. End-tidal anesthetic agent monitoring provides a more accurate estimate of blood (and hence brain) concentrations of volatile anesthetics. Unfortunately, no convenient monitors exist for depth of anesthesia, or online methods for measuring intravenous anesthetics, so assessment of adequacy of anesthesia is more difficult. Inaccurate titration of intravenous agents can cause a patient to be underanesthetized (i.e., experiencing intraoperative recall) or excessively anesthetized with postoperative sedation or cardiorespiratory depression. In addition, significant interpatient biologic variability exists in anesthetic and analgesic requirements for intravenous agents. Another disadvantage of intravenous anesthesia is the need for specialized infusion pumps, and a second intravenous infusion line is needed. The clinical effects of intravenous drugs are terminated by elimination or redistribution of the drug, which depends on the patient's overall health. In addition, patients can have reactions to intravenous agents that are not dose related (e.g., erythema, urticaria anaphylaxis, pain on injection). Finally, only limited information from well-controlled clinical trials addresses optimal dosages and combinations of intravenous agents for various types of surgical procedures.

In today's cost-conscious health care environment, new methods and drugs will be required to prove not only efficacy and safety, but also improved outcome and cost-effectiveness (6). Hourly costs of low-flow desflurane, sevoflurane, and isoflurane are similar (7). Comparing the costs of maintaining anesthesia for 1 hour with desflurane or propofol would suggest that propofol is roughly four times more expensive (8). Comparing inpatient charges at the University of Utah Medical Center, sufentanil is six times more expensive than fentanyl, and an induction dose of propofol is at least three times more expensive than thiopental. Capitated contracts more than likely will steer anesthesiologists toward the least expensive technique unless other methods of cost analysis demonstrate an improved outcome with the more costly drugs. Pharmacoeconomic analyses are being applied to anesthetic drugs and techniques. For intravenous techniques to be utilized more widely, the results of cost-effective or cost-to-benefit analyses will have to be favorable (8).

The currently available fentanyl analogs, including alfentanil and sufentanil, are pharmacodynamically similar, acting at the opioid receptors. They are associated with troublesome side effects, including respiratory depression, ileus, nausea, vomiting, bradycardia, difficulty in voiding, and muscular rigidity. Even though the fentanyl compounds are pharmacokinetically superior to morphine and meperidine, they are still relatively long acting and thus can delay emergence from anesthesia and contribute to postoperative complications. Current opioid research is focused on shorter-acting opioid compounds that are more easily titratable (e.g., remifentanil).

Even though drug concentrations are usually measured in the plasma, the plasma is not the site of anesthetic drug effect. The latter is often referred to as the "biophase," in which specific receptors and enzymes come in contact with the drug. Distribution time is needed for intravenous drugs to pass from the plasma to the biophase site. Plasma concentrations are not reflective of the effect site until the plasma and biophase concentrations are in equilibrium. The rate of drug equilibration depends on the speed of drug delivery to the tissues relative to the capacity of the tissue to take up the drug and the rate of drug penetration into cellular membranes. It is not yet feasible to measure concentrations of a drug at its site of action, but once equilibration occurs, the drug concentration in the biophase is proportional to its concentration in plasma. The $t_{1/2}$ k_{e0} value represents the delay between the peak drug blood level and the peak pharmacodynamic effect. The shorter the $t_{1/2}$ k_{e0}, the faster the onset of action. Using electroencephalographic (EEG) frequency changes or an experimental pain model, alfentanil was found to have a time to peak effect of 1.4 minutes versus 3.6 minutes for fentanyl (9).

To achieve and maintain a drug effect rapidly using an infusion, the bolus-elimination-transfer (BET) scheme is useful. The BET scheme consists of an initial loading bolus (B), a constant infusion rate to replace drug that has been eliminated (E), and an exponentially declining infusion rate to compensate for transfer (T) of drug to peripheral compartments. The transfer of drug to peripheral compartments has varying rates of distribution, analogous to the inhalation agents. As drug accumulates in the so-called peripheral compartments, decreasing the infusion rate is required to maintain plasma concentrations in the therapeutic window. The therapeutic window is defined as the plasma concentration necessary for the drug to exert the desired pharmacodynamic effect.

When an infusion is stopped, the decrease in plasma concentration depends on elimination and redistribution of the drug. The elimination half-life values represent the time for a 50% decrease in the plasma concentration during the elimination phase. The elimination half-life does not incorporate the influence of redistribution effects. Context-sensitive half-time defines the time for a 50% decrease in the plasma concentration after steady-state infusions of varying durations. With anesthetics that have multicompartmental pharmacokinetics, redistribution from peripheral-to-central (plasma) compartments can be a significant contributor to the central compartment drug elimination.

These models are not ideal, and many biologic variables (e.g., age, body weight, and gender) appear to significantly influence these models. Population studies of plasma effective site concentrations have varied as much as 60% (9). Whether these marked differences in theoretic concentrations have clinically meaningful implications remains to be proven. In 1968, Kruger-Theimer proposed a pharmacokinetic model of continuous infusion drug delivery (10). Because the infusion calculations are complex and need to be performed frequently, only in the last 10 years, with the use of sophisticated computer technology, have pharmacokinetic-based infusion drug delivery systems become available. Automated drug delivery systems based on pharmacokinetic measurements are called model-based or open-loop delivery systems, with no feedback signal from the patient required. These pharmacokinetic-based devices titrate the drug infusion based on theoretical plasma concentrations. Errors in open-loop infusions are expected when patients have altered drug distribution or metabolism. Pharmacodynamic-based (or closed-loop) delivery systems use feedback signals (e.g., median frequency EEG measurements) for alfentanil infusions (11). However, many of the physiologic measurements used to control a closed-loop infusion are nonlinear and are influenced by other physiologic processes. A good example is a nitroprusside-blood pressure closed-loop system that may be greatly altered by hyper- or hypovolemia. Manual infusions require the anesthesiologist to vary the infusion rate, depending on whether anesthesia is adequate or inadequate. Automated drug-delivery systems may assist the clinician to titrate drug infusions more carefully during the perioperative period.

Continuous infusion techniques appear to have some distinct advantages over intermittent bolus dosing methods (12-15). The most convincing data supporting the use of continuous infusions relate to more optimal hemodynamic control and a decrease in the total drug requirement. The decreased drug dosage may contribute to more rapid recovery and fewer perioperative side effects (14, 15). Computer-assisted continuous infusion (CACI) can predict present and future anesthetic blood levels, regardless of the length of anesthesia (13). However, preliminary studies with these devices have shown that CACI has a predictive accuracy of only about 30%.

As mentioned earlier, the pharmacodynamic characteristics of fentanyl, sufentanil, and alfentanil are similar. However, their pharmacokinetic properties are different. Fentanyl accumulates in the body, resulting in a progressively increasing context-sensitive half-time. Sufentanil also gradually accumulates, but to a lesser degree than fentanyl. Sufentanil has the shortest half-time for opioid infusions, lasting 10 hours or less. Alfentanil shows the most stable infusion characteristics with no further increase in half-time after 200 minutes. Another important difference among the fentanyl analogs is the time to peak effective biophase concentration after a bolus dose, the so-called $t_{1/2}$ k_{e0} value, which is independent of the opioid's potency. Alfentanil has the most rapid onset of pharmacodynamic effect, followed by fentanyl, and then sufentanil.

Similar pharmacokinetic measurements have also been performed for the sedative hypnotics. The $t_{1/2}$ k_{e0} value for propofol is 1 to 2 minutes, whereas midazolam's $t_{1/2}$ k_{e0} is 2 to 4 minutes (11). Because the elimination phase of propofol is shorter than that of midazolam, a bolus of propofol is much shorter lasting than a bolus of midazolam. The context-sensitive half-time of propofol is also much shorter than midazolam's, contributing to more rapid recovery following termination of a propofol infusion.

Midazolam is more rapidly and extensively metabolized by hepatic microsomal enzymes than diazepam and lorazepam. In addition, the metabolites of midazolam have minimal central nervous system (CNS) activity. Midazolam has the unique property of being water soluble at an acid pH, but at normal body pH, it is one of the most lipid soluble of all the available benzodiazepines. As a result, midazolam is prepared and distributed in an acid aqueous solution. This preparation allows for pain-free intravenous injection. Following intravenous injection, the compound undergoes an intramolecular rearrangement that allows the development of a more rapid peak biophase site concentration, compared with diazepam or lorazepam. Future injectable anesthetics may focus on similar beneficial pharmacokinetic profiles that can be altered by pH.

Flumazenil is a benzodiazepine antagonist that is useful for reversal of benzodiazepine sedation and overdose (16). Recovery times after TIVA are decreased with flumazenil, and recovery after a midazolam-isoflurane anesthetic regimen with flumazenil reversal is similar to that after a propofol-isoflurane anesthetic regimen (17). Flumazenil has also been shown to decrease midazolam-induced sedation and tidal volume significantly, but decreases in respiratory rate and carbon dioxide responsiveness are unchanged (18). However, the role of flumazenil in anesthetic practice is yet to be determined.

The pharmacodynamic and pharmacokinetic characteristics of porpofol make it ideally suited for both short and long infusions in the operating room. Studies have shown this agent to be a useful alternative to fentanyl, thiopental, and enflurane for cardiac surgery (19). It has also been approved by the United States Food and Drug Administration (FDA) for pediatric patients and for use outside the operating room. The infusion rates of propofol needed to sedate patients in the intensive care unit (ICU) (12.5 to 50 μg/kg/min) are less than those required for the operating room, ranging from 25 to 100 μg/kg/min. Patients have been maintained on propofol infusions for ICU sedation for up to 2 weeks (20). Conventional opioid and midazolam infusions do not provide the rapid emergence associated with propofol sedation. Propofol in subanesthetic doses, 10 to 20 μg/kg/min, can effectively treat chemotherapy-induced nausea and vomiting (21). Postoperative nausea and vomiting have also been effectively treated with propofol boluses of 10 to 20 mg (22).

The use of continuous infusions of intravenous sedatives and analgesics can provide significant advantages in the postoperative period. Several studies have suggested a correlation between postoperative morbidity and elevations in catecholamines and pain after major vascular and cardiac surgery (23). Patients receiving sufentanil experience less elevation of these stress-responding hormones and have fewer complications during and after cardiac surgery than patients receiving isoflurane and morphine. More aggressive postoperative analgesia after major abdominal surgery may shorten recovery times and reduce postoperative complications. For example, Anand and associates randomized children having congenital heart surgery into three groups (24). The first group had a halothane anesthetic with morphine and diazepam postoperatively. The second group had a high-dose sufentanil anesthetic, followed by morphine and diazepam postoperatively. The third group had a high-dose sufentanil anesthetic, and the sufentanil infusion was maintained for several days postoperatively. In this high-risk pediatric population, the last technique was associated with significantly lower mortality and fewer ICU stays. The cost and benefit of these innovative approaches need to be evaluated and compared with more standard techniques.

Other new methods of using intravenous anesthetics and analgesics include propofol and sufentanil infusions after cardiac surgery (25). These techniques have been shown to improve control of hemodynamics and may be associated with less myocardial ischemia. With propofol, patients awaken and are extubated earlier, compared with patients receiving high-dose opioid techniques. Intraoperative patient-controlled sedation and analgesia are other new methods utilized during local and regional anesthesia (26, 27). With computerized drug delivery systems, patients can titrate propofol or midazolam to their desired level of sedation while the infusion pump monitors their vital signs; it is an ideal closed system (28).

Fentanyl and its newer analogs have significantly higher therapeutic indices than the traditional opioid analgesics morphine and meperidine. The fentanyl compounds do not have ideal pharmacokinetic characteristics for variable-length infusions. Moreover, a new opioid analgesic may change concerns regarding the use of opioid infusions. Remifentanil is a potent μ agonist with pharmacodynamic effects similar to those of existing opioid analgesics. Although remifentanil's potency appears to be similar to that of fentanyl and of alfentanil, it has an ester linkage that is hydrolyzed by nonspecific tissue esterases, resulting in rapid metabolic breakdown. Its volume of distribution is small, making it a unique narcotic. Remifentanil does not release histamine, and its major metabolite is approximately 1:1000 as potent as the parent compound. Remifentanil's $t_{1/2}$ k_{e0} is even shorter than that of alfentanil. More important, the clearance of this agent appears to have no correlation with age, body weight, and gender (unlike other opioids). Pharmacokinetic data suggest that remifentanil reaches steady-state concentrations within 10 minutes, and the context-sensitive half-time is independent of its infusion duration. Investigators are not certain how postoperative analgesic requirements will be met when using remifentanil during the intraoperative period. Perhaps remifentanil infusions will be continued into the early postoperative period (e.g., ICU). Remifentanil will probably be our first truly predictable opioid and the next important intravenous drug introduced into clinical practice. Depending on its side effect profile, remifentanil may shift anesthetic balance toward relatively higher opioid and lower hypnotic concentrations. Trefentanil is another investigational opioid with similar pharmacokinetic properties.

Eltanolone, an investigational sedative-hypnotic induction and maintenance anesthetic, is also under clinical investigation. Eltanolone, a metabolite of progesterone, activates the γ-aminobutyric acid (GABA) receptor and has a high therapeutic index. An anesthetic induction dose of eltanolone (0.5 to 1 mg/kg) decreases blood pressure by 20 to 30% without changing heart rate. The decrease in blood pressure appears to be due to mild afterload reduction and myocardial depression. Thus, eltanolone is likely to preserve the myocardial oxygen supply-demand ratio. It does not irritate veins when it is given as a bolus for induction of anesthesia, but it does produce some excitatory movements. Initial recovery from eltanolone anesthesia is slower than after propofol, but once patients awaken, the recovery profile parallels that of propofol. Unpublished reports indicate that eltanolone has a context-sensitive half-time of 20 to 30 minutes after a 1- to 3-hour infusion. Despite its advantages (e.g., lack of pain on injection, hemodynamic stability), enthusiasm for the drug is lacking because it appears to have a slower onset and recovery compared with propofol.

Anesthesia may be viewed as a quantal phenomenon. Either the patient is adequately or inadequately anesthetized. Movement, changes in ventilatory pattern, diaphoresis, lacrimation, tachycardia, and hypertension are relevant, but no single feature is specific enough to infer that the patient is unconscious. Because little or no change occurs in autonomic function with intravenous anesthetic and analgesics, it can be difficult to avoid "overdosing" or underdosing patients. When using opioids as the primary anesthetic agent, some clinicians administer the drug until the patient reaches a rigid, narcotized state as an end point to ensure unconsciousness. The lack of a direct measure of anesthetic effect on the CNS is a disadvantage when using intravenous anesthetic techniques. A monitor of depth of anesthesia should be sensitive enough to detect inadequate anesthesia and analgesia and to predict recovery time following the end of anesthesia and the adequacy of analgesia in the immediate postoperative period. A CNS monitor should be independent of the anesthetic technique and should provide a reasonable correlation of the depth of anesthesia with the anesthetic concentration at the site of action in the CNS.

Early attempts at developing a monitor of depth of anesthesia have proved no better than traditional autonomic signs (e.g., lower esophageal contractility, facial muscle tone). Although therapeutic blood levels of many intravenous anesthetics and analgesics have been defined during surgery (29, 30), obtaining blood concentrations of intravenous anesthetics in real time is expensive and is not clinically feasible at the present time. As technology improves, these measurements may become a clinical reality in the future.

The EEG can measure summed neuronal synaptic activity, and it has been used to assess the effects of intravenous anesthetics. Studies suggest that the EEG may be useful in monitoring levels of consciousness with sedative-hypnotic drugs (31, 32). Complex EEG analytic methods, such as bispectral (BIS) analysis, also appear to correlate with end-tidal concentrations of isoflurane and plasma concentrations of midazolam and alfentanil during anesthesia. Preliminary studies suggest that one can predict when a patient will recover from a given anesthetic technique (33). An EEG-BIS value below 70 suggests a low risk of recall; a value below 60 is consistent with an unconscious state. The clinical value of the EEG-BIS value in improving intraoperative anesthetic conditions and clinical outcome is yet to be determined. Some practitioners believe that it may be more useful as a sedation monitor for patients in the ICU who are paralyzed for long periods of time. However, other clinicians believe that it will become a useful technique for providing sedation with a closed-loop approach.

In 1991, the cost of developing a new drug from discovery to FDA approval was $231 million, and the average time required was 12 years. In 1995, it still took 12 years after a drug was discovered to obtain FDA approval; however, the cost was over $280 million. Current sales of all anesthetics probably generate $600 to $800 million per year. Although these numbers sound large, they pale when compared with the annual sales of H_2-receptor blockers and many cardiovascular drugs, each of which exceed a billion dollars a year. The anesthetic drug market is not large enough to develop new drugs constantly, so future drug development will more than likely use existing drugs and deliver them using novel methods, routes, techniques, as well as drug combinations. The goals of these new approaches will be to increase the efficacy of drug delivery, to decrease the costs of drugs and delivery systems, to improve safety, and to decrease side effects by providing more stable drug delivery with fewer peaks and valleys in the plasma concentrations, thereby improving convenience of administering drugs and patient compliance in taking medication. By using preexisting drugs, the cost of the new trials and the time to FDA approval should be reduced. One innovative method of using preexisting drugs may be specific drug combinations that improve the therapeutic indice and pharmacologic action of a particular drug. When 4-aminopyridine is added to an opioid analgesic, the therapeutic index is increased 100-fold because it leads to a reduction in respiratory depression.

Clonidine is a selective partial α-adrenergic agonist, roughly 200:1 α_2:α_1. When clonidine is administered with any anesthetic agent, it attenuates increases in plasma catecholamine levels, potentiating the opioid analgesic effect and thereby decreasing the narcotic dose requirements, reducing opioid-related side effects and postoperative recovery times. Dexmedetomidine is an investigational α_2 agonist that is an order of magnitude more selective than clonidine. Sedation and anxiolysis are the most consistent effects of α_2 agonists. Although clonidine is "only" able to reduce the anesthetic requirement by 50% (because of its α_1 activation), dexmedetomidine is able to reduce it by 90% in animals, indicating that this agent may be capable of producing an subanesthetic state by virtue of its potent α_2 activity. Dexmedetomidine is currently in phase III studies for perioperative use to improve intraoperative hemodynamic stability and to reduce anesthetic and analgesic requirements during and after surgery.

An increasingly popular method of using preexisting drugs involves the use of combinations of peripheral nerve blocks, tissue infiltration of local anesthetics, or wound instillation with intravenous sedation (34). Common side effects of nausea, vomiting, dizziness, lethargy, and residual sympathetic blockade are avoided. The risk of aspiration pneumonitis is minimized, postanesthesia nursing care may be decreased, and residual analgesia is provided in the early postoperative period. Up to 60% of the cases at selected ambulatory centers are performed with these so-called monitored anesthesia care techniques. Perhaps as more anesthetists become familiar with peripheral nerve blocks, these techniques will become more popular. Parenteral absorption is the most effective method of administering many anesthetic and analgesic drugs. Intramuscular (and subcutaneous) injection is painful, requires trained personnel, and necessitates a set schedule that may have unpredictable results. Intravenous administration requires a patent vein. By using novel routes of drug administration (i.e., dermal, nasal, rectal, and transmucosal techniques), it may be possible to achieve the foregoing goals.

Patients and physicians alike strive to have specific substances (i.e., magic bullets) that do exactly what is wanted for as long as is wanted, without any adverse side effects. Current drugs are more specific and potent, because of the availability of computerized receptor pharmacology. Because of toxic metabolites and unpredictable deleterious side effects that occur away from the desired site of action, many of these "designer drugs" are still not ideal. The future of anesthetic drug development may lie in the concept of drug focusing, that is, limiting an anesthetic's action to specific receptor sites. Drugs would be "steered" to targeted cells, tissues, or organs by nonpharmacologic methods. Onset and termination of drug action would be measured in microseconds. One way of focusing existing receptor-specific drugs would be by encapsulating them in lipid vehicles. These drug bags then could be made site selective by lysing the bags with microwave, ultrasonic, or other waves that increase the temperature at the site of action by 1 to 2°C. Another technique would involve the production of microspheres that would contain a measured amount of a drug that would stimulate μ, GABA, or local anesthetic receptors. These microspheres would be steered directly to the receptor sites in the CNS. This method could involve the use of monoclonal antibodies.

Manipulating endogenous peptides may be another novel method of providing anesthesia and analgesia. These peptides have extremely high therapeutic indices, and the potential benefits of manipulating endogenous peptides (e.g., endorphins, enkephalins) have been shown by Nadar-Djalal and colleagues (35). These investigators examined the preoperative levels of endorphin and meta-enkephalin in patients having prostate surgery and found that higher CSF levels of endorphin and meta-enkephalin at the start of surgery correlated with a decreased requirement for morphine postoperatively. Other studies have revealed a peptide in brain tissue responsible for inducing hibernation. When hibernation trigger factor is isolated and injected into nonhibernating species, it can produce sleep with profound decreases in temperature, oxygen consumption, and heart and respiratory rates. These "hibernating" effects are reversible with the opioid antagonist naloxone. The potential benefits of endogenous peptide manipulation, with few or no adverse systemic effects are exciting.

The concept of producing anesthesia by nonpharmacologic methods is not new. Two hundred years B.C., electric eels were used to decrease phantom limb pain. Acupuncture and acupressure have been used for many years for similar reasons. Transcutaneous electrical nerve stimulation and percutaneous electrical nerve stimulation are effective in the treatment of both acute and chronic pain conditions. Investigators have suggested that specific receptor site drug actions can be electrically provoked without the presence of the agonist drug. This finding infers that it should be possible to influence (i.e., depress or activate) receptor activity using focused energy sources. In 1971, investigators demonstrated that externally applied electrical fields could alter polarization in brain tissue (36). Noninvasive methods that can favorably influence receptors and central peptides may have profound anesthetic and nonanesthetic implications.

In the 1950s through the 1970s, anesthetic and pain research concentrated on whole-organ physiology and pharmacology. In the 1980s and 1990s, the emphasis of research has been on molecular physiology and pharmacology. Anesthesia research has also concentrated on obtaining pharmacokinetic and pharmacodynamic data relating to specific drugs. Future research will need to define fundamental molecular mechanisms of anesthetic drug actions and interactions. Regardless of advances in future research, several caveats will have to be addressed. Is it possible that the hurdle will be too high, given the small anesthesia market, to demand that a new drug have better pharmacokinetics, and pharmacodynamic properties, enhanced safety profile, and fewer side effects, as well as economic advantages? It will be important to develop simpler and improved drug delivery systems. Intravenous anesthesia will move slowly until this barrier is overcome. Outside of academic institutions, intravenous anesthesia has not yet had a marked impact on anesthetic practice. It is often used without pumps and is commonly supplemented with inhalation anesthetic agents. Currently, CACI appears to have more limited applications for administering intravenous anesthetics compared with muscle relaxants and sedative-amnestic drugs. A CACI-controlled propofol infusion pump is on the horizon (Diprafusor™); however, CACI will only be accepted if the physician retains the ability to control the drug infusion. For this technique to achieve widespread acceptance, practitioners will need to think in terms of drug levels rather than dosages. Anesthesia machines and carts will become anesthetic "workstations," equipped with prefilled syringes and simple programmable pumps. Future drug development will more than likely involve using more centrally-active adjunctive drugs, like dexmedetomidine and adenosine, as well as development of ester-linked drugs (e.g., esmolol, mivacurium, remifentanil). A shorter-acting, more easily titratable benzodiazepine (e.g., Ro48-6791) and muscle relaxant (ORG 9487) should be available in the near future. The ability to clone μ, κ, and δ opiate receptors and GABA receptors should facilitate the development of more specific agonist and antagonist drugs. Spinal cord research should concentrate on preemptive analgesia, analgesia monitoring, and highly selective μ agonists with minimal systemic side effects. Noninvasive drug delivery routes and patient-controlled delivery systems may play a prominent role in the future. Thus, the stage is set for the next millennium to provide us with anesthetic techniques beyond our wildest expectations!

REFERENCES

1. White PF, Way WL, Trevor AJ. Ketamine: its pharmacology and therapeutic uses. Anesthesiology 1982;56:119–136.
2. Smith I, White PF. Anesthetic considerations for laparoscopic surgery. Semin Laparosc Surg 1994;1:198–206.
3. Riverso P, Launo C, Bonilauri M, et al. Blood levels of cortisol and prolactin: are they indices of the degree of protection against surgical stress? Minerva Anestesiol 1992;58:1315–1317.
4. Marais ML, Maher MW, Wetchler BV, et al. Reduced demands on recovery room resources with propofol (Diprivan) compared to thiopental-isoflurane. Anesthesiol Rev 1989;16:29–40.
5. Van Hemelrijck J, White PF. Non-opioid intravenous anesthetics. In: Barash PG, Cullen BF, Stoelting RK, eds. Clinical anesthesia. Philadelphia: JB Lippincott, 1995.
6. Watcha MF, White PF. Economics of anesthetic practice. Anesthesiology (in press).
7. Dershwitz M. How can the costs of anesthesia be decreased? In: Apfelbaum JL, ed. Intravenous anesthesia today. Yardley, PA: The Medicine Group, 1994:4–9.
8. Rosenberg MK, Bridge P, Brown M. Cost comparison: a desflurane- versus a propofol-based general anesthetic technique. Anesth Analg 1994;79:852–855.
9. Shafer SL, Kern SE, Stanski DR. The scientific basis of infusion techniques in anesthesia. North Reading, MA: Bard Med-Systems Division, CR Bard, 1990.
10. Kruger-Thiemer. Continuous intravenous infusion and multicompartment accumulation. Eur J Pharmacol 1968;4:317–324.
11. Schwilden H, Stoeckel H. Closed-loop feedback controlled administration of alfentanil during alfentanil-nitrous oxide anaesthesia. Br J Anaesth 1993;70:389–393.
12. Newson C, Joshi G, Victory R, White PF. Comparison of propofol administration techniques during monitored anesthesia care. Anesth Analg 1995;81:486–491.
13. Reves JG, Croughwell ND, Jacobs J, et al. Continuous infusion of fentanyl and midazolam for cardiac surgery. Anesth Analg 1990;70:S323.
14. White PF. Use of continuous infusion versus intermittent bolus administration of fentanyl or ketamine during outpatient anesthesia. Anesthesiology 1983;59:294–300.
15. White PF. Patient-controlled analgesia: a new approach to the management of postoperative pain. Semin Anesth 1985;4:255–266.
16. White PF, Shafer A, Boyle WA, et al. Benzodiazepine antagonism does not provoke a stress response. Anesthesiology 1989; 70:636–639.
17. Jensen AG, Møller JT, Lybecker H, Hansen PA. A random trial comparing recovery after midazolam-alfentanil anesthesia with and without reversal with flumazenil, and standardized neurolept anesthesia for major gynecologic surgery. J Clin Anesth 1995;7:63–70.
18. Mora CT, Torjman M, White PF. Sedative and ventilatory effects of midazolam infusion: effect of flumazenil reversal. Can J Anaesth 1995;42:677–684.
19. Mora CT, Duke C, Torjman MC, White PF. Effect of anesthetic technique on the hemodynamic response and recovery profile after coronary revascularization. Anesth Analg 1995;81:900–910.
20. Boyle WA, Shear JM, White PF, Schuller D. Long-term sedative infusion in the intensive care unit: propofol versus midazolam. J Drug Dev 1991;4:43–45.
21. Scher CS, Amar D, McDowall RH, et al. Use of propofol for the prevention of chemotherapy-induced nausea and emesis in oncology patients. Can J Anaesth 1992;39:170–172.
22. Borgeat A, Wilder-Smith OH, Saiah M, et al. Subhypnotic doses of propofol possess direct antiemetic properties. Anesth Analg 1992;74:539–541.
23. Mangano DT. Postoperative myocardial ischemia: therapeutic trials using extensive analgesia following surgery. Anesthesiology 1992;76:342–353.
24. Anand KJS, Philbin D, Hickey PR. Halothane-morphine compared with high-dose sufentanil for anesthesia and postoperative analgesia in neonatal cardiac surgery. N Engl J Med 1992; 326:1–9.
25. Hall RI, Murphy JT, Landymore R, et al. Myocardial metabolic and hemodynamic changes during propofol anesthesia for cardiac surgery in patients with reduced ventricular function. Anesth Analg 1993;77:680–689.
26. Zelcer J, White PF, Paull JD, Chester S. Intraoperative PCA: a comparison with alfentanil bolus and infusion techniques during outpatient monitored anesthesia care. Anesth Analg 1992; 75:41–44.
27. Ghouri AF, Taylor E, White PF. Patient-controlled sedation: a comparison of midazolam, propofol and alfentanil during local anesthesia. J Clin Anesth 1992;4:476–479.
28. Glass PSA. Intravenous anesthesia: new drugs and techniques. Paper presented at the American Society of Anesthesiologists Refresher Course, San Francisco, 1994.
29. Bailey PL, Stanley TH. Intravenous opioid anesthesia. In: Miller RD, ed. Anesthesia. New York: Churchill Livingstone, 1994: 291–387.
30. Reves JG, Glass PSA, Lubarsky DA. Nonbarbiturate intravenous anesthetics. In: Miller RD, ed. Anesthesia. New York: Churchill Livingstone, 1994:247–289.
31. Liu J, Singh H, White PF. EEG bispectral analysis predicts the depth of midazolam-induced sedation. Anesthesiology 1996; 84:64–69.
32. Liu J, Singh H, White PF. EEG bispectral index predicts intraoperative recall and depth of propofol-induced sedation. Anesthesiology 1996;84:64–69.
33. Kearse L, Rosow C, Sebel P, et al. The bispectral index correlates with sedation/hypnosis and recall: comparison using multiple agents. Anesthesiology 1995;83:A506.
34. White PF. Ambulatory anesthesia and surgery: past, present and future. In: White PF, ed. Ambulatory anesthesia and surgery. Philadelphia: WB Saunders, 1996.
35. Anonymous. Higher levels of endogenous peptides in CSF found to correlate with less patient pain. Anesthesiol News 1995;Feb:29.
36. Stanley TH. Anesthesiology in the 21st century: analgesic, sedative and anesthetic focusing. Int J Clin Monit Comput 1986; 3:21–25.

INDEX

Page numbers in *italics* indicate figures; page numbers with *t* indicate tables.

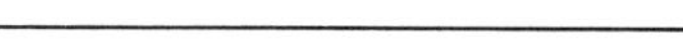